Third Edition

Current
C A N C E R
Therapeutics

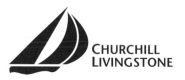

John M. Kirkwood, MD

Professor and Chief, Division of Medical Oncology, University of Pittsburgh School of Medicine
Chief, Melanoma Center, University of Pittsburgh Cancer Institute, Pittsburgh, Pennsylvania

Michael T. Lotze, MD

Professor, Departments of Surgery, Molecular Genetics, and Biochemistry, University of Pittsburgh,
University of Pittsburgh Cancer Institute, Pittsburgh, Pennsylvania

Joyce M. Yasko, PhD

Professor, School of Nursing, University of Pittsburgh
Associate Director, Clinical and Network Programs, University of Pittsburgh Cancer Institute, Pittsburgh, Pennsylvania

With 62 contributors

CHURCHILL LIVINGSTONE

Developed by Current Medicine, Inc., Philadelphia

CURRENT MEDICINE, INC.
400 Market Street
Suite 700
Philadelphia, PA 19106

DIRECTOR OF PRODUCT DEVELOPMENT: *Lori J. Bainbridge*
DEVELOPMENTAL EDITOR: *Scott Thomas Hurd*
ASSISTANT EDITOR: *Jennifer Schafhauser*
ART DIRECTOR: *Paul Fennessy*
DESIGNER: *Christine Keller-Quirk, Patrick Whelan*
ILLUSTRATION DIRECTOR: *Ann Saydlowski*
ILLUSTRATOR: *Debra Wertz*
PRODUCTION: *Lori Holland and Amy Watts*

Although every effort has been made to ensure that drug doses and other information are presented accurately in this publication, the ultimate responsibility rests with the prescribing physician. Neither the publishers nor the authors can be held responsible for errors or for any consequences arising from the use of information contained herein. Products mentioned in this publication should be used in accordance with the prescribing information prepared by the manufacturers. No claims or endorsements are made for any drug or compound at present under clinical investigation.

ISBN: 0-443-06527-6
ISSN: 1074-2816

Printed in the United States of America by Edwards Brothers, Inc.
5 4 3 2 1

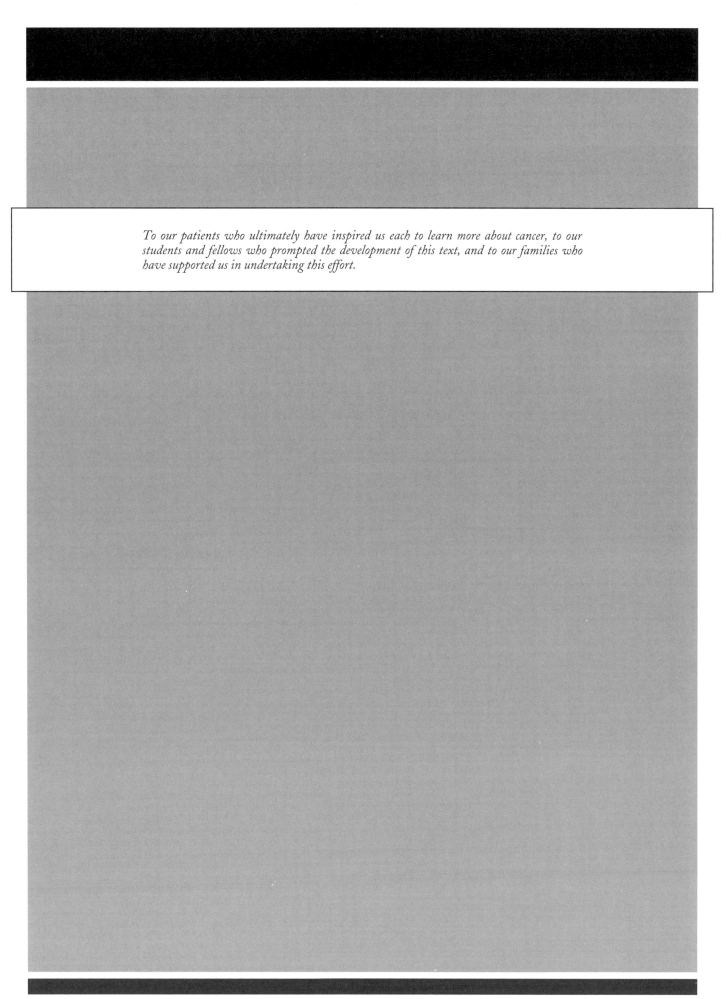

To our patients who ultimately have inspired us each to learn more about cancer, to our students and fellows who prompted the development of this text, and to our families who have supported us in undertaking this effort.

CONTRIBUTORS

JAMES L. ABBRUZZESE, MD
Professor of Medicine
Department of Gastrointestinal Medical
   Oncology and Digestive Diseases
University of Texas, M.D. Anderson
   Cancer Center
Houston, Texas

SANJIV S. AGARWALA, MD
Assistant Professor
Department of Medicine
University of Pittsburgh
Pittsburgh, Pennsylvania

EDWIN ALYEA, MD
Instructor in Medicine
Department of Adult Oncology
Harvard Medical School
Boston, Massachusetts

ROBERT J. AMDUR, MD
Associate Professor
Department of Medicine
Dartmouth University Medical School;
Chief
Section of Radiation Oncology
Dartmouth-Hitchcock Medical Center
Lebanon, New Hampshire

JANET A. AMICO, MD
Professor
Department of Medicine
Division of Endocrinology
University of Pittsburgh
Pittsburgh, Pennsylvania

MICHAEL B. ATKINS, MD
Associate Professor
Harvard Medical School;
Director
Melanoma and Biologic Therapy
   Programs
Division of Hematology/Oncology
Beth Israel Deaconess Medical Center
Boston, Massachusetts

JOSEPH BAAR, MD, PhD
Assistant Professor
Department of Medicine and Surgery
University of Pittsburgh;
University of Pittsburgh Cancer Institute
Pittsburgh, Pennsylvania

DAVID L. BARTLETT, MD
Senior Investigator
Surgery Branch
National Cancer Institute, National
   Institutes of Health
Bethesda, Maryland

JULIE G. BEITZ, MD
Food and Drug Administration
Rockville, Maryland

JAMES R. BERENSON, MD
Professor of Medicine
Department of Hematology/Oncology
UCLA School of Medicine;
West Los Angeles Veteran's Affairs
   Medical Center
Los Angeles, California

RONALD H. BLUM, MD
Professor
Department of Medicine
New York Medical College;
Medical Director
Saint Vincent's Comprehensive Cancer
   Center
New York City, New York

MICHAEL E. BOZIK, MD
Fellow in Neuro-oncology
Brain Tumor Center
Pittsburgh Cancer Institute
Pittsburgh, Pennsylvania

PAUL A. BUNN Jr., MD
Grohne Stapp Professor and Director
University of Colorado Cancer Center
University of Colorado School of
   Medicine;
University Hospital
Denver, Colorado

JUDY H. CHIAO, MD
Food and Drug Administration
Rockville, Maryland

BERNARD F. COLE, PhD
Assistant Professor
Department of Community and Family
   Medicine
Dartmouth University Medical School
Lebanon, New Hampshire

ROBERT J. DeLAP, MD, PhD
Food and Drug Administration
Rockville, Maryland

GERARD M. DOHERTY, MD
Assistant Professor
Department of Surgery
Washington University School of
   Medicine
St. Louis, Missouri

AFSHIN DOWLATI, MD
Hematology/Oncology Clinical Fellow
Department of Medicine
Case Western Reserve University;
Clinical Fellow
Department of Hematology/Oncology
University Hospitals of Cleveland
Cleveland, Ohio

MARC S. ERNSTOFF, MD
Professor
Department of Medicine
Dartmouth University Medical School;
Chief
Section of Hematology/Oncology
Dartmouth-Hitchcock Medical Center
Lebanon, New Hampshire

YUMAN FONG, MD
Assistant Professor of Surgery and Cell
   Biology and Anatomy
Cornell University Medical Center
New York City, New York

RICHARD D. GELBER, PhD
Professor
Department of Pediatrics
Harvard Medical School;
Dana-Farber Cancer Institute
Boston, Massachusetts

SHARI GELBER, MS
Frontier Science and Technology
   Research Foundation
Brookline, Massachusetts

STANTON L. GERSON, MD
Professor
Department of Medicine
Case Western Reserve University;
University Hospitals of Cleveland
Cleveland, Ohio

MARK R. GILBERT, MD
Assistant Professor
Department of Neurosurgery,
   Neurology, and Medicine
University of Pittsburgh;
University of Pittsburgh Medical Center
Pittsburgh, Pennsylvania

MICHAEL S. GORDON, MD
Associate Professor of Medicine
Department of Medicine
Indiana University School of Medicine;
University Hospital
Indianapolis, Indiana

CONTRIBUTORS

JEAN L. GREM, MD
Navy Medical Oncology Branch
National Cancer Institute, National
  Institutes of Health
Bethesda, Maryland

J. MICHAEL HAMILTON, MD
Navy Medical Oncology Branch
National Cancer Institute, National
  Institutes of Health
Bethesda, Maryland

JOHN A. HEANEY, MD, BCH
Professor
Department of Surgery
Dartmouth University Medical School;
Chief
Section of Urology
Dartmouth-Hitchcock Medical Center
Lebanon, New Hampshire

I. CRAIG HENDERSON, MD
Adjunct Professor of Medicine
University of California, San Francisco
San Francisco, California

HOWARD HOCHSTER, MD
Associate Professor of Clinical Medicine
Department of Medicine
New York University School of
  Medicine;
New York University Medical Center
New York City, New York

JEAN L. HOLLEY, MD
Associate Professor
Department of Medicine
University of Rochester;
Nephrology Unit
University of Rochester Medical Center
Rochester, New York

SANDRA J. HORNING, MD
Associate Professor
Department of Medicine
Division of Oncology
Stanford University;
Stanford University Medical Center
Stanford, California

DAVID T. KIANG, MD, PHD
Professor
Department of Medicine
University of Minnesota;
Fairview–University Medical Center
Minneapolis, Minnesota

JOHN M. KIRKWOOD, MD
Professor and Chief
Division of Medical Oncology
University of Pittsburgh School of
  Medicine;
Chief
Melanoma Center
University of Pittsburgh Cancer Institute
Pittsburgh, Pennsylvania

BARRY C. LEMBERSKY, MD
Assistant Professor of Medicine
Department of Human Oncology
Allegheny University of Health Sciences;
Allegheny Cancer Center
Pittsburgh, Pennsylvania

MICHAEL T. LOTZE, MD
Professor
Departments of Surgery, Molecular
  Genetics, and Biochemisty
University of Pittsburgh;
University of Pittsburgh Cancer Institute
Pittsburgh, Pennsylvania

JENNIFER LOWNEY, MD
Research Fellow
Department of Surgery
Washington University School of
  Medicine
St. Louis, Missouri

STEPHEN F. LOWRY, MD
Chairman
Department of Surgery
Robert Wood Johnson Medical School
University of Medicine and Dentistry of
  New Jersey
New Brunswick, New Jersey

DAVID F. McDERMOTT, MD
Instructor in Medicine
Department of Medicine
Harvard Medical School;
Beth Israel Deaconess Medical Center
Boston, Massachusetts

CRAIG H. MOSKOWITZ, MD
Instructor
Department of Medicine
Cornell University;
Clinical Associate Attending
Memorial Sloan-Kettering Cancer
  Center
New York City, New York

CAROL S. PORTLOCK, MD
Associate Professor of Medicine
Department of Medicine
Cornell University;
Clinical Associate Attending
Memorial Sloan-Kettering Cancer
  Center
New York City, New York

RAMESH K. RAMANATHAN, MD
Assistant Professor
Department of Medical Oncology
University of Pittsburgh Medical School;
University of Pittsburgh Cancer Institute
Pittsburgh, Pennsylvania

BLANCHE RASMUSSEN, PHD
Cancer Center Pharmacist
University of Nebraska Medical Center
Omaha, Nebraska

SCOT C. REMICK, MD
Associate Professor
Department of Medicine
Case Western Reserve University;
Program Leader
Developmental Therapeutics
University Hospitals of Cleveland
Cleveland, Ohio

JEROME RITZ, MD
Professor of Medicine
Department of Adult Oncology
Harvard Medical School;
Dana-Farber Cancer Institute
Boston, Massachussetts

**LINDA BARRY ROBERTSON, RN, MSN,
OCN, CCRC**
Adjunct Faculty
University of Pittsburgh School of
  Nursing;
University of Pittsburgh Medical Center
  Health Systems
University of Pittsburgh Cancer Institute
Pittsburgh, Pennsylvania

JOSHUA T. RUBIN, MD
Associate Professor
Department of Surgery
University of Pittsburgh;
University of Pittsburgh Medical Center
Pittsburgh, Pennsylvania

JOHN C. RUCKDESCHEL, MD
Professor of Medicine and Director
H. Lee Moffitt Cancer Center and
  Research Institute
University of South Florida
Tampa, Florida

CONTRIBUTORS

SUSAN A. SAJER, MD
Assistant Professor of Medicine
Tufts University School of Medicine
Boston, Massachussetts;
Emerson Hospital
Concord, Massachussetts

HUBERT SCHEFER, MD
Division of Oncology
Department of Medicine
Kantonsspital
Lucerne, Switzerland

DAVID SCHIFF, MD
Assistant Professor
Department of Neurosurgery,
  Neurology, and Medicine
University of Pittsburgh;
University of Pittsburgh Medical Center
Pittsburgh, Pennsylvania

ARIEL F. SORIANO, MD
Clincal Fellow
University of Colorado Cancer Center
University of Colorado School of
  Medicine;
University Hospital
Denver, Colorado

ROGER STUPP, MD
Attending Physician
Multidisciplinary Center for Oncology
University Hospital Center of Vaud
Lausanne, Switzerland

MARGARET A. TEMPERO, MD
Professor
Department of Internal Medicine
University of Nebraska;
Deputy Director and Interim Director
University of Nebraska Medical
  Center/Eppley Cancer Center
Omaha, Nebraska

CHRISTOPHER TRETTER, MD, CM
Instructor
Department of Medicine
Dartmouth University Medical School;
Clinical Fellow
Department of Hematology/Oncology
Dartmouth-Hitchcock Medical Center
Lebanon, New Hampshire

DEBASISH TRIPATHY, MD
Associate Clinical Professor
Department of Medicine
University of California, San Francisco
San Francisco, California

IRFAN A. VAZIRI, MD
Fellow
Department of Internal Medicine
Hematology/Oncology Section
University of Nebraska;
University of Nebraska Medical Center
Omaha, Nebraska

EVERETT E. VOKES, MD
Professor
Department of Medicine
Section of Hematology/Oncology
University of Chicago Pritzker School of
  Medicine;
Director of Clinical Affairs
University of Chicago Cancer Research
  Center
Chicago, Illinois

MATTHEW VOLM, MD
Clinical Instructor
Department of Medicine
New York University School of
  Medicine;
Bellevue Hospital Center
New York City, New York

SCOTT WADLER, MD
Professor
Department of Oncology
Albert Einstein College of Medicine
Montefiore Medical Center
Bronx, New York

ALAN R. YUEN, MD
Assistant Professor
Department of Medicine
Stanford University;
Stanford University Medical Center
Stanford, California

HERBERT J. ZEH, MD
Clinical Associate
Surgery Branch
National Cancer Institute, National
  Institutes of Health
Bethesda, Maryland

INTRODUCTION

As this book enters its third edition, the evolution of new therapies to clinical acceptance is accelerating, driven by a more enlightened drug-approval process and by expanded funding for basic and clinical research. Although we are gratified at this development, we are humbled by the slow translation of current knowledge of cancer biology into real benefits for our patients. Recent approvals of new biologic therapies for refractory tumors, such as melanoma, suggest that these may improve both the cure of early disease and the survival of patients with more advanced tumors that have been refractory to all approaches with conventional drugs [1,2]. There is evidence that local therapies with surgery can be made substantially more precise, less debilitating, and less expensive [3]; there is also evidence to show that established local tools of radiotherapy can improve survival in diseases such as breast cancer [4,5]. The ability to move therapies into regional approaches for selected patients [6,7] suggests the possibility that advances will occur not just with new agents but also with more imaginative and refined application of older therapies as we understand how to maximize their therapeutic gain and limit their systemic toxicity.

The advances in our understanding of the process of cancer and more rational and effective means to apply old and new tools to treat and ultimately prevent this disease will certainly be highlighted in future editions of this text.

REFERENCES

1. Evans WE, Relling MV, Rodman JH, *et al.*: Conventional compared with individualized chemotherapy for childhood acute lymphoblastic leukemia. *N Engl J Med* 1998, 338:499–505.

2. Kirkwood JM, Strawderman MH, Ernstoff ML, *et al.*: Interferon alfa-2b adjuvant therapy of high risk resected cutaneous melanoma: the Eastern Cooperative Oncology Group Trial EST 1684. *J Clin Oncol* 1996, 14:7–17.

3. Reintgen D, Balch C, Kirkwood J: Recent advances in the care of the patient with malignant melanoma. *Ann Surg* 1997, 225:1–14.

4. Overgaard M, Hansen PS, Overgaard J, *et al.*: Postoperative radiotherapy in high-risk premenopausal women with breast cancer who receive adjuvant chemotherapy. Danish Breast Cancer Cooperative Group 82b Trial. *N Engl J Med* 1997, 337:949–955.

5. Ragaz J, Jackson SM, Le N, *et al.*: Adjuvant radiotherapy and chemotherapy in node-positive premenopausal women with breast cancer. *N Engl J Med* 1997, 337:956–962.

6. Alberts DS, Liu PY, Hannigan EV, *et al.*: Intraperitoneal cisplatin plus intravenous cyclophosphamide versus intravenous cisplatin plus intravenous cyclophosphamide for stage III ovarian cancer. *N Engl J Med* 1996, 335:1950–1955.

7. Lotze MT, Rubin JT: *Regional Therapy of Advanced Cancer.* Philadelphia: JB Lippincott; 1997.

CONTENTS

CHAPTER 1: ALKYLATING AGENTS
Stanton L. Gerson

Alkylating agents form the backbone of many anticancer regimens and are used in both conventional and high-dose therapy settings. The biologic and chemical activities of the nitrogen mustards were studied extensively between the World Wars. Because of their vesicant activity on the skin, eyes, and respiratory tract, the mustards also were studied for their effects on lymphosarcomas in mice during World War II. This led to the start of clinical studies, in 1942, and kicked off the era of modern cancer chemotherapy [1].

Alkylating agents are polyfunctional compounds that have the ability to substitute alkyl groups for hydrogen ions. These compounds react with phosphate, amino, hydroxyl, sulfhydryl, carboxyl, and imidazole groups, which are part of the molecular make-up of the body. In neutral or alkaline solution, these drugs ionize and produce positively charged ions that attach to susceptible nuclear proteins, with the most likely site of alkylation being the N-7 position of guanine. This alkylation reaction leads to abnormal base pairing, cleaving of the imidazole ring of guanine, cross-linking of DNA, depurination of DNA, and interference with DNA replication, transcription of RNA, and the disruption of nucleic acid function. These actions lead to an interruption in the normal cell functions of both cancerous and normal tissues [1,2]. Cytotoxicity, in large part, is due to DNA alkylation at N or O. Disruption of DNA synthesis by the DNA adducts formed (particularly crosslinks or induction of apoptosis during the process of DNA repair) represents predominant mechanisms of cytotoxicity.

The alkylating agents are cell cycle phase–nonspecific agents because they exert their activity independently of the specific phase of the cell cycle. The nitrogen mustards and alkyl alkone sulfonates are most effective against cells in the G_1 or M phase. Nitrosoureas, nitrogen mustards, and aziridines impair progression from the G_1 and S phases to the M phase.

CLASSES

The alkylating agents traditionally are divided into five classes; however, the platinum-containing compounds have been added as a sixth class owing to their ability to bind to DNA and produce cross-links in the DNA helix. The traditional classes of alkylators include the bischloroethylamines (nitrogen mustards), the aziridines (ethylenimines), the alkyl alkone sulfonates, the nitrosoureas, and the nonclassical alkylating agents [1–4].

The bischloroethylamines, commonly referred to as the nitrogen mustards, include mechlorethamine, melphalan, chlorambucil, cyclophosphamide, ifosfamide, and uracil mustard. Thiotepa is a member of the aziridine class. Busulfan belongs to the alkyl alkone sulfonate class. Carmustine, lomustine, and streptozocin are members of the nitrosourea family. The nonclassical alkylating

Table 1-1. Classes of Alkylating Agents and Mechanisms of Action

Alkylating Agent	Trade Name	Manufacturer	Dosage Forms
Bischloroethylamines (nitrogen mustards)*†			
Chlorambucil	Leukeran	Glaxo-Wellcome	PO
Cyclophosphamide	Cytoxan	Mead Johnson Oncology	PO, IV
	Neosar	Adria	IV
Ifosfamide	Ifex	Mead Johnson Oncology	IV
Mechlorethamine	Mustargen	Merck, Sharpe, & Dohme	IV
Melphalan	Alkeran	Glaxo-Wellcome	PO, IV
Uracil mustard	Uracil Mustard	Upjohn	PO
Aziridines*			
Thiotepa	Thioplex	Immunex	IV
Alkyl alkone sulfonates*			
Busulfan	Myleran	Glaxo-Wellcome	PO
Nitrosoureas†			
Carmustine	BiCNU	Bristol-Myers Oncology	IV
Lomustine	CeeNU	Bristol-Myers Oncology	PO
Streptozocin	Zanosar	Upjohn	IV
Nonclassic Alkylating Agents‡			
Altretamine	Hexalen	US Bioscience	PO
Dacarbazine	DTIC	Dome	IV
Procarbazine	Matulane	Roche	PO
Platinum Compounds§			
Carboplatin	Paraplatin	Bristol-Myers Oncology	IV
Cisplatin	Platinol	Bristol-Myers Oncology	IV

*Interfere with DNA replication and transcription and DNA crosslinks.
†Alkylation of DNA, RNA, DNA crosslinks, and methylate DNA.
‡Alkylation; inhibition of DNA, RNA, and protein synthesis.
§Formation of interstrand and intrastrand DNA cross-links.

agents include procarbazine, dacarbazine, and altretamine (formerly called hexamethylmelamine). Carboplatin and cisplatin are the platinum compounds that exhibit alkylating activity.

Table 1-1 lists the mechanisms of action for each class of alkylating agents as well as the trade name, manufacturer, and dosage forms for each member of the class.

PHARMACOKINETICS

As shown in Table 1-2, most of the alkylating agents are hepatically metabolized prior to renal excretion. Active metabolites are formed in the liver from cyclophosphamide, ifosfamide, chlorambucil, and carboplatin [3,5–7]. Melphalan is uniquely cleared by hydrolysis to monohydroxy- and dihydroxymelphalan. Cisplatin and mechlorethamine are not metabolized prior to renal elimination. Carmustine primarily is cleared by the kidneys but a small portion is eliminated from the lungs [8,9].

The half-lives of the alkylators range from 10 minutes for procarbazine up to 290 hours for cisplatin. No half-life is given for mechlorethamine because it undergoes rapid chemical transformation in body fluids until the drug is no longer present in active form within a few minutes after administration. Dacarbazine, lomustine, streptozocin, and thiotepa have both initial and terminal phase half-lives [10].

APPROVED INDICATIONS

The alkylating agents are active against a wide variety of neoplastic diseases, with significant activity in the treatment of leukemias and lymphomas as well as many solid tumors. This group of drugs is routinely used in the treatment of acute and chronic leukemias; Hodgkin's disease; non-Hodgkin's lymphoma; multiple myeloma; primary brain tumors; carcinomas of the breast, ovaries, testes, lungs, bladder, cervix, head, and neck, and malignant melanoma [4,5,11–14].

A list of the indications for the alkylating agents is included in Table 1-3.

DOSAGES

Dosages of the alkylating agents are varied. Many of the drugs are used not only as single-agent therapy but as a part of combination regimens that include other antineoplastic agents. Clinicians should

Table 1-2. Pharmacokinetics of the Alkylating Agents

Agent	Half-life	Metabolism	Elimination
Bischloroethylamines			
Chlorambucil	90 min (parent drug)	Liver to active metabolites	Renal
Cyclophosphamide	145 min (metabolite)	Liver to active metabolites	Renal
Ifosfamide	4–6.5 h (parent drug)	Liver to active metabolites	Renal
Mechlorethamine	7–14 h (parent drug)	—	Renal
Melphalan	—	Hydrolysis	Chemical hydrolysis to
	Oral–90 min		monohydroxy- and
	IV — 6–10 min (initial)		dihydroxymelphalan;
	40–75 min (terminal)		low renal clearance
Aziridines			
Thiotepa	10 min (initial)	Liver to active metabolites	Renal (60%)
	125 min (terminal)		
Alkyl alkone sulfonates			
Busulfan	1.5–2.6 h	Liver	Renal
Nitrosoureas			
Carmustine	α — 6.1 min	Liver	Renal (60%–70%)
	β — 21.5 min		Lungs (6%–7%)
Lomustine	6 h (initial plasma)	Liver to active metabolites	Renal
	1–2 d (second plasma)		
Streptozocin	5 min (initial)	Liver and kidneys	Renal (60%–70%)
	35–40 min (terminal)		
Nonclassic alkylating agents			
Altretamine	3–10 h	Liver to active metabolites	Renal
Daacarbazine	19–55 min (initial phase)	Liver	Renal
	5–7.2 h (terminal phase)	Liver	Renal
Procarbazine	10 min	Liver and kidneys	Renal (70%)
Platinum Compounds			
Carboplatin	α (free drug) — 90 min	Liver to active metabolites	Renal
	β (free drug) — 180 min		
	β (free platinum) — 90 min		
Cisplatin	α — 20 min	—	Renal (unchanged)
	β — 48–70 min		
	γ — 24 h		

refer to the individual drug monographs for a more complete list of dosing regimens and for adjustments to dosing based on other factors.

TOXICITIES

The major toxicity common to all of the alkylating agents is myelosuppression. Gastrointestinal adverse effects of variable severity occur commonly and various organ toxicities are associated with specific compounds [3,4].

Leukopenia, thrombocytopenia, and anemia are all commonly occurring hematologic toxicities due to the effect of these drugs on the hematopoietic system. Hematologic toxicity is dose-related, cumulative, and can lead to treatment cycle delay or dosage reductions. Although the problem is usually reversible following discontinuation of the alkylator, long-term administration of the alkylating agents can lead to severe and prolonged duration of suppression of the bone marrow. The oral agents, chlorambucil, melphalan, busulfan, lomustine, altretamine, and procarbazine, have slower onset of hematologic toxicity, taking anywhere from 3 to 6 weeks for decreases in blood counts to appear. Nadirs for the IV administered alkylators appear within 1 or 2 weeks and persist for 1 or 2 weeks after discontinuing drug therapy. Prophylactic colony-stimulating factor use may be indicated.

A CBC including hematocrit, hemoglobin, platelets, and total and differential leukocyte counts should be obtained weekly throughout the treatment course to allow the physician to monitor for significant hematologic changes. Other serum chemistries, such as BUN, creatinine, SGPT, SGOT, lactate dehydrogenase, and bilirubin should be obtained at periodic intervals to monitor for adverse effects on liver and kidney function.

Patients being treated for lymphomas and leukemias who have high tumor burdens are especially subject to hyperuricemia. Hyperuricemia is caused by extensive purine catabolism that accompanies rapid cellular destruction and is not a specific toxicity of the drug. Because hyperuricemia is associated with rapid tumor lysis, patients being treated with chlorambucil, cyclophosphamide, mechlorethamine, uracil mustard, busulfan, carboplatin, and cisplatin should have serum uric acid levels monitored throughout the course of therapy.

Treatment of severe hematologic toxicity includes supportive therapy with platelet and erythrocyte transfusions and appropriate antibiotics for febrile neutropenia. Patients who have elevated serum uric acid levels should be treated with allopurinol and advised to increase their oral fluid intake.

Antineoplastic agents, including the alkylators, are toxic to rapidly proliferating cells. Because the gastrointestinal mucosa turns over rapidly, it is susceptible to these agents. Nausea and vomiting are the most common adverse gastrointestinal effects seen with this group of drugs. Stomatitis and anorexia also occur. These adverse effects can lead to decreased nutritional intake.

The gastrointestinal effects can be minimized by prescribing appropriate antiemetic agents as a part of the chemotherapy regimen and providing patients with orally or rectally administered antiemetics to use at home to combat delayed-onset emesis. Adequate fluid is essential to prevent complications associated with dehydration due to loss of excessive fluid volume. Electrolyte replacement may be necessary for patients with severe emesis or diarrhea.

Table 1-3. Approved Indications for Alkylating Agents

Alkylating Agent	Approved Indications
Bischloroethylamines	
Chlorambucil	Chronic lymphocytic leukemia, malignant lymphomas, lymphosarcoma, giant follicular lymphoma, Hodgkin's disease
Cyclophosphamide	Acute lymphocytic leukemia, acute myelocytic leukemia, chronic myelocytic leukemia, chronic lymphoncytic leukemia, acute monocytic leukemia, Hodgkin's and non-Hodgkin's lymphoma, carcinoma of the breast and ovary, multiple myeloma, mycosis fungoides, Burkitt's lymphoma, neuroblastoma, retinoblastoma
Ifosfamide	Third-line therapy for germ cell testicular tumors
Mechlorethamine	Palliative treatment of stage III and IV Hodgkin's disease, lymphosarcoma, chronic myelocytic leukemia, chornic lymphocytic leukemia, polycythemia vera, mycosis fungoides, bronchogenic carcinoma, palliative intraperitoneal treatment of metastatic carcinoma
Melphalan	Palliative treatment of multiple myeloma and nonresectable epithelial ovarian carcinoma
Uracil mustard	Palliative treatment of chonic lymphocytic leukemia, chronic myelocytic leukemia, non-Hodgkin's lymphomas, mycosis fungoides, early polycythemia vera
Aziridines	
Thiotepa	Intravesical treatment of tumors of the bladder, palliative treatment of adenocarcinoma of the breast or ovary, intrathecal treatment of meningeal neoplasms
Alkyl alkone sulfonates	
Busulfan	Chronic myelogenous leukemia, severe thrombocytosis, polycythemia vera
Nitrosoureas	
Carmustine	Palliative treatment of primary and metastatic brain tumors, multiple myeloma, disseminated Hodgkin's disease, non-Hodgkin's lymphomas
Lomustine	Palliative treatment of primary and metastatic brain tumors, disseminated Hodgkin's disease
Streptozocin	Metastatic islet cell carcinoma of the pancreas
Nonclassic alkylating agents	
Altretamine	Palliative treatment of persistent or recurrent ovarian cancer
Dacarbazine	Malignant melanoma, Hodgkin's disease
Procarbazine	Advanced Hodgkin's disease
Platinum compounds	
Carboplatin	Advanced ovarian carcinoma
Cisplatin	Metastatic testicular tumors, metastatic ovarian tumors, advanced bladder carcinoma

ALKYLATING AGENTS

Hemorrhagic cystitis is a major toxicity of ifosfamide as well as high-dose cyclophosphamide therapy and is caused by concentration of the metabolite acrolein in the bladder [3,4,11,15–18]. A urinalysis should be obtained and examined for microscopic hematuria prior to each course of treatment, especially with ifosfamide. To help prevent this complication, patients should be adequately hydrated prior to the start of the ifosfamide or cyclophosphamide infusion. Mesna, a uroprotective agent, should be administered in an intravenous dosage equal to 20% of the ifosfamide dosage (weight/weight) at the time of ifosfamide administration and repeated 4 and 8 hours after each dose of ifosfamide. Other mesna dosing schedules also may be used in patients receiving either ifosfamide or high-dose cyclophosphamide.

Patients receiving ifosfamide or high-dose cyclophosphamide therapy on an outpatient basis should be advised to increase their oral fluid intake and to void every 2 hours during the day and once at night on the days they receive their chemotherapy treatments to decrease the risk of hemorrhagic cystitis.

Table 1-4 lists the hematologic, gastrointestinal, and other major toxicities associated with the alkylating agents [2,11,15–21,41].

INVESTIGATIONAL AGENTS

Temozolomide and fotemustine are alkylating agents currently undergoing investigational study (Table 1-5). Temozolomide, an

Table 1-4. Major Toxicities of the Alkylating Agents

Alkylating Agent	Hematologic	Gastrointestinal	Other
Bischloroethylamines			
Chlorambucil	Leukopenia, thrombocytopenia	Nausea, vomiting, diarrhea, gastric discomfort (doses>20 mg)	Hyperuricemia*
Cyclophosphamide	Leukopenia, anemia, thrombocytopenia	Nausea, vomiting, anorexia	Hemorrhagic cystitis, alopecia, hyperuricemia*
Ifosfamide	Leukopenia, thrombocytopenia	Nausea, vomiting	Hemorrhagic cystitis, alopecia
Mechlorethamine	Leukopenia, anemia, thrombocytopenia, hemorrhagic diathesis	Nausea, vomiting	Thrombophlebitis, headache, weakness, hyperuricemia*
Melphalan	Leukopenia, thrombocytopenia	Nausea, vomiting (infrequently PO, more IV), mucositis	
Uracil mustard	Leukopenia, thrombocytopenia	Nausea, vomiting, anorexia, diarrhea, epigastric distress	Hyperuricemia*
Aziridines			
Thiotepa	Leukopenia, anemia, thrombocytopenia, pancytopenia	Nausea, vomiting, anorexia (infrequently), diarrhea	Pain at injection site, headache, dizziness
Alkyl alkone sulfonates			
Busulfan	Leukopenia, anemia, thrombocytopenia	Nausea, vomiting, diarrhea (infrequently)	Hyperuricemia*
Nitrosoureas			
Carmustine	Leukopenia, anemia, thrombocytopenia	Nausea, vomiting	Hepatotoxicity, pulmonary infiltrates
Lomustine	Leukopenia, anemia, thrombocytopenia with prolonged therapy	Nausea, vomiting	
Streptozocin	Mild to moderate leukopenia, anemia, thrombocytopenia	Nausea, vomiting	Nephrotoxicity, pain at injection site
Nonclassic Alkylating Agents			
Altretamine	Leukopenia, anemia, thrombocytopenia	Nausea, vomiting	Peripheral neuropathy
Dacarbazine	Leukopenia, thrombocytopenia	Nausea, vomiting, anorexia	Pain at injection site, fever, myalgia, malaise, hypocalcemia, hypotension (high doses)
Procarbazine	Leukopenia, anemia, thrombocytopenia	Nausea, vomiting, anorexia, stomatitis	
Platinum Compounds			
Carboplatin	Leukopenia, anemia, thrombocytopenia	Nausea, vomiting	Peripheral neuropathies, ototoxicity
Cisplatin	Leukopenia, anemia, thrombocytopenia	Nausea, vomiting	Nephrotoxicity, hypomagnesemia, hypocalcemia, hypokalemia, ototoxicity, peripheral neuropathy, hyperuricemia*

*Hyperuricemia is most often associated with leukemia and lymphoma in patients who have a high tumor burden and is not necessarily an adverse effect of the drug.

Table 1-5. Investigational Alkylating Agents

Agent	Class	Investigational Uses
Temozolomide	Nonclassical alkylator	Primary brain tumors, malignant melanoma, mycosis fungoides, high-grade recurrent astrocytoma
Fotemustine	Nitrosourea	Colorectal cancer, metastatic malignant melanoma, non–small cell lung cancer, high-grade gliomas

imidazotetrazine derivative, is an oral nonclassical alkylator that has activity against primary brain tumors, malignant melanoma, mycosis fungoides, and high-grade recurrent astrocytoma. Doses of 750–1000 mg/m² divided equally over 5 days have been used. The major toxicities of temozolomide are leukopenia and thrombocytopenia, mild to moderate nausea and vomiting, and rarely alopecia or skin rash [22–28].

Fotemustine, an amino acid–linked chloroethyl nitrosourea, has activity against disseminated malignant melanoma. It also has been studied in colorectal cancer, non–small cell lung cancer, and high-grade gliomas. Doses of 100 to 500 mg/m² in a variety of treatment regimens have been investigated. Leukopenia, thrombocytopenia, anemia, central nervous system toxicity, and transient liver chemistry abnormalities are the major reported toxicities of fotemustine [29–34].

COST ANALYSIS

The cost of treating cancer patients with the alkylating agents varies based on the treatment course selected, doses of the alkylating agents, and number of cycles of therapy.

Two key mechanisms are 1) high levels of O6-alkylguanine-DNA alkyltransferase for resistance to nitrosoureas [35], and 2) glutathione and glutathione-s transformed for alkylating agents [36]. DNA repair processes explain most of the resistance. Recently, tumor defects in mismatch repair have been associated with platinum- and methylating-agent resistance [37,38].

MECHANISMS OF RESISTANCE

Resistance to antineoplastic agents is the major cause of treatment failure for many cancer patients. Increasing dosages of drugs may be required to levels where toxicities are prohibitive. Alternatively, changing the treatment to a non–cross-resistant drug or combination of drugs that will be effective against the particular neoplasm is required. Resistance is either primary (natural) or acquired. Primary resistance results when innate resistance is selected out from natural cell lines. Acquired resistance results from drug-induced adaptation or mutation of neoplastic cells. Acquired resistance may be due to decreased intracellular concentrations of the drug, increased degradation of the active compound, decreased conversion of the drug to the active form, changes in cellular metabolism and utilization of separate metabolic pathways, and increased activity or concentration of target enzymes within the cell. Among the alkylating agents, cross-resistance has been reported with carmustine and lomustine.

AREAS OF RESEARCH ACTIVITY

As oncologists strive to improve the treatment of cancer, research studies continue with many drugs being studied for possible new indications [6,39–40]. The alkylating agents, although among the oldest antineoplastic agents, continue to be studied for possible new indications, both alone and in combination with other antineoplastics.

Among the alkylators, ifosfamide and dacarbazine are being examined in the treatment of soft tissue sarcomas. Mechlorethamine and carmustine have been studied for topical application in the treatment of mycosis fungoides [7]. Cyclophosphamide is being studied in small cell lung carcinoma and in carcinomas of the gastrointestinal tract, endometrium, testes, prostate, and bladder and in renal cell carcinoma. Streptozocin has shown activity in metastatic carcinoid tumors and in metastatic colorectal cancer. Cisplatin has shown activity in metastatic squamous cell carcinomas of the head and neck and cervix, and in non–small cell lung carcinoma. Temozolomide shows promising activity in anaplastic astrocytomas and melanoma.

High-dose chemotherapy is being increasingly utilized with hematopoietic cellular support (eg, bone marrow or peripheral blood progenitor cell transfusion and colony-stimulating factor use). Cyclophosphamide, carmustine, carboplatin, cisplatin, melphalan, and thiotepa are among the alkylators that have been used in this approach to cancer chemotherapy [8,39–45]. Recently, a potent inhibitor of O6-alkylguanine-DNA alkyltransferase, O6-benzylguanine, has been identified that potentiates the anti-tumor efficacy of nitrosoureas and methylating agents such as temozolomide [46]. It has now entered phase 1 and 2 clinical trials [47]. In addition, d,l-Buthionine-S,R-sulfoximine (L-BSO) has been identified as an inhibitor of the synthesis if glutathione resulting in increased cytotoxicity of many alkylating agents [36,48]. It also has entered phase 1 and 2 clinical trials [49]. Both represent a new class of mechanism-based agents designed to overcome tumor drug resistance.

REFERENCES

1. Calabresi P, Rall T, Nies A, Palmer T. In *Goodman and Gilman's The Pharmacological Basis of Therapeutics*, edn 8 Edited by Gilman A, Rall T, Nies A, Palmer T. New York: Pergamon Press, 1990:1202–1276.

2. Chabner BA, Collins JM, eds: *Cancer Chemotherapy: Principles and Practice*. Philadelphia: JB Lippincott, 1990.

3. Black DJ, Livingston RB: Antineoplastic drugs in 1990: a review (Part I). *Drugs* 1990, 39:489–501.

4. Black DJ, Livingston RB: Antineoplastic drugs in 1990: a review (Part II). *Drugs* 1990, 39:652–673.

5. Alberts DS: Clinical pharmacology of carboplatin. *Semin Oncol* 1990, 7(Suppl):6–9.

6. Whitmore WF, Yagoda Y: Chemotherapy in the management of bladder tumors. *Drugs* 1989, 38:301–312.

7. Zackheim HS, Epstein EH, Carin WR: Topical carmustine (BCNU) for cutaneous T-cell lymphoma: a 15-year experience in 143 patients. *J Am Acad Dermatol* 1990, 22(Part 1):802–810.

8. Henner WD, Peters WP, Eden JP: Pharmacokinetics and immediate effects of high-dose carmustine in man. *Cancer Treat Rep* 1986, 70:877–880.

9. Jones RB, Matthes S, Dufton C, *et al.*: Pharmacokinetic/pharmacodynamic interactions of intensive cyclophosphamide, cisplatin, and BCNU in patients with breast cancer. *Breast Cancer Res Treat* 1993, 26:S11–17.

10. Cohen BG, Egorin MJ, Kohlhepp EA, *et al.*: Human plasma pharmacokinetics and urinary excretion of thiotepa and its metabolites. *Cancer Treat Rep* 1986, 70:859–864.

11. Dechant KL, Brogden RN, Pillington T, Faulds D: Ifosfamide/mesna: a review of antineoplastic activity, pharmacokinetic properties, and therapeutic efficacy in cancer. *Drugs* 1991, 42:428–467.

12. Gad E, Mawla N, *et al.*: Ifosfamide, methotrexate, and 5-fluorouracil: effective combination in resistant breast cancer. *Cancer Chemother Pharmacol* 1990, 26(Suppl):S85–S86.

13. Hansen LA, Hughes TE: Altretamine. DICP, *Ann Pharmacother* 1991, 25:146–152.

14. Loehrer PJ, Einhorn LH: Cisplatin. *Ann Inter Med* 1984, 100:704–713.

15. Dorr RT: Ifosfamide and cyclophosphamide: review and appraisal. 1992.

16. Frasier LH, Kanekal S, Kehrer JP: Cyclophosphamide toxicity: characterizing and avoiding the problem. *Drugs* 1991, 42:781–795.

17. Sanchiz F, Milla A: High-dose ifosfamide and mesna in advanced breast cancer. *Cancer Chemother Pharmacol* 1990, 26(Suppl):S91–S92.

18. Thigpen T, Lambath BW, Vance RB: Ifosfamide in the management of gynecologic cancers. *Semin Oncol* 1990, 17(Suppl 4): 11–18.

19. Finley RS, Fortner CL, Grove WR: Cisplatin nephrotoxicity: a summary of preventative interventions. *Drug Intelligence Clin Pharma* 1985, 19:362–367.

20. Kris MG, Gralla RJ, Clark RA, *et al.*: Incidence, course, and severity of delayed nausea and vomiting following the administration of high-dose cisplatin. *J Clin Oncol* 1985, 3:1379–1384.

21. Smith AC: The pulmonary toxicity of nitrosoureas. *Pharmacol Therapeutics* 1989, 41:443–460.

22. Brada M, Moore S, Judson I, *et al.*: A phase I study of SCH52365 in adult patients with advanced cancer. *Proc Am Soc Clin Oncol* 1995, 14:470. Abstract.

23. Eckardt JR, Weiss GR, Burris HA: Phase I and pharmacokinetic trial of SCH52365 given orally daily x 5 days. *Proc Am Soc Clin Oncol* 1995, 14:1759.

24. Newlands ES, Stevens MF, Wedge SR, *et al.*: Temozolomide: a review of its discovery, chemical properties, pre-clinical development and clinical trials. *Cancer Treat Rev* 1997, 23:35-61.

25. Newlands ES, O'Reilly SM, Glaser MG, *et al.*: The Charing Cross Hospital experience with temozolomide in patients with gliomas. *Eur J Cancer* 1996, 13:2236-2241.

26. O'Reilly SM, Newlands ES, Glaser MG, *et al.*: Temozolomide: a new oral cytotoxic chemotherapeutic agent with promising activity against primary brain tumors. *Euro J Cancer* 1993, 29A:940–942.

27. Patel M, McCully C, Godwin K, Balis F: Plasma and cerebrospinal fluid pharmacokinetics of temozolomide. *Proc Am Soc Clin Oncol* 1995, 14:461. Abstract.

28. Stevens MFG, Newland ES: From triazines and triazenes to temozolomide. *Euro J Cancer* 1993, 29A:1045–1047.

29. Antico J, Pascon G, Turjansky L, *et al.*: Phase II study of fotemustine in gliomas: preliminary report. *Proc Am Soc Oncol* 1995, 14:151. Abstract.

30. Fishchel JL: Tamoxifen enhances the cytotoxic effects of the nitrosourea fotemustine: results of human melanoma cell lines. *Euro J Cancer* 1993, 29A:2269–2273.

31. Khayat D, Berille J, Gerard B, *et al.*: Fotemustine in the treatment of brain primary tumors and metastases. *Cancer Invest* 1994, 12:414–420.

32. Riviere A, LeCesne A, Berille J, *et al.*: Cisplatin-fotemustine combination in inoperable non-small lung cancer: preliminary report of a French multicenter phase II trial. *Euro J Cancer* 1994, 30A:587–590.

33. Rougier P, Chabot GG, Bonneterre J, *et al.*: Phase II and pharmacokinetics study of fotemustine in inoperable colorectal cancer. *Euro J Cancer* 1993, 29A:288–289.

34. Trachand B, Lucas C, Biron F, *et al.*: Phase I pharmacokinetics study of high dose fotemustine and its metabolite 2-chloroethanol in patients with high-grade gliomas. *Cancer Chemother Pharmacol* 1993, 32:46–52.

35. Pegg AE, Dolan ME, Moschel RC: Structure, function, and inhibition of O6-alkylguanine-DNA alkyltransferase. *Prog Nucleic Acid Res Mol Biol* 1995, 51:167-223.

36. Skapek SX, Colvin OM, Griffith OW, *et al.*: Enhanced melphalan cytotoxicity following buthionine sulfoximine-mediated glutathione depletion in a human medulloblastoma xenograft in athymic mice. *Cancer Res* 1988, 48:2764-2767.

37. Liu L, Markowitz S, Gerson SL: Mismatch repair mutations override alkyltransferase in conferring resistance to temozolomide but not to 1,3-bis (2-chloroethyl) nitrosourea. *Cancer Res* 1996, 56:5375-5379.

38. Fink D, Zheng H, Nebel S, *et al.*: In vitro and in vivo resistance to cisplatin in cells that have lost DNA mismatch repair. *Cancer Res* 1997, 57:1841-1845.

39. Calvert AH, Newell DR, Gore HE: Future directions with carboplatin: can therapeutic monitoring, high dose administration, and hematologic support with growth factors expand the spectrum compared with cisplatin? *Semin Oncol* 1992, 19(Suppl 2):155–163.

40. Batts CN: Adjuvant intravesical therapy for superficial bladder cancer. *Ann Pharmacother* 1992, 26:1270–1276.

41. Corden BJ, Fine RL, Ozols RF, Collins JM: Clinical pharmacology of high-dose cisplatin. *Cancer Chemother Pharmacol* 1985, 14:38–41.

42. Ackland SP, Choi K, Ratain MJ: Human plasma pharmacokinetics following administration of high-dose thiotepa and cyclophosphamide. *J Clin Oncol* 1988, 6:1192–1196.

43. Bishop JF: Current experience with high-dose carboplatin therapy. *Semin Oncol* 1992, 19(Suppl):150–154.

44. Rohaly J: The use of busulfan therapy in bone marrow transplantation. *Cancer Nursing* 1989, 12:144–152.

45. Antman, K, Eder JP, Elias A, *et al.*: High-dose thiotepa alone and in combination regimens with bone marrow support. *Semin Oncol* 1990, 17:33-38.

46. Dolan, ME, Stine L, Mitchell RB, *et al.*: Modulation of mammalian O6-alkylguanine-DNA alkyltransferase in vivo by O6-benzylguanine and its effect on the sensitivity of a human glioma tumor to 1-(2-chloroethyl)-3-(4-methylcyclohexyl)-1-nitrosourea. *Cancer Commun* 1990, 2:371-377.

47. Gerson SL, Willson JK: O6-alkylguanine-DNA alkyltransferase. A target for the modulation of drug resistance. *Hematol Oncol Clin North Am* 1995, 9:431-450.

48. Du, DL, Volpe DA, Grieshaber CK, Murphy M Jr: Effects of L-phenylalanine mustard and L-buthionine sulfoximine on murine and human hematopoietic progenitor cells in vitro. *Cancer Res* 1990, 50:4038-4043.

49. Lacreta, FP, Brennan JM, Hamilton TC, *et al.*: Stereoselective pharmacokinetics of L-buthionine SR-sulfoximine in patients with cancer. *Drug Metab Dispos* 1994, 22:835-842.

50. Lazarus, HM, Crilley P, Ciobanu N, *et al.*: High-dose carmustine, etoposide, and cisplatin and autologous bone marrow transplantation for relapsed and refractory lymphoma. *J Clin Oncol* 1992, 10:1682-1689.

51. Jones, RB, Matthes S, Shpall EJ, *et al.*: Acute lung injury following treatment with high-dose cyclophosphamide, cisplatin, and carmustine: pharmacodynamic evaluation of carmustine. *J Natl Cancer Inst* 1993, 85:640-647.

ALTRETAMINE

Altretamine (also known as hexamethylmelamine) is an antineoplastic agent structurally similar to triethylenemelamine, a known alkylating agent. The mechanism of action is unknown. It has been postulated that altretamine may act as an alkylator or as an antimetabolite. Altretamine is activated via hepatic microsomal enzymes to cytotoxic intermediates, which may bind to microsomal proteins and DNA. The National Cancer Institute developed altretamine ~18 y ago. The United States Food and Drug Administration approved the drug for market in 1991.

DOSAGE AND ADMINISTRATION

Usual dose is 4–12 mg/kg PO in divided daily doses for 21–90 d, or 240–320 mg/m² PO in divided daily doses for 14–21 d; doses are repeated every 6 wk

SPECIAL PRECAUTIONS

All cytotoxic drugs may be embryotoxic or teratogenic; use with caution in pregnant or nursing patients

TOXICITIES

GI: nausea and vomiting occur in approximately 50%–70% of patients and are usually considered dose-limiting; anorexia, abdominal cramps, and diarrhea also have been reported; **CNS:** neurologic side effects are reported in 20% of patients, including paresthesias, numbness, sleep disturbances, confusion, hallucinations, seizures, and Parkinsonian-like syndrome with ataxia; **Hematologic:** mild leukopenia and thrombocytopenia; **Miscellaneous:** alopecia, rash, and pruritus

INDICATIONS

FDA-approved: Treatment of advanced ovarian cancer; Clinical studies show activity in metastatic breast cancer, refractory lymphoma, pancreatic adenocarcinoma, and colorectal, cervical, and endometrial cancers; **investigational uses:** treatment of small cell and non–small cell lung cancer

PHARMACOKINETICS

Absorption—the micronized capsule form exhibits enhanced gastrointestinal absorption; however, oral absorption is extremely variable; peak plasma concentrations can occur from 0.5–3 h after administration; **Distribution**—altretamine is minimally protein bound and highly lipid-soluble; it tends to distribute in tissues with a high lipid content, such as the omentum and subcutaneous tissues; the parent drug does not cross the blood—brain barrier to a significant extent; altretamine metabolites may be more protein bound and also cross the blood–brain barrier more readily. Therefore, the CNS side effects may be due to the metabolites, not the parent drug; **Metabolism**—altretamine is extensively metabolized in the liver; extrahepatic metabolism also may occur; **Elimination**—the elimination half-life varies from 3–10 h; primarily eliminated in the urine as metabolites; a small amount may be excreted through the lungs as expired air and in the feces

DRUG INTERACTIONS

Cimetidine increases the toxicity of altretamine by prolonging its half-life by 29%–80%; phenobarbital may induce the metabolism of altretamine and reduce its antitumor activity; monoamine oxidase inhibitors may result in severe orthostatic hypotension

RESPONSE RATES

When altretamine is used as single-agent treatment for ovarian cancer, response rates of 20%–30% have been reported; in combination with cyclophosphamide, doxorubicin and melphalan response rates increased, ranging from 20%–80% (including complete and partial responses); single-agent therapy for small cell and non—small cell lung cancer ranges from 4%–42%; adding altretamine to cytotoxic agents known to be active against small cell lung cancer produced widely variable results, 7%–94%

PATIENT MONITORING

CBC, including differential leukocyte count and platelet count, should be performed during therapy to monitor for leukopenia and thrombocytopenia; complete neurologic exam should be performed on a routine basis; health care professionals responsible for monitoring patients on altretamine therapy should be familiar with the broad spectrum of other adverse effects that can occur, albeit less commonly, with this treatment

NURSING INTERVENTIONS

Monitor treatment tolerance, weight, and nutritional status; nausea and vomiting are common especially with high doses; appropriate antiemetics should be administered and daily doses should be divided into a four times a day schedule (after meals and at bedtime); neurotoxicity may be decreased by concomitant administration of 100 mg of pyridoxine

PATIENT INFORMATION

Call the doctor immediately if intractable nausea and vomiting occur, unusual bruising or bleeding occurs, fevers above 101°F occur; it is important to continue medication despite nausea and vomiting; GI effects can be controlled so the medication will be better tolerated—please report vomiting episodes that occur soon after the oral dose is taken; take after meals; report signs and symptoms of neurotoxicity

FORMULATION

Available as Hexalen (Applied Analytical Industries, Wilmington, NC, distributed by US Bioscience, West Conshohocken, PA) 50-mg hard gelatin capsules; stored at room temperature.

BUSULFAN

Busulfan is an oral alkylating agent that is cell cycle nonspecific and forms interstrand DNA crosslinks. It interferes with DNA replication and transcription of RNA and ultimately results in the disruption of nucleic acid function. Busulfan is primarily used to control chronic myelogenous leukemia because of its selective depression of granulocytopoiesis at low doses. At higher doses the effect on all three hematopoietic cell lines is increased.

DOSAGE AND ADMINISTRATION

Chronic myelogenous leukemia: 0.06 mg/kg or 1.8 mg/m^2 is recommended for both children and adults; therapy varies among clinicians and can be intermittent or continuous (most clinicians discontinue therapy when leukocyte counts decrease to ≤ 10,000/mm^3 and resume therapy when leukocyte counts reach 50,000/mm^3); **Bone marrow transplant preparatory regimens:** high-dose busulfan, 16 mg/kg total dose (4 mg/kg/d for 4 d) (also used in a variety of refractory cancers experimentally)

SPECIAL PRECAUTIONS

Life-threatening pancytopenia can occur with busulfan therapy (extensive monitoring of hematologic parameters is warranted); a rare but life-threatening hepatic venoocclusive disease has been reported with very high dose busulfan; contraindicated in patients with known hypersensitivity to the drug; contraindicated in patients whose chronic myelogenous leukemia has demonstrated resistance to this therapy; all cytotoxic drugs may be embryotoxic or teratogenic; busulfan therapy can cause widespread epithelial dysplasia, chromosomal aberrations, and germ cell aplasia; should be avoided in pregnant and nursing patients

INDICATIONS

FDA-approved: Palliative treatment of chronic myelogenous leukemias; **Clinical studies show activity in** other myeloproliferative disorders including severe thrombocytosis and polycythemia vera; myelofibrosis; and, in high doses, as a component of marrow-ablative conditioning regimens prior to bone marrow transplant for the treatment of malignant and nonmalignant conditions; now used as third-line treatment of chronic myelogenous leukemias after interferon-α and hydroxyurea and in combination with cyclophosphamide in preparative regimens for myeloablative therapy prior to autologous and allogeneic transplantation of bone marrow, peripheral blood, progenitor cell and cord blood

PHARMACOKINETICS

Absorption: rapidly and completely absorbed from the GI tract with measurable blood concentrations obtained within 0.5–2 h after oral administration; **Distribution:** cleared rapidly from the plasma; it is not known whether the drug is distributed into cerebrospinal fluid or into breast milk; **Metabolism:** extensively metabolized by the liver, with 12 metabolites being isolated to date; most of the metabolites have not been identified and it is not known if they possess cytotoxic activity; **Elimination:** ~10%–50% of the dose is excreted in the urine as metabolites within 24 h; monitoring peak blood levels during high-dose therapy is advised to decrease the incidence of venoocclusive disease

DRUG INTERACTIONS

Additive myelosuppression can occur when busulfan is combined with other cytotoxic drugs; hepatoxicity has been reported with the concomitant use of busulfan and thioguanine (more studies are needed to validate this interaction); phenytoin may significantly decrease the clearance of busulfan

RESPONSE RATES

Response rates of 90% have been reported in patients with previously untreated chronic myelogenous leukemia while taking busulfan; although not curative, hematologic remission with regression or stabilization of organomegaly has been noted with relief of symptoms; busulfan is less effective in patients with chronic myelogenous leukemia who lack the Philadelphia chromosome

BUSULFAN (Continued)

TOXICITIES

Hematologic: major dose-related adverse effect is bone marrow suppression (usually reversible but some patients can be very sensitive to the drug and experience an abrupt onset of possibly irreversible toxicity); severe leukopenia, anemia, and thrombocytopenia usually occur approximately 10 d after therapy and can continue 1–2 wk; severe toxicity due to overdose may be prolonged with complete recovery taking 1 mo–2 y; bone marrow fibrosis and chronic aplasia have been reported with busulfan administration; secondary neoplasia is possible

Pulmonary: a syndrome called *busulfan lung* is rare and can occur after long-term therapy; this syndrome is manifested by bronchopulmonary dysplasia with a diffuse interstitial pulmonary fibrosis and is characterized by persistent cough, fever, rales, and dyspnea; discontinuance of busulfan and administration of corticosteroids may improve symptoms and minimize permanent lung damage; in some patients the syndrome progresses to respiratory insufficiency despite intervention, and deaths usually occur within 6 mo

Metabolic: hyperuricemia may occur when the leukemia cell count is rapidly reduced; an Addison-like adrenal insufficiency syndrome is apparent in a small number of patients after long-term therapy

CNS: dizziness, blurred vision, loss of consciousness, and intermittent muscle twitching; myoclonic and generalized tonic-clonic seizures have occurred especially with high-dose therapy; prophylactic anticonvulsant administration has been employed during high-dose therapy for marrow-ablative conditioning regimens prior to bone marrow transplant

Infertility: germinal aplasia and sterility have been reported in rats but not humans; ovarian suppression and amenorrhea with menopausal symptoms commonly occur during busulfan therapy in premenopausal women; ovarian fibrosis and atrophy also have occurred; interferes with spermatogenesis and causes impotence, sterility, azoospermia, and testicular atrophy in male humans

Miscellaneous: mild gynecomastia, cheilosis, glossitis, hepatic dysfunction and cholestatic jaundice, porphyria cutanea tarda, melanoderma, urticaria, rashes, dryness of skin and mucous membranes, anhidrosis, alopecia, cataracts, hemorrhagic cystitis, and fatigue are rare; nausea, vomiting, diarrhea, anorexia, and weight loss are infrequent; venooclusive disease has been seen in high-dose therapy accompanied by hyperbilirubinemia, weight gain, ascites, and hepatic injury

PATIENT MONITORING

A CBC, including differential leukocyte count and platelet count, is generally obtained weekly; leukocyte count generally will not decrease for 10–15 d—this delay should not be interpreted as resistance to the drug nor should the dose be increased; because the effects of busulfan will continue to decrease leukocyte count after discontinuance, the drug should be withheld when leukocyte counts have fallen between 10,000–15,000/mm^3; treatment should be resumed once leukocyte count increases again to ≥ 50,000/mm^3; signs of persistent cough and progressive dyspnea should be carefully monitored; monitor for symptoms of adrenal insufficiency, such as abrupt weakness, unusual fatigue, anorexia, weight loss, nausea and vomiting, and melanoderma; monitoring busulfan serum concentrations and subsequently adjusting the dose may lessen the toxicities observed with high-dose therapy used in bone marrow transplant; health care professionals responsible for monitoring patients on busulfan therapy should be familiar with the broad spectrum of other adverse effects that can occur, albeit less commonly, with this treatment

NURSING INTERVENTIONS

Monitor treatment tolerance, weight, and nutritional status; assure that appropriate lab tests are conducted to monitor for hematologic effects as well as for hyperuricemia and renal function; explain to the patient the importance of weekly blood count monitoring

PATIENT INFORMATION

Call the doctor immediately if the following occurs: unusual bruising or bleeding, temperature over 101°F, sore throat, or other signs of infection; let the doctor or nurse know if you are experiencing a persistent cough or having difficulty breathing; continue to take medication despite the nausea and vomiting; continued monitoring of blood counts is very important and should not be missed; do not take aspirin-containing products they may increase the chance of bleeding; if you forget your because medication, take it as soon as you remember within 24 h of the missed dose (if it has been more than 24 h since the dose was missed, do not take an extra dose but continue with the next regularly scheduled dose)

FORMULATION

Available as Myleran (Glaxo Wellcome Co., Research Triangle Park, NC) 2-mg scored tablets each containing the inactive ingredients magnesium stearate and sodium chloride.

CARBOPLATIN

Carboplatin is a second-generation platinum compound that may be classified as a nonclassical alkylating agent and is cell cycle nonspecific. Carboplatin and cisplatin have similar spectrums of activity. This second-generation platinum is used primarily for the treatment of ovarian cancer but also has shown promise in the treatment of seminomas, squamous cell carcinomas of the head and neck, and small cell lung cancer. Carboplatin, "the kinder platinum," is similar to cisplatin but was developed in an attempt to decrease the severe side effects of cisplatin. Nephrotoxicity, ototoxicity, neurotoxicity, and dose-limiting nausea and vomiting are lessened with carboplatin therapy. The major dose-limiting toxicity of carboplatin is myelosuppression. Like cisplatin, carboplatin is a cytotoxic platinum complex that reacts with nucleophilic sites on DNA. This causes interstrand and intrastrand cross-links and DNA-protein cross-links, which inhibits DNA, RNA, and protein synthesis.

DOSAGE AND ADMINISTRATION

Many clinicians routinely use the Calvert formula to dose carboplatin instead of the standard dosing schema mentioned above. This formula is based on a target area under the curve (AUC), the average being 7 mg/mL/min (4–11 mg/mL/min) and the patient's glomerular filtration rate (GFR, mL/min), because the original Calvert formula measured GFR with ^{51}Cr-labeled EDTA. Modifications using estimated creatinine clearance have been used but are less accurate at predicting the actual AUC. Target AUC depends on the patient's previous treatment history, concomitant chemotherapy, and disease state. The Calvert formula is: Total Dose = target AUC times (GFR + 25). Intraperitoneal doses of 200–650 mg/m^2 have been used. High-dose carboplatin (800–2000 mg/m^2) has been used investigationally with and without bone marrow support. Doses higher than 2000 mg/m^2 have been associated with hepatic toxicity. There is no therapeutic difference between 24-h continuous infusion and bolus dosing. Bolus dosing may be more convenient and does not require hospital admittance.

SPECIAL PRECAUTIONS

Myelosuppression is the major dose-limiting toxicity of carboplatin; monitoring for leukopenia, anemia, and thrombocytopenia should be continued throughout therapy; thrombocytopenia can be more severe than leukopenia and anemia; all cytotoxic drugs may be embryotoxic or teratogenic; use with caution in pregnant or nursing patients; contraindicated in patients with a history of severe allergic reactions to cisplatin or other platinum-containing compounds, or mannitol

INDICATIONS

FDA-approved: Initial and secondary treatment of advanced ovarian cancer; clinical studies show activity in lung cancers, squamous cell cancers of the head and neck, gastrointestinal cancer, and testicular cancer

PHARMACOKINETICS

Absorption: AUC increases proportionally with the dose of carboplatin; when administered intraperitoneally, plasma concentrations are approximately one fifth of the peritoneal dose; **Distribution:** 24 h after administration, tissue concentrations of carboplatin can be detected in the kidneys, liver, skin, and ileum; very low concentrations can be found in the spleen, lung, muscle, heart, testes, brain, fat, and bone marrow; 10%–18% of plasma carboplatin is protein bound shortly after bolus administration (some studies have shown protein binding as high as 40%–87% 24 h after carboplatin administration); the volume of distribution has been measured as 16–20 L; **Metabolism:** limited information available; it has been reported that carboplatin is metabolized into highly reactive diamine metabolites that may be similar to cisplatin metabolites; **Elimination:** renal clearance is the main route of excretion of carboplatin and its metabolites; within the first 24 h, 58%–77% of the administered dose is excreted as free platinum and approximately 32% is excreted as unchanged carboplatin; the plasma elimination half lives of carboplatin and free platinum are approximately 3 and 6 h, respectively; renal and total body clearance can be compromised in older or renally impaired patients

DRUG INTERACTIONS

If carboplatin is given concurrently with **nephrotoxic drugs**, myelosuppression and renal toxicity can be enhanced

RESPONSE RATES

Response rates of 25%–28% have been reported in the treatment of ovarian cancer with carboplatin alone in patients previously treated with cisplatin: this may indicate that the two platinum agents are not completely cross-resistant; patients not previously treated with cisplatin achieved responses of 85% with carboplatin; when carboplatin is used in combination with other cytotoxic drugs (*ie*, cyclophosphamide, doxorubicin, 5-fluorouracil, and cisplatin), complete and partial response rates are seen in 30%–83% of patients; intraperitoneal carboplatin has produced 53% response rates in patients previously treated with cisplatin

Varied response rates to carboplatin have been reported in small cell lung cancer and non–small cell lung cancer; responses are usually much higher in patients who have not been previously treated; responses of 0%–60% have been reported in patients with small cell lung cancer treated with carboplatin alone; the combinations of carboplatin with other cytotoxic drugs exhibits slightly improved responses of 50%–77%; in non–small cell lung cancer, combination therapy has produced response rates of 40%–56%

(Continued on next page)

CARBOPLATIN (Continued)

TOXICITIES

Hematologic: dose-limiting thrombocytopenia can occur in 37%–80% of patients receiving carboplatin; contributing factors include increased age, renal impairment, and concurrent and previous chemotherapy; the extent of myelosuppression appears to be proportional to area under the curve (AUC) of ultrafilterable platinum; leukopenia and anemia have been reported in 27%–38% of patients who receive carboplatin alone; myelosuppression is reversible but severity may be cumulative with repeated doses

GI: mild and manageable nausea and vomiting (dose-dependent but rarely dose-limiting); delayed GI toxicity can occur 6–12 h after carboplatin is administered

Renal: although less common than cisplatin, nephrotoxicity can occur with carboplatin therapy, usually caused by chronic tubular damage

Miscellaneous: alopecia is mild but can increase in severity with cumulative therapy; usually mild and infrequent: abnormal liver function tests, mild neurotoxicity, hypersensitivity, stomatitis, mucositis, and flu-like syndrome; with high-dose regimens used in autologous bone marrow transplant, hepatotoxicity, severe renal dysfunction, and severe nausea, vomiting, and electrolyte wasting have been reported

DOSAGE AND ADMINISTRATION*

Treatment Schedule	Dosage, mg/m^2		
	Adults		**Children**
	Previous Therapy	**No Previous Therapy**	
Bolus every 4 wk	240–270	350–450	560
24 h coninuous infusion every 4–5 wk	240	320	
Weekly bolus for 4 consecutive wk with 2 wk of rest	100	125	175
Bolus for 5 consecutive days every 4–6 wk	77	100	

*_It is preferred to use the Calvert dosing formula to individualize dosing based on patient GFR._

RENAL DOSAGE ADJUSTMENT

Baseline Creatinine Clearance, mL/min	Recommended Dose on Day 1, mg/m^2
41–59	250
16–40	200

Dosage adjustment in older or renally impaired patients is recommended. Renal dosage adjustment should only be used for initial therapy. Doses for subsequent courses should be based on hematologic parameters.

HEMATOLOGIC DOSE ADJUSTMENT

Platelets	Neurtrophils	Adjusted Dose (From Prior Course)
>100,000	>2000	125%
50–100,000	500–2000	No adjustemtn
<50,000	<500	75%

RESPONSE RATES *(Continued)*

Low response rates averaging 25% are reported when carboplatin is used alone in the treatment of squamous cell carcinoma of the head and neck; when combined with 5-fluorouracil, response rates increase to 62%–92%

Carboplatin alone has demonstrated poor results in the treatment of gastrointestinal cancers; in combination with 5-fluorouracil response rates increase

Promising responses of 84%–86% in patients with seminomatous testicular cancer have been reported; these responses include both previously treated and untreated patients; however, very poor results are reported in the treatment of nonseminomatous testicular cancer

PATIENT MONITORING

CBC, including differential leukocyte count, platelet count, and hemoglobin and hematocrit should be obtained during therapy to monitor for leukopenia, thrombocytopenia, and anemia; routine serum chemistries, especially serum creatinine, should be obtained regularly to monitor electrolyte status and renal function; although the occurrence is infrequent, neurotoxicity is reported—a complete neurologic examination should be performed at the beginning of and then intermittently through therapy; health care professionals responsible for monitoring patients on carboplatin therapy should be familiar with the less common adverse effects that can occur with therapy

NURSING INTERVENTIONS

Monitor treatment tolerance, weight, nutritional status; ensure that appropriate lab tests are conducted to monitor for leukopenia, thrombocytopenia, anemia, and renal function; nausea and vomiting are usually mild to moderate—appropriate antiemetics should be given for management; fluid hydration should be given concurrently; notify physician of uncommon adverse events such as hypersensitivity reactions and skin rashes

PATIENT INFORMATION

Call the doctor immediately if intractable nausea and vomiting occur, unusual bruising and bleeding occur, temperature over 101°F; avoid exposure to people with infections; continue hydration by drinking several glasses of water for 1 or 2 d after therapy

FORMULATION

Available as Paraplatin (Bristol-Myers Oncology Division, Princeton, NJ) in 50-, 150-, and 450-mg vials

Carboplatin is available as a sterile, lyophilized white powder for injection containing equal parts of carboplatin and mannitol; unopened vials should be stored at room temperature and protected from light; the drug must be reconstituted with either sterile water for injection, 0.9% sodium chloride, or dextrose 5% and water yielding a concentration of 10 mg/mL; the reconstituted solution is stable for 8 h and should be discarded because the drug contains no antibacterial preservative; after reconstitution, carboplatin may be further diluted in 0.9% sodium chloride or dextrose 5% water and should be given a 24-h expiration; carboplatin can be infused over 30 or 60 min or 24 h; during preparation and administration, aluminum needles and administration sets should not be used (when carboplatin comes in contact with aluminum the interaction will form a precipitate and result in loss of potency of the drug).

CARMUSTINE

Carmustine (also known a BiCNU or BCNU) is a nitrosourea derivative that has demonstrated cytotoxic activity against a wide variety of malignancies. As with other alkylating agents, carmustine is considered to be cell cycle nonspecific. Active metabolites are responsible for the alkylation, DNA crosslink formation, and carbamoylation activity that interferes with DNA, RNA, and protein synthesis. Cross-resistance between carmustine and lomustine has occurred. Tumors expressing high O6-alkylguanine-DNA alkyltransferase are resistant. Carmustine and its metabolites are distributed rapidly into the cerebrospinal fluid. Nitrosoureas as a class tend to be highly lipophilic, thus enhancing their ability to cross the blood–brain barrier and to be used in the treatment of meningeal leukemias and brain tumors. The long-term use of nitrosoureas has been associated with profound cumulative myelosuppression and renal failure (especially with methyl-CCNU, used investigationally only) with lesions similar to radiation-induced nephritis.

Topical preparations of carmustine have been used to treat mycosis fungoides (cutaneous T-cell lymphoma, or CTCL). Historically topical nitrogen mustard (mechlorethamine) has been used for mycosis fungoides. The mechanism of action is unknown because the alkylating action of mechlorethamine is dissipated shortly after it is dissolved in water but the anti-CTCL activity still remains. The mechanism of action of topical carmustine is similarly unknown.

DOSAGE AND ADMINISTRATION

Adult doses ranging from 30–200 mg/m^2 have been used; may be given as a single slow infusion or divided into multiple infusions over 2–5 d every 6 wk; repeat doses should not be given until leukocyte count is > 4000/mm^3, absolute neutrophil count is < 1500/mm^3, and platelet count is > 100,000/mm^3; doses up to 600 mg/m^2 (as a single dose or divided over 3 d) are used in single-agent or combination therapy in autologous bone marrow transplant protocols for breast cancer or advanced neoplasms [43].

The manufacturer suggests adjusting subsequent doses according to previous treatment nadirs.

NADIR AFTER PRIOR DOSAGE (CELLS/MM^3)

Leukocytes	Platelets	Amount of Prior Dose to be Given, %
> 4000	< 100,000	100
3000–3999	75,000–99,999	100
2000–2999	25,000–74,999	70
< 2000	<25,000	50

Some clinicians use absolute neutrophil count (ANC) as the basis of dose adjustment; in which case, reduce the dose by 2.5% for an ANC at nadir of < 1000/mm^3 and by 50% for an ANC < 500/mm^3.

Carmustine is applied topically for mycosis fungoides in a hydroalcoholic solution or ointment in concentrations of 0.05%–0.4%. Topical carmustine is applied once or twice a day. Carmustine can also be given intralesionally at concentrations of 0.1%–0.2% for the management of persistent papules or small nodules associated with mycosis fungoides.

INDICATIONS

FDA-approved: Palliative treatment of primary and metastatic brain tumors; used in combination with prednisone and other cytotoxic agents in the treatment of multiple myeloma; used in combination with other chemotherapeutic agents for the treatment of disseminated Hodgkin's disease and non-Hodgkin's lymphoma; clinical studies show activity in carcinoma of the lung, carcinoma of the GI tract, breast carcinoma, Ewing's sarcoma, malignant melanoma, Burkitt's lymphoma; as a topical formulation, carmustine has been shown to have activity in mycosis fungoides

PHARMACOKINETICS

Absorption: not absorbed across the GI tract; absorption from topical application is apparent; **Distribution:** cleared rapidly from the plasma; carmustine and its metabolites rapidly cross the blood–brain barrier; cerebrospinal fluid concentrations of metabolites have been reported to be 15%–70% of the concurrent plasma concentrations; plasma carmustine is ~77% protein bound; is also distributed in breast milk; **Metabolism/Elimination—** rapidly metabolized by the liver; approximately 60%–70% of carmustine and its metabolites are excreted in the urine within 96 h, 6%–7% are excreted as carbon dioxide by the lungs, and 1% is excreted in the feces; average plasma half-life is 22 min; volume of distribution reported in some studies has been as high as 5.1 L/kg; researchers have discovered great patient-to-patient variation in plasma clearance of carmustine—factors causing such variation may include the percent of body fat, serum lipid concentration, and sample collection; some enterohepatic circulation is believed to occur

DRUG INTERACTIONS

Concomitant use of cimetidine and carmustine can result in increased bone marrow toxicity

RESPONSE RATES

When used as a single agent for brain tumors, objective response rates occur in ~50% of patients; similar response rates are reported with carmustine-containing chemotherapy combinations

The use of carmustine and prednisone in multiple myeloma has produced response rates of 39%, as opposed to a response rate of 11% when carmustine is used alone

Response rates of 50% have been demonstrated in patients with advanced Hodgkin's disease refractory to other established treatments; carmustine has been used as a substitute for mechlorethamine in MOPP therapy

For patients with non-Hodgkin's lymphoma, a 28% response rate has been reported using carmustine alone

Carmustine is considered inferior to dacarbazine in the treatment of malignant melanoma; although response rates of 30% have been reported in the treatment of malignant melanoma, carmustine-containing combinations have failed to produce adequate CNS response

A 21% response rate has been reported with carmustine in the treatment of solid tumors: lung, breast, and GI tract

(Continued on next page)

CARMUSTINE (Continued)

SPECIAL PRECAUTIONS

Because of the prolonged myelosuppression, treatment should not be given more often than every 6 wk; blood counts should be performed weekly for 6–8 wk after administration of carmustine; pulmonary toxicity appears to be related to cumulative dose; pulmonary function tests should be performed prior to therapy, and follow-up tests should be performed if patient becomes symptomatic and particularly after cumulative doses of 400 mg/m^2 or more; drug accumulation may occur in patients with hepatic or renal dysfunction; therefore, routine monitoring of liver and renal function should be performed; carmustine is contraindicated in patients who have demonstrated previous hypersensitivity to the drug; safety and efficacy in children has not been established; all cytotoxic drugs may be embryotoxic or teratogenic; use with caution in pregnant and nursing patients; carmustine has been shown to affect the fertility of male rats receiving higher than usual human doses

TOXICITIES

Hematologic: delayed cumulative hematologic toxicity is the major dose limiting adverse effect; leukocyte nadir occurs first at approximately 15 d after therapy, then a second, lower nadir occurs at approximately 4–6 wk and persists for 1–2 wk after carmustine administration; the degree of leukopenia depends on previous exposure to chemotherapy and can vary among patients; thrombocytopenia is usually the most severe hematologic effect, occurring about 4 wk after therapy and persisting 1–2 wk; anemia can occur but generally is less frequent and less severe than the other hematologic toxicities; bone marrow aplasia occurs at doses of ≥ 600 mg/m^2; rarely, acute leukemias and bone marrow dysplasias have been reported with long-term therapy; **GI:** moderate to severe nausea and vomiting beginning minutes to 2 h after IV administration and lasting 4–6 h after is common; diarrhea, esophagitis, anorexia, and dysphagia occur less frequently; **Pulmonary:** pulmonary infiltrates or fibrosis can be common in patients who have received cumulative doses > 400 mg/m^2; pulmonary toxicity can be progressive and fatal, and its onset may be delayed; oxygen exposure increases the risk of pulmonary fibrosis and should be limited; early use of corticosteroids may prevent fibrosis; **Hepatic:** generally mild and reversible hepatotoxicity has been reported in up to 26% of patients; incidence of hepatic dysfunction may increase with high-dose therapy; **Miscellaneous:** renal toxicity is rare but can occur in patients who have received cumulative doses > 600 mg/m^2; significant hypotension can occur, especially with high-dose therapy; tachycardia and hypotension are associated with intense flushing of the skin of the face and upper chest (this reaction can persist for several hours after the infusion is completed and is believed to be due to the combination of carmustine itself and the alcohol used to reconstitute the drug); dementia has been reported with high-dose regimens; burning at the site of injection; after topical application, dermatologic effects have occurred such as severe dermatitis, petechiae, hyperpigmentation, telangiectasia, and hypersensitivity reactions (occur rarely); mild bone marrow depression incidence is < 10%

RESPONSE RATES (Continued)

Good results have been described in the treatment of mycosis fungoides with topical carmustine; in studies comparing the use of carmustine versus nitrogen mustard, efficacy of the two agents appeared to be equal, with carmustine causing less hypersensitivity reactions and topical side effects; 5-y survival rates are approximately 30% with carmustine depending on the stage of the disease at the time of treatment; in high doses (400–600 mg/m^2), carmustine is effective in combination therapy for refractory breast cancer, non-Hodgkin's lymphoma, Hodgkin's disease, and glioma [50,51]

PATIENT MONITORING

CBC, including differential leukocyte count and platelet count, is generally obtained weekly for 6–8 wk after administration of carmustine to monitor for leukopenia, thrombocytopenia, and anemia—some clinicians suggest waiting 2–3 wk after therapy before obtaining the first CBC and then following up with weekly labs until blood counts are normal or appropriate for subsequent treatment, usually within 6–8 wk; monitor renal, hepatic, and pulmonary status; health care professionals responsible for monitoring patients receiving carmustine therapy should be familiar with the broad spectrum of other adverse effects that can occur, albeit less commonly, with this treatment; pulmonary toxicity may be increased by long radiation

NURSING INTERVENTIONS

Monitor treatment tolerance, weight, and nutritional status; educate patients about neutropenic precautions and self-care at home; wear gloves while administering carmustine and avoid contact with the skin (hyperpigmentation of the skin is common after accidental contact); do not mix with other drugs during IV administration; if pain occurs at the infusion site, dilute solution further or slow the infusion rate; carmustine is considered an irritant—if extravasation occurs, stop infusion immediately and infiltrate the area with injections of 0.5 mEq/mL sodium bicarbonate solution; nausea and vomiting are common (give appropriate antiemetics); intense facial and upper chest flushing may occur due to the alcohol used during reconstitution—this will resolve within 2–4 h and can usually be minimized by slowing the infusion; along with the flushing, significant hypotension (particularly with high-dose therapy) can occur; therefore, blood pressure should be monitored during and after the infusion

PATIENT INFORMATION

Call the doctor immediately if the following occurs: unusual bruising or bleeding, temperature over 101°F, sore throat, or other signs of infection; avoid aspirin and nonsteroidal antiinflammatory agents; avoid exposure to people with infections; follow-up blood counts are essential when receiving carmustine therapy

FORMULATION

Available as BiCNU (Bristol-Myers Oncology Division, Princeton, NJ) 100-mg vial; the drug should appear as dry flakes or as a dry, congealed mass; the drug should be stored at 2–8°C; if an oily film has formed in the vial, the drug has decomposed due to warm temperatures and should be discarded; carmustine powder should be reconstituted with 3 mL dehydrated alcohol provided by the manufacturer followed by 27 mL sterile water for injection; the reconstituted solution must be further diluted in either normal saline or 5% dextrose and water before administration; solutions of 0.2 mg/mL in glass containers are stable for 4–8 h when refrigerated and protected from light; plastic IV bags should not be used due to instability; patients with central IV catheters can tolerate carmustine solutions in a total volume of 250 mL; patients with peripheral IV lines should have the solutions further diluted with a total volume of 500 mL; for preparation of the topical solution, reconstitute a 100-mg vial as per the manufacturer, add the reconstituted drug to a 60-mL light-resistant bottle, and fill it to a total volume of 50 mL with 95% alcohol (concentration = 2 mg/mL); the prepared solution has a shelf-life of 2–3 mo when kept at 4°C.

CHLORAMBUCIL

Chlorambucil is a bifunctional alkylating agent of the nitrogen mustard type. It is a cell cycle nonspecific antineoplastic agent that is cytotoxic to nonproliferating cells. Its antineoplastic activity occurs from the formation of an unstable ethyleneimmonium ion, which then alkylates or binds with intracellular structures. The cytotoxicity of chlorambucil is due to cross-linking of strands of DNA and RNA and to inhibition of protein synthesis. Additionally, chlorambucil is metabolized to phenylacetic acid mustard, which is also a bifunctional alkylating agent. Phenylacetic acid mustard has shown antineoplastic activity in some human cell lines approximately equal to that of chlorambucil. Chlorambucil also has immunosuppressant activity. It has the slowest onset of activity and the least toxicity of the classic nitrogen mustard type agents.

DOSAGE AND ADMINISTRATION

Chlorambucil is used alone or in combination with other agents such as prednisone. The incidence and severity of side effects may be altered in combination regimens. Most patients require dose reductions sometime during therapy. **Chronic lymphocytic leukemia:** *Remission induction*—0.1–0.2 mg/kg (4–10 mg total) daily for 3–6 wk (given as single or divided doses); *Maintenance*—2–4 mg daily; *Intermittent or pulse therapy*—1.5–2 mg/kg every month; 0.4 mg/kg every 2 wk, increasing by 0.1-mg/kg increments to toxicity or remission; **Hodgkin's and non-Hodgkin's lymphoma:** 0.1–0.2 mg/kg/d or 0.4 mg/kg every 2 wk, increased by 0.1-mg/kg increments to toxicity or remission (duration of therapy is usually 6–12 mo); **immunosuppressant for nephrotic syndrome:** 0.1–0.2 mg/kg/d in a single dose for 8–12 wk.

If lymphocytic infiltration of the bone marrow is present or the bone marrow is hypoplastic, do not exceed a dose of 0.1 mg/kg/d; chlorambucil dose should be adjusted to patient response and the dose reduced if there is an abrupt decrease in leukocyte count; short courses of treatment are safer than continuous maintenance therapy although both methods of treatment are effective.

Dose adjustments for organ dysfunction: no information.

SPECIAL PRECAUTIONS

Do not give at full dosage prior to 4 wk after a full course of radiation therapy or chemotherapy because of the vulnerability of the bone marrow to damage; may treat with a reduced dose if pretherapy leukocyte or platelet counts are depressed from bone marrow disease process prior to institution of therapy; follow patients carefully to avoid life-threatening damage to the bone marrow—decrease dosage if leukocyte or platelet counts fall below normal values; use with caution in patients with a history of seizures or a history of hypersensitivity to the drug; safe and effective use in pediatric patients has not been fully established—it has been used if the potential benefits outweigh the risks

INDICATIONS

FDA-approved: Palliation for chronic lymphocytic leukemia (CLL), malignant lymphomas, lymphosarcoma, giant follicular lymphoma, and Hodgkin's disease; clinical trials show activity in hairy cell leukemia, acute histiocytosis X, autoimmune hepatic anemias, advanced breast cancer, nonseminomatous testicular carcinoma, multiple myeloma, mycosis fungoides, Wegener's granulomatosis, sarcoidosis, macroglobulinemia, polycythemia vera, ovarian cancer, nephrotic syndrome, and thrombocythemia

PHARMACOKINETICS

Absorption: rapidly absorbed from the GI tract with peak plasma levels reached in 1 h; oral bioavailability is estimated to be 50%; **Distribution:** chlorambucil and its metabolites are extensively protein bound (99%) to plasma proteins (primarily albumin); it is not known if chlorambucil crosses the blood–brain barrier, although some adverse CNS effects have been reported; chlorambucil apparently crosses the placenta; it is unknown if the drug or its metabolites are distributed into breast milk; **Metabolism:** extensively metabolized in the liver and its primary metabolite, phenylacetic acid mustard, is pharmacologically active; **Elimination:** reported plasma half-lives of the parent drug and phenylacetic acid are 90 and 145 min, respectively; chlorambucil is excreted via the kidneys almost completely as its metabolites; < 1% is excreted as unchanged chlorambucil or phenylacetic acid mustard; most of the drug is excreted as the monohydroxy and dihydroxy derivatives

DRUG INTERACTIONS

Chlorambucil toxicity is potentiated by barbiturates, possibly by inducing hepatic activation of chlorambucil (discontinue barbiturate if possible); probenecid, sulfinpyrazone, bone marrow depressants, and immunosuppressants also have clinically significant interactions with chlorambucil

RESPONSE RATES

CLL: a decrease in lymphocyte count and lymphadenopathy generally are seen over a minimum of 3–12 mo of therapy; response rates to chlorambucil as a single agent range from 64%–75%; in combination with prednisone, response rates of 38%–87% are reported; recent studies indicate similar responses with fludarabine, and combination therapy has been proposed.

Hodgkin's disease: chlorambucil in combination with vinblastine, procarbazine, and prednisone (Ch1VPP) has been used as a substitute for MOPP therapy, yielding response rates of 70%–89%

Malignant lymphomas: chlorambucil used alone in the treatment of non-Hodgkin's lymphoma has produced complete response rates of 10%–15% and partial response of 40%–70%; intermittent regimens of chlorambucil to treat nodular lymphocytic lymphomas have produced complete responses of 60%–70%

CHLORAMBUCIL (Continued)

TOXICITIES

Hematologic: hematologic effects are the major dose-limiting side effects of chlorambucil; for continuous treatment courses, leukopenia usually appears after the third week of therapy and generally will last between 2–4 wk after discontinuation of therapy; after administration of a single high-dose treatment, leukocyte and platelet nadirs will occur between 7–14 d and will recover in approximately 2–3 wk; thrombocytopenia may continue longer than leukopenia; bone marrow suppression usually is reversible up to a cumulative dose of 6.5 mg/kg in a single-treatment course; acute leukemias and bone marrow dysplasias have been reported with long-term therapy; **GI:** nausea and vomiting (mild), diarrhea, oral ulceration, anorexia, and abdominal pain; **Hepatic:** hepatotoxicity including jaundice, hepatic necrosis, and cirrhosis have rarely been reported; **Pulmonary:** bronchopulmonary dysplasia, pulmonary fibrosis, and interstitial pneumonia (pulmonary effects are rare and occur usually with prolonged therapy); **Reproductive:** sterility (high incidence) in prepubertal and pubertal males, azoospermia, and amenorrhea; **CNS:** tremors, muscular twitching, confusion, agitation, ataxia, flaccid paresis, hallucinations (rare), and seizures; **Miscellaneous:** drug fever, skin hypersensitivity, peripheral neuropathy, sterile cystitis, keratitis, hyperuricemia, and uric acid nephropathy

PATIENT MONITORING

CBC, including hematocrit, hemoglobin, platelet count, and total leukocyte counts should be obtained at periodic intervals (every 2 wk) throughout therapy; other lab tests such as SGPT, SGOT, lactate dehydrogenase and serum uric acid levels are recommended prior to therapy and at periodic intervals; monitor for incidence of leukopenia and thrombocytopenia as these parameters are used to individualize dosage

NURSING INTERVENTIONS

Monitor treatment tolerance, weight, nutritional status; administer antiemetics as necessary; educate patient about most common side effects of chlorambucil, neutropenic precautions, and self-care at home; hyperuricemia can be prevented by adequate hydration and the administration of allopurinol; if patient is unable to swallow tablets, an aqueous suspension can be made from the tablets at a concentration of 2 mg/mL

PATIENT INFORMATION

Call the doctor immediately if vomiting occurs shortly after the dose is taken or a sore throat, fever, or any unusual bruising or bleeding develops; take tablets on an empty stomach; the total daily dose can be taken at one time; chlorambucil may cause permanent or temporary sterility; avoid aspirin and nonsteroidal antiinflammatory agents; avoid exposure to people with infections; follow-up blood counts are essential when receiving chlorambucil therapy

FORMULATION

Available as Leukeran (Glaxo-Wellcome, Research Triangle Park, NC) 2-mg sugar-coated tablets in bottles of 50 tablets; should be stored in a well-closed, light-resistant container at 15–30°C; an oral solution containing 2 mg/mL can be extemporaneously prepared from the tablets using a suspending agent and a syrup; the suspension is stable for 7 d at 5°C.

CISPLATIN

Discovered accidentally in 1965 during experiments examining the effects of electricity on the growth of *Escherichia coli*, cisplatin was the first heavy metal compound shown to have antineoplastic activity. During phase I trials cisplatin was nearly discarded due to its extreme gastrointestinal and renal toxicities. However, responses reported with testicular cancer showed promise and researchers developed mechanisms to decrease toxicity.

The mechanism of action of cisplatin is similar to alkylating agents and it is therefore considered a nonclassical alkylator. The *cis*, not the *trans*, isomer of cisplatin is the active moiety. In the relatively high chloride concentrations of plasma, the cisplatin complex is un-ionized and able to pass through cell membranes. In the presence of low chloride concentrations, intracellularly, the chloride ligands of the complex are displaced by water and produce the positively charged platinum compound, which is toxic and probably the active form of the drug. The *cis* isomer forms intrastrand and interstrand cross-links between guanine-guanine pairs of DNA and inhibits synthesis. Cisplatin, to a lesser extent, binds to RNA and protein, ultimately inhibiting synthesis. Other cytotoxic activity may include tumor immunogenicity, and the drug has immunosuppressive, radiosensitizing, and antimicrobial properties.

DOSAGE AND ADMINISTRATION

Testicular cancer: usually used in combination with other cytotoxic drugs such as bleomycin and vinblastine; 20–40 mg/m^2 of cisplatin daily for 5 d *or* 120 mg/m^2 as a single dose every 3–4 wk

Ovarian cancer: usually used in combination with doxorubicin; 30–120 mg/m^2 as a single dose every 3–4 wk

Bladder cancer: 50–70 mg/m^2 as a single dose every 3–4 wk *or* 1 mg/kg once a week for 6 wk then every 3 wk thereafter

Head and neck cancer, cervical cancer, non–small cell lung cancer: treatment varies in dosing schedule and whether single-agent or combination therapy is used; doses range from 50–120 mg/m^2 every 3–6 wk

Bladder cancer, malignant melanoma, osteogenic sarcoma: intraarterial dosing is usually reserved for treatment of regionally confined malignancies such as advanced bladder cancer, malignant melanoma, and osteogenic sarcoma, in doses ranging from 75–150 mg/m^2 as a single dose every 2–5 wk for 1–4 courses

Advanced ovarian carcinoma, carcinoid tumors, and mesotheliomas: intraperitoneal dosing of cisplatin is used primarily in the treatment of advanced ovarian carcinoma, carcinoid tumors, and mesotheliomas, which may or may not be associated with malignant ascites, in doses ranging from 60–270 mg/m^2

Pediatric osteogenic sarcoma or neuroblastoma: reported doses are 90 mg/m^2 once every 3 wk or 30 mg/m^2 once a week

Recurrent pediatric brain tumors: 60 mg/m^2 daily for 2 d every 3–4 wk

High-dose therapy: doses up to 40 mg/m^2 daily × 5 are used in patients receiving combination high-dose therapy for lymphoma

Dose adjustments for renal impairment: clinicians recommend avoiding treatment in patients with a serum creatinine ≥ 1.5 or a creatinine clearance (CLcr) of < 50 mL/min; other guidelines suggest reducing dose to 75% of the usual in patients with CLcr of 10–50 mL/min and 50% of usual in patients with CLcr < 10 mL/min

INDICATIONS

FDA-approved: Treatment of metastatic testicular and ovarian tumors and advanced bladder cancer; clinical studies show activity in head and neck cancer, cervical carcinoma, lung cancer, osteogenic sarcoma, neuroblastoma, recurrent brain tumors, advanced esophageal carcinoma, advanced prostatic carcinoma, malignant melanoma, endometrial cancer, penile carcinoma, breast carcinoma, advanced Hodgkin's disease, malignant lymphomas, advanced soft tissue and bone sarcomas, refractory choriocarcinoma, metastatic adrenal carcinoma, malignant thymoma, medullary carcinoma of the thyroid, and gastric carcinoma

PHARMACOKINETICS

Absorption: cisplatin is not administered orally or intramuscularly; when given by the intraperitoneal route, 50% to 100% of the drug is absorbed systemically.

Distribution: after administration of cisplatin, the platinum compound is widely distributed into the tissues exhibiting high concentrations in the kidneys, liver, and prostate; platinum concentrations also can be found in the bladder, muscle, testes, pancreas, spleen, the small and large intestines, adrenals, heart, lungs, lymph nodes, thyroid, gallbladder, thymus, cerebrum, cerebellum, ovaries, and uterus; platinum can accumulate in the tissues and be detected for up to 6 mo after the last dose of cisplatin; the volume of distribution is estimated between 20–80 L; cisplatin is rapidly distributed into pleural effusions and ascitic fluid; it is not known if platinum distributes into breast milk or crosses the placenta; platinum-containing products generally do not penetrate the CNS; low platinum concentrations have been found in tumors of the brain but seldom in healthy brain tissue; cisplatin is extensively and irreversibly protein bound to plasma and tissue proteins—protein binding measures ≥90%

Metabolism: unclear; the drug may undergo some enterohepatic circulation

Elimination: cisplatin is primarily excreted unchanged in the urine; total elimination tends to decrease with time; initial phase half-life is ~25–79 min, whereas a terminal phase half-life of 73–290 h has been reported; hemodialysis minimally removes cisplatin and its platinum-containing products

DRUG INTERACTIONS

The administration of other nephrotoxic drugs, such as aminoglycosides and amphotericin should be avoided (unless clearly indicated) for at least 2 wk after treatment with cisplatin, although evidence of synergistic toxicity is lacking; however, concurrent administration increases the risk of nephrotoxicity and acute renal failure significantly; ototoxicity may be exacerbated by the concomitant administration of the other ototoxic drugs, such as aminoglycosides and diuretics; a synergistic antineoplastic effect has been reported with cisplatin and etoposide; other possibly synergistic agents include bleomycin, doxorubicin, 5-fluorouracil, methotrexate, vinblastine, and vincristine; cisplatin may alter the renal clearance of some drugs as a result of drug-induced nephrotoxicity, thus possibly causing increased systemic toxicity of the renally cleared drug; there may be a possible drug interaction with cisplatin and anticonvulsant drugs—anticonvulsant plasma levels have been reported to be subtherapeutic during cisplatin therapy

RESPONSE RATES

Testicular neoplasms: cisplatin is one of the most active agents used in the treatment of nonseminomatous testicular carcinoma; although cisplatin can be used as a single agent, combination therapy including cisplatin, bleomycin, and vinblastine

(Continued on next page)

CISPLATIN (Continued)

SPECIAL PRECAUTIONS

Safety and efficacy of cisplatin in children has not been established—however, cisplatin therapy has shown encouraging results in the treatment of pediatric osteogenic sarcoma, neuroblastoma, and recurrent brain tumors; cisplatin may be mutagenic and carcinogenic but a direct causal relationship has not been fully elucidated; all cytotoxic drugs may be embryotoxic or teratogenic; use with caution in pregnant or nursing patients; contraindicated in patients who have experienced hypersensitivity reactions to platinum-containing compounds

TOXICITIES

Renal: nephrotoxicity is dose-related and can be severe without appropriate hydration, renal toxicity is associated with increased serum creatinine, BUN, serum uric acid, or decrease in creatinine clearance and glomerular filtration rate; cisplatin-induced renal toxicity is directly associated with renal tubular damage; nephrotoxicity typically appears during the second week after administration of the drug, or within several days after high-dose therapy; renal impairment is usually reversible when associated with low- to moderate-dose regimens but high-dose and repeated therapy may cause irreversible renal insufficiency; recovery generally occurs within 2–4 wk

Electrolyte: due to cisplatin-induced renal tubular dysfunction, electrolyte disturbances are common; hypomagnesemia, hypokalemia, hypocalcemia, hypophosphatemia, and hyponatremia can occur and may persist for several weeks; hypomagnesemia and hypocalcemia can be delayed in onset up to 3–4 wk after therapy

GI: moderate to severe nausea and vomiting are dose-related and may be intractable, especially with rapid infusion of high doses; GI disturbances begin within 1 h of starting cisplatin and can last 8–12 h after administration; delayed nausea and vomiting can occur for up to 5 d and are difficult to manage; anorexia often occurs due to the delayed nausea and vomiting; diarrhea occurs rarely but may increase in frequency when cisplatin is combined with other cytotoxic agents or when high-dose therapy is used

Otic: ototoxicity is usually manifested by tinnitus or high-frequency hearing loss (ototoxicity is reported in up to 31% of patients receiving usual doses); it also may be related to administration time, rapid infusions causing more hearing loss than slow infusions over 1–3 h or 24 h; audiogram abnormalities can be both unilateral and bilateral and may be more severe in children than in adults

Nervous system: neurotoxicity is usually characterized by peripheral neuropathies, including sensory (paresthesias) and motor (gait); neuronal impairment typically is associated with prolonged therapy (4–7 mo) but can occur after single doses; peripheral neuropathy can be irreversible but in most patients it can be partially or completely reversible after discontinuation of the cisplatin; tonic-clonic seizures, slurred speech, loss of taste, memory loss, and intention tremor have also been reported; recovery may take 4–12 mo

Hematologic: leukopenia, thrombocytopenia, and anemia are usually mild to moderate and occur in approximately 25%–30% of patients; an increased incidence of myelosuppression can occur in patients who have been heavily pretreated with cisplatin or other antineoplastic agents; leukocyte and platelet nadirs usually appear 18–23 d after cisplatin therapy with levels returning to baseline by day 39; anemia is suspected to be caused by myelosuppression, decreased erythropoiesis, and hemolysis; acute leukemia has been reported but is rare

(Continued on next page)

RESPONSE RATES *(Continued)*

provides improved responses; patients with stage III disseminated disease receiving combination therapy usually achieve complete remissions ranging from 60%–70%; response rates are higher in patients with minimal stage III disease; disease-free remissions for > 2 y are considered cure; combination of cisplatin and etoposide also has been used in disseminated disease, producing complete remissions of 50%; in seminoma testis and extragonadal germ cell tumors, cisplatin alone or in combination therapy can produce response rates similar to those reported in the treatment of nonseminomatous testicular carcinoma

Cisplatin alone can produce objective responses of 25%–33% in the treatment of advanced ovarian carcinoma refractory to prior chemotherapy or radiation therapy; complete responses are rare; patients who were previously untreated usually achieve increased response rates; combination therapy with doxorubicin can produce overall response rates of 35%–80%; other combinations with cisplatin, cyclophosphamide, and doxorubicin yield improved response rates of 50%–85%—using this three-drug combination and adding altretamine produces response rates of 50%–95%

Intraperitoneal administration of cisplatin for the treatment of advanced ovarian cancers produces varied response rates

Partial response rates lasting 5–7 mo are produced in about one third of bladder cancer patients when treated with cisplatin alone; the superiority of combination cisplatin-based therapy is not established; slightly higher response rates have been reported when cisplatin is combined with cyclophosphamide or with methotrexate and vinblastine

Cisplatin has been reported to produce 30% response rates in patients with metastatic squamous cell carcinoma of the head and neck; several cisplatin-based treatment combinations have been used but most studies are uncontrolled and results are varied

Response rates of 25%–50% have been reported in the treatment of recurrent or advanced squamous cell carcinoma of the cervix. The role of combination therapy has not been established

Lung cancer: cisplatin is one of the more active chemotherapy agents in the treatment of non–small cell carcinoma; objective responses of 15%–20% have been reported with cisplatin therapy; cisplatin-based combinations with cyclophosphamide and doxorubicin or etoposide and vinblastine or vinorelbine have produced slightly increased response rates of 25%–50%; cisplatin alone produces very poor responses in patients with small cell lung carcinoma; when cisplatin is combined with etoposide-containing regimens, high but varied response rates have been produced; median survival after treatment usually averages 12–16 mo

Lymphoma: the combination of cisplatin, carmustine, and etoposide in high doses with autologous progenitor cell infusion has shown a 4% long-term remission in patients with recurrent or refractory disease

PATIENT MONITORING

Renal function should be monitored frequently—the manufacturer recommends avoiding subsequent treatment until renal function has returned to normal; complete serum chemistries should be obtained to monitor electrolyte status, paying particular attention to serum magnesium, potassium, sodium, and calcium concentrations—electrolytes should be supplemented as needed; because cisplatin-induced ototoxicity is cumulative, audiometry should be performed prior to initial and repeated therapies—many clinicians suggest withholding cisplatin until audiometric determinations are within normal limits; neurologic exams should be performed routinely; CBC, including leukocyte count differential and platelet count, should be obtained every week or every other week to monitor for leukopenia, anemia, and thrombocytopenia

CISPLATIN (Continued)

TOXICITIES (Continued)

Sensitivity reactions: anaphylactoid reactions usually occur after at least five doses of cisplatin; the mechanism of the hypersensitivity is not known but may be immune mediated; these reactions manifest as facial edema, flushing, wheezing, and respiratory difficulty, tachycardia, and hypotension and will appear within minutes after IV administration; mild hypersensitivity reactions such as urticarial or nonspecific maculopapular rashes, recurrent dermatitis, and erythema

Ocular: optic neuritis, papilledema, and cerebral blindness have been reported

Cardiovascular: bradycardia, left bundle branch block, ST-T wave changes with congestive heart failure, postural hypotension, and hypertension have all been reported but are considered rare; these effects may be due to cisplatin directly or due to electrolyte changes during cisplatin therapy

Miscellaneous: hepatic effects of mild and transient elevations of serum AST (SGOT) and ALT (SGPT) concentrations occur rarely; local effects such as phlebitis and, rarely, severe cellulitis with fibrosis or skin necrosis after extravasation have been reported; the incidence of the following is infrequent: hyperuricemia (due to drug-induced nephrotoxicity), mild alopecia, myalgia, pyrexia, gingival platinum line, aspermia, and syndrome of inappropriate antidiuretic hormone secretion

NURSING INTERVENTIONS

Anaphylactic-like reactions have been reported to occur within minutes of cisplatin administration; these reactions usually occur in patients who have been previously exposed to platinum-containing compounds; antihistamines, epinephrine, oxygen, and corticosteroids should be readily available in case of anaphylaxis

Monitor treatment tolerance, weight, and nutritional status; nausea and vomiting occur in ≥ 90% of patients receiving cisplatin; appropriate antiemetics such as metoclopramide (2 or 3 mg/kg) or serotonin antagonists in combination with dexamethasone or lorazepam or diphenhydramine should be used; phenothiazine antiemetics (*ie*, prochlorperazine) usually are not effective

Extensive hydration is successful in preventing or decreasing the occurrence and severity of renal toxicity—there are several effective methods of hydration, all routinely include the following: before administering cisplatin, maintain urine output at 100–150 mL/h using 1–2 L of D5W 1/2 NS or 0.9% sodium chloride supplemented with potassium or magnesium; use IV furosemide if urine output is not satisfactory; 12.5 g mannitol can be added to the cisplatin IV bag or given IV push before the cisplatin is administered to maintain appropriate urine output during the infusion; and post-hydration equaling 1–2 L of fluid should be used; hydration should be modified in patients with cardiovascular compromise

Ensure that appropriate labs are drawn to monitor electrolyte status, renal function, and hematologic parameters

Do not use aluminum-containing IV administration sets with cisplatin (aluminum will interact with cisplatin causing a precipitate to form with loss of potency)

Cisplatin is not a vesicant but can cause tissue irritation if extravasated; extent of tissue damage is concentration dependent; fibrosis and necrosis have been reported

When cisplatin is administered intraperitoneally, remember that much of the drug is systemically absorbed and can cause the same side effects; appropriate antiemetics and monitoring of electrolyte, renal, and hematologic status are still warranted

Monitor for ototoxicity and neurotoxicity at each visit

PATIENT INFORMATION

Call the doctor immediately if unusual bruising or bleeding occurs; temperature of ≥ 101°F; intractable nausea and vomiting occur; hearing loss occurs; or numbness or tingling in hands or feet occur; avoid exposure to people with infections; maintain adequate fluid intake for several days after receiving cisplatin, especially if nausea and vomiting are persistent—this will decrease the incidence of kidney damage and dehydration

FORMULATION

Available as an aqueous solution of 1 mg/mL in 50- and 100-mg vials (Platinol-AQ, Bristol-Myers Squibb Oncology Division, Princeton, NJ)

Cisplatin solution for injection should be protected from light and stored at 15–25°C; cisplatin in multiple vials is stable up to 28 d in the dark; refrigeration of the powder and the reconstituted solution should be avoided due to precipitate formation; if cisplatin is accidentally stored in the refrigerator, the precipitate will dissolve at room temperature and no loss of potency is apparent; cisplatin can be further diluted in sodium chloride–containing IV solutions and are stable from 24–72 h; commonly used IV solutions are dextrose 5% and water (D5W) with 0.9% or 0.45% sodium chloride (NS or 1/2 NS) or varied concentrations of sodium chloride solutions; cisplatin is not compatible with sodium bicarbonate; the use of aluminum needles should be avoided in the preparation of cisplatin.

The information here is provided as guidance only. Prescribers should always consult the manufacturer's current prescribing information.

18

CYCLOPHOSPHAMIDE

Cyclophosphamide is a cell cycle nonspecific alkylating agent of the nitrogen mustard type. It is a prodrug, metabolized in the liver to active metabolites that alkylate nucleic acids. Cyclophosphamide prevents cell division by cross-linking DNA and RNA strands, resulting in an imbalance of growth within the cell, leading to cell death. Cyclophosphamide also has phosphorylating properties that enhance its cytotoxicity and it possesses significant immunosuppressive activity.

DOSAGE AND ADMINISTRATION

Cyclophosphamide is administered over a wide dosing range depending on the disease process being treated. It may be administered orally or parenterally, alone or in combination with other agents, as a part of a chemotherapy regimen. It can be given to both adults and children.

Adults: 50–100 mg/m^2 PO × 10–14 d; 50–1000 mg/m^2 as a single IV dose on d 1 and 8 (or every 14–21 d); *High-dose therapy*—2000–7000 mg/m^2 over 1–4 d; 1875 mg/m^2/d × 3 d × 1 course; 50 mg/kg/d × 4 d; *Maintenance dose*—1–5 mg/kg PO daily; 10–15 mg/kg IV q 7–10 d; 3–5 mg/kg IV twice weekly; **Children:** 2–8 mg/kg or 60–250 mg/m^2 PO or IV qd × 6 d (divide PO dosages; IV doses are given once a week); *Maintenance dose*—2–5 mg/kg or 50–150 mg/m^2 PO twice weekly; **Dosage adjustment in organ dysfunction:** patients with compromised renal function may show significantly prolonged retention of active alkylating metabolites, but no dosage adjustment is necessary; *High-dose therapy*—addition of mesna will reduce the complication of hemorrhagic cystitis; administer mesna at 20% dose equivalence of cyclophosphamide concurrently and repeat 4, 8, and 12 h later; alternatively, give 100% dose equivalency as a 24-h infusion at the start of the cyclophosphamide infusion

INDICATIONS

FDA-approved: Cyclophosphamide is used alone or in combination with other drugs in the treatment of the following malignancies: ALL, AML, CML, CLL, acute monocytic leukemia, Hodgkin's or non-Hodgkin's lymphoma, carcinoma of the ovary or breast, multiple myeloma, Burkitt's lymphoma, neuroblastoma, retinoblastoma; cyclophosphamide is also used as an immuno-suppressant in the following conditions: polymyositis, rheumatoid arthritis, Wegener's agranulomatosis, and nephrotic syndrome in children; clinical studies show activity in bronchogenic carcinoma, small cell lung carcinoma, rhabdomyosarcoma, Ewing's sarcoma, carcinomas of the GI tract, endometrium, testes, prostate, bladder, and renal cell, Wilm's tumor, squamous cell tumors of the cervix, head, and neck; it also has been used as an immunosuppressant to control rejection following kidney, heart, liver, and bone marrow transplants

PHARMACOKINETICS

Absorption: almost completely absorbed from the GI tract in doses < 100 mg; higher doses are 75% absorbed; cyclophosphamide is administered both orally and parenterally; **Distribution:** throughout the body, with minimal amounts found in saliva, sweat, and synovial fluid; crosses the blood–brain barrier to a limited extent but not enough to treat meningeal leukemia; active metabolites are approximately 50% bound to plasma proteins; **Metabolism:** metabolized to 4-hydroxycyclophosphamide, by hepatic microsomal enzymes, which is then able to cross cellular membranes and subsequently is metabolized to the active alkylating species; this metabolite is further metabolized to activate the alkylating moieties phosphoramide mustard and nornitrogen mustard and inactive metabolites; **Excretion:** primarily in the urine with 15%–30% as unchanged drug; acrolein is thought to be the metabolite that is most responsible for causing hemorrhagic cystitis; plasma half-life of the parent compound is 4–6.5 h; however, drug can be detected in the plasma for up to 72 h after administration

DRUG INTERACTIONS

Barbiturates, phenytoin, and chloral hydrate alter the metabolism of cyclophosphamide, leading to an increase in toxic metabolites; ondansetron may increase clearance of cyclophosphamide and increase formation of active metabolites; effects of other antiemetics have not been studied; corticosteroids initially inhibit cyclophosphamide activation, leading to a decreased antineoplastic effect; cyclophosphamide can potentiate the cardiotoxic effects of doxorubicin; interactions with probenecid, chloramphenicol, sulfinpyrazone, bone marrow depressants, radiation therapy, cocaine, and cytarabine all have some clinical significance; the interaction with allopurinol is controversial; allopurinol can increase the cyclophosphamide level and prolong the half-life of cyclophosphamide, leading to an increase in the side effects; the use of these two drugs in combination should be followed closely.

RESPONSE RATES

Hodgkin's disease: 60% objective response rate when treated with cyclophosphamide alone
Lymphoma: 10%–20% complete response and 40%–70% objective response rate with cyclophosphamide alone; when used as part of a combination regimen, the complete response rate rose to 50%
Burkitt's lymphoma: 90% complete response rate with cyclophosphamide alone
Multiple myeloma: 30% objective response rate
ALL: 20%–40% objective response rate
AML: 10% objective response rate
Neuroblastoma: 65% objective response rate
Ovarian cancer: 60% objective response rate
Breast cancer: 35% objective response rate with cyclophosphamide alone; up to 90% objective response in combination therapy
High-dose therapy: 30%–50% response rates in patients with active disease when used in combination therapy for lymphoma, myeloma, breast cancer, and chronic myelogenous leukemias
Progenitor cell transplantations: used with busulfan and other agents as preparation prior to cell reinfusion for autologous and allogenic progenitor cell transplants for leukemias (acute and chronic) and lymphomas

CYCLOPHOSPHAMIDE (Continued)

SPECIAL PRECAUTIONS

As with all cytotoxic drugs, use with caution in myelosuppressed patients or patients with infection due to the potential for severe immunosuppression; use with caution in patients with renal impairment; hemorrhagic myocarditis may occur within 1 wk after therapy in patients receiving high-dose cyclophosphamide; all cytotoxic drugs may be embryotoxic or teratogenic; use with caution in pregnant or nursing patients; cyclophosphamide is excreted in breast milk

TOXICITIES

Hematologic: leukopenia, bone marrow depression, thrombocytopenia, anemia; **GI:** nausea (increased incidence in high-dose regimens), vomiting, diarrhea, anorexia; **Dermatologic:** skin rash, hives, itching, increased sweating, redness, swelling, and pain at the injection site; **Renal and genitourinary:** uric acid nephropathy, hemorrhagic cystitis, nephrotoxicity, hyperuricemia (especially when used as therapy for leukemias and lymphomas); **Cardiac:** acute myopericarditis (with doses > 5 g/m^2, but rarely at lower doses); **Pulmonary:** pneumonitis, interstitial pulmonary fibrosis; **Miscellaneous:** hyperglycemia, alopecia, hepatitis, syndrome of inappropriate diuretic hormone secretion, azoospermia

PATIENT MONITORING

CBC, including hematocrit, hemoglobin, platelet count, and total and differential leukocyte counts should be obtained weekly; other serum chemistries such as BUN, serum creatinine, SGPT, SGOT, lactate dehydrogenase, and serum bilirubin should be obtained at periodic intervals throughout treatment; urinary output and specific gravity determinations are recommended following high-dose IV administration; urine should be examined for microscopic hematuria prior to and during therapy

NURSING INTERVENTIONS

Monitor treatment tolerance, weight, nutritional status; encourage good oral hygiene; administer antiemetics as necessary; encourage the patient to increase fluid intake and to void every 2 h to avoid development of hemorrhagic cystitis; educate patient regarding side effects of cyclophosphamide, and when to notify the physician; educate patient regarding care of central venous access devices; educate patient regarding self-care at home

PATIENT INFORMATION

Advise patient to avoid use of aspirin and nonsteroidal antiinflammatory agents; neutropenic precautions should be observed following treatment to reduce the risk of infection; explain side effects of cyclophosphamide (alopecia is a common side effect); stress ample fluid intake (up to 3 L/d) and to void every 2 h to reduce the risk of hemorrhagic cystitis; oral doses may be divided and given with or after a meal to lessen nausea; cyclophosphamide may be given with cold foods to improve tolerance; notify physician if blood is present in the urine

FORMULATION

Oral tablets available as Cytoxan (Bristol-Myers Oncology Division, Princeton, NJ); injection form available as Cytoxan (Bristol-Myers Oncology Division), as Neosar (Elkins-Sinn, Adria Laboratories, Dublin, OH), and as Endoxan (Asta-Werke) Available as oral tablets containing 25 or 50 mg of cyclophosphamide per tablet and as an injection in vials of 100 mg, 200 mg, 500 mg, 1 g, and 2 g of powder for reconstitution; the tablets and injection should be stored at temperatures not to exceed 25°C; the injection may be reconstituted with sterile water for injection with the resulting concentration equal to 20 mg/mL for all vial sizes; the reconstituted solution is stable for 24 h at room temperature and for 6 d under refrigeration; it is compatible with 5% dextrose in water, 5% dextrose and 0.9% sodium chloride injection, 5% dextrose and Ringer's injection, lactated Ringer's injection, 0.45% sodium chloride injection, and sodium lactate injection; an oral solution may be extemporaneously prepared from the injection using aromatic elixir, NF as a diluent and vehicle; the concentration range is 1–5 mg/mL; it should be stored tightly sealed in the refrigerator and is stable for up to 14 d.

DACARBAZINE

Dacarbazine (also known as DTIC) is a cell cycle nonspecific alkylating agent that is a synthetic analogue of the naturally occurring purine precursor, 5-amino-1H-imidazole-4-carboxamide. It is believed to exert its cytotoxic activity by three mechanisms: 1) formation of methylating carbonium ions leading to DNA alkylation at O6 of guanine; 2) antimetabolite activity as a false precursor for purine synthesis; and 3) binding with sulfhydryl groups in proteins. Cytotoxicity appears predominantly due to recognition of a methyl guanine by the mismatch repair system, resulting in apoptotic cell death. Dacarbazine is metabolized in the liver to an active hydroxylated and N-dimethylated species. Exposure to light also can lead to formation of an active moiety, which can contribute to cytotoxicity.

DOSAGE AND ADMINISTRATION

Dacarbazine is administered parenterally alone or in combination with other agents as part of a chemotherapy regimen. **Malignant melanoma:** 2–4.5 mg/kg/d x 10 d, every 28 d; up to 250 mg/m^2/d x 5 days, every 21 d; dosage regimens of 400–500 mg/m^2 on d 1 and 2 every 3–4 wk also have been used **Hodgkin's disease (in combination with doxorubicin, bleomycin, and vinblastine):** 150 mg/m^2 x 5 d, every 4 wk; 375 mg/m^2 on d 1, repeated every 15 d, in combination with other agents **Dosage adjustment for organ dysfunction:** may be needed in patients with renal or hepatic impairment receiving repeated courses; dacarbazine therapy should be temporarily suspended if leukocyte counts fall below 3000/mm^3, absolute neutrophil count < 1000 mm^3, and platelet counts fall below 100,000/mm^3; given the frequency of nausea and vomiting, adequate antiemetics should be coadministered

INDICATIONS

FDA-approved: Used in the treatment of malignant melanoma and Hodgkin's lymphoma; dacarbazine is rarely used as a single agent in the treatment of Hodgkin's lymphoma; combination therapy with doxorubicin, bleomycin, vinblastine, and dacarbazine (ABVD) is clearly superior to single-agent therapy; clinical studies show activity in treatment of soft-tissue sarcomas (leiomyosarcoma, fibrosarcoma, rhabdomyosarcoma), neuroblastoma, and malignant glucagonoma

PHARMACOKINETICS

Absorption: not absorbed across the GI tract; **Distribution:** localizes in body tissues, especially the liver; crosses the blood–brain barrier to a limited extent; low plasma-protein binding, approximately 20%; exhibits poor cerebrospinal fluid penetration; **Metabolism:** rapid oxidative metabolism by the liver to several compounds, some of which are active; **Elimination:** biphasic elimination with initial phase half-life of 19 min and terminal phase half-life of 5 h in patients with normal renal and hepatic function; in patients with renal or hepatic impairment, the initial phase half-life is 55 min and the terminal phase half-life is 7.2 h; 30%–45% of a dose is excreted in the urine within 6 h, about half as unchanged dacarbazine and half as metabolites

DRUG INTERACTIONS

Barbiturates and phenytoin increase the metabolism of dacarbazine leading to a decrease in activity; reports of enhanced efficacy of dacarbazine in combination with bacillus Calmette-Guérin (BCG) immunotherapy in advanced malignant melanoma are controversial; dacarbazine is physically incompatible with solutions containing hydrocortisone sodium succinate

RESPONSE RATES

About 20% of metastatic malignant melanoma patients obtain an objective response of > 50% reduction in measurable tumor mass; dacarbazine in the combination regimen (ABVD) is used as a second-line therapy in advanced Hodgkin's disease after relapse with MOPP (mechlorethamine, vincristine, procarbazine, and prednisone) therapy—3-y survival rates of approximately 60% have been reported with ABVD alone; regimens alternating MOPP and ABVD have not significantly improved survival rates compared with using ABVD alone

PATIENT MONITORING

CBC, including hematocrit, hemoglobin, platelets, and total and differential leukocyte counts, should be obtained weekly to monitor for hematologic changes; hematologic toxicity (leukocyte count < 3000/mm^3 and a platelet count < 100,000 mm^2) may require delaying treatment; other serum chemistries such as BUN, creatinine, SGPT, SGOT, lactate dehydrogenase, bilirubin, and uric acid should be obtained at periodic intervals throughout treatment; monitor temperature daily

DACARBAZINE (Continued)

SPECIAL PRECAUTIONS

Because of its severe hematologic effects, leukocyte, erythrocyte, and platelet counts should be performed prior to and at regular intervals; dacarbazine has been reported to cause anaphylactic reactions and should not be administered to patients who have demonstrated hypersensitivity to the drug; all cytotoxic drugs may be embryotoxic or teratogenic; use with caution in pregnant or nursing patients

TOXICITIES

Hematologic: dose-limiting bone marrow depression, leukopenia, thrombocytopenia, and anemia occur with nadirs between 2–4 wk; the occurrence of acute leukemias has been reported but is considered rare; **GI:** severe nausea and vomiting occur within 1–3 h after therapy in 90% of patients; usually subsiding approximately 12 h after completion of therapy; anorexia, stomatitis, and diarrhea have been reported rarely; **Dermatologic:** phototoxicity, urticaria, and alopecia; **CNS:** confusion, lethargy, blurred vision, seizures, and headache; **Local:** pain, burning, and irritation at the injection site; extravasation can cause tissue damage and severe pain; **Miscellaneous:** flu-like syndrome (fever, myalgia, malaise), numbness and flushing of the face; hypotension can be a dose-limiting toxicity; the citrate salt drug formulation can cause hypocalcemia

NURSING INTERVENTIONS

Monitor treatment tolerance, weight, nutritional status; encourage good oral hygiene; educate patients about neutropenic precautions and self-care at home; care should be taken to avoid extravasation—dacarbazine can be given IV push over 1–2 min or further diluted in D5W or normal saline to a total volume of 100, 250, or 500 mL; further dilution and a slower infusion rate can decrease the pain at the injection site; dacarbazine is considered an irritant and rarely causes extravasation necrosis—if extravasation occurs, treat by applying ice to relieve burning sensation, local pain, and irritation; nausea and vomiting are common—appropriate antiemetics should be given; the oral intake of food and fluids should be avoided 4–6 h before treatment due to the high incidence of nausea and vomiting; some clinicians suggest hydrating the patient 1 h before treatment to avoid dehydration from vomiting

PATIENT INFORMATION

Avoid the use of aspirin and nonsteroidal antiinflammatory agents; call if any moderate or severe adverse effects develop such as sore throat, fever ≥ 101°F, or unusual bruising or bleeding; avoid sun exposure and exposure to sunlamps for at least 2 d posttreatment; avoid exposure to people with infections; treat flu-like symptoms with acetaminophen; maintain good nutrition—modify eating patterns, use dietary supplements as needed to maintain adequate caloric intake

FORMULATION

Available as DTIC-Dome (Bayer Pharmaceutical Division, West Haven, CT).

FOTEMUSTINE

Fotemustine, a chloroethylnitrosourea compound, was synthesized and developed by the Servier Research Institute. Fotemustine is a lipophilic chemical structure with a phosphonoalanine group grafted onto a nitrosourea radical. Chloroethylnitrosoureas are the most active agents in brain tumors and may be used with radiotherapy for added efficacy.

DOSAGE AND ADMINISTRATION

In phase II clinical trials the dosage recommendation is 100 mg/m^2 IV over 1 h, weekly for 3 consecutive wk followed by a 5 wk rest period. If response or stabilization of disease occurs after the initial dose a maintenance dose of 100 mg/m^2 every 3 wk is suggested; high-dose regimens with autologous bone marrow transplant consist of total doses of 500–1000 mg/m^2; intraarterial infusions are given through the carotid or vertebrobasilar artery (the artery supplying the tumor), at 100–200 mg every 6 wk

SPECIAL PRECAUTIONS

Myelosuppression is the major toxicity of fotemustine; monitoring for leukopenia, thrombocytopenia, and anemia should be continued throughout therapy; all cytotoxic drugs may be embryotoxic or teratogenic; investigational agents should not be used in pregnant or nursing patients

TOXICITIES

Hematologic: grade III and IV reversible leukopenia, thrombocytopenia, and anemia have been observed at several doses; no aplasia-related deaths have been reported; **GI:** mild nausea, vomiting, and epigastric pain; abnormal liver function tests have been noted in 22% of treated patients but no hepatotoxicity has been observed; **CNS:** CNS toxicity has been reported with intraarterial administration; mild to severe ocular pain during the infusion, depending on the dose; severe loss of vision, blindness, and encephalopathy-related neurotoxicity have been observed with intraarterial administration; **Miscellaneous:** rare allergic reaction (fever and rash) during the infusion; rare supravenous hyperpigmentation

INDICATIONS

FDA-approved: none—fotemustine is an investigational agent in phase II clinical trials.

Clinical studies have shown activity in recurrent malignant glioma, brain metastases of non–small cell lung cancer and malignant melanoma, and colon cancer

PHARMACOKINETICS

Absorption: not given by the oral or intramuscular route at this time; **Distribution:** rapid distribution into the brain tissue occurs, representing approximately 17%–30% of the concomitant plasma concentration; volume of distribution is estimated at 33 L/m^2; **Metabolism:** limited information available; chemical degradation of fotemustine to an active metabolite, 2-chloroethanol; **Elimination:** short elimination half-life of ≤ 20 min; total body clearance ranges from 8.96–83.49 L/h; parent drug and metabolite are renally eliminated with urinary metabolite measuring 50%–60% of the delivered dose

DRUG INTERACTIONS

Fotemustine toxicity may be enhanced if given with other myelosuppressive drugs and therapies; fotemustine given in combination with tamoxifen may have synergistic cytotoxicity

RESPONSE RATES

Objective response rates of 24% are reported in patients with melanoma; these studies also revealed a 25% (8.3%–60%) median response rate of brain metastases in these patients; studies are ongoing using fotemustine in combination with dacarbazine, cisplatin, and tamoxifen to increase response rates; in patients with recurrent malignant gliomas, a 26.3% objective response is reported; fotemustine combined with radiotherapy may increase response rates to 29%; a 16.7% response rate has been shown in brain metastases of non–small cell lung cancer; studies are ongoing in this patient population combining cisplatin and fotemustine; only 7% partial response has been reported with colorectal cancer

PATIENT MONITORING

CBC, including differential leukocyte count, platelet count, and hemoglobin and hematocrit should be obtained to monitor for leukopenia, thrombocytopenia, and anemia; if an intraarterial infusion is used, monitor for sudden change or loss in vision and headache; monitor liver chemistries intermittently; health care professionals responsible for monitoring patients on fotemustine therapy should be familiar with the less common adverse effects that can occur with therapy

NURSING INTERVENTIONS

Monitor treatment tolerance, weight, nutritional status; ensure that appropriate lab tests are conducted to monitor for leukopenia, thrombocytopenia, and anemia; ensure appropriate documentation and notify physician of all adverse effects and patient complaints in patients receiving investigational drugs; ensure that a consent form is signed by the patient to receive investigational drugs; nausea and vomiting are mild to moderate—appropriate antiemetics should be given

PATIENT INFORMATION

Call the doctor immediately if intractable nausea and vomiting, unusual bruising and bleeding, temperature over 101°F, change or loss in vision, or severe headache occurs; avoid exposure to people with infections

FORMULATION

Fotemustine for injection is mixed in 50–250 mL of 5% dextrose in water (D5W) and protected from light. IV infusion is over 1 h. Intraarterial and intrahepatic infusions are also mixed in D5W and given over 4 h.

IFOSFAMIDE

Ifosfamide is a cell cycle nonspecific alkylating agent of the nitrogen mustard type. It is a synthetic analogue of cyclophosphamide that must be activated by hepatic microsomal enzymes to exert its antineoplastic effect. It is hydroxylated to 4-hydroxyifosfamide (an active metabolite) and then metabolized to 4-ketoifosfamide and to 4-carboxyifosfamide (neither of which is cytotoxic). The active metabolites interact with DNA, forming cross-linking strands of both DNA and RNA as well as inhibiting protein synthesis.

DOSAGE AND ADMINISTRATION

Many dosage schedules and regimens exist for ifosfamide. It may be used alone or in combination with other agents. Dose fractionation, vigorous hydration, and the administration of the uroprotector mesna should be part of the therapeutic regimen to decrease the risk of hemorrhagic cystitis.

Non-Hodgkin's lymphoma: 700–1000 mg/m^2/d x 5 d, repeated q 3 wk;
Nonseminomatous germ cell tumors: 1.2 g/m^2/d x 3 d, repeated q 3 wk;
Non–small cell lung cancer: 2400 mg/m^2/d x 3d, repeated q 3 wk; **Advanced lung cancer:** up to 5000 mg/m^2 as a single dose **Non–small cell cancer:** 2400 mg/m^2/d x 3d; repeat q 3 wk.

Ifosfamide should be given with the uroprotective agent, mesna, for the prophylaxis of ifosfamide-induced hemorrhagic cystitis. Mesna is given as an IV bolus in a dosage equal to 20% of the ifosfamide dosage (weight/weight) at the time of ifosfamide administration and 4 and 8 h after each dose of ifosfamide. Alternatively, mesna may begin at 100% of the ifosfamide dose as a 24-h continuous infusion. Mesna can be given orally by doubling the IV dose and mixing in juice, soda, or milk immediately prior to administration of the mesna dose.

INDICATIONS

FDA-approved: Third-line therapy for germ-cell testicular tumors; clinical studies show activity in treatment of soft tissue sarcomas, Ewing's sarcoma, Hodgkin's and non-Hodgkin's lymphoma, carcinoma of the breast, lung, pancreas, and ovaries, ALL, and CLL

PHARMACOKINETICS

Absorption: not administered orally; **Distribution:** crosses the blood–brain barrier but its metabolites do not; **Metabolism:** 50% of a dose is metabolized in the liver; doses of 3.8–5 g/m^2 have a biphasic decay and a half-life of 15 h; doses of 1.6–2.4 g/m^2 have a monophasic decay and a half-life of 7 h; **Elimination:** 70%–86% of a dose is renally excreted, with 61% excreted unchanged at single doses of 5 g/m^2 and 12%–18% excreted unchanged at doses of 1.2–2.4 g/m^2; plasma elimination half-life is approximately 14 h

DRUG INTERACTIONS

Phenobarbital, phenytoin, and chloral hydrate may increase ifosfamide activity due to induction of microsomal enzymes; corticosteroids inhibit these enzymes, leading to decreased ifosfamide activity; allopurinol increases the activity and bone marrow toxicity of ifosfamide; bone marrow depressants, radiation therapy, and live virus vaccines also have the potential for clinically significant interactions with ifosfamide; in the kidney, mesna interacts with the urotoxic ifosfamide metabolites, acrolein and 4-hydroxyifosfamide, resulting in the detoxification of these metabolites

IFOSFAMIDE (Continued)

SPECIAL PRECAUTIONS

Use with caution in elderly patients due to age-related renal function impairment; contraindicated in patients who have demonstrated a previous hypersensitivity to ifosfamide; do not administer to patients with leukocyte count < 2000 µL or platelet counts below 50,000 µL; all cytotoxic drugs may be embryotoxic or teratogenic; use with caution in pregnant and nursing patients; breast-feeding is not recommended because ifosfamide is excreted in breast milk

TOXICITIES

Hematologic: severe myelosuppression that is dose-related and dose-limiting is frequently observed, especially when given in combination with other antineoplastic agents; leukopenia and thrombocytopenia are the most common; **GI:** nausea and vomiting are most common; anorexia, diarrhea, and in some cases constipation may occur; **CNS:** lethargy, confusion, hallucinations, encephalopathy; **Renal:** hemorrhagic cystitis is the most frequent; others are dysuria, urinary frequency and renal insufficiency; **Pulmonary:** cough, shortness of breath; **Miscellaneous:** phlebitis, infection, hepatotoxicity, alopecia

RESPONSE RATES

Nonseminomatous germ cell tumors (in combination with cisplatin and etoposide or vinblastine): 21% complete response rate

Nonseminomatous germ cell tumors (in combination with etoposide, cisplatin, and mesna): 26% complete response rate

Bulky seminoma (in combination with cisplatin and vinblastine): 87% complete response rate

Small cell lung cancer (in combination with etoposide and radiation therapy): 76% complete response and 14% partial response

Recurrent or disseminated lung cancer treated with high-dose ifosfamide: 33% response rate

Non–small cell lung cancer treated with ifosfamide alone: 24% response rate

Non–oat cell lung cancer treated with ifosfamide alone: 30% response rate

Advanced non–small cell lung cancer (in combination with cisplatin and etoposide): 26% response rate

Advanced non–small lung cancer (in combination regimen with cyclophosphamide): 38% response rate (7% complete response rate)

PATIENT MONITORING

CBC should be obtained weekly and should include hematocrit, hemoglobin, platelet count, and total and differential leukocyte counts; other serum chemistries such as BUN, serum creatinine, SGPT, SGOT, lactate dehydrogenase, and serum bilirubin should be obtained at periodic intervals; the urine should be examined for microscopic hematuria prior to each course of treatment

NURSING INTERVENTIONS

Monitor treatment tolerance, weight, nutritional status; encourage good oral hygiene; administer antiemetics as necessary; encourage patient to increase fluid intake to prevent hemorrhagic cystitis; encourage patient to void every 2 h during the day and once at night to decrease the risk of hemorrhagic cystitis; educate patient regarding care of central venous access devices and self-care at home

PATIENT INFORMATION

Avoid the use of aspirin and nonsteroidal antiinflammatory agents; ensure adequate fluid intake and frequent voiding; continue therapy in spite of nausea and vomiting; notify doctor if you see blood in the urine or have clinical signs of infection; maintain good nutrition—modify eating patterns and use dietary supplements as needed to maintain adequate caloric intake

FORMULATION

Available as Ifex (Bristol-Myers Oncology Division, Princeton, NJ) in a combination package with mesna.

LOMUSTINE

Lomustine (also known as CeeNU and CCNU) is a nitrosourea derivative that has demonstrated cytotoxic activity against a wide variation of malignancies. As with other alkylating agents, lomustine is considered to be cell cycle nonspecific. Within 1 to 6 hours after oral administration of lomustine, peak metabolite concentrations occur. These metabolites are responsible for the alkylation and carbamoylation activity, which interfere with DNA, RNA, and protein synthesis. Cross-resistance between lomustine and carmustine has occurred. Lomustine and its metabolites are widely distributed in the body. Nitrosoureas as a class tend to be highly lipophilic, thus enhancing their ability to cross the blood–brain barrier and to be used in the treatment of meningeal leukemias and brain tumors. The long-term use of nitrosoureas has been associated with profound cumulative myelosuppression and renal failure (especially with methyl-CCNU) with lesions similar to radiation-induced nephritis.

DOSAGE AND ADMINISTRATION

For adults and children 75–130 mg/m^2 by mouth once every 6–8 wk. Repeated doses should not be given until leukocyte count is > 4000/mm^3 and platelet count is > 100,000/mm^3.

The manufacturer suggests adjusting subsequent doses according to previous treatment nadirs.

NADIR AFTER PRIOR DOSE (CELLS/MM³)

Leukocytes	Platelets	Amount of Prior Dose to be Given (%)
> 4000	< 100,000	100
3000–3999	75,000–99,999	100
2000–2999	25,000–74,999	70
< 2000	<25,000	50

Some clinicians use absolute neutrophil count (ANC) as the basis of dose adjustment; in which case, reduce the dose by 2.5% for an ANC at nadir of < 1000/mm^3 and by 50% for an ANC < 500/mm^3.

INDICATIONS

FDA-approved: Palliative treatment of primary and metastatic brain tumors; used in combination regimens for the treatment of disseminated Hodgkin's disease in disease refractory to other established treatment regimens; clinical studies show activity in bronchiogenic carcinoma, non-Hodgkin's lymphoma, malignant melanoma, breast carcinoma, renal cell carcinoma, and carcinoma of the GI tract

PHARMACOKINETICS

Absorption: rapidly absorbed from the GI tract; oral bioavailability is considered high (60%–90%); **Distribution:** widely distributed; lomustine and its metabolites rapidly cross the blood–brain barrier; cerebrospinal fluid concentrations of metabolites have been reported to be 15%–50% or greater than concurrent plasma concentrations; **Metabolism and elimination:** oral dose is completely metabolized within 1 h after administration; half-life of the metabolites is biphasic; initial plasma half-life is 6 h; second plasma half-life is 1–2 d; 15%–20% of the metabolites may remain in the body for 5 d after oral administration; lomustine is excreted completely in the urine as metabolites within 4–5 d

DRUG INTERACTIONS

Interactions with phenobarbital and cimetidine have been described, although the significance is controversial; cimetidine has been reported to potentiate the neutropenic side effects of lomustine; phenobarbital is a hepatic microsomal enzyme inducer and may decrease the effects of nitrosoureas

RESPONSE RATES

Precise response rates for patients with refractory Hodgkin's disease have not been established; some studies in a limited number of patients with brain tumors have demonstrated a partial response rate of 40%

PATIENT MONITORING

CBC, including differential leukocyte count and platelet count, is generally obtained weekly for 6–8 wk after the oral administration of lomustine to monitor for leukopenia, thrombocytopenia, and anemia; some clinicians suggest waiting 2–3 wk after therapy before obtaining the first CBC and then following up with weekly labs until blood counts are normal or appropriate for subsequent treatment, usually within 6–8 wk; monitor renal and hepatic status; health care professionals responsible for monitoring patients on lomustine therapy should be familiar with the broad spectrum of other adverse effects that can occur, albeit less commonly, with this treatment

LOMUSTINE (Continued)

SPECIAL PRECAUTIONS

Because of the prolonged myelosuppression, treatment should not be given more often than every 6 wk; blood counts should be performed weekly and for 6–8 wk after administration; contraindicated in patients who have demonstrated previous hypersensitivity to the drug; all cytotoxic drugs may be embryotoxic or teratogenic; use with caution in pregnant and nursing patients

TOXICITIES

Hematologic: delayed hematologic toxicity is the major dose-limiting adverse effect; leukocyte nadirs occur first at approximately 15 d after therapy, then a second, lower nadir occurs at approximately 6 wk and persists for 1–2 wk after an oral dose; the degree of leukopenia depends on previous exposure to chemotherapy and can vary among patients; thrombocytopenia generally occurs about 4 wk after therapy and persists approximately 1–2 wk; refractory anemia, acute leukemias, and bone marrow dysplasias have been reported with long-term therapy; **GI:** mild to moderate nausea and vomiting occur beginning 4–5 h after administration of oral lomustine and can last up to 24 h; anorexia often occurs 2–3 d following therapy; stomatitis has occurred infrequently; **CNS:** lethargy, ataxia, and dysarthria occur rarely; **Miscellaneous:** mild hepatotoxicity evidenced by transient elevation in liver enzymes; nephrotoxicity and progressive azotemia are uncommon at total doses < 1000 mg/m^2; pulmonary fibrosis is uncommon at total doses of < 1000 mg/m^2; alopecia

NURSING INTERVENTIONS

Monitor treatment tolerance, weight, and nutritional status; administer antiemetics if necessary; educate patient about neutropenic precautions and self-care at home

PATIENT INFORMATION

Call the doctor immediately if vomiting occurs shortly after the dose is taken, or a sore throat or fever or any unusual bruising or bleeding develops; the medication should be taken on an empty stomach, 2–4 h after meals; anorexia may persist for 2–3 d after the dose is given; avoid aspirin and nonsteroidal antiinflammatory agents; avoid exposure to people with infections

FORMULATION

Available as CeeNU (Bristol-Myers Oncology Division, Princeton, NJ); available as 10-, 40-, and 100-mg capsules; also available as a dose kit containing a total of 300 mg (two 10-mg capsules, two 40-mg capsules, and two 100-mg capsules)

Store in tightly closed containers at a temperature < 40°C.

MECHLORETHAMINE

Mechlorethamine hydrochloride, also known as nitrogen mustard, is a nitrogen analogue of sulfur mustard. It is a bifunctional alkylating agent that interferes with DNA replication and transcription of RNA in rapidly proliferating cells, eventually resulting in disruption of nucleic acid function. Mechlorethamine also possesses weak immunosuppressive activity. The drug is cell cycle nonspecific. Its cytotoxic activity is most pronounced on rapidly proliferating cells. The activity of mechlorethamine is due to the transfer of an alkyl group to cellular constituents such as phosphate, amino, hydroxyl, sulfhydryl, carboxyl, and imidazole groups. In neutral or alkaline solution, the drug is ionized to produce a positively charged carbonium ion, which then attaches to susceptible nuclear proteins at the N-7 position of guanine, a nucleoside found in DNA. This leads to abnormal base pairing of guanine with thymine, cleaving of the imidazole ring of guanine, cross-linking of DNA, and depurination of DNA. Mechlorethamine also inhibits glycolysis, respiration, and RNA-directed protein synthesis.

DOSAGE AND ADMINISTRATION

Mechlorethamine is used in combination with other agents. The drug may be given as follows: 0.4 mg/kg for each course either as a single dose or in 2–4 divided doses of 0.1–0.2 mg/kg/d; or 6 mg/m² on d 1 and 8, repeated every 28 d, for 6 cycles as part of a combination regimen; or 6 mg/m² on d 1 and 8, repeated every other month as part of a combination regimen.

Dose adjustment for myelosuppression: delay treatment 1 wk for absolute neutrophil count (ANC) < 1500/mm³ or platelet count < 100,000/mm³ at time of treatment; after the 1-wk delay, reduce subsequent dose 25% for ANC of 1000–1500/mm³ or platelets of 75,000–100,000/mm³; hold treatment an additional week for patients with values below these.

INDICATIONS

FDA-approved: Palliative treatment of Hodgkin's disease (stage III and IV), lymphosarcoma, chronic myelocytic leukemia, chronic lymphocytic leukemia, polycythemia vera, mycosis fungoides, bronchogenic carcinoma, palliative intraperitoneal treatment of metastatic carcinoma; clinical studies show activity in topical application on cutaneous lymphoma, mycosis fungoides, and psoriasis

PHARMACOKINETICS

Absorption: incompletely absorbed following intracavitary administration due to rapid chemical transformation in water or body fluids, so that the drug is no longer present in the active form a few minutes after administration; **Metabolism:** 0.01% of an IV dose is excreted unchanged in the urine; **Elimination:** apparently renal

DRUG INTERACTIONS

Adjust the doses of uricosuric agents because mechlorethamine raises the blood uric acid concentration; patients on blood dyscrasia–causing medications should have their mechlorethamine dosage adjusted based on their blood counts; use mechlorethamine with extreme caution, if at all, in any patient who is receiving radiation therapy; mechlorethamine may increase the likelihood of infections following the use of live virus vaccines (avoid these in patients receiving immunosuppressive therapy)

RESPONSE RATES

70%–80% of previously untreated patients with advanced Hodgkin's disease showed a complete response while receiving MOPP therapy; of this group, 60%–70% will remain disease-free at 10 y, and cures in these patients are likely; the use of mechloroethamine in other clinical settings has been supplanted by other agents

PATIENT MONITORING

Patients should be monitored throughout their course of treatment; hematocrit and hemoglobin status should be followed as well as platelet counts and total (or differential) leukocyte counts; audiometric testing is warranted at periodic intervals in patients receiving high doses of mechlorethamine; other lab tests that should be followed include SGPT, SGOT, serum bilirubin, lactate dehydrogenase, and uric acid concentrations; radiographic examination is recommended to detect reaccumulation of fluid after intracavitary administration

MECHLORETHAMINE (Continued)

SPECIAL PRECAUTIONS

Mechlorethamine is highly toxic and has a low therapeutic index; avoid inhalation of dust and vapors and contact of the drug with skin or mucous membranes; can predispose the patient to bacterial, viral, or fungal infection due to its immunosuppressive activity; use with extreme caution in patients with leukopenia, thrombocytopenia, or anemia caused by infiltration of the bone marrow with malignant cells; chronic lymphocytic leukemia patients appear to be especially sensitive to the hematopoietic effects of mechlorethamine and should receive the drug with caution if at all; can lead to hematologic complications if combined with irradiation; in the event of extravasation, aspirate as much as possible and neutralize the area with 1/6-molar sterile, isotonic sodium thiosulfate and apply cold compresses for 6–12 h; breast-feeding is not recommended because of the risks to the infant (it is not known whether the drug is excreted in breast milk); if skin contact occurs, irrigate the affected area immediately with large amounts of water for 15 min, then irrigate with a 2% sodium thiosulfate solution

TOXICITIES

Hematologic: lymphocytopenia, granulocytopenia (occurs 6–8 d after treatment and lasts for 10 d–3 wk), agranulocytosis, thrombocytopenia, severe leukopenia, anemia, hemorrhagic diathesis; depression of the hematopoietic system may be found up to 50 d or more after starting therapy; **GI:** nausea, vomiting (onset 1–3 h after use), diarrhea, jaundice, anorexia; **Dermatologic:** maculopapular skin eruptions, alopecia, erythema multiforme; **Reproductive:** delayed menses, oligomenorrhea, temporary or permanent amenorrhea, impaired spermatogenesis, azoospermia, total germinal aplasia; **Local toxicity:** thrombosis, thrombophlebitis, extravasation; **Miscellaneous:** weakness, vertigo, tinnitus, diminished hearing, chromosomal abnormalities

NURSING INTERVENTIONS

Monitor treatment tolerance, weight, nutritional status; administer antiemetics as necessary to control delayed-onset nausea and vomiting; educate patient regarding care of central venous access devices and self-care at home

PATIENT INFORMATION

Avoid use of aspirin and nonsteroidal antiinflammatory agents; call if any moderate or severe adverse effects develop, particularly nausea or fever, or other signs of serious infection; maintain good nutrition and adequate fluid intake—modify eating patterns, use dietary supplements as needed to maintain adequate caloric intake; if the drug is to be applied topically (either ointment or topical solution), shower and rinse carefully just before application unless otherwise directed; wear rubber or plastic gloves when applying; mechlorethamine should be applied more lightly to the groin, inside the elbow, and behind the knees; avoid contact with the eyes, nose, and mouth

FORMULATION

Available as Mustargen (Merck, West Point, PA)
Available in vials containing 10 mg of mechlorethamine triturated with 100 mg of sodium chloride; unopened vials are stored at room temperature and protected from light; mechlorethamine is reconstituted with 10 mL of sterile water for injection or 0.9% sodium chloride for injection; the resultant solution contains 1 mg/mL of mechlorethamine; a topical solution can be made by diluting mechlorethamine 10 mg in 60 mL of sterile water; to prepare the topical ointment, dissolve 10 mg of mechlorethamine in 1 mL of sterile water for injection and blend into 100 g of soft white paraffin.

MELPHALAN

Melphalan, also known as L-phenylalanine mustard, L-PAM, or L-sarcolysin, is a bifunctional alkylating agent that is a phenylalanine derivative of nitrogen mustard. It is a cell cycle nonspecific agent. Because it is an alkylator of the bischlorethamine type, its antineoplastic activity occurs due to the formation of an unstable ethyleneimmonium ion. This unstable ion alkylates with many intracellular molecular components including nucleic acids. The result is cross-linking of strands of DNA (at the N-7 position of guanine) and RNA and disruption of cellular division leading to cellular death. Melphalan also inhibits protein synthesis and exhibits immunosuppressant activity. It is active against both resting and rapidly dividing tumor cells.

DOSAGE AND ADMINISTRATION

Melphalan is used either alone or in combination with other drugs in various chemotherapy regimens. The following regimens have been used in specific carcinomas.

Multiple myeloma: usual oral dose is 6 mg qd adjusted on the basis of weekly blood counts; 10 mg/d x 7–10 d with maintenance dose of 2 mg/d when leukocytes > 4000 and platelets > 100,000; 0.15 mg/kg/d for 7 d, off for 3 wk, then maintenance dose of 0.05 mg/kg/d; 7 mg/m^2 or 0.25 mg/kg/d x 5 d every 5–6 wk; 16 mg/m^2 IV q 2 wk x 4 doses, then, after recovery from toxicity, at 4-wk intervals; **ovarian carcinoma:** 0.2 mg/kg/d x 5 d every 4–5 wk; **high-dose regimens:** 30–40 mg/m^2 IV q 21 d; 120–200 mg/m^2 IV x 1 dose with hematopoietic cellular support

Dosage adjustment in organ dysfunction: patients with BUN ≥ 30 mg/dL should be monitored closely and IV dosage reductions of 50% should be made; in patients with moderate to severe renal impairment, current data do not support an absolute recommendation on oral dosage reduction, but it may be prudent to initially decrease the dose

SPECIAL PRECAUTIONS

Use with caution in patients who have had prior radiation or chemotherapy; use with caution in elderly patients due to age-related renal impairment; all cytotoxic drugs may be embryotoxic or teratogenic; use with caution in pregnant or nursing patients

TOXICITIES

Hematologic: bone marrow suppression, leukopenia, thrombocytopenia, and hemolytic anemia are most common; leukocyte and platelet nadirs usually occur 2–3 wk posttreatment with recovery in 4–5 wk; irreversible bone marrow failure has been reported; **GI:** nausea, vomiting, diarrhea, oral ulceration (dose-dependent, common with high-dose regimens), esophagitis; **Dermatologic:** skin hypersensitivity, allergic reaction hyperpigmentation; **Pulmonary:** pulmonary fibrosis, interstitial pneumonitis; **Renal:** proteinuria, elevated SGT and BUN; **Miscellaneous:** vasculitis, fever, chill, cough, hoarseness, alopecia, hematuria

INDICATIONS

FDA-approved: Palliative treatment of multiple myeloma and nonresectable epithelial ovarian carcinoma; clinical studies show activity in carcinoma of the breast and testes

PHARMACOKINETICS

Absorption: oral doses variably and incompletely absorbed in the GI tract; **Distribution:** rapidly and widely distributed in total body water; initial plasma protein binding is 50%–60% and increases to 80%–90% over time; ~30% is irreversibly bound; penetration across the blood–brain barrier is low; **Metabolism:** deactivated in body fluids and tissues by the process of hydrolysis; plasma half-life is 90 min for oral dosing and biphasic for IV dosing with an initial half-life of 6–10 min and a terminal half-life of 40–75 min; **Elimination:** eliminated from the plasma primarily by chemical hydrolysis to monohydroxy- and dihydroxymelphalan; renal clearance is apparently low

DRUG INTERACTIONS

Concomitant administration with cimetidine, famotidine, nizatidine, and ranitidine has reduced the bioavailability of oral melphalan because these drugs increase gastric pH; severe renal failure has occurred in patients receiving high-dose melphalan and cyclosporine; use with caution with other bone marrow depressants and live virus vaccines

RESPONSE RATES

Melphalan is not curative but can prolong survival of patients with multiple myeloma; it may take 3–12 mo of therapy to evaluate response to the drug; an objective response occurs in 30%–50% of ovarian carcinoma patients taking melphalan alone (combination regimens appear to be more effective); in high-dose regimens, melphalan at doses of 120–200 mg/m^2 is associated with complete remission rates of 30%–50% in patients with myeloma and delayed recurrence of disease when compared with conventional therapy in selected patients

PATIENT MONITORING

CBC, including hemoglobin, platelets, and total and differential leukocyte counts, should be obtained weekly; BUN, serum creatinine, and serum uric acid combinations should be obtained prior to therapy and monthly throughout the course of therapy

NURSING INTERVENTIONS

Monitor treatment tolerance, weight, nutritional status; encourage good oral hygiene; administer antiemetics as necessary; educate patient regarding side effects of melphalan and when to notify the physician; educate patient regarding self-care at home

PATIENT INFORMATION

Avoid use of aspirin and nonsteroidal antiinflammatory agents; oral dose may be taken all at one time and should be given on an empty stomach because food decreases absorption; continue taking melphalan even though you may have some nausea and vomiting; notify the doctor if any signs or symptoms of infection or bleeding develop

FORMULATION

Available as Alkeran (Glaxo-Wellcome, Research Triangle Park, NC) Tablet is supplied in 2-mg bottles of 50 scored tablets; injection form contains a 50-mg single-use vial of melphalan and a 10-mL vial of sterile diluent; should be stored in well-closed, light-resistant container at 15°–30°C. Melphalan should be dispensed in a glass container. Melphalan injection is available in 50-mg glass vials and should be protected from light and stored at 15°–30°C. Melphalan is reconstituted with 10 mL of the supplied sterile diluent. The resulting solution has a concentration of 5 mg/mL of melphalan. The drug should be further diluted in 0.9% sodium chloride injection, USP to a concentration not greater than 0.45 mg/mL and administered over a minimum of 15 min. Complete administration should be accomplished within 60 minutes of reconstitution. The reconstituted solution should not be refrigerated because a precipitate forms.

PROCARBAZINE

Procarbazine, a 1-methyl-2-benzyl derivative of hydrazine, is used in combination therapy for the treatment of lymphomas and primary brain cancers. It has very little activity in solid tumors. Its major activity is found in the treatment of Hodgkin's disease. Procarbazine, considered a nonclassic alkylator, is a prodrug that is metabolized to form numerous active intermediates and methylates DNA at O6 of guanine. It acts by inhibiting the incorporation of thymidine, deoxycytidine, formate, adenine, and 4-amino-5-imidazole carboxylamide into DNA, inhibiting RNA synthesis and inhibiting protein synthesis. Studies have shown procarbazine to inhibit mitosis, particularly in the S and G_2 phases, making the drug cell cycle phase specific. The cytotoxic effects of procarbazine are limited to tissues with high rates of cellular proliferation, and these effects are most evident in cells actively synthesizing DNA because O6-methylgaunine lesions are recognized by mismatch repair, resulting in cell death. Procarbazine also has monoamine oxidase–inhibiting properties.

DOSAGE AND ADMINISTRATION

Procarbazine is administered orally. Dosage must be individualized based on clinical and hematologic response, and on patient's body weight. In patients with abnormal fluid retention, the patient's ideal body weight should be used to calculate the dosage.

Single agent: 50–200 mg/d for 10–20 d, *or* 50 mg initially, then add 50 mg daily up to a maximum of 300 mg daily, or 2–4 mg/kg/d x 1 wk, then 4–6 mg/kg/d until maximum response is achieved.

Maintenance dose: 1–2 mg/kg/d

As component of MOPP therapy for advanced Hodgkin's disease: 100 mg/m² on d 1–14 of 28-d cycle (usually given for minimum of 6 cycles or as many cycles as needed to achieve a complete remission plus 2 or 3 additional cycles as consolidation therapy)

Pediatric dose: 50 mg/m² qd x 1 wk, then 100 mg/m² qd; *pediatric maintenance dose*—50 mg/m²

SPECIAL PRECAUTIONS

Hypersensitivity to procarbazine; inadequate marrow reserve; G6PD deficiency; pregnant or nursing patients; interrupt therapy if the leukocyte count is reduced to ≤ 4000/mm³, if the platelet count falls to ≤ 100,000/mm³, or if hemorrhagic or bleeding tendencies occur

TOXICITIES

Hematologic: bone marrow depression (leukopenia, anemia, thrombocytopenia), pancytopenia, eosinophilia, hemolytic anemia, petechiae, purpura, epistaxis, hemoptysis; **GI:** nausea, vomiting, hepatic dysfunction, jaundice, stomatitis, hematemesis, diarrhea, dysphagia, anorexia, abdominal pain, constipation, dry mouth; **Neurologic:** coma, convulsions, neuropathy, ataxia, paresthesia, nystagmus, headache, dizziness, diminished reflexes, unsteadiness, falling, foot drop, drowsiness, hallucinations, depression, nervousness, confusion, nightmares; **Cardiovascular:** hypotension, tachycardia, syncope; **Respiratory:** pneumonitis, pleural effusion, cough; **Dermatologic:** herpes, dermatitis, pruritus, alopecia, urticaria, flushing; **Miscellaneous:** papilledema, photophobia, diplopia, hematuria, urinary frequency, nocturia, pain, tremors, hearing loss, weakness, fatigue, edema, chills

INDICATIONS

FDA-approved: stage III and IV Hodgkin's disease; clinical studies show activity in non-Hodgkin's lymphomas, mycosis fungoides, brain tumors, small cell lung carcinoma

PHARMACOKINETICS

Absorption: rapidly and nearly completely absorbed from the GI tract; peak plasma concentrations attained within 1 h; **Distribution:** liver, kidneys, intestinal wall, skin; crosses blood–brain barrier and distributes into the cerebrospinal fluid; **Metabolism:** primarily in the liver; **Elimination:** 25%–42% excreted as unchanged drug or as *N*-isopropyl-terephathalmic acid; **Half-life**—10 min

DRUG AND FOOD INTERACTIONS

Barbiturates, antihistamines, opiates, hypotensive agents, phenothiazines, sympathomimetics, local anesthetics, tricyclic antidepressants, and drugs and food with high tyramine content; such as cheese, bananas, tea, coffee, wine, dark beer, cola drinks

RESPONSE RATES

Previously untreated patients with advanced Hodgkin's disease receiving MOPP therapy, 70%–80%; in patients with brain cancer, procarbazine used in combination with CCNU and vincristine improves survival after radiation

PATIENT MONITORING

Bone marrow studies prior to therapy and 2–8 wk after initiation of therapy; hemoglobin, hematocrit, leukocyte and differential counts and reticulocyte and platelet determinations prior to therapy and every 3–4 d thereafter; urinalysis, serum transaminase, serum alkaline phosphatase, BUN obtained prior to therapy and weekly during therapy

NURSING INTERVENTIONS

Monitor treatment tolerance, weight, nutritional status; ensure appropriate lab tests are conducted to monitor for hematologic and hepatic abnormalities

PATIENT INFORMATION

Call physician immediately if intractable nausea or vomiting or fever above 101°C occur; report vomiting episodes that occur soon after taking an oral dose

FORMULATION

Available as Matulane (Roche Laboratories, Nutley, NJ) 50-mg capsules; store in well-closed container at 15°–30°C.

STREPTOZOCIN

Streptozocin is an antineoplastic antibiotic produced by *Streptomyces achromogenes*. As an antibiotic, streptozocin has activity against gram-positive and gram-negative bacteria but its cytotoxicity limits its use as an antibiotic. Streptozocin exhibits alkylating action in vivo by decomposing into reactive methylcarbonium ions that methylates DNA at O6 of guanine and exerts its cytotoxic effect by activation of mismatch repair, resulting in apoptosis. Although streptozocin blocks progression of cells into mitosis, it also blocks other sites of the cell cycle and is referred to as cell cycle nonspecific. The presence of D-glucopyranose moiety explains streptozocin's enhanced uptake by pancreatic islet cells. No other alkylating agent contains a sugar moiety.

DOSAGE AND ADMINISTRATION

The usual dose is 500 mg/m^2/d for 5 d every 6 wk; single doses exceeding 1.5 g/m^2 are not recommended due to the increased risk of azotemia; **Dosage adjustment for renal impairment:** patients with a creatinine clearance between 10–50 mL/min should receive 75% of the normal dose; patients with creatinine clearances < 10 mL/min should receive 50% of the normal dose

SPECIAL PRECAUTIONS

Because streptozocin-induced nephrotoxicity may be irreversible and fatal, routine monitoring of renal function is highly recommended; weekly CBCs and liver function tests should be performed; no information available on the use of streptozocin in children; all cytotoxic drugs may be embryotoxic or teratogenic; use with caution in pregnant or nursing patients

INDICATIONS

FDA-approved: Drug of choice for treating pancreatic islet cell carcinoma; clinical studies show activity in malignant carcinoid tumors, lung cancer, squamous cell carcinoma of the oral cavity, synovial sarcoma, adenocarcinoma of the gallbladder, colorectal cancer, malignant Zollinger-Ellison tumors, and Hodgkin's disease

PHARMACOKINETICS

Absorption: oral absorption of streptozocin is poor (< 20%) and the drug is not active when given orally; **Distribution:** protein binding has not been determined; after IV and intraperitoneal administration, streptozocin and its metabolites are rapidly distributed mainly into the liver, kidneys, intestine, and pancreas; although the drug has not been shown to cross the blood–brain barrier, metabolite concentrations in the cerebrospinal fluid equal to the plasma concentrations have been detected; **Metabolism:** extensively metabolized in the liver and kidneys; **Elimination:** biphasic, with an initial half-life of 5 min and a terminal half-life of 35–40 min; in patients with normal renal and hepatic function, approximately 60%–70% of the dose is excreted in the urine as metabolites; 10%–20% of the dose is eliminated unchanged as the parent drug; the drug can also be eliminated in expired air and feces (5% and 1%, respectively)

DRUG INTERACTIONS

Because streptozocin causes a significant amount of nephrotoxicity, the cumulative effect of other nephrotoxic drugs should be avoided; phenytoin has been reported to decrease the cytotoxic effects of streptozocin on beta cells to the pancreas—therefore, concomitant administration of phenytoin and streptozocin when treating pancreatic islet cell carcinoma should be avoided; streptozocin may prolong the elimination half-life of doxorubicin—if used together, the dose of doxorubicin should be decreased

RESPONSE RATES

Response rates of 35%–60% with streptozocin alone and in combination with 5-fluorouracil have been demonstrated in patients with pancreatic islet cell carcinoma; combination therapy may be slightly better than single-agent therapy; when used alone for the palliative treatment of metastatic carcinoid tumor, responses have been partial and of short duration; combination therapy with cyclophosphamide produced evidence of biochemical response and measurable tumor regression in 26% of patients; combination therapy with 5-fluorouracil produced similar responses in 33% of patients

STREPTOZOCIN (Continued)

TOXICITIES

Renal: renal toxicity is the most serious and dose-limiting adverse effect, occurring in approximately 25%–75% of patients; glomerular and renal tubular dysfunction may be manifested by azotemia, anuria, proteinuria, hypophosphatemia, hyperchloremia, and proximal renal tubular acidosis; the first signs of renal abnormalities usually appear as hypophosphatemia and mild proteinuria; increases in BUN and serum creatinine occur later in therapy; histologic changes in the kidneys can occur; the mechanism of streptozocin-induced nephrotoxicity may be the direct effect of the drug and its metabolites on the renal tubular epithelium; some clinicians suggest that adequate hydration may decrease the concentration of the drug and its metabolites in the kidneys and lessen the adverse effect; this is controversial and not clearly established; nephrogenic diabetes insipidus has also been reported; **GI:** severe nausea and vomiting occur in most patients receiving streptozocin—may be dose-limiting and become progressively worse over a 5-d treatment schedule; mild diarrhea may occur; **Hematologic:** mild to moderate myelosuppression is evidenced, with leukocyte and platelet nadirs occurring within 1–2 wk; **Hepatic:** transient and mild increases in serum concentrations of liver enzymes, lactate dehydrogenase or alkaline phosphatase occur in 25% of streptozocin-treated patients; **Metabolic:** hypoglycemia in patients with insulinoma may be severe but transient; hyperglycemia is uncommon in normal and diabetic patients because normal beta cells are usually insensitive to streptozocin's effect; **Local:** streptozocin is considered an irritant and severe necrosis has been reported after extravasation; **Miscellaneous:** confusion, lethargy, depression, and fever

PATIENT MONITORING

Renal function should be assessed in all patients prior to and during therapy; urinalyses and routine serum chemistries should be obtained; attention to BUN, serum creatinine, and electrolyte concentrations should be determined; CBC, including differential leukocyte count and platelet count, should be performed weekly to monitor for neutropenia, thrombocytopenia, and anemia; health care professionals responsible for monitoring patients on streptozocin therapy should be familiar with the broad spectrum of other adverse effects that can occur, albeit less commonly, with this treatment

NURSING INTERVENTIONS

Monitor treatment tolerance, weight, and nutritional status; streptozocin can be administered by rapid IV push or by IV infusion over 15 min–6 h; nausea and vomiting will occur in ≥ 90% of patients—appropriate antiemetics should be administered; wear gloves when administering streptozocin; the drug is considered an irritant and extravasation should be avoided; keep dextrose 50% at the bedside due to the risk of hypoglycemia from sudden release of insulin; test urine for protein and glucose; proteinuria is one of the first signs of renal toxicity

PATIENT INFORMATION

Call the doctor immediately if intractable nausea and vomiting occur, unusual bruising or bleeding occurs, fever above 101°F; avoid people with infections; fluid intake should be increased during therapy with streptozocin to reduce the potential for renal toxicity; diabetic patients should perform intensive glucose monitoring while being treated with streptozocin

FORMULATION

Available as Zanosar (Upjohn Company, Kalamazoo, MI)
1-g vials of powder for injection.

TEMOZOLOMIDE

Temozolomide is an imidazotetrazine derivative developed in 1980 after many of its ancestor molecules, discovered in the 1960s, produced profound toxicities. Mitozolomide, the monochloroethyltriazene derivative, demonstrated dose-limiting thrombocytopenia in phase I studies. During phase II trials the recommended and reduced doses continued to be too toxic. The myelosuppression of mitozolomide was determined to be due to the monochloroethyltriazene decomposition. A second generation of imidazotetrazines was explored and temozolomide, the 3-methyl congener, was incorporated in the phase I and II trials. Temozolomide is a prodrug that undergoes ring-opening at physiologic pH to monomethytriazene (MTIC). Dacarbazine also converts to MTIC by metabolic *N*-demethylation. The suggested mechanism of action of this nonclassical alkylating agent is probably a methylation reaction at the O^6 position of guanine residues by the reactive species MTIC, with additional alkylation occurring at the N-7 position. Recognition of the O6-methylguanine lesions by mismatch repair enzymes leads to strand breaks, single-strand patches, and induction of apoptosis.

DOSAGE AND ADMINISTRATION

The activity of temozolomide is very schedule dependent. Single bolus doses demonstrated limited clinical activity with various tumor types. The current recommended dose for continued phase II trials is 750–1000 mg/m^2 split over 5 d. The divided dose over 5 d every 4 wk has shown enhanced tumor activity compared with the single-dose regimens. Dose reduction to 500 mg/m^2 may be needed for patients who have been heavily pretreated.

SPECIAL PRECAUTIONS

Myelosuppression is the major dose-limiting toxicity of temozolomide; monitoring for leukopenia and thrombocytopenia should continue throughout therapy; all cytotoxic drugs may be embryotoxic or teratogenic; investigational agents should not be used in pregnant or nursing patients

TOXICITIES

Hematologic: dose-limiting thrombocytopenia (and occasionally leukopenia) occur at approximately 1 g/m^2; patients who have been heavily pretreated with chemotherapy or radiotherapy have a greater risk of myelosuppression; **GI:** mild to moderate nausea and vomiting; **Miscellaneous:** rare alopecia, mild erythematous skin rash, renal toxicity, constipation, and headaches

INDICATIONS

FDA-approved: none; temozolomide is an investigational agent in phase I and II clinical trials. Clinical studies have shown activity in malignant melanoma, recurrent high-grade astrocytomas, mycosis fungoides

PHARMACOKINETICS

Absorption: area under the curve (AUC) increases linearly with increases in dose; when first synthesized, temozolomide was administered by IV infusion over 1 h; owing to the extensive preparation of the IV formulation, oral capsules were developed; temozolomide capsules are rapidly absorbed; oral bioavailability is very good with some studies reporting similar AUC for both IV and oral administration; **Distribution:** peak plasma concentrations of 3.3 to 15.3 µg/mL are reached within 60 m; steady-state volume of distribution is 13 ± 6 L/m^2; cerebrospinal fluid to plasma concentration ratio is 29% ± 8%, therefore achieving adequate penetrating through the blood±brain barrier; there is no accumulation of drug from d 1 to d 5 of therapy; **Metabolism:** limited information available; temozolomide undergoes ring-opening under physiologic pH to monomethytriazene; there is some suggestion of enterohepatic recirculation; **Elimination:** half-life is biexponential with alpha half-life being 1 h and beta-half life of 8–9 h; total body clearance is 32 mL/min/m^2; there is much less interpatient variability than with dacarbazine

DRUG INTERACTIONS

Temozolomide toxicity may be enhanced if given with other myelosuppressive drugs or therapies

RESPONSE RATES

Response rates, both complete and partial, of 17% have been reported in the treatment of metastatic melanoma; varied responses have been reported in patients with high-grade astrocytomas and mycosis fungoides (patient numbers in most trials so far are small)

PATIENT MONITORING

CBC, including differential leukocyte count and platelet count, should be obtained during therapy to monitor for leukopenia and thrombocytopenia; health care professionals responsible for monitoring patients on temozolomide therapy should be familiar with the less common adverse effects that can occur with therapy

NURSING INTERVENTIONS

Monitor treatment tolerance, weight, nutritional status; ensure that appropriate lab tests are conducted to monitor leukopenia and thrombocytopenia; ensure appropriate documentation and notify physician of all adverse effects and patient complaints in patients receiving investigational drugs; ensure that a consent form is signed by the patient to receive investigational drugs; nausea and vomiting are mild to moderate; appropriate antiemetics should be given

PATIENT INFORMATION

Call the doctor immediately if intractable nausea and vomiting occur or if vomiting occurs after taking the temozolomide capsules, unusual bruising and bleeding occurs, or temperature over 101°F occurs; avoid exposure to people with infections

FORMULATION

Available as Temedal (Schering-Plough, Kenilworth, NJ)
Hard gelatin capsules containing 20, 50, 100, and 250 mg are available for phase I and II trials; still investigational.

THIOTEPA

Thiotepa is a synthetic polyfunctional alkylating agent that also possesses some immunosuppressive activity. Thiotepa interferes with DNA replication and transcription of RNA and ultimately results in the disruption of nucleic acid function. This alkylating agent has been in clinical use for more than 30 years. It can be administered by several different routes and is primarily used as an intravesical instillation for bladder carcinoma. Recently, several studies have investigated the value of thiotepa in high doses to treat several tumor types such as chronic leukemia, Hodgkin's disease, non-Hodgkin's lymphoma, breast and ovarian carcinoma, and melanoma.

DOSAGE AND ADMINISTRATION

Thiotepa can be administered by several different routes including IV, intrapleural, intraperitoneal, intrapericardial, intratumor, intramuscular, intrathecal, and ophthalmic instillation.

Intravesical instillation for superficial bladder tumors: the recommended dose is 30–60 mg in 30 to 60 mL of sterile water instilled by a catheter into the bladder and retained for 2 h; the patient should be repositioned every 15 min for maximum area contact; the treatment course is once a week for 4 wk then once a month for 1 y, as long as the patient remains tumor-free

Intratumor injection: Initial doses of 0.6–0.8 mg/kg administered directly into the tumor; a maintenance dose of 0.07–0.8 mg/kg can be administered every 1–4 wk

Intracavitary and intrapericardial: for intracavitary infusions, doses of 0.6–0.8 mg/kg every week; intrapericardial doses of 15–30 mg have been administered

Conventional doses used for breast, lung, and ovarian cancers, lymphomas and Hodgkin's disease: 0.2 mg/kg IV daily for 5 d repeated every 2–4 wk; or 0.3–0.4 mg/kg IV every 1–4 wk

High dose therapies: 60 to 475 mg/m^2 with or without autologous marrow transplantation; 180 to 1575 mg/m^2 with autologous marrow transplantation

Intrathecal administration: 1 to 10 mg/m^2 once or twice a week as a 1 mg/mL concentration

Ophthalmic instillation: to prevent pterygium recurrence, a 0.05% solution of thiotepa in Ringer's injection instilled into the eye every 3 h during waking hours for 6 to 8 wk postoperatively

SPECIAL PRECAUTIONS

Avoid in patients who have experienced hypersensitivity reactions to the drug; all cytotoxic drugs may be embryotoxic or teratogenic; use with caution in pregnant or nursing patients

INDICATIONS

FDA-approved: Used intravesically in the treatment of superficial tumors of the bladder such as transitional cell carcinoma, papilloma, and carcinoma in situ; clinical studies have shown activity in breast cancer, Hodgkin's disease, non-Hodgkin's lymphoma, chronic leukemias, lung cancer, ovarian cancer, malignant melanoma, and pterygium

PHARMACOKINETICS

Absorption: incompletely absorbed from the GI tract; absorption through serous membranes ranges from 10% to almost 100%; **Distribution:** thiotepa is very lipophilic and penetrates the CNS readily; it is extensively and rapidly distributed to all tissues of the body, exhibiting an average volume of distribution of 0.7 L/kg; it is not known whether thiotepa distributes into breast milk; **Metabolism:** extensively metabolized in the liver; primary active metabolite is trimethylene phosphoramide (TEPA); this metabolite may possess more potent cytotoxic activity than thiotepa; other metabolites may exist but are undefined at this time; **Excretion:** exhibits a biexponential half-life, with an alpha half-life of approximately 10 min and a beta half-life of about 125 min; total clearance ranges from 150–500 mL/h/kg depending on the dose and patient parameters; approximately 60% of the IV dose is excreted in the urine within 24–72 h; TEPA excretion is slower than thiotepa

DRUG INTERACTIONS

The concomitant use of thiotepa and succinylcholine may cause prolonged respirations and apnea; thiotepa inhibits the activity of pseudocholinesterase, the enzyme that deactivates succinylcholine; in theory, thiotepa may inhibit the metabolism of other drugs; however, this has not been extensively evaluated in humans

RESPONSE RATES

Complete responses of 38% and partial responses of 24% have been reported in patients with superficial bladder tumors; recurrence rates decrease when thiotepa is used in combination with tumor resection or fulguration; when used as palliative treatment in breast and ovarian carcinomas and in high-dose therapy regimens, response rates of 20%–30% and 30%–50%, respectively, have been reported.

THIOTEPA (Continued)

TOXICITIES

Hematologic: leukopenia is the major adverse effect of thiotepa; effects are usually dose-related and cumulative; leukocyte nadir is typically 10–14 d but has been reported to occur at approximately 30 d; manufacturer recommends discontinuing therapy if leukocyte counts fall to 3000/mm^3 and platelet counts fall < 150,000/mm^3; thiotepa can be absorbed through serous membranes—therefore, intracavitary and intravesical instillation can cause systemic hematologic effects; the development of secondary malignancies can occur with thiotepa administration; **GI:** nausea, vomiting, and anorexia occur infrequently at usual doses; high-dose regimens significantly increase the incidence of nausea, vomiting, mucositis, esophagitis, and diarrhea; **CNS:** headache and dizziness with IV administration has been reported; at high doses, CNS toxicity can become dose-limiting; mild to moderate cognitive dysfunction becomes apparent at doses of 1125 mg/m^2; cognitive dysfunction is exhibited by the inability to follow simple commands or perform coordinated tasks; demyelination has been reported; **Dermatologic:** usually absent or mild consisting of allergic reaction type hives, rash, and pruritus; high-dose therapy has been reported to produce a novel skin toxicity described as generalized erythema or a maculopapular, nonpruritic rash associated with dry desquamation; a bronzing of the skin was also noticed several days following therapy; some alopecia has been reported; **Miscellaneous:** intravesical administration can produce lower abdominal pain, vesical irritability, hematuria, and rarely hemorrhagic chemical cystitis; intrathecal administration can be associated with lower extremity weakness and pain; transient elevations (< 10-fold) in liver function tests have been reported with high-dose thiotepa; amenorrhea and impaired spermatogenesis have occurred

PATIENT MONITORING

CBC, including differentia leukocyte count and platelet count, should be performed weekly during therapy and for at least 3 wk after therapy; when treating patients with a high tumor burden, uric acid concentrations should be monitored and allopurinol should be given to decrease the risk of tumor lysis syndrome; a complete neurologic exam should be performed at the beginning and intermittently throughout therapy to evaluate cognitive function; health care professionals responsible for monitoring patients on thiotepa therapy should be familiar with the broad spectrum of other adverse effects that can occur, albeit less commonly, with this treatment

NURSING INTERVENTIONS

Monitor treatment tolerance, weight, and nutritional status; thiotepa is not a vesicant and can be given by several routes—procaine 2% or epinephrine 1:1000, or both, can be mixed with thiotepa and used for local administration; administer antiemetics when appropriate, especially when giving high-dose thiotepa; evaluate cognitive function, coordination, and mental status at each visit

PATIENT INFORMATION

Call the doctor immediately if sore throat, unusual bruising or bleeding, or fever above 101°F occurs; avoid people with infections; do not drink fluids for 8–10 h before bladder installation of thiotepa; hair loss is normal and will grow back after therapy has ended; inform the doctor of any loss of memory or coordination

FORMULATION

Available as Thioplex (Immunex, Seattle, WA) parenteral for injection in a 15-mg vial; each vial also contains 80 mg of sodium chloride and 50 mg of sodium bicarbonate so that following reconstitution with sterile water for injection, solutions of the drug are isotonic; thiotepa sterile lyophilized powder for injection and reconstituted solutions of the drug should be stored at 2–8°C and protected from light; thiotepa powder for injection should be reconstituted with 1.5 mL sterile water for injection to yield a concentration of approximately 10 mg/mL; the reconstituted injection is stable for 8 h at 2–8°C; solutions that are grossly opaque or contain a precipitate should not be used; when intrathecal injections are intended, preservative-free 0.9% sodium chloride should be used; the reconstituted powder can be further diluted in 0.9% sodium chloride, dextrose 5% and water, Ringer's, and lactated Ringer's solutions.

The antitumor antibiotics are a diverse group of drugs that are grouped together by virtue of the fact that they are produced in a manner similar to antibiotics as a modification of natural products and because they are effective in a variety of human tumors. Novel antitumor antibiotics are being developed based on rational design from an increasing knowledge of structure-activity relationships. The major class of drugs in this group are the anthracyclines, which include doxorubicin, daunorubicin, and their analogues; epirubicin and idarubicin; and the unique anthracycline mitoxantrone, an anthracenedione. The anthracyclines are therapeutic across a range of neoplastic diseases, including carcinomas (of the breast, lung, stomach, and thyroid), lymphomas, myelogenous leukemias, myelomas, and sarcomas.

ANTHRACYCLINES

The anthracyclines comprise a series of large ring structures attached to a daunosamine sugar. The compounds differ in the nature of the side chain (ketone versus ketol), the stereochemistry of the attached sugar, and the presence or absence of a methoxy side group on the ring structure. The planar semiquinone ring facilitates intercalation into DNA; this is a key event because incorporation of the anthracycline creates the local conditions critical to its cytotoxicity.

MECHANISM OF ACTION

Interference with the action of DNA topoisomerase II in regions of transcriptionally active DNA is the most widely cited and generally accepted mechanism of action for the anthracyclines (Table 2-1). This enzyme acts by binding to DNA and nicking one of its strands, thus allowing the supercoiled macromolecule to relax as the opposite strand passes through the break. The enzyme then reanneals the broken ends. Anthracyclines are thought to act by stabilizing the topoisomerase–DNA complex in the cleaved configuration. This event not only maintains the single-strand breaks but also helps to create further double-strand breaks. During mitosis, topoisomerase II levels rise rapidly, and the cell becomes more vulnerable to the effects of doxorubicin, thus possibly accounting for selective effects on rapidly dividing tumors.

The ability of these drugs to generate free radicals, which are cytotoxic to both normal and malignant tissues, has attracted much attention. Doxorubicin, as well as the other anthracyclines, is highly reactive with heavy metal ions, such as Cu^{2+} and Al^{3+}. Following entry into the cell, free drug in the cytosol is thought to bind ferric (Fe^{3+}) iron, which then generates highly reactive hydroxyl radical species by a one-electron reduction of the hydroxyquinone structure. The drug–iron complex binds to cell membranes and causes oxidative cell damage; most tissues possess adequate defenses against this type of event (in the form of superoxide dismutase, glutathione, and so on) and are able to repair the damage. Cardiac tissue, however, is notably deficient in this respect and is highly vulnerable to oxidative attack. The cardiotoxicity caused by anthracyclines is not the result of a particular affinity for cardiac tissue but rather the result of a deficiency in host protective factors.

This rich and varied organometallic chemistry also carries several practical implications. The ketol side chain of doxorubicin and its analogues is highly susceptible to oxidation by iron with its resultant destruction, whereas the ketone side chain of daunorubicin and its analogues lacks this reactivity. Therefore, doxorubicin is much less stable than daunorubicin when reconstituted in aqueous solution because iron is a frequent contaminant of many buffers and glassware items. For similar reasons, contact with metal surfaces and objects (*eg*, syringe needles or aluminum foil) should not be prolonged.

PHARMACOKINETICS

Following intravenous bolus injection, doxorubicin and the anthracyclines leave the central pharmacokinetic compartment rapidly and distribute to the peripheral tissues, except the brain, in direct proportion to the DNA content of the peripheral tissue. The anthracyclines are metabolized in the liver and excreted in the bile (Table 2-2). One controversial area has been whether the dose of doxorubicin should be reduced in the face of abnormal liver function. Opinion is divided on this point; however, the conservative recommendation is to adjust the drug dose downward for an elevated bilirubin level.

Table 2-1. Mechanisms of Action of Antineoplastic Antibiotics

Agent	Mechanisms
Doxorubicin	Topoisomerase II inhibition, free-radical formation, direct membrane interactions, DNA-RNA intercalation
Daunorubicin	Topoisomerase II inhibition, free-radical formation, direct membrane interactions, DNA-RNA intercalation
Idarubicin	Free-radical generation
Mitoxantrone	Single/double-stranded DNA breaks, cell membrane and mitochondrial lipid peroxidation, inhibition of glutathione synthesis
Dactinomycin	DNA intercalation, DNA-directed RNA synthesis inhibition
Bleomycin	Oxygen-derived free-radical generation, DNA intercalation, single/double-strand DNA breaks
Mitomycin C	Oxygen-derived free-radical generation, DNA alkylation, cross-linking of DNA strands, single-strand DNA breaks
Plicamycin	DNA binding, RNA synthesis inhibition, single-strand DNA breaks

Table 2-2. Pharmacokinetics of Antineoplastic Antibiotics

Drug	Half-life, h	Total Body Clearance	Route of Excretion
Bleomycin	2–4 (IV) 3 (intrapleural) 5 (intraperitoneal)	3 l/mL/m^2	50%–70% renal
Dactinomycin	36–48	Unknown	Possibly 15% hepatic, 20%–30% renal
Daunorubicin	20	34–67 l/mL/m^2	40% hepatic, 10% renal
Doxorubicin	16–24	15–30 l/mL/m^2	40%–50% hepatic, 5%–10% renal
Idarubicin	10–30	30–60 l/mL/m^2	5% renal
Mitomycin C	1–2	30 l/mL	9%–20% renal
Mitoxantrone	23–47	13–34 l/mL/m^2	40%–50% hepatic, 5%–10% renal
Plicamycin	Unknown	Unknown	?50% renal

TOXICITIES

The primary toxicity of the anthracyclines is myelosuppression (Table 2-3), especially granulocytopenia, usually with the maximal effectiveness seen at approximately day 10 from the start of administration on an intermittent schedule. Mucositis often accompanies the granulocytopenia, and the severity correlates with the degree of myelosuppression. Total alopecia occurs approximately 3 weeks after the administration of full-dose anthracyclines. Anthracyclines are potent vesicants; therefore, care must be taken to avoid extravasation injury.

Anthracycline cardiac toxicity is potentially significant. An acute pericardial–myocardial toxicity has been reported associated with higher single doses, is clinically apparent with transient decrease in ejection fraction and electrocardiogram changes characteristic of pericarditis, and is usually self-limited. The chronic cardiac toxicity is a dilated cardiomyopathy that can lead to congestive heart failure. Serial radionuclide-gated cardiac-function studies are of proven value in detecting cardiomyopathy prior to the clinical manifestations of congestive heart failure. The incidence increases with increasing cumulative doses in excess of 450 mg/m^2. Cardiomyopathy may occur at lower cumulative doses in patients who have had prior mediastinal radiation, preexisting cardiomyopathy, or concurrent cyclophosphamide. The incidence of cardiomyopathy may be lower in patients receiving a prolonged infusion of doxorubicin.

Dexrazoxane (Zinecard Pharmacia & Upjohn, Kalamazoo, MI) has been approved for reducing the incidence and severity of cardiomyopathy associated with doxorubicin administration in women with metastatic breast cancer who have received a cumulative dose of greater than 300 mg/m^2 [1]. Clinical studies are underway to test cardioprotection in other clinical settings. The approved indication for dexrazoxane is limited to those women being treated for metastatic breast cancer who have had a cumulative doxorubicin dose of 300 mg/m^2 and in whom the physician judges that there is additional benefit of continued doxorubicin therapy. The recommended dose is based on a ratio of 10:1 dexrazoxane to doxorubicin to be given as an intravenous infusion within 30 minutes of the doxorubicin intravenous injection.

The success of dexrazoxane, a cardioprotective agent, is based on protection from free-radical generation. Dexrazoxane is a metal-chelating agent, as is ethylenediaminetetraacetic acid, which is lipid soluble and able to diffuse across the cell membrane. Once inside the cell, it is hydrolyzed to form a highly active metal-chelating agent that binds with iron and removes it from the cardiac myocyte, protecting the cell from oxidative injury.

The sugar moiety of both doxorubicin and daunorubicin binds to heparin, and concomitant administration of an anthracycline and heparin can hasten clearance of doxorubicin. Both anthracyclines are associated with a radiation recall phenomenon, in which previously irradiated tissue becomes more susceptible to anthracycline-induced toxicity than would normal tissue. In patients with Hodgkin's disease and breast and small cell lung cancer, recall becomes a significant problem because these patients are often treated with chest or mediastinal radiation therapy as well as anthracycline-based chemotherapy.

MITOMYCIN C

MECHANISM OF ACTION

In contrast to the anthracyclines, mitomycin C is a prodrug and requires metabolic activation to realize its cytotoxic potential [2,3]. Three different chemically active sites have been identified, although the precise mechanisms by which activation occurs in vivo are unclear. The quinone structure easily forms highly reactive semiquinone intermediates by chemical reduction, which can then bind to DNA and form an alkylated DNA adduct. Alternatively, reductive activation also can form highly toxic oxygen free-radical intermediates that attack cell membranes and subcellular structures. The urethane ring and the Cl carbon also can be activated to form alkylating moieties.

Mitomycin C is considered the prototypical bioreductive alkylating agent, and the predominant mode of action is thought to be alkylation of DNA at the N-6 position of adenine or at the N-2 or O-6 positions of guanine by one of the active metabolites mentioned above. The drug has been moderately successful in the treatment of breast, non–small cell lung, gastric, pancreatic, colorectal, cervical, prostate, and superficial bladder cancers.

PHARMACOKINETICS

Activation to the reactive species can occur in all tissues; mitomycin C is cleared rapidly from the circulation following initial intravenous injection and distributes to total body water. It demonstrates pharmacokinetic behavior consistent with a two-compartment linear

Table 2-3. Toxicities of Antineoplastic Antibiotics

Toxicity	Bleomycin	Dactinomycin	Daunorubicin	Doxorubicin	Idarubicin	Mitomycin C	Mitoxantrone	Plicamycin
Myelosuppression	—	X	X	X	X	X	X	X
Nausea, vomiting	—	X	X	X	X	X	X	X
Stomatitis, alopecia	X	X	X	X	X	X	X	—
Extravasation necrosis	—	X	X	X	X	X	—	X
Pulmonary	X	—	—	—	—	X	—	—
Renal	—	—	—	—	—	X	—	X
Hepatic	—	X	—	—	—	—	—	X
Skin	X	X	X	X	X	—	—	—
Hemolysis	—	—	—	—	—	—	—	—
Cardiac	—	—	X	X	X	X	X	X
Fever	X	X	—	—	—	—	X	X

model, with a β-elimination half-life of approximately 1 hour. Thus, significant drug levels will remain in the body for approximately 4 hours following an intravenous bolus administration.

TOXICITIES

Unlike other chemotherapeutic agents, the myelosuppression associated with mitomycin C is delayed, occurring approximately 4 weeks after treatment, suggesting that mitomycin acts on hematopoietic stem cells. Thrombocytopenia is often more severe than leukopenia or anemia. Mitomycin toxicities are cumulative with progressively more severe myelosuppression. Mitomycin is a potent vesicant, and precautions should be taken to avoid extravasation during administration of this drug.

Among the dose-limiting toxicities unique to mitomycin C is a vasculitis that encompasses a spectrum of disease, including hemolytic–uremic syndrome and venoocclusive disease. Interstitial pneumonitis and cardiac failure also occur. Approximately 200 patients treated with mitomycin C have developed a syndrome that includes renal failure and hemolysis. This development seems to be dose related, with most cases occurring after cumulative doses of 50 mg/m² have been given. Although the etiology of this syndrome is unknown, an autoimmune mechanism has been postulated; the fact that red blood cell transfusions can aggravate the hemolytic process supports this notion. Treatment is mainly supportive and consists of hemodialysis, avoidance of red cell transfusions, and the use of various immunosuppressive agents. The use of a staphylococcal protein A immunoperfusion column has been reported to be of benefit.

Pulmonary toxicity appears to be idiosyncratic, potentiated by exposure to vinca alkaloids and radiation. Clinically, it is similar to that produced by other antineoplastics agents and is characterized by progressive pulmonary fibrosis mediated by free radical mechanisms. When given in combination with doxorubicin, mitomycin can act synergistically to increase cardiotoxicity, a possible consequence of both agents producing free radicals. Regardless of the mechanisms by which these increased toxicities are produced, caution is indicated when administering mitomycin in combination with anthracyclines.

BLEOMYCIN

MECHANISM OF ACTION

Bleomycin is a mixture of polypeptides, all with a common structural component called bleomycinic acid. Bleomycin A_2 is the predominant species; a series of analogues based on purified forms of the various polypeptides are in development. Like the anthracyclines, bleomycin chelates iron and forms an activated complex, which then binds the guanine bases in the DNA. Once formed, the DNA–bleomycin–iron adduct catalyzes the reduction of molecular oxygen to form highly reactive free-radical species that cause DNA strand scission in the linker regions between nucleosomes. Thus, bleomycin causes not only DNA-strand cleavage but also actual chromosomal breaks that can be seen microscopically.

Bleomycin is a phase-specific agent that is most active in mitosis and G_2 phases of the cell cycle. Further supporting the concept of schedule dependency is the in vitro finding that both cell death and DNA-strand breaks increase proportionally with the length of drug

exposure, up to 6 hours. Thus, bleomycin may be better administered by continuous infusion rather than by intravenous bolus.

PHARMACOKINETICS

Following intravenous injection in patients with normal renal function, bleomycin distributes to the peripheral compartment with an α half-life of approximately 30 minutes, and then is more slowly excreted with a β half-life of between 2 and 4 hours. In the case of patients with impaired renal function, the terminal elimination half-life is extended significantly; several authorities recommend decreasing the dose of bleomycin with creatinine clearances of less than 35 mL/min/m².

TOXICITIES

Bleomycin is toxic to lung tissue. This toxicity has either a diffuse or nodular radiographic pattern, follows a course of relentless pulmonary fibrosis and insufficiency, and appears to be similar to the "final common pathway" noted for a number of other pulmonary toxins. The incidence of this complication increases with cumulative doses over 250 U, reaching 10% at total doses of 450 U. Elderly patients (> 70 y), patients with underling pulmonary disease, and patients previously exposed to pulmonary or mediastinal irradiation appear to be at increased risk. Treatment is mainly supportive. In regard to the mechanism of the pulmonary toxicity, it is of interest that bleomycin is degraded by hydrolysis; the aminohydrolases responsible for this are found in low concentrations in lung tissue and in skin. These tissues are particularly susceptible to bleomycin-induced injury and may be examples of injury due to a lack of host protective factors rather than to tissue tropism of the drug itself.

Cutaneous manifestations of bleomycin appear as erythematous, hyperpigmenting, or desquamating reactions, typically occurring on the pressure points and skin creases. Frank ulcerations occasionally occur. These changes affect the flexor surfaces and areas of prior exposure to radiation. A dermatographic response also occurs. Vascular changes in the form of Raynaud's phenomenon has also been reported [4]. An acute idiosyncratic reaction consisting of confusion, faintness, fever, chills, and wheezing has been reported in patients with lymphoma receiving more than 25 U/m². This syndrome may progress to cardiorespiratory collapse and usually occurs after the first or second dose. Other side effects of drug administration include fever (occurring up to 48 h after infusion) and hyperbilirubinemia.

Perioperative management of patients who have previously received bleomycin is a vexing problem because there is evidence suggesting that high inspired fractions of oxygen can potentiate or exacerbate bleomycin-induced pulmonary toxicity [5]. The clinical picture and physical findings of dyspnea, tachypnea, dry cough, and rales should prompt the performance of baseline arterial blood gas testing and chest radiography. If results are abnormal, then pulmonary function testing with DLCO should be pursued. If these tests are abnormal, or in the presence of other pulmonary risk factors, regional anesthesia should be considered, if feasible. If general anesthesia cannot be avoided, the best guidelines call for continuous oxygen saturation analysis and intermittent arterial blood gas sampling intraoperatively. For oxygen management, a brief period of 100% oxygen should be administered immediately prior to the induction of anesthesia, with subsequent inhaled concentrations kept at the minimum level necessary. Close monitoring of the patient's volume status and gas exchange is crucial both intra- and postoperatively, and mechanical ventilation may be required postoperatively to assure adequate oxygenation [5].

DACTINOMYCIN

MECHANISM OF ACTION

Dactinomycin (or actinomycin D), one of the first chemotherapeutic agents to be introduced into general use, has a structure similar to the anthracyclines in that it consists of a planar, multiring phenoxazone moiety with two substituents. In this case, two identical cyclic polypeptide arms are attached to the aromatic rings. The planar nature of the phenoxazone structure allows actinomycin to intercalate itself between DNA base pairs while the polypeptide rings lie within the minor groove; the overall effect is to bind together the two complementary strands of DNA, preventing the synthesis of the corresponding RNA molecules. At low concentrations, actinomycin mainly inhibits DNA-directed RNA synthesis, whereas at high concentrations, both RNA transcription and DNA replication are affected.

PHARMACOKINETICS

Unlike many other chemotherapeutic agents, dactinomycin freely diffuses into the cell and distributes rapidly to the peripheral tissues. It has an elimination half-life of approximately 36 hours, mainly due to slow release from tissue- and DNA-binding sites. The drug is not significantly metabolized and is excreted unchanged into both bile and urine.

TOXICITIES

The dose-limiting toxicity of dactinomycin is primarily myelosuppression, although nausea, vomiting, diarrhea, and mucositis also occur. It can also cause a radiation recall phenomenon by inhibiting DNA repair mechanisms. The organs most prone to this effect are the skin and the gastrointestinal tract, although late effects can be seen in the lungs and the liver.

Dactinomycin has been used extensively in the treatment of gestational trophoblastic disease, Wilms' tumor, and other pediatric malignancies.

PLICAMYCIN

Although used originally in the treatment of Paget's disease and embryonal cell carcinoma of the testis, plicamycin is now used primarily in the management of hypercalcemia due to malignancy. With the advent of newer agents, such as gallium nitrate and etidronate, however, use of the drug for this indication is also declining.

The mechanism of action involves inhibition of RNA synthesis but definitive molecular pharmacology studies have not been done. Likewise, because the drug was developed and marketed in the 1960s, contemporary pharmacokinetics are not available. The dose-limiting toxicity is a diffuse hemorrhagic syndrome, which occurs with a dose-related incidence of approximately 5% to 10%. Other side effects of hepatotoxicity and renal toxicity are seen in high-dose regimens.

REFERENCES

1. Speyer JL, Green MD, Zeleniuch-Jacquette A, *et al.*: ICRF-187 permits longer treatment with doxorubicin in women with breast cancer. *J Clin Oncol* 1992, 10:117–127.

2. Verwij J, Pinedo HM: Mitomycin C: mechanism of action, usefulness and limitations. *Anticancer Drugs* 1990, 1:5–13.

3. Verweij J, Pinedo HM: Mitomycin C. *Cancer Chemother Biol Resp Mod* 1991, 12:59–65.

4. Vogelzang NJ, Bosl GJ, Johnson K, *et al.*: Raynaud's phenomenon: a common toxicity after combination chemotherapy for testicular cancer. *Ann Intern Med* 1981, 95:288–292.

5. Waid-Jones MI, Coursin DB: Perioperative considerations for patients treated with bleomycin. *Chest* 1991, 99:993–999.

6. Calero F, Rodriguez-Escudero F, Jimeno J, *et al.*: Single agent epirubicin in squamous cell cervical cancer. *Acta Oncol* 1991, 30:325–327.

7. Calero F, Asins-Codoñer, Jimeno J, *et al.*: Epirubicin in advanced endometrial adenocarcinoma: a phase II study of the Grup Ginecologico Español para el Tratamiento Oncologico (GGETO). *Eur J Cancer* 1991, 27:864–866.

8. Nielsen D, Dombernowsky P, Skovsgaard T, *et al.*: Epirubicin or epirubicin and vindesine in advanced breast cancer: a phase III study. *Ann Oncol* 1990, 1:275–280.

9. Wade JR, Kelman AW, Kerr DJ, *et al.*: Variability in the pharmacokinetics of epirubicin: a population analysis. *Cancer Chemother Pharmacol* 1992, 29:391–395.

10. Berman E, Heller G, Santorsa J, *et al.*: Results of a randomized trial comparing idarubicin and cytosine arabinoside with daunorubicin and cytosine arabinoside in adult patients with newly diagnosed acute myelogenous leukemia. *Blood* 1991, 77:1666–1674.

11. Vogler WR, Velez-Garcia E, Weiner RS, *et al.*: A phase III trial comparing idarubicin and daunorubicin in combination with cytarabine in acute myelogenous leukemia: a Southeastern Cancer Study Group study. *J Clin Oncol* 1991; 10:1103–1111.

12. Mandelli F, Petti MC, Ardia A, *et al.*: A randomised clinical trial comparing idarubicin and cytarabine to daunorubicin and cytarabine in the treatment of acute non-lymphoid leukemia. *Eur J Cancer* 1991, 27:750–755.

13. Nissen NI, Hansen SW: High activity of daily-schedule mitoxantrone in newly-diagnosed low-grade non-Hodgkin's lymphomas: a 5-year follow-up. *Sem Oncol* 1990, 17:10–13.

14. Cowan JD, Neidhart J, McClure S, *et al.*: Randomized trial of doxorubicin, bisantrene, and mitoxantrone in advanced breast cancer: a Southwest Oncology Group study. *J Nat Cancer Inst* 1991, 83:1077–1084.

15. Tannock IF, Osaba D, Stocker MR, *et al.*: Chemotherapy with mitoxantrone plus prednisone or prednisone alone for symptomatic hormone-resistant prostate cancer: a Canadian randomized trial with palliative end points. *J Clin Oncol* 1996, 14:1756–1764.

BLEOMYCIN

Bleomycin is a mixture of fungal polypeptides isolated from *Streptomyces verticullus* that creates DNA-strand breaks. Because bleomycin is cleared mainly through the kidneys, caution is advised in using this drug in the presence of impaired renal function, although no data exist on which to base specific dosing recommendations. Usually, the drug is given by intravenous infusion, but it is also used frequently in the setting of intracavitary instillation for sclerosis of the pleural or peritoneal cavities. Fever may occur in the immediate peri-infusion period, and occasional instances of hypersensitivity reactions have been reported. In combination chemotherapy protocols, bleomycin is most commonly used with cisplatin and etoposide as an essential part of the PEB regimen for testicular cancer.

Raynaud's phenomenon has been described as a complication of bleomycin therapy when given as part of combination chemotherapy regimens for testicular cancer. Speculated causal mechanisms have included arterial obstruction, increased neuromuscular instability due to hypomagnesemia, and sympathetic hyperreactivity. However, no single mechanism has been proven. Fortunately, the problem remains localized to the digits and causes little life- or limb-threatening morbidity.

DOSAGE AND ADMINISTRATION

Equipment and medication necessary for treatment of a possible anaphylactic reaction should be readily available at each administration. Test dose of 1–2 U given 2–4 h prior to therapy is frequently recommended. Some clinicians recommend premedication with acetaminophen, steroids, and diphenhydramine hydrochloride to reduce fever and risk of anaphylaxis.

Intravenous administration: 10–20 U/m²/wk IV **or** 15 U/m² continuous infusion over 24 h for 4–5 d. Maintenance dose for Hodgkin's disease: 1 U/d **or** 5 U/wk until completion of therapy; **Regional arterial infusion:** 30–60 U/d over 1–24 h; **Intrapleural injection:** 15–120 U in 100 mL 0.9% NS injection, instilled and removed after 24 h; **Intraperitoneal injection:** 60–120 U (base) in 100 mL 0.9% NS injection, instilled and removed after 24 h; **Intralesional injection:** 0.2–0.8 U (base) (according to lesion size) one or more times at intervals of 2–4 wk, up to a maximum total dose of 2 U, using a solution of 15 U of bleomycin in 15 mL of 0.9% NS injection or water for injection

DOSAGE MODIFICATIONS: Cumulative doses should not exceed 250–450 U (less in patients with risk factors mentioned above or with renal impairment, < 35 mL/min/m²). When given intrapleurally or intraperitoneally, half of the intracavitary dose should be counted toward this total.

SPECIAL PRECAUTIONS

Pediatric patients; patients > 70 y of age (increased risk of pulmonary toxicity and decline in renal function warrant dose reduction); patients who smoke; pregnant and nursing patients; potential for perioperative pulmonary complications.
Conditions requiring special considerations: herpes zoster, chickenpox, hepatic functional impairment, Raynaud's phenomenon, peripheral vascular disease

TOXICITIES

Degree of Severity	Frequent	Occasional	Rare
Need acute medical attention	Fever and chills, pulmonary toxicity, stomatitis	Hypersensitivity reaction	Hepatotoxicity, pleuropericarditis, renal and vascular toxicity
Medical attention if persistent/bothersome	Skin changes, vomiting, loss of appetite	Weight loss	
Less need for medical attention		Alopecia	
Medical attention if occurring after withdrawal		Shortness of breath, cough	

INDICATIONS

FDA-approved: Hodgkin's disease, non-Hodgkin's lymphoma, head and neck, laryngeal, cervical, penile, skin, and vulvar carcinoma; clinical studies show activity in paralaryngeal carcinoma, osteosarcoma, malignant pleural and peritoneal effusions, germ cell and ovarian tumors, mycosis fungoides, testicular carcinoma

PHARMACOKINETICS

Distribution: 45% absorbed into the systemic circulation following intrapleural or intraperitoneal administration; **Protein binding:** < 1%; **Metabolism:** unknown, although degradative pathways involve aminohydrolases. Enzyme activity is high in liver, kidneys, bone marrow, and lymph nodes, low in skin and lungs; **Half-life:** (with normal renal function) α, 0.25 h; β, 2–4 h; increases exponentially as creatinine clearance decreases; **Excretion:** 60%–70% renal

DRUG INTERACTIONS

Oxygen therapy, cisplatin, vincristine, lomustine, digoxin, phenytoin

PATIENT MONITORING

Obtain chest radiograph, pulmonary function tests (including FVC and DLCO), BUN, serum creatinine, hematocrit or hemoglobin, platelet count, total and/or differential leukocyte count, serum alanine aminotransferase (SGPT) concentrations, serum aspartate aminotransferase (SGOT), serum bilirubin, serum lactate dehydrogenase; check patient's mouth for ulceration and lungs for rales, decreased breath sounds, or evidence of restrictive lung disease before administration of each dose

PATIENT INFORMATION

Patient should stop smoking due to pulmonary toxicity; continue medication despite stomach upset; careful attention and monitoring are required if surgery (including dental) or emergency treatment is needed; watch for the development of shortness of breath, cough, oral ulcerations and pain, fever, or chills

NURSING INTERVENTION

Administer acetaminophen on routine basis

FORMULATION

Available as Blenoxane®, Bristol Laboratories Oncology Products, Princeton, NJ
Stored at 2°–8°C and protected from light.

DACTINOMYCIN

Although it is one of the first antineoplastic agents, dactinomycin (or actinomycin D) is rarely used in current practice. Responses have been noted in patients with Wilms' tumor, Ewing's sarcoma, embryonal rhabdomyosarcoma, and gestational choriocarcinoma. Its action is via DNA intercalation, and it is rapidly distributed to tissues and DNA. Clearance is slow, however, mainly due to a slow rate of release from tissue compartments and occurs through the biliary and renal routes.

DOSAGE AND ADMINISTRATION

The dosage of dactinomycin is calculated in micrograms. The usual adult dosage is 500 µg (0.5 mg) daily IV for a maximum of 5 d. The dosage for adults or children should not exceed 15 µg/kg or 400–600 µg/m^2 (if body surface area) daily IV for 5 d. Calculation in obese patients should be on the basis of surface area an effort to relate dose to lean body mass.

SPECIAL PRECAUTIONS

Precautions should be used with infants (especially those < 6 mo), patients with previous exposure to cytotoxic drugs and radiation therapy, or pregnant and nursing patients. Lower doses are recommended. Active herpes zoster or herpes varicella are relative contraindications. Obese patients should receive a lower dose based on body surface area rather than solely on body weight and be observed daily for toxicity.

TOXICITIES

Degree of Severity	Frequent	Occasional	Rare
Need acute medical attention	Anemia, leukopenia, thrombocytopenia, pharyngitis		Anaphylaxis, uric acid nephropathy, hyperuricemia, phlebitis, cellulitis
Medical attention if persistent/bothersome	Skin rash/acne, fatigue		
Less need for medical attention	Nausea/vomiting, darkening/redness of skin, alopecia		
Medical attention if occurring after withdrawal	Bone marrow depression, GI ulceration, esophagitis	Ulcerative stomatitis, hepatotoxicity	

INDICATIONS

FDA-approved: Ewing's sarcoma, sarcoma botryoides, trophoblastic tumors, endometrial carcinoma, testicular carcinoma, Wilm's tumor, rhabdomyosarcoma; clinical studies show activity in ovarian carcinoma, Kaposi's sarcoma, osteosarcoma, malignant melanoma

PHARMACOKINETICS

Distribution: does not cross the blood–brain barrier; distributes particularly to bone marrow/tumor cells, subaxillary gland, liver, and kidney; **Protein binding:** extensive, to tissues; **Half-life:** 36 h; **Excretion:** 50% biliary/fecal, 10% renal (both unchanged); 30% dose in urine/feces within 1 wk

DRUG INTERACTIONS

Allopurinol, colchicine, sulfinpyrazone, bone marrow depressants, radiation therapy, blood dyscrasia-causing medications, vaccines, probenecid, doxorubicin, vitamin K

PATIENT MONITORING

Examine patient's mouth for ulceration; monitor hematocrit or hemoglobin, platelet count, total or differential leukocyte count, serum alanine aminotransferase (SGPT) concentrations, serum aspartate aminotransferase (SGOT), serum bilirubin, serum lactate dehydrogenase, and serum uric acid

NURSING INTERVENTIONS

Avoid contact with soft tissues; if given directly into vein, use one sterile needle for reconstituting and withdrawing dose from vial, another for administration; if extravasation occurs, stop immediately and administer remaining dose by another vein; to prevent hyperuricemia and hyperuricuria, give IV fluid therapy and allopurinol (4–5 d) during severe oral toxicity (*ie*, patient unable to drink)

PATIENT INFORMATION

Patient should take each medication at correct time and continue despite stomach upset; avoid immunization unless approved by physician; maintain ample fluid intake; call physician if unusual bleeding, bruising, or black, tarry stools, blood in urine or stools, fever, chills, cough/hoarseness, lower back side pain and painful/difficult urination, or pinpoint red spots on skin occur; call physician immediately if redness, pain, or swelling occurs at injection site; use caution with dental hygiene; avoid trauma to mucosal surfaces of eyes, nose, mouth; avoid activities or situations where bruising is likely to occur; avoid exposure to persons with bacterial infections

FORMULATION

Cosmegen®, Merck Co., Westpoint, PA
Vials of 500 µg (0.5 mg). Stored at 15°–30°C and protected from light.

DAUNORUBICIN

With the licensing of idarubicin for the treatment of acute myelogenous leukemia, daunorubicin is viewed by many as an alternative anthracycline for use in remission and maintenance for acute myelogenous leukemia. Daunorubicin had been recommended over doxorubicin because of the reduced mortality in CALGB studies.

DOSAGE AND ADMINISTRATION

Courses cannot be administered more frequently than every 21 d, to allow bone marrow to recover.

Acute lymphocytic leukemia: 45 mg/m² IV d 1, 2, 3 of a 32-d course in combination with vincristine, prednisone, and l-asparaginase

Acute nonlymphocytic leukemia: 45 mg/m² IV d 1, 2, 3 of first course and d 1, 2 of second course in combination with cytarabine

DOSAGE MODIFICATIONS: Limit total lifetime dosage to 550 mg (base)/m² or 450 mg (base)/m² in patients who have received previous chest radiation therapy. In acute leukemia, agent may be administered despite presence of thrombocytopenia and bleeding; stoppage of bleeding and increase in platelet count have occurred during treatment in some cases, and platelet transfusions are useful in others.

SPECIAL PRECAUTIONS

Pediatric patients

Geriatric patients, particularly those with age-related bone marrow depression and renal impairment

Patients with inadequate bone marrow reserves

Pregnant and nursing patients

Conditions requiring special consideration: bone marrow depression, chickenpox, herpes zoster, gout, urate renal stones, heart disease, herpes/renal impairment, infection, tumor cell infiltration of the bone marrow

TOXICITIES

Degree of Severity	Frequent	Occasional	Rare
Need medical attention	Esophagitis, infection, leukopenia, thrombocytopenia	GI ulceration, uric acid nephropathy, extravasation, cellulitis, tissue necrosis, hyperuricemia, cardiotoxicity	Cardiotoxicity/pericarditis—myocarditis, allergic reaction
Medical attention if persistent/bothersome		Stomatitis	Diarrhea
Less need for acute medical attention	Nausea/vomiting, alopecia, reddish urine		Darkening/redness of skin
Medical attention if occurring after withdrawal	Irregular heartbeat, shortness of breath	Edema in lower extremities	

INDICATIONS

FDA-approved: erythroleukemia, acute lymphocytic leukemia, acute myelocytic leukemia, acute monocytic leukemia; clinical show activity in neuroblastoma, non-Hodgkin's lymphomas, chronic myelocytic leukemia, Wilm's tumor, Ewing's sarcoma

PHARMACOKINETICS

Distribution: rapid, especially to major organs; does not cross blood–brain barrier; **Half-life:** 45 min; **Excretion:** prolonged; 25% (active) in urine, 40% biliary

DRUG INTERACTIONS

Allopurinol, colchicine, probenecid, sulfinpyrazone, blood dyscrasia-causing medications, radiation therapy, doxorubicin, hepatotoxic medications, vaccines, bone marrow depressants

PATIENT MONITORING

Monitor with chest radiography, echocardiography, ECG, radionuclide angiography determination of ejection fraction, hematocrit or hemoglobin, platelet count, total or differential leukocyte count, serum alanine aminotransferase, serum aspartate aminotransferase (SGOT) concentrations, serum bilirubin, serum lactate dehydrogenase, serum uric acid

NURSING INTERVENTIONS

If extravasation occurs (local burning stinging), stop injection and resume in an alternate vein; maintain oral hydration and (if necessary) administer allopurinol; avoid inhalation of doxorubicin or exposure to the skin (use gloves)

PATIENT INFORMATION

Patient should consume medication despite stomach upset; avoid immunization unless approved by physician; avoid exposure to those who have taken oral poliovirus vaccine; call physician immediately if unusual bleeding or bruising, black, tarry stools, blood in urine or stools, or pinpoint red spots on skin occur; use caution with dental hygiene tools; avoid trauma to mucosal surfaces of eyes, nose, mouth; call physician immediately if redness, pain, or swelling occurs at injection site; urine may turn red during the first 24–48 h after therapy

FORMULATION

Available as Cerubidine®, Wyeth-Ayerst Laboratories, Philadelphia, PA
Vials containing 20 mg (base) (21.4 mg as HCl). Stored at 15°–30°C and protected from light.

DOXORUBICIN

Doxorubicin is the standard anthracycline for use against nonhematologic tumors. Dexrazoxane (Zinecard) for injection has been approved for use in reducing the incidence and severity of myocardiopathy associated with doxorubicin administration.

DOSAGE AND ADMINISTRATION

60–75 mg/m^2 IV, repeated every 21 d; **or** 25–30 mg/m^2/d IV on 2–3 consecutive d, repeated every 3–4 wk; **or** 20 mg/m^2/wk IV.

DOSAGE MODIFICATIONS: Doxorubicin doses must be reduced in the setting of hepatocellular dysfunction. The myocardial toxicity manifested in its most severe form is a potentially fatal congestive heart failure that may occur either during therapy or months to years after termination of therapy. The probability of developing impaired myocardial function based on the combined index of clinical symptoms and fall in left ventricular injection fraction (LVEF) is estimated to be 1%–2% at the cumulative dose of 300 mg/m^2, 3%–5% at 400 mg/m^2, 5%–8% at 450 mg/m^2 and 6%–20% at 500 mg/m^2. The risk of developing congestion heart failure increases rapidly with increasing cumulative doses of doxorubicin in excess of 450 mg/m^2. The toxicity may occur at lower cumulative doses in patients with prior mediastinal irradiation or high concurrent cyclophosphamide or with preexisting heart disease.

SPECIAL PRECAUTIONS

Pediatric patients (cardiotoxicity more frequent in those < 2 y)
Elderly patients (cardiotoxicity more frequent in those > 70 y)
Pregnant and nursing patients
Conditions requiring special considerations: bone marrow depression, heart disease, herpes zoster, hepatic function impairment, gout, tumor cell infiltration of the bone marrow, urate renal stones, chickenpox

TOXICITIES

Degree of Severity	Frequent	Occasional	Rare
Need medical attention	Esophagitis, leukopenia, infection	Uric acid nephropathy, GI ulceration, tissue necrosis, cellulitis congestive, cardiotoxicity, postradiation erythema, recall; extravasation, hyperuricemia, thrombocytopenia, phlebosclerosis	Anaphylaxis, allergic reaction, cardiac arrhythmia
Medical attention if persistent/bothersome	Stomatitis	Diarrhea	
Less need for acute medical attention	Nausea/vomiting, alopecia	Darkening of soles, palms, or nails; reddish urine	
Medical attention if occurring after withdrawal	Possible cardiotoxicity: fast/irregular heartbeat	Shortness of breath, peripheral edema	

INDICATIONS

FDA-approved: acute lymphocyte leukemia, acute myelocytic leukemia, neuroblastoma, ovarian carcinoma, thyroid carcinoma, Wilm's tumor, lung carcinoma, gastric carcinoma, Hodgkin's lymphomas, non-Hodgkin's lymphomas, soft tissue sarcomas, osteosarcoma; clinical studies show activity in head and neck, cervical, hepatic, pancreatic, prostatic, testicular, and endometrial carcinoma, germ cell and ovarian tumors, Ewing's sarcoma, multiple myeloma

PHARMACOKINETICS

Metabolism: rapid (within 1 h); hepatic, with one active metabolite; **Half-life:** doxorubicin: α phase, 0.6 h; β phase, 16.7 h; metabolites: α phase, 3.3 h; β phase, 31.7 h; **Excretion:** 50% biliary (unchanged); 23% as adramycinol; < 10% renal

DRUG INTERACTIONS

Allopurinol, colchicine, probenecid, sulfinpyrazone, radiation therapy, hepatotoxic medications, streptozocin, vaccines, bone marrow depressants, daunorubicin, mitomycin C, dactinomycin, cyclophosphamide, blood dyscrasia-causing medications, digoxin, verapamil

PATIENT MONITORING

Examine patient's mouth for ulceration before each dose; monitor chest radiography, echocardiography, ECG, radionuclide angiographic determination of ejection fraction, hematocrit or hemoglobin, platelet count, total or differential leukocyte count, serum alanine aminotransferase (SGPT) concentrations, serum aspartate aminotransferase (SGOT), serum bilirubin, serum lactate dehydrogenase, serum uric acid

NURSING INTERVENTIONS

Maintain ample fluid intake and increase in urine output; avoid inhalation of doxorubicin or exposure to the skin (use gloves)

PATIENT INFORMATION

Patient should continue medication despite stomach upset; avoid immunization unless approved by physician; avoid exposure to those who have taken oral poliovirus vaccine; call physician immediately if unusual bleeding or bruising, black, tarry stools, blood in urine or stools, or pinpoint red spots on skin occurs; call physician immediately if redness, pain, or swelling occurs at injection site; use caution with dental hygiene; avoid trauma to mucosal surfaces of eyes, nose, mouth; urine may turn red during the first 24–48 h after therapy

FORMULATIONS

Available as Adriamycin PFS and RDF®, Pharmacia Inc., Dublin, OH; Doxorubicin Hydrochloride, Astra USA, Westboro, MA; Rubex®, Mead-Johnson Oncology Products, Princeton, NJ
Vials of 10-, 20-, 50-, 100-, 150-, and 200-mg doxorubicin hydrochloride for injection. Stored at 15°–30°C and protected from light.

EPIRUBICIN

Epirubicin is a stereoisomer of doxorubicin, differing only in the orientation of the 4'-hydroxyl group in the amino sugar. The drug is available commercially in Europe. It differs in its catabolic pathway from doxorubicin in that it is conjugated with glucuronic acid, and this reaction is thought to account for its shorter half-life and lessened cardiotoxicity relative to doxorubicin. Indeed, its dose-limiting toxicity is myelosuppression, with neutropenia being most prominent.

Epirubicin has been used in phase II testing in cervical cancer [6], endometrial cancer [7], and advanced breast cancer [8], with response rates ranging from 18.5%–26%. Population pharmacokinetic analysis shows that it follows a two-compartment model and that age and sex significantly influence the clearance rates of the drug [9].

DOSAGE AND ADMINISTRATION

75–90 mg/m^2 IV, repeated every 21 d, may be given in divided doses over 2 d; limit cumulative dosage to 700 mg/m^2

DOSAGE MODIFICATIONS: *When given as part of combination protocols in elderly patients or in patients with prior chemo/radiation therapy, dose should be reduced, although no guidelines are available. Reduce dose by 50% in patients with liver metastases or abnormal liver function tests.*

SPECIAL PRECAUTIONS

Pediatric patients (cardiotoxicity more frequent in those < 2 y)
Elderly patients (cardiotoxicity more frequent in those > 70 y)
Patients with inadequate bone marrow reserves
Pregnant/nursing patients
Conditions requiring special considerations: bone marrow depression, heart disease, herpes zoster, hepatic function impairment, gout, tumor cell infiltration of the bone marrow, urate renal stones, chickenpox

TOXICITIES

Degree of Severity	Frequent	Occasional	Rare
Need acute medical attention	Esophagitis, leukopenia, infection	Uric acid nephropathy, GI ulceration, tissue necrosis, cellulitis, cardiotoxicity, postradiation erythema, recall; extravasation, hyperuricemia, thrombocytopenia, phlebosclerosis	Anaphylaxis, allergic reaction
Medical attention if persistent/bothersome	Stomatitis	Diarrhea	
Less need for medical attention	Nausea/vomiting, alopecia	Darkening of soles, palms, or nails; reddish urine	
Medical attention if occurring after withdrawal	Possible cardiotoxicity: fast/irregular heartbeat	Shortness of breath, peripheral edema	

INDICATIONS

Clinical studies show activity in breast carcinoma, acute myelogenous leukemia, non-Hodgkin's lymphoma, GI tract carcinoma

PHARMACOKINETICS

Metabolism: rapid, hepatic, with one active metabolite; **Half-life:** α phase, 0.6 h; β phase, 40 h; **Excretion:** mainly biliary

PATIENT MONITORING

Examine patient's mouth for ulceration before each dose; monitor chest radiography, echocardiography, ECG, radionuclide angiography determination of ejection fraction, hematocrit or hemoglobin, platelet count, total or differential leukocyte count, serum alanine aminotransferase (SGPT) concentrations, serum aspartate aminotransferase (SGOT), serum bilirubin, serum lactate dehydrogenase, serum uric acid

NURSING INTERVENTIONS

Maintain ample fluid intake and increase in urine output; avoid inhalation or exposure to the skin (use gloves)

PATIENT INFORMATION

Patient should continue medication despite stomach upset; avoid immunization unless approved by physician; avoid exposure to those who have taken oral poliovirus vaccine; call physician immediately if unusual bleeding or bruising; black, tarry stools, blood in urine or stools, or pinpoint red spots on skin occurs; call physician immediately if redness, pain, or swelling occurs at injection site; use caution with dental hygiene avoid trauma to mucosal surfaces of eyes, nose, mouth

AVAILABILITY

Epirubicin is not commercially available in the United States.

IDARUBICIN

A stereoisomer of daunorubicin, idarubicin is a less cardiotoxic substitute for daunorubicin in treatment protocols for acute myelogenous leukemia (AML). Like daunorubicin, it is metabolized to an active hydroxylated metabolite (1,3-dihydroidarubicin). A long elimination half-life (twice that of idarubicin) for idarubicinol allows for the maintenance of cytotoxic concentrations for prolonged periods of time.

Idarubicin is thought by most to be the anthracycline of choice for the induction of remission in AML. Prospective phase III randomized trails comparing idarubicin to daunorubicin demonstrate that idarubicin is superior in the percent of complete response and remission duration [11,12].

DOSAGE AND ADMINISTRATION

12 mg/m^2/d IV for 3 d as single agent. In combination with cytosine arabinoside, 100 mg/m^2/d continuous IV infusion for 7 d **or** single dose of 25 mg/m^2 IV followed by 200 mg/m^2/d continuous IV infusion for 5 d. Give dose slowly (over 10–15 min) into the tubing of a freely running IV infusion of 0.9% NaCl injection USP or 5% dextrose injection USP.

SPECIAL PRECAUTIONS

Pediatric patients (cardiotoxicity more frequent in those < 2 y)
Elderly patients (cardiotoxicity more frequent in those ≥ 70 y)
Patients with inadequate bone marrow reserves
Pregnant and nursing patients
Conditions requiring special considerations: bone marrow depression, heart disease, herpes zoster, hepatic function impairment, gout, tumor cell infiltration of the bone marrow, urate renal stones, chickenpox

TOXICITIES

Degree of Severity	Frequent	Occasional	Rare
Need acute medical attention	Esophagitis, leukopenia, infection	Uric acid nephropathy, GI ulceration, tissue necrosis, cellulitis, cardiotoxicity, postradiation erythema, recall; extravasation, hyperuricemia, thrombocytopenia, phlebosclerosis	Anaphylaxis, allergic reaction
Medical attention if persistent/bothersome	Stomatitis	Diarrhea	
Less need for medical attention	Nausea/vomiting, alopecia	Darkening of soles, palms, or nails; reddish urine	
Medical attention if occurring after withdrawal	Possible cardiotoxicity: fast/irregular heartbeat	Shortness of breath, peripheral edema	

INDICATIONS

FDA-approved: acute myeloid leukemia in combination with other antileukemic drugs; clinical studies show activity in the treatment of lymphoma and an array of solid tumors, but the role of idarubicin has not been validated by controlled clinical trails

PHARMACOKINETICS

Metabolism: rapid, hepatic, with one active metabolite; **Protein binding:** 97%, although it is concentration-dependent; **Half-life:** 14–35 h with oral dosing, 12–27 h with IV dosing; **Excretion:** 15% biliary (unchanged); 15% renal

DRUG INTERACTIONS

Allopurinol, colchicine, probenecid, sulfinpyrazone, radiation therapy, hepatotoxic medications, streptozocin, vaccines, bone marrow depressants, daunorubicin, mitomycin C, dactinomycin, cyclophosphamide, blood dyscrasia-causing medications

PATIENT MONITORING

Examine patient's mouth for ulceration before each dose; monitor chest radiography, echocardiography, ECG, radionuclide angiographic determination of ejection fraction, hematocrit or hemoglobin, platelet count, total or differential leukocyte count, serum alanine aminotransferase (SGPT) concentrations, serum aspartate aminotransferase (SGOT), serum bilirubin, serum lactate dehydrogenase, serum uric acid

NURSING INTERVENTIONS

Maintain ample fluid intake and increase in urine output; avoid inhalation or exposure to the skin (use gloves)

PATIENT INFORMATION

Patient should continue medication despite stomach upset; avoid immunization unless approved by physician; avoid exposure to those who have taken oral poliovirus vaccine; call physician immediately if unusual bleeding or bruising, black, tarry stools, blood in urine or stools, or pinpoint red spots on skin occur; call doctor immediately if redness, pain, or swelling occurs at injection site; use caution with dental hygiene; avoid trauma to mucosal surfaces of eyes, nose, mouth

FORMULATIONS

Available as Idamycin®, Pharmacia Inc., Dublin, OH Vials of 5- and 10-mg idarubicin hydrochloride. Stored at controlled room temperature (59°–86°F).

MITOMYCIN C

Mitomycin C is a bioreductive alkylating agent requiring in vivo activation to the cytotoxic species. The primary side effects are delayed myelosuppression and injury due to extravasation. Occasional cases of vasculitis with manifestations ranging from hemolytic–uremic syndrome to lethal venoocclusive disease have been observed. Because of the potential for vascular toxicity, total cumulative doses should not exceed 50 mg/m^2. When given in combination with an anthracycline, mitomycin C can enhance the cardiotoxic effect of the anthracycline. Mitomycin C can also produce an interstitial pneumonitis.

Response rates of 16% to 30% have been noted when mitomycin C is given as a single agent for treatment of a variety of gastrointestinal tract, pancreatic, breast, genitourinary tract, and non–small cell lung cancers [1]. Recent studies have investigated the use of mitomycin C as a radiosensitizing agent; although extensive experience is lacking, this approach seems to hold promise.

DOSAGE AND ADMINISTRATION

10–20 mg/m^2 IV as a single dose, repeated every 6–8 wk

DOSAGE MODIFICATIONS: Myelosuppression usually occurs approximately 4 wk following treatment. If leukocytes are 2000–2999/mm^3 and platelets are 25,000–74,999/mm^3, reduce dose by 30%; if leukocytes are < 2000/mm^3 and platelets are < 25,000/mm^3, reduce dose by 50%. No repeat dose should be given until leukocyte count has returned to 4000/mm^3 and platelet count to 100,000/mm^3. Limit doses to 20 mg/m^2. Greater doses increase the risk of toxicity and show no increased effect. Do not administer cumulative doses of > 50 mg/m^2.

SPECIAL PRECAUTIONS

Geriatric patients (caution with those with age-related renal impairment)
Patients who have had previous cytotoxic drug or radiation therapy
Pregnant and nursing patients
Conditions requiring special consideration: bone marrow depression, chickenpox, herpes zoster, coagulation disorders, infection, renal impairment

TOXICITIES

Degree of Severity	Frequent	Occasional
Need medical attention		Numbness/tingling in extremities
Medical attention if persistent/ bothersome	Anorexia	Skin rash, fatigue
Less need for medical attention	Nausea/vomiting	Purple-colored bands on nails, alopecia
Medical attention if occurring after withdrawal	Bone marrow depression, hemolytic-uremic syndrome	

INDICATIONS

FDA-approved: gastric and pancreatic carcinoma; clinical studies show activity in colorectal, breast, head and neck, bladder, biliary, lung, and cervical carcinoma, chronic myelocytic leukemia

PHARMACOKINETICS

Distribution: does not cross blood–brain barrier; particularly concentrated in kidney, tongue, muscle, heart, and lung tissue; **Metabolism:** hepatic, some in other tissues and kidney; **Half-life:** initial, 5–15 min; terminal, about 50 min; **Excretion:** renal (10% unchanged); small amounts in bile and feces

DRUG INTERACTIONS

Blood dyscrasia-causing medications, bone marrow depressants, radiation therapy, vaccines, doxorubicin

PATIENT MONITORING

Monitor blood urea nitrogen, serum creatinine, hematocrit or hemoglobin, observe for fragmented red blood cells on peripheral blood smears, platelet count, total or differential leukocyte count; monitor renal and hematologic function for several months after therapy (possible hemolytic–uremic syndrome)

NURSING INTERVENTIONS

If extravasation occurs, stop injection immediately and resume in alternate site (surgical excision of original area may be necessary); although a variety of interventions have been proposed for known extravasations, none is proven to be of benefit

PATIENT INFORMATION

Patient should continue medication despite stomach upset; avoid immunization unless approved by physician; avoid exposure to those who have taken oral poliovirus vaccine; call physician immediately if unusual bleeding or bruising, black, tarry stools, blood in urine or stools, or pinpoint red spots on skin occur; call physician immediately if redness, pain, or swelling occurs at injection site; use caution with dental hygiene; avoid trauma to mucosal surfaces of eyes, nose, mouth

FORMULATION

Available as Mutamycin®, Bristol Laboratories Oncology Products, Princeton, NJ
Vials of 5, 20, and 40 mg. Stored at 15°–30°C and protected from light.

MITOXANTRONE

Mitoxantrone is a substituted anthracenedione, related to a group of compounds found in nature that have been used for centuries as dyes and laxatives. It exerts a cycle-specific cytotoxic effect on cells, with most activity on cells in the G1 and G2 phases by binding to G-C-base-pair–rich regions and causing DNA strand breaks. A variety of possible mechanisms of action have been advanced, including free radical formation, steric hindrance with topoisomerase II action, and prostaglandin interference.

Mitoxantrone in combination with other antileukemic drugs is indicated in the initial therapy of acute nonleukocytic leukemia based on pivotal trails demonstrating equivalency to daunorubicin based regimens. Direct comparisons of mitoxantrone to idarubicin are ongoing. Mitoxantrone has definite therapeutic activity in non-Hodgkin's and Hodgkin's lymphoma both as first-line and in recurrent and refractory clinical settings [13]. Studies in breast cancer demonstrate that mitoxantrone is also an active drug alone or in combination, but the substitution of mitoxantrone for doxorubicin is not warranted in most clinical settings [14].

Mitoxantrone is indicated for the treatment of advanced prostate cancer based on a randomized trial that showed improved pain control in hormone-resistant patients treated with mixoxantrone and prednisone compared with patients treated with prednisone alone. The mitoxantrone did not have a significant impact on overall survival, well being, or measured global quality of life [15].

DOSAGE AND ADMINISTRATION

14 mg/m² IV every 21 d (introduce slowly into tubing of freely running IV infusion of 0.9% sodium chloride or 5% dextrose injection over period not less than 3 min)

DOSAGE MODIFICATIONS: *Lower initial dose (12 mg [base]/m²) recommended in patients with inadequate bone marrow reserves. Subsequent doses only appropriate when leukocyte and platelet counts recover from previous dose. Reduce dosage if severe bone marrow depression occurs.*

SPECIAL PRECAUTIONS

Geriatric patients
Patients with inadequate bone marrow reserves
Pregnant and nursing patients
Conditions requiring special consideration: bone marrow depression, chickenpox, herpes zoster, gout, urate renal stones, heart disease, hepatic impairment, infection

TOXICITIES

Degree of Severity	Frequent	Occasional	Rare
Need acute medical attention	GI bleeding, stomach pain, cough, shortness of breath, arrhythmias, leukopenia/infection (usually asymptomatic) stomatitis/mucositis	Seizures, CHF, thrombocytopenia (usually asymptomatic), renal failure, conjuctivitis	Allergic reaction, extravasation, local irritation/plebitis
Medical attention if persistent/bothersome	Diarrhea, headache	Jaundice	
Less need for medical attention	Nausea/vomiting, alopecia, blue-green urine	Blue color in whites of eyes	

INDICATIONS

FDA-approved: acute myelocytic, acute promyelocytic, acute monocytic, and acute erythroid leukemias, clinical studies show activity in breast and hepatic carcinoma, non-Hodgkin's lymphoma

PHARMACOKINETICS

Distribution: rapid and extensive; concentrated in the thyroid, liver, heart, red blood cells, pleural fluid, kidneys; **Metabolism**: hepatic; **Protein binding**: high, 78%; **Half-life**: mean, 5.8 d; range, 2.3–13.0 d; **Excretion**: 25% biliary/fecal (maximum, in 5 d); 6%–11% renal (unchanged); extensive tissue absorption and binding for dose (thought to be gradually released)

DRUG INTERACTIONS

Allopurinol, colchicine, probenecid, daunorubicin, doxorubicin, heparin, vaccines, sulfinpyrazone, blood dyscrasia-causing medication, radiation therapy to mediastinal area

PATIENT MONITORING

Monitor chest radiography, echocardiography, ECG, radionuclide angiographic determination of ejection fraction, hematocrit or hemoglobin, platelet count; total or differential leukocyte count, serum alanine aminotransferase (SGPT) concentrations, serum aspartate aminotransferase (SGOT), serum bilirubin; serum lactate dehydrogenase, serum uric acid

NURSING INTERVENTIONS

Do not administer intrathecally (paralysis has occurred); concentrate must be diluted prior to administration; administer additional course only after toxic effects of first course have subsided; alleviate volume depletion and dehydration before initiation of therapy; if extravasation occurs, discontinue infusion and resume in alternate site

PATIENT INFORMATION

Patient should call physician immediately if pregnancy is suspected; continue medication despite stomach upset; avoid both salicylate-containing medications and immunizations unless approved by physician; avoid exposure to those who have taken oral poliovirus vaccine; call physician immediately if unusual bleeding or bruising, black, tarry stools, blood in urine or stools, or pinpoint red spots on skin occur; call physician immediately if redness, pain, or swelling occurs at injection site; use caution with dental hygiene; avoid trauma to mucosal surfaces of eyes, nose, mouth

FORMULATION

Available as Novantrone®, Immunex Corporation, Seattle, WA
2 mg (base)mL. Stored at 15°–30°C and protected from freezing.

PLICAMYCIN

This antibiotic, known previously as mithramycin, was originally used in the treatment of testicular cancer. It is now almost exclusively reserved for the management of hypercalcemia. Very little is known of its pharmacokinetics and tissue distribution. The side effect profile is marked by several potentially serious, and unusual, events. It can cause a diffuse hemorrhagic syndrome, probably similar to disseminated intravascular coagulation, characterized by thrombocytopenia and impaired production of factors II, V, VII, and X. As a consequence, the prothrombin time is lengthened. Death can occur from refractory gastrointestinal hemorrhage. Substantial nephro- and hepatotoxicity also have been reported, although the mechanisms of these actions are unclear.

Other side effects can include fever, myalgia, headache, and the induction of a hypercoagulable state. Plicamycin's only indication as a cytotoxic agent is testicular cancer. Much lower doses than those required for antineoplastic activity are effective in treating hypercalcemia.

DOSAGE AND ADMINISTRATION

Antineoplastic: 25–30 μg (0.025–0.03 mg)/kg/d IV infusion, over 4–6 h, for 8–10 d unless significant toxicities occur, **or** 25–50 μg (0.025–0.05 mg)/kg/d every other day for up to 8 doses or until toxicity requires discontinuation. Additional courses of therapy may be administered at 1-mo intervals.

Antihypercalcemic: Initially 15–25 μg (0.015–0.025 mg)/kg/d IV infusion, over a period of 4–6 h for 3–4 d. Repeat at 1 wk (or more) intervals, if necessary, until desired response.

DOSAGE MODIFICATIONS: *Doses > 30 μg (0.03 mg)/kg and/or duration of therapy exceeding 10 d increase risk of hemorrhagic diathesis. Alternate-day schedule has been shown to decrease toxicity potential. Delayed toxicity may occur as late as 72 h after discontinuation with daily administration but does not occur when alternate-day schedule is used.*

SPECIAL PRECAUTIONS

Patients with previous cytotoxic drug or radiation therapy or general debilitation
Pregnant and nursing patients
Patients with renal dysfunction
Contraindications: blood dyscrasias, including thrombocytopathy and thrombocytopenia, chickenpox, herpes zoster, coagulation disorders or increased susceptibility to bleeding

TOXICITIES

Degree of Severity	Frequent	Occasional
Need acute medical attention		Pain/swelling at injection site, fever
Medical attention if persistent/bothersome	Diarrhea, irritation/soreness of mouth	Mental depression, headache, fatigue
Less need for medical attention	Nausea/vomiting, anorexia	Drowsiness
Medical attention if occurring after withdrawal	Vomiting of blood, unusual bleeding/bruising	Sore throat and fever
Symptom of toxicity	GI bleeding, thrombocytopenia, leukopenia	Petechial bleeding, toxic epidermal necrolysis, nosebleed/other bleeding

INDICATIONS
FDA-approved: testicular carcinoma, hypercalcemia (associated with neoplasms), hypercalciuria (associated with neoplasms); **clinical studies show activity in:** Paget's disease of bone (unaccepted)

PHARMACOKINETICS
Distribution: concentrated in Kupffer cells of liver, in renal tubular cells, and along formed bone surfaces; may localize in areas of active bone resorption; crosses blood–brain barrier; enters cerebrospinal fluid; **Onset of action:** reduction of plasma calcium within 24–48 h; **Excretion:** renal

DRUG INTERACTIONS
Estrogen, heparin, thrombolytic agents, NSAIDs, aspirin, bone marrow depressants, nephrotoxic medications, hepatotoxic medications, sulfinpyrazone, anticoagulants, live vaccines, dextran, dipyridamole, valproic acid

PATIENT MONITORING
Bleeding and prothrombin time determinations, complete and differential blood count, platelet count, hepatic and renal function determinations, serum calcium, serum phosphorus, serum potassium

NURSING INTERVENTIONS
Alleviate volume depletion/dehydration before initiation of therapy; give antiemetics prior to and during treatment; avoid rapid direct infusion; if extravasation occurs, apply cold pack immediately—with swelling, apply moderate heat to aid in dispersing medication from site, with cellulitis, discontinue infusion and resume in alternate site

PATIENT INFORMATION
Patient should continue medication despite stomach upset; avoid both salicylate-containing medications and immunization unless approved by physician; avoid exposure to those who have taken oral poliovirus vaccine; call physician immediately if unusual bleeding or bruising, black, tarry stools, blood in urine or stools, or pinpoint red spots on skin occur; call physician immediately if redness, pain, or swelling occurs at injection site; use caution with dental hygiene; avoid trauma to mucosal surfaces of nose, eyes, mouth

FORMULATION
Available as Mithracin®, Miles Pharmaceutical Division, West Haven, CT
2500 μg (2.5 mg). Stored at 2°–8°C protected from light.

CHAPTER 3: ANTIMETABOLIC AGENTS
Judy Chiao, Julie Beitz, Robert J. DeLap

The antimetabolites constitute a large group of anticancer drugs that interfere with metabolic processes vital to the physiology and proliferation of cancer cells. The major classes of the antimetabolites are the antifols, the purine analogues, and the pyrimidine analogues [1–4].

Antimetabolites have been used in cancer treatment since 1948, when Sidney Farber first reported that aminopterin (an antifol related to methotrexate) produced temporary remissions in children with acute lymphoblastic leukemia. The use of methotrexate in women with gestational trophoblastic neoplasia in the late 1950s demonstrated, for the first time, that chemotherapy could cure patients with metastatic cancer. The fluoropyrimidines were the first drugs found to have useful clinical activity in the treatment of gastrointestinal malignancies, and they continue to be important in the management of patients with several common forms of cancer. Insights gained from laboratory studies of the fluoropyrimidines have recently led to the development of new, more effective treatment regimens for advanced colorectal cancer.

Recent years have seen the discovery of important new antimetabolites, including fludarabine phosphate (a purine antimetabolite with substantial activity in lymphoid malignancies) [5] and 2-chlorodeoxyadenosine (which may cure a high percentage of patients with hairy cell leukemia with a single course of therapy) [6]. Although modern molecular biology and immunology have opened new frontiers for cancer research, it is clear that antimetabolites will continue to play a major role in cancer treatment for the foreseeable future.

PHARMACOLOGY AND PHARMACOKINETICS
Actively proliferating cancer cells must continually synthesize large quantities of nucleic acids, proteins, lipids, and other vital cellular constituents. Almost all of the antimetabolites in clinical use inhibit the synthesis of purine or pyrimidine nucleotides (needed for DNA synthesis) or directly inhibit the enzymes of DNA replication. Many antimetabolites also interfere with the synthesis of ribonucleotides and RNA, and some antimetabolites (eg, methotrexate) may affect amino acid metabolism and protein synthesis as well (Table 3-1). The effects of a given antimetabolite

on different organs, tissues, and cell types can vary greatly due to nuances in cellular metabolism. For example, normal bone marrow is rich in purines, and these purines are actively salvaged and reutilized by normal progenitor cells in the marrow. Therefore, it is not surprising that many purine antimetabolites (eg, thioguanine) are toxic to the bone marrow and particularly effective against malignancies of bone marrow origin (ie, leukemias).

When metabolic pathways for synthesis of vital cellular constituents are blocked by antimetabolites, cancer cells temporarily may stop proliferating (enter a quiescent or noncycling state, a cytostatic effect of treatment). Alternatively, cancer cells that continue to proliferate—even when cellular constituents required for proliferation have been depleted by antimetabolite treatment—can be destroyed (a cytotoxic treatment result). Thus, by interfering with the synthesis of vital cellular constituents, antimetabolites can delay or arrest the growth of cancers.

Antimetabolites also may affect the growth of cancers by other mechanisms. For example, several antimetabolites have been shown to induce terminal differentiation in certain cancer cell lines maintained in vitro. In this process, actively proliferating, poorly differentiated cancer cells acquire the phenotype of mature, differentiated, nonproliferating cells. Antimetabolites also have been shown to trigger apoptosis (or programmed cell death) in some cancer cell lines [7]. Finally, some antimetabolites are known to have effects on the immune system and may alter immune responses to cancer in treated patients.

Table 3-2 describes the route of elimination and elimination half-lives for antimetabolic agents that are marketed in the United States for use in cancer treatment. Table 3-3 lists the FDA-approved cancer treatment indications for these agents.

ADVERSE EFFECTS
Many of the adverse effects of antimetabolite treatment result from suppression of cellular proliferation in mitotically active tissues, such as the bone marrow or gastrointestinal mucosa. Patients treated with these agents commonly experience bone marrow suppression, stomatitis, diarrhea, and hair loss (Table 3-4). As noted previously, however, there are significant metabolic differences among these normal tissues, and the precise pattern and severity of treatment toxicities observed can

Table 3-1. Classes and Mechanisms of Action of Antimetabolites

Generic Name	Class	Primary Pharmacologic Actions
Fluorouracil (5-FU)	Pyrimidine analogue	Thymidylate synthase inhibition; incorporation into RNA
Floxuridine (5-FUdR)	Pyrimidine deoxynucleoside analogue	Thymidylate synthase inhibition
Methotrexate	Antifol	Dihydrofolate reductase inhibition
Leucovorin	Reduced folate (vitamin)	Enhanced thymidylate synthase inhibition (with 5-FU or 5-FUdR); "rescue" from antimetabolic effects of antifols
Hydroxyurea	Synthetic antimetabolite	Ribonucleotide reductase inhibition
Thioguanine (6-TG)	Purine analogue	Inhibition of purine nucleotide biosynthesis; incorporation into DNA
Mercaptopurine (6-MP)	Purine analogue	Inhibition of purine nucleotide biosynthesis
Cytarabine	Pyrimidine deoxynucleoside analogue	Incorporation into DNA; inhibition of DNA synthesis
Pentostatin	Purine deoxynucleoside analogue	Adenosine deaminase inhibitor
Fludarabine phosphate	Purine deoxynucleoside analogue	Ribonucleotide reductase and DNA synthesis inhibition
Cladribine (2-CDA)	Purine deoxynucleoside analogue	Ribonucleotide reductase and DNA synthesis inhibition
Asparaginase	Enzyme	Asparagine (amino acid) depletion
Gemcitabine	Pyrimidine deoxynucleoside analogue	Incorporation into DNA; inhibition of DNA synthesis

Table 3-2. Pharmacokinetics

Generic Name	Route of Elimination	Elimination Half-Life
Fluorouracil (5-FU)	Metabolic	6–20 min
Floxuridine (5-FUdR)	Metabolic	3–20 min, IV infusion; 70%–90% first-pass clearance, hepatic artery infusion
Methotrexate	Renal	Primary, 3–10 h (low dose) or 10–15 h (high dose)
Leucovorin	Metabolic	Parent compound, 1 h; active 5-methyl metabolite, 4–7 h
Hydroxyurea	Primarily renal	3.5–4.5 h
Thioguanine (6-TG)	Metabolic	25–240 min
Mercaptopurine (6-MP)	Metabolic	90 min
Cytarabine	Metabolic	7–20 min
Pentostatin	Renal	2.5–6.0 h
Fludarabine phosphate	Primarily renal	Active metabolite, 10 h
Cladribine (2-CDA)	Renal	5.7–19.7 h
Asparaginase	Metabolic	8–30 h (IV); 39–49 h (IM)
Gemcitabine	Metabolic	32–94 min (short IV infusion); 245–638 (long IV infusion)

Table 3-3. FDA-Approved Indications

Generic Name	Approved Cancer Indications
Fluorouracil (5-FU)	Carcinomas of colon, rectum, breast, stomach, and pancreas
Floxuridine (5-FUdR)	Hepatic arterial infusion, for liver metastases from gastrointestinal adenocarcinomas
Methotrexate	Choriocarcinoma and gestational trophoblastic disease; acute lymphocytic leukemia; meningeal leukemia; breast cancer; squamous head and neck cancers; mycosis fungoides; lung cancer; non-Hodgkin's lymphoma; osteogenic sarcoma
Leucovorin	Advanced colorectal cancer (with 5-FU); "rescue" following high dose methotrexate for osteosarcoma; "rescue" following methotrexate overdose
Hydroxyurea	Ovarian adenocarcinoma; malignant melanoma; chronic myelocytic leukemia; with radiation therapy for squamous head and neck cancers (radiation sensitizer)
Thioguanine (6-TG)	Acute nonlymphocytic leukemias; chronic myelocytic leukemia (alternative to busulfan)
Mercaptopurine (6-MP)	Acute lymphocytic leukemia; acute nonlymphoytic leukemias
Cytarabine	Acute nonlymphocytic leukemia; acute lyphocytic leukemia; blast phase of chronic myelocytic leukemia; meningeal leukemia
Pentostatin	Hairy cell leukemia
Fludarabine phosphate	Chronic lymphocytic leukemia
Cladribine (2-CDA)	Hairy cell leukemia
Asparaginase	Acute lymphocytic leukemia (induction therapy)
Gemcitabine	Locally advanced or metastatic pancreatic cancer

vary greatly depending on the antimetabolite administered, the schedule of administration, and nutritional and other factors.

In addition, many antimetabolites can produce adverse effects that appear to be unrelated to their antiproliferative effects. These effects are more commonly seen at high drug doses and may affect tissues that are not mitotically active. Examples include neurotoxicity seen with high-dose cytosine arabinoside and high-dose methotrexate treatment.

Gonadal function is usually suppressed in patients receiving cytotoxic chemotherapy [8]. Low doses of methotrexate, as used in the treatment of psoriasis, appear to have little effect on gonadal function, but this drug is clearly embryotoxic and teratogenic. Cytosine arabinoside has been shown to produce reversible inhibition of spermatogenesis. With the advent of modern combination chemotherapy regimens, few recent data are available regarding the effects of other individual antimetabolites on gonadal function. Available laboratory and clinical data suggest, however, that the effects of other antimetabolites on gonadal function are less severe and more reversible than, for example, the effects of nitrogen mustard and other DNA alkylating agents.

The administration of antimetabolites in pregnant women deserves special comment. It is sometimes stated that administration of antimetabolites is contraindicated in pregnancy (primarily due to the risk of teratogenesis), whereas other anticancer medications, such as alkylating agents and anthracyclines, may be used with caution. There is, in fact, no laboratory or clinical evidence supporting the concept that antimetabolites *as a class* are more mutagenic or teratogenic than are other cytotoxic anticancer agents. The only antimetabolites known to be significant human teratogens are the antifols (methotrexate, aminopterin, and related compounds). This is consistent with the known teratogenicity of folate deficiency in pregnancy. Clearly, all cytotoxic drugs must be regarded as potentially teratogenic and embryotoxic, and administration of cytotoxic drugs should be avoided in pregnancy whenever possible. However, there is presently no persuasive evidence that antimetabolites other than methotrexate carry a significantly greater risk to the human fetus compared with the risks associated with other classes of cytotoxic drugs.

MECHANISMS OF RESISTANCE

Cancer cells may overcome the cytotoxic and cytostatic effects of antimetabolite chemotherapy by a variety of mechanisms, including allosteric, pathophysiologic, and cell cycle control mechanisms. A comprehensive discussion of all known mechanisms of cancer cell resistance to each of the antimetabolites in clinical use is beyond the scope of this review. Instead, important classes of resistance mechanisms are discussed, using the known mechanisms of resistance to the fluoropyrimidines as examples.

Fluorouracil, the most commonly administered fluoropyrimidine, has several antimetabolic effects on cancer cells, including inhibition of the enzyme thymidylate synthase by the fluorouracil metabolite fluorodeoxyuridine monophosphate (this blocks de novo synthesis of thymidine nucleotides, required for DNA synthesis and repair); misincorporation of fluorodeoxyuridine nucleotides into DNA, in place of thymidine nucleotides (resulting in structural damage to DNA); and interference with RNA synthesis and processing. Inhibition of thymidylate synthase may be the most important mechanism of anticancer action for fluorouracil and other fluoropyrimidines. Inhibition of this enzyme can deplete cellular levels of thymidine nucleotides, which can result in destruction of cancer cells, in the DNA synthetic S phase of the cell cycle.

Cellular levels of vital cellular constituents, such as thymidine nucleotides, are controlled automatically and precisely by a series of allosteric (homeostatic or feedback-control) mechanisms. Inhibition of thymidylate synthase and depletion of cellular thymidine nucleotide levels, as produced by fluorouracil treatment, leads to automatic compensatory increases in the activity of several other key enzymes of the de novo and salvage pathways for thymidine nucleotide synthesis. The increased activity of these other enzymes (*eg*, aspartate carbamoyltransferase, ribonucleotide reductase, thymidine kinase) results in production of high levels of the normal substrate for the thymidylate synthase reaction (deoxyuridine monophosphate), which can competitively overcome the inhibition of this enzyme by the fluorouracil metabolite fluorodeoxyuridine monophosphate; and production of more thymidine nucleotides by the thymidine salvage pathway (which uses preformed thymidine), thus bypassing the de novo pathway inhibition produced by fluorouracil.

Cancer cells also exhibit pathophysiologic mechanisms of resistance to antimetabolites. For example, the gene for thymidylate synthase may be amplified in fluorouracil-resistant cancer cells. TS protein content can also increase through accelerated translation. Free TS protein is known to be capable of repressing the translation of its own mRNA through a process known as translational auto regulation. After TS protein is bound to the ternary complex, it is no longer able to suppress its mRNA translation, and thus the rate of new TS protein synthesis increases. The cancer cells may thus produce higher levels of this enzyme, and it becomes much more difficult to adequately inhibit this enzyme with fluorouracil treatment. Alternatively, cancer cells may acquire a mutation in the gene for thymidylate synthase, rendering this enzyme resistant to inhibition by fluorouracil treatment.

Finally, even if thymidine nucleotide levels are successfully depleted by fluorouracil treatment, cancer cells may evade the cytotoxic consequences of thymidine nucleotide depletion via cell cycle control mechanisms. The progression of cells through the cell cycle is regulated tightly by cyclins and other cell-cycle regulatory elements. Cells that are thymidine nucleotide deficient may arrest (stop cycling) at the G_1-S interface and may not proceed into the DNA synthetic S phase of the cell cycle, in which thymidine nucleotide depletion is lethal, until thymidine nucleotide levels are restored.

To make further progress in the use of antimetabolites in cancer treatment, it will be important to fully understand the mechanisms of cancer cell resistance to antimetabolites and to incorporate this understanding in the design of new antimetabolite chemotherapy regimens.

BIOCHEMICAL MODULATION

Biochemical modulation refers to the use of antimetabolites in multidrug regimens that are designed to enhance the efficacy of antimetabolites and overcome known mechanisms of cancer cell resistance to these agents. As noted earlier, laboratory studies of antimetabolites have continued to yield new insights into the mechanisms of action of these drugs and the mechanisms of cancer cell resistance [9]. These laboratory studies have further indicated that certain drug combinations could yield enhanced clinical efficacy in cancer treatment. Fluorouracil and leucovorin combination treatment regimens for colorectal cancer represent the most successful clinical application of biochemical modulation research to date.

Based on studies of the mechanism of thymidylate synthase inhibition by the fluoropyrimidines, Santi and coworkers first suggested that leucovorin could enhance the efficacy of fluorouracil [10]. Their observations ultimately led to the clinical finding that fluorouracil and leucovorin combination regimens are modestly superior to fluorouracil alone in the treatment of advanced colorectal cancer [11]. The clinical success of this relatively simple biochemical modulation, which modifies only one of the many mechanisms now known to be operative in the resistance of cancer cells to fluorouracil, has stimulated a substantial resurgence in clinical and laboratory biochemical

modulation research. More complex drug combination regimens, which target critical metabolic pathways at multiple points, are undergoing laboratory and clinical evaluation at a number of cancer research centers around the world. Whereas these more complex, multidrug regimens can be expected to inhibit the targeted metabolic pathways more effectively, the ultimate clinical success of these regimens will be determined by their degree of selectivity.

SELECTIVITY

Bacterial infections usually are treated easily and successfully because normal host immune defenses efficiently recognize and clear bacteria, and bacterial metabolism and human metabolism differ sufficiently to allow for use of selective antimetabolites (antibiotics), which interfere with critical bacterial metabolic pathways but do not have significant adverse effects on the patient. In contrast, cancer cells are immunologically and metabolically very similar to nonmalignant cells of the cancer patient; therefore, selective destruction of cancer cells with systemic chemical or biologic treatment is much more problematic. It is clear, however, that some forms of cancer can be cured with systemic therapy. At least in some patients, selective destruction of cancer cells can be achieved with systemic therapy.

Commonly considered mechanisms for the selective destruction of cancer cells emphasize known or presumed immunologic, metabolic, and kinetic differences between cancer cells and normal cells. Biologic agents with immunomodulating properties have been shown to produce useful antitumor responses in some patients by enhancing immune recognition and destruction of tumor cells (see Chapter 5). Antimetabolites are not known to have any therapeutically useful immunomodulatory anticancer activity, although research is continuing into possible roles for combinations of antimetabolites and biologic agents in cancer treatment.

Inherent metabolic differences between cancer cells and nonneoplastic cells may account for some of the selectivity observed with antimetabolites in cancer treatment. For example, useful clinical remissions can sometimes be obtained, with little clinical toxicity, in patients with colorectal cancer who are treated with prolonged continuous infusions of fluorouracil, suggesting that tumor cells sometimes have a greater innate sensitivity to fluorouracil than normal gastrointestinal mucosal cells (or other normal cells). The precise metabolic differences allowing for this selectivity are unclear, but they may relate to toxic effects of imbalances in deoxynucleotide levels that may follow fluorouracil treatment. Unfortunately, it appears that cancer cells usually do not have metabolic features that can be selectively targeted with antimetabolites. Rather, cancer cells commonly have (or develop) metabolic capabilities that confer decreased susceptibility to antimetabolites (compared to nonneoplastic cells).

Kinetic differences between cancer cells and normal cells may account for much of the clinical selectivity observed with current antimetabolite chemotherapy regimens. Antimetabolites are selectively toxic to proliferating cells and typically produce few toxic effects in nonproliferating cells and tissues. Cancers characteristically exhibit a much higher rate of proliferation than normal cells and tissues even when compared with mitotically active tissues, such as the bone marrow and gastrointestinal mucosa and thus are inherently more susceptible to antimetabolites. Cancers also characteristically exhibit a high rate of cell loss. Normally, cellular proliferation exceeds the rate of cell loss in a growing tumor. Periodic antimetabolite treatment may serve to alter this balance, leading to stabilization or regression of tumors (until the cancer develops resistance to the antimetabolite treatment regimen).

Table 3-4. Antimetabolite Toxicities

Generic Name	Primary Toxic Effects
Fluorouracil	Mucositis, diarrhea, myelosuppression
Floxuridine (5-FUdR)	Chemical hepatitis, sclerosing cholangitis (hepatic arterial infusion)
Methotrexate	Mucositis, diarrhea, myelosuppression
Leucovorin	Increases 5-FU toxicities; decreases methotrexate toxicities
Hydroxyurea	Myelosuppression
Thiguanine (6-TG)	Myelosuppression
Mercaptopurine (6-MP)	Myelosuppression
Cytarabine	Myelosuppression, nausea, vomiting, diarrhea, mucositis; neurotoxicty at high doses
Pentostatin	Nephrotoxicity, neurotoxicity, myelosuppression, immunosuppression
Fludarabine phosphate	Myelosuppression, immunosuppression, neurotoxicity at high doses
Cladribine (2-CDA)	Myelosuppression, fever, immunosuppression
Asparaginase	Hypersensitivity reactions
Gemcitabine	Myelosuppression

Table 3-5. Selected New Antimetabolites Under Study in Cancer Treatment

Generic or Common Name	Pharmacologic Actions	Potential Primary Indications
ZD 1694	Thymidylate synthase inhibitor	Colorectal cancer
Trimetrexate	Dihydrofolate reductase inhibitor	Colorectal cancer (combined with fluororacil and leucovorin)
Edatrexate	Dihydrofolate reductase inhibitor	Breast cancer (with paclitaxel)

AREAS OF RESEARCH ACTIVITY

Many research centers are continuing to investigate the biochemical mechanisms of action and resistance of antimetabolite chemotherapy. Clinical studies are beginning to incorporate measures of in vivo biochemical effects of antimetabolite therapy (*eg*, determining inhibition of a targeted enzyme in a patient's tumor by posttreatment biopsy or using nuclear magnetic resonance spectroscopy to monitor drug uptake and retention in tumors) [12]. This research will clearly enhance our understanding of the failure of current antimetabolite chemotherapy regimens to control cancer growth in many patients and may lead to more effective use of these drugs in new biochemical modulation treatment regimens.

Another area of research activity relates to circadian patterns of cellular metabolic and mitotic activity and the possibility that these patterns may differ between malignant and normal cells. For example, if normal proliferating gastrointestinal cells enter the DNA synthetic S phase primarily in the morning hours, whereas proliferating cells of gastrointestinal malignancies enter the DNA synthetic S phase throughout the day, then it would make sense to administer S-phase–selective antimetabolites to patients with these malignancies at times other than the morning hours [13,14]. Because most antimetabolites have narrow therapeutic indices in cancer treatment, careful attention to details (*eg*, the timing of administration) that may enhance the selectivity of these drugs is critical.

A number of new antimetabolic agents are being evaluated in clinical trials in cancer patients. Promising results have been obtained with ZD 1694, trimetrexate (marketed in the United States for a noncancer indication, *Pneumocystis carinii* penumonia), and edatrexate (Table 3-5) [15,16].

Finally, laboratory and clinical studies have repeatedly shown that combinations of antimetabolites with biologic agents (*eg*, the interferons, other chemotherapeutic agents, or radiation therapy) can result in synergistic anticancer activity. Research into the mechanisms of these synergistic interactions is continuing, and numerous clinical studies are further evaluating a variety of combination treatment regimens.

REFERENCES

1. Chabner BA, Collins JM (eds): *Cancer Chemotherapy: Principles and Practice.* Philadelphia: JB Lippincott; 1990.

2. Chen AP, Grem JL: Antimetabolites. *Curr Opin Oncol* 1992, 4:1089–1098.

3. Cheson BD: New antimetabolites in the treatment of human malignancies. *Sem Oncol* 1992, 19:695–706.

4. Clarke SJ, Jackman AL, Harrap KR: Antimetabolites in cancer chemotherapy. *Adv Exp Biol Med* 1991, 309A:7–13.

5. Keating MJ, Kantarjian H, Talpaz M, *et al.*: Fludarabine: a new agent with major activity against chronic lymphocytic leukemia. *Blood* 1989, 74:19–25.

6. Piro LD, Carrera CJ, Carson DA, *et al.*: Lasting remissions in hairy-cell leukemia induced by a single infusion of 2-chlorodeoxyadenosine. *N Engl J Med* 1990, 322:1117–1121.

7. Darry MA, Behnke CA, Eastman A: Activation of programmed cell death (apoptosis) by cisplatin, other anticancer drugs, toxins, and hyperthermia. *Biochem Pharmacol* 1990, 40:2353–2362.

8. Averette H, Boike G, Jarrell M: Effects of cancer chemotherapy on gonadal function and reproductive capacity. *CA Can J Clin* 1990, 40:199–209.

9. Grem JL, Chu E, Boarman D, *et al.*: Biochemical modulation of fluorouracil with leucovorin and interferon: preclinical and clinical investigations. *Sem Oncol* 1992, 2(suppl 3):36–44.

10. Ullman B, Lee M, Martin DW, Santi DV: Cytotoxicity of 5-fluoro-2´-deoxyuridine: requirement for reduced folate cofactors and antagonism by methotrexate. *Proc Nat Acad Sci USA* 1978, 75:980–983.

11. Poon MA, O'Connell MJ, Wieand HS, *et al.*: Biochemical modulation of fluorouracil with leucovorin: confirmatory evidence of improved therapeutic efficacy in advanced colorectal cancer. *J Clin Oncol* 1991, 9:1967–1972.

12. Presant C, Wolf W, Albright MJ, *et al.*: Human tumor fluorouracil trapping: Clinical correlations of *in vivo* ^{19}F nuclear magnetic resonance spectroscopy pharmacokinetics. *J Clin Oncol* 1990, 8:1868–1873.

13. Buchi KN, Moore JG, Hrushesky WJ, *et al.*: Circadian rhythm of cellular proliferation in the human rectal mucosa. *Gastroenterology* 1991, 101:410–415.

14. Von Roemeling R, Hrushesky WJ: Circadian patterning of continuous floxuridine infusion reduces toxicity and allows higher dose intensity in patients with widespread cancer. *J Clin Oncol* 1989, 7:1710–1719.

15. Takimoto CH, Allegra CJ: New antifolates in clinical development. *Oncology* 1995, 9:649–665.

16. DeVita VT, Hellman S, Rosenberg SA (eds): *Cancer: Principles and Practice of Oncology.* Philadelphia: JB Lipponcott; 1997.

ASPARAGINASE

Asparaginase (or L-asparaginase) is an enzyme that catalyzes the hydrolysis of asparagine (a nonessential amino acid) to aspartic acid and ammonia. Although most normal cells can synthesize all asparagine required for cellular protein synthesis, some cancer cells are dependent on exogenous asparagine to support cellular protein synthesis and proliferation. Asparaginase acts to deplete plasma levels of asparagine, thus depriving susceptible cancer cells of this nutrient. Clinically, asparaginase has useful activity in the treatment of acute lymphocytic leukemia and may have some activity in treatment of lymphomas. Asparaginase also blocks the cytotoxic effects of methotrexate and, thus, can be used as a rescue agent following high-dose methotrexate administration.

The clinical usefulness of asparaginase is limited due to the frequent development of hypersensitivity reactions with repeated courses of treatment. Pegasparaginase, a modified version of asparaginase, is now commercially available for treatment of patients who are hypersensitive to the native form of asparaginase. If necessary, patients hypersensitive to the commercially available formulation can be treated with an investigational one derived from *Erwinia carotovora* (available from the National Cancer Institute for treatment of acute lymphocytic leukemia).

DOSAGE AND ADMINISTRATION

Acute lymphocytic leukemia (in remission-induction combination chemotherapy only; repeated or prolonged use should be avoided):
6000 U/m^2/d (IM injection) for 10 d **or** 500 U/kg (IV) every 10 d **or** 12,000 U/m^2 (IM injection) on d 2, 4, 7, 9, 11, 14
ONCASPAR (pegasparaginase): 2500 IU/m^2 every 14 d IM (preferred) or IV
Pegasparaginase is also approved for use as part of a maintenance regimen

SPECIAL PRECAUTIONS

Hypersensitivity reactions; pregnant and nursing patients

TOXICITIES

Hypersensitivity: urticaria, chills, fever, rash, anaphylaxis
GI: anorexia, nausea, vomiting; elevated serum levels of hepatic enzymes, usually transient; lethal acute hepatic failure (rare); pancreatitis in 5%, with pancreatic insufficiency and hyperglycemia (rarely severe)
Neurologic: headache, lethargy, depression, confusion; obtundation, coma, seizures (rare)
Hematologic: transient myelosuppression (rare)
Miscellaneous: Decreased serum albumin levels; decreased plasma levels of fibrinogen and vitamin K–dependent clotting factors; decreased levels of antithrombin III; proteinuria; renal insufficiency, oliguric renal failure (rare)

INDICATIONS

FDA-approved: acute lymphocytic leukemia (in remission-induction therapy); clinical studies show activity in as rescue agent following administration of high-dose methotrexate

PHARMACOKINETICS

Absorption: oral bioavailability very low (administered IM or IV); **Distribution**: plasma volume, little penetration into CSF; **Elimination**: metabolic (degraded by proteolytic enzymes); **Half-life**: 8–30 h (IV); 39–49 h (IM); serum levels of asparagine undetectable within minutes of injection, remain low days after treatment; **Adjustments for organ dysfunction**: unnecessary for renal dysfunction; use with caution in patients with hepatic dysfunction

DRUG INTERACTIONS

Methotrexate; cytarabine; vincristine

RESPONSE RATES

Pediatric ALL (induction phase, combination chemotherapy): complete remission in most patients; cure rate approximately 50%

PATIENT MONITORING

Be prepared for hypersensitivity reactions; monitor vital signs for 1 h following administration; follow-up monitoring of symptoms, hematology, serum chemistry panel, PT, PTT, amylase, glucose

NURSING INTERVENTIONS

Monitor weight, nutritional status; encourage good oral hygiene; give antiemetics, and mouthwashes and other adjuncts as needed for stomatitis

PATIENT INFORMATION

Patient should avoid use of aspirin or nonsteroidal anti-inflammatory agents; call physician if fever or other signs of serious infection develop; maintain good nutrition

FORMULATION

Available as ELSPAR® Merck & Co., West Point, PA 10-mL vials containing 10,000 IU lyophilized preservative-free *E. coli* asparaginase. Store at 2°–8°C.
Pegasparaginase is available as ONCASPAR® Rhone-Poulenc-Rorer, Collegeville, PA 5-mL vials containing 3750 IU preservative-free modified *E. coli* asparaginase. Store at 2°–8°C.

CLADRIBINE

2-Chlorodeoxyadenosine (2-CDA) or cladribine is a synthetic analogue of the naturally occurring purine nucleoside, deoxyadenosine. Like deoxyadenosine, cladribine is enzymatically converted to active nucleotide metabolites by cellular kinases, and reconverted to the nucleoside parent compound by 5′-nucleotidase. Unlike deoxyadenosine, cladribine is resistant to inactivation by the enzyme adenosine deaminase. Substantial levels of cladribine nucleotides can accumulate in lymphocytes, which have a particularly high ratio of (activating) kinases to (inactivating) 5′-nucleotidase.

The active nucleotide metabolites of cladribine interfere with several vital cellular metabolic processes. Inhibition of ribonucleotide reductase by the triphosphate of cladribine results in depletion and imbalances of cellular deoxyribonucleotide pools. The triphosphate metabolite of cladribine is also an inhibitor of DNA polymerases and can itself be incorporated into DNA. In addition, cells exposed to cladribine exhibit decreased RNA synthesis and an increase in DNA double-strand breaks. Finally, cellular levels of the key cofactor nicotinamide-adenine dinucleotide (NAD) may be depleted, as NAD is consumed in the synthesis of poly (ADP-ribose), which occurs in response to DNA damage. Most of these antimetabolic effects of cladribine are selectively cytotoxic to proliferating cells in the DNA-synthetic S phase of the cell cycle. However, depletion of NAD is cytotoxic to resting cells as well.

In clinical studies cladribine has demonstrated remarkable activity against hairy cell leukemia and substantial activity against other lymphoid malignancies.

DOSAGE AND ADMINISTRATION

Hairy cell leukemia: 0.1 mg/kg/d × 7 d (continuous IV infusion); one course sufficient); or 0.12 mg/kg/d × 5 d (IV over 2 h)
Chronic lymphocytic leukemia: 0.05–0.2 mg/kg/d × 7 d (continuous IV infusion; repeat up to 4 courses)

SPECIAL PRECAUTIONS

Pregnant/nursing patients

TOXICITIES

Hematologic: lymphopenia; anemia; neutropenia and thrombocytopenia (mild at low doses; dose-limiting at high doses; may be cumulative); immunosuppression
GI: occasional nausea, vomiting (mild), diarrhea, elevated serum levels of liver enzymes
Miscellaneous: fever; neurotoxicity at high doses

INDICATIONS

FDA-approved: hairy cell leukemia; clinical studies show activity in chronic lymphocytic leukemia, low-grade non-Hodgkin's lymphomas, cutaneous T-cell lymphomas, Waldenstrom's disease

PHARMACOKINETICS

Absorption: limited data; oral bioavailability may be low and erratic (acid labile); **Distribution**: concentration in cerebrospinal fluid is 25% of that in plasma in patients with CNS disease and exceeds plasma concentrations in patients with meningeal disease; **Elimination**: primarily renal; **Half-life**: 5.7–19.7 h; **Dose adjustments for organ dysfunction**: unknown, use cautiously in patients with renal dysfunction

RESPONSE RATES

Hairy cell leukemia: complete remission rate 75%–85% (relapses are uncommon; 14% at median 33-mo follow-up)
Chronic lymphocytic leukemia, low-grade non-Hodgkin's lymphoma, cutaneous T-cell lymphoma (previously treated): partial remission rates 40%–50%; Waldenstrom's disease: overall response rate 79% (complete remission rate 10%)

PATIENT MONITORING

Vital signs, symptoms, examination, hematology, serum chemistry panel

NURSING INTERVENTIONS

Monitor weight, nutritional status; encourage good oral hygiene; give antiemetics, and mouthwashes and other adjuncts as needed; administer antipyretics for fever

PATIENT INFORMATION

Patient should avoid use of aspirin or nonsteroidal anti-inflammatory agents; call physician if fever or other signs of serious infection develop; maintain good nutrition

FORMULATION

Available as LEUSTATIN® (cladribine), Ortho Biotech, Raritan, NJ
Preservative-free 10-mg vials (1 mg/mL solution). Stored at 2°–8°C and protected from light.

CYTARABINE

Cytarabine (cytosine arabinoside or ara-C) acts pharmacologically as a deoxycytidine analogue and has several effects on DNA metabolism. Cellular kinases convert ara-C to active nucleotide metabolites; the triphosphate metabolite (araCTP) inhibits enzymes of DNA synthesis and repair and is incorporated into DNA. Incorporation of araCTP interferes with DNA template function and causes chain termination; this appears to be the primary mechanism of ara-C cytotoxicity. Other antimetabolic and biologic effects of ara-C include inhibition of ribonucleotide reductase and promotion of differentiation of leukemic cells in vitro. Finally, several cytarabine metabolites, including araCDP-choline, araCMP, and araCTP, can inhibit metabolic pathways of glycoprotein and glycolipid synthesis and thus may affect the structure and function of cell membranes.

Deaminases convert ara-C and its active nucleotide metabolites to inactive uridine arabinoside and nucleotides thereof. There is evidence that cells sensitive to the cytotoxic effects of ara-C have higher levels of activating enzymes, or lower levels of inactivating enzymes, than do resistant cells. Pilot studies have suggested that formation and retention of araCTP in leukemic cells may correlate with clinical response to ara-C.

DOSAGE AND ADMINISTRATION

Acute leukemia (usually with anthracycline): 100 mg/m^2/d (bolus IV injection) every 12 h × 5–7 d **or** 100 mg/m^2/d (continuous IV infusion) × 5–7 d **or** 3 g/m^2 (IV infusion over 1 h) every 12 h × 4–8 doses
Leukemic meningitis: 30 mg/m^2 (intrathecal) repeated every 4 d until negative CSF cytology, then one additional dose

SPECIAL PRECAUTIONS

Patients over 50: severe neurotoxicity, GI toxicity, hepatotoxicity with high-dose ara-C; pregnant and nursing patients

TOXICITIES

Hematologic: neutropenia, thrombocytopenia, anemia (reversible)
GI: anorexia, nausea, vomiting; oral, esophageal, GI mucositis and ulceration (possibly severe, prolonged, with gastrointestinal bleeding); abdominal pain, ileus, diarrhea (possibly severe); reversible intrahepatic cholestasis (common, mild); pancreatitis
Neurologic: neurotoxicity (at high doses); patients with renal dysfunction have a higher incidence of neurotoxicity
Dermatologic: rash
Miscellaneous: fever, conjunctivitis, anaphylaxis (rare)
Intrathecal: nausea, vomiting, fever; paraparesis, paraplegia, leukoencephalopathy (rare)
Intermediate (1 g/m^2) **or high-dose** (≥ 3 g/m^2): cerebellar dysfunction, dementia, obtundation, coma, seizures, personality changes (usually reversible); severe GI ulceration; pneumatosis cystoides intestinalis and peritonitis; bowel necrosis; jaundice; pulmonary edema; interstitial pneumonitis; hemorrhagic conjunctivitis; severe skin rash with desquamation; alopecia totalis; cardiomyopathy; pancreatitis

INDICATIONS

FDA-approved: remission induction in acute nonlymphocytic leukemia, acute lymphocytic leukemia, blast phase of chronic myelocytic leukemia, meningeal leukemia; clinical studies show activity in non-Hodgkin's lymphomas

PHARMACOKINETICS

Absorption: oral bioavailability very low;
Distribution: CSF concentration 20%–40% of plasma concentration at steady state); **Elimination:** metabolic (deaminases); **Half-life:** 7–20 min; clearance prolonged with high-dose ara-C; **Adjustments for organ dysfunction:** use intermediate- and high-dose regimens with caution in patients with preexisting hepatic dysfunction or renal insufficiency

DRUG INTERACTIONS

Methotrexate, thioguanine, mercaptopurine, hydroxyurea, thymidine, cisplatin, cyclophosphamide, etoposide, digoxin, gentamicin

RESPONSE RATES

Adult acute nonlymphocytic leukemia (with an anthracycline): complete remission rate 40%–75%, cure rate 5%–15%

PATIENT MONITORING

Vital signs, symptoms (mucositis, abdominal pain, diarrhea), examination, hematology (weekly; daily in leukemia induction therapy), serum chemistry panel

NURSING INTERVENTIONS

Monitor weight, nutritional status; encourage good oral hygiene; give antiemetics; mouthwashes and other adjuncts; and antidiarrheals as needed; evaluate for bacterial etiology if diarrhea is severe

PATIENT INFORMATION

Patient should avoid use of aspirin or nonsteroidal antiinflammatory agents; call physician if fever or other signs of serious infection develop; avoid excessive sun exposure; maintain good nutrition

FORMULATION

Available as Cytosar-U®, The Upjohn Company, Kalamazoo, MI
100-mg, 500-mg, 1-g, and 2-g vials of cytarabine powder. Store at 15°–30°C.

FLOXURIDINE

Floxuridine (fluorodeoxyuridine or 5-FUDR) is a synthetic analogue of the naturally occurring pyrimidine nucleoside, deoxyuridine. Inhibition of thymidylate synthase (TS) by 5-fluorodeoxyuridine monophosphate (FdUMP), an active metabolite of floxuridine, is believed to be the primary mechanism of anticancer efficacy of this drug. Because 5-FUDR is a direct precursor of FdUMP, this drug may act more selectively as a thymidylate synthase inhibitor than 5-FU (fluorouracil). However, 5-FUDR also can be enzymatically hydrolyzed (to 5-FU). Depending on the precise route and schedule of administration selected, the pharmacologic effects of 5-FUDR may thus closely resemble (or differ from) those observed with fluorouracil administration.

Floxuridine commonly is administered via hepatic arterial infusion to patients who have liver metastases from gastrointestinal malignancies. Compared with 5-FU, 5-FUDR is more water-soluble and more potent, permitting outpatient administration using small, implanted continuous infusion pumps. Also, the high first-pass hepatic metabolism of 5-FUDR results in less systemic exposure and less systemic toxicity. Randomized clinical trials have shown that hepatic arterial 5-FUDR can yield significantly higher objective response rates and a significantly delayed progression of liver metastases compared with systemic fluoropyrimidine treatment.

DOSAGE AND ADMINISTRATION

Hepatic arterial continuous infusion: 0.1–0.6 mg/kg/d × 14 d, repeat every 28 d
IV continuous infusion: 0.1–0.15 mg/kg/d × 14 d, repeat every 28 d
IP administration: 1–2 g/m²/d × 3 d, repeat every 21 d

SPECIAL PRECAUTIONS

Arterial catheter misplacement, dislodgement and migration; chemical hepatitis; pregnant and nursing patients

TOXICITIES

With hepatic arterial infusions:
Hematologic: neutropenia (rare)
Hepatic: abnormal liver functions, sclerosing cholangitis, acalculous cholecystitis, biliary sclerosis in 8%–21%
Other GI: anorexia (common), nausea, vomiting (mild), oral mucositis (rare), diarrhea; epigastric pain, gastritis, ulcers
Neurologic: headache, confusion, cerebellar ataxia (rare)
Dermatologic: alopecia (rare), dermatitis, pruritus, rash
Cardiovascular: myocardial ischemia (rare), angina
Catheter complications: arterial ischemia, perforation of vessel, dislodgement of catheter, catheter occlusion, thrombosis, infection

INDICATIONS

FDA-approved: hepatic arterial infusion for palliative management of hepatic metastases from gastrointestinal adenocarcinomas

PHARMACOKINETICS

Absorption: oral bioavailability limited, variable; **Distribution**: no data regarding CNS penetration; **Elimination**: metabolized 70%–90% first-pass in liver; **Systemic half-life**: 3–20 min; **Adjustments for organ dysfunction**: reduce dose or hold for abnormal liver function tests

DRUG INTERACTIONS

Leucovorin (increased hepatotoxicity)

RESPONSE RATES

Colorectal cancer with liver metastases: 40%–50%

PATIENT MONITORING

Monitor vital signs, symptoms (abdominal pain, nausea, vomiting, diarrhea—verify hepatic artery catheter placement; mucositis—interrupt treatment); examination; hematology; serum chemistry panel (significant hepatic enzyme elevations—interrupt treatment)

NURSING INTERVENTIONS

Monitor weight, nutritional status; encourage good oral hygiene; give antiemetics; mouthwashes and other adjuncts; antidiarrheals as needed; educate patients on care of vascular access devices and home infusion pumps

PATIENT INFORMATION

Patient should avoid use of aspirin or nonsteroidal anti-inflammatory agents; call physician if any moderate or severe diarrhea, fever, or other signs of serious infection develop; avoid excessive sun exposure; maintain good nutrition

FORMULATION

Available as FUDR®, Roche Laboratories, Nutley, NJ 500-mg vials containing lyophilized powder. Stored at 15°–30°C and protected from light.

FLUDARABINE PHOSPHATE

Fludarabine phosphate (2-fluoro-ara-AMP) is a synthetic analogue of the naturally occurring purine nucleotide, deoxyadenosine monophosphate, and is a fluorinated nucleotide analogue of the antiviral agent vidarabine. Compared with vidarabine, the fluorine substitution renders 2-fluoro-ara-AMP relatively resistant to inactivation by the enzyme adenosine deaminase, and the phosphate moiety enhances aqueous solubility. Following intravenous infusion, fludarabine phosphate is rapidly dephosphorylated to 2-fluoro-ara-A; intracellularly, 2-fluoro-ara-A is rephosphorylated to the active triphosphate, 2-fluoro-ara-ATP. This triphosphate metabolite is an inhibitor of several key enzymes in deoxyribonucleotide metabolism and DNA synthesis, including ribonucleotide reductase, DNA polymerase alpha, and DNA primase. Interestingly, fludarabine phosphate also has been shown to stimulate the activity of natural killer cells in in vitro studies.

Fludarabine phosphate has been shown to be effective in the treatment of chronic lymphocytic leukemia and other lymphoid malignancies, but has little or no activity against solid tumors. High doses of this drug can produce profound toxicities, including a distinctive syndrome of progressive neurotoxicity, characterized by delayed onset of progressive encephalopathy with cortical blindness and eventual death. Fortunately, standard doses appear to pose little risk of this catastrophic syndrome, even with repeated dosing.

DOSAGE AND ADMINISTRATION

Chronic lymphocytic leukemia: 25 mg/m^2/d (30-min IV infusion) $\times$ 5 consecutive d, repeat at 28-d intervals to maximal response and for three more cycles, then discontinue

SPECIAL PRECAUTIONS

Pregnant and nursing patients

TOXICITIES

Hematologic: neutropenia, thrombocytopenia, anemia (possibly severe and cumulative)
GI: anorexia, nausea, vomiting; stomatitis, diarrhea, GI bleeding (uncommon); abnormal liver function (occasional)
Neurologic: at recommended doses—weakness, agitation, confusion, visual disturbances, coma (rare), peripheral neuropathy; at high doses—delayed dementia, cortical blindness, coma, death (onset 21–60 d after last dose)
Pulmonary: possible increased susceptibility to pneumonia; pulmonary hypersensitivity reactions (dyspnea, cough, interstitial infiltrate)
Flu-like: malaise, fatigue, fever, chills
Miscellaneous: increased frequency of serious opportunistic infections (*Pneumocystis carinii*, *Listeria monocytogenes*, cryptococcus); tumor lysis syndrome (with hyperuricemia, hyperphosphatemia, hypocalcemia, hyperkalemia, urate crystalluria, renal failure); edema; rash; autoimmune hemolytic anemia

INDICATIONS

FDA-approved: chronic lymphocytic leukemia; clinical studies show activity in low-grade non-Hodgkin's lymphomas; macroglobulinemia; mycosis fungoides, Hodgkin's disease (possibly)

PHARMACOKINETICS

Absorption: insufficient data; **Distribution**: insufficient data; **Elimination**: renal; **Half-life**: 10 h; **Adjustments for organ dysfunction**: use with caution in patients with renal insufficiency

DRUG INTERACTIONS

Pentostatin (possibly lethal), dipyridamole

RESPONSE RATES

Chronic lymphocytic leukemia: in previously treated patients, complete response rate 10%–15%, overall response rate 32%–57%; with no prior chemotherapy, complete response rate 33%, overall response rate 79%; **Low-grade non-Hodgkin's lymphomas**: overall response rate 67%

PATIENT MONITORING

Vital signs, symptoms, examination, hematology, serum chemistry panel; bone marrow examination for persistent cytopenias

NURSING INTERVENTIONS

Monitor weight, nutritional status; encourage good oral hygiene; give antiemetics, and mouthwashes and other adjuncts as needed for stomatitis; consider IV gammaglobulin to reduce frequent bacterial infections in chronic lymphocytic leukemia; give antidiarrheals as needed, evaluate for infectious etiology if diarrhea is persistent or severe

PATIENT INFORMATION

Patient should avoid use of aspirin or nonsteroidal antiinflammatory agents; call physician if fever or other signs of serious infection develop; maintain good nutrition

FORMULATION

Available as FLUDARA®, Berlex Laboratories, Richmond, CA
50-mg vials. Stored at 2°–8°C.

FLUOROURACIL

Fluorouracil (5-FU) is a synthetic analogue of the naturally occurring pyrimidine, uracil. Several active metabolites of 5-FU have pharmacologic effects on the synthesis and function of cellular DNA and RNA. Inhibition of thymidylate synthase (TS) by 5-fluorodeoxyuridine monophosphate (FdUMP) is believed to be the primary mechanism of anticancer efficacy of 5-FU. Other active metabolites include 5-fluorouridine triphosphate (FUTP) and 5-fluorodeoxyuridine triphosphate (FdUTP). FUTP is misincorporated into RNA and may affect several aspects of RNA stability and function. Similarly, FdUTP can be misincorporated into cellular DNA (in place of thymidine triphosphate); the level of this misincorporation may be enhanced by the depletion of normal thymidine nucleotides, resulting from thymidylate synthase inhibition by FdUMP. Fluorodeoxyuridine nucleotides that have been misincorporated into DNA are recognized and cleaved by a glycosylase, yielding apyrimidinic sites in the DNA double helix and leading to DNA strand breaks.

Numerous pharmacologic interactions have been observed between 5-FU and other drugs commonly administered to cancer patients. Clinically, leucovorin has been shown to significantly enhance both the toxicity and the anticancer activity of fluorouracil.

DOSAGE AND ADMINISTRATION

Solid tumors: 500 mg/m^2/d (bolus IV injection) × 5 d, repeated at 4–5 wk intervals **or** 1000 mg/m^2/d (continuous IV infusion) × 5 d, repeated every 4 wk **or** 500–600 mg/m^2 (bolus IV injection), repeated weekly × 6 wk **or** 300 mg/m^2/d (continuous IV infusion) × 4 wk or longer
In combination with leucovorin: 5-FU dose usually must be reduced 25%–33%

SPECIAL PRECAUTIONS

Severe diarrhea (especially in elderly patients and with leucovorin or interferon α); patients with dihydropyrimidine dehydrogenase deficiency; pregnant and nursing patients

TOXICITIES

Hematologic: neutropenia, occasional thrombocytopenia (reversible)
GI: anorexia, nausea, vomiting (mild); oral, esophageal, GI mucositis and ulceration; diarrhea (sometimes severe), heartburn, taste alterations
Neurologic: cerebellar ataxia (can be irreversible), obtundation, disorientation, confusion, euphoria, nystagmus, headache; seizures (with leucovorin); acute neurotoxicity with progressive obtundation, hypotension, death (with high doses)
Dermatologic: hand-foot syndrome, rash, dry skin, fissuring, nail changes and loss, photosensitivity, alopecia, hyperpigmentation
Cardiovascular: myocardial ischemia, angina, infarction
Laboratory abnormalities: elevation of alkaline phosphatase, transaminase, and bilirubin (with levamisole, mild and reversible)
Miscellaneous: epistaxis, conjunctivitis, generalized allergic reactions (very rare)

INDICATIONS

FDA-approved: palliative management of carcinomas of the colon, rectum, breast, stomach, and pancreas; clinical studies show activity in head and neck carcinomas; as a radiosensitizer, in the adjuvant treatment of adenocarcinoma of the rectum, esophageal cancer, and head and neck cancer (organ preservation)

PHARMACOKINETICS

Absorption: oral bioavailability low, variable; **Distribution:** readily penetrates the CNS and malignant effusions, crosses the placenta; **Elimination:** metabolism (dihydropyrimidine dehydrogenase); **Half-life:** 6–20 min; **Adjustments for hepatic or renal dysfunction:** unnecessary

DRUG INTERACTIONS

Leucovorin, interferon alpha, interferon gamma, methotrexate, allopurinol, PALA, uridine, thymidine, dipyridamole, hydroxyurea, levamisole

RESPONSE RATES

Colorectal cancer: partial remissions 10%–20%; 30%–40% with leucovorin; **Head and neck squamous cancers:** partial remissions 10%–20%; **Breast cancer:** partial remissions 10%–20%; **Gastric cancer:** partial remissions 10%–15%

PATIENT MONITORING

Vital signs, symptoms (mucositis, diarrhea), examination, hematology, serum chemistry panel

NURSING INTERVENTIONS

Monitor weight, nutritional status; encourage good oral hygiene; give antiemetics as necessary; mouthwashes and other adjuncts for stomatitis; antidiarrheals for mild diarrhea (inform physician); educate on care of central venous access devices and home infusion pumps

PATIENT INFORMATION

Patient should avoid use of aspirin or nonsteroidal antiinflammatory agents. Call physician if any moderate or severe diarrhea, fever, or other signs of serious infection develop. Avoid excessive sun exposure; maintain good nutrition

FORMULATION

Available as Fluorouracil (Roche Laboratories, Nutley, NJ; Adria Laboratories, Dublin, OH; and other manufacturers)
500-mg ampules (50 mg/mL); 10-mL and 100-mL vials (50 mg/mL). Stored at 15°–30°C and protected from light. Administer undiluted, or dilute with 5% dextrose in water or 0.9% sodium chloride.

GEMCITABINE

Gemcitabine (2'-deoxy-2',2'-difluorocytidine monohydrochloride) is a nucleoside analogue that exhibits cell cycle specificity by affecting cells undergoing DNA synthesis (S-phase) and by blocking the progression of cells through the G_1/S-phase boundary. Gemcitabine is metabolized intracellularly by deoxycytidine kinase to the active forms of diphosphate and triphosphate nucleosides. Gemcitabine diphosphate inhibits ribonucleotide reductase, which catalyzes reactions and generates deoxynucleoside triphosphates for DNA synthesis. The reduction in the intracellular concentration of deoxycytidine triphosphate (dCTP) facilitates the incorporation of gemcitabine triphosphate into DNA. Further chain elongation is terminated after gemcitabine triphosphate and one additional nucleotide are incorporated into the growing DNA strands. DNA polymerase epsilon is unable to remove the incorporated gemcitabine triphosphate.

Gemcitabine is rapidly metabolized to an inactive uridine derivative (dFdU) by cytidine deaminase. However, in comparison with ara-C, gemcitabine has greater membrane permeability and enzyme affinity as well as considerably longer intracellular retention.

DOSAGE AND ADMINISTRATION

Locally advanced or metastatic pancreatic cancer: 1000 mg/m² IV over 30 min weekly × 7 wk, followed by 2 wk of rest; then 1000 mg/m² IV weekly × 3 every 4 wk

SPECIAL PRECAUTIONS

Pregnant and nursing patients

TOXICITIES

Hematologic: anemia, neutropenia, thrombocytopenia
GI: nausea, vomiting (mild), diarrhea, stomatitis
Dermatologic: rash
Miscellaneous: fever, hemolytic uremic syndrome (rare), flu-like symptoms, dyspnea, peripheral edema, noncardiogenic pulmonary edema (rare, fatal)

INDICATIONS

FDA-approved: first-line therapy for locally advanced or metastatic pancreatic cancer; clinical studies show activity in lung cancer

PHARMACOKINETICS

Absorption: no data; **Distribution:** Volume of distribution significantly influenced by duration of infusion and gender; clearance influenced by age and gender; **Half-life:** 32–94 min (short IV infusion); 245–638 minutes (long IV infusion); **Adjustment for organ dysfunction:** use with caution in patients with renal or hepatic dysfunction

RESPONSE RATE

Pancreatic cancer: 22.2% clinical benefit response (defined as a ≥ 50% reduction in pain or analgesic use, improvement in performance status, or ≥ 7% weight gain)

PATIENT MONITORING

Vital signs, symptoms, examination, hematology prior to each dose, liver and renal function

NURSING INTERVENTIONS

Monitor weight, nutritional status; encourage good oral hygiene; antidiarrheals as needed; evaluate for bacterial etiology if diarrhea is severe

PATIENT INFORMATION

Patient should avoid use of aspirin or nonsteroidal anti-inflammatory agents; call physician if fever or other signs of infection develop

FORMULATION

Available as Gemzar® Eli Lilly and Company, Indianapolis, IN
200-mg , 1000-mg vials of Gemzar lyophilized powder. Stored at 20°–25°C.

HYDROXYUREA

The anticancer effects of hydroxyurea appear to be related to inhibition of ribonucleotide reductase. Clinically, this agent is used primarily in the treatment of chronic myelocytic leukemia and related myeloproliferative disorders. Although hydroxyurea is also approved for use in malignant melanoma and ovarian cancer, there is currently little evidence that this drug has any significant activity in solid tumors. However, potentially synergistic interactions between hydroxyurea and other drugs that affect pyrimidine nucleotide biosynthesis and DNA metabolism (*eg*, methotrexate, the fluoropyrimidines, and cytarabine) have been identified in laboratory studies, and rationally designed combinations of hydroxyurea with other drugs continue to be the subject of numerous clinical investigations. Hydroxyurea can stimulate hemoglobin F production, and it is being investigated as a useful agent in treating sickle cell disease

DOSAGE AND ADMINISTRATION
800–1200 mg/m²/d PO daily **or** 2000–3200 mg/m² PO every 3 d

SPECIAL PRECAUTIONS
Pregnant and nursing patients

TOXICITIES
Hematologic: neutropenia (reversible) thrombocytopenia, anemia
GI: anorexia, nausea, vomiting (mild); oral, esophageal, GI mucositis and ulceration; constipation, diarrhea; liver function abnormalities (rarely progressing to jaundice)
Dermatologic: hyperpigmentation, erythema of face and hands, diffuse maculopapular rash, dry skin, thinning of skin, nail changes, alopecia (rare)
Neurologic: headache, drowsiness, dizziness, confusion (mild)
Miscellaneous: transient renal function abnormalities, radiation recall reactions

INDICATIONS
FDA-approved: ovarian adenocarcinoma, malignant melanoma, and chronic myelocytic leukemia; concurrently with radiation therapy for squamous carcinomas of the head and neck; clinical studies show activity in acute nonlymphocytic leukemia and essential thrombocytosis (acute control of dangerously elevated cell counts, pending initiation of standard cytarabine-based treatment regimens); polycythemia vera; as a radiosensitizer, in locally advanced cancer of the uterine cervix

PHARMACOKINETICS
Absorption: high oral availability; **Distribution**: readily penetrates the CNS and malignant effusions (excreted in significant quantities in breast milk); **Elimination**: primarily renal; **Half-life**: 3.5–4.5 hr; **Adjustments for organ dysfunction**: intitial reduced doses to patients with renal dysfunction recommended

DRUG INTERACTIONS
Cytarabine, fluorouracil, methotrexate

RESPONSE RATES
Chronic myelocytic leukemia: reduction of leukocyte count in over 75% of patients

PATIENT MONITORING
Vital signs, symptoms (mucositis, diarrhea), examination, hematology (weekly), serum chemistry panel

NURSING INTERVENTIONS
Monitor weight, nutritional status; encourage good oral hygiene; give antiemetics; mouthwashes and other adjuncts for stomatitis; antidiarrheals as needed

PATIENT INFORMATION
Patient should avoid use of aspirin or nonsteroidal antiinflammatory agents; call physician if fever or other signs of serious infection develop; avoid excessive sun exposure

FORMULATION
Hydrea® Bristol-Myers Oncology Division, Princeton, NJ; also available as Hydroxyurea capsules, Roxane Laboratories, Inc., Columbus, OH 500-mg capsules. Stored at 15°–30°C in tightly sealed container.

LEUCOVORIN

Leucovorin (5-formyl-tetrahydrofolate) is a reduced folate that can be readily transformed to all folates required for cellular metabolism. Thus, it serves as an effective antidote for methotrexate and other antifols and can be used to reduce the adverse effects caused by these drugs. Preliminary data indicate that leucovorin will serve as an antidote for newer, investigational antifols, including trimetrexate, piritrexim, and edatrexate. In contrast, leucovorin increases the toxicity and enhances the efficacy of the fluoropyrimidines; the leucovorin metabolite, 5,10-methylene-tetrahydrofolate, enhances the inhibition of the enzyme thymidylate synthase produced by fluorodeoxyuridine monophosphate, an active metabolite of the fluoropyrimidines.

DOSAGE AND ADMINISTRATION

Methotrexate rescue: beginning 6–24 h after methotrexate therapy, administer leucovorin 15 mg IV or PO every 6 h for ~10 doses (until methotrexate level is 0.05 µmol/L). Start rescue no later than 24 h after high-dose methotrexate. Higher leucovorin doses and longer treatment may be required if methotrexate clearance is abnormal (see manufacturer's guidelines).

With fluorouracil (for colorectal cancer): leucovorin 20 mg/m^2 followed by 425 mg/m^2 fluorouracil **or** leucovorin 200 mg/m^2 followed by 370 mg/m^2 fluorouracil daily for 5 d. Alternate regimen: leucovorin 500 mg/m^2 IV infusion over 2 h with fluorouracil injection (500–600 mg/m^2) at midpoint of leucovorin infusion; repeat weekly for 6 wk.

SPECIAL PRECAUTIONS

None

TOXICITIES

Allergic: sensitization (possibly)
Neurologic: seizures (with 5-FU)

INDICATIONS

FDA-approved: antidote for overdose of methotrexate or other folic acid antagonists; osteosarcoma (adjuvant chemotherapy, with high-dose methotrexate); advanced colorectal cancer (with 5-FU); clinical studies show activity in advanced breast cancer (with 5-FU)

PHARMACOKINETICS

Absorption: high bioavailability at oral doses up to 40 mg, less at higher doses; **Distribution:** negligible CSF penetration, (approximately 1% of systemic levels); **Elimination:** metabolized and excreted renally; **Half-life:** 1 hr (parent compound) and 4–7 h (active 5-methyl-tetrahydrofolate metabolite); **Adjustments for organ dysfunction:** unnecessary

DRUG INTERACTIONS

Fluoropyrimidines, methotrexate, edatrexate, trimetrexate, piritrexim, iododeoxyuridine

RESPONSE RATES

See page on methotrexate; *see* chapter on lower gastrointestinal cancer

PATIENT MONITORING

None required for single-agent leucovorin

NURSING INTERVENTIONS

None required for single-agent leucovorin (see pages on methotrexate and 5-FU for combination therapy)

PATIENT INFORMATION

No specific information required for single-agent leucovorin

FORMULATION

Available from Immunex, Seattle, WA; Wellcovorin®, Burroughs Wellcome Co., Research Triangle Park, NC; Elkins-Sinn, Cherry Hill, NJ; and Cetus, Oncology Corporation, Emeryville, CA. 5-mg, 10-mg, 15-mg, and 25-mg tablets; 50-mg, 100-mg, and 350-mg vials of cryodessicated powder. Stored at 15°–30°C and protected from light.

METHOTREXATE

Methotrexate, a synthetic analogue of folic acid, is a potent inhibitor of dihydrofolate reductase (DHFR), a key enzyme in folate metabolism. Inhibition of DHFR results in depletion of cellular reduced folates and interferes with vital cellular enzymes that require reduced folate cofactors (including enzymes of thymidylate and purine synthesis and amino acid metabolism). Inside the cell, methotrexate is metabolized to active polyglutamate metabolites, which inhibit DHFR and several other cellular enzymes, including enzymes that catalyze formyl transfer reactions in purine biosynthesis. Active polyglutamate metabolites of methotrexate may be retained by cells for long periods of time; hence, the antimetabolic effects of this drug may persist long after circulating levels of methotrexate are undetectable.

Leucovorin can reverse most of the antimetabolic effects produced by methotrexate and thus can rescue both normal and malignant cells from the cytotoxic effects of methotrexate. Used appropriately, leucovorin can enhance the therapeutic index of methotrexate by controlling and limiting the toxicity of higher doses of methotrexate. Pharmacologic interactions may also occur between methotrexate and many other drugs commonly administered to cancer patients. Clinically, the combination of methotrexate and fluorouracil has been extensively evaluated; available data suggest therapeutic synergy for treatment schedules in which fluorouracil administration follows methotrexate administration.

DOSAGE AND ADMINISTRATION

Solid tumors: 30–40 mg/m²/wk (IV infusion) **or** 3–12 g/m² as a 4–6 h (IV infusion) with leucovorin rescue beginning at 6–24 h, repeated weekly × 2–3 wk
Oral regimens: 15–30 mg (total dose) PO, repeated weekly (usually used for psoriasis, rheumatoid arthritis); 2.5–10.0 mg (total dose) PO daily (used for mycosis fungoides)
Intrathecal administration: Dose according to age (< 1 y, 6 mg; 1 y, 8 mg; 2 y, 10 mg; 3 y or older, 12 mg); repeat administration 1–2 times weekly, until CSF cytology has been negative for malignant cells for 1 wk; consider periodic maintenance therapy

SPECIAL PRECAUTIONS

Patients with pleural effusions, ascites, impaired renal function (may delay clearance, increase toxicity); pregnant and nursing patients; patients with poor nutritional status; patients on high-dose regimens; recent nitrous oxide anesthesia

TOXICITIES

Hematologic: neutropenia, anemia thrombocytopenia (occasional, reversible)
GI: anorexia, nausea, vomiting, diarrhea; oral, esophageal, GI mucositis and ulceration; transient abnormalities in serum levels of liver enzymes; cirrhosis, hepatic failure (rare)
Neurologic: headache, drowsiness, dizziness; with high doses, acute confusion, obtundation, seizures, encephalopathy, leukoencephalopathy; with intrathecal administration, chronic dementia, acute chemical arachnoiditis (rare, possible severe)
Dermatologic: rash, pruritus, urticaria, pigmentary changes, photosensitivity, alopecia, acne, skin necrosis, exfoliative dermatitis
Pulmonary: interstitial pneumonitis, *Pneumocystis carinii* pneumonia
Cardiovascular: pericarditis, pericardial effusion, hypotension, thromboembolic events
Renal: acute renal failure (especially with high doses), hyperuricemia
Miscellaneous: anaphylaxis (rare), radiation recall, osteopathy, other opportunistic infections, malignant lymphoma (rare)

INDICATIONS

FDA-approved: choriocarcinoma and gestational trophoblastic disease, ALL, meningeal leukemia, breast cancer, squamous head and neck cancers, mycosis fungoides, lung cancer, non-Hodgkin's lymphomas, osteogenic sarcoma; clinical studies show activity in carcinoma of the bladder, post-transplantation immunosuppression

PHARMACOKINETICS

Absorption: 60% oral bioavailability (for doses up to 30 mg) significant interindividual variability in pediatric leukemic patients (23%–95%); **Distribution**: 1%–3% penetration into CSF, slow penetrating, slow release from pleural effusions or ascites; **Elimination**: 80%–90% renal; **Half-life**: 3–10 h (at or below 30 mg/m²); 10–15 h (high doses); **Adjustments for renal insufficiency (creatinine clearance < 40 mL/min; or, for high-dose regimens, creatinine clearance < 60 mL/min)**: do not administer

DRUG INTERACTIONS

Leucovorin, 5FU, ara-C, asparaginase, carboxypeptidase, thiopurines, colchicine, nitrous oxide, probenecid, aspirin, NSAID, sulfonamides, triamterene, trimethoprim, pyrimethamine, penicillins, retinoids

RESPONSE RATES

Choriocarcinoma and gestational trophoblastic disease: generally curative; **Pediatric ALL**: response to combination regimens with methotrexate 90%; cured 50%; **Breast cancer**: with cyclophosphamide and 5-FU, 30%–50% remission; **Squamous head and neck cancers**: partial remissions in 30%; **Mycosis fungoides**: complete response rate 40%–50%; **Osteogenic sarcoma**: cure rate of nonmetastatic disease 50%–60% with adjuvant combination therapy

PATIENT MONITORING

Vital signs, symptoms, examination, hematology, serum chemistry panel; with high doses, closely monitor renal function, urine output, urine pH, serum electrolytes, serum methotrexate levels

NURSING INTERVENTIONS

Monitor weight, nutritional status; encourage good oral hygiene; give antiemetics: with high doses, monitor fluid intake and output, assess patient's oral intake and ability to take leucovorin rescue as instructed post-discharge

PATIENT INFORMATION

Patient should avoid use of aspirin or NSAIDs; call physician if moderate or severe adverse effects develop

FORMULATION

Available from Immunex, Seattle, WA; Folex®, Adria Labs, Dublin, OH; Mexate®, Bristol-Myers Oncology Division, Princeton, NJ; 50-, 100-, 200-, and 250-mg vials containing 25-mg/mL preservative-free solution; 50-mg and 250-mg vials containing 25-mg/mL preservative-protected solution; 20-mg, 50-mg, and 1-g vials of methotrexate; 2.5-mg tablets. Stored at 15°–30°C and protected from light.

MERCAPTOPURINE

Mercaptopurine (6-mercaptopurine or 6-MP) is a thiopurine that has been in clinical use as an antileukemic drug since the 1950s. Mercaptopurine is enzymatically converted to 6-thioinosine monophosphate (6-TIMP) by a purine salvage enzyme, hypoxanthine-guanine phosphoribosyltransferase (HGPRT). Although 6-TIMP is a relatively poor substrate for cellular enzymes and accumulates to significant levels in 6-MP-treated cells, 6-TIMP can be converted to a variety of other metabolites, including the corresponding ribonucleoside and deoxyribonucleoside di- and triphosphates, 6-methylmercaptopurine and its nucleotides, and 6-thioguanine nucleotides. The 6-TIMP metabolite of mercaptopurine inhibits several enzymes important in purine biosynthesis; 6-thiodeoxyguanosine triphosphate formed from 6-MP can be incorporated into DNA and can produce DNA strand breaks; and the many other metabolites of 6-MP produce additional antimetabolic effects. It is not yet clear which mechanisms account for the anti-cancer activity of mercaptopurine.

Relationships among the thiopurines in clinical use (mercaptopurine, thioguanine, and azathioprine) are discussed in the section on thioguanine.

DOSAGE AND ADMINISTRATION

Acute lymphoblastic leukemia: 50–75 mg/m^2/d for 30–36 mo (maintenance chemotherapy, with methotrexate)

Acute nonlymphocytic leukemia: 500 mg/m^2/d IV (using investigational IV formulation) $\times$ 5 d (in induction combination chemotherapy)

SPECIAL PRECAUTIONS

Pregnant and nursing patients; patients receiving allopurinol (reduce doses at least 50%)

TOXICITIES

Hematologic: neutropenia, thrombocytopenia, anemia (reversible, dose-related)
GI: anorexia, nausea, vomiting, diarrhea, (mild); oral, esophageal, GI mucositis and ulceration; reversible cholestatic jaundice; hepatic necrosis (rare)
Dermatologic: rash, hyperpigmentation
Miscellaneous: fever, pancreatitis (rare), hematuria and crystalluria with high IV doses

INDICATIONS

FDA-approved: acute lymphocytic leukemia, acute nonlymphocytic leukemias; clinical studies show activity in chronic myelocytic leukemia

PHARMACOKINETICS

Absorption: oral bioavailability (approx 16%), erratic, extensive first-pass metabolism in intestinal mucosa and liver; **Distribution:** no CSF penetration; **Elimination:** via metabolism (xanthine oxidase, other pathways); **Half-life:** 1.5 h; **Adjustments for organ dysfunction:** insufficient data

DRUG INTERACTIONS

Allopurinol, methotrexate, tiazofurin, trimethoprim-sulfamethoxazole, coumadin

RESPONSE RATES

Not applicable (used in maintenance phase treatment following complete remission of pediatric ALL; overall cure rate 50%)

PATIENT MONITORING

Vital signs, symptoms (mucositis, diarrhea), examination, hematology (weekly), serum chemistry panel

NURSING INTERVENTIONS

Monitor weight, nutritional status; encourage good oral hygiene; given antiemetics; mouthwashes and other adjuncts for somatitis; antidiarrheals as needed

PATIENT INFORMATION

Patient should avoid use of aspirin or nonsteroidal anti-inflammatory agents; call physician if fever or other signs of serious infection develop; avoid excessive sun exposure; maintain good nutrition

FORMULATION

Available as Purinethol®, Burroughs Wellcome Co., Research Triangle Park, NC
50-mg tablets. Stored at 15°–25°C in a dry place. Investigators with NCI-approved research protocols can obtain investigational tablet (10 mg) and IV formulations from the Pharmaceutical Resources Branch, National Cancer Institute
50-mL vials containing 500-mg mercaptopurine (sodium salt), lyophilized powder. Store unopened vials at room temperature (22°–25°C).

PENTOSTATIN

Pentostatin (2´-deoxycoformycin or DCF) is a purine deoxynucleoside analogue isolated from fermentation cultures of *Streptomyces antibioticus*. Pentostatin is a potent inhibitor of the enzyme adenosine deaminase, which hydrolyzes adenosine to inosine. The pharmacologic actions of pentostatin are believed to be mediated by the accumulation of adenine nucleotides, which can occur when adenosine hydrolysis is blocked. High intracellular levels of deoxyadenosine triphosphate can inhibit the activity of the enzyme ribonucleotide reductase, resulting in depletion of levels of other cellular deoxyribonucleotides. High levels of deoxyadenosine nucleotides can also inhibit the enzyme S-adenosylhomocysteine hydrolase, thus interfering with cellular methylation pathways and causing accumulation of S-adenosylhomocysteine, a toxic metabolite. Cells such as lymphocytes that have low levels of the nucleotide-cleaving enzyme 5´-nucleotidase may be particularly sensitive to these antimetabolic effects of pentostatin. Other known antimetabolic effects of pentostatin include inhibition of RNA synthesis and misincorporation of the triphosphate metabolite of pentostatin into cellular DNA.

In initial phase I studies using high doses of pentostatin, toxicities were frequently observed, with limited evidence of clinical efficacy. However, subsequent research has shown that this agent is highly active against hairy cell leukemia (a B-cell lymphoid neoplasm), has activity in other lymphoid malignancies as well, and can be used safely and effectively at lower doses. Pentostatin is not active in the treatment of solid tumors, and significant immunosuppression occurs as an adverse effect even at low doses of pentostatin.

DOSAGE AND ADMINISTRATION

Hairy cell leukemia: pretreat with allopurinol (300 mg/d) × 7 d. Then pentostatin (4 mg/m^2) once every 2 wk until complete response, followed by two additional doses, or to maximum of 12 mo. If no partial response by 6 mo, change to alternate treatment. Adjust dose if creatinine clearance is less than 60 mL/min.

SPECIAL PRECAUTIONS

Opportunistic (eg, *Pneumocystis carinii*) and severe infections
Pregnant/nursing patients

TOXICITIES

Hematologic: lymphopenia (particularly T cells), neutropenia, thrombocytopenia, immunosuppression (possibly severe and prolonged); infectious complications (common, including opportunistic infections)
Neurologic: anxiety, depression, confusion, lethargy, obtundation, coma, seizures
Renal: azotemia, acute renal failure, long-term residual impairment (possible)
Dermatologic: rash (possibly severe and increased with continued treatment)
GI: anorexia, nausea, vomiting (not severe), stomatitis, elevations in liver function tests (reversible)
Miscellaneous: fever, pneumonitis, myalgias, arthralgias, pleuritis, peritonitis, pericarditis, keratoconjunctivitis

INDICATIONS

FDA-approved: untreated or interferon α–refractory hairy cell leukemia; clinical studies show activity in T- and B-cell lymphomas, acute lymphoblastic leukemia, chronic lymphocytic leukemia, mycosis fungoides, Sézary syndrome, Waldenstrom's macroglobulinemia; **Possible activity:** multiple myeloma, Hodgkin's lymphomas

PHARMACOKINETICS

Absorption: insufficient data; **Distribution:** insufficient data on CNS penetration; **Elimination:** renal; **Half-life;** 2.5–6 h; **Adjustments for organ dysfunction:** delayed elimination of pentostatin with renal dysfunction; patients should have a creatinine clearance ≥ 60 mL/min

DRUG INTERACTIONS

Fludarabine phosphate, vidarabine

RESPONSE RATES

Hairy cell leukemia (untreated): 68% complete response in blood and marrow plus 5% partial response; **Hairy cell leukemia (refractory to interferon α):** 58%–85% complete response plus 4%–28% partial response

PATIENT MONITORING

Vital signs, symptoms, examination, hematology, serum chemistry panel; creatinine clearance pretreatment and during treatment; bone marrow examination for persistent cytopenias

NURSING INTERVENTIONS

Monitor weight, nutritional status; encourage good oral hygiene; give antiemetics as necessary; give mouthwashes and other adjuncts as needed for stomatitis; give antidiarrheals as needed; evaluate for infectious etiology if diarrhea is persistent or severe

PATIENT INFORMATION

Patient should avoid use of aspirin or nonsteroidal anti-inflammatory agents; call physician if fever or other signs of serious infection develop; maintain good nutrition

FORMULATION

Available as NIPENT® Parke-Davis, Morris Plains, NJ 10-mg vials of lyophilized powder. Stored at 2°–8°C.

THIOGUANINE

Thioguanine (6-thioguanine or 6-TG) a purine analogue, has been in clinical use as an antileukemic drug since the 1950s. Thioguanine is activated to 6-thioguanosine monophosphate by a purine salvage enzyme, hypoxanthine-guanine phosphoribosyltransferase (HGPRT). This ribonucleotide can be phosphorylated further by cellular kinases to generate thioguanosine di- and triphosphates or reduced (via the action of the enzyme ribonucleotide reductase) to generate thioguanine deoxyribonucleotides. Thioguanine and its metabolites produce numerous antimetabolic effects in cells, and it is not clear which mechanism(s) accounts for the anticancer activity of this drug.

The thiopurines are active agents in the treatment of acute and chronic leukemias and may have modest activity in the treatment of non-Hodgkin's lymphomas, but they have demonstrated no significant clinical activity against solid tumors. For historic reasons, azathioprine is used as an immunosuppressive, 6-thioguanine is used primarily in treatment of nonlymphocytic leukemias, and 6-mercaptopurine is used primarily in treatment of lymphocytic leukemias. Although clinical comparative studies have not been performed, it is likely that any of these drugs could be used for any of these indications, with comparable results. The only clinically significant pharmacologic difference among these three drugs is that the metabolic elimination of thioguanine is *not* significantly affected by allopurinol; hence, thioguanine doses need not be adjusted in patients receiving allopurinol.

DOSAGE AND ADMINISTRATION

Acute leukemia (in combination chemotherapy): 75–200 mg/m^2/d × 5 to 7 d in one or two divided oral doses

SPECIAL PRECAUTIONS

Pregnancy and nursing patients; hepatic impairment

TOXICITIES

Hematologic: neutropenia, thrombocytopenia, anemia (reversible, dose-related)
GI: anorexia, nausea, vomiting (mild), diarrhea; oral, esophageal, GI mucositis and ulceration; cholestatic jaundice
Dermatologic: rash, hyperpigmentation

INDICATIONS

FDA-approved: acute nonlymphocyctic leukemias; chronic myelocyctic leukemia (alternative to busulfan); clinical studies show activity in acute lymphocyctic leukmeia

PHARMACOKINETICS

Absorption: limited oral bioavailability (approximately 30%), highly variable (food intake reduces bioavailability); **Distribution**: does not penetrate CNS; **Elimination**: metabolism (methylation); **Half-life**: 25–240 min; **Adjustments for organ dysfunction**: insufficient data, use with caution in hepatic impairment

DRUG INTERACTIONS

Methotrexate, other antifols, tiazofurin

RESPONSE RATES

Adult acute nonlymphocyctic leukemia (with cytosine arabinoside and daunorubicin or doxorubicin): complete remission rate 40%–75%; cure rate 5%–10%

PATIENT MONITORING

Vital signs, symptoms (mucositis, diarrhea), examination, hematology (weekly or daily in leukemia induction therapy), serum chemistry panel

NURSING INTERVENTIONS

Monitor weight, nutritional status; encourage good oral hygiene; give antiemetics; mouthwashes and other adjuncts for stomatitis; antidiarrheals as needed

PATIENT INFORMATION

Patient should avoid use of aspirin or nonsteroidal anti-inflammatory agents; call physician if fever or other signs of serious infection develop; avoid excessive sun exposure; maintain good nutrition

FORMULATIONS

Available as Tabloid® from Burroughs Wellcome Co., Triangle Research Park, NC
40-mg tablets. Stored at 15°–25°C in a dry place.
Investigators with NCI-approved research protocols can obtain the investigational IV formulation from the Pharmaceutical Resources Branch, National Cancer Institute.
Investigational IV formulation, 10-mL vials containing 75-mg thioguanine (base), lyophilized powder. Unopened vials are refrigerated (2°–8°C), but are also stable at room temperature (22°–25°C).

The conventional treatment of cancer includes chemotherapy, radiation therapy, or surgery used singly or in combination. A fourth modality, biologic therapy, uses biologic reagents to elicit tumor regression. The biotherapeutic pharmacopeia includes recombinant cytokines, some of which possess profound immunomodulatory and antitumor activity, including interleukin-2 (aldesleukin) and interferon α (IFN α). The cytokines IL-4 and IL-12 are being evaluated. Other recombinant cytokines, termed colony stimulating factors (CSF), exert profound effects on hematopoiesis and immune function. They include erythropoietin (epoietin α), granulocyte-CSF (filgrastim), and granulocyte, macrophage-CSF (sargramostim). Although they do not have antitumor activity, these recombinant proteins have been shown to blunt chemotherapy-induced myelopoietic toxicity, and they have become useful adjuvants to bone marrow transplantation.

Other immunomodulating reagents with demonstrated antitumor activity include bacillus Calmette-Guérin and levamisole. Although the levamisole is not a biologic reagent, both reagents purportedly mediate their antitumor effects through immune modulation. Octreotide is a long-acting octapeptide that mimics the effects of the naturally occurring hormone somatostatin. Its pleiotropic effects include antiproliferative activity against several types of tumor. Additional anticancer biologic reagents, including IL-1, IL-4, IL-6, IL-7, and IL-12, as well as adoptively transferred lymphoid cells, are being evaluated for clinical efficacy but will not be discussed because of their experimental nature.

ALDESLEUKIN

Aldesleukin, or interleukin 2 (IL-2), is a T-cell growth factor that is central to T-cell–mediated immune responses [1,2]. It is a hydrophobic, 15kD, 133 amino acid glycoprotein that is elaborated primarily by activated CD4+ T lymphocytes. Its production is regulated at the transcriptional level by signals transduced across the plasma cell membrane when a mature T cell encounters its cognate antigen in concert with secondary signals provided by accessory cells. Aldesleukin is the recombinant protein elaborated by *Escherichia coli* that contain the human IL-2 gene. The cysteine residue at position 125 is substituted in the recombinant product by similar space-occupying amino acids to avoid aggregation and disulfide exchange leading to the accumulation of less active forms.

Aldesleukin has been approved for the treatment of patients with metastatic renal cell carcinoma and metastatic malignant melanoma. Aldesleukin has also been used in patients with HIV infection.

Renal Cell Carcinoma

In an update of 255 patients with metastatic renal cell carcinoma treated in a total of seven phase II clinical trials with high-dose aldesleukin (600,000 or 720,000 IU/kg every 8 h IV), an overall response rate of 15% (8% partial and 7% complete responses) has been reported [3,4]. The overall median duration of response was 54.0 months, the median survival for all patients was 16.3 months, and 10% to 20% of patients were estimated to be alive 5 to 10 years following treatment. However, because of the toxicity associated with the administration of high-dose IL-2, other dosing regimens have been evaluated in this disease. Examples of administration of low-dose IL-2 [5], IL-2 by continuous IV [6–9], subcutaneous administration [10,11], or in combination with IFN α with or without 5-Fluorouracil [12,13] has resulted in response rates ranging from

14% to 29%. Toxicities associated with these regimens have generally been less severe than those associated with high-dose IL-2. Studies to determine which dosing regimen of IL-2 is optimal for the treatment of metastatic renal cell carcinoma are ongoing. An updated report of an ongoing prospective randomized comparison of high-dose (720,000 IU/kg q8h) versus low-dose (72,000 IU/kg q8h) bolus intravenous IL-2 versus outpatient subcutaneous IL-2 (wk 1: 250,000 IU/kg/d for 5 d; wk 2–6: 125,000 IU/kg/d for 5 d) has reported response rates of 16%, 4%, and 11%, respectively [14].

Malignant Melanoma

An updated report on the treatment of 134 patients with metastatic melanoma with high-dose aldesleukin (720,000 IU/kg every 8 h IV) has resulted in overall response rates of 17% in patients with metastatic melanoma, with a significant number of durable complete responders (7%) [16,17]. As in renal cell carcinoma, other dosing regimens, such as continuous infusion or in combination with IFN α with or without chemotherapy [17–23], have been evaluated in metastatic melanoma. It appears that clinical responses in patients treated with less dose-intensive regimens are comparable to those with high-dose aldesleukin but of shorter duration.

HIV

Trials of aldesleukin by continuous intravenous or subcutaneous administration (with or without antiviral agents) in patients with HIV have demonstrated reproducible increases in CD4+ T-cell numbers without concomitant increases in viral load [24]. Improved CD4+ T-cell function has also been shown to be positively correlated with administration of aldesleukin as assessed by delayed-type hypersensitivity reactivity. Although these results are encouraging, evidence of a correlation between improved CD4+ T-cell number and function and patient survival remains to be determined.

Although combinations of IL-2 with other agents (*eg*, immune modulators [25] or the adoptive transfer of IL-2 expanded tumor infiltrating lymphocytes [6]) continue to be tested, the prolonged response durations of high-dose IL-2 lasting as long as 10 years have yet to be exceeded. Other novel strategies for the use of IL-2 (*eg*, for the treatment of malignant effusions [26], hematologic malignancies [27], or after bone marrow or stem-cell transplantation for hematologic or solid malignancies [28–32]) continue to be tested as well.

MECHANISM OF ACTION

Interleukin 2 plays a central role in T-cell activation. It is requisite for cell-cycle progression from G1 to S phase and the subsequent T-cell proliferation that is the sine qua non of cell-mediated immune responses. The effects of IL-2 are mediated through a heterotrimeric receptor (IL-2R) that may take many cell-surface forms based on which of its three subunits are expressed. The IL-2 receptor I chain (IL-2RI), also referred to as p55, CD25, or Tac, has low affinity for IL-2 ($Kd \approx 10\text{-}8$ M) and is not constitutively expressed. The J chain of the IL-2R, or p75, is a 70 to 75 Kd, 525 amino acid molecule with intermediate affinity for IL-2 ($Kd \approx 10\text{-}9$ M). IL-2RJ is expressed by monocytes, some mature CD4+ and CD8+ T cells, and large granular lymphocytes (LGL). It is also expressed in concert with IL-2RI on a subset of CD16-NK cells. In the presence of large concentrations of IL-2, the IL-2RJ chain is capable of signal transduction. The high affinity IL-2R ($Kd \approx 10^{-11}$ M) is a noncovalently linked heterotrimer consisting of the I, J, and K subunits.

Ligation of the high- or the intermediate-affinity IL-2R with IL-2 leads to internalization of the complex and a cascade of genetic events that activates a cell. Large granular lymphocytes proliferate and develop lymphokine-activated killer (LAK) activity. The cytotoxic activity of monocytes and CD8+ T cells is stimulated as well. Activated B cells are induced to proliferate and elaborate secretory rather than membranous IgM. T cells that express the high-affinity IL-2R undergo cell division following exposure to IL-2. The ability of IL-2-stimulated mononuclear cells to elaborate IFN γ, TNF α, IL-6, and IL-1 accounts for additional pleiotropic effects. Although IL-2 has been shown to downregulate the help provided by CD4+ T cells to humoral effector cells in certain models, the net effect on immune function is stimulatory.

The selective antitumor effects seen in some patients treated with aldesleukin are believed to be the result of a cell-mediated immune response that discriminates between self and nonself. This suggests that antigenic differences exist between some cancers and normal cells. There is compelling evidence derived from both murine models and clinical trials that this immune response is primarily T-cell mediated.

MECHANISMS OF RESISTANCE

At least 70% of patients with renal cell carcinoma who are treated with IL-2 have no measurable clinical response to therapy. The majority of patients who manifest treatment-related tumor regression eventually develop progressive disease despite retreatment. Although responses have been reported in patients with metastatic melanoma, colorectal carcinoma, ovarian cancer, lymphoma, and lung cancer, these responses have been transient or infrequent. The mechanisms that underlie this apparent escape from immune-mediated tumor regression have not been elucidated. Antigenic heterogeneity within a tumor may allow for the outgrowth of antigenically distinct clones that are not recognized by the immune system. Alternatively, defects in cell trafficking or tumor-cell susceptibility to lysis may develop that lead to unchecked tumor progression. Definition of the mechanisms of resistance await a better understanding of the mechanisms of response [33]. Although antibodies route to IL-2 have been identified in some patients receiving IL-2, especially by the subcutaneous route [34], it does not appear that this causes a change in the effectiveness of IL-2 treatment.

ADVERSE EFFECTS

The supraphysiologic doses of IL-2 that have been used for therapy are associated with a myriad of side effects, which are most likely mediated by other cytokines (TNF α in particular). Hematologic toxicity, including anemia requiring transfusion, and thrombocytopenia less than 20,000, have been observed in 60% and about 15% of treatment courses, respectively. Effects on the kidney include oliguria and decreased fractional excretion of sodium associated with rising serum creatinine and blood urea nitrogen in most patients. These can be managed successfully in most patients with the intravenous administration of volume expanders and dopamine infusions (2–3 μg/kg/min). Renal toxicity resolves in nearly all instances within several days. Cardiovascular toxicity includes increased heart rate, and myocardial depression manifests by decreased ejection fraction. Elevations of adrenocorticotropic hormone, endorphins, growth hormone, prolactin, and glucocorticoids have been observed in treated patients. Some patients develop clinically overt hypothyroidism that requires long-term thyroid hormone replacement therapy. Nearly all patients develop a vascular leak syndrome that is associated with egress of intravascular fluid into the soft tissues, where it remains sequestered until therapy ends. This redistribution of fluid probably contributes to the hypotension observed in most treated patients and can be managed effectively with vigorous fluid resuscitation using volume as crystalloid [35]. The volume of administered fluid is limited in some patients by noncardiogenic pulmonary edema secondary to capillary leak. In these patients, phenylephrine can be used to support the blood pressure in lieu of volume expansion, often while the patient remains on a conventional ward.

INTERFERONS

The interferons include more than 20 antigenically discrete but related immunomodulatory proteins [36,37]. They differ in their physic properties but manifest similar effects on the immune system, albeit to different degrees and with some exceptions. In spite of the profound immunomodulatory and antiproliferative effects manifest by the interferons, their use as single agents ostensibly has had limited impact on the treatment of solid tumors [38].

Interferon α, also referred to as leukocyte interferon, includes more than 23 related subtypes with overlapping activities. These are elaborated primarily by macrophages, large granular lymphocytes, and B cells following exposure to viruses, double-stranded RNA, tumor necrosis factor α (TNF), and IL-1. Most of the naturally occurring IFN α subtypes are composed of 166 amino acids and have molecular weights between 18,000 and 20,000. Their structure is that of an α-helix that is stabilized by disulfide bonds between cysteine residues at positions 1, 29, 99, and 139. The IFN α gene, located on chromosome 9, is constitutively transcribed in some cell types and may confer a degree of protection against viral infection.

Natural IFN α (IFN α-n3, Alferon) is prepared from pooled human leukocytes that have been induced by infection with the avian Sendai virus (Purdue Frederick). The specific composition of this preparation has not been elucidated. Recombinant IFN-α is available in the United States as IFN α-2a (Roferon A, Hoffmann-LaRoche) and IFN α-2b (Inferon A, Schering-Plough). These two recombinant cytokines differ from natural IFN-α in that amino acid 44 has been deleted and amino acid 23 has been replaced by lysine (IFN α-2a) or arginine (IFN α-2b). The half lives of IFN α-2a and IFN α-2b differ slightly after intravenous administration and are 5 (3.7–8.5) and 2 to 3 (0.5–3) hours, respectively.

Interferon β (fibroblast interferon) is a 166 amino acid glycoprotein that shares 30% homology with IFN α. The predominant sources of IFN β in vivo are fibroblasts and epithelial cells. Its production is upregulated by the same stimuli that induce the production of IFN α. Both IFN α and IFN β share a common cell-surface receptor. Unlike most naturally occurring IFN α subtypes, IFN β is N-glycosylated, its functional unit is a dimer, its α-helical content is less than 50%, and there is only one molecular species that is encoded by a gene located on chromosome 9. Recombinant IFN β (Betaseron, Cetus Corporation) is a nonglycosylated analogue in which cysteine has been replaced by serine at position 17 to maintain stability. Its activity is similar to that of the naturally occurring protein. It has not been approved for clinical use.

Interferon γ (type II or immune interferon) is a 143 amino acid glycoprotein that shares little homology to the type I interferons α and β. It is encoded by a gene on chromosome 12 and is made predomi-

The information here is provided as guidance only. Prescribers should always consult the manufacturer's current prescribing information.

68

nantly by CD4+ and CD8+ T cells, NK cells, and macrophages following exposure to antigen, mitogen, or IL-2. The dimeric molecule interacts with a unique, high-affinity, cell-surface receptor that is specific for IFN γ. There are an estimated 1000 receptors per cell with perhaps higher numbers on some tumor cells. IFN γ has been approved by the United States Food and Drug Administration (FDA) for the treatment of chronic granulomatous disease. In addition to natural IFN γ, several recombinant products are available from Genentech, Biogen, Schering-Plough, and Amgen. Differences in the N-terminal sequences and the number of amino acids account for variable pharmacokinetics and bioavailability between these products.

IFN α has demonstrated activity against many solid and hematologic malignancies. The latter appear to be particularly sensitive. An 80% to 90% response rate has been observed among patients with hairy cell leukemia treated with IFN α. Complete response in the bone marrow is rare, however, and most patients eventually relapse with the median time to clinically significant hematologic deterioration being 18 to 24 months. Benefits of therapy include a decrease in the incidence of serious infection and a reduced requirement for blood products. Survival appears to be prolonged compared with historical controls.

The hematologic response among patients with chronic myelogenous leukemia who are treated within 1 year of diagnosis is 50% to 70%. Despite an associated 20% complete cytogenetic response rate that appears to be durable, a survival benefit has not been demonstrated. The role of IFN in the treatment of other hematologic malignancies appears to be limited with the exception of essential thrombocythemia in which response rates approaching 80% have been observed.

Adjuvant therapy of melanoma with IFN α has been approved by the FDA. Kaposi's sarcoma is the only other solid tumor that has been approved by the FDA. The use of high doses ($> 20 \times 10^6$ U/m^2/d) administered intramuscularly or subcutaneously is associated with a response rate of 30% among treated patients without B symptoms and prior opportunistic infection and with CD4+ lymphocyte counts greater than 200. Half of these responses are complete and durable. Several other solid tumors manifest some degree of sensitivity to interferons. These include renal cell carcinoma, malignant melanoma, carcinoid tumor, malignant endocrine pancreatic tumors, basal cell carcinoma, and superficial bladder cancer.

MECHANISM OF ACTION

The interferons have been investigated intensely as anticancer agents because of their pleiotropic effects on immune reactivity, cell differentiation, and the rate of cell proliferation. These effects are mediated through the ligation of cell-surface receptors that are specific for the interferons. About 1000 high-affinity receptors, consisting of two separate chains, are present on most cells and interact with both IFN α and IFN β. IFN γ interacts with a different receptor heterodimer. Following receptor binding, incompletely understood cytoplasmic events ensue that lead to alterations in gene transcription and, as a result, the generation of regulatory enzymes and oncogenes that underlie the biologic effects of IFN.

Interferons retard proliferation of both normal and malignant cells by prolonging all stages of the cell cycle. Some cellular protooncogenes, including c-myc, c-fos, c-ras, and c-src are downregulated, suggesting that this effect is mediated in part at the transcriptional level. The action of growth factors, including platelet-derived growth factor, epidermal growth factor, fibroblast growth factor, insulin, and macrophage-colony stimulating factor is also antago-

nized. Three interferon-induced enzymes that also could account for the observed antiproliferative effects are 2',5'-oligoadenylate synthetase, protein kinase, and indolamine 2,3 dioxygenase.

Interferons modulate immune reactivity by enhancing target-cell immunogenicity and activating immune effector cells. Major histocompatability complex class I antigen expression is upregulated by all 3 classes of IFN. The expression of some tumor-associated antigens, such as carcinoembryonic antigen and TAG-72, also is enhanced. These alterations in cell-surface antigen expression are thought to render tumors more susceptible to immune recognition. Direct effects on immune reactivity include enhanced cytotoxic T-cell activity, macrophage and NK-cell activation, induction of B-cell immunoglobulin production, and enhanced NK-cell–mediated antibody-dependent cellular cytotoxicity (ADCC). Effects on cellular differentiation and angiogenesis may contribute indirectly.

MECHANISMS OF RESISTANCE

The clinical responses associated with the use of IFN α, which are dramatic in some hematologic malignancies, suggest that some neoplastic cells are much more sensitive to IFN than are normal cells. This could be accounted for by antigenic differences that exist between some cancers and normal cells or differences in cell-cycle kinetics. Resistance to IFN is poorly understood. At the cellular level, freshly isolated tumor cells demonstrate a range of sensitivity to IFN that does not correlate with tumor cell type. Resistance in vitro is not necessarily accompanied by changes in the number of cell-surface receptors. A better understanding of resistance awaits elucidation of the mechanisms underlying tumor regression.

ADVERSE EFFECTS

Therapy with IFN-α is usually well tolerated. Fewer than 10% of patients discontinue treatment as a result of severe toxicity. The most common adverse effect is a flu-like syndrome, occurring in as many as 98% of treated patients and consisting of fever (40%–98%), chills (40%–65%), myalgias (30%–75%), headache (20%–70%), malaise (50%–95%), and arthralgias (5%–24%). Fever may be as high as 40°C and occurs within 6 hours of a dose. Chills may be severe. Pretreatment with acetaminophen or nonsteroidal antiinflammatory drugs can attenuate these toxicities, which become less severe with continued therapy. Adverse hematologic effects are mild and include neutropenia, anemia, and thrombocytopenia. Some patients manifest elevated serum concentrations of AST and ALT. Other gastrointestinal side effects include nausea, vomiting, diarrhea, and a metallic taste. Dyspnea, alopecia, rashes, proteinuria, thyroid dysfunction, and edema also have been reported.

BIOCHEMICAL MODULATION

Synergistic interactions between IFN and other anticancer agents have been well documented [39]. Antiproliferative synergy against transformed cell lines has been demonstrated for IFN α and IFN γ. Their immune potentiating effects on NK cells also are enhanced in combination. Synergistic effects also are seen with combinations of IFN α and IL-2 at lower doses [13,18–23].

IFN α has been observed to enhance the efficacy of many cancer chemotherapeutics, including 5-FU, cis-platinum, cyclophosphamide, and doxorubicin. This may be a result of altered pharmacokinetics. IFN α–mediated inhibition of the cytochrome P450 system may delay the metabolism of doxorubicin and cyclophosphamide. The clearance of 5-FU also is inhibited by unknown mechanisms. It is also possible that the antitumor immune response generated by IFN may compliment the pharmacologic tumor debulking characteristic of chemotherapy by eradicating microscopic residual disease.

Melanoma has been reported to respond favorably to IFN α treatment and has been given in higher dose regiments as an adjuvant following surgical excision of nodal metastatic disease [40–43]. In a randomized controlled study of IFN α-2b in patients with high-risk stage IIb or stage III melanoma, it has been demonstrated that high-dose IFN α-2b significantly prolonged both relapse-free survival and overall survival in comparison with untreated patients [41]. As a result, IFN α-2b has been approved by the FDA for the adjuvant treatment of high-risk melanomas. With IFN α available, novel application in the combination treatment of malignant neuroendocrine tumors [44] with 5-FU and as a treatment for cutaneous T-cell lymphomas [45] have been proposed. Further applications, particularly in combination with more conventional therapeutics, are forthcoming.

BACILLUS CALMETTE-GUÉRIN

The history of immunotherapy is replete with examples of attempted cancer therapy using agents that were casually observed to augment immunoreactivity. The panoply of agents has included lectins, viable or nonviable bacteria, and bacterial products. No well-executed trials demonstrated any clinical advantage to the use of these agents until recently.

Bacillus Calmette-Guérin is a live, attenuated strain of *Mycobacterium bovis* with nonspecific, immunostimulating properties [46]. Intradermal administration of bacillus Calmette-Guérin in some animal models has been demonstrated to restore immunocompetence and protect against infection and malignancy. The mechanism responsible for these systemic effects is unknown, although they have been attributed to reticuloendothelial cell activation [46], decreased suppressor cell activity, macrophage and lymphocyte activation.

A number of trials have demonstrated prolonged disease-free survival, prolonged survival, delayed tumor progression, and eradication of carcinoma in situ of the urinary bladder among patients treated with intravesical bacillus Calmette-Guérin after transurethral resection (TUR) compared with patients treated with TUR alone [47]. Papillary carcinoma and carcinoma in situ of the bladder seem particularly well suited for local therapy with bacillus Calmette-Guérin because of the minimal tumor burden remaining after TUR, the ease of exposing all at-risk surfaces to treatment, the immunocompetence of most patients, and the ease of follow-up evaluation.

MECHANISM OF ACTION

Bacillus Calmette-Guérin is a nonspecific immunostimulant that is believed to exert its antitumor effect through the induction of a DTH-like response. According to this paradigm, tumor cells are destroyed as innocent bystanders, either directly by activated macrophages and lymphoid cells, or indirectly by the local secretion of cytokines. These nonspecific immune effectors represent a reaction to components of the bacillus cell wall. Rare regional responses, which are characterized by regression of some uninjected tumors, suggest that specific antitumor immunity is induced in some treated patients. This, however, has been difficult to prove.

MECHANISMS OF RESISTANCE

Clinical experience has defined criteria that are associated with a low likelihood of response to therapy with bacillus Calmette-Guérin. These relate primarily to tumor size and patient immunocompetence. Large tumors are unlikely to regress. The reason for this observed inverse relationship between tumor size and response to therapy is not known; however, tumor vasculature is believed to play a role. This observation has led to the use of intravesical bacillus Calmette-Guérin as an adjuvant to transurethral resection of tumors rather than as a primary mode of therapy. It is also applied to the treatment of carcinoma in situ for the same reason.

ADVERSE EFFECTS

The risk of developing toxicity depends in large measure on the integrity of intravesical and systemic immunity. Impairment of either one of these can lead to dissemination of viable organisms and overwhelming mycobacterial infection. Patients who are receiving systemic steroids, bone marrow depressants, or radiation therapy or who have compromised immune systems for any other reason should not be treated. Local factors that predispose to disseminated infection include ongoing urinary tract infection and healing bladder mucosal injury secondary to instrumentation.

Other adverse manifestations of therapy include those related to local effects on the bladder. Urinary symptoms, which include dysuria, frequency, urgency, and decreased bladder capacity, are a result of bladder irritation and usually do not occur until the third course of treatment. Systemic symptoms, including fever, malaise, and chills may be due to hypersensitivity and resolve after 1 to 3 days.

Patients who are immunocompromised at the time of therapy also are unlikely to respond. This is not surprising even in light of our limited understanding of the mechanism of response, which probably involves immune effectors that have been nonspecifically activated by bacillus Calmette-Guérin. Commonly encountered causes of immunosuppression in these patients include previous chemotherapy and radiation therapy, use of corticosteroids, poor nutrition, or advanced disease.

LEVAMISOLE

Levamisole is an immunomodulatory drug that initially was developed as an anthelminthic agent [48]. The anthelminthic effect has been shown to be mediated by inhibition of a unique succinate dehydrogenase-fumarate system that serves as a terminal electron acceptor in the generation of adenosine triphosphate. This effectively paralyzes treated worms.

The immunologic effects of levamisole in vitro are protean and include enhancement of polymorphonuclear and mononuclear phagocytosis and chemotaxis. Lymphocyte proliferation in response to mitogens and cytotoxic activity also are enhanced. B-cell and NK-cell function appear to be unaffected. A direct antitumor effect has not been demonstrated [49].

The results of studies designed to evaluate the immunologic effects of levamisole in animals and humans are conflicting and have provided little insight into the design of future clinical trials. In 1989, the North Central Cancer Treatment Group (NCCTG) reported that adjuvant therapy of colorectal cancer with levamisole and 5-FU may be of benefit. This combination was based on the presumption that enhanced immunoreactivity engendered by levamisole would contribute to the minimal effects of 5-FU in eliminating microscopic disease. A subsequent intergroup trial conducted by the Eastern Cooperative Oncology Group, the NCCTG, the Southwest Oncology Group, and the Mayo Clinic corroborated these findings [50]. There was a statistically significant prolongation of disease-free and overall survival among patients with stage III disease who were treated with the combination of levamisole, 50 mg every 8 hours, and 5-FU, 450 mg/m^2/day for 1 year. The observed toxicity was generally that expected with 5-FU. In a final report of this trial [51], 5-year follow-up of 929 patients revealed a 40% reduction in recurrence rate and a 33% reduction in death rate in the group of patients treated with 5-FU and levamisole. These results have been questioned on the basis of the experimental design, which did not include a 5-FU control arm. However, concomitant 5-FU and levamisole represent standard therapy for patients with node-positive colorectal carcinoma who have undergone curative resection.

MECHANISM OF ACTION

Levamisole alone has not consistently demonstrated antitumor activity. It is not known whether levamisole mediates a salutary effect by reversing the immunosuppression associated with 5-FU or whether it biochemically modulates the anticancer activity of 5-FU [52]. Levamisole is a heterocyclic compound that is purported to exert immunomodulatory effects through either its imidazole or thiazol rings. The cytoplasmic or cell-wall targets for this molecule are not known. Neither are the mechanisms by which subsequent biochemical events within the cell are effected. One theory holds that the sulfhydryl group leads to glutathione repletion. Others have suggested that cholinergic-like effects of the imidazole ring underlie the observed enhancement of IL-2–induced T-cell proliferation. It is known that levamisole increases the level of cytoplasmic cGMP and reciprocally decreases levels of cAMP in treated lymphocytes. It may increase the intracellular calcium concentration as well. Decreased cell-membrane adenylate cyclase activity also has been observed. Whether these findings are relevant to the observed immunomodulatory effects is not known.

MECHANISMS OF RESISTANCE

Evasion of a levamisole-induced immune response is one mechanism by which cancer cells may overcome the effects of levamisole and 5-FU. However, clinically exploitable antigenic differences between colon cancer and normal cells have yet to be demonstrated. Resistance also may arise through modulation of the levels of certain vital intracellular constituents. For example, gene duplication or a compensatory increase in the activity of certain enzymes may lead to elevated levels of thymidylate synthetase. This could partially overcome the detrimental effect 5-FU exerts on DNA and RNA synthesis and repair.

ADVERSE EFFECTS

Adverse reactions to levamisole generally are mild. Agranulocytosis, which is usually reversible following discontinuation of treatment, rarely has been reported. This may be accompanied by a flu-like syndrome. Neutropenia, thrombocytopenia, and anemia occur frequently in patients treated with levamisole and 5-FU in combination. Almost all patients treated with levamisole and 5-FU experience toxicity that is otherwise associated with 5-FU alone. Other rare toxi-

cities include rashes, myalgia, arthralgia, and renal failure. Central nervous system toxicity includes confusion, convulsions, hallucinations, impaired concentration, and an encaphalopathic syndrome. Fatigue and altered taste sensation also have been reported.

COLONY-STIMULATING FACTORS

The colony-stimulating factors (CSF), like the interleukins from which they have been arbitrarily distinguished, are cytokines that control hematopoiesis and possess intrinsic immunomodulatory activity. These glycoproteins are elaborated by a variety of cell types, including T cells, B cells, NK cells, granulocytes, macrophages, vascular endothelial cells, smooth muscle cells, and fibroblasts. Some are produced constitutively and probably maintain steady-state levels of circulating cells. Their elaboration can be induced by a variety of physiologic stimuli, including mononuclear cell-derived cytokines, bacterial endotoxin, and hypoxemia.

The CSFs exert their effects at several stages of blood-cell development [53–55]. Multi-CSF (IL-3), and steel factor (*c-kit* ligand) act on the pluripotent stem cell, as do more differentiated cells in multiple lineages. Granulocyte, macrophage-CSF (GM-CSF) acts a little later in blood cell development, probably in concert with IL-3 and steel factor. Monocyte-CSF (M-CSF), granulocyte-CSF (G-CSF), and erythropoietin act on more differentiated cells and are more lineage specific, as their names imply. The picture that has emerged is one characterized by multiple regulatory proteins with overlapping functions that interact with one another within the stromal microenvironment of the bone marrow. Their effects are mediated either directly, through cell surface receptors, or indirectly, through the induction of other cytokines. The outcome is hematopoietic homeostasis that gives way to adaptive increases in the levels of circulating mature and immature cells during periods of stress.

Three CSFs have been approved for clinical use. Erythropoietin (Epoietin α) is a 166 amino acid glycoprotein that serves as an obligate growth factor for red blood cell progenitors [56–59]. It is made primarily by peritubular cells within the kidney in response to an oxygen-sensing heme protein. The liver contributes a fraction to the total amount of circulating protein, as well. Under normal conditions the serum level of erythropoietin ranges from 4 to 24 mU/mL. There is an inverse correlation between serum erythropoietin level and hemoglobin concentration below 10.5 g. Levels may rise as high as 10,000 Mu/mL in response to profound anemia. A normal response to a specific degree of anemia is difficult to define owing to large variations from the mean that have been observed.

Patients undergoing chemotherapy, radiation therapy, or whose bone marrow is replaced by tumor may develop anemia that is difficult to manage. Some of these patients have lower erythropoietin levels than patients with comparable degrees of iron deficiency anemia, and the inverse correlation between serum hemoglobin concentration and erythropoietin may be attenuated. The administration of epoietin-α between courses of chemotherapy has been observed to reduce the transfusion requirement of some patients, including those with solid tumors, lymphoma, and multiple myeloma [56–59]. Patients whose pretreatment erythropoietin level is greater than 500 Mu/mL are unlikely to respond to epoietin-α.

Granulocyte-CSF is a 174 amino acid glycoprotein that is produced by mononuclear phagocytes, endothelial cells, fibroblasts, and neutrophils [60,61]. G-CSF is central to the control of circulating blood neutrophil numbers, during both times of health and infection. G-CSF also has profound effects on mature granulocyte function. Phase III studies have evaluated the efficacy of recombinant G-CSF (filgrastim) in patients with solid tumors who are treated with myelosuppressive chemotherapy. Patients treated with filgrastim have manifested less profound and less persistent neutropenia, decreased incidence of neutropenic fever, and fewer culture-positive infections. This has translated to a decreased use of antibiotics and shorter hospital stays.

Granulocyte, macrophage colony-stimulating factor is a 127 amino acid protein with a molecular weight that ranges from 18 to 22 Kd due to variable glycosylation [62]. It stimulates the growth and differentiation of cells committed to the neutrophil and macrophage lineages. It also synergizes with other CSFs to stimulate multipotential progenitor cells. Randomized, placebo-controlled trials of recombinant GM-CSF (sargramostim) after bone marrow transplantation have revealed shorter periods of neutropenia and fewer infectious complications among treated patients. This has been associated with shorter hospital stays for treated patients.

The availability of reagents that augment the in vivo production of erythrocytes and granulocytes may have profound implications for the palliation and treatment of cancer [63,64]. Anemia associated with malignancy and chemotherapy may be debilitating. Red blood cell transfusion is associated with a small risk of serious infection as well as a variety of immune-mediated transfusion reactions. Many chemotherapeutics also cause life-threatening bone marrow toxicity manifest as granulocytopenia or thrombocytopenia. The risk of infection and bleeding associated with these dose-limiting toxicities is significant, and the impact on treatment efficacy may be substantial [65–68].

MECHANISM OF ACTION

Each of the CSFs mediate their effects by binding to specific cell-surface receptors that share structural characteristics with those of other CSFs and interleukins. High-affinity receptors unique for each growth factor have been identified. Together they constitute the cytokine receptor family, which includes the receptors for erythropoietin, G-CSF, GM-CSF, IL-2J, IL-3, IL-4, IL-5, IL-6, IL-7, prolactin, and growth hormone. All share amino acid sequences that may be functionally important.

Receptor activation leads to the modulation of second messengers, which then initiate a cascade of cytoplasmic events culminating in increased gene transcription. This is probably mediated by nuclear proteins that release cytokine promotors from inhibition. CSF-specific signal transduction pathways remain to be completely defined, but protein kinase C and elevated levels of intracellular calcium are thought to be involved.

The cellular distribution of receptors determines the effect of each CSF. The receptors for GM-CSF are found on pluripotent progenitors as well as on more differentiated cells of the macrophage and granulocyte lineages. This accounts for its effects on many mature lineages, including neutrophils, eosinophils, basophils, macrophages, and Langerhans cells, and its effects on most blast-forming and colony-forming unit precursors. Receptors for erythropoietin and G-CSF are distributed on more mature cells in a lineage-restricted fashion, which accounts for their effects being confined mainly to red blood cells and neutrophils, respectively. Receptors for G- and GM-CSF also are present on endothelial cells. The pleiotropic effects of GM-CSF may be due, in part, to

the release of other cytokines.

Effects of filgrastim include decreased transit time of granulocytes from the mitotic to the postmitotic compartment with more rapid release of mature granulocytes from the bone marrow. Mature granulocytes are primed to produce superoxide, and their migration is enhanced. Antibody-dependent cellular cytotoxic activity, immunoglobulin A–mediated phagocytosis, and release of inflammatory mediators is also augmented. The net effect is to increase the number of mature, circulating granulocytes and to enhance their function.

Sargramostim shares many of these properties with filgrastim. It also enhances the cytotoxic activity of mature eosinophils and macrophages. The macrophages develop tumoricidal activity, as well. The circulating half-life of neutrophils is prolonged. A role for GM-CSF in wound healing is suggested by its augmentation of vascular endothelial cell migration.

ADVERSE EFFECTS

Therapy with filgrastim is rarely associated with clinical toxicity. Mild bone marrow discomfort, which responds to treatment with acetaminophen, occurs in 20% of treated patients. Exacerbation of preexisting cutaneous inflammatory disorders, including eczema and vasculitis, have been observed. This resolves with discontinuation of filgrastim. Prolonged therapy has been associated with splenomegaly in few patients. This is a result of extramedullary hematopoiesis. Serum uric acid and LDH also may become elevated, reflecting increased cell turnover.

Sargramostim produces dose-dependent toxicities, some of which may be mediated through the release of other cytokines. Side effects seen in patients treated with high doses ($1000~\mu g/m^2$) include thrombosis, pleural or pericardial effusion, peripheral edema, headache, and a flu-like syndrome. Lower, clinically effective, doses are better tolerated but may be associated with malaise, anorexia, fever, chills, arthralgias, myalgias, headache, and edema. A first-pass effect, characterized by respiratory distress, has been seen in some patients coincident with the first dose of sargramostim. This may require steroids, if severe, and unrecognized cases may require mechanical ventilation. Induction of cell-surface adhesion molecules on circulating granulocytes by sargramostim or release of cytokines from alveolar macrophages may underlie this toxicity.

Therapy with epoietin-α is well tolerated and is associated with a very low incidence of clinically significant toxicity at therapeutic doses. Preexisting hypertension may be exacerbated and should be well controlled before instituting therapy. Some patients may experience arthralgias. The propensity for central venous catheters to become occluded by thrombus is increased.

OCTREOTIDE

Octreotide (SMS 201-995) is a long-acting, synthetic octapeptide with pharmacologic actions that mimic those of the naturally occurring, 14 amino-acid hormone somatostatin (SMS 14) [69,70]. Other naturally occurring analogues have been identified, including prosomatostatin (SMS 28) and preprosomatostatins (SMS 128). This family of peptides generally exerts inhibitory effects on a variety of organ systems. It downregulates the release of growth hormone, prolactin, and all gastrointestinal hormones. It inhibits gastric acid secretion, gastrointestinal motility, intestinal absorption, pancreatic secretion, and portal blood flow. The secretion of gastroenteropancreatic peptides, including insulin, vasoactive intestinal peptide, gastrin, and glucagon, also are reduced. Interest in octreotide as an anticancer agent has been stimulated by its documented antiproliferative activity against many tumor cell lines. However, the mechanism underlying this effect has not been fully elucidated.

The half-life of the naturally-occurring hormone somatostatin is so ephemeral (half-life = 3 min) that it is of no clinical use. The D amino-acid substitutions of octreotide and other synthetic analogues, such as the octapeptide Somatuline (Ipsen International, Paris, France), confer resistance to serum peptidases, prolonging their half lives. The half-life of octreotide is about 60 minutes after intravenous administration and 2 hours after subcutaneous injection. Although a formulation for oral use has been developed, its use is limited by very poor bioavailability.

Octreotide acetate has been approved for use as an agent to palliate patients who suffer diarrhea as a result of carcinoid syndrome or VIPoma. It has demonstrated clinical efficacy in the treatment of other hypersecretory disorders, including insulinoma, glucagonoma, Zollinger-Ellison syndrome, acromegaly, and pancreatic ascites. It also has proven to be a useful adjunct in the management of enterocutaneous and pancreaticocutaneous fistulae. Its use as an anticancer agent remains investigational.

MECHANISM OF ACTION

Octreotide exerts its pleiotropic effects through cell-surface receptors that vary in their affinity for different somatostatin analogues. They are widely distributed throughout the body and have been demonstrated on cells that compose the central nervous system, the gastrointestinal tract, the exocrine glands, and the kidneys. These receptors also have been detected in human meningioma, breast carcinoma, and carcinoid tumors.

Octreotide's antiproliferative effects are thought to be mediated in several ways. It inhibits and reduces the levels of several growth factors that have been associated with tumor growth, including epidermal growth factor, platelet-derived growth factor, fibroblast growth factor, transforming growth factor-α, and bombesin. Octreotide also possesses direct antiproliferative effects that are poorly understood. Receptor binding also may be associated with dephosphorylation of cell membrane proteins that are necessary for proliferation. Stimulation of the reticuloendothelial system may be responsible, in part, for the antitumor effects of octreotide that have been observed in murine models.

ADVERSE EFFECTS

The therapeutic index for octreotide is wide, and serious toxicity is unusual. Nausea, diarrhea, and abdominal discomfort have been observed in about 5% to 10% of treated patients. Less common side effects (< 2%) include headache, dizziness, flushing, fatigue, hypoglycemia, and hyperglycemia. There is a risk of cholelithiasis as a result of changes in bile composition and gall bladder contractility, but this has been observed in fewer than 1% of treated patients.

RETINOIDS

Retinoids are a family of structurally and functionally related molecules that exercise a profound effect on cell growth and differentiation

[71–75]. This class of compounds includes all-trans-retinol (vitamin A), which is obtained primarily through the conversion of dietary precursors, including retinal palmitate and beta-carotene. Conversion occurs within the intestinal lumen and enterocytes, respectively. The conversion of carotenoids to retinol is tightly regulated so that ingestion of excessive amounts of beta-carotene do not produce hypervitaminosis A. Retinol is transported in chylomicrons through intestinal lymph. It is taken up by hepatocytes and transferred to stellate cells within the liver. These cells contain about 80% of the body's store of vitamin A, and they maintain plasma levels at about 2 –M.

Retinol, secreted by stellate cells complexed with a binding protein, is reversibly bound further to transthyretin, a protein that protects vitamin A from loss through glomerular filtration. The mechanism by which target tissues take up retinol remains an enigma. Many of its effects are thought to be mediated by its intracellular conversion to all-trans retinoic acid (tretinoin). Another metabolite of vitamin A with therapeutic potential is 13-*cis*-retinoic acid (isotretinoin).

Retinoids are essential to embryonic development, epithelial cell differentiation, and growth. They may be requisite for immunologic integrity because they have been shown to enhance certain cell-mediated immune responses, augment IL-2–induced LAK-cell generation, and upregulate macrophage phagocytic activity. Vitamin A also plays an important role in vision, reproduction, and hematopoiesis.

Retinoids possess antineoplastic activity and may have some clinical value in the treatment of a variety of malignancies. Transient complete remissions are associated with the use of single-agent tretinoin in most patients with acute promyelocytic leukemia. The role of concomitant chemotherapy remains to be defined. Isotretinoin has induced complete clinical responses in about 50% of patients with basal cell and squamous cell carcinoma of the skin [74]. Tumor regression has been seen less frequently among treated patients with mycosis fungoides.

Retinoids prevent the development of tumors in a variety of animal models. This has led to several chemoprevention trials in patients at high risk for malignancy. Isotretinoin has been associated with a decreased tumor frequency among treated patients with xeroderma pigmentosum. This effect lasted only as long as treatment was continued. Among patients with treated head and neck cancer, isotretinoin is associated with a lower frequency of secondary aerodigestive malignancy. Unfortunately, the incidence of tumor recurrence appears to be unaffected and as many as 33% of patients required discontinuation of therapy due to intolerable toxicity.

MECHANISM OF ACTION

Retinol and retinoic acid are bound within the cell cytoplasm by proteins whose function is unclear. Retinoic acid is then transported to the nucleus, where it is complexed by any of 3 receptors. These share substantial homology and are members of the steroid-thyroid superfamily of nuclear receptors. Retinoic acid receptor (RAR) α is widely distributed throughout the body. The distribution of RAR β is more limited, and RAR γ is expressed almost exclusively in high levels by epithelial cells of the skin and oral mucosa.

Retinoic acid mediates many of its effects through the induction of gene expression. The RA-RAR complexes bind to specific DNA sequences termed *retinoic acid response elements*. Some of these sequences encode DNA binding proteins that regulate the transcription of genes encoding proteins that are necessary for cell growth and differentiation. Retinoic acid–responsive genes also include those for epidermal growth factor receptor, vasoactive intestinal peptide receptor, and melanocyte stimulating hormone receptor. Direct effects of retinoic acid include a detergent-like effect on cell membranes that results in decreased membrane stability. Lysosomal membranes also may be disrupted.

Antitumor activity may be mediated by any of several proposed mechanisms. Retinoic acid has been shown to induce cell differentiation. This is evident for some human acute myeloid leukemia, melanoma, neuroblastoma, and teratocarcinoma tumor cell lines. These effects are enhanced by some cytokines, including IFN-α, tumor necrosis factor α (TNF α), and G-CSF. Retinoic acid also reverses squamous metaplasia in vitamin A deficient animals. These observations have served as the basis for chemoprevention trials.

A number of tumor cell lines respond to retinoic acid with growth inhibition. This may be mediated by a direct effect of retinoic acid on the cells or in a paracrine fashion through the induction of transforming growth factor β (TGF β) expression. The latter also may be responsible for the induction of apoptosis, which has been associated with the use of retinoic acid. Growth inhibitory effects of retinoic acid are enhanced by IFN α and IFN γ.

MECHANISMS OF RESISTANCE

Resistance to the antitumor effects of retinoids is not understood. Some observations suggest that this has a pharmacokinetic basis. Specifically, plasma levels of tretinoin decline during prolonged therapy. This may be a result of homeostatic mechanisms that regulate retinoid metabolism because it is not reversed by dose escalation.

ADVERSE EFFECTS

The spectrum of toxicity differs between tretinoin and isotretinoin. Both are teratogenic, and their use in women who are pregnant or who may become pregnant is contraindicated. It is recommended that these drugs should not be used in women of childbearing age unless they understand the risks and are capable of following mandatory contraceptive measures. These include the use of effective contraception for 1 month before, during, and after therapy.

The most frequent complication associated with both drugs is cheilitis, which occurs in 90% of treated patients. Xerosis is seen in about 50% of patients. This may be complicated by conjunctivitis, epistaxis, and pruritus. Rash, thinning hair, photosensitivity, and nail changes are seen less frequently. Gastrointestinal morbidity includes nausea and vomiting, which is seen in 20% to 30% of patients. The onset of inflammatory bowel disease has been associated temporally with the use of retinoids, although a cause and effect relationship has not been established. Headache frequently is associated with the use of tretinoin but is uncommon among patients treated with isotretinoin. Other neurologic toxicities are rare and include fatigue, depression, and pseudotumor cerebri. Moderate musculoskeletal symptoms are seen in about 15% of treated patients.

An unusual and potentially fatal complication of therapy with tretinoin has been seen among patients who have acute promyelocytic leukemia. This syndrome includes respiratory distress, fever, pulmonary infiltrates, pleural and pericardial effusions, edema, and myocardial depression. This is almost invariably associated with hyperleukocytosis. Resolution of this syndrome has been associated with the use of dexamethasone, 10 mg intravenously twice daily.

Metabolic effects include hypertriglyceridemia, hepatic transaminasemia, hyperglycemia, hyperuricemia, hypercholesterolemia, and decreased high density lipoproteins. These effects are reversible on discontinuation of therapy.

NEW AGENTS

As shown in Table 4-1, there are many new agents under evaluation that have yet to be approved by the FDA. This includes the retinoic acid derivatives as well as new cytokines, such as IL-4 [76], IL-6 [77], and IL-12 [78,79]. Anecdotal responses have been observed with all of these agents. New agents under evaluation to support platelets include IL-3 [80], IL-11, and thrombopoietin. Although no antibody preparation has been approved for treatment of cancer, the murine monoclonal antibody 17-1A has demonstrated efficacy as an adjuvant therapy for patients with resected colorectal cancer [81], which needs to be confirmed in prospective studies.

Table 4-1. Agents Being Studied

Agent	Dose/Route	Supplier	Mechanism of Action	Pharmacokinetics (Half-life)
Interleukin 3	1000 μg/m²/d	Immunex	Increase hematopoietic precursors	18.8–52.9 min
Interleukin 4	0.25–5 μg/kg/d SC	Schering	Enhance immunity; induce apoptosis	8–48 min
Interleukin 10	1–25 μg/kg/d SC	Schering	Allow emigration of CD8+ cells; inhibit macrophages; prevent apoptosis some cells	60 min
Interleukin 11	Not reported	Genetics Institute	Increased platelet count; gut protection	Not reported
Interleukin 12	10–100 ng/kg/d SC, IV	Genetics Institute, Roche	Antiangiogenesis; enhance immunity	5–8 h
17-1A	100–500 mg	Centocor	Antibody-dependent cellular cytotoxicity	8–24 h
PIXY 321		Immunex	GM-CSF/IL-3 fusion; enhance myelopoiesis	
Transretinoic acid	45 mg/m²/d PO	Roche	Alone or with α-interferon for the treatment of various malignancies (acute promyelocytic leukemia)	4 h
13-cis-retinoic acid	1–3 mg/kg/d PO	Roche	Prevention of second malignancies in patients with previously diagnosed head and neck cancer	10–20 h
Stem cell factor	Not reported	Amgen	Promotes bone marrow reconstitution	Not reported

REFERENCES

1. Rubin JT: Interleukin-2: its biology and clinical application in patients with cancer. *Cancer Invest* 1993, 11:460–472.

2. Lotze MT: Biologic therapy with interleukin-2: preclinical studies. In *The Biologic Therapy of Cancer, edn 2.* Edited by DeVita V, Hellman S, Rosenberg S. Philadelphia: JB Lippincott, 1991:207–234.

3. Fyfe G, Fisher RI, Rosenberg SA, *et al.*: Results of treatment of 255 patients with metastatic renal cell carcinoma who received high-dose recombinant interleukin-2 therapy. *J Clin Oncol* 1995, 13:688–696.

4. Fisher RI, Rosenberg SA, Sznol M, *et al.*: High-dose aldesleukin in renal cell carcinoma: long-term survival update. *Cancer J Sci Am* 1997, 3:S70–S72.

5. Yang JC, Topalian SL, Parkinson D, *et al.*: Randomized comparison of high-dose and low-dose intravenous interleukin-2 for the therapy of metastatic renal cell carcinoma: an interim report. *J Clin Oncol* 1994, 12:1572–1576.

6. West WH, Tauer KW, Yanelli, JR, *et al.*: Constant-infusion recombinant interleukin-2 in adoptive immunotherapy of advanced cancer. *N Engl J Med* 1987, 316:898–905.

7. Palmer PA, Vinke J, Evers P, *et al.*: Continuous infusion of recombinant interleukin-2 with or without autologous lymphokine activated killer cells for the treatment of advanced renal cell carcinoma. *Eur J Cancer* 1992, 28A:1038–1044.

8. Gold PJ, Thompson JA, Markowitz DR: Metastatic renal cell carcinoma: long-term survival after therapy with high-dose continuous infusion interleukin-2. *Cancer J Sci Am* 1997, 3:S85–S91.

9. Vlasveld LT, Hekman A, Vyth-Dreese FA, *et al.*: A phase I study of prolonged continuous infusion of low dose recombinant interleukin-2 in melanoma and renal cell cancer, part II: immunological aspects. *Br J Cancer* 1993, 68:559–567.

10. Sleijfer DT, Janssen RA, Buter J, *et al.*: Phase II study of subcutaneous IL-2 in unselected patients with advanced renal cell cancer on an outpatient basis. *J Clin Oncol* 1992, 10:1119–1123.

11. Lissoni P, Barni S, Ardizzoia A, *et al.*: Prognostic factors of the clinical response to subcutaneous immunotherapy with interleukin-2 alone in patients with metastatic renal cell carcinoma. *Oncology* 1994, 51:59–62.

12. Dutcher JP, Atkins M, Fisher R, *et al.*: Interleukin-2-based therapy for metastatic renal cell cancer: the Cytokine Working Group experience, 1989-1997. *Cancer J Sci Am* 1997, 3:S73–S78.

13. Atzpodien J, Lopez JE, Kirchner H, *et al.*: Multi-institutional home therapy trial of recombinant human interleukin-2 and interferon a-2 in progressive metastatic renal cell carcinoma. *J Clin Oncol* 1995, 13:497–501.

14. Yang JC, Rosenberg SA: An ongoing prospective randomized comparison of interleukin-2 regimens for the treatment of metastatic renal cell carcinoma. *Cancer J Sci Am* 1997, 3:S79–S84.

15. Rosenberg SA, Yang JC, Topalian SL, *et al.*: Treatment of 283 consecutive patients with metastatic melanoma or renal cell cancer using high-dose bolus interleukin-2. *JAMA* 1994, 271:907–913.

16. Rosenberg SA: Keynote address: Perspectives on the use of interleukin-2 in cancer treatment. *Cancer J Sci Am* 1997, 3:S2–S6.

17. Legha SS, Gianan MA, Plager C, *et al.*: Evaluation of interleukin-2 administered by continuous infusion in patients with metastatic melanoma. *Cancer* 1996, 77:89–96.

18. Keilholz U, Scheibenbogen C, Tilgen W, *et al.*: Interferon-a and interleukin-2 in the treatment of metastatic melanoma: comparison of two phase II trials. *Cancer* 1993, 72:607–614.

19. Marincola FM, White DE, Wise AP, Rosenberg SA. Combination therapy with interferon a-2a and interleukin-2 for the treatment of metastatic cancer. *J Clin Oncol* 1995, 13:1110–1122.

20. Keilholz U, Scheibembogen C, Möhler T, *et al.*: Addition of dacarbazine or cisplatin to interferon-a/interleukin-2 in metastatic melanoma: toxicity and immunological effects. *Melanoma Res* 1995, 5:283–287.

21. Antoine EC, Benhammouda A, Bernard A, *et al.*: Salpêtrière hospital experience with biochemotherapy in metastatic melanoma. *Cancer J Sci Am* 1997, 3:S16–S21.

22. Keilholz U, Stoter G, Punt CJA, *et al.*: Recombinant interleukin-2-based treatments for advanced melanoma: the experience of the European Organization for Research and Treatment of Cancer Melanoma Cooperative Group. *Cancer J Sci Am* 1997, 3:S22–S28.

23. Thompson JA, Gold PJ, Markowitz DR, *et al.*: Updated analysis of an outpatient chemoimmunotherapy regimen for treating metastatic melanoma. *Cancer J Sci Am* 1997, 3:S29–S34.

24. Kovacs JA, Baseler M, Dewar RJ, *et al.*: Increases in CD4 T lymphocytes with intermittent courses of interleukin-2 in patients with human immunodeficiency virus infection. A preliminary study. *N Engl J Med* 1995, 332:567–575.

25. Holmlund JT, Kopp WC, Wiltrout RH, *et al.*: A phase I clinical trial of glavone-8-acetic acid in combination with interleukin-2. *J Natl Cancer Inst* 1995, 87:134–136.

26. Astoul P, Bertault-Peres P, Durand A, *et al.*: Pharmacokinetics of intrapleural recombinant interleukin-2 in immunotherapy for malignant pleural effusion. *Cancer* 1994, 73:308–313.

27. Fefer A: Interleukin-2 in the treatment of hematologic malignances. *Cancer J Sci Am* 1997, 3:S35–S36.

28. Mazumder A: Experimental evidence of interleukin-2 activity in bone marrow transplantation. *Cancer J Sci Am* 1997, 3:S37–S42.

29. Meloni G, Vignetti M, Pogliani E, *et al.*: Interleukin-2 therapy in relapsed acute myelogenous leukemia. *Cancer J Sci Am* 1997, 3:S43–S47.

30. Fefer A, Robinson N, Benyunes MC, *et al.*: Interleukin-2 therapy after bone marrow or stem cell transplantation for hematologic malignancies. *Cancer J Sci Am* 1997, 3:S48–S53.

31. van Besien K, Margolin K, Champlin R, *et al.*: Activity of interleukin-2 in non-Hodgkin's lymphoma following transplantation of interleukin-2-activated autologous bone marrow or stem cells. *Cancer J Sci Am* 1997, 3:S54–S58.

32. Slavin S, Nagler A: Cytokine-mediated immunotherapy following autologous bone marrow transplantation in lymphoma and evidence of interleukin-2-induced immunomodulation in allogeneic transplants. *Cancer J Sci Am* 1997, 3:S59–S67.

33. Schwartzentruber DJ: In vitro predictors of clinical response in patients receiving interleukin-2–based immunotherapy. *Curr Opin Oncol* 1993, 5:1055–1058.

34. Scharenberg JGM, Stam AGM, von Blomberg BME, *et al.*: The development of anti-interleukin-2 (IL-2) antibodies in cancer patients treated with recombinant IL-2. *Eur J Cancer* 1994, 30:1804–1809.

35. Pockaj BA, Yang JC, Lotze MT, *et al.*: A prospective randomized trial evaluating colloid versus crystalloid resuscitation in the treatment of the vascular leak syndrome associated with interleukin-2 therapy. *J Immunother* 1994, 15:22–28.

36. DeVita VT, Hellman S, Rosenberg SA: *The Biologic Therapy of Cancer.* Philadelphia: JB Lippincott, 1991.

37. Itri LM: The interferons. *Cancer* 1992, 70:940–945.

38. Wadler S: The role of interferons in the treatment of solid tumors. *Cancer* 1992, 70:949–958.

39. Wadler S, Schwartz EL: Principles in the biomodulation of cytotoxic drugs by interferons. *Semin Oncol* 1992, 19(suppl):45–48.

40. Kirkwood JM. Biologic therapy with interferon-α and J: clinical applications; melanoma. In *Biologic Therapy of Cancer, edn 2*. Edited by DeVita V, Hellman S, Rosenberg S. Philadelphia: JB Lippincott, 1995:388–410.

41. Kirkwood JM, Strawderman MH, Ernstoff MX, *et al*.: Interferon α-2B adjuvant therapy of high-risk resected cutaneous melanoma: the Eastern Cooperative Oncology Group Trial EST 1684. *J Clin Oncl*, 1996.

42. Cascinelli N, Bufalino R, Morabito A, MacKie R: Results of adjuvant interferon study in WHO melanoma programme. *Lancet* 1994, 343:913–914.

43. Cascinelli N: Evaluation of efficacy of adjuvant rIFNI 2A in melanoma patients with regional node metastases. *Proc ASCO* 1995, 14:410.

44. Andreyev HJN, Scott-Mackie P, Cunningham D, *et al*.: Phase II study of continuous infusion fluorouracil and interferon α-2b in the palliation of malignnanat neuroendocrine tumors. *J Clin Oncol* 1995, 13:1486–1492.

45. Kuzel TM, Roenigk HH, Samuelson E, *et al*.: Effectiveness of interferon α-2a combined with phototherapy for mycosis fungoides and the Sézary syndrome. *J Clin Oncol* 1995, 13:257–263.

46. Pryor K, Goddard J, Goldstein D, *et al*.: Bacillus Calmette-Guérin (BCG) enhances monocyte- and lymphocyte-mediated bladder tumour cell killing. *Br J Cancer* 1995, 71:801–7.

47. Lamm DL, Blumenstein BA, Crawford ED, *et al*.: A randomized trial of intravesical doxorubicin and immunotherapy with bacille Calmette-Guérin for transitional cell carcinoma of the bladder. *N Engl J Med* 1991, 325:1205–1210.

48. Janssen PAJ: Levamisole as an adjuvant in cancer treatment. *J Clin Pharmacol* 1991, 31:396–400.

49. Stevenson HC, Green I, Hamilton JM, *et al*.: Levamisole: known effects on the immune system, clinical results, and future applications to the treatment of cancer. *J Clin Oncol* 1991, 9:2052–2066.

50. Moertel CG, Fleming TR, MacDonald JS, et al: Levamisole and fluorouracil for adjuvant therapy of resected colon carcinoma. *N Engl J Med* 1990, 322:352–358.

51. Moertel CG, Fleming TR, Macdonald JS, *et al*.: Fluorouracil plus levamisole as effective adjuvant therapy after resection of stage III colon carcinoma: a final report. *Ann Int Med* 1995, 122:321–326.

52. Schiller JH, Witt PL: Levamisole: clinical and biological effects. *Biol Ther Cancer Updates* 1992, 2:1–14.

53. Crosier PS, Clark SC: Basic biology of the hematopoietic growth factors. *Semin Oncol* 1992, 19:349–361.

54. Brugger W, Rosenthal FM, Kanz L, *et al*.: Clinical role of colony stimulating factors. *Acta Haematol* 1991, 86:138–147.

55. St. Onge J, Jacobson RJ: The role of hematopoietic growth factors in the treatment of neoplastic diseases. *Semin Hematol* 1992, 29(suppl):53–63.

56. Spivak JL: The application of recombinant erythropoietin in anemic patients with cancer. *Semin Oncol* 1992, 19(suppl):25–28.

57. Erslev AJ: The therapeutic role of recombinant erythropoietin in anemic patients with intact endogenous production of erythropoietin. *Semin Oncol* 1992, 19(suppl):14–18.

58. Henry DH, Brooks BJ Jr, Case DC, *et al*.: Recombinant human erythropoietin therapy for anemic cancer patients receiving cisplatin chemotherapy. *Cancer J Sci Am* 1995, 1:252–260.

59. Welch RS, James RD, Wilkinson PM, *et al*.: Recombinant human erythropoietin and platinum-based chemotherapy in advanced ovarian cancer. *Cancer J Sci Am* 1995, 1:261–266.

60. Glaspy JA, Golde DW: Granulocyte colony-stimulating factor (G-CSF): preclinical and clinical studies. *Semin Oncol* 1992, 19:386–394.

61. Gabrilove JL: Granulocyte colony-stimulating factor and granulocyte-macrophage colony-stimulating factor in chemotherapy. *Biol Ther Cancer Updates* 1992, 2:1–11.

62. Demetri GD, Antman KHS: Granulocyte-macrophage colony-stimulating factor (GM-CSF): preclinical and clinical investigations. *Semin Oncol* 1992, 19:362–385.

63. Neidhart JA: Hematopoietic colony-stimulating factors. Uses in combination with standard chemotherapeutic regimens and in support of dose intensification. *Cancer* 1992, 70:913–920.

64. Quesenberry PJ: Biomodulation of chemotherapy-induced myelosuppression. *Semin Oncol* 1992, 19(suppl):8–13.

65. Bunn P, Crowley J, Kelly K, *et al*.: Chemoradiotherapy with or without granulocyte-macrophage colony-stimulating factor in the treatment of limited-stage small-cell lung cancer: a prospective Phase III randomized study of the Southwest Oncology Group. *J Clin Oncol* 1995, 13:1632–1641.

66. Rowe JM, Anderson JW, Mazza JJ, *et al*.: A randomized placebo-controlled phase III study of granulocyte-macrophage colony-stimulating factor in adult patients (> 55 to 70 years of age) with acute myelogenous leukemia: a study of the Eastern Cooperative Oncology Group (E1490). *Blood* 1995, 86:457–462.

67. Broxmeyer HE, Benninger L, Patel S, *et al*.: Kinetic response of human marrow myeloid progenitor cell to in vivo treatment of patients with granulocyte colony-stimulating factor is different from the response to treatment with granulocyte-macrophage colony-stimulating factor. *Exp Hematol* 1994, 22:100–106.

68. Grem JL, McAtee N, Murphy R, *et al*.: Phase I and pharmacokinetic study of recombinant human granulocyte-macrophage colony-stimulating factor given in combination with fluorouracil plus calcium leucovorin in metastatic gastrointestinal adenocarcinoma. *J Clin Oncol* 1994, 12:560–568.

69. Evers MB, Parekh D, Townsend CM, *et al*.: Somatostatin and analogues in the treatment of cancer. *Ann Surg* 1991, 213:190–198.

70. Parmar H, Bogden A, Mollard M, *et al*.: Somatostatin and somatostatin analogues in oncology. *Cancer Treat Rev* 1989, 16:95–115.

71. Smith MA, Parkinson DR, Cheson BD, *et al*.: Retinoids in cancer therapy. *J Clin Oncol* 1992, 10:839–864.

72. Hofmann SL: Retinoids—differentiation agents for cancer treatment and prevention. *Am J Med Sci* 1992, 304:202–213.

73. Greenberg ER, Baron JA, Stukel TA: A clinical trial of beta carotene to prevent basal-cell and squamous-cell cancers of the skin. *N Engl J Med* 1990, 323:189–195.

74. Tangrea JA, Edwards BK, Taylor PR: Long-term therapy with low-dose isoretinoin for prevention of basal cell carcinoma: a multicenter clinical trial. *J Natl Cancer Inst* 1992, 84:328–332.

75. Holdener EE, Bollag W: Retinoids. *Curr Opin Oncol* 1993, 5:1059–1066.

76. Lotze MT: Role of IL-4 in the antitumor response in H. In *Interleukin-4*. Edited by Spits. New York: Raven Press, 1992:237–262.

77. Weber J, Gunn H, Yang J, *et al*.: A phase I trial of intravenous interleukin-6 in patients with advanced cancer. *J Immunother* 1994, 15:292–302.

78. Zeh HJ, Tahara H, Lotze MT: Interleukin-12. In *Cytokine Handbook*. Edited by Thomsom A. London: Academic Press; 1994:342–371.

79. Nastala CL, Edington H, Storkus W, *et al*.: Recombinant interleukin-12 induces tumor regression in murine models: interferon-γ but not nitric oxide dependent effects. *J Immunol* 1994, 153:1697–1706.

80. Kurzrock R, Talpaz M, Estrov Z, *et al*. Phase I study of recombinant interleukin-3 in patients with bone marrow failure. *J Clin Oncol* 1991, 9:1241–1250.

81. Riethmüller G, Schneider-Gödicke E, Schlimok G, *et al*.: Randomized trial of monoclonal antibody for adjuvant therapy of resected Duke's C colorectal carcinoma. *Lancet* 1994, 343:117–83.

ALDESLEUKIN

Aldesleukin is a highly purified lymphokine produced by genetically engineered *E. coli*. It differs from native IL-2 in that it is not glycosylated, it does not have an N-terminal alanine, and cysteine 125 has been replaced by serine. Aldesleukin possesses the same immunoregulatory capacity as natural IL-2. Some of its effects include T-cell and NK cell activation, the generation of LAK activity, and induction of interferon γ production by macrophages.

The systemic administration of IL-2 to patients with selected malignancies has been associated with tumor regression. IL-2 is potentially active against renal cell carcinoma and metastatic melanoma, with response rates of ~20% [3–23]. Its use with adoptively transferred lymphocytes, chemotherapeutics, other cytokines, and other biologic agents is under investigation.

SPECIAL PRECAUTIONS

Patients should be evaluated carefully for significant cardiac, pulmonary, hepatic, or renal dysfunction prior to therapy. Patients with these impairments are at a very high risk of treatment-limiting morbidity and mortality at the recommended dose of IL-2.

Patients with untreated brain metastases should not receive IL-2 owing to the early onset of treatment-related central nervous system (CNS) toxicity.

Preexisting infection should be adequately treated prior to therapy.

Reversible renal and hepatic dysfunction is commonly associated with therapy. Concomitant medications should be used with caution.

The effect of IL-2 on fertility is not known. There is no meaningful experience with the use of IL-2 in pregnant women.

IL-2 should be used with caution in patients with gastrointestinal or genitourinary tract bleeding because of the risk of treatment-related thrombocytopenia.

Patients whose tumors encroach on the spinal canal are at risk of spinal cord injury due to IL-2-induced swelling of the tumor.

Patients should not be retreated with IL-2 if they suffered angina or myocardial infarction during initial treatment.

Enhanced cellular immune function may increase the risk of allograft rejection in transplant recipients treated with IL-2.

INDICATIONS

FDA-approved: metastatic renal cell carcinoma and metastatic malignant melanoma; clinical studies show that activity in response rates among patients with metastatic renal cell carcinoma and metastatic melanoma are ~20%; responses also have been observed in patients with non-Hodgkin's lymphoma and colorectal carcinoma

PHARMACOKINETICS

Following a short IV infusion, IL-2 rapidly distributes to the extravascular space with preferential uptake by the liver, kidneys, and lungs; very little IL-2 penetrates the CNS; the serum distribution and elimination half-life are 13 min and 85 min, respectively; IL-2 is cleared from the circulation by glomerular filtration and peritubular extraction; it is metabolized in the cells of the proximal renal tubules with very little bioactive protein appearing in the urine; the mean clearance rate, about 270 mL/min, is not affected by rising serum creatinine

DRUG INTERACTIONS

IL-2 may cause reversible hepatic and renal dysfunction; drugs that are metabolized by either of these routes may require modification of their dosage during IL-2 therapy; for the same reason, nephrotoxic and hepatotoxic drugs should be used with caution; IL-2 has been used concomitantly with TNF, IFN α, cyclophosphamide, IL-4, radiation therapy, LAK cells, and tumor infiltrating lymphocytes (TILs) to enhance its efficacy. There is no proven benefit to the use of IL-2 in combination with any of these agents over IL-2 alone

RESPONSE RATES

~20% of patients with metastatic renal cell carcinoma who have a good performance status (ECOG 0-1) manifest a partial or complete response to IL-2 therapy; among patients with metastatic melanoma, about 20% of patients respond to therapy; complete responses are durable and may last as long as several years

PATIENT MONITORING

IL-2 must be administered in a hospital where patients can be monitored closely for the development of toxicity; this requires vital signs immediately before each dose and then every 4 h afterward or more frequently depending on the clinical status of the patient; hypotension, tachycardia, and cardiac dysrhythmias are frequent complications of treatment; urine output must be measured and recorded accurately because of the high incidence of oliguria; oxygen saturation should be checked if the patient develops symptoms of hypoxemia; daily or more frequent physical examinations are important to assess patients for capillary leak syndrome, organ hypoperfusion, CNS toxicity, sepsis, pulmonary edema, and stomatitis; blood should be collected at least daily to evaluate renal function, hepatic function, serum magnesium, phosphorus, calcium, electrolytes, CPK, and blood counts; the clinical suspicion of hypothyroidism after therapy should prompt a biochemical evaluation of thyroid function; patients should be transferred to a setting in which they can be closely monitored if they develop hypoxemia, disorientation, or hypotension and oliguria that requires the use of vasopressors

ALDESLEUKIN (Continued)

TOXICITIES

Cardiovascular: both ventricular and supraventricular dysrhythmias have been associated with the use of IL-2. Myocardial infarction has been seen in ~2% of treated patients. Myocarditis also has been described. Hypotension frequently is seen in treated patients and is thought to be due to a capillary leak syndrome

Pulmonary: noncardiogenic pulmonary edema thought to be secondary to a capillary leak syndrome has been observed in most patients. This is accompanied by dyspnea in about 50% of patients and, rarely, reversible respiratory failure. The capillary leak syndrome also may contribute to the development of ascites and pleural effusions that can contribute to shortness of breath

Renal: reversible oliguria occurs in the majority of treated patients and is accompanied by elevations of BUN and creatinine; ~1% of patients require dialysis until their renal function improves

CNS: mental status changes occur in few patients, although the contribution of concomitantly administered psychotropic drugs is unclear; subtle disorientation or impaired cognitive function may precede more profound CNS impairment. This may lead to coma

Dermatologic: pruritus occurs in as many as 50% of patients. Exfoliative dermatitis may occur following treatment; dry skin may be a persistent problem for about 10% of treated patients; hair loss also has been observed

GI: nausea, vomiting, and diarrhea occur in most patients. Stomatitis occurs less frequently; patients rarely may suffer life-threatening intestinal perforation, which requires emergency surgical repair

Musculoskeletal: fewer than 50% of treated patients develop reversible arthralgia and myalgia

Hematologic: anemia, thrombocytopenia, leukopenia, and eosinophilia are common during treatment; rebound lymphocytosis frequently is seen after cessation of IL-2; impaired neutrophil function is associated with an increased incidence of central venous catheter–associated *Staphylococcus aureus* infection

Capillary leak syndrome: this is seen in nearly all treated patients. It is, in part, responsible for hypotension and decreased organ profusion that often occurs. It also is responsible for the development of noncardiogenic pulmonary edema, ascites, pleural effusions, and anasarca.

Miscellaneous: fever and rigors commonly are seen 1–2 h after a dose of IL-2; ~10% of treated patients develop hypothyroidism. Frequent laboratory abnormalities include hypophosphatemia, hypomagnesemia, metabolic acidosis, hepatic transaminasemia, and hyperbilirubinemia.

DOSAGE AND ADMINISTRATION

A dose of 600,000 IU/kg (0.037 mg/kg) is administered intravenously over 15 min every 8 h; each course of therapy consists of 2 cycles, neither one exceeding 14 doses, and administered 7–10 d apart; decisions to withhold doses or terminate a cycle of treatment are made based on the clinical status of the patient; the median number of doses is 20 out of a possible 28; patients who manifest evidence of tumor regression 2 mo after treatment should be retreated if there are no contraindications

NURSING INTERVENTIONS

Dose-limiting toxicities often can be controlled if treated early; patients should be evaluated frequently for nausea, vomiting, diarrhea, and stomatitis; patients should be encouraged to use bicarbonate mouthwash regularly; regular doses of antiemetics and antidiarrheal medications should be initiated coincident with the onset of these toxicities; patients should be evaluated for the onset of rigors 1–2 h after each dose of IL-2; symptomatic treatment includes warm blankets and intravenous meperidine; vital signs and urine output should be monitored closely owing to the frequent occurrence of hypotension, dysrhythmias, and oliguria; a Foley catheter should be placed to accurately monitor urine output, if necessary; patients' mental status should be evaluated regularly; central venous lines should be dressed according to standard protocols; the skin entry site should be monitored for evidence of infection at the time of dressing changes and coincident with the onset of fevers that are not temporally related to doses of IL-2; pruritus is common and can be controlled with diphenhydramine or hydroxyzine

PATIENT INFORMATION

IL-2 may sensitize the skin to solar radiation; patients should be warned to avoid direct sunlight or to wear sunscreen, a hat, long-sleeved shirts, and long pants; patients should refrain from driving until fully recovered; symptoms of hypothyroidism should be reported if they occur; patients should be instructed to use emollients to manage dry skin

PREPARATION AND STORAGE

Each vial contains 22×10^6 IU (1.3 mg) of lyophilized IL-2 with dodecyl sulfate as a solubilizing agent; the contents of each vial should be reconstituted with 1.2 mL of preservative-free, sterile water for injection; when adding the water, it should be directed toward the side of the vial and mix by swirling, not shaking to avoid creating foam; reconstituted in this fashion, each milliliter contains 18×10^6 IU of IL-2; the dose of IL-2 should be diluted with 50 mL of 5% dextrose for injection in a plastic IV administration bag; vials are for single use only; unopened vials and reconstituted drug should be stored at 2°–8°C; once reconstituted, IL-2 should be administered within 48 h

FORMULATIONS

IL-2 is marketed as Proleukin by Cetus Corporation.

BACILLUS CALMETTE-GUÉRIN

Bacillus Calmette-Guérin is a live, attenuated strain of *M. bovis* that has demonstrated efficacy in the treatment of primary or recurrent in situ carcinoma of the urinary bladder. The mechanism of this therapeutic effect is unknown but it is thought to be immune mediated.

SPECIAL PRECAUTIONS

Immunosuppressed patients are at risk of developing systemic mycobacterial sepsis. Patients with ongoing infection should not be treated until the infection is adequately treated.

Urinary tract infection increases the risk of developing disseminated mycobacterial infection and is associated with increased severity of bladder irritation.

Bacillus Calmette-Guérin may sensitize patients to mycobacteria, leading to false-positive PPD reactivity. It may be useful to skin test patients prior to initiating therapy.

Patients with small bladder capacity are at increased risk of developing severe local inflammatory reactions to bacillus Calmette-Guérin.

It is not known whether bacillus Calmette-Guérin causes fetal harm or is excreted in breast milk.

Patients in whom bladder catheterization was traumatic should have their treatment deferred for 1–2 wk. Similarly, treatments should be delayed 1–2 wk following transurethral resection of bladder tumors.

TOXICITY

Genitourinary: Dysuria, urinary frequency, hematuria, and urinary urgency may occur in as many as 40% of treated patients. Severe reactions occur less frequently. Most bladder toxicity occurs after the third installation, begins within 2 to 4 hours of therapy, and persists for only 1–3 d. Less frequent side effects include bladder cramps, nocturia, passage of urinary debris, and urethritis.
Gastrointestinal: Nausea, vomiting, diarrhea, anorexia, and mild abdominal pain may develop in few treated patients.
Systemic: Systemic side effects are common and include fever, malaise, and chills. These symptoms usually resolve within 3 d.
Miscellaneous: Less frequent side effects include anemia, neutropenia, allergic reactions, systemic infection, hepatitis, and hepatic granuloma.

INDICATIONS

FDA-approved: primary and relapsed carcinoma in situ of the urinary bladder

DRUG INTERACTIONS

Immunosuppressive or myelosuppressive drugs or radiation therapy may abrogate the response to bacillus Calmette-Guérin or may predispose treated patients to the development of disseminated bacillus Calmette-Guérin infection

RESPONSE RATES

In one study, a complete response rate of 75% was reported. Median time to treatment failure was 48 m, and median time to death was 2 y; in another study, 75% of treated patients manifested a complete clinical response; after a median follow-up of 4 y, about 40% of them had relapsed and 13% had died of other diseases; two of the former patients responded to another course of treatment

PATIENT MONITORING

Patients should be monitored for symptoms of systemic bacillus Calmette-Guérin infection, including fever greater than 39°C, fever greater than 38°C that lasts 2 or more days, severe malaise, and cough; fever, chills, and malaise also may represent hypersensitivity reactions, which may respond to antihistamines; patients should also be monitored for the development of bladder inflammation which can be managed with phenazopyridine, propantheline, or oxybutynin; irritative bladder symptoms may also indicate urinary tract infection, which should be ruled out

NURSING INTERVENTIONS

Bacillus Calmette-Guérin contains a viable, attenuated mycobacteria and should be handled as infectious; all material that comes into contact with bacillus Calmette-Guérin should be placed into plastic bags that have been labeled "Infectious Waste" and disposed of accordingly; urine voided within 6 h of treatment should be disinfected with approximately equal volumes of undiluted household bleach for 15 min before flushing; bacillus Calmette-Guérin should not be handled by immunocompromised people; health-care personnel should consider wearing gown and gloves while handling bacillus Calmette-Guérin; nurses should closely monitor patients for symptoms of bladder irritation, urinary tract infection, and systemic bacillus Calmette-Guérin infection, which would include fever and cough

BACILLUS CALMETTE-GUÉRIN (Continued)

DOSAGE AND ADMINISTRATION

Therapy should begin 7–14 d after bladder biopsy or transurethral resection of bladder tumors. One of several published protocols follows [25]. A bladder catheter should be placed in sterile fashion. Reconstituted bacillus Calmette-Guérin should be instilled slowly by gravity after the bladder has been drained of all urine. The catheter should then be withdrawn and the patient assisted in lying for 15 min in each of 4 positions: prone, supine, right side down, and left side down. The patient should try to delay voiding for another hour while up and about. After no more than 2 h, the patient should empty the bladder while seated. Treatment should be delayed at least 1 wk if bladder catheterization is thought to have been traumatic.

Thera-Cys: The contents of 3 vials (27 mg/vial) reconstituted with the diluent provided and further diluted with 50 mL of sterile, preservative-free saline (53 mL total) are administered for each treatment. This dose should be repeated at 3, 6, 12, 18, and 24 mo.

TICE bacillus Calmette-Guérin: One ampule (50 mg) suspended in 50 mL of sterile, preservative-free saline, should be instilled weekly for 6 wk and then monthly for 6 to 12 mo.

PATIENT INFORMATION

Patients should be instructed to report signs or symptoms of systemic bacillus Calmette-Guérin infection and bladder irritation; women should avoid becoming pregnant while being treated; patients should be instructed to disinfect all urine voided within 6 h of treatment

PREPARATION AND STORAGE

Bacillus Calmette-Guérin and its diluent should be protected from light and stored at temperatures between 2° and 8°C; bacillus Calmette-Guérin should be administered within 2 h of reconstitution. Thera-Cys (Connaught) is available in vials containing 27 mg ($3.4 \pm 3 \times 10^8$ CFU/vial); bacillus Calmette-Guérin should be reconstituted with the accompanying diluent (1 mL/vial); the contents of 3 vials reconstituted in 3 mL are further diluted with 50 mL of sterile, preservative-free saline prior to administration

TICE bacillus Calmette-Guérin (Organon) is available in 2-mL ampules containing 50 mg ($1–8 \times 10^6$ CFU); the contents of one ampule should be reconstituted with 1 mL of sterile, preservative-free saline and then suspended in an additional 49 mL

FORMULATIONS

TICE bacillus Calmette-Guérin is marketed by Organon; Thera-cys is marketed by Connaught; both are freeze-dried suspensions of bacillus Calmette-Guérin.

LEVAMISOLE

Levamisole originally was developed as an anthelminthic agent. This effect is mediated by its inhibition of a helminth-specific electron transport system. Levamisole exerts anticholinergic and immunomodulatory activity in humans. Effects on the immune system include enhanced T-cell activation and proliferation, augmented macrophage activity, increased neutrophil chemotaxis, and enhanced antibody formation. Two clinical trials have demonstrated a statistically significant prolongation of disease-free and overall survival among patients who were treated with adjuvant levamisole and 5-FU following resection of Duke's C colon carcinoma. The mechanism of this effect is unknown, and the results of these studies have been questioned owing to the omission of an 5-FU control group.

SPECIAL PRECAUTIONS

Levamisole has been associated with increased plasma levels of phenytoin. Epileptics treated with this drug should have their phenytoin levels closely monitored. The safety of levamisole in pregnant or nursing women has not been established.

TOXICITY

Hematologic: agranulocytosis, which is usually reversible following discontinuation of treatment, has rarely been reported; neutropenia, thrombocytopenia, and anemia occur frequently in patients treated with both levamisole and 5-FU; almost all patients treated with levamisole and 5-FU experience toxicity that is otherwise associated with 5-FU alone
Dermatologic: rashes occur in ~2% of treated patients
Musculoskeletal: myalgia and arthralgia occur in 2% of treated patients
Genitourinary: renal failure is a rare complication of treatment
CNS: these toxicities are rare and include confusion, convulsions, hallucinations, impaired concentration, and an encaphalopathic syndrome
Miscellaneous: a flu-like syndrome may accompany the onset of agranulocytosis

DOSAGE AND ADMINISTRATION

Treatment with levamisole should begin within 7–30 d of surgery, as follows [25]. Levamisole, 50 mg, should be administered orally every 8 h for 3 d. This should be repeated every 14 d. 5-FU should be started concomitantly with a cycle of levamisole between 21–35 d postoperatively. 5-FU should be administered at a dose of 450 mg/m^2/d by rapid IV bolus daily for 5 d. This should be followed after 28 d by weekly doses of 5-FU, 450 mg/m^2/week. Therapy should be continued for 1 y. If mild stomatitis or diarrhea develop during weekly treatment, the next dose of 5-FU should be deferred until these toxicities resolve. If they are moderate to severe, the dose of 5-FU should be reduced by 20% when it is resumed. Other dose modifications of 5-FU should be made according to established protocols. Otherwise the following set of guidelines may be followed:

If WBC = 2, 500–3500/mm^3, defer 5-FU until WBC > 33,500/mm^3

If WBC < 2500/mm^3, defer 5-FU until WBC > 33,500/mm^3; resume at 80% of the dose if WBC < 2500/mm^3 for ≥10 d, discontinue levamisole

If platelet < 100,000, defer both drugs

INDICATIONS

FDA-approved: use in combination with 5-FU for adjuvant treatment of Duke's C colon cancer following surgical resection

PHARMACOKINETICS

Rapidly absorbed from the GI tract after oral administration; extensively metabolized in the liver, and the metabolites are excreted mainly by the kidneys (70% over 3 d) with lesser amounts appearing in the stool; 5% of the drug appears unchanged in the urine; plasma elimination half-life is 3–4 h; the effect of 5-FU on the pharmacokinetics of levamisole and use in patients with hepatic insufficiency have not been studied

DRUG INTERACTIONS

When used with alcoholic beverages, levamisole may induce a disulfuran-like reaction; coadministration of levamisole and 5-FU has led to an elevation of blood phenytoin levels

RESPONSE RATES

Use of adjuvant levamisole and 5-FU in patients with Duke's C colon cancer has been associated with about a 30% reduction in recurrence rate and death rate; the significance of these results has been questioned in light of the absence of a 5-FU control arm

PATIENT MONITORING

Patients should have a baseline CBC with differential and platelet count, serum electrolytes, and liver function tests performed; perform weekly CBC with differential and platelet count prior to each dose of 5-FU; monitor electrolytes and liver function studies monthly; monitor for mucositis and diarrhea, and modify the dose of 5-FU accordingly; phenytoin levels should be evaluated regularly in patients who take this medication

NURSING INTERVENTIONS

Treatment tolerance, weight, and nutrition should be monitored; patients should be instructed regarding oral hygiene; stomatitis may be managed with a variety of preparations, including combinations of Benadryl, a magnesium-based preparation, and viscous lidocaine; oral candidiasis should be ruled out; diarrhea should be treated aggressively, particularly in the aged; hospitalization may be required

PATIENT INFORMATION

Patients should be instructed to immediately report flu-like symptoms; the use of alcohol should be avoided; women should be advised not to become pregnant; nursing should be discontinued

PREPARATION AND STORAGE

Levamisole is available as 50-mg tablets; these should be stored at room temperature

FORMULATIONS

Levamisole is marketed as Ergamisol by Janssen.

FILGRASTIM

Granulocyte colony-stimulating factor (G-CSF) is a 174 amino acid glycoprotein that serves as an obligate factor in maintaining adequate numbers of circulating polymorphonuclear leukocytes (PMN). It targets granulocyte precursors, which are induced to proliferate when G-CSF binds to its cell-surface receptor. PMN chemotaxis, phagocytosis, and intracellular killing through enhanced generation of reactive oxygen intermediates also are augmented.

Filgrastim is the recombinant glycoprotein that has been expressed in *E. coli* containing the human gene. It is well tolerated and has been shown to be of benefit in the setting of chemotherapy-induced neutropenia. Its use after myelosuppressive chemotherapy has been associated with decreases in duration of neutropenia, frequency of infection, incidence of neutropenic fever, and use of antibiotics. Because receptors for G-CSF have been found on small cell lung carcinoma lines, there is a risk that filgrastim may serve as a growth factor for this and other solid tumors. No clinically evident tumor progression has been noted, however.

SPECIAL PRECAUTIONS

Patients with atherosclerotic cardiovascular disease may be at slightly greater risk of myocardial infarction when treated with filgrastim.

Septic patients are at risk of developing adult respiratory distress syndrome due to the pulmonary sequestration of PMN.

The safety of filgrastim in pregnant or nursing women has not been established.

The possibility that filgrastim could serve as a growth factor for any tumor type, particularly myeloid malignancies, has not been excluded unequivocally.

TOXICITY

Hematologic: there is a small risk of excessive leukocytosis (WBC > 100,000/mm^3) associated with therapeutic doses of filgrastim
Cardiovascular: transient decreases in blood pressure rarely may be observed
Musculoskeletal: mild to moderate medullary bone pain may be associated with therapy
Reticuloendothelial: clinically evident splenomegaly has been noted in 3% of patients who are treated chronically with filgrastim
Dermatologic: preexisting inflammatory conditions, such as eczema or vasculitis, may be exacerbated by therapy
Miscellaneous: reversible, mild elevations of LDH and alkaline phosphatase have been noted

DOSAGE AND ADMINISTRATION

Filgrastim should not be administered during or within 24 h of chemotherapy; a dose of 5 μg/kg/d should be administered as a daily SC or IV injection [25]; the former route may be more effective; doses may be increased incrementally by 5 μg/kg for each chemotherapy cycle depending on the response during the previous cycle; treatment should be continued until the WBC reaches 10,000/mm^3 after the chemotherapy-induced nadir; the duration of therapy will depend on the severity of myelotoxicity; one must be careful to avoid premature termination of treatment based on a frequently observed initial increase in WBC that is due to the release of WBC stores

INDICATIONS

FDA-approved: patients with nonmyeloid malignancies who have severe neutropenia as a consequence of myelosuppressive anticancer drugs

PHARMACOKINETICS

Peak plasma levels of filgrastim are attained within 2–8 h of SC injection; the elimination half-life is about 3.5 h; half-lives are similar for SC or IV administration

DRUG INTERACTIONS

There is a risk that filgrastim could sensitize myeloid progenitors to the toxic effects of chemotherapy by increasing the rate of their proliferation

PATIENT MONITORING

The WBC should be evaluated twice weekly to avoid excessive leukocytosis and assess response to therapy; treatment should be stopped when the WBC reaches 10,000/mm^3 following the expected chemotherapy-induced WBC nadir; platelet counts also should be monitored to not overlook concomitant effects of chemotherapy

NURSING INTERVENTIONS

Patients who can be treated at home require training in the self-administration of filgrastim; they should be instructed in the safe disposal of needles, drug vials, and syringes after each dose

PATIENT INFORMATION

Patients may experience mild bone pain that can be managed with acetaminophen; patients should avoid using aspirin and nonsteroidal antiinflammatory drugs because thrombocytopenia may accompany chemotherapy; patients should be instructed to discard unused drug and used needles and syringes after each dose

PREPARATION AND STORAGE

Filgrastim is available at a concentration of 300 μg/mL in 1 mL and 1.6 mL single-dose vials; the formulation also contains acetate, mannitol, Tween, and sodium; vials should be stored at 2°–8°C and warmed to room temperature for no more than 6 h prior to use; unused drug and drug left at room temperature for more than 6 h should be discarded; vials should not be agitated

FORMULATIONS

Filgrastim is marketed as Neupogen by Amgen.

SARGRAMOSTIM

Sargramostim is a 127 amino acid recombinant, human granulocyte macrophage-stimulating factor (GM-CSF) that is produced in a yeast expression system. It differs from the natural glycoprotein by the substitution of leucine at amino acid position 23. The carbohydrate moiety also may differ. Sargramostim affects progenitors of multiple lineages, including granulocytes, monocytes, eosinophils, megakaryocytes, and erythrocytes. Its effect on these immature cells requires other CFSs, including erythropoietin. Sargramostim's greatest effect is on lineage-committed granulocyte and monocyte precursors. In addition to increasing the number of circulating PMN and monocytes, it enhances their function.

SPECIAL PRECAUTIONS

Patients with a history of cardiac disease are at slightly increased risk of developing supraventricular dysrhythmias. Dyspnea may occur during infusion of sargramostim. This is thought to be secondary to pulmonary sequestration of granulocytes; therefore, patients with preexisting hypoxemic lung disease should be treated with caution. Treatment may be associated with fluid retention that could exacerbate preexisting pericardial effusion, plural effusion, or congestive heart failure. Sargramostim may exacerbate preexisting hepatic or renal dysfunction. The safety of this drug in pregnant or nursing women has not been established. Use of sargramostim in patients with acute myelocytic leukemia and myelodysplastic syndrome is not recommended due to the risk that it may serve as a growth factor for abnormal myeloid cells. Sargramostim should not be administered within 24 hours of chemotherapy or within 12 hours of radiation therapy. Their concomitant use also is proscribed. The effect of sargramostim on myeloid reconstitution after bone marrow transplantation may be blunted in patients who have previously been treated with intensive chemotherapy or radiation therapy. Patients with excessive myeloid blasts in the bone marrow or peripheral blood (> 10%) should not be treated.

TOXICITY

Cardiovascular: patients with preexisting heart disease are at risk for the development of supraventricular tachydysrhythmias. These tend to be transient. Fluid retention may exacerbate congestive heart failure and pericardial effusion. Hypotension, flushing, and syncope have been associated with the first dose of sargramostim.
Respiratory: dyspnea may occur as a result of the pulmonary sequestration of granulocytes; this may exacerbate preexisting lung disease.
Immunologic: ~3% of treated patients will develop neutralizing antibodies to sargramostim; the effect this has on hematopoiesis is unknown
Renal: preexisting renal disease may be exacerbated
Hepatic: preexisting liver disease may be exacerbated
Hematologic: reversible thrombocytosis and leukocytosis have occurred
Musculoskeletal: medullary bone pain of mild to moderate severity may be experienced
Gastrointestinal: patient may experience diarrhea
Miscellaneous: a flu-like syndrome may occur, which is characterized by headache, asthenia, fever, and myalgia

DOSAGE AND ADMINISTRATION

Myeloid reconstitution after autologous bone marrow transplantation [25]: 250 µg/m²/d administered as a single, daily 2-h IV infusion for 21 d. Begin treatment 2–4 h after marrow infusion but no less than 24 h after chemotherapy or 12 h after radiation therapy.

Bone marrow transplant failure or engraftment delay [25]: 250 µg/m²/d administered as a single, daily 2-h IV infusion for 14 d. Repeat after 7 d if engraftment has not occurred. A third 14-d course of treatment, 500 µg/m², can be given after 7 d if engraftment still has not occurred. Further therapy, however, would not be useful.

In both case the drug should be discontinued if blast cells appear or disease progression occurs. If severe drug reactions occur, the dose may be decreased or delayed until the reaction abates.

INDICATIONS

FDA-approved: Myeloid reconstitution after autologous bone marrow transplantation, bone marrow transplantation failure, or bone marrow transplant engraftment delay; **Off-label:** myelodysplastic syndrome; HIV-positive patients treated with zidovudine; to decrease the nadir of leukopenia secondary to chemotherapy; to decrease myelosuppression in preleukemic patients; to correct neutropenia in patients with aplastic anemia; and to treat neutropenia in recipients of organ transplants in order to reduce the incidence of damage to the transplanted organ

PHARMACOKINETICS

The serum concentration approaches 23,000 pg/mL after a dose of 250 µg/m² given by a 2-h IV infusion; the α half-life is about 15 min; the β half-life is about 2 h; absorption is good after SC administration with peak serum levels observed about 2 h after injection

DRUG INTERACTIONS

Lithium and corticosteroids may potentiate the myeloproliferative effects of sargramostim

PATIENT MONITORING

To avoid complications of excessive leukocytosis, CBCs should be performed twice weekly; patients with preexisting renal or hepatic dysfunction should have twice weekly evaluation of renal and hepatic function

NURSING INTERVENTIONS

The flu-like syndrome associated with treatment may be more tolerable if sargramostim is administered in the evening; acetaminophen, given concomitantly, also may be helpful; monitor for evidence of adverse reactions, including flushing, dyspnea, and hypotension

PATIENT INFORMATION

Patients should report signs of fluid retention, including weight gain and edema; patients with preexisting heart or lung disease should be particularly wary of this side effect

PREPARATION AND STORAGE

Sargramostim is available in single-dose vials containing either 250 µg or 500 µg of preservative-free, lyophilized recombinant GM-CSF; this should be reconstituted with 1 mL of preservative-free sterile water for injection; unused drug should be discarded; during reconstitution, the sterile water should be directed at the side of the vial, and the solution should be swirled, not shaken, to avoid foaming; the final dilution should be made with 0.9% sodium chloride for injection if the final concentration is < 10 µg/mL, the final dilution should be made with 0.1% human albumin in sodium chloride; an in-line membrane filter should not be used when infusing the drug; sargramostim should be administered as soon as possible within 6 h of reconstitution; unopened vials and reconstituted drug should be stored at 2°–8°C

FORMULATIONS

Sargramostim is marketed as Leukine (Immunex) and Prokine (Hoechst-Roussel).

EPOETIN α (ERYTHROPOIETIN, EPO)

Erythropoietin is a 166 amino acid glycoprotein that is an obligatory growth factor for erythroid progenitors. It is produced predominantly by the kidney in response to decreased tissue oxygen tension as sensed by a heme-like protein in the renal tubules. The recombinant product is made by gene-modified mammalian cells that contain the human gene.

The anemia associated with cancer is thought to be due in part to a blunted response to erythropoietin. This can be overcome to some extent by administering epoetin α, although it is unclear whether transfusion requirements or quality of life are significantly affected.

SPECIAL PRECAUTIONS

Patients with uncontrolled hypertension should not be treated until their blood pressure is well controlled
Patients with preexisting vascular disease may be at increased risk of thrombotic events
Epoetin α may exacerbate preexisting porphyria
The safe use of epoetin α in pregnant or nursing women has not been established

TOXICITY

Epoetin α is generally well tolerated, even at high doses
Cardiovascular: erythropoietin may exacerbate preexisting hypertension
Musculoskeletal: some patients may experience mild arthralgias
Miscellaneous: there is an increased incidence of thrombosis of venous access devices

DOSAGE AND ADMINISTRATION

Guidelines have been most firmly established for the treatment of anemia associated with chronic renal failure and the use of AZT in HIV-infected patients [25]. Serum iron studies should be assessed prior to starting treatment, and deficits should be corrected with oral iron preparations. Determine the endogenous erythropoietin level. Data suggests that patients whose levels are greater than 500 mU/mL are unlikely to respond to therapy.

For the treatment of cancer-associated or chemotherapy-associated anemia, a dose of 100 U/kg should be administered SC three times a week for 8 wk. The hematocrit should be assessed regularly, and the dose of epoetin α should be adjusted based on this value.

Epoetin α is also useful preoperatively for increasing the volume of blood that a patient may store for autologous transfusion. One regimen employs 600 U/kg IV twice weekly for 3 wk. Surgery is then performed about 1 month after phlebotomy.

INDICATIONS

FDA-approved: Anemia associated with chronic renal failure or the use of AZT in HIV-infected patients; **Off-label:** cancer-related or chemotherapy-related anemia; epoetin α also has been used preoperatively to enhance the volume of donated blood for autologous transfusion

PHARMACOKINETICS

The circulating half-life of epoetin α is 3–10 h; detectable plasma levels are maintained for at least 24 h after a therapeutic dose; peak serum levels appear between 5 and 24 h after a SC dose

DRUG INTERACTIONS

None

PATIENT MONITORING

Blood pressure should be evaluated regularly because of the risk of hypertension associated with the use epoetin α; response to therapy should be assessed with twice weekly hematocrits; when the hematocrit surpasses 30%, the dosage should be decreased by a total of 25 U/kg; if the hematocrit approaches or surpasses 36%, doses of epoetin α should be withheld until the value decreases to the target range of 30%–33%.; treatment should then be resumed at a dose that is 25 U/kg less than the preceding dose; if the response to 100 U/kg is not satisfactory within 8 wk, the dose can be increased by 50 U/kg to 100 U/kg administered thrice weekly; patients who do not respond to 300 U/kg three times per week over 8 wk are unlikely to respond to higher doses; at this point, other causes of anemia should also be evaluated, such as iron deficiency, bleeding, and hemolysis
Prior to beginning therapy, transferrin saturation, serum iron, total iron binding capacity, and serum ferritin should be assessed; therapy with oral iron preparations should be initiated if iron stores are low; prior to therapy, the endogenous erythropoietin level also should be measured; data suggest that patients with levels > 500 mU/mL are unlikely to respond to treatment

NURSING INTERVENTIONS

Central venous catheters should be well flushed due to the increased risk of thrombosis; the perfusion of the lower legs should be evaluated in patients with significant peripheral vascular disease because of the risk of spontaneous thrombosis; patients who develop arthralgia can be treated with acetaminophen

PATIENT INFORMATION

Patients who are taking concomitant iron should be instructed about the possible side effects of this drug; the incidence of epoetin α–associated toxicity is very low; patients should understand that arthralgias may be associated with treatment and they can be treated with acetaminophen

PREPARATION AND STORAGE

Epoetin α is supplied in 1-mL vials containing 2000 U, 3000 U, 4000 U, or 10,000 U; there are 2.5 mg of human albumin per vial and no preservatives; the vials should be stored at 2° to 8°C; vials should not be shaken because this may denature the epoetin α, rendering it inactive; each vial should be used for 1 dose only, and any unused epoetin α should be discarded

FORMULATIONS

Epoetin α is marketed as Epogen (Amgen) and Procrit (Ortho Biotech).

The information here is provided as guidance only. Prescribers should always consult the manufacturer's current prescribing information.

84

OCTREOTIDE (SOMATOSTATIN ANALOGUE SMS 201-995)

Octreotide is a long-acting somatostatin analogue, the effects of which are pleiotropic and generally inhibitory. Its activity is mediated through binding to widely distributed cell-surface receptors. These have been identified on the cells of some tumor types, suggesting that they may be susceptible to the inhibitory effects of octreotide. Antitumor efficacy also is suggested by its ability to downregulate the activity of myriad growth factors, its direct antiproliferative effects on some tumor-cell lines, and its stimulation of reticuloendothelial activity.

The therapeutic index of octreotide is wide. It has demonstrated activity against some symptoms associated with hypersecretory neuroendocrine tumors. Its inhibitory effects on GI function are useful in the management of enterocutaneous fistulae. Its use in the treatment of cancer, however, remains investigational.

SPECIAL PRECAUTIONS

The half-life of octreotide may be increased in patients with renal dysfunction who require dialysis.

Nursing women and women who are pregnant should use this drug with caution. It is not known whether this drug is excreted in milk. The teratogenic potential in humans has not been investigated adequately.

Diabetics may have to adjust their dose of insulin or sulfonylureas when treated concomitantly with octreotide.

Transplant patients who are taking cyclosporine should be monitored closely. Octreotide has been associated with a decrease in the blood levels of cyclosporine and may have contributed to organ rejection in 1 patient.

TOXICITY

Gastrointestinal: nausea, diarrhea, or abdominal discomfort may occur in 5%–10% of treated patients; other GI effects, including cholelithiasis, are unusual.
Endocrine: hyperglycemia or hypoglycemia have occurred in ~2% of treated patients; other endocrine effects are unusual.
Soft Tissue: pain at the injection site has occurred in ~5% of treated patients.

DOSAGE AND ADMINISTRATION

SC injection is the preferred route of administration due to its prolonged half life; the initial recommended dosage is 50 µg once or twice daily [25]; dosage adjustment may be required thereafter to achieve control of symptoms; this should be done gradually over several weeks; patients with carcinoid syndrome or VIPoma may be treated more aggressively; daily doses of 200–300 µg given in 2–4 divided doses are recommended during the initial 2 wk of therapy; doses above 450 µg/d usually are not required, although occasional patients have needed doses as high as 1500 µg/d.

INDICATIONS

FDA-approved: Symptomatic treatment of patients with carcinoid syndrome or VIPoma in whom diarrhea, electrolyte abnormalities, and flushing may be improved

PHARMACOKINETICS

Absorption after SC injection is rapid and complete; distribution from plasma occurs quickly with an α half-life of about 10 min; circulating octreotide is bound to lipoprotein and albumin in a concentration-independent manner; elimination half-life is about 100 min, and duration of action may be as long as 12 h; the role of the liver on metabolism of octreotide is unknown; 30% of a dose is excreted unchanged in the urine

DRUG INTERACTIONS

Octreotide has been associated with both hyperglycemia and hypoglycemia; adjustment of the dose of insulin or sulfonylureas may be required; the drug may lower the level of cyclosporine; monitor transplant patients closely

PATIENT MONITORING

Monitor clinical biochemical effects in patients with carcinoid syndrome by measurement of serum serotonin and substance P; monitor urinary 5-hydroxyindole acetic acid (5-HIAA) and thyroid function; patients with VIPoma can be monitored by measurement of serum vasoactive intestinal peptide (VIP); diabetics, in particular, should be monitored for hyperglycemia and hypoglycemia

Fat malabsorption may be exacerbated by octreotide; selected patients should be periodically evaluated with 72-h fecal fat and serum carotene determinations; patients undergoing prolonged therapy should have periodic ultrasound examinations of the gall bladder and biliary tree; transplant patients who are treated with cyclosporine should have their dose carefully evaluated because of the possibility that octreotide may lower serum levels and precipitate organ rejection

NURSING INTERVENTIONS

Patients should be assessed for signs and symptoms of hyperglycemia, hypoglycemia, and hypothyroidism; patients who can be treated at home will require training in the self-administration of octreotide; they should be instructed in the safe disposal of needles, drug vials, and syringes; multiple injections at the same site within short periods of time should be avoided; the drug should not be used if discoloration or particulates develop

PREPARATION AND STORAGE

Octreotide is available in 1-mL ampules that contain either 0.05 mg, 0.1 mg, or 0.5 mg; a patient home starter kit is also available; ampules can be stored at room temperature for the day that they will be used; otherwise, they should be refrigerated at 2°–8°C

FORMULATIONS

Octreotide is marketed as Sandostatin by Sandoz.

The information here is provided as guidance only. Prescribers should always consult the manufacturer's current prescribing information.

RETINOIDS

Retinoids are a family of structurally and functionally related molecules that exercise a profound effect on cell growth and differentiation. This class of compounds includes all-*trans*-retinol (vitamin A); its metabolites, all-*trans*-retinoic acid (tretinoin) and 13-*cis*-retinoic acid (isotretinoin); and beta carotene. Retinoids possess antineoplastic activity and may have some clinical value in the treatment of acute promyelocytic leukemia, basal cell and squamous cell carcinoma of the skin, and mycosis fungoides. The efficacy of retinoic acid in the treatment of these and other malignancies is being investigated.

Retinoids prevent the development of tumors in a variety of animal models. This has led to several chemoprevention trials in patients at high risk for malignancy. Isotretinoin has been associated with a lower frequency of secondary aerodigestive tumors among patients with surgically treated squamous cell carcinoma of the head and neck.

SPECIAL PRECAUTIONS

Both tretinoin and isotretinoin are teratogenic. Their use in women who are pregnant or who may become pregnant is contraindicated. It is recommended that these drugs should not be used in women of childbearing age unless they understand the risks and are capable of following mandatory contraceptive measures. These include the use of effective contraception for 1 mo before, during, and after therapy.

It is not known whether these drugs are excreted in breast milk. Therefore, their use in nursing mothers is contraindicated.

Patients at risk for hypertriglyceridemia, including those with diabetes mellitus, obesity, increased alcohol intake, and a positive family history, should use these drugs with caution. The effect of treatment on serum lipids should be assessed periodically.

Diabetic patients may require adjustment of their hypoglycemic medications during therapy.

The commercially available formulation of isotretinoin (Accutane) contains parabens. Patients who are allergic to this drug should not use Accutane.

INDICATIONS
FDA-approved: *Oene vulgaris*

PHARMACOKINETICS
Peak plasma levels of isotretinoin occur about 3 h after an oral dose; in adults with normal renal function, its elimination profile is biphasic with a terminal-phase half-life that varies from 7–40 h; both tretinoin and isotretinoin are metabolized by cytochrome P-450-dependent hydroxylation; they undergo conjugation with glucuronide and are secreted in the bile; ~70% of an oral dose is excreted in the urine and feces in equal proportions; unlike retinol, the metabolites tretinoin and isotretinoin do not accumulate within the liver and cause hepatic damage as a sequelae of prolonged consumption

DRUG INTERACTIONS
Minocycline and tetracycline have been associated with the development of pseudotumor cerebri in patients who are also being treated with retinoic acid; concomitant use of vitamin A should be avoided; topical dermatologics may potentiate the drying effects; ethanol may potentiate the hypertriglyceridemia associated with treatment

PATIENT MONITORING
Women of childbearing age should have a negative serum pregnancy test within 2 wk of beginning therapy; a monthly pregnancy testing should be performed; monitor patients for the development of headache, nausea, vomiting, or visual disturbances—if these symptoms occur, patients should be evaluated for papilledema or ophthalmologic disorders; a baseline lipid profile should be obtained; this should be repeated once or twice weekly until the lipid response to therapy has been determined, usually 8 wk; other blood tests that should be followed include glucose, liver function studies, uric acid, cholesterol, complete blood counts, and platelet counts

RETINOIDS (Continued)

TOXICITY

Dermatologic: cheilitis and xerosis occur frequently and may lead to pruritus, conjunctivitis, blepharitis, and epistaxis; thinning of the hair and brittle nails have been reported

GI: dry mouth, nausea, and vomiting are commonly observed; the onset of inflammatory bowel disease has been associated temporally with administration of retinoic acid

Ophthalmic: conjunctivitis occurs in ~40% of treated patients; optic neuritis, corneal opacities, and photophobia occur rarely

CNS: fatigue and headache are uncommon complications of therapy with isotretinoin; these toxicities frequently are associated with the administration of tretinoin; pseudotumor cerebri has occurred during therapy with retinoic acid

Musculoskeletal: moderate musculoskeletal symptoms occur in ~15% of treated patients

Metabolic: reversible hypertriglyceridemia, hyperglycemia, hyperuricemia, and hypercholesterolemia may occur; elevations of AST, ALT, LDH are seen in ~10% of treated patients

DOSAGE AND ADMINISTRATION

Both isotretinoin and tretinoin should be administered orally, preferably with food; the use of these drugs for the treatment and prevention of cancer remains investigational; therefore, the optimal doses have not been defined; clinical responses among patients with acute promyelocytic leukemia have been associated with tretinoin, 45 mg/m^2/d; doses of isotretinoin associated with clinical response among patients with solid tumors have ranged from 1–3 mg/kg/d.

NURSING INTERVENTIONS

Women of childbearing age should be counseled frequently about contraception; 2 methods of contraception should be used simultaneously unless abstinence is practiced

Decreased night vision may accompany therapy with retinoids; patients should be made aware of this and should be warned to exercise caution when driving at night

Monitor patients for signs and symptoms of inflammatory bowel disease, including abdominal pain, diarrhea, and rectal bleeding; treatment should be discontinued if this occurs; retinoic acid may cause photosensitivity, and patients should be cautioned to avoid significant exposure to the sun and to wear sunscreen

Patients should be instructed not to donate blood for at least 30 d after the discontinuation of therapy owing to the teratogenic potential of retinoic acid

Patients with diabetes mellitus should be made aware that their insulin or antihyperglycemic medications may require adjustment

Patients should be instructed to take their medication with meals and avoid crushing the capsules

Concomitant use of vitamin A supplements and benzoyl peroxide should be avoided

Patients should be instructed to minimize their intake of ethanol

PREPARATION AND STORAGE

Isotretinoin is available as capsules containing either 10, 20, or 30 mg of drug as a suspension in soybean oil; the capsules also contain parabens, EDTA, and glycerin; isotretinoin is photosensitive and should be stored at 15°–30°C in light-resistant containers; the capsules are stable for 2 y after their manufacture

FORMULATIONS

Isotretinoin is marketed as Accutane by Roche; Tretinoin is also made by Roche but is not commercially available.

Hormones play a pivotal role in regulating the growth and development of their target organs. Various hormonal agents have been used in the treatment of tumors originating from these target organs, namely the breast, uterus, ovary, and prostate.

MECHANISM OF ACTION

Estrogens, androgens, and progestins exert their function mainly through their respective receptors. After binding to the receptors in high affinity, the steroids alter the configuration of receptor molecules and make them capable of binding to a segment of DNA template called hormone response element, where they regulate gene transcription and control the cellular growth and function [1].

Tamoxifen may affect cancer cell growth through mechanisms other than the steroid receptor pathway, such as through the protein kinase C system, by inhibition of ornithine decarboxylase and polyamine [2], by suppression of the plasma level of insulin-like growth factor [3], by modulation of the multidrug resistance gene *MDR*, or through antiangiogenesis [4].

COMPLEXED CELLULAR REGULATION UNDER HORMONES

It is a complex system that governs the growth of normal and cancerous cells. The endocrine function is under a tight feedback loop of autoregulation within one type of hormone as well as under interregulation between hormones. The former can best be illustrated using the case of pharmacologic dosages of estrogen that downregulate the estrogen receptors. As for interhormonal regulation, estrogens promote the production of progesterone receptor, whereas progestins downregulate the estrogen receptors.

There is also a second level of fine tuning at the site of local microenvironment, where the cellular functions are mediated through paracrine effects of various growth factors [5]. Estrogen supports the breast cancer growth through an enhanced production of transforming growth factor-α and an inhibition of transforming growth factor-β. Hormonal therapy aims to disrupt this regulatory pathway. Tamoxifen, progestins, and ovariectomy act to reverse the effects of estrogen on growth-factor production. Various modalities of endocrine therapy can be classified arbitrarily as additive, ablative, competitive, and inhibitive (Table 5-1).

APOPTOSIS AS A MECHANISM OF ANTITUMOR EFFECTS

It is well documented that the antitumor effects of many endocrine therapies are mediated through the process of apoptosis (programmed cell death). Deprivation of hormones by orchiectomy or ovariectomy induces apoptosis of tumor cells in prostate and breast cancer, respectively [6]. Both antiestrogen and antiprogestin acts through competitive mechanisms to achieve tumor regression through the apoptotic process [7].

TISSUE-SPECIFIC RESPONSE TO TAMOXIFEN

Although the action of tamoxifen in humans is mainly an antiestrogenic effect, tamoxifen also possesses estrogenic effect depending on the type and condition of target tissues. In breast cancer, tamoxifen acts mainly as an antiestrogen. In vaginal epithelium, endometrium, and skeletal bones, however, tamoxifen acts like estrogen. This differential function explains why tamoxifen inhibits breast cancer growth while increasing the risk of endometrial cancer. It also explains why tamoxifen, instead of causing osteoporosis, promotes mineral bone formation, as estrogens do. When breast cancer relapses following a tamoxifen response, some of the metabolites of tamoxifen become predominantly estrogen-like in promoting tumor growth. Under such conditions, tamoxifen withdrawal may induce another round of tumor regression.

INDICATIONS FOR HORMONAL THERAPY

The types of cancers that have shown responses to hormonal agents are listed in Table 5-2. Because the major action of hormones is mediated through steroid receptors, theoretically only receptor-positive tumor cells will respond to this modality of therapy. Indeed, 60% of receptor-positive breast cancers responded to first-line hormonal therapy; less than 10% of receptor-negative tumors responded. Prostate cancer cells are usually androgen-dependent and respond to androgen deprivation, either by orchiectomy or by a combination of antiandrogen (flutamide) and a luteinizing hormone–releasing hormone (LH-RH) analogue. The presence of steroid receptors in ovarian and uterine cancers is less frequent than their presence in breast and prostate cancers. However, even in receptor-positive tumors, the response of ovarian and uterine cancer to hormonal agents is at best modest or rare.

There is no clear rational basis for treating renal cell cancer or melanoma with hormonal therapy because no genuine steroid receptor has been found in these two types of cancer. Unlike hamster kidney cancer, human renal cell carcinoma is hormonally independent. The estrogen receptors previously reported in melanoma are actually tyrosinase. However, because tamoxifen plays multiple roles

Table 5-1. Categories of Current Endocrine Therapy

Additive	Competitive
Estrogens	Antiestrogens
Progestins	Antiandrogens
Androgens	Antiprogestins
Ablative	Inhibitive
Ovariectomy	Aromatase inhibitors
	LH-RH analogues

Table 5-2. Type of Tumor Subjected to Hormonal Therapy

High Probability of Response (40%–80%)	Low Probability of Response (10%–30%)	Rare Response (< 10%)
Steroid receptor-positive	Endometrial cancer	Steroid receptor-negative
Breast cancer		Breast cancer
Prostate cancer		Prostate cancer
Meningioma		Ovarian cancer
		Renal cell cancer
Tamoxifen and chemotherapy		
Melanoma		

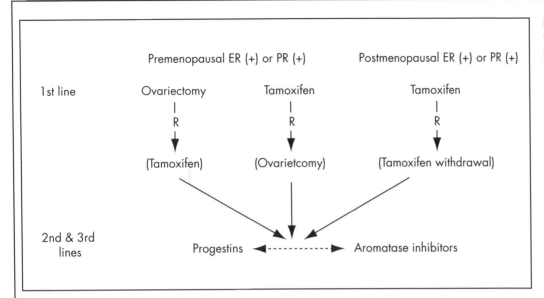

FIGURE 5-1.

Sequential hormonal therapy in advanced breast cancer. ER(+) — estrogen-receptor—positive; PR(+) — progesterone-receptor—positive; R — responders.

other than that of estrogen-receptor mediation, the response rate of melanoma to combination chemotherapy has been reported in one uncontrolled study to be improved from 10% without tamoxifen to 51% with tamoxifen [8]. This has not been borne out in a randomized controlled trial of the ECOG.

FLARE FOLLOWING HORMONAL THERAPY

Flare has been observed with every known hormonal therapy. The frequent manifestations are an abrupt increase of bony pain, erythema around skin lesions, and induced hypercalcemia. However, evidence of actual increase of tumor growth is lacking. In some cases, the flare may be a good prognostic sign that the tumor is hormonally responsive. Therefore, by an adequate control of pain or hypercalcemia, a continued use of the hormonal agent may result in tumor regression. This practice is especially important and prudent in the use of LH-RH analogue for prostate cancer, in which an initial increase of the blood androgen level and bone pain is frequently inevitable.

DURATION OF TREATMENT

Because of the cytostatic effects on tumor cells from most hormonal agents, a minimal period of 2 months of continuous treatment is needed to adequately determine the efficacy of these agents.

COMBINED OR SEQUENTIAL USE OF HORMONAL THERAPY

As described earlier, when cancer cell growth is dependent on hormones, there are many ways to interrupt such dependency: by removing or reducing the hormone source or by blocking the hormonal action at the receptor site. Therefore, a combined hormone approach makes sense and has been used for treatment of advanced prostate cancer (LH-RH analogue plus flutamide) [9]. The results of such combination approaches in breast cancer are less convincing; specifically, such an approach does not translate

into a survival advantage. It is recommended, therefore, that hormone therapy in breast cancer be used in sequence (Fig. 5-1).

COMBINED HORMONAL THERAPY AND CHEMOTHERAPY

A combination of hormonal therapy and chemotherapy is also logical because these two modalities have different mechanisms of antitumor action and different types of side effects. Clinical studies around the world have not shown benefit for such a combination, especially in terms of the duration of response or survival in patients with breast cancer [10]. Therefore, for palliative purposes in advanced breast cancer, sequential application of hormonal therapy and chemotherapy to achieve a prolonged control of the disease is advised (Fig. 5-2).

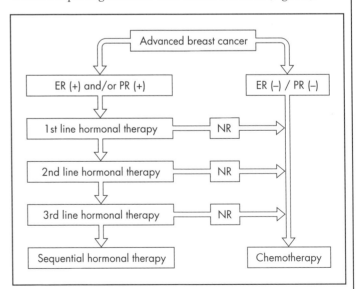

FIGURE 5-2.

Treatment for advanced breast cancer.

NEW DEVELOPMENTS

There is an impressive number of new hormonal agents added in the 1997 roster for the management of malignant diseases. Most of the new agents belong to the category of antiestrogens (toremifene, raloxifene), antiandrogens (bicalutamide, nilutamide), and aromatase inhibitors (anastrozole , tetrazole). In general, these new agents do not seem to advance the therapeutic indexes; rather a marked improvement is achieved in compliance (eg, once-daily dose) as well as in the reduction of untoward side effects.

A major recent thrust is the development of new hormonal agents in at least two frontiers. A great deal attention was focused on the tissue-specific response to antiestrogens as alluded to previously. Recent findings suggest that the binding of estrogen receptor to DNA-response elements involves various cellular adapter proteins that confer the tissue-specificity [12]. Based on this concept, a new class of compounds known as SERMs (selective estrogen-receptor modulators) are being developed. The antiestrogen raloxifene is one of the products that acts as an estrogen agonist on bone tissues and serum lipids but behaves as estrogen antagonist in the breast and uterine tissues [13]. Although raloxifene is still under investigation for the treatment of breast cancer, it has already been approved by the FDA in December 1997 for marketing for the prevention of osteoporosis. The other exciting frontier is the ongoing research into the use of human chorionic gonadotropin for the treatment of AIDS-related Kaposi's sarcoma [14].

REFERENCES

1. Baxter JD, Funder JW: Hormone receptors. *N Engl J Med* 1979, 301:1149–1161.

2. Thomas T, Trend B, Butterfield JR, *et al.*: Regulation of ornithine decarboxylase gene expression in MCF-7 breast cancer cells by antiestrogens. *Cancer Res* 1989, 49:5852–5857.

3. Winston R, Kao PC, Kiang DT: Regulation of insulin-like growth factors by antiestrogen. *Breast Cancer Res Treat* 1994, 31:107–115.

4. Gagliardi A, Collins DC: Inhibition of angiogenesis by antiestrogens. *Cancer Res* 1993, 53:533–535.

5. Lippman ME, Dickson RB, Bates S, *et al.*: Autocrine and paracrine growth regulation of human breast cancer. *Breast Cancer Res Treat* 1986, 7:59–71.

6. Buttyan R: Genetic response of prostate cells to androgen deprivation: insights into the cellular mechanism of apoptosis. In *Apoptosis: The Molecular Basis of Death*. Edited by Tomei LD, Cope FO. Plainview, NY: Cold Spring Harbor Laboratory Press; 1991:157–173.

7. Bardon S, Vignon F, Montcourrier PHR: Steroid receptor-mediated cytotoxicity of an antiestrogen and an antiprogestin in breast cancer cells. *Cancer Res* 1987, 47:1441–1448.

8. McClay EF, McClay MET: Tamoxifen: is it useful in the treatment of patients with metastatic melanoma? *J Clin Oncol* 1994, 12:617–626.

9. Crawford ED, Eisenberger MA, McLeod DG, *et al.*: A controlled trial of leuprolide with and without flutamide in prostatic carcinoma. *N Engl J Med* 1989, 321:419–424.

10. Rausch DJ, Kiang DT: Interaction between endocrine and cytotoxic therapy. In *Endocrine Therapy in Cancer*. Edited by Stoll BA. Basel, Switzerland: Karger; 1988:102–118.

11. Eisenhauer EA, Pritchard KI, Perrault D, *et al.*: Phase II study of mifepristone (RU486) in previously untreated patients (PTS) with metastatic breast cancer (BC): a trial of the NCI Canada Clinical Trials Group. *Proc Amer Soc Clin Oncology* 1995; 14:114.

12. Yang NN, Venugopalan M, Hardikar S, *et. al.*: Identification of an estrogen response element activated by metabolites of 17 beta-estradiol and raloxifene. *Science* 1996, 273:1222–1225.

13. Delmas PD, Bjarnason NH, Mitlak BH, *et. al.*: Effects of raloxifene on bone mineral density, serum cholesterol concentrations, and uterine endometrium in postmenopausal women. *N Engl J Med* 1997, 337:1641–1647.

14. Gill PS, Lunardi-Ishkandar Y, Louie S, *et. al.*: The effects of preparations of human chorionic gonadotropin on AIDS-related Kaposi's sarcoma. *N Engl J Med* 1996, 335:1261–1269.

AMINOGLUTETHIMIDE

EFFICACY AND USAGE

Aminoglutethimide has been referred to casually as a medical adrenalectomy. The role of this agent in therapy for breast cancer is attributed to its action as inhibitor of the enzyme aromatase. Aromatase catalyzes the conversion of testosterone to estradiol and the conversion of androstenedione to estrone. This enzyme is present in the adrenal cortex and extraglandular peripheral tissues, including adipose and breast cancer tissues.

DOSAGE AND ADMINISTRATION

250 mg two to four times daily with hydrocortisone 20-mg bid supplement

SPECIAL PRECAUTIONS

Given its similarity to the sedative glutethimide, severe sedation may occur especially in elderly patients

TOXICITIES

Side effects are unpredictable and occur in 50% of patients; skin (morbilliform maculopapular) rashes are most common (30%), followed by lethargy and somnolence; thrombocytopenia and leukopenia are less common; others include hypothyroidism, hypotension, and flu-like syndrome

INDICATIONS

FDA-approved: Second- or third-line endocrine therapy for advanced breast cancer in post-menopausal patients

CONTRAINDICATIONS

History of hypersensitivity to glutethimide

PHARMACOKINETICS

Addition of hydrocortisone is necessary to suppress a reflex rise in ACTH levels, which could act to overcome the blockade in steroid synthesis caused by aminoglutethimide

DRUG INTERACTIONS

Aminoglutethimide binds to cytochrome p450 enzymes and may increase the clearance rate of warfarin, antipyrine, theophylline, digitoxin, and tamoxifen

RESPONSE RATES

Third-line therapy for breast cancer—~30% in patients who previously responded to endocrine therapy

NURSING INTERVENTIONS

Carefully monitor for side effects, especially mental status

PATIENT INFORMATION

Patient should check for skin rashes and drowsiness

AVAILABILITY

Available as Cytadren by Ciba Pharmaceutical Co., Summit, NJ; 250-mg tablets that may be stored in light-protected container at room temperature.

DIETHYLSTILBESTROL

EFFICACY AND USAGE

Diethylstilbestrol is a synthetic estrogen used for breast cancer and prostate cancer treatment. Because of its dichotomous effects on breast cancer—tumor flare at physiological doses and regression at pharmacologic doses—the dosage for breast cancer should be in the pharmacologic range. On the contrary, the dosage used for prostate cancer should be low in order to prevent cardiovascular complications. The suppression of serum androgens may be measured to document the adequacy of dosage.

DOSAGE AND ADMINISTRATION

Breast cancer: 5 mg three times daily
Prostate cancer: 1–3 mg daily

SPECIAL PRECAUTIONS

Pregnant patients; patients with poor liver or renal function, congestive heart failure, gallbladder disease, endometrial problems, or history of thrombophlebitis or embolism

TOXICITIES

GI: nausea and vomiting, cholestatic jaundice, and increased gallbladder disease; **Cardiovascular:** exacerbation of congestive heart failure and thromboembolism; **GU:** vaginal bleeding and candidiasis, cystitis-like symptoms; **Metabolic:** hypercalcemia and fluid retention; **CNS:** headache, migraine, and mental depression; **Skin:** pigmentation of nipple and axillae; **Breasts:** gynecomastia in males; **Tumor flare:** 5%–10%

INDICATIONS

FDA-approved: for postmenopausal female patients or male patients with advanced breast cancer and for patients with metastatic prostate cancer

CONTRAINDICATIONS

Pregnancy, active thrombophlebitis, known or suspected estrogen-dependent malignancy

PHARMACOKINETICS

Absorption: relatively complete; **Binding to serum hormone binding globulin:** 40%–50%; **Blood levels:** 0.15–6.0 mg/mL after administration at 1 mg three times daily; **Metabolism:** hepatic biotransformation and biliary excretion

DRUG INTERACTIONS

None directly; however, estrogen decreases the prothrombin time, impairs glucose tolerance, and increases the thyroid-binding globulin

RESPONSE RATES

Approximately 30% of postmenopausal breast cancers and 55%–60% of estrogen receptor–positive cancers will respond; the response rate in male breast cancer is similar to that in female breast cancer; the objective response rate in prostate cancer is ~65%; if subjective pain relief is included as responders, the total response rate could be up to 85%

NURSING INTERVENTIONS

Carefully monitor and document signs and symptoms

PATIENT INFORMATION

Patient should be aware of increased risk of endometrial carcinoma, carcinogenic effects on fetus during pregnancy, and all the potential side effects listed above

AVAILABILITY

Distributed by Eli Lilly and Co., Indianapolis, IN; 0.1-, 0.25-, 0.5-, 1-, 2-, 5-, and 10-mg tablets stored in light-protected container at room temperature.

FLUOXYMESTEROL

EFFICACY AND USAGE

Fluoxymesterol is a synthetic steroid hormone used for the treatment of advanced breast cancer. The response rate is lower than that of tamoxifen. It is frequently used as a third-line therapy. The erythropoietic effects may provide a sense of well-being in anemic patients.

DOSAGE AND ADMINISTRATION

10 mg twice daily orally

SPECIAL PRECAUTIONS

Masculinization effects and, occasionally, induced hypercalcemia

TOXICITIES

GU: virilization, amenorrhea, and irregular menstrual periods; **GI**: nausea, cholestatic jaundice; **Hematologic**: suppression of clotting factors, and polycythemia; **CNS**: increased libido, headache, anxiety, aggressiveness, and depression; **Skin**: acne and hirsutism

INDICATIONS

FDA-approved: advanced breast cancer

CONTRAINDICATIONS

Known hypersensitivity to the drug, suspected prostate cancer, pregnancy, or serious cardiac, hepatic, or renal disease

PHARMACOKINETICS

Absorption: rapid; **Biotransformation**: in liver; **Half-life**: 9.2 h; **Excretion**: 90% in urine after being glucuronidated

DRUG INTERACTIONS

Increases the sensitivity to anticoagulants, decreasing the requirement for insulin and interfering with laboratory testing for thyroid function

RESPONSE RATES

Breast cancer: 15%–25%

NURSING INTERVENTIONS

Monitor and document signs and symptoms

PATIENT INFORMATION

Causes masculinization, hoarseness, acne, and changes in menstrual periods

AVAILABILITY

Distributed as Halotestin by Upjohn Co., Kalamazoo, MI; 2-, 5-, and 10-mg tablets.

FLUTAMIDE

EFFICACY AND USAGE

Flutamide is a nonsteroid antiandrogen. It is used in combination with LH-RH analogue for the treatment of metastatic prostate cancer. The drug blocks the androgenic action at its target site.

DOSAGE AND ADMINISTRATION

250 mg every 8 h orally

SPECIAL PRECAUTIONS

Patients with hepatic toxicity with elevation of hepatic transaminases and cholestatic jaundice

TOXICITIES

Most frequent: hot flushes, impotence, and loss of libido; **GI**—nausea, vomiting; **Cardiovascular**—hypertension and edema; **CNS**—drowsiness, depression, and anxiety; **Hematologic** (occasionally)—anemia, leukopenia, thrombocytopenia

INDICATIONS

FDA-approved: advanced prostate cancer

CONTRAINDICATIONS

Liver function impairment

PHARMACOKINETICS

Absorption: it is rapidly orally absorbed; **Metabolism**: its biologic metabolites reach a maximal plasma level in 2 h and a steady-state level in 9.6 h; **Plasma half-life**: ~8 h; **Excretion**: mainly in the urine

DRUG INTERACTIONS

Increased prothrombin time in patients on long-term warfarin

RESPONSE RATES

Flutamide is frequently used in combination with an LH-RH analogue, which suppresses the production of testicular androgens. The overall response rate for the combination therapy is about 70%, and the drug provides a significantly prolonged survival compared with LH-RH alone (36 versus 28 mo)

NURSING INTERVENTIONS

Monitor signs and symptoms

PATIENT INFORMATION

May cause hepatic injury such as cholestatic jaundice and the patient may need more frequent monitoring of prothrombin time while on warfarin

AVAILABILITY

Supplied by Schering Corporation, Kenilworth, NJ, as Eulexin; 125-mg capsules stored at room temperature and protected from heat and moisture.

GOSERELIN ACETATE

Goserelin is a synthetic decapeptide analogue of LH-RH with a much prolonged half-life and 100 times greater potency than that of the natural releasing hormone. Therefore, it downregulates the LH-RH receptors and reduces the release of gonadotropic hormones, which in turn results in a decrease in blood testosterone or estrogen levels. Thus, the functional result of LH-RH analogue therapy is equivalent to medical castration.

DOSAGE AND ADMINISTRATION

A depot dose of 3.6 mg/implant given subcutaneously every 4 wk

SPECIAL PRECAUTIONS

Patients with hypersensitivity to LH-RH; initial exacerbation of symptoms from prostate cancer; pregnant nursing patients

TOXICITIES

Endocrine: sexual dysfunction; **Respiratory**: bronchitis; **Cardiovascular**: hot flushes, arrhythmias, hypertension; **CNS**: depression, anxiety, headache; **GI**: constipation, diarrhea, dyspepsia

INDICATIONS

FDA-approved: advanced prostate cancer and premenopausal breast cancer

CONTRAINDICATIONS

Pregnant nursing patients
History of hypersensitivity to LH-RH

PHARMACOKINETICS

Absorption: very slow; **Peak blood level**: achieved in 12–15 d following a single dose (3.6-mg) injection; **Action**: following goserelin therapy, the mean serum estradiol or testosterone values fall into the range of castrated level within 2–3 wk; **Elimination**: the drug is excreted through both urine and hepatic metabolism, and there is no drug accumulation on an every-28-d schedule

DRUG INTERACTIONS

None

RESPONSE RATES

Advanced prostate cancer: in combination with flutamide, 70%; **Pre- and perimenopausal receptor-positive breast cancer**: 45%

NURSING INTERVENTIONS

Monitor signs and symptoms

PATIENT INFORMATION

Because of the initial, but transient, surge of blood testosterone level, patient may experience exacerbation of bone pain at metastatic sites of prostate cancer or urethral obstruction; patient may experience hot flushes and sexual dysfunctions

AVAILABILITY

Supplied by Zeneca Pharmaceutics, Wilmington, DE; under the trade name of Zoladex; 3.6-mg disposable syringe device. Stored at room temperature of < 25°C.

KETOCONAZOLE

EFFICACY AND USAGE

Ketoconazole is a synthetic imidazole with antifungal action. It inhibits the synthesis of ergosterol, a vital membranous component of fungal cells. Because of its inhibition of testosterone synthesis, ketoconazole is also used for the treatment of advanced prostate cancer.

DOSAGE AND ADMINISTRATION

400 mg every 8 h in order to sustain the androgen suppression

SPECIAL PRECAUTIONS

Patients with hypersensitivity to the drug; at high dosage, decreases the ACTH-induced corticosteroid level

TOXICITIES

Hepatic toxicity and hypersensitivity; in patients treated with 1200 mg daily for prostate cancer, death within 2 wk from unknown mechanism was observed

INDICATIONS

Used for advanced prostate cancer but is not approved by the FDA

CONTRAINDICATIONS

Coadministration with terfenadine, astemizole, cisapride, and oral triazolam

PHARMACOKINETICS

Absorption: rapid; **Peak blood level**: reached within 1–2 h; **Half-life**: biphasic with initial 2 h during the first 10 h then 8 h thereafter; **Plasma binding**: 99% to albumin; **Metabolism**: converts into inactive metabolites; **Excretion**: the major route is via bile; **CNS penetration**: poor

DRUG INTERACTIONS

Inhibits the metabolism of the drugs listed in the Contraindications section above and increases their blood level, resulting in cardiac arrhythmia including ventricular tachycardia; may enhance the anticoagulant effect of warfarin; should not be given concomitantly with rifampin or isoniazid; interacts with cyclosporine and methylprednisolone; concomitant administration with miconazole (another imidazole) may potentiate the hypoglycemia episodes; antacids, anticholinergics, and H_2-blockers reduce the dissolution and absorption of ketoconazole

RESPONSE RATES

Difficult to assess the tumor response rate; most study series included pain relief as response

NURSING INTERVENTIONS

Closely monitor the signs and symptoms and determine the potential interaction with other medications; for overdose: gastric lavage with sodium bicarbonate

PATIENT INFORMATION

Take the medication with a meal and avoid alcohol consumption

AVAILABILITY

Supplied as Nizoral by Janssen Pharmaceutica, Titusville, NJ; 200-mg tablets. Requires acidity for dissolution; store at room temperature.

LEUPROLIDE

EFFICACY AND USAGE

Leuprolide acetate is a synthetic nonapeptide analogue of naturally LH-RH. It desensitizes the LH-RH receptor and reduces the production of gonadotropic hormones. It acts as medical castration in reducing testosterone in males and estrogens in females. It has been used for the treatment of advanced prostate cancer and breast cancer.

DOSAGE AND ADMINISTRATION

7.5-mg depot administered intramuscularly every month or 22.5-mg depot every 3 mo under the supervision of a physician

SPECIAL PRECAUTIONS

Hypersensitivity to the agent and tumor flare may occur owing to an initial surge of blood testosterone or estrogen levels in the beginning of therapy

TOXICITIES

Endocrine: sexual dysfunction; **Respiratory:** bronchitis; **Cardiovascular:** hot flushes, arrhythmias, hypertension; **CNS:** depression, anxiety, headache; **GI:** constipation, diarrhea, dyspepsia

INDICATIONS

FDA-approved: palliative treatment of advanced prostate cancer and of premenopausal advanced breast cancer

CONTRAINDICATIONS

History of hypersensitivity to the drug
Pregnant nursing patients

PHARMACOKINETICS

Bioavailability: 90%; **Metabolism, distribution, and excretion:** not fully determined

DRUG INTERACTIONS

None reported

RESPONSE RATES

40–45% response rates have been observed in premenopausal patients with estrogen receptor–positive advanced breast cancer. The response rates of prostate cancer to leuprolide vs leuprolide/flutamide are not significantly different; however, the median survival is in favor of the combination (36 versus 28 mo)

NURSING INTERVENTIONS

Monitor signs and symptoms

PATIENT INFORMATION

Hypersensitivity and sexual dysfunction may occur

AVAILABILITY

Supplied as Lupron depot from TAP Pharmaceuticals, Deerfield, IL; 3.75-mg, 7.5-mg, and 22.5-mg depot formulations for IM injection. Store at room temperature. Protect from freezing.

MEGESTROL ACETATE

EFFICACY AND USAGE

Megestrol acetate is a synthetic progestational drug used in the treatment of advanced breast cancer and endometrial cancer. At higher dosages, it is also used to improve anorexia and cachexia in cancer and AIDS patients. Progestins have significant antiestrogenic effect through either the conversion of estradiol to a less active estrone or downregulation of estrogen receptors.

DOSAGE AND ADMINISTRATION

Breast and endometrial cancer: 40 mg tablet four times daily PO; **cachexia/anorexia:** 400–800 mg of PO suspension daily in divided doses

SPECIAL PRECAUTIONS

Weight gain in obese patients; patients with history of thromboembolic episodes

TOXICITIES

In general, the drug is well tolerated; **Metabolic:** weight gain, hypercalcemia; **Cardiovascular:** thromboembolic episodes, hypertension, dyspnea; **GI:** nausea, vomiting

INDICATIONS

FDA-approved: advanced breast cancer, endometrial cancer, and cancer-related cachexia

CONTRAINDICATIONS

Early stage of pregnancy

PHARMACOKINETICS

Oral bioavailability: 97%; **Peak plasma levels:** in 2–3 h; **Half-life:** biphasic with a terminal half-life of 15–20 h; **Metabolism:** in liver; **Excretion:** majority in urine

DRUG INTERACTIONS

Decreases the clearance of warfarin

RESPONSE RATES

Approximately 60% of steroid receptor–positive breast cancer respond to megestrol; response rate is higher in tumors with positive progesterone receptors; the response rate in endometrial cancer is ~30%

NURSING INTERVENTIONS

Monitor signs and symptoms

PATIENT INFORMATION

Patient should be aware of the effects of weight gain and thromboembolic episodes and the need to avoid pregnancy

AVAILABILITY

Supplied as Megace from Bristol-Myers-Squibb Co., Princeton, NJ; 20- and 40-mg tablets to be stored at room temperature. Also available in 40-mg micronized megestrol acetate per milliliter oral suspension to be stored at < 25°C.

MIFEPRISTONE

EFFICACY AND USAGE

Mifepristone is a synthetic derivative of progesterone. It acts as an antiprogestin and antiglucocorticoid. It has anti-tumor effect on rat mammary tumors and human breast cancer and meningioma cell lines. Clinical trials in Europe have shown tumor regression from mifepristone in human breast cancers and unresectable meningioma. It should be noted that about 72% of meningiomas are progesterone-receptor positive.

DOSAGE AND ADMINISTRATION

100 mg to 200 mg twice daily

SPECIAL PRECAUTIONS

Pregnant patients

TOXICITIES

In general, it is well tolerated; **Major side effects:** nausea, anorexia, hot flushes, dizziness, lethargy, gynecomastia in male patients

INDICATIONS

Clinical studies show modest activity in palliative treatment for advanced breast cancer and unresectable meningioma

CONTRAINDICATIONS

Pregnant patients

PHARMACOKINETICS

Half-life: 20 h

DRUG INTERACTIONS

None reported

RESPONSE RATES

Mifepristone showed minimal activity against breast cancer in two small European trials; preliminary results from a recent Canadian phase II study also showed a modest antitumor activity; partial responses observed in only 2 of 22 patients [11]; the response rate for meningioma was reported to be ~30%–40%

NURSING INTERVENTIONS

Monitor and document signs and symptoms

PATIENT INFORMATION

Should not be used in patients who are pregnant or planning for conception

AVAILABILITY

50- and 200-mg tablets from Roussel-Uclaf, France; stored at room temperature.

TAMOXIFEN

EFFICACY AND USAGE

Tamoxifen is a nonsteroidal antiestrogen that exerts its effect on breast cancer by competitively inhibiting the binding of estrogen to estrogen receptors. Tamoxifen has been used in combination with chemotherapeutic agents for cancers other than breast in origin, such as melanoma.

DOSAGE AND ADMINISTRATION

20 mg daily

SPECIAL PRECAUTIONS

Barrier forms of contraception should be considered in premenopausal patients because tamoxifen may initially induce ovulation; close monitoring of endometrium is required in prolonged use of tamoxifen for early detection of endometrial cancer

TOXICITIES

Vascular: hot flushes, lightheadedness, thromboembolism; **Gynecologic:** vaginal bleeding, altered menses, ovarian cyst, increased incidence of endometrial cancer; **GI:** nausea, vomiting, anorexia; **Metabolic:** hypercalcemia; **CNS:** emotional instability, depression; **Ophthalmologic:** at prolonged high dosage, visual disturbance (macular retinopathy and corneal opacity)

INDICATIONS

FDA-approved: female and male advanced breast cancer; adjuvant therapy after surgical removal of primary breast cancer lesion; in combination with chemotherapy, tamoxifen has been used for other cancer, such as melanoma

CONTRAINDICATIONS

Known hypersensitivity to tamoxifen; pregnant patients

PHARMACOKINETICS

Absorption: well-absorbed; **Plasma peak level:** 4–7 h; **Metabolism:** hydroxylation or N-oxidation to active metabolites; **Half-life:** biphasic, initially 9–12 h, later 7 d; **Excretion:** mainly in the feces

DRUG INTERACTIONS

Tamoxifen is a cytostatic drug that blocks the cell cycle at the late G_1 phase; therefore, it may attenuate cytotoxicity of many chemotherapeutic agents such as 5-fluorouracil and doxorubicin

RESPONSE RATES

When tamoxifen is used as first-line hormonal therapy, ~60% of steroid receptor–positive female and male breast cancers respond; in the treatment of melanoma, adding tamoxifen to combination chemotherapy increases the response rate significantly from 10% to 51%

NURSING INTERVENTIONS

Monitor and document signs and symptoms

PATIENT INFORMATION

Barrier form of contraception in premenopausal patients, and frequent gynecologic examination for early detection of endometrial cancer

AVAILABILITY

Supplied as Nolvadex by Zeneca Pharmaceutics, Wilmington, DE, and available in generic form; 10-mg and 20-mg tablets to be stored at room temperature and protected from heat and light.

ANASTROZOLE

EFFICACY AND USAGE

Anastrozole is a newer nonsteroidal aromatase inhibitor for the treatment of post-menopausal breast cancer. It specifically suppresses the enzyme that converts androgens to estrogens, with no effect on corticosteroid or aldosterone synthesis.

DOSAGE AND ADMINISTRATION

1 mg daily orally

SPECIAL PRECAUTIONS

Anastrozole should not be administered in pregnant woman and should be closely monitored for side effects in patients with impaired liver function

TOXICITIES

The drug is generally well tolerated; the main side effects are gastrointestinal disturbance, headache, hot flashes, and edema; incidence of rashes and central nervous system symptoms (*eg*, lethargy) may occur but much less often than with the first-generation aromatase inhibitors

INDICATIONS

For advanced breast cancer in postmenopausal patients, especially those with estrogen-receptor–positive tumors and a prior history of response to tamoxifen

CONTRAINDICATIONS

None known

PHARMACOKINETICS

Anastrozole is well absorbed and bound to plasma proteins; it is metabolized in liver and excreted mainly through the biliary tract; it reaches the steady-state level at ~7 d with a half-life of 50 h in postmenopausal women

DRUG INTERACTIONS

Although anastrozole inhibits reactions catalyzed by certain P450 enzymes, it does not have known inter-actions with other drugs

RESPONSE RATES

In patients having prior treatment with tamoxifen for advanced breast cancer, approximately one-third had either an objective response (10%) or stable disease (24%), with an overall median time to progression of 21 wk

NURSING INTERVENTIONS

In patients with poor liver function, the side effects of anastrozole should be closely monitored

PATIENT INFORMATION

In premenopausal patient, pregnancy test should be done prior to receiving anastrozole

AVAILABILITY

Distributed as Arimidex by Zeneca Pharmaceuticals, Wilmington, DE., in 1-mg tablets stored in room temperature between 20° to 25°C.

BICALUTAMIDE

EFFICACY AND USAGE

Bicalutamide is a nonsteroidal "pure" antiandrogen used in the treatment of advance prostate cancer. It competitively binds to androgen receptors and inhibits the action of androgens.

DOSAGE AND ADMINISTRATION

50 mg daily orally

SPECIAL PRECAUTIONS

In patients with moderate to severe hepatic impairment

TOXICITIES

Most common side effects include hot flushes, bone pain, hematuria, and gastrointestinal symptoms (diarrhea)

INDICATIONS

A combination with an LH-RH analogue for the treatment of advanced prostate cancer

CONTRAINDICATIONS

In patients who had a prior history of a hypersensitivity reaction to this drug

PHARMACOKINETICS

Bicalutamide is well absorbed orally and not affected by the food intake; the active component (R-enantiomer) is highly protein bound; it reaches its maximal plasma level by 19 h and a steady-state level by 1 mo. It is metabolized mainly in the liver by glucuronidation and excreted in feces and urine with a half-life of ~6–7 d

DRUG INTERACTIONS

May interact with coumarin at its protein-binding sites

RESPONSE RATES

The response and survival of patients with advanced prostate cancer treated with bicalutamide monotherapy is inferior to that treated with castration; tumors that progress from bicalutamide monotherapy have a high-level amplification of the androgen receptor gene; therefore, bicalutamide should be used in combination with a LH-RH analogue for total androgen blockade; for bicalutamide in combination with LH-RH, the median time to treatment failure in prostate cancer is 97 wk

NURSING INTERVENTIONS

Closely monitor the side effects in patients with impaired liver function; adjust coumarin dosages according the prothrombin time

PATIENT INFORMATION

Bicalutamide should be started simultaneously with an LH-RH analog; it may cause gynecomastia and breast pain

AVAILABILITY

Supplied as Casodex by Zenaca Pharmaceuticals, Wilmington, DE; 50-mg tablets stored at room temperature.

LETROZOLE

EFFICACY AND USAGE

Letrozole is a newer selective and potent aromatase inhibitor. The circulating estrogens decrease by more than 95% within 2 wk of daily doses of letrozole, with no change in aldosterone or clinically significant changes in cortisol levels. It is used for the treatment of advanced breast cancer in postmenopausal patients with disease progression following antiestrogen therapy.

DOSAGE AND ADMINISTRATION

2.5 mg daily orally

SPECIAL PRECAUTIONS

Should not be used in pregnant woman

TOXICITIES

Letrozole is well tolerated; transient thrombocytopenia and elevation of liver transaminases have been reported; other minor side effects are fatigue, nausea, vomiting, musculoskeletal pain, headache, hypertension, dyspnea, hot flashes, and depression

INDICATIONS

Used as a second- and third-line hormonal therapy for advanced breast cancer

CONTRAINDICATIONS

In pregnant woman or patients with known hypersensitivity to this drug

PHARMACOKINETICS

Letrozole is rapidly and completely absorbed through the oral route and reaches a steady-state blood level by 2–6 wk; it is metabolized through the glucuronidation pathway and excreted (90%) in urine with a elimination half-life of 2 d

DRUG INTERACTIONS

None recorded

RESPONSE RATES

Objective response to letrozole as a second- and third-line hormonal therapy in patients with advanced breast cancer are ~24% and ~22%, respectively

NURSING INTERVENTIONS

Monitor the liver function tests in patients with impaired liver function

PATIENT INFORMATION

Be aware of those symptoms that may be derived from estrogen depletion or potential side effects

AVAILABILITY

Distributed as Femara by Novartis Pharmaceuticals Corp., East Hanover, NJ; 2.5-mg tablets stored at room temperature.

NILUTAMIDE

EFFICACY AND USAGE

Nilutamide is a nonsteroidal antiandrogen used in conjunction with surgical castration for advance prostate cancer

DOSAGE AND ADMINISTRATION

300 mg daily orally for the first month, then 150 mg daily orally

SPECIAL PRECAUTIONS

Be aware of the untoward side effects mentioned in the Toxicities section

TOXICITIES

Hot flushes, diarrhea, visual disturbance (dark adaptation), interstitial pneumonitis (2% up to 17% in a small study), and hepatitis (1%) with liver function abnormalities; the inhibition of the mitochondrial respiratory chain and adenosine triphosphate formation by nilutamide may contribute to the aforementioned untoward, sometimes serious, toxicities.

INDICATIONS

Nilutamide should be used in combination with castration for metastatic prostate cancer; it should be started simultaneously with castration

CONTRAINDICATIONS

For patients with severe impairment of liver function and respiratory insufficiency or patients with history of hypersensitivities to this drug

PHARMACOKINETICS

Nilutamide is rapidly and completely absorbed through the oral route; ~84% of the drug is bound to plasma proteins; the steady-state plasma concentration is reached within 2–4 wk; the drug is extensively metabolized and mainly excreted through the kidneys; the plasma elimination half-life is ~50–60 h

DRUG INTERACTIONS

Intolerance to ethanol consumption (hot flashes, malaise, and hypotension); interaction with drugs (noticeably, vitamin K antagonists, phenytoin, theophylline, and others) that are metabolized via the P450 system

RESPONSE RATES

Comparing nilutamide/orchiectomy combination therapy with orchiectomy alone, the response rates were 40%–50% vs 24%–33%; progression-free survival was 21 mo vs 15 mo, and overall survival was 37 mo vs 30 mo. The improvement of bone pain and prostate-specific antigen is also in favor of the combination; however, no data is currently available to compare nilutamide with other newer antiandrogen (*eg*, bicalutamide) in a combination modality with orchiectomy or with LH-RH analog

NURSING INTERVENTIONS

Patient should have a chest radiograph taken before initiation of nilutamide and have liver functions closely monitored; be aware of those drugs that may interact with nilutamide, and monitor the drug level closely

PATIENT INFORMATION

Patients should be aware of possible visual disturbance (delayed adaptation to dark) and should be cautious about driving at night; patients should also be informed about the symptoms of interstitial pneumonitis and potential deterioration of liver functions

AVAILABILITY

Available as Nilandron by Hoechst Marion Roussel, Inc., Kansas City, MO; 50-mg tablets stored at room temperature and protected from light.

TOREMIFENE

EFFICACY AND USAGE

Toremifene is a newer nonsteroidal antiestrogen used for the treatment of advanced breast cancer in patients with steroid-receptor–positive or unknown tumors. It claims to have less incidence of endometrial cancer (yet to be proven) and less tumorigenic effects in a rodent hepatic model.

DOSAGE AND ADMINISTRATION

60 mg daily orally

SPECIAL PRECAUTIONS

Should be cautious in patients with severe renal and hepatic insufficiency; drug-related hypercalcemia may occur

TOXICITIES

The most common adverse events are hot flashes, nausea, vaginal discharge or bleeding, and dizziness; other minor ones are anorexia, headache, diarrhea, vaginitis, rash, pruritus, depression, and insomnia; thromboembolic events (3%), elevated liver function tests (19%), and hypercalcemia (3%) have also been observed

INDICATIONS

FDA-approved: for the treatment of advanced breast cancer in postmenopausal patients

CONTRAINDICATIONS

Should not be used in pregnant patients

PHARMACOKINETICS

Toremifene is well absorbed after oral administration; the steady state blood level could be reached in 4–6 wk; the drug is mainly metabolized through the cytochrome P450 system in liver and is excreted in feces; the elimination half-life is ~5 d

DRUG INTERACTIONS

May interact with coumarin and cytochrome P450 inducers (phenobarbital, phenytoin) or inhibitors (ketoconazole)

RESPONSE RATES

As a first-line hormonal therapy for estrogen-receptor–positive or unknown advanced breast cancer, the response rates (21%–31%) in various randomized trials are comparable to that of tamoxifen (19%–37%); the time to progression and overall survival are also comparable

NURSING INTERVENTIONS

Monitoring prothrombin time and adjusting the coumarin dosage

PATIENT INFORMATION

Should not be used in pregnant woman

AVAILABILITY

Distributed as Fareston from Schering Corp., Kenilworth, NJ; 60-mg tablets stored at room temperature and protected from heat and light.

CHAPTER 6: PLANT-DERIVED AGENTS
Sanjiv S. Agarwala

Substances derived from plants have been used to treat cancer for over 200 years. The oldest known plant-derived chemotherapeutic agent was colchicine, which was shown to bind to the mitotic spindle and lead to mitotic arrest. The alkaloids vincristine and vinblastine, which were discovered in the late 1950s, are widely used plant-derived chemotherapeutic agents. Vindesine (desacetyl vinblastine) is another vinca alkaloid derived from vinblastine and displays similar activity. Although it has shown efficacy in a number of malignancies, particularly non–small cell lung cancer, it is not yet approved for use in the United States. Vinzolidine and vinorelbine are two newer semisynthetic compounds that have aroused considerable interest and are being tested vigorously in clinical trials. Paclitaxel and docetaxel belong to a new class of agents, the taxanes, one of the most important classes of antineoplastic drugs to emerge over the last two decades. The epipodophyllotoxins, etoposide (VP-16) and teniposide (VM-26), are semisynthetic compounds derived from podophyllotoxin, a plant product. Yet another group of plant-derived agents includes camptothecin (CPT) and its derivatives, topotecan and irinotecan (CPT-11). A brief overview follows these classes and the key agents in each.

SOURCES

Extracts of the common periwinkle plant (*Vinca rosea linn*) were initially tested for their potential hypoglycemic properties and were found serendipitously to cause bone marrow suppression in rats. This led to the extraction of vincristine and vinblastine, the naturally occurring chemotherapeutic alkaloids. Vinorelbine tartrate is a semisynthetic agent developed to improve the therapeutic index of vinblastine. Podophyllotoxin is derived from the May apple or mandrake plant. Its two clinically useful semisynthetic derivatives are the epipodophyllotoxins etoposide and teniposide.

Paclitaxel (Taxol; Bristol-Myers, Princeton, NJ) originally isolated in 1971, is a diterpene obtained from the bark of *Taxus brevifolia* (Western Yew tree). Docetaxel (Taxotere; Rhone-Poulenc Rorer, Collegeville, PA) is a semisynthetic compound derived from a noncytotoxic precursor (10-deacetyl baccatin III) that is extracted from the needles of *Taxus baccata-L* (European Yew tree). Because these needles are a constantly renewable source of the drug, production and supply should be easier than it has been for paclitaxel.

Camptothecan is a plant alkaloid isolated from the Chinese tree *Camptotheca acuminata*. This compound is too toxic for clinical use, but two promising derivatives of CPT, topotecan and irinotecan, have been synthesized.

MECHANISM OF ACTION

The vinca alkaloids and the taxanes are unique among chemotherapy drugs in that they do not target DNA. Vincristine, vinblastine, and vinorelbine exert their effects by selectively binding to tubulin. Tubulins are structural proteins that are an integral part of eukaryotic cells and the major component of the mitotic spindle. Microtubules of the mitotic spindle are responsible for separation of the chromosomes during mitosis. The vinca alkaloids, by binding to tubulin, inhibit microtubule assembly and are therefore cell-cycle dependent, causing arrest in the G_2 and M phases of the cell cycle.

Separate binding sites have been isolated for colchicine, the vinca alkaloids, and the taxanes. Two sites of vinca alkaloid binding have been described: a high-affinity binding site responsible for polymerization of tubulin and a low-affinity binding site responsible for microtubular unwinding and spiral formation. The vinca alkaloids also may alter the structure and function of lipid membranes by virtue of their hydrophobic properties and lead to cellular disruption.

Paclitaxel and docetaxel, on the other hand, alter the dynamics of microtubules. Under normal circumstances, microtubules form through polymerization of α and β subunits and require guanine triphosphate and microtubule-associated proteins (MAP) for this process. In the presence of paclitaxel, polymerization occurs in the absence of guanosine triphosphate and MAP. The normal equilibrium of microtubule assembly and disassembly is shifted toward microtubule assembly and the cell is thereby "frozen" in the G_2 and M phases of the cell cycle [1]. The specific binding site for paclitaxel is the microtubule, unlike the vinca alkaloids, which bind to unpolymerized tubulin. Paclitaxel also stimulates release of tumor necrosis factor and interleukin-1, which may contribute to antitumor activity.

Although podophyllotoxin itself acts on microtubules to inhibit their polymerization, its two clinically useful derivatives, the epipodophyllotoxins etoposide and teniposide, act on DNA. Their target is the nuclear enzyme DNA topoisomerase II, the enzyme responsible for catalyzing the separation of daughter DNA strands prior to miosis [2]. By inhibiting this enzyme, these drugs lead to permanent cross-linking of DNA strands and, consequently, cell death.

DRUG RESISTANCE

Drug resistance is of particular relevance to this class of agents because of the phenomenon of cross-resistance, whereby resistance to one of these drugs is often associated with resistance to other naturally derived chemotherapy drugs. These include the vinca alkaloids, the podophyllotoxins, the taxanes, and the DNA intercalators (daunorubicin, doxorubicin, mitoxantrone), but not the antimetabolites or alkylating agents. The most widely studied mechanism of this multidrug resistant (*mdr*) phenotype has to do with a membrane protein known as P-glycoprotein (P170), found in high concentrations in drug-resistant cells. This protein is encoded by the *mdr-1* gene and is thought to function as a membrane efflux pump that actively extrudes chemotherapeutic drugs from the interior of the cell by an energy (ATP)-dependent mechanism, leading to decreased intracellular drug concentration. It is present in small quantities in drug-sensitive cells, and amplification of the *mdr-1* gene is the basis for the increased expression of this protein. The degree of resistance correlates with the P-glycoprotein content of the cell. Cells resistant to chemotherapy due to increased P-glycoprotein show homogeneously staining chromosomal regions or double-minute chromosomes on cytogenetic analysis. Overexpression of P-glycoprotein is the major mode of acquired drug resistance of plant-derived chemotherapy agents.

P-glycoprotein bears significant homology to a number of ATP-binding proteins in bacteria, suggesting that it functions as general transport protein. This is further borne out by the fact that significant amounts of P-glycoprotein are found in various epithelial tissues, such as colonic mucosa and renal tubular epithelium. The *mdr-1* gene has been found to be overexpressed in many tumor types that are traditionally resistant to chemotherapy. Certain classes of drugs, particularly the calcium channel blockers (*eg*, verapamil, quinidine), actively compete for binding to P170. This has led to efforts to modulate or circumvent this resistance by combining these agents with chemotherapeutic agents [3].

Another less well-described mechanism for resistance to the vinca alkaloids involves genetically mediated mutations of the α and β subunits of tubulin. As a consequence, binding of the alkaloid to the tubulin substrate is decreased [4]. A number of mechanisms have been proposed to explain resistance to etoposide. Alterations in membrane transport occur, leading to decreased drug uptake and enhanced efflux; the latter may be mediated through P-glycoprotein and the *mdr* gene. Mutations of the topoisomerase II gene leading to decreased synthesis of the enzyme have been demonstrated in a P388 cell line. Different isoenzymes of topoisomerase II with differing sensitivity to drugs have been described; less sensitive isoenzymes may be present or preferentially synthesized in drug-resistant cells. Resistance to etoposide is accompanied by resistance to teniposide, but not to the vinca alkaloids.

Two types of paclitaxel-resistant cell lines have been described. One of the phenotypes isolated is resistant to multiple drugs due to increased drug efflux through a mechanism similar to the classic P-glycoprotein–mediated multidrug resistance phenotype. The other cell line resistant to paclitaxel exhibits mutations in either the α or β subunit of tubulin. Interestingly, these cells may actually require paclitaxel for growth in that they are unable to form mitotic spindles in its absence.

PHARMACOKINETICS

The pharmacokinetics of the vinca alkaloids depend on the route of administration. When given by the traditional intravenous (IV) bolus method, they exhibit a triphasic pattern of plasma clearance with a terminal half-life of approximately 24 hours [5]. They are rapidly taken up by various tissues, including platelets, which may account for the initial rapid clearance from circulation; the drug is then slowly released from these sites, leading to the prolonged terminal phase. These drugs are actively metabolized in the liver, which is the primary mode of excretion. Dose reduction of 50% is recommended in patients with a serum bilirubin of 3 mg/dL or higher. The administration of these drugs by continuous IV infusion may lead to higher steady-state concentrations than can be achieved by bolus therapy [6]. Vinorelbine also has been given orally; bioavailability by this route is approximately 30%.

Etoposide can be given both orally and IV. The oral bioavailability is approximately 50%, with peak concentrations occurring approximately 1 hour after administration. Absorption is not affected by food. IV injection leads to peak plasma concentrations of 30 μg/mL, with biphasic clearance and a terminal half-life of approximately 8 hours that is independent of both dose and mode of administration (bolus versus continuous infusion). Teniposide exhibits biphasic or triphasic plasma clearance with a terminal half-life of approximately 40 hours. Both agents are highly protein bound. Etoposide is metabolized in the liver. Approximately 40% of etoposide is excreted unchanged in the urine, which necessitates dose reduction in renal insufficiency. Teniposide is metabolized to inactive metabolites before it is excreted in the urine; therefore, dose reduction is unnecessary in the setting of renal insufficiency. Neither agent penetrates the cerebrospinal fluid to any significant degree.

The pharmacokinetics of paclitaxel have been investigated following 1-, 3-, 6-, 24-, and 96-hour infusions. Paclitaxel plasma concentrations decline in biphasic manner following IV administration, implying initial rapid distribution and elimination followed by a subsequent slow efflux from the peripheral compartment. When paclitaxel is administered in a 3-hour infusion, a significant nonlinear relationship exists between the dose-administered and the measured plasma paclitaxel C_{max} and the area under the curve. These nonlinear relationships are less pronounced with the 24-hour infusion [7]. The major metabolic pathway is hydroxylation by the cytochrome P450 enzyme system in the liver with formation of 6α-hydroxylpaclitaxel. Biliary excretion accounts for about 25% of the administered dose in humans. Eighty-nine percent to 98% of the drug is bound to plasma proteins [8].

TOXICITY

Although similar in structure, the vinca alkaloids display markedly different spectrums of clinical toxicity. Much of the toxicity induced by vincristine can be explained by its action on microtubules. Microtubules are ubiquitous structures found in diverse cell types, both dividing and nondividing. For example, microtubules are involved in neuronal transport; neurotoxicity, dose limiting for vincristine, may result as a direct consequence of this inhibition of neuronal function. Disruption of the microtubular structure of platelet membranes may lead to altered platelet function. The dose-limiting toxicity of vinblastine is myelosuppression. Vindesine causes neurotoxicity similar to that of vincristine and leukopenia without thrombocytopenia.

Paclitaxel causes dose-limiting neutropenia with relative sparing of the other hematopoietic cell lines. Interestingly, identical doses of paclitaxel cause markedly less myelosuppression when delivered by 3-hour than by 24-hour infusion. This phenomenon has been correlated with the time at which plasma concentrations of paclitaxel are 0.05 μmol/L or more [7]. Type 1 hypersensitivity reactions related to the Cremaphor-EL vehicle have largely been prevented by appropriate premedication with corticosteroids and histamine receptor (H1/H2) antagonists. The toxicity profile of docetaxel is similar.

The major toxicity of the epipodophyllotoxins is hematologic (neutropenia and thrombocytopenia). Other side effects include transient hepatic enzyme abnormalities, alopecia, allergic reactions, and peripheral neuropathy. Further details are provided on the individual drug pages in this chapter.

EFFICACY AND USE

The vinca alkaloids have been widely incorporated into several combination chemotherapy protocols. This usage is based on their distinct mechanism of action and their lack of nonoverlapping toxicity with the alkylators and antimetabolites. For instance, the dose-limiting neurologic toxicity of vincristine makes it an attractive candidate for incorporation into regimens using myelosuppressive drugs. Vincristine is used in the treatment of the leukemias, Hodgkin's and non-Hodgkin's lymphoma, and the childhood tumors neuroblastoma, rhabdomyosarcoma, and Wilms' tumor. Vinblastine is used against the lymphomas, testicular cancer, renal cell carcinoma, mycosis fungoides, and Kaposi's sarcoma [9]. Vinorelbine is effective against non–small cell lung cancer (NSCLC) and has been approved by the Food and Drug Administration (FDA) for this use in the United States.

Paclitaxel has undergone intensive investigation in a number of phase I and II trials, and has demonstrated activity against ovarian carcinoma refractory to other agents, breast carcinoma, non–small cell lung carcinoma, and melanoma. Docetaxel has shown promising activity against advanced breast cancer, NSCLC, and ovarian cancer. Etoposide is active against a wide range of neoplasms, of which small cell lung cancer, testicular cancer, and NSCLC are most responsive. It has also shown promise in various hematologic malignancies, including acute myeloid leukemia. Teniposide is an investigational agent that is active in combination with cytarabine against acute myeloid leukemia and other pediatric hematologic malignancies. Other tumors against which this agent is active include non-Hodgkin's lymphoma, bladder cancer, and small cell lung cancer.

NEWER AGENTS

A number of new plant-derived agents have been synthesized and extensively investigated. The following summarizes some of the current research in this arena.

Camptothecin is a plant alkaloid derived from the Chinese tree *Camptotheca acuminata*. Camptothecin inhibits the mammalian enzyme, DNA topoisomerase I. Topoisomerases are nuclear enzymes, which as their name suggests are necessary for appropriate topography of DNA. Two topoisomerases have been identified: one produces single-strand breaks (type I) and the other, double-strand breaks (type II). Camptothecin and its derivatives inhibit topoisomerase I, causing single-strand breaks in DNA and RNA, and they are maximally cytotoxic on cells in the S phase of the cell cycle.

Despite demonstrating significant antitumor activity in vitro, camptothecin proved too toxic for clinical use, due to severe unpredictable myelosuppression, hemorrhagic cystitis, and diarrhea. Topotecan is a semisynthetic analogue of camptothecin with improved water solubility. It undergoes pH-dependent hydrolysis to the active lactone form. Clearance from plasma is biexponential, with renal elimination the major route of excretion. The dose-limit-ing toxicity in phase I studies was neutropenia. Topotecan has recently been approved for second-line treatment of ovarian cancer.

Irinotecan is another semisynthetic analogue of camptothecin that showed promise both in vitro and in vivo. Its mechanism of action is similar to that of camptothecin. It acts as a prodrug, its major metabolite being 7-ethyl-10-hydroxycamptothecin (SN-38), a compound with a 300–1000-fold greater cytotoxic activity than the parent drug. Following IV administration, plasma levels of both irinotecan and SN-38 decline biexponentially. Dose-limiting toxicity is diarrhea, which is thought to be due to a cholinergic effect. If diarrhea is controlled using high doses of loperamide, granulocytopenia becomes dose-limiting [10]. It has shown activity in 5-fluorouracil-refractory colon cancer, advanced lung cancer (combined with cisplatin), and pancreatic cancer. Unlike topotecan, irinotecan is not affected by the multidrug resistance (P-glycoprotein) phenotype. Irinotecan has recently gained approval for use in 5-flourouracil refractory metastatic colorectal cancer.

The combination of topoisomerase inhibitors has been reported to be synergistic with cisplatin, possibly due to the potential for topoisomerase I inhibitors to interfere with cisplatin-induced DNA damage. Similarly, these drugs also may enhance the cytotoxic effects of ionizing radiation by inhibiting DNA repair. This hypothesis needs to be explored in clinical trials. Also notable is the fact that although concomitant administration of topoisomerase I and II inhibitors is antagonistic, sequential use may be additive. This effect may be related to the observed upregulation of intracellular topoisomerase II levels after exposure to topoisomerase I inhibitors. In this regard, two phase I studies—one combining etoposide with irinotecan and the other with topotecan—showed promising results in patients with lung cancer.

REFERENCES

1. Schiff PB, Fant J, Horwitz SB: Promotion of microtubule assembly in vitro by taxol. *Nature* 1979, 277:665–667.
2. Wozniak AJ, Ross WE: DNA damage as a basis for 4′-dimethylepipodo-phyllotoxin-9-(4,6-O-ethylidene-β-D-glucopyranoside) (etoposide) cytotoxicity. *Cancer Res* 1983, 43:120–124.
3. Beck WT: Multidrug resistance and its circumvention. *Eur J Cancer* 1990, 26:513–515.
4. Cabral FR, Brady RC, Schibler MJ: A mechanism of cellular resistance to drugs that interfere with microtubule assembly. *Ann N Y Acad Sci* 1986, 466:745–756.
5. Nelson RL: The comparative clinical pharmacology and pharmacokinetics of vindesine, vincristine, and vinblastine in human patients with cancer. *Med Pediatr Oncol* 1982, 10:115–127.
6. Wiernik PH, Schwartz EL, Straumann JJ, *et al.*: Phase I clinical and pharmacokinetic study of taxol. *Cancer Res* 1987, 47:2486–2493.
7. Gianni L, Kearns CM, Giani A, *et al.*: Nonlinear pharmacokinetic and metabolism of paclitaxel and its pharmacokinetic/pharmacodynamic relationships to humans. *J Clin Oncol* 1995, 13:180–190.
8. Clark PI, Slevin ML: The clinical pharmacology of etoposide and teniposide. *Clin Pharmacokinet* 1987, 12:223–252.
9. Rowinsky EK, Donehower RC: The clinical pharmacology and use of antimicrotubule agents in cancer chemotherapeutics. *Pharmacol Ther* 1991, 52:35–84.
10. Abigerges D, Chabot GG, Armand JP, *et al.*: Phase I and pharmacologic studies of the camptothecin analog irinotecan administered every 3 weeks in cancer patients. *J Clin Oncol* 1995, 13:210–221.

11. Madoc-Jones H, Mauro F: Interphase action of vinblastine and vincristine: differences in their lethal action through the mitotic cycle of cultured mammalian cells. *J Cell Physiol* 1968, 72:185–196.
12. Jackson DV, Bender RA: Cytotoxic thresholds of vincristine in a murine and human leukemia cell line *in vitro*. *Cancer Res* 1979, 39:4346–4349.
13. Greco FA, Johnson DH, Hainsworth JD: Chronic daily administration of oral etoposide. *Semin Oncol* 1990, 17(suppl):71–74.
14. Schacter L: Etoposide phosphate: what, why, where, and how. *Semin Oncol* 1996, 23(suppl 13):1–7.
15. O'Dwyer PJ, LaCreta FP, Daugherty JP, *et al.*: Phase I pharmacokinetic study of intraperitoneal etoposide [abstract]. *Cancer Res* 1991, 51:2041–2046.
16. Porter LL III, Johnson DH, Hainsworth JD, *et al.*: Cisplatin and etoposide combination chemotherapy for refractory small cell carcinoma of the lung. *Cancer Treat Rep* 1985, 69:479–481.
17. Wilson WH, Berg SL, Bryant G, *et al.*: Paclitaxel in doxorubicin-refractory or mitoxantrone-refractory breast cancer: a phase I/II trial of 96-hour infusion. *J Clin Oncol* 1994, 12:1621–1629.
18. Rowinsky EK, Eisenhauer EA, Chaudhry V, *et al.*: Clinical toxicities encountered with paclitaxel (Taxol). *Semin Oncol* 1993, 20(suppl):1–15.
19. Rowinsky EK, Gilbert MR, McGuire WP, *et al.*: Sequences of taxol and cisplatin; a phase I and pharmacologic study. *J Clin Oncol* 1991, 9:1692–1703.
20. Hanauske AR, Degen D, Hilsensbeck SG, *et al.*: Effects of taxotere and taxol on in vitro colony formation of freshly explanted human tumour cells. *Anticancer Drugs* 1992, 3:121–124.

VINCRISTINE

Vincristine is an alkaloid derived from *Vinca rosea linn*, the common periwinkle. It is a dimeric compound formed from two multiringed units, vindoline and catharanthine, that are joined by a carbon–carbon bridge. It is available as vincristine sulfate and has a molecular weight of 923. Its major mechanism of action appears to be the arrest of cells as they enter metaphase by binding to tubulin.

DOSAGE AND ADMINISTRATION

IV bolus: usually administered as a component of combination chemotherapy regimens at a dose of 1.4 mg/m^2 IV bolus over 1 min at weekly intervals
IV continuous infusion: low, sustained concentrations inhibit the formation of microtubules in vitro [11]; this and other similar data [12] have led to the use of a low-dose, continuous infusion of vincristine in clinical protocols; the superiority of this method of administration remains to be confirmed in the clinical setting

SPECIAL PRECAUTIONS

Patients with liver disease, particularly those with obstructive jaundice, are at greatest risk for adverse reactions and especially neurotoxicity (a dose reduction is indicated when the serum bilirubin is ≥ 3 mg/dL); neurotoxicity may be manifested as obstipation in elderly patients, for whom prophylactic cathartics or stool softeners are indicated; because it is a strong vesicant, this drug must be given through a free-flowing IV line only; special care is needed to avoid extravasation (*see* Nursing Interventions next page)

INDICATIONS

FDA-approved: acute lymphoblastic leukemia in children and adults, lymphoma (both Hodgkin's and non-Hodgkin's), and the childhood tumors; Wilms' tumor, Ewing's sarcoma, and rhabdomyosarcoma; clinical studies show activity in small cell lung cancer, multiple myeloma, and breast cancer

PHARMACOKINETICS

Absorption: not given by the oral route due to poor absorption and increased toxicity; **Distribution and clearance:** the drug undergoes triphasic serum clearance when given by bolus IV injection; it is rapidly taken up by various tissues, including platelets and other formed elements of blood and then slowly released; peak plasma concentrations are about 500 nM and steady-state concentrations between 1–2 nM; terminal half-life is longer than that of the other vinca alkaloids, area under the serum vincristine concentration–time curve is increased following continuous IV infusion; penetration into the cerebrospinal fluid is insignificant and levels are 20–30-fold less than those obtained in the serum; distribution into breast milk is unknown; **Elimination:** hepatic metabolism and excretion in the bile is the major mode of elimination; up to 70% is excreted in the feces and most of this is as a result of biliary excretion; biliary concentrations may exceed plasma levels by a factor of ≥ 100; ~15% is excreted unchanged in the urine

DRUG INTERACTIONS

Drugs that interfere with hepatic clearance may increase serum levels of vincristine; of note is the drug **asparaginase**, which along with vincristine forms a component of chemotherapy protocols for treatment of ALL; vincristine may increase blood and tissue levels of **methotrexate**; it may also decrease the bioavailability of **digoxin** by an unknown mechanism

RESPONSE RATES

ALL: complete remission (CR) rates of 90% in combination regimens; **Hodgkin's disease:** vincristine is part of the MOPP regimen (mechlorethamine, oncovin, procarbazine, prednisone) with CRs in 70%–80% of patients; approximately two thirds of these will be disease-free for 10 y and presumably cured; **Childhood tumors:** when combined with cyclophosphamide, responses have been noted in up to 100% of children with neuroblastoma; response rates of 80%–90% are seen in rhabdomyosarcoma and Wilms' tumor, again in combination with other drugs

VINCRISTINE (Continued)

TOXICITIES

Neurologic: this is dose-limiting and most commonly manifests as a mixed (sensorimotor) neuropathy; the earliest symptoms are numbness and paresthesias in the toes and fingers and the earliest objective clinical sign is the loss of the ankle jerk reflex—these symptoms and signs by themselves do not mandate dose reduction; at higher doses, painful paresthesias, muscle cramps, and ataxia occur and dose reduction or drug discontinuation is recommended; foot or wrist drop due to extensor muscle weakness is a late manifestation and is usually irreversible.

Autonomic neuropathy can present as unexplained abdominal pain, severe constipation, and ileus, particularly in older patients; involvement of nerves that innervate the bladder sometimes causes urinary retention and incontinence; cranial nerve involvement can lead to hoarseness, diplopia, and facial weakness; occasionally, headache and jaw pain occur, which usually resolve with continued therapy; depression, confusion, and other alterations in mental status also occur; intrathecal injection of vincristine is fatal.

The pathologic lesions underlying the nerve damage are both axonal degeneration and demyelination, with the former predominating; this selective axonal involvement may explain the early loss of deep tendon reflexes, which are mediated through unmyelinated nerves.

Dermatologic: reversible alopecia occurs in ~20% of patients; skin rashes are rare.

Endocrine: the syndrome of inappropriate antidiuretic hormone excretion occurs rarely.

Hematologic: much less pronounced effects on the bone marrow as compared with vinblastine; occasional leukopenia or thrombocytopenia can occur; paradoxically, vincristine may cause an increase in the platelet count by stimulating the endoreduplication of megakaryocytes.

Cardiovascular: occasional hypotension or hypertension may occur.

PATIENT MONITORING

Clinical: neurologic assessment for toxicity—earliest sign is the loss of the Achilles tendon reflex (therapy need not be stopped at this point but careful observation for further signs of peripheral neuropathy is indicated); **Laboratory:** liver functions, especially if abnormal to start with; dose reduction if serum bilirubin increases to ≥ 3 mg/dL

NURSING INTERVENTIONS

Care is required to avoid extravasation during administration; if this does occur, local application of moderate heat together with hyaluronidase may decrease necrosis

PATIENT INFORMATION

Information regarding potential neurotoxicity; if footdrop occurs, use caution while driving

FORMULATIONS

Available as Oncovin (Eli Lilly, Indianapolis, IN), Vincasar PFS (preservative free) (Adria Laboratories, Dublin, OH), Vincristine Sulfate Injection (Lymphomed, Deerfield, IL)
Vials containing 1 mg/mL of drug, stored at 2°–8°C and protected from light.

VINBLASTINE

Vinblastine is formulated as a vinblastine sulfate, an alkaloid also isolated from *Vinca rosea linn*. It differs from vincristine by one alkyl group. Its mechanism of action is similar to that of vincristine in that it arrests cells as they enter metaphase by binding to tubulin.

DOSAGE AND ADMINISTRATION

The usual starting dose is 3.7 mg/m² (5 mg in an average-sized adult). This may be increased gradually depending on the nadir leukocyte count, to a maximum recommended dose of 18.5 mg/m²; most patients are unable to tolerate more than 10–12 mg/wk. The drug is given at weekly intervals and therapy should be withheld until the leukocyte count is 4×10^9/L. When used as part of the ABVD (doxorubicin, bleomycin, vinblastine, dacarbazine) regimen for Hodgkin's disease, the dose is 6 mg/m².

Unlike vincristine, this drug is not usually given as a continuous 24-h infusion, because up to 10% of activity may be lost over this period when the drug is stored at room temperature. This may be due to interaction with the infusion device. For routine administration, vinblastine is reconstituted in sterile saline to a concentration of 1 mg/mL and administered as a 1-min bolus through a free-flowing IV line with care to avoid extravasation.

SPECIAL PRECAUTIONS

Elderly, cachectic patients; patients who have had prior chemotherapy or radiation (risk of leukopenia); patients with elevated liver enzymes or serum bilirubin; extreme irritant to tissues; free-flowing IV line only; precautions against extravasation; corneal ulceration possible on eye contact

TOXICITIES

Hematologic: myelosuppression (dose-limiting); leukopenia most common with nadir counts about a week after administration with recovery in 7–14 d; thrombocytopenia and anemia are less frequent; **Gastrointestinal:** nausea and vomiting are common but are easily controlled; abdominal pain, constipation, and ileus occur; mucositis of the oral and pharyngeal membranes occurs frequently; **Dermatologic:** alopecia occurs, but is usually partial and reversible; **Neurologic:** sensorimotor neuropathy (similar but less frequent than with vincristine and only occurs at high doses); autonomic neuropathy (*see* GI toxicity); **Cardiovascular:** hypertension occurs more commonly than does hypotension; Raynaud's phenomenon (late and prolonged side effect usually with combination chemotherapy); **Endocrine:** syndrome of inappropriate antidiuretic hormone secretion can occur

INDICATIONS

FDA-approved: Hodgkin's disease, testicular cancer, choriocarcinoma, non–small cell lung cancer, bladder carcinoma, head and neck and cervical cancer; *palliative therapy* for choriocarcinoma, breast cancer, Kaposi's sarcoma, mycosis fungoides

PHARMACOKINETICS

Absorption: not administered orally due to erratic absorption through the GI tract; **Distribution and clearance:** rapidly taken up by tissues including erythrocytes and platelets; it is highly protein bound (80%) and clearance from plasma is triphasic; a rapid distribution phase (~5 min) is followed by a β phase of 60–90 min; the terminal half-life is approximately 25 h; it does not penetrate into the cerebrospinal fluid; **Elimination:** metabolism is mainly hepatic and dose reduction is indicated in patients with altered liver function; < 20% excreted in the urine

DRUG INTERACTIONS

Lasparaginase, methotrexate, digoxin, phenytoin

RESPONSE RATES

Hodgkin's disease (with ABVD regimen): response rates of 50%–80%, CRs of 10%–30%; **Advanced nonseminomatous germ cell tumors of the testis** (with PBV [cisplatin, bleomycin, vinblastine] regimen): produced dramatic cures in patients (largely replaced by BEP [bleomycin, etoposide, platinum] regimen)

PATIENT MONITORING

A leukocyte count is mandatory before treatment and weekly thereafter, to monitor myelosuppression; treatment should be withheld for nadir leukocyte counts of < 4000/mm³; liver functions are checked at initiation of treatment and a 50% dose reduction is indicated for a serum bilirubin of ≥ 3 mg/dL

NURSING INTERVENTIONS

Precautions against and treatment for extravasation: aspirate venous blood into the syringe before and after administration as an added safety measure, to ensure line placement; if extravasation does occur, attempt to aspirate any residual drug, apply local heat to the affected area, and inject 150 mg of hyaluronidase subcutaneously around the injection site (may diminish the chances of skin necrosis or cellulitis)

PATIENT INFORMATION

Due to the increased risks of potentially life-threatening infection secondary to leukopenia, notify the physician at the first signs of an infection

FORMULATION

Available as Vinblastine Sulfate Injection (Lymphomed, Deerfield, IL), Velban (Eli Lilly, Indianapolis, IN), Velsar (Adria Laboratories, Dublin, OH), Vinblastine Sulfate Sterile (Cetus Oncology, Emeryville, CA)
Vials of 10 mg of lyophilized powder, stored at room temperature and protected from light.

ETOPOSIDE

Etoposide is a derivative of podophyllotoxin, an ancient substance that was used in the 19th century as a topical agent for the treatment of skin cancers. Podophyllotoxin itself is extracted from the American mandrake or *Podophyllum peltatum*. Chemically it is a β-glycoside of podophyllotoxin, with a molecular weight of 588, with reduced toxicity and greater therapeutic efficacy than the parent compound.

Podophyllotoxin is an antimitotic agent that, like the vinca alkaloids, binds to tubulin, but at a site distinct to that occupied by the latter. It originally was thought that its derivatives, etoposide and tenoposide, also exerted their neoplastic activity through mitotic inhibition. However, their major mechanism of action is now known to be interference with DNA synthesis by interaction with the enzyme topoisomerase II. Topoisomerase II is responsible for "untangling" daughter chromosomes during mitosis. During this process it causes transient DNA strand breaks. These breaks are then resealed by this same enzyme. It is this resealing that is inhibited by the podophyllotoxin derivatives, leading to permanent DNA strand breakage. Maximal cytotoxic effect occurs on cells in the G_2 and S phases; this may be due to the decreased topoisomerase content of resting cells. Another postulated mechanism of action is the formation of toxic free radicals, with consequent cytotoxicity. Prolonged low-dose exposure to etoposide may be more important than intermittent bolus doses; which accounts for the interest in long-term low-dose oral administration [13]. Etoposide phosphate (Etophos; Bristol Myers Squibb, Princeton, NJ) is a water soluble derivative of etoposide that has recently become commercially available [14]. The lack of water solubility of etoposide requires its formulation in polyethylene glycol, ethanol and polysorbate. The maximum recommended concentration is 0.4 mg/mL which necessitates administration of large volumes of fluids for the higher doses used in bone marrow transplantation, and also limits its use as a continuous infusion. Etoposide phosphate, on the other hand, is a water soluble prodrug that is rapidly and completely converted to etoposide 5-30 minutes after IV administration. It is pharmacokinetically and therapeutically equivalent to etoposide and can be given by bolus at high concentrations or by continuous IV infusion.

DOSAGE AND ADMINISTRATION

IV: *testicular cancer*—100 mg/m²/d × 5 d every 3 wk as part of BEP (bleomycin, etoposide, cisplatin) regimen; *small cell lung cancer*—usually 80 mg/m²/d X 3 d in combination with cisplatin; *Kaposi's sarcoma*—150 mg/m²/d IV for 3 d every 4 wk (*Note*: this can be given at higher doses with autologous bone marrow support.)
Oral: *Small cell lung cancer*—50 mg/d for 21 d; repeat cycle every 28–35 d
Hold treatment if absolute neutrophil count < 500/mm³ or platelets < 500,000/mm³

SPECIAL PRECAUTIONS

Anaphylaxis and analphylactoid reactions can occur following IV administration; appropriate measures and equipment should be available prior to drug administration; close monitoring for myelosuppression; patients with impaired renal function

INDICATIONS

FDA-approved: testicular cancer, small cell lung cancer; clinical studies show activity in Kaposi's sarcoma, peritoneal metastases

PHARMACOKINETICS

IV: it is highly bound to plasma proteins with a steady-state volume of distribution of 7–20 L/m²; its elimination is biphasic with a distribution half-life of 90 min, and a terminal half-life of 3–12 h; ~30%–40% of the dose is excreted unchanged in the urine; dose reduction may thus be indicated in patients with significantly compromised renal function; only ~2% is excreted in the bile; the site of metabolism of the remainder has not yet been determined; its major urinary metabolite is a hydroxy acid metabolic obtained after opening the lactone ring; other metabolites such as etoposide aglycon and glucuronide conjugates have been detected in small quantities in the urine—none of these appear to have any significant antineoplastic activity; cerebrospinal fluid penetration is poor (< 5%) unless given at doses of ≥ 400 mg/m²; **Oral:** peak plasma concentrations are attained 1–4 h after oral administration; absorption is not affected by food; oral bioavailability is ~50%, but is variable between patients; individualization of oral therapy is thus necessary for optimal therapeutic effect; **Other:** etoposide has been given by intraperitoneal infusion for the treatment of peritoneal metastases; the maximum tolerated dose using this approach is 700 mg/m², with myelosuppression and peritonitis being dose limiting [15]

DRUG INTERACTIONS

Both clinical and laboratory evidence indicate that etoposide synergizes with cisplatinum [16]; other commonly used agents with reported synergy include cyclophosphamide, vincristine, ara-C, and 5-fluorouracil

RESPONSE RATES

Nonseminomatous testicular germ cell cancer (as single agent): response rates of 35% in patients, both de novo and in those with refractory disease—in combination regimen, 61% complete response rate; **Stage II seminoma** (in cisplatin-based regimens): complete response rate of 61%; **Small cell lung cancer** (as single agent): response rates of 30%–35%—in combination with cisplatin, response rates of approximately 50% in previously treated patients; **Non–small cell lung cancer** (with cisplatin): response rates of up to 40%; **Non–Hodgkin's lymphoma and Hodgkin's disease:** objective response rates of 30%–40% in previously treated non-Hodgkin's lymphoma of unfavorable histology; **Metastatic carcinoma of unknown primary site** (*with cisplatin*): 73% response rate in 78 evaluable patients (31% were complete)

ETOPOSIDE (Continued)

TOXICITIES

Hematologic: leukopenia is dose limiting and may be severe; nadir counts occur in 7–14 d, with recovery by the third to fourth week of treatment; thrombocytopenia and anemia are less common; there is no cumulative bone marrow toxicity.
GI: moderately severe nausea and vomiting are a frequent (30%–40%) complication but easily controlled by commonly used antiemetic drugs; a 5-d continuous infusion may cause less nausea and vomiting; diarrhea and stomatitis occur in up to 10% of patients; stomatitis is frequent at higher doses and is, in fact, the nonhematologic dose-limiting toxicity of this agent; GI toxicity is greater with oral administration; **Anaphylaxis:** following IV administration (reduces rate of infusion);
Cardiovascular: transient hypotension unrelated to allergic reactions may occur and is more common in the elderly; (reduce rate of infusion); **Dermatologic:** reversible alopecia is frequent (70%); pruritus, hyperpigmentation, and radiation recall dermatitis have been reported; **Neurologic:** mixed (sensorimotor) neuropathy in 1%–2% (greater frequency when administered concomitantly with vincristine or other neurotoxic agents); **Other:** dystonic reactions, radiation recall, and phlebitis have been reported

PATIENT MONITORING

Careful observation for possible anaphylactoid reactions; if hypotension occurs, the infusion should be discontinued and appropriate measures taken for the therapy of anaphylaxis; hematologic function is monitored before and then frequently during therapy; a minimum of a pretreatment CBC and platelet count, repeated twice weekly during treatment, and before each subsequent dose, should be performed

NURSING INTERVENTIONS

Observation for anaphylaxis as above: IV administration should be slow (over at least 30–60 min; etoposide is a vesicant and care should be taken to prevent extravasation; wear protective gloves during handling

PATIENT INFORMATION

Inform a physician if any signs of infection develop

FORMULATIONS

Available as VePesid (Bristol-Myers Oncology Division, Princeton, NJ)
Multiple-use vials of 20 mg/mL, stored at room temperature; 50-mg capsules; stored at 2°–8°C.

TENIPOSIDE

This agent is similar to etoposide and shares a common source and mechanism of action. The structure of teniposide differs only by the substitution of a thenylidene group for the methyl group on the glucopyranoside sugar. Although the synthesis of this agent preceded that of etoposide, it is not approved for use in this country except as a second-line agent in the treatment of acute lymphoblastic leukemia (ALL) in children. It has been widely tested and extensively used in Europe.

DOSAGE AND ADMINISTRATION

ALL in children: 165–250 mg/m^2 slow IV infusion (30–60 min) to avoid reactions or hypotension; **Bladder carcinoma:** 50 mg/30–50 mL of sterile water or 0.9% sodium chloride instilled directly into bladder

SPECIAL PRECAUTIONS

Dose reduction may be indicated in patients with hepatic and renal impairment; patients who have been heavily pretreated with myelosuppressive agents or irradiation

TOXICITIES

Hematologic: leukopenia is dose-limiting; nadirs occur at ~7–10 d and recovery by 21 d; mild thrombocytopenia; **GI:** moderate nausea and vomiting, stomatitis, diarrhea, and mucositis; **Cardiovascular:** hypotension with rapid infusion (probably due to the Cremaphor diluent); decreased with slower infusion rates (> 30 min)

INDICATIONS

FDA-approved: childhood ALL as a second-line agent

PHARMACOKINETICS

Distribution: 8–30 L/m^2 volume; **Absorption:** limited penetration into cerebrospinal fluid; **Half-life:** bi- or triphasic plasma clearance, 6- to 8-h terminal half-life; **Protein-binding:** more than etoposide and more completely metabolized; **Metabolism:** uncertain; **Elimination:** 10%–20% unchanged in the urine

RESPONSE RATES

ALL in children refractory to other agents: effective in combination with cytosine arabinoside; **Hodgkin's and non-Hodgkin's lymphoma:** response rates of about 30%; **Other responsive malignancies:** acute myeloid leukemia, small cell lung cancer, carcinoma of the bladder, neuroblastoma

PATIENT MONITORING

Observe closely for anaphylactoid reactions (discontinue if hypotension occurs); monitor hematologic function before and frequently during therapy; monitor CBC and platelet counts twice weekly

NURSING INTERVENTIONS

Administer by slow IV infusion; avoid extravasation; wear protective gloves during handling

FORMULATION

Available as Vumon (Bristol-Myers Oncology Division, Princeton, NJ)
Vials of 10 mg/mL concentration for injection, stored at room temperature.

PACLITAXEL

Paclitaxel is the prototype of the taxanes, a new and important group of antineo-plastic agents. It was isolated in 1969 and its structure was described in 1971. It is a complex diterpene with a taxane ring system and C-13 side-chain that is necessary for its cytotoxic activity in mammalian cells. It was derived originally from the bark of the Pacific or Western yew tree, a comparatively rare and ancient inhabitant of the forests of the Pacific northwest. Isolation of the precursor of paclitaxel (10-deacetyl baccatin III) from the needles and twigs of the Himalayan yew (*Taxus baccata*) has allowed the semisynthetic production of paclitaxel from totally renewable resources. The FDA approved the production of semisynthetic paclitaxel in 1995, and this form of the drug has replaced the original, which was derived from the bark of *Taxus brevifolia*.

Its unique mechanism of action as a promoter of microtubule assembly distinguishes paclitaxel from the vinca alkaloids and other tubulin-interacting drugs. All aspects of tubulin polymerization are enhanced at concentrations as low as 0.05 μmol/L. By stabilizing the microtubule and preventing its disassembly, paclitaxel causes tubulin-microtubule disequilibrium; this eventually leads to cell death. Morphologically, paclitaxel-treated cells display multiple bundles of disorganized microtubules during the cell cycle as well as multiple asters of microtubules during mitosis. These microtubular bundles interact with other cellular organelles, including myosin, the Golgi apparatus, and smooth and rough endoplasmic reticulum. Due to the widespread presence of microtubules in various cell types, paclitaxel perturbs multiple cellular functions, including fibroblast activity, leukocyte migration, and sperm motility. The clinical significance of these observations is unknown. Paclitaxel also may enhance the cytotoxic effects of radiation.

DOSAGE AND ADMINISTRATION

Three-hour IV infusion: *breast cancer*—175 mg/m^2 every 3 wk; *ovarian cancer*—135 mg/m^2 or 175 mg/m^2 every 3 wk; *AIDS-related Kaposi's sarcoma (KS)*—135 mg/m^2 every 3 wk **or** 100 mg/m^2 (over 3 h) every 2 wk (*see* Special Precautions); **Other infusion schedules:** can be administered as a continuous 24-h infusion; it is also being tested as 96-hour continuous infusion and as a 1-h infusion (weekly and 3-weekly); **Intraperitoneal:** experimental, abdominal pain is dose limiting at > 125 mg/m^2; may be pharmacokinetically advantageous

SPECIAL PRECAUTIONS

Hypersensitivity and hypotensive reactions: premedicate with adequate doses of corticosteroids (dexamethasone 20 mg PO 12 and 6 h prior to infusion), H1 antagonists (diphenhydramine 50 mg IV 30 min prior to infusion), and H2 antagonists (cimetidine 300 mg or ranitidine 50 mg IV 30 min prior to infusion); administer only under close supervision and with appropriate resuscitation equipment available; due to the immunosuppressed status of AIDS-related KS, dexamethasone dose should be reduced to 10 mg PO for two doses; **Neutropenia:** contraindicated if neutrophil counts are < 1500/mm^3; for AIDS-related KS, absolute neutrophil count should be > 1000 cells/mm^2

INDICATIONS

FDA-approved: metastatic ovarian cancer after failure of first-line chemotherapy; metastatic or relapsed breast cancer after failure of combination chemotherapy (anthracycline based) or relapse within 6 mo of adjuvant chemotherapy; AIDS-related KS (approved June 1997); **Other:** currently under investigation as combination therapy with doxorubicin, 5-fluorouracil, cisplatin, and carboplatin and with cyclophosphamide for breast, lung, and head and neck cancer and other malignancies

PHARMACOKINETICS

Peak plasma concentrations: 0.6–13 μM depending on dose and schedule; **Distribution:** mean central volume of distribution (VD$_c$) 13.8 L/m^2 (range, 8.6–19.2 L/m^2); mean steady state volume of distribution (VD$_{ss}$) 87 L/m^2 (range, 48–182 L/m^2); **Protein-binding:** 95%–98%; **Half-life:** biphasic; mean α half-life 0.34 h; mean β half-life 4.9 h; **Tissue distribution:** has been detected in ascitic fluid but not in cerebrospinal fluid; **Elimination:** 5%–10% recovered unchanged in the urine; major metabolite is 6α-hydroxypaclitaxel, formed in the liver cytochrome P-450 system; overall liver metabolism about 25%

DRUG INTERACTIONS

Cisplatin: mean paclitaxel clearance rates are lower when given following cisplatin as compared with the reverse sequence [19]; the postulated mechanism is interference with the cytochrome P-450 system by cisplatin; **Ketoconazole:** based on in vitro data demonstrating possible inhibition of paclitaxel metabolism by ketoconazole, the manufacturer recommends caution when using these two agents concomitantly; **Doxorubicin:** plasma levels of doxorubicin may be increased when used in combination with paclitaxel

RESPONSE RATES

Ovarian cancer: phase II studies have shown a 24%–45% response rate in patients with platinum-resistant, and 41%–50% response rate in platinum-sensitive disease, respectively; a recently completed trial comparing cisplatin combined with either paclitaxel or cyclophosphamide in previously untreated patients showed significantly improved partial response, complete response and pathologic response rates for the paclitaxel arm; **Breast cancer:** objective responses of 56%–62% have been noted in previously treated patients; combination regimens with doxorubicin and cyclophosphamide are under investigation; **Non–small cell lung cancer:** response rates of 34%–40% in previously untreated patients; **Small cell lung cancer:** response rate of 34% in previously untreated patients with extensive-stage disease; **Head and neck cancer:** phase II trial using paclitaxel 250 mg/m^2 with granulocyte colony-stimulating factor (GCSF) support showed a 41% response rate in 17 previously untreated patients; **Esophageal carcinoma:** 32% response rate in 50 patients with squamous and adenocarcinomas of the esophagus using paclitaxel with GCSF (median duration of response 17 wk); **Melanoma:** partial responses in 4 of 12 patients in an early phase I study; 4 of 28 responses seen in a phase II study (1 complete response); **Bladder cancer:** response rates of 42%–56% in small phase II studies (previously untreated patients)

PACLITAXEL (Continued)

TOXICITIES

Myelosuppression: neutropenia (dose-limiting and more severe when administered by 24-h infusion [18]); anemia and thrombocytopenia (less common); **Cardiovascular:** arrhythmias, transient bradycardia (3% of patients), hypotension (up to 12% of patients); usually require no treatment; not correlated with previous anthracycline therapy [12]; **Hypersensitivity reactions:** manifesting as hypotension (see Special Precautions), bronchospasm, and urticaria (related to the Cremaphor-EL vehicle and are histamine mediated); **Neurotoxicity:** frequency and severity of neurologic manifestations are dose-dependent but not influenced by infusion duration; peripheral neuropathy observed in 60% (3% severe); preexisting neuropathy is not a contraindication for therapy; **GI:** anorexia, nausea, and vomiting (uncommon and not severe); mucositis is dose dependent; **Dermatologic:** alopecia (nearly universal at doses of > 130 mg/m^2); reversible, but in contrast to other antineoplastic agents, involves all body hair sites, such as the axillary and pubic hair, eyelashes, and eyebrows

PATIENT MONITORING

Monitor carefully for neutropenia; subsequent treatment cycles are generally withheld until the neutrophil count is > 1500 cells/mm^3; dose reduction by 20% is recommended for severe neutropenia (absolute neutrophil count < 500/mm^3); observe carefully for the development of hypersensitivity reactions or peripheral neuropathy

NURSING INTERVENTION

Observation for toxicity, particularly immediate hypersensitivity reactions as outlined above; care against extravasation is important—although not a vesicant, paclitaxel can lead to local pain, erythema, and swelling immediately following extravasation; it generally responds well to local measures and does not lead to necrosis or sclerosis; the Cremaphor vehicle is a surfactant and has been shown to leach plastic from polyvinyl chloride plastic bags; paclitaxel infusions should thus be prepared in glass bottles and infused through polyethylene-lined (non–polyvinyl chloride) infusion sets; it should be infused through an in-line filter with a microporous membrane (≈ 0.22 microns)

PATIENT INFORMATION

Be aware of possible hypersensitivity reactions and neutropenia

FORMULATIONS

Available as Taxol (Bristol-Myers Oncology Division, Princeton, NJ)
30 mg/5 mL single-dose vials; 100 mg/16.7 mL multidose vials.

TOPOTECAN

Topotecan is a semisynthetic, water soluble analogue of camptothecin, a plant alkaloid derived from *Camptotheca acuminata*, a tree indigenous to China. Camptothecin proved to be too toxic for clinical use, and following elucidation of its unique mechanism of action, the semisynthetic analogue topotecan was developed. Unlike the other commercially available camptothecin analogue (irinotecan), topotecan is not a pro-drug and is clinically active in the lactone form.

Topotecan is a potent reversible inhibitor of the nuclear enzyme DNA topoisomerase I (topo-1), which is responsible for "relaxation" of supercoiled double-stranded DNA by creating single-stranded breaks through which another DNA strand can pass during transcription. Topo-1 then reseals the break allowing DNA replication to occur. Inhibition of topo-1 leads to the formation of stable DNA-topoisomerase complexes, with eventual formation of irreversible double-stranded DNA breaks, leading to apoptosis and cell death. Topotecan is most lethal during the S-phase of the cell cycle, which also implies possibly greater efficacy with prolonged continuous exposure to the drug. However, thus far, this has not been borne out in clinical practice.

DOSAGE AND ADMINISTRATION

Recommended dose is 1.5 mg/m^2 by IV infusion over 30 min daily for 5 consecutive d, starting on d 1 of a 21-d course; as the median time to response may be delayed for as long as 8–12 wk, a minimum of four courses of treatment is recommended; if severe neutropenia occurs (absolute neutrophil count [ANC] < 500/mm^3), dosage should be reduced by 0.25 mg/m^2 for subsequent courses. Topotecan has also been tested in higher dosages (2 mg/m^2) with the same schedule and as a 21-d continuous infusion; to date, no advantage for the latter route of administration is apparent.

SPECIAL PRECAUTIONS

Hematologic: adequate bone marrow function is essential, and treatment should not be initiated for neutrophils < 1500/mm^3 and platelets < 100,000/mm^3. Blood counts should be monitored frequently and re-treatment should be held till ANC > 1000/mm^3 and platelets > 100,000/mm^3; **Renal:** for moderate renal insufficiency (creatinine clearance, 20–39 mL/min), a dosage reduction to 0.75 mg/m^2 is recommended; not recommended for patients with creatinine clearance of < 20 mL/min; **Other:** contraindicated in women who are pregnant or nursing

INDICATIONS

FDA-approved: metastatic ovarian carcinoma after failure of initial or subsequent therapy; **Experimental:** currently being tested as a component of first line therapy of ovarian cancer in combination with cisplatin, paclitaxel, and G-CSF; has activity in breast and colon cancer and in small cell lung cancer (SCLC) and non–small cell lung cancer (NSCLC); may also be useful as a radiation sensitizer

PHARMACOKINETICS

Half-life—topotecan exhibits linear pharmacokinetics following short IV infusions, terminal half-life 2–3 h; **Protein binding**—20%–35%; **Metabolism**—rapidly metabolized by nonenzymatic hydrolysis to less active carboxylate; liver microsomal system acts as minor metabolic pathway; **CSF penetration**—32% of plasma concentration in a pediatric study; **Elimination**—mainly (30%–40%) excreted by the kidneys

DRUG INTERACTIONS

Cisplatin: myelosuppression is more severe when topotecan is given in combination with cisplatin; concomitant administration of topotecan 1.25 mg/mm^2 and cisplatin 50 mg/m^2 led to neutropenia for 12 d in one phase I study and neutropenic death in one patient; this effect is worse if cisplatin is administered prior to topotecan, presumably due to cisplatin-induced reduction in renal clearance
Paclitaxel: myelosuppression with the combination is more severe, even with G-CSF support; dose-limiting neutropenia and thrombocytopenia in a Gynecologic Oncology Group phase I study at a dose of topotecan 0.75 mg/mm^2 daily $\times$ 5 with paclitaxel 135 mg/m^2 by 24-h infusion with G-CSF support
G-CSF: concomitant administration of topotecan and G-CSF may prolong the duration of neutropenia; G-CSF should only be started on d 6 at least 24 h after completion of topotecan infusion

TOPOTECAN (Continued)

TOXICITIES

Neutropenia: this was dose-limiting toxicity in most studies (ANC ≤ 500/mm^3 for > 5 d) and occurred in about 40% of courses; the ANC nadir occurs at ~d 11 with recovery by d 21; prophylactic G-CSF was given in 27% of courses after the first cycle but is not recommended routinely; neutropenic fever or sepsis occurred in about 25% of patients; septic death occurred in 0.7%; **Thrombocytopenia:** (platelets ≤ 25,000/mm^3) occurs in ~25% of patients and < 10% of courses; platelet nadirs occur at ~d 15 and last a median of 5 d; platelet transfusions were required in 13% of patients in clinical trials; **Anemia:** grade 3 or 4 anemia (hemoglobin < 8 g/dL) occurred in 40% of patients; transfusions were needed in 56% of patients; **Gastrointestinal:** nausea and vomiting in 50%–75% of patients; diarrhea in 40%; **Alopecia:** total alopecia in 42% of patients; **Central nervous system:** headache in 20% of patients; grade 1 paraesthesia in < 10%.

RESPONSE RATES

Refractory metastatic ovarian cancer: in 454 patients who had failed one or two platinum-based regimens, response rates ranged from 13.3%–20.5% (complete plus partial); was found to be equivalent to paclitaxel in a phase III randomized trial in this patient population but with a higher incidence of myelosuppression and febrile neutropenia; response rates are lower (5.9%; CI: 0.7%–19.7%) in patients who are truly platinum refractory (no response or progression during cisplatin therapy); **SCLC:** response rates of 39% documented in one study of untreated patients with extensive stage SCLC, using 2 mg/m^2/d for 5 d; median duration of response was 4.8 mo; grade 3–4 neutropenia and thrombocytopenia occurred in 29% and 38%, respectively, despite routine use of G-CSF; with standard 1.5 mg/m^2/d X 5 dosing, response rates varied from 10%–33%; phase III trials of topotecan in addition to standard regimens in SCLC are underway; **NSCLC:** may be less active; response rates range from 0%–15%; **Colorectal cancer:** response rates of 7%–10% in two phase II studies of untreated metastatic colorectal cancer; myelosuppression was dose limiting; **Hematologic malignancies:** promising activity shown in myelodysplastic syndromes. response rate of 27% obtained in 22 patients at a dose of 2 mg/m^2 over 24 h as a 5-d continuous infusion; of note, 8 of these 22 patients also became cytogenetic normal; similar results have been seen in chronic myelomonocytic leukemia; toxicity in these studies was considerable (myelosuppression, mucositis); also being tested in acute leukemia and chronic myelogenous leukemia; **Other:** currently undergoing evaluation in metastatic breast cancer and pediatric malignancies (neuroblastoma, rhabdomyosarcoma).

PATIENT MONITORING

Laboratory: hematologic parameters (hemoglobin, ANC, and platelets) prior to treatment and weekly during therapy; initiate therapy if ANC > 1500/mm^3 and platelets > 100,000/mm^3; withhold re-treatment unless ANC > 1000/mm^3 and platelets > 100,000/mm^3; **Mutagenicity:** camptothecin derivatives may theoretically increase the incidence of secondary malignancies; clinical monitoring should be considered in long-term survivors.

NURSING INTERVENTIONS

Standard precautions for chemotherapy administration; extravasation has been associated with only mild local reactions.

PATIENT INFORMATION

Topotecan may be harmful to the unborn fetus; precautions against pregnancy should be taken while on treatment; information regarding potential for neutropenia and fever should be provided.

FORMULATIONS

Available as Hycamtin (SmithKline Beecham, Philadelphia, PA)
4-mg (base) single-dose vials; each vial should be reconstituted with 4 mL sterile water for injection, which is then diluted in either a 0.9% NaCl or a 5% dextrose solution.

IRINOTECAN

Irinotecan (CPT-11) is a semisynthetic analogue of camptothecin with improved water solubility. Like its parent compound, irinotecan is an S-phase–specific inhibitor of DNA topoisomerase-I (topo-1). Topo-1 catalyzes the relaxation of the DNA molecule by introducing a transient break in one of the two strands of DNA. Inhibition of the enzyme leads to the stabilization of cleavable complexes formed by the enzyme and the DNA molecule, preventing the repair of the break caused by topo-1. This leads to the formation of single- and double-stranded DNA breaks and cell death by apoptosis. Irinotecan was the first drug in its class to be approved for clinical use.

Irinotecan acts as a prodrug and undergoes rapid partial conversion to its active metabolite, SN-38 (7-ethyl-1-hydroxy-camptothecin) through hydrolysis by cellular carboxyl esterase. SN-38 is 250 to 1000 times more potent than the parent compound. This reaction occurs in several body tissues, including the liver and the gastrointestinal tract. In equilibrium, it exists in two forms: an active lactone form favored at acidic pH and an inactive carboxyl form. In the plasma, SN-38 is found mainly in the lactone form.

DOSAGE AND ADMINISTRATION

Recommended starting dose: 125 mg/m^2 IV infusion over 90 min; one treatment course comprises 125 mg/m^2 once weekly for 4 wk followed by a 2-wk rest; the dose may be adjusted up to 150 mg/m^2 or down to 50 mg/m^2 depending upon patient tolerance; if tolerated, courses may be continued until disease progression; **In Europe:** the drug has been used at a dose of 350 mg/m^2 as a 30–90 min infusion once every 3 wk; other investigational schedules include once every 2 wk, once every 4 wk, and as a 5-d continuous infusion

SPECIAL PRECAUTIONS

IV administration: take care to avoid extravasation; flushing with sterile water and application of ice are recommended in case of extravasation; **diarrhea:** *early*—diarrhea, abdominal cramping, or diaphoresis occurring within 24 h of irinotecan administration should be treated with 0.25–1.0 mg atropine IV, unless clinically contraindicated; *late*—diarrhea occurring later than 24 h after administration should be treated with 4 mg of loperamide PO at the first sign of increased bowel frequency or loose stools, followed by 2 mg every 2 h until patient is diarrhea free for at least 12 h; elderly patients or those who have received prior pelvic or abdominal radiation are at increased risk of adverse events and should be closely monitored; **Hepatic dysfunction:** contraindicated if serum bilirubin > 2 mg/dL or transaminases > 3 times normal without liver metastases and > 5 times normal with liver metastases

INDICATIONS

FDA-approved: patients with metastatic colorectal carcinoma with disease progression, recurrence, or lack of response to 5-fluorouracil–based chemotherapy

PHARMACOKINETICS

Absorption: usually administered IV; **Peak plasma concentration:** with 350 mg/m^2 bolus, the mean peak of irinotecan plasma concentration is 7.7 µg/mL and 56 ng/mL for SN-38; AUC of irinotecan, but not SN-38, increases linearly with dose; maximum concentrations are seen in 1 h following a 90-min infusion; **Half-life:** mean terminal half-life is 8.8 h for irinotecan and 11.6 h for SN-38; **Protein binding:** irinotecan, 65%; SN-38, 95%; **Metabolism and excretion:** conversion of irinotecan to SN-38 occurs by carboxylesterase enzymes, primarily in the liver; glucuronidation of SN-38 occurs in the liver; total hepatic excretion is 25%–50%; urinary excretion is < 20%

DRUG INTERACTIONS

Potential for greater myelosuppression if used with other chemotherapeutic agents; caution in patients who have received prior abdominal/pelvic radiation

RESPONSE RATES

Metastatic colorectal cancer: European phase II study demonstrated response rates of 18.8% (chemotherapy naive patients) and 17.7% (previously treated patients) at a dose of 350 mg/m^2 once every 3 wk; median duration of response was 9.1 mo, and median survival was 10.6 mo; a recent North Central Cancer Treatment Group (US) phase II study of 121 patients at a dose of 125 mg/m^2 × 4 wk, followed by a 2-wk rest reported response rates of 13.3% in previously treated patients and 25.8% in previously untreated patients; **Non–small cell lung cancer:** phase II studies in Japan reported response rates of 31%–34% (previously untreated patients); response rates of 42%–54% were reported in combination therapy with cisplatin; neutropenia and diarrhea are dose limiting in these studies; overall response rates were 21.3% in a Japanese phase II study with etoposide and G-CSF; **Gastric cancer:** phase I-II study from Japan reported a response rate of 41.7% in 24 patients in combination with cisplatin; **Other:** irinotecan has shown activity against leukemia, non-Hodgkin's lymphoma, and ovarian, cervical, and small cell lung cancer

PATIENT MONITORING

Hematologic: CBC with differential and platelets prior to each dose; consider dose reduction by 25 mg/m for grade 2 toxicity and 50 mg/m^2 for grade 3 or 4 toxicity; withhold treatment until absolute neutrophil count is > 1500/mm^3 and platelets are > 100,000/mm^3; **Diarrhea (early and late):** treatment should be withheld until diarrhea is resolved; for grade 3 (7–9 stools/d), reduce dose by 25 mg/m^2 and for grade 4 (> 10 stools/d), reduce dose by 50 mg/m^2

IRINOTECAN (Continued)

TOXICITIES

Gastrointestinal: diarrhea can occur early (within 24 h) or late (after 24 h); median time to onset of late diarrhea is about 11 d; factors that increase the risk of grade 3 or 4 diarrhea include a starting dose of 125 mg/m^2 as opposed to 100 mg/m^2, age > 65 y, and prior abdominal/pelvic irradiation (*see* Special Precautions for treatment); nausea and vomiting is uncommon with antiemetics (dexamethasone with 5-HT antagonist); **Hematologic:** leukopenia and neutropenia are common; neutropenic fever occurred in 3% of patients in clinical trials; thrombocytopenia and anemia are less common; **Hepatic:** grade 3–4 elevation of transaminases occur in ~10% of a patients, particularly in those with liver metastases; **Alopecia:** uncommon

NURSING INTERVENTIONS

Irinotecan should be diluted in a 5% dextrose or a 0.9% NaCl solution prior to administration; observation for early abdominal cramps, diaphoresis, or early diarrhea; *see* Special Precautions.

PATIENT INFORMATION

Diarrhea: strict instructions on loperamide schedule for late diarrhea (*see* Special Precautions); instruct patient to call physician if diarrhea does not resolve; avoid usage of drugs with laxative properties; **Pregnancy and breast feeding:** female patients should use birth control and avoid nursing while on treatment.

FORMULATION

Available as Camptosar (Pharmacia and Upjohn, Kalamazoo, MI)
5-mL single-dose vial containing 20 mg/mL irinotecan for IV injection.

DOCETAXEL

Docetaxel (RP 65976, NSC 628503) is a semisynthetic derivative of 10-deacetyl baccatin III, a precursor of paclitaxel. It is extracted from the needles of the European yew, *Taxus baccata*, an abundantly available and renewable source. Its mechanism of action is similar to that of paclitaxel, promoting microtubule assembly and stabilization, arresting cells in the M phase of the cell cycle. In experimental systems, it has shown more potent activity on microtubules than paclitaxel. In a head-to-head comparison against a variety of human tumors, in vitro docetaxel was more cytotoxic than paclitaxel (1.3- to 12-fold) [20]. In addition, cross-resistance between these two agents is incomplete. Docetaxel represents the second antineoplastic agent of the taxane family to gain FDA approval for the treatment of metastatic breast cancer. It is currently undergoing extensive evaluation in other malignancies as a single agent and in combination.

DOSAGE AND ADMINISTRATION

The recommended phase II dose is 100 mg/m^2 given as a 1-h IV infusion, once every 3 wk; determination of the appropriate dose in combination regimens is ongoing

SPECIAL PRECAUTIONS

Hypersensitivity and fluid retention: all patients should be premedicated with corticosteroids to reduce the incidence of hypersensitivity and fluid retention; a recommended regimen is 8 mg of dexamethasone twice daily, starting 1 day prior to docetaxel administration; patients should be observed closely for signs of hypersensitivity, and appropriate resuscitative measures should be close at hand; **Hepatic:** should be avoided if bilirubin is > the upper limit of normal (ULN), if transaminases is > 1.5 times ULN, and if alkaline phosphatase is > 2.5 times ULN; toxicity of docetaxel is significantly higher in these situations; **Neutropenia:** hold if absolute neutrophil count is < 1500/mm^3

INDICATIONS

FDA-approved: locally advanced or metastatic breast cancer that has progressed during anthracycline-based therapy or relapsed following anthracycline-based adjuvant therapy; shows activity in ovarian, lung (small and non–small cell), and head and neck cancers

PHARMACOKINETICS

Peak plasma concentrations: (after 100 mg/m^2 1-h infusion) 3.6 µg/mL; AUC=4.7 µg/mL; **Half-life:** biphasic at lower doses, triphasic at doses > 85 mg/m^2; **Elimination half-life:** ~12 h; **Protein binding:** 97%; **Elimination:** mainly fecal excretion; < 9% excreted in urine

DRUG INTERACTIONS

Inducers of p450 liver enzymes, such as phenytoin, may accelerate docetaxel metabolism, but the clinical significance of this is unknown

RESPONSE RATES

Metastatic breast cancer: in 7 studies involving 283 patients, response rates of 56% (chemotherapy-naive patients) and 49% (previously treated patients); response rates in patients with true anthracycline resistance was 41% in three trials (higher than that observed with paclitaxel); **Non–small cell lung cancer:** response rates in 160 patients with newly diagnosed non–small cell lung cancer treated at 100 mg/m^2 in five phase II trials was 27% with a median survival of 9 mo; response rates in platinum-resistant/refractory patients was 17%; ongoing trials are testing combinations with cisplatin, carboplatin, vinorelbine, and gemcitabine; **Ovarian cancer:** activity demonstrated in both platinum-sensitive and platinum-refractory tumors

PATIENT MONITORING

Hematologic: weekly complete blood and absolute neutrophil counts to determine neutrophil nadir; patients with grade 4 neutropenia lasting more than 1 wk or those with neutropenic fever should have their dose reduced from 100 mg/m^2 to 75 mg/m^2; **Hypersensitivity:** close observation of patients, particularly after first two infusions; **Weight gain:** should be monitored at each visit; **Neurologic:** check for signs and symptoms of peripheral neuropathy; if severe, consider 25% dose reduction

DOCETAXEL (Continued)

TOXICITIES

Myelosuppression: neutropenia is dose-limiting; grade 4 neutropenia occurs in almost 100% of patients treated at 100 mg/m^2; thrombocytopenia and anemia are uncommon; **Hypersensitivity reactions:** observed in 17% of patients in phase I and II studies; routine premedication with steroids is recommended; **Dermatologic:** localized macular or maculopapular eruptions occur, particularly on hands and feet; nail changes (hypo- or hyperpigmentation and onycholysis) have been reported; alopecia reported in > 60% of patients; **Fluid retention:** edema, weight gain, pleural and pericardial effusions, and ascites may occur; incidence of severe fluid retention is about 2%; median weight gain is about 2 kg; completely reversible at median of 29 wk; **GI:** nausea and vomiting are easily controlled with standard antiemetics; diarrhea (31%) and stomatitis (20%) in phase II trials; **Neurotoxicity:** peripheral neuropathy in 12%; mainly mild to moderate paresthesias; **Asthenia:** severe in 11% of patients

NURSING INTERVENTIONS

Transfer diluent to appropriate vial of docetaxel concentrate and then add to NaCl or 5% dextrose solution to produce a final concentration of 0.3–0.9 mg/mL; administer as a 1-h IV infusion; precautions and monitoring for hypersensitivity reactions (*see* Patient Monitoring); minimize contact of undiluted concentrate with plastic or PVC equipment; infusion-site reactions are uncommon and mild

PATIENT INFORMATION

Strict regimen of steroids to prevent hypersensitivity; information on neutropenia and appropriate precautions; information regarding edema and weight gain; patients may experience temporary worsening of performance status while on therapy, even if responding

FORMULATION

Available as Taxotere (Rhone-Poulenc Rorer, Collegeville, PA) for injection concentrate 20-mg and 80-mg single-dose vials with accompanying diluent.

VINORELBINE

Vinorelbine is a unique semisynthetic vinca alkaloid derived from the leaves of the periwinkle plant, first synthesized in 1978. It differs from the natural vinca alkaloids by an eight- as opposed to a nine-member catharanthine ring; in contrast, the other vincas are modified at the vindoline ring. This unique structure may be responsible for its greater microtubule specificity and antitumor activity. It is a classic antitubulin in that it causes mitotic arrest of cells in the G_2 and M phases of the cell cycle by inhibiting tubulin assembly. It does this at lower concentrations than the other vinca alkaloids and at concentrations that spare axonal microtubules. This suggests that vinorelbine may have lower neurotoxicity and greater specificity for cancer cells.

DOSAGE AND ADMINISTRATION

IV: 30 mg/m^2 over 6–10 min once every week; the same dose and schedule can be used in combination with cisplatin, 120 mg/m^2 (given on d 1 and 29); **Oral:** a liquid-filled soft gelatin capsule has been tested at doses of 60–100 mg/m^2/d; this form is not yet commercially available

SPECIAL PRECAUTIONS

Should be administered with caution in patients with compromised bone marrow reserve (prior radiation or chemotherapy); granulocyte counts should be $\geq$ 1000 cells/mm^3 prior to administration; acute shortness of breath and bronchospasm have been an infrequent complication following IV administration; facilities for supplemental oxygen, bronchodilators, and corticosteroids should be at hand; dose modification is recommended for hepatic insufficiency: for bilirubin 2.1–3 mg/dL, the dose is 15 mg/m^2; for bilirubin > 3 mg/dL, the dose is 7.5 mg/m^2

TOXICITIES

Myelosuppression: neutropenia is dose-limiting. Nadirs occur in 7–10 d; it is noncumulative and reversible; infectious complications and septic deaths are rare. Anemia and thrombocytopenia are infrequent; **Neurologic:** mild to moderate peripheral neuropathy occurs in about 25% of patients; loss of deep tendon reflexes occurs in about 5%; **GI:** mild to moderate nausea and vomiting occur in about a third of patients and are easily controlled with standard antiemetics; constipation also occurs in about a third of patients but paralytic ileus is extremely rare; mild diarrhea and stomatitis have been reported; **Dermatologic:** alopecia reported in 10% of patients; **Hepatic:** transient, reversible elevations of hepatic transaminases occur; **Pulmonary:** dyspnea and bronchospasm reported in 1%–3% of patients (see Precautions); **Cardiovascular:** approximately 6% of patients experienced chest pain with or without electrocardiographic changes (most had underlying cardiac disease)

INDICATIONS

FDA-approved: stage IV non–small cell lung cancer (NSCLC), either as a single agent or in combination with cisplatin; stage III NSCLC in combination with cisplatin; clinical studies show activity in metastatic breast cancer, both pretreated and previously untreated patients, Hodgkin's and non-Hodgkin's lymphoma, ovarian cancer

PHARMACOKINETICS

Absorption—oral bioavailability 27% ± 12%; **Peak plasma concentrations**—1088 ng/mL following 30 mg/m^2 IV bolus; 114 ± 43 ng/mL following 100 mg/m^2 oral gelatin capsule; T$_{max}$ 1.49 h following oral administration; highly protein-bound; **Half-life:** triphasic plasma decay following IV and oral administration; terminal phase is 28–44 h (IV), 18 h (oral), and reflects prolonged slow efflux from the peripheral compartment; **Volume of distribution**—25.4–40.1 L/kg; **Elimination**—major site of metabolism is the liver; deacetylvinorelbine, a metabolite, may possess antitumor activity; 18% excreted in urine, 46% in the feces

DRUG INTERACTIONS

Mitomycin: acute pulmonary reactions reported when given with this agent; **cisplatin:** no pharmacokinetic interaction but incidence and severity of neutropenia are higher

RESPONSE RATES

NSCLC (advanced, unresectable): objective response rate of 33% as a single agent in previously untreated patients; in a European multicenter, phase III trial, the combination of vinorelbine plus cisplatin was significantly superior (response rate 28%, median survival 40 wk) to vindesine plus cisplatin (response rate 19%, median survival 32 wk); in a US phase II/III multicenter trial, vinorelbine was superior (response rate 18%, median survival 30 wk) to 5-fluorouracil plus leucovorin (response rate 7%, median survival 22 wk); a response rate of 15% and a median survival of 29 wk were seen in 162 patients with stage IV NSCLC treated with oral vinorelbine at 60–100 mg/m^2/d; **Breast cancer:** overall response rate of 46% in patients with advanced breast cancer in an early phase II study; response rate of 78% reported in combination with doxorubicin; **Hodgkin's disease and non-Hodgkin's lymphoma:** response rates of 34% and 38%, respectively; **Ovarian cancer:** response rate of 17% in heavily pretreated patients

PATIENT MONITORING

Monitor for neutropenia and hepatic function abnormalities; blood counts should be checked prior to administration of each dose

NURSING INTERVENTIONS

Dilute in a syringe or IV bag using 5% dextrose or 0.9% sodium chloride injection; administer over 6–10 min into the side-port of a freely flowing IV; flush with 75–125 mL of the diluent; it is a strong vesicant and care must be taken to avoid extravasation; injection site reactions (erythema, pain, discoloration) occur in up to one third of patients; chemical phlebitis occurs in 10%; avoid eye contamination

PATIENT INFORMATION

Inform patient about the risk for neutropenia and subsequent infectious complications; women of child-bearing potential should be advised against pregnancy

FORMULATION

Available as Navelbine (Burroughs Wellcome, Research Triangle Park, NC) 10- or 50-mg/5 mL single-use vials.

ETIOLOGY AND RISK FACTORS

The incidence of breast cancer in the United States has been rising steadily during the past few decades. Early detection through patient screening and self-examination accounts for only part of this trend. The death rate and incidence of advanced breast cancer have remained stable, while the number of early stage, particularly node-negative, and in situ lesions has increased. This trend may be due in part to earlier detection, improvement in surgical and radiation therapy techniques, and the increasing use of systemic adjuvant therapy. Approximately 182,000 new cases and 44,000 deaths from breast cancer are seen yearly in the United States [1]. Risk factors for the development of breast cancer include older age, immediate family history of breast cancer at a young age or bilateral breast cancer, early menarche, late menopause, nulliparity, the use of prolonged, high doses of conjugated estrogens, exposure to ionizing radiation at a young age, and a past history of atypical hyperplasia, in situ or invasive carcinoma (Table 7-1) [2]. Familial risk is likely due to inherited genetic abnormalities, although some of these may only confer a slight elevation or risk (incomplete penetrance). Two recently identified genes, BRCA-1 and BRCA-2, are likely to account for a majority of families with inherited predisposition to breast or breast and ovarian cancer [3]. Dietary risks from high-fat or low-fiber diets, however, have been hard to demonstrate.

SCREENING FOR BREAST CANCER

The modalities of breast self examination, examination by a physician, and screening mammography are used to detect breast cancer owing to the assumption that therapy at an earlier stage will improve outcome. This approach is supported by the known relationship of survival to stage of disease. Of these modalities, only the use of mammography has been shown to decrease mortality due to breast cancer. Randomized trials comparing mammography every 1 to 2 years to routine physical examinations have shown relative reductions in breast cancer-related mortality in the range of 25% to 30% [4]. These trials initially showed a mortality benefit only in women over 50 years of age, but longer follow-up and pooled analyses of trials are now showing mortality reductions in women between 40 and 50 years of age as well. In this group, however, the higher ratio of normal biopsies to cancers diagnosed reflects the lower positive predictive value because breast cancer is less prevalent in younger women. Furthermore, mammograms may be less sensitive in younger women as a result of increased breast tissue density; a false reassurance from a negative mammogram may result. Guidelines for screening are listed in Table 7-2. Any suspicious palpable breast mass should be evaluated with close observation and biopsy if there is no resolution or immediate biopsy regardless of mammographic findings. Fine needle aspiration is of acceptable accuracy if the operator and cytopathologist are experienced; otherwise, excisional biopsy should be performed in these cases.

Nonpalpable mammographic abnormalities, particularly spiculated densities, clustered microcalcifications, and new mammographic densities and calcifications, can be evaluated with a mammographically or ultrasound-directed excisional or stereotactic core biopsy. In some cases, mammographic abnormalities are best assessed by additional views, magnifications, or ultrasound to exclude a cyst.

STAGING AND PROGNOSIS

Patients presenting with a palpable breast lesion, new breast asymmetry, or mammographic abnormalities (including microcalcifications, dominant mass, significant architectural distortion or asymmetric density) should undergo a biopsy. Fine-needle aspiration performed and interpreted by an experienced pathologist has a positive predictive value of close to 100%, although negative predictive values ranging from 87% to 99% may warrant examination of additional tissue based on the situation [5]. Excisional biopsy, or needle localization for nonpalpable mammographic abnormalities, can also be carried out, with suitable tissue preparation for histopathologic examination and measurement of hormone receptor content.

Full surgical TNM staging should be determined for all invasive tumors after partial or complete mastectomy and axillary lymph node dissection (Table 7-3). Apart from the measurement of hormone receptor content, no clear consensus exists on how to base clinical decisions on other tumor parameters such as ploidy, S-phase percent, cathepsin D, epidermal growth factor receptor, or HER2/*neu* oncogene expression; therefore, these determinations need not be performed outside of the investigative setting. Preoperative staging should include a complete blood count, serum measurements of liver function, and a chest radiograph. Radionuclide bone scintigraphy and liver scan are of low yield in asymptomatic stage I disease but may be considered in more advanced stages.

THERAPY FOR IN SITU BREAST CANCER

Carcinoma in situ is a preinvasive lesion within breast ducts without penetration of the basement membrane and the potential for metastases. Historically, these have been treated with wide local excision, and local recurrence rates ranging from 10% to 20% have been reported. These recurrence can be either in situ or invasive carcinoma. Lobular carcinoma in situ is not believed to require full surgi-

Table 7-1. Risk Factors for the Development of Breast Cancer
Age
Family history of breast cancer
(especially if less than age 50 y, or bilateral breast cancer)
Prior breast cancer, in situ cancer, or atypical hyperplasia
Nulliparity or first pregnancy after age 30 y
Early menarche and late menopause
Prolonged use of high-dose estrogens
High alcohol intake
Exposure to radiation younger than age 30 y

Table 7-2. Recommendation for Screening and Early Detection
Monthly self-examination beginning at age 20 y
Mammograms every year beginning at age 40 y
Mammograms every 1–2 y after age 50 y
For high familial risk or BRCA 1/2-positive, yearly mammogram beginning 5 y prior to age of youngest relative with breast cancer

cal excision, yet is a marker of high risk for subsequent breast cancer in either breast. Ductal carcinoma in situ (also termed intraductal carcinoma), generally is treated with wide local excision, and the addition of radiation therapy has been shown to reduce the likelihood of local recurrence (both in situ and invasive), especially in high-risk lesions, which include those of large size and high grade histology [5]. The role of systemic treatment, such as tamoxifen for in situ breast cancer, has not yet been determined.

THERAPY FOR PRIMARY DISEASE

Primary local therapy for patients with clinical stage I and II disease can be accomplished with either a modified radical mastectomy or partial mastectomy followed by external beam irradiation. Local and distant recurrence rates are equal with either approach if negative margins are accomplished with breast-conserving surgery [7]. Axillary lymph node dissection is necessary for staging as such information is needed to choose the appropriate adjuvant therapy, although there is

Table 7-3. Staging of Breast Cancer

Primary Tumor	Criteria	
Tx	Primary tumor size cannot be assessed	
Tis	Carcinoma in situ	
T1		
T1a	< 0.5 cm	
T1b	0.5–1.0 cm	
T1c	> 1.0–2.0 cm	
T2	> 2–5 cm	
T3	> 5 cm	
T4	Tumor of any size fixed to the chest wall or skin	
T4a	Fixation to chest wall only	
T4b	Edema (*peau d'orange*), ulceration of skin, satellite skin nodules	
T4c	Both T4a and T4b	
T4d	Inflammatory changes	
Nodes		
Nx	Regional lymph nodes cannot be assessed	
N0	No regional lymph node metastases	
N1	Involved, movable ipsilateral axillary lymph nodes	
N2	Involved, fixed ipsilateral axillary lymph nodes	
N3	Involved, ipsilateral internal mammary lymph nodes	
Metastases		
Mx	Metastases cannot be assessed	
M0	No metastases	
M1	Distant metastases present, including nonregional (ie, ipsilateral supraclavicular) lymph nodes	
Stage	**TNM Staging**	**5-Y Survival (%)**
I	T1N0	95
IIA	T2N0, T0N1, T1N1, T2N0	86
IIB	T2N1, T3N0	70
IIIA	T0–3N2, T3N1	52
IIIB	T4N0–3M0, T0–4N3M0	49
IV	Any M1	17

From Beahrs et al. [26]; with permission.

conflicting evidence as to whether or not lymph node dissection reduces distant recurrences or improves survival. Sentinel node identification and analysis using color dye or radionuclide tracer injected into the tumor or tumor bed can be used to spare a node dissection if the sentinel node is negative for tumor. This may lower morbidity of node dissection, including the low risk of chronic lymphedema. Postmastectomy radiation has recently been shown to improve not only local recurrence but distant recurrence rates and overall survival in patients with node-positive breast cancer [8,9]. At this time, accepted indications for postmastectomy radiation include close or positive margins not amenable to further surgical resection, large primary tumor < 5 cm, and more than four axillary nodes (the value of radiation for fewer nodes involved remains controversial). Locally advanced (stage III) disease is generally treated with initial induction chemotherapy, followed by mastectomy, radiotherapy, or both. Primary therapy, including mastectomy or radiotherapy for metastatic disease, can improve local control but does not affect survival. This approach may be suitable for patients with large primary lesions who have a good functional status; it is sometimes facilitated after an initial response to hormonal therapy or chemotherapy.

ADJUVANT THERAPY FOR REGIONAL DISEASE

The single most powerful predictor of relapse in operable breast cancer (stages I and II) is the presence of axillary nodal involvement. Multiple randomized trials have demonstrated the benefit of cytotoxic and hormonal therapy in lowering or delaying the recurrence of breast cancer and improving 5- and 10-year overall survival in certain subsets of patients. An overview analysis, including data from 133 such trials, has recently been published [10]. Relative reductions in annual rates of recurrence and death of 25% and 17%, respectively, were seen with tamoxifen treatment compared to similar treatment without tamoxifen. Treatment with polychemotherapy compared to similar treatment without polychemotherapy yielded relative reductions of 28% and 17%. Therefore, the absolute benefit that patients derive from therapy in terms of reductions of recurrence or death risk at 5 and 10 years is proportional to the overall risk of recurrence and death. Patients at low risk (*eg*, those with negative nodes and small tumors) may benefit from therapy, but the small difference in outcome or risk afforded by treatment may not be justified when balanced against the short- and long-term side effects.

Node-Positive Patients

Outcome among node-positive patients in the overview analysis has confirmed the findings of many individual trials. A significant reduction in mortality was seen with tamoxifen treatment among women aged over 50 years with node-positive disease; the benefit was nearly doubled for patients with tumors classified as estrogen receptor (ER) rich (≥ 10 fmol/mg) compared to ER poor. Indirect comparisons suggested that 2 to 5 years of tamoxifen therapy was superior to 1 year. The addition of chemotherapy to tamoxifen in older women reduced the odds of recurrence, but not the mortality rate. Only one study has demonstrated a survival benefit from the addition of chemotherapy to tamoxifen [11], and further trials are underway to address this controversial issue. For women younger than 50 years old, the analysis found a significant reduction in mortality rates with chemotherapy. In the chemotherapy trials, results with combination chemotherapy regimens were superior to those with single agents, but there was no advantage to long-term administration (≥ 12 mo) over short-term administration (≤ 6 mo). The CMF combination regimen was the most represented in the analysis. No benefit was seen with the addition of tamoxifen to chemotherapy among women aged under 50.

There is as of yet no firm evidence that adjuvant chemotherapy regimens other than standard CMF provide a greater advantage for node-positive patients. Although doxorubicin-containing regimens produce superior response rates in metastatic breast cancer, few trials have directly assessed anthracycline content in the adjuvant setting. A comparison of CMF to CAF has not demonstrated a difference in outcome [12]. Alternatively, doxorubicin-based regimens have been examined in order to shorten the duration of chemotherapy without compromising effectiveness. Short, intensive doxorubicin and cyclophosphamide (AC) was found to be equally effective as standard oral CMF [13]. AC treatment required less than half the total time of treatment and one third the number of health professional visits as standard CMF, but it was accompanied by more vomiting and greater hair loss.

The roles of total dose and dose density (defined as the amount of drug administered per unit of time) beyond conventional ranges are currently being studied. Preliminary results from one such trial that randomized patients to low-, moderate-, and high-dose CAF revealed a significant survival difference between low and moderate or high doses, but no difference between moderate and high doses [14]. However, because the low doses used in this study are lower than conventional CAF, this difference may be more indicative of a threshhold effect, signifying a minimal effective dose necessary to delay recurrence. Another study showed a superiority of sequential compared with alternating doxorubicin followed by CMF in patients with more than three lymph nodes, yet no standard arm was included in this study [15]. This illustrates that not only specific agents and doses but also dose density and sequence may be important factors in achieving sufficient cell kill to alter clinical outcome. Recently completed and ongoing trials are assessing the use of other classes of chemotherapeutic agents, such as taxanes, as well as the role of combination compared with sequential agents and different dose densities.

In summary, adjuvant chemotherapy is indicated in women younger than 50 years old with positive axillary lymph nodes. Chemotherapy may also provide a benefit in women over 50 years of age when added to tamoxifen. Standard oral CMF for 6 months remains the standard regimen, while shorter, more intensive AC for 4 cycles is an alternative for patients who prefer shorter treatment times and fewer clinic visits, at the cost of greater toxicities [13]. The use of more intense doxorubicin-containing regimens, dose intensification, multiagent sequential therapy, or chemohormonal therapy remains investigational. Therefore, current recommendations for adjuvant therapy for node-positive patients include tamoxifen administration for 2 to 5 years with the consideration of adding chemotherapy for women aged over 50 and CMF or AC polychemotherapy for 6 months for women aged under 50. Additionally, the use of tamoxifen in patients under age 50 and chemotherapy in older women remain experimental and are being evaluated in ongoing trials. The use of chemotherapy in women over the age of 70 years has not been well studied.

Node-Negative Patients

Due to the comparatively low 10-year recurrence rate of about 30% among node-negative patients, large numbers of patients must be studied to detect significant outcome differences. It has therefore been difficult to demonstrate a benefit of systemic adjuvant therapy from earlier trials within this subset of patients. In 1990, a National Institutes of Health Consensus Conference recommended the consideration of adjuvant hormonal or cytotoxic therapy for some patients with node-negative breast cancer, although no criteria were provided on whom to treat. This was based on the findings of four trials limited to node-negative patients that differed considerably in design yet all demonstrated small but significant improvements in relapse-free (but not overall) survival among treated patients compared to those receiving no treatment. The Intergroup Study included ER-negative patients with tumors of any size and ER-positive patients with tumors greater than 3 cm; the treatment group received CMF plus prednisone [16]. In the Ludwig V Study, the treated group received a single cycle of perioperative intravenous CMF and leucovorin [17], whereas the National Surgical Adjuvant Bowel and Breast Project Group treated ER-positive patients with tamoxifen (10 mg twice a day) and ER-negative patients with sequential methotrexate and 5-fluorouracil for 12 cycles [18,19].

At this time, it appears that hormonal therapy is appropriate for patients with node-negative, hormone receptor–positive (ER- or PR-positive) tumors regardless of age, although the number of very young patients (< 40 y) included in these trials is very small. Preliminary results of a study comparing tamoxifen alone with tamoxifen plus chemotherapy for this patient population does show a small relapse-free (but not overall) survival advantage from the addition of chemotherapy [20]. For patients with node-negative, hormone receptor–negative (both ER- and PR-negative) tumors, CMF chemotherapy (or MF only for women > 50 y of age) is appropriate. For women over 70 years of age, chemotherapy has not yet been well studied, so tamoxifen may be appropriate regardless of hormone receptor status. As mentioned earlier, the absolute benefit in terms or reduction in risk of relapse or death is proportional to the overall risk, so that individualized decisions need to be made with low-risk cancers. A new generation of studies has recently been completed to assess the independent values of cytotoxic and hormonal therapy, as well as the relative merits of alkylating and doxorubicin-based regimens. Considerable variability in outcome exists within node-negative patients, and a greater absolute benefit of therapy may be derived from high-risk patients, whereas the the potential long-term risks of hormonal and cytotoxic therapy must be weighed against the smaller benefit in low-risk patients [21]. Further risk stratification based on tumor size, hormone receptor content, and other indices, including DNA ploidy, S-phase percent, and HER2/*neu* expression, may help select appropriate candidates for treatment [22]. However, such approaches need to be validated prospectively before they can be incorporated into standard clinical practice [23], and so far, only a gene-based assay for HER2/*neu* gene amplification has been approved to help stratify risk for patients with node-negative breast cancer.

THERAPY FOR ADVANCED DISEASE

Locally Advanced Breast Cancer

Locally advanced breast cancer generally encompasses stage III disease, defined by the presence of a large primary tumor (> 5 cm) or bulky ipsilateral axillary or internal mammary nodes (N2 or N3). Surgery alone results in low long-term survival rates, whereas the addition of radiation therapy appears to lower the incidence of local, but not distant recurrence. The advent of preoperative induction chemotherapy followed by definitive local therapy (mastectomy, radiation therapy, or both) has resulted in improved disease-free and overall survival times compared to historical controls, although few randomized, comparative trials have been performed. The largest such trial reported improvement in local recurrence, but not distant recurrence or survival, with endocrine or cytotoxic therapies added to radiation therapy compared to radiation therapy alone [24]. When combined with chemotherapy, the local control modalities of mastectomy versus radiation therapy have resulted in equal relapse-free and overall survival rates in a randomized trial [25]. Recently published series using doxorubicin-containing induction regimens, such as FAC (due to this agent's superior response rate in metastatic breast cancer), followed by either radiation therapy, mastectomy, or both, followed by additional chemotherapy, have yielded complete response rates (at the time of surgery) of 58% to 100%, 3- to 5-year relapse-free survival rates of 20% to 73% and local recurrence rates of 13% to 38%.

Inflammatory breast cancer is identified by the clinical appearance of a diffuse erythema, *peau d'orange* (edema), and ridging in the skin overlying the tumor or by histopathologic evidence of tumor emboli within dermal lymphatics [26]. Strategies similar to those used for locally advanced breast cancer have yielded similar or slightly lower response and survival rates [27]. Due to the small number of patients that present with locally advanced or inflammatory breast cancer, the optimal treatment has not been defined by a series of controlled, randomized studies. A reasonable approach includes initial hormonal treatment (in ER-positive, older patients) or combination chemotherapy such as CMF or CAF (in ER-negative, younger patients) for two to four cycles or until a plateau in the response is reached, followed by modified radical mastectomy or radiation therapy, and then additional chemotherapy. The role of dose intensification (with or without bone marrow support), optimal agents, duration of use, and sequence of modalities remains undetermined.

Metastatic Breast Cancer

Of the approximately 45,000 deaths in the United States due to breast cancer, virtually all are associated with progressive metastatic disease. Although metastatic breast cancer is not curable with any current modality, the length and quality of life of patients with relapsed or

newly diagnosed disseminated breast cancer upon presentation vary greatly. The median survival rate from time of presentation of 2 to 3.5 years has been reported, with 25% to 35% of patients living beyond 5 years and up to 10% living beyond 10 years [28]. Factors associated with a more favorable prognosis include longer interval from initial diagnosis to recurrence, older age, lower number of involved sites, sites limited to bone or soft tissue, ER-positive disease, and low histologic grade. The effect of any therapy on survival is modest at best. Therefore, the timing of therapy and the selection of agents should reflect therapeutic goals whose benefits outweigh the toxicity of treatment. In general, palliation of organ-specific symptoms related to tumor or a rapid clinical course suggestive of impending multiorgan involvement would be a greater impetus for systemic therapy, whereas local therapy, such as radiation of an isolated symptomatic boney lesion or close observation of asymptomatic patients with few sites of involvement, may be more appropriate.

Endocrine Therapy

Approximately one third of unselected patients with metastatic breast cancer (and two thirds of those with ER-positive tumors) will respond to endocrine manipulation [29]. Endocrine agents are best used as initial therapy in patients with ER-positive tumors in older patients, and in those exhibiting low-burden, predominantly nonvisceral disease. These modalities yield equivalent results, with the possible exception of androgens and corticosteroids alone resulting in slightly lower response rates (Table 7-4). For premenopausal patients, oophorectomy or tamoxifen treatment may be considered first, followed by progestin or androgen treatment in the event of progression.

First-line endocrine therapy for postmenopausal patients generally consists of tamoxifen, followed by a progestin, an aromatase inhibitor, or androgen upon progression. Ablative therapies, such as adrenalectomy and hypophysectomy, are not used today due to surgical risks and complications. There is no evidence that doses higher than those listed in Table 7-4 for tamoxifen, megestrol acetate, fluoxymesterone, or aromatase inhibitors are more effective. Only a few studies have demonstrated superior response rates when using combinations of these agents, and generally there has not been an improvement in median survival rates [28]. The median duration of response to any of these endocrine therapies is between 1 and 2 years. Response rates and durations of response are less with retreatment with a second or third agent upon progression. There is no evidence that combination hormonal treatment results in greater response rates. Although chemohormonal treatment may lead to higher response rates compared to hormonal treatment alone, a survival benefit has not been demonstrated [28]. Furthermore, in ER-positive patients with metastatic breast cancer, response rates to hormonal therapy and chemotherapy are equal as initial therapy. The roles of newer antiestrogens, aromatase inhibitors, luteinizing hormone-releasing hormone analogues, antiprogestins, and somatostatin analogues are under investigation (*see* Chapter 5 for further discussion).

Chemotherapy

About two thirds of all patients with metastatic breast cancer will have a response to some form of chemotherapy, although complete response rates in the range of 5% to 25% have been reported in most trials. The median duration of response to chemotherapy is 6 to 12 months [28]. Previous phase II trials have demonstrated single-agent response rates of 27% to 33% for the four drugs considered to be the

Table 7-4. Endocrine Therapy for Metastatic Breast Cancer

Endocrine Maneuver	Setting	Dose
Ablative oophorectomy	Premenopausal	
Competitive antiestrogen Tamoxifen	Premenopausal (esp ER-positive) Postmenopausal	20 mg/d
Progestin Megestrol acetate	Any age	40 mg qid
Aromatase inhibitor Anastrazole Letrozol	Postmenopausal	250 or 500 mg bid
Estrogen Diethylstilbesterol Ethinyl estradiol Conjugated estrogen	Postmenopausal	5 mg tid 1 mg tid 2.5 mg tid
Androgen Fluoxymesterone Anastrazole Letrozole	Any age	10 mg bid 1 mg/d 2.5 mg/d

most active in patients with metastatic breast cancer: doxorubicin, cyclophosphamide, methotrexate, and 5-fluorouracil [28]. Combination chemotherapy can achieve higher response rates, albeit at the cost of greater toxicity. Therefore, the most widely used combinations in the treatment of metastatic breast cancer are CMF and CAF. Doxorubicin, taken as a single agent, is a less toxic alternative, especially in patients previously exposed to CMF, to which no cross resistance exists. Although doxorubicin-containing regimens, such as CAF, appear to result in superior response rates compared to doxorubicin alone, the difference in survival time is modest and it is accompanied by higher toxicity. In the responding patients, the duration of therapy for optimal palliation and survival is not clear. Comparative studies that have examined regimens of increasing dose intensity have failed to show a benefit, except in those trials in which the lower doses were less intensive than standard CMF or CAF [30]. Two studies that randomized patients to receive intermittent chemotherapy (3 to 6 cycles) and retreatment at time of progression versus continuous or longer term (18 cycles) therapy demonstrated increased response rates and better quality of life, but no or only marginal improvement in survival rates [31, 32].

It should be emphasized that cumulative doses of doxorubicin exceeding 450 mg/m^2 are associated with significant cardiotoxicity [33]; therefore, doxorubicin should not be given beyond this total dose, avoided entirely in patients with clinical evidence of congestive cardiomyopathy, and used with caution (perhaps accompanied by frequent measurement of ejection fraction [EF] and withheld for EF < 40% or a fall of more than 10%–20% from baseline) in patients at risk for cardiac disease or those approaching toxic cumulative doses. Likewise, systemic side effects need to be monitored, with therapy modified or adjusted accordingly (see protocol).

Salvage chemotherapy for refractory patients generally results in lower response rates and durations of response compared to those for front-line therapy. There are few comparative trials to guide the clinician in the most appropriate regimen. Patients who have not received an anthracycline can be treated with doxorubicin as a single agent or a combination regimen (AC or CAF). Paclitaxel (Taxol) has shown significant activity as initial and salvage therapy, including in patients refractory to doxorubicin or other anthracycline drugs [34]. Paclitaxel can be used as a single agent and has been shown to result in a slightly better response rate and time to progression in combination with doxorubicin [35]. Another taxane, docetaxel (Taxotere) is also effective in the salvage setting [36]. Other single agents with activity in the salvage setting include vinorelbine (not velbine), mitomycin C, and vinblastine, yielding response rates of 25% to 30% [28]. Although many small uncontrolled trials have examined combinations including these and other drugs, the latter are associated with increased toxicity and direct comparative studies are lacking. There are no definitive data on the merit of combination or sequential chemohormonal regimens. The roles of other active agents, including platinum, etoposide, mitoxantrone, and 5-fluorouracil with leucovorin modulation as well myeloablative regimens with peripheral stem cell or bone marrow support and subablative therapy with recombinant hematopoietic growth factors, are under investigation.

NEW TECHNOLOGY AND THE ROLE OF CLINICAL TRIALS

New approaches in breast cancer include new cytotoxic agents from synthetic and natural sources that emerge from drug screening programs and demonstrate activity in breast cancer cell lines in vitro and in animal models without limiting toxicities. Phase I toxicity and phase II efficacy human studies generally include patients with advanced breast cancer, and there has been a recent trend to include asymptomatic patients who may have not yet been treated with standard chemotherapy. This is due to the absence of curative or definitively life-prolonging conventional therapy. Dose intensification, including high-dose chemotherapy with various chemotherapeutic agents and bone marrow or stem cell support remains investigational and many variables (*eg*, the dose and agents, methods of marrow or stem cell purging, and the use of tandem [multiple sequential] transplant) continue to be studied. However, one small randomized study did find an improved response rate, time to progression, and survival benefit with high-dose therapy and bone marrow transplant compared with standard-dose chemotherapy [37]. Newer biologic approaches of rationally designed drugs that interfere with known phenotypic characteristics of carcinogenesis increasingly are reaching the clinical trial stage (Table 7-5).

Table 7-5. New Therapeutic Approaches

Designed or Screened Biologic Agents
Adoptive immunotherapy (cytokine modulation)
Active immunotherapy (vaccines)
Passive immunotherapy (monoclonal antibodies)
Immunotoxins
Antiangiogenesis agents
Oncogene-directed
Growth factor-directed and cell signaling modulators
Steroid hormone antagonists and antagonists
Inhibitors of cell cycling (cyclin-dependent kinase inhibitors)
Modulators of apoptosis
Anticarcinogenesis (chemopreventative) agents
   Retinoids and retinoid-receptor superfamily pathway modulators
   Polyphenolics
   Kinase inhibitors (genestein, bryostatins)
   Steroid hormone antagonists and antagonists

New Chemotherapeutic Agents
New DNA intercalators (amonafide)
Topoisomerase I inhibitors (topotecan)
Inhibitors of microtubule assembly (vinca-like drugs, *eg*, vinorelbine)
Inhibitors of tubule disassembly (taxanoids, *eg*, taxotere)
Liposomal chemotherapy
Antimetabolites

New Approaches to Improve Effects of Adjuvant Therapy
Dose intensification (growth factor and stem cell support)
Modulation of dose sequence and dose density
Integration of taxanes (paclitaxel, docetaxel)
Combinations with hormonal or biological therapy
New prognostic factors to improve outcome or improve patient selection for adjuvant therapy

As treatment with higher response rates are identified in patients with advanced breast cancer, some are incorporated into clinical trials in the adjuvant setting in order to improve on the reduction in recurrence and death. Most trials in the adjuvant setting are investigating changes in dose and sequence of standard chemotherapeutic agents. Escalation of doses of cyclophosphamide and doxorubicin, introduction of paclitaxel, and the use of high-dose therapy with bone marrow or stem cell support are being assessed in comparative studies. An uncovering of scientific misconduct with the deliberate entry of ineligible patients onto National Surgical Adjuvant Bowel and Bladder Project studies was not believed to have altered the results or conclusion [38]. The heterogeneity of patients with breast cancer as well as random error and occasional misconduct underscores the need to design and conduct studies of sufficient size and statistical power. Furthermore, improvements in outcome due to new regimens or agents are likely to be small enough to require well-designed, randomized studies before being accepted as standard therapy.

Newer biologic agents being tested primarily in patients with metastatic breast cancer include vaccines, angiogenesis inhibitors, kinase inhibitors, and other novel compounds that are targeting specific pathways thought to be pivotal to the oncogenesis. One example is an agonistic antibody to the HER2/*neu* membrane tyrosine kinase receptor that has been shown to have activity in patients with HER2/*neu*-overexpressing tumors and has also been shown to prolong time to disease progression when used with chemotherapy [39]. The number of such new compounds entering clinical trials is growing rapidly and some of these may soon be tested in an adjuvant setting as well.

REFERENCES

1. Parker SL, Tong T, Bolden S, *et al.*: Cancer statistics, 1997. *CA* 1997, 47:5–27.

2. Henderson IC: Risk factors for breast cancer development. *Cancer (suppl)* 1993, 71:2127–2140.

3. Struewing JP, Hartge P, Wacholder S, *et al.*: The risk of cancer associated with specific mutations of BRCA1 and BRCA2 among Ashkenazi Jews. *New Engl J Med* 1997, 336:1401–1408.

4. Kerlikowske K, Grady D, Rubin SM, *et al.*: Efficacy of screening mammography. A meta-analysis. *JAMA* 1995, 273:149–154.

5. Harris JR, Lippmann ME, Veronesi U, *et al.*: Breast cancer. *N Engl J Med* 1992, 327:319–328.

6. Fisher ER, Constantino J, Fisher B, *et al.*: Pathologic findings from the National Surgical Adjuvant Breast Project (NSAPB) Protocol B-17. Intraductal carcinoma (ductal carcinoma in situ). The National Surgical Adjuvant Breast and Bowel project Collaborating Investigators. *Cancer* 1995, 75:1310–9.

7. Fisher B, Redmond C, Poisson R, *et al.*: Eight year results of a randomized clinical trial comparing total mastectomy and lumpectomy with or without irradiation in the treatment of breast cancer. *N Engl J Med* 1989, 320:822–828.

8. Ragaz J, Jackson SM, Le N, *et al.*: Adjuvant radiotherapy and chemotherapy in node-positive premenopausal women with breast cancer. *New Engl J Med* 1997, 337:956–962.

9. Overgaard M, Hansen PS, Overgaard J, *et al.*: Postoperative radiotherapy in high-risk premenopausal women with breast cancer who receive adjuvant chemotherapy. *New Engl J Med* 1997, 337:949–955.

10. Early Breast Cancer Trialists' Collaborative Group: systemic treatment of early breast cancer by hormonal, cytotoxic, or immune therapy. *Lancet* 1992, 339:1–15, 71–85.

11. Fisher B, Redmond C, Legault-Poisson S, *et al.*: Postoperative chemotherapy and tamoxifen compared with tamoxifen alone in the treatment of positive-node breast cancer patients aged 50 years or older with tumors resposive to tamoxifen: Results from NSABP B-16. *J Clin Oncol* 1990, 8:1005–1018.

12. Carpenter JT, Velez-Garcia E, Aron BS, *et al.*: Five-year results of a randomized comparison of cyclophosphamide, doxorubicin (Adriamycin) and fluorouracil (CAF) vs. cyclophosphamide, methotrexate and fluorouracil (CMF) for node-positive carcinoma: A Southeastern Cancer Study Group Study. *Proc ASCO* 1994, 13:66.

13. Fisher B, Brown AM, Dimitrov NV, *et al.*: Two months of doxorubicin-cyclophosphamide with and without interval reinduction therapy compared with 6 months of cyclophosphamide, methotrexate and fluorouracil in positive-node breast cancer patients with tamoxifen-nonresponsive tumors: results from the National Surgical Adjuvant Breast and Bowel Project B-15. *J Clin Oncol* 1990, 8:1483–1496.

14. Wood WC, Budman DR, Korzun AH, *et al.*: Dose and dose intensity of adjuvant chemotherapy for stage II, node-positive breast carcinoma. *N Engl J Med* 1994, 330:1253–1259.

15. Bonadonna G, Zambetti M, Valagussa P: Sequential or altering doxorubicin and CMF regimens in breast cancer with more than three positive nodes. *JAMA* 1995, 273:542–547.

16. Mansour EG, Gray R, Shatila AH, *et al.*: Efficacy of adjuvant chemotherapy in high-risk node-negative breast cancer. *N Engl J Med* 1989, 320:485–490.

17. The Ludwig Breast Cancer Study Group: Prolonged disease-free survival after one course of perioperative adjuvant chemotherapy for node-negative breast cancer. *N Engl J Med* 1989, 320:491–496.

18. Fisher B, Constantino J, Redmond C, *et al.*: A randomized clinical trial evaluating tamoxifen in the treatment of patients with node-negative breast cancer who have estrogen-receptor-positive tumors. *N Engl J Med* 1989, 320:479–484.

19. Fisher B, Dignam J, Mamounas EP, *et al.*: Sequential methotrexate and fluorouracil for the treatment of node-negative breast cancer patients with estrogen receptor-negative tumors: eight-year results from National Surgical Adjuvant Breast and Bowel Project (NSABP) B-13 and first report of findings from NSABP B-19 comparing methotrexate and fluorouracil with conventional cyclophosphamide, methotrexate, and fluorouracil. *J Clin Oncol* 1996, 14:1982–1992.

20. Fisher B, Dignam J, Wolmark, *et al.*: Tamoxifen and chemotherapy for lymph node-negative, estrogen receptor–positive breast cancer. *J Natl Cancer Inst* 1997, 89:1673–1682.

21. Curtis RE, John MA, Boice JD, *et al.*: Risk of leukemia after chemotherapy and radiation treatment for breast cancer. *N Engl J Med* 1992, 326:1745–1751.

22. Gasparini G, Pozza F, Harris, AL: Evaluating the potential usefulness of new prognostic and predictive indicators in node-negative breast cancer patients. *J Natl Cancer Inst* 1993, 85:1206–1219.

23. Henderson IC: Breast cancer therapy—The price for success. *New Engl J Med* 1992, 326:1774–1775.

24. Rubens RD, Bartelink H, Engelsman E, *et al.*: The contribution of cytotoxic and endocrine treatment to radiotherapy. An EORTC Breast Cancer Co-operative trial (10792). *Eur J Cancer Clin Oncol* 1989, 25:667–678.

25. Perloff M, Lesnick GJ, Korzun A, *et al.*: Combination chemotherapy with mastectomy or radiation for stage III breast carcinoma: a Cancer and Leukemia Group B study. *J Clin Oncol* 1988, 6:261–269.

26. Beahrs OH, Henson DE, Hutter RVP, *et al.*: Manual for Staging of Cancer, 4th ed. Philadelphia: JB Lippincott; 1992:149–154.

27. Jaiyesimi IA, Buzdar AU, Hortobagyi G: Inflammatory breast cancer: A review. *J Clin Oncol* 1992, 10:1014–1024.

28. Henderson IC, Harris JR: Principles in the management of metastatic disease. In Harris JR, Hellman S, Henderson IC, *et al.* (eds): Breast Diseases. Philadelphia: JB Lippincott; 1991,547–679.

29. Glauber JG, Kiang DT: The changing role of hormonal therapy in advanced breast cancer. *Sem Oncol* 1992, 19:308–316.

30. Sledge GW, Antman KH: Progress in chemotherapy for metastatic breast cancer. *Sem Oncol* 1992, 19:317–332.

31. Coates A, Gebski V, Bishop JF, *et al.*: Improving the quality of life during chemotherapy for advanced breast cancer. A comparison of intermittent and continuous treatment strategies. *N Engl J Med* 1987, 317:1490–1495.

32. Ejlerten B, Pfeiffer P, Pederson D, *et al.*: Diminished efficacy by reducing duration of CEF from 18 to 6 months in the treatment of metastatic breast cancer. *Proc ASCO* 1990, 9:23.

33. Von Hoff DD, Layard MW, Basa P, *et al.*: Risk factors for doxorubicin-induced congestive heart failure. *Ann Intern Med* 1979, 91:710–717.

34. Seidman AD: Single-agent use of Taxol (paclitaxel) in breast cancer. *Ann Oncol* 1994, 5 Suppl 6:S17–22.

35. Sledge GW, Neuberg D, Ingle S, *et al.*: Phase III trial of doxorubicin vs. paclitaxel vs. doxorubicin plus paclitaxel as first-line therapy for metastatic breast cancer: an Intergroup trial. *Proc Am Soc Clin Oncol* 1997, 16:1a.

36. Valero V: Docetaxel as single-agent therapy in metastatic breast cancer: clinical efficacy. *Semin Oncol* 1997, 4(suppl 13):11–18.

37. Bezwoda WR, Seymour L, Dansey RD, *et al.*: High-dose chemotherapy with hematopoietic rescue as primary treatment for metastatic breast cancer: a randomized trial. *J Clin Oncol* 1995, 13:2483–2489.

38. Sondik EJ, Reanalyses of NSABP studies. National Surgical Adjuvant Breast and Bowel Project. *J Natl Cancer Inst* 1994, 8:655.

39. Baselga J, Tripathy D, Mendelsohn J, *et al.*: Phase II study of weekly intravenous recombinant humanized anti-p185[HER2/neu] monoclonal antibody in patients with HER2/neu overexpressing metastatic breast cancer. *J Clin Oncol* 1996, 14:737–744.

CMF
Cyclophosphamide, Methotrexate, and 5-Fluorouracil

Cyclophosphamide is an alkylating agent that inhibits DNA replication and is therefore toxic to dividing cells. Methotrexate is an antimetabolite that inhibits dihydrofolate reductase and the subsequent generation of thymidine necessary for DNA synthesis. 5-Fluorouracil (5-FU) is likewise an antimetabolite that blocks the methylation of deoxyuridylate to thymidylate, inhibiting the synthesis of RNA and DNA. This combination of agents is used because the agents possess different modes of action and are noncross-resistant and can therefore eradicate resistant clones.

DOSAGE AND SCHEDULING

	Day													
Cyclophosphamide 100 mg/m² PO daily d 1–14														
MTX 40 mg/m² IV, d 1,8														
5-FU 600 mg/m² IV, d 1,8														
CBC, lytes, Cr, LFT														
Day	1	2	3	4	5	6	7	8	9	10	11	12	13	14

6 cycles for adjuvant therapy.

DOSAGE MODIFICATIONS: *50% of cyclophosphamide, MTX, or 5-FU for WBC < 3.5k, platelet 75–100k; hold therapy for WBC < 2.5k, platelet< 75k. Use 75% MTX for creatinine clearance < 50 mL/min, 50% if < 25 mL/min.*

RECENT EXPERIENCES AND RESPONSE RATES

Study	Evaluable Patients, *n*	Dosage/Schedule	Response for Metastatic Disease, %
Valagussa *et al.*, Proc Am Soc Clin Oncol 1983, 2:111	53	C 100 mg/m² PO d 1–14 M 40 mg/m² IV d 1, 8 F 600 mg/m² IV d 1, 8	53
Canellos *et al.*, Cancer 1976, 38: 1882-1886	93	C 100 mg/m² PO d 1–14 M 60 mg/m² IV d 1, 8 F 600 mg/m² IV d 1,8	53
Muss *et al.*, Arch Int Med 1977, 137: 1711-1714	38	C 10 mg/kg IV d 1, 5 mg/kg IV d 15 then q 7 d M 0.2 mg/kg IV d 1, 0.1 mg/kg IV d 15 then q 7 d F 12 mg/kg IV d 1, 10 mg/kg d 15 then q 7 d	34
Aisner *et al.*, J Clin Oncol 1987, 5: 1523-1533	99	C 100 mg/m² PO d 1–14 M 40 mg/m² IV d 1, 8 F 500 mg/m² IV d 1, 8	37
Creech *et al.*, Cancer 1975 35:1101-1107	46	C 50 mg/m² PO d 1–14 M 25 mg/m² IV d 1, 8 F 500 mg/m² IV d 1, 8	46

CANDIDATES FOR TREATMENT
Adjuvant treatment of premenopausal node-positive and selected node-negative patients, metastatic disease in patients with aggressive visceral disease or failed initial hormonal therapy

SPECIAL PRECAUTIONS
Enhanced leukopenia and skin toxicity with concommitant radiation therapy

ALTERNATIVE THERAPIES
CAF or AC combination chemotherapy for adjuvant therapy; CAF or single-agent doxorubicin for metastatic disease

TOXICITIES
Cyclophosphamide: nausea, vomiting, anorexia, fatigue, cystitis, leukopenia, anemia, thrombocytopenia, alopecia, pigment changes in skin and nails; pulmonary fibrosis, hepatitis, renal tubular necrosis (rare); **Methotrexate:** nausea, vomiting, mouth sores, fatigue, dermatitis, leukopenia, hepatitis; interstitial pneumonitis, renal tubular damage (rare); **5-FU:** nausea, vomiting, anorexia, diarrhea, abdominal cramps, mouth sores, dermatitis, hyperpigmentation, photosensitivity, phlebitis, increased tearing of eyes, leukopenia, anemia; vascular complications including heart attack and stroke (rare)

DRUG INTERACTIONS
Cyclophosphamide: phenobarbital; **methotrexate:** nonsteroidal anti-inflammatory agents, sulfa drugs, nonabsorbable antibiotics; **5-FU:** interferon, leucovorin

NURSING INTERVENTIONS
Give antiemetic (usually prochlorperazine and/or lorazapam) and evaluate blood counts and sometimes renal and hepatic function prior to administration

PATIENT INFORMATION
Patient should immediately report severe mucositis, chest pain, shortness of breath, signs of infection (fever, chills, dysuria), diarrhea, and abdominal cramps. High fluid intake is necessary while taking cyclophosphamide.

CAF
Cyclophosphamide, Doxorubicin, and 5-Fluorouracil

Doxorubicin is an anthacycline whose mode of action is inhibition of mitosis by intercalation of DNA. Although there is no clear evidence that this combination of drugs is superior to CMF in the adjuvant setting, it is clear that it is more toxic. In metastatic breast cancer, CAF is associated with a higher rate and duration of response, but no difference in the overall survival rate. Due to doxorubicin's superior single-agent activity in metastatic breast cancer, this regimen is commonly used in high-risk stage II and in stage III and IV breast cancers (see discussion on CMF).

DOSAGE AND SCHEDULING

ORAL CYCLOPHOSPHAMIDE REGIMEN

		Day
Cyclophosphamide 100 mg/m² PO daily days 1–14	██████████████████	
Doxo 30 mg/m² IV, d 1,8	■ ■	
5-FU 500 mg/m² IV, d 1,8	■ ■	
CBC, lytes, Cr, LFT	□ □	
Day	1 2 3 4 5 6 7 8 9 10 11 12 13 14	

IV CYCLOPHOSPHAMIDE REGIMEN

Cyclo 500 mg/m² IV	■
Doxo 50 mg/m² IV	■
5-FU 500 mg/m² IV, d 1,8	■ ■
CBC, lytes, Cr, LFT	□ □
Day	1 2 3 4 5 6 7 8

DOSAGE MODIFICATIONS: Use 50% of cyclophosphamide, 5-FU, or doxorubicin for WBC < 3.5k, platelet 75-100k; hold therapy for WBC < 3.5k platelet < 75k. Use 50% doxorubicin for bilirubin 1.5–3.0 mg/dL, 25% dose for > 30 mg/dL.

RECENT EXPERIENCES AND RESPONSE RATES

Study	Evaluable Patients, n	Dosage/Schedule	Response for Metastatic Disease, %
Kardinal et al., Breast Cancer Res Treat 1983 3:365–372	116	C 100mg/m² PO d 1-14 A 25 mg/m² IV d 1,8 F 500 mg/m² IV d 1,8 q 4 wk	51
Tranum et al., Cancer 1978, 41:2078–2083	105	C 400 mg/m² IV d 1 A 40 mg/m² IV d 1 F 400 mg/m² IV d 1,8 q 3 wk	49
Smalley et al., Cancer 1977, 40:625-632	59	C 500 mg/m² IV d 1 A 50 mg/m² IV d 1 F 500 mg/m² IV d 1 q 3 wk	64
Tormey et al., Cancer Clin Trials 1979, 2:247–256	46	C 100 mg/m² PO d 1-14 A 30 mg/m² IV d 1,8 F 500 mg/m² IV d 1,8 q 4 wk	52
Vogel et al., J Clin Oncol 1984, 2:643–651	66	C 500 mg/m² IV d 1 A 50 mg/m² IV d 1 F 500 mg/m² IV d 1 q 3 wk	29
Bull et al., Cancer 1978, 41:1649–1657	38	C 100 mg/m² PO d 1-14 A 30 mg/m² IV d 1,8 F 500 mg/m² IV d 1,8 q 4 wk	82

CANDIDATES FOR TREATMENT
Adjuvant treatment of premenopausal, node-positive patients and patients with locally advanced disease; metastatic disease in patients with aggressive visceral disease or failed initial hormonal therapy

SPECIAL PRECAUTIONS
Patients undergoing radiotherapy; cardiotoxicity with cumulative doxorubicin > 450 mg/m², further enhanced with concommitant radiotherapy; extravasation of doxorubicin, a vesicant, may lead to tissue necrosis; it should be administered by experienced personnel through large peripheral or central vein

ALTERNATIVE THERAPIES
CMF or AC combination chemotherapy for adjuvant therapy; CMF or single-agent doxorubicin for metastatic disease

TOXICITIES
Cyclophosphamide: nausea, vomiting, anorexia, fatigue, cystitis, leukopenia, anemia, thrombocytopenia, alopecia, pigment changes in skin and nails; pulmonary fibrosis, hepatitis, renal tubular necrosis (rare); **Doxorubicin**: nausea, vomiting, anorexia, mucositis, alopecia, onycholysis, extravasation reaction, anaphylaxis (rare); congestive cardiomyopathy (with high doses); **5-FU**: nausea, vomiting, anorexia, diarrhea, abdominal cramps, mouth sores, dermatitis, hyperpigmentation, photosensitivity, phlebitis, increased tearing of eyes, leukopenia, anemia; vascular complications including myocardial infarction and stroke (rare)

DRUG INTERACTIONS
Cyclophosphamide: phenobarbital; **Doxorubicin**: cyclophosphamide, 6-mercaptopurine; **5-FU**: interferon, leucovorin

NURSING INTERVENTIONS
Give antiemetic and evaluate blood counts and renal and hepatic function prior to administration

PATIENT INFORMATION
Patient should report severe mucositis, chest pain, shortness of breath, diarrhea and abdominal cramps, signs of infection, skin redness, or pain at infusion site immediately. High fluid intake is necessary while taking cyclophosphamide.

AC
Doxorubicin and Cyclophosphamide

In the NSABP B-15, the AC regimen was used in the adjuvant setting for node-positive women. The rates for relapse-free and overall survival were equivalent to those with standard CMF. However, the AC regimen was delivered in half the total time with one third the office visits, but at the expense of more vomiting and alopecia. (*See* discussions on CMF and CAF.)

DOSAGE AND SCHEDULING

Cyclo 600 mg/m² IV	■							
Doxo 60 mg/m² IV	■							
CBC, lytes, Cr, LFT	☐							
Day	1	2	3	4	5	6	7	

Cycle q 3 wk × 4 cycles.

DOSAGE MODIFICATIONS: *Dose is withheld if granulocytes are < 1000 and platelets < 100,000. If fever accompanies neutropenia, reduce subsequent AC dose by 25% or consider full doses with recombinant G-CSF. Use 50% doxorubicin for bilirubin 1.5–3.0 mg/dL, 25% dose for 30 mg/dL.*

RECENT EXPERIENCE AND RESPONSE RATES

Study	Evaluable Patients, n	Dosage/Schedule	3-Y Disease-Free Survival, %
Fisher *et al.*, J Clin Oncol 1990, 8:1483-1496	535	Doxo 60 mg/m² iv q 3 wk × 4 cycles	68
		Cyclo 600 mg/m² iv q 3 wk × 4 cycles	

CANDIDATES FOR TREATMENT
Adjuvant treatment of node-positive patients

SPECIAL PRECAUTIONS
Enhanced toxicity with radiotherapy. Cardiotoxicity with cumulative doxorubicin > 450 mg/m², further enhanced with concommitant radiotherapy; extravasation of doxorubicin, a vesicant, may lead to tissue necrosis; it should be administered by experienced personnel through large peripheral or central vein

ALTERNATIVE THERAPIES
CMF or CAF combination chemotherapy

TOXICITIES
Cyclophosphamide: nausea, vomiting, anorexia, fatigue, cystitis, leukopenia, anemia, thrombocytopenia, alopecia, pigment changes in skin and nails; pulmonary fibrosis, hepatitis, renal tubular necrosis (rare); **Doxorubicin**: nausea, vomiting, anorexia, mucositis, alopecia, onycholysis, extravasation reaction, anaphylaxis (rare)

DRUG INTERACTIONS
Cyclophosphamide: phenobarbital; **Doxorubicin**: cyclophosphamide, 6-mercaptopurine

NURSING INTERVENTIONS
Give antiemetic and evaluate blood counts and renal and hepatic function prior to administration

PATIENT INFORMATION
Patient should report severe mucositis, chest pain, shortness of breath, diarrhea and abdominal cramps, skin redness, signs of infection, or pain at infusion site immediately. High fluid intake is necessary while taking cyclophosphamide.

VATH
Vinblastine, Doxorubicin, Thiotepa, and Fluoxymesterone

VATH is a doxorubicin-based combination commonly used as second-line chemotherapy for metastatic breast cancer, especially if the patient has not had prior exposure to doxorubicin. Single-agent regimens are preferable because no randomized comparative trials have been performed to compare this to other less-toxic single-agent regimens.

DOSAGE AND SCHEDULING

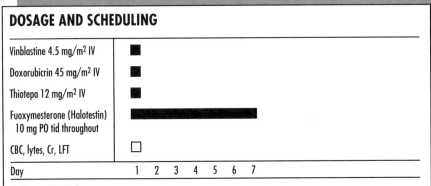

	Day 1 2 3 4 5 6 7
Vinblastine 4.5 mg/m² IV	
Doxorubicrin 45 mg/m² IV	
Thiotepa 12 mg/m² IV	
Fuoxymesterone (Halotestin) 10 mg PO tid throughout	
CBC, lytes, Cr, LFT	

Cycle every 21–28 days

DOSAGE MODIFICATIONS: *Delay vinblastine if neutrophil count < 2000, platelet count < 120,000; 50% doxorubicin or vinblastine if total bilirubin 1.5–3.0 mg/dL; 25%, > 3.0 mg/dL.*

RECENT EXPERIENCE AND RESPONSE RATES

Study	Evaluable Patients, *n*	Dosage/Schedule	Response for Metastatic Disease, %*
Perloff *et al.*, Cancer 1978, 42:2534-2537	19	V 2.25 mg/m² IV d 1,5 A 11.25 mg/m² IV d 1,5 T 6 mg/m² IV d 1 H 30 mg PO q d continuous q 4 wk	52
Hart *et al.*, Cancer 1981, 48:1522-1527	29	V 4.5 mg/m² IV d 1 A 45 mg/m² IV d 1 T 12 mg/m² IV d 1 H 20 mg PO q d continuous q 3 wk	45
Skeel *et al.*, Cancer 1989, 64:1393-1399	84	V 4.5 mg/m² IV d 1 A 45 mg/m² IV d 1 T 12 mg/m² IV d 1 H 20 mg PO q d continuous q 3 wk	38

*No patients had received doxorubicin prior to therapy

CANDIDATES FOR TREATMENT
Recurrent or metastatic breast cancer in those patients who have failed first- or second-line therapy and have no prior exposure to doxorubicin

SPECIAL PRECAUTIONS
Administer through large or central vein. Enhanced marrow suppression with concommitant radiotherapy

ALTERNATIVE THERAPIES
Single-agent doxorubicin, vinblastine or mitomycin C

TOXICITIES
Drug combination: nausea, vomiting, anorexia, mucositis, alopecia, onycholysis, extravasation reaction, anaphylaxis (rare), myalgias, parathesias, neutropenia, anemia, thrombocytopenia.
Fluoxymesterone: hirsutism and cholestatic jaundice

DRUG INTERACTIONS
Cyclophosphamide, 6-mercaptopurine (doxorubicin)

NURSING INTERVENTIONS
Give antiemetic and evaluate blood counts and renal and hepatic function prior to administration

PATIENT INFORMATION
Patient should report any redness or pain at infusion site. Severe headaches, confusion, nausea, vomiting, fever, and signs of infection should be reported immediately.

MITOMYCIN C AND VINBLASTINE

The combination of mitomycin C and vinblastine is used as second-line therapy for metastatic breast cancer. No comparative trials assessing this regimen over either single agent have been reported. It is possible that this combination is associated with a higher response rate at the cost of greater toxicity, particularly myelosuppression, given the known single-agent toxicities.

DOSAGE AND SCHEDULING

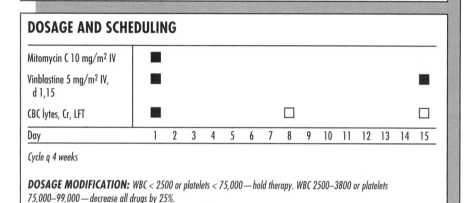

Mitomycin C 10 mg/m² IV	■														
Vinblastine 5 mg/m² IV, d 1,15	■														■
CBC lytes, Cr, LFT	■							□							□
Day	1	2	3	4	5	6	7	8	9	10	11	12	13	14	15

Cycle q 4 weeks

DOSAGE MODIFICATION: *WBC < 2500 or platelets < 75,000 — hold therapy. WBC 2500–3800 or platelets 75,000–99,000 — decrease all drugs by 25%.*

RECENT EXPERIENCES AND RESPONSE RATES

Study	Evaluable Patients, *n*	Dosage/Schedule	Response for Metastatic Disease, %
Denefrio *et al.,* Cancer Treat Rep 1978, 62:2113–2115	14	M 6 mg/m² IV d 1 V 5 mg/m² IV d 1 q 2 wk	7
Konits *et al.,* Cancer 1981,48:1295–1298	303	M 20 mg/m² IV d 1 V 0.15 mg/mg IV d 1 q 3 wk	40
Garewal *et al.,* J Clin Oncol 1983, 1:772–775	22	M 10 mgm² IV d 1 V 5 mg/m² IV d 1 q 2 wk	32

CANDIDATES FOR TREATMENT

Recurrent or metastatic breast cancer in patients who have failed doxorubicin or other first- or second-line therapy containing doxorubicin

SPECIAL PRECAUTIONS

Patients with hepatic insufficiency; extravasation of vinblastine, a vesicant, may lead to tissue necrosis

ALTERNATIVE THERAPIES

Doxorubicin or VATH in patients not previously exposed to doxorubicin; single-agent mitomycin C or vinblastine

TOXICITIES

Drug combination: fevers, nausea, vomiting, anorexia, anemia, prolonged leukopenia, thrombocytopenia, hemolytic uremic syndrome, rare pulmonary fibrosis, renal toxicity, peripheral paresthesias, neuropathy, constipation and rare ileus

DRUG INTERACTIONS

None known

NURSING INTERVENTIONS

Give antiemetic and evaluate blood counts and renal and hepatic function prior to administration

PATIENT INFORMATION

Patient should report any redness or pain at infusion site. Severe headaches, confusion, nausea, vomiting, fever, and signs of infection should be reported immediately.

PACLITAXEL

Paclitaxel is indicated as a single agent for the treatment of metastatic (stage IV) breast cancer after progression of combination chemotherapy for metastatic disease or after relapse within 6 mo of adjuvant therapy. Prior therapy should have included an anthracycline unless clinically contraindicated.

DOSAGE AND SCHEDULING

PREMEDICATE WITH DEXAMETHASONE 20 MG PO AT 12 AND 6 H PRIOR TO INFUSION AND WITH DIPHENHYDRAMINE 50 MG IV AND CIMETIDINE 300 MG IV 30 MIN PRIOR TO INFUSION

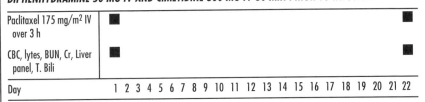

Paclitaxel 175 mg/m² IV over 3 h	■																					■	
CBC, lytes, BUN, Cr, Liver panel, T. Bili	■																					■	
Day	1	2	3	4	5	6	7	8	9	10	11	12	13	14	15	16	17	18	19	20	21	22	

Cycle every 3 wk

DOSAGE MODIFICATIONS: Do not administer for pretreatment neutrophil count < 1500. For severe posttreatment neutropenia (neutrophil count < 500 for ≥ 7 d), reduce subsequent paclitaxel dose by 20%. Reduce dose for elevated liver enzymes or elevated bilirubin (firm guidelines are not published).

RECENT EXPERIENCES AND RESPONSE RATES

Study	Evaluable patients, *n*	Dosage/Schedule (every 3 wk)	Response for metastatic disease, %
Abrams *et al., J Clin Oncol* 1995, 13:2056	172	175 mg/m² IV over 24 h	23
Nabholtz *et al., J Clin Oncol* 1996, 14:1858	227	135 mg/m² IV over 3 h	22
Nabholtz *et al., J Clin Oncol* 1996, 14:1858	223	175 mg/m² IV over 3 h	29
Seidman *et al., J Clin Oncol* 1995, 13:1152	76	200–250 mg/m² IV over 24 h	33
Sledge *et al., Proc Am Soc Clin Oncol* 1997, 16:1a	266	175 mg/m² IV over 24 h	33

CANDIDATES FOR TREATMENT

Paclitaxel is indicated as a single agent for the treatment of metastatic (stage IV) breast cancer after progression of combination chemotherapy for metastatic disease or after relapse within 6 mo of adjuvant therapy; prior therapy should have included an anthracycline unless clinically contraindicated

SPECIAL PRECAUTIONS

Administer through large or central vein; enhanced toxicities with prior or concomitant radiation; reduce dose with liver function test abnormalities

ALTERNATIVE THERAPIES

Doxorubicin, docetaxel

TOXICITIES

Neutropenia, anemia, thrombocytopenia, peripheral neuropathy, alopecia, nausea, vomiting, myalgia, asthenia, mucositis, rare hypersensitivity reaction, rare bradycardia, rare motor neuropathy and coordination problems

DRUG INTERACTIONS

None known

NURSING INTERVENTIONS

Use appropriate premedications and antiemetics (paclitaxel is considered low to moderately emetogenic); check laboratory values (especially blood counts and liver function) prior to administration; inform patients of toxicities

PATIENT INFORMATION

Patients should report and bleeding, fevers, or severe mucositis.

DOCETAXEL

Docetaxel is indicated as a single agent for the treatment of metastatic (stage IV) or locally advanced (stage III) breast cancer after progression during anthracycline-containing chemotherapy for patients with metastatic disease or for those who have relapsed during anthracycline-containing adjuvant therapy.

DOSAGE AND SCHEDULING

MEDICATE WITH DEXAMETHASONE 8 MG PO TWICE DAILY FOR 5 D, BEGINNING 1 D PRIOR TO INFUSION

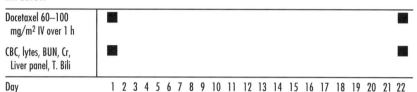

Docetaxel 60–100 mg/m² IV over 1 h	■ ■
CBC, lytes, BUN, Cr, Liver panel, T. Bili	■ ■
Day	1 2 3 4 5 6 7 8 9 10 11 12 13 14 15 16 17 18 19 20 21 22

Cycle every 3 wk

DOSAGE MODIFICATIONS: *Do not administer for pretreatment neutrophil count < 1500. For severe posttreatment neutropenia (neutrophil count < 500 for ≥ 7 d) or febrile neutropenia, reduce subsequent docetaxel dose by 25%. Do not use if total bilirubin is elevated or if SGPT or SGOT is > 1.5 times institutional norm concomitant with alkaline phosphatase > 2.5 times institutional norm.*

RECENT EXPERIENCE AND RESPONSE RATES

Study	Evaluable patients, *n*	Dosage/Schedule (every 3 wk)	Response for metastatic disease, %
Chevallier *et al., J Clin Oncol* 1995, 13:314	31	100 mg/m² IV over 1 h	68
Dieras *et al., Br J Cancer* 1996, 74:650	31	75 mg/m² IV over 1 h	52
Hudis *et al., J Clin Oncol* 1996, 14:58	37	100 mg/m² IV over 1 h	64
Ravdin *et al., J Clin Oncol* 1995, 13:2879	35	100 mg/m² IV over 1 h	58
Piccart *et al., Eur J Cancer* 1994, 30A(suppl 2):24	52	50 mg/m² IV over 1 h, day 1, 8	33
Chan *et al., Breast Cancer Res Treat* 1997, 46:23a	161	100 mg/m² IV over 1 h	47

CANDIDATES FOR TREATMENT

Docetaxel is indicated as a single agent for the treatment of metastatic (stage IV) or locally advanced (stage III) breast cancer after progression during anthracycline-containing chemotherapy for patients with metastatic disease or for those who have relapsed during anthracycline-containing adjuvant therapy

SPECIAL PRECAUTIONS

Administer through large or central vein; enhanced toxicities with prior or concomitant radiation

ALTERNATIVE THERAPIES

Paclitaxel, mitomycin, vinblastine

TOXICITIES

Neutropenia, anemia, thrombocytopenia, peripheral neuropathy, alopecia, fluid retention/edema, asthenia, nausea, vomiting, myalgia, mucositis, rare hypersensitivity reaction, rare bradycardia, rare motor neuropathy and coordination problems

DRUG INTERACTIONS

Cyclosporine, terfenadine, ketoconazole, erythromycin

NURSING INTERVENTIONS

Use appropriate premedications and antiemetics (docetaxel is considered moderately emetogenic); check laboratory values (especially blood counts and liver function) prior to administration; inform patients of toxicities

PATIENT INFORMATION

Patients should report bleeding, fevers, or severe mucositis.

Malignancies of the upper gastrointestinal tract pose substantial challenges for therapy. In most cases, surgery remains the mainstay of therapy and is the only known curative therapeutic modality for this group of diseases. However, the 5-year survival rates remain low and ranges from 3% for pancreatic adenocarcinoma to 15% for gastric cancer. These statistics have stimulated interest in alternate forms of management for these malignancies. Experience with chemotherapy and radiation therapy, often as combined-modality treatment with or without surgery, is growing. This chapter compares a variety of chemotherapeutic approaches within each disease group and highlights selected chemotherapy regimens that are in common use or that have unique applications in upper gastrointestinal tract cancer (Tables 8-1 and 8-2).

ESOPHAGEAL CANCER

In 1998, 12,500 new cases of esophageal carcinoma are expected to be diagnosed in the United States, with men having more than a twofold increase in risk compared with women. For unknown reasons, the incidence of adenocarcinoma of the esophagus is increasing at a rate faster than that of nearly any other cancer. The overall 5-year survival has never exceeded 10% [1]. Locoregional or systemic spread of disease is often attributed to the lack of anatomic barriers to dissemination. The esophagus does not have a serosa to provide a natural defense for local invasion, and this organ is rich in submucosal lymphatics, which probably allow longitudinal spread from the primary site. Autopsy findings from patients who have recently undergone surgery for squamous cell carcinoma of the esophagus have demonstrated a high incidence of unsuspected early metastatic disease.

THERAPY FOR ADVANCED DISEASE

Single-agent chemotherapy is now rarely used for advanced disease. Agents with adequate activity include bleomycin, mitomycin C, doxorubicin, cisplatin, carboplatin, plant alkaloids, 5-fluorouracil (5-FU), lomustine, ifosfamide, mitoguazone, methotrexate, and the relatively newer agents paclitaxel and vindesine. Paclitaxel as a single agent has been reported to produce a response rate of 34% and 28% in patients with adenocarcinoma and squamous cell carcinoma, respectively [2]. The best response rates are achieved with a combination of chemotherapeutic agents; however, there have been no randomized trials comparing and, thus, confirming the superiority of combination regimens over single-agent therapy. The most commonly used combination chemotherapy regimen is 5-FU and cisplatin, which can produce an objective response rate as high as 42% [3]. Other agents in cisplatin-containing combinations have included etoposide, epirubicin with protracted-infusion 5-FU, and interferon with 5-FU. These combinations have shown encouraging response rates of up to 65% [4–6].

THERAPY FOR LOCALLY UNRESECTABLE DISEASE

Perhaps the most vigorously tested role of combination chemotherapy in esophageal cancer has been in the multimodality management of local or regional disease. In the past, radiation therapy had been the mainstay of therapy as palliation for patients who were believed to have disease that could not be resected with reasonable chance for cure (T4,M1 disease) (Table 8-3). The relief of dysphagia in these patients is excellent, with reported palliative responses of up to 80%. However, it is now well established that even a small change in tumor size can lead to marked improvement in swallowing function, resulting from a decrease in the resistance to flow (based on the law of LaPlace). This may explain why the high palliative rate observed with radiation therapy alone has not resulted in significant changes in median survival. A variety of studies have assessed the safety, feasibility, and regression rates of combination chemotherapy and radiation for patients with locally unresectable disease. The mainstay of drug therapy in this setting has been 5-FU combined with other radiation-sensitizing drugs, such as cisplatin or mitomycin. Pilot experiences with this approach have shown encouragingly high 2-year survival rates. In some cases, durable complete responses have been observed [7]. An additional intriguing report of this approach in the treatment of patients with adenocarcinoma of the esophagus and gastroesophageal junction involved a

Table 8-1. Risk Factors for Cancers of the Upper Gastrointestinal Tract

Esophagus	*Pancreas*
Exposure to nitrosamines	Cigarette smoking
Cigarette smoking	Exposure to beta-naphthylamine, benzidine
Excessive alcohol use	Chronic pancreatitis
Lye ingestion	Family history
Achalasia	
Barrett's mucosa	*Liver*
Tylosis	Hepatitis B carrier state
Infection with transforming viruses (HPV, HSV, CMV, EBV)	Chronic liver disease (chronic active hepatitis, cirrhosis)
Plummer Vinson Syndrome	Exposure to mycotoxin, ionizing radiation, steroid hormones, arsenic
Mycotoxin	*Bile Ducts*
	Sclerosing cholangitis
Stomach	Parasitic infections
Achlorhydria	Use of steroid hormones
Helicobacter pylori infection	
Previous gastrectomy, Billroth II procedures	
Family history	

CMV—cytomegalovirus; EBV—Epstein–Barr virus; HPV—human papillomavirus; HSV—herpes simplex virus.

Table 8-2. General Guidelines for Prevention and Early Detection of Cancers of the Upper Gastrointestinal Tract

Prevention	Early Detection
Avoid cigarette smoking	Esophagus
Use alcohol in moderation	Annual upper gastrointestinal endoscopy in patients with known Barrett's mucosa, tylosis, or history of caustic esophageal injury
Eat a low-fat diet, rich in fresh fruit and vegetables	Hepatoma
Avoid exposure to occupational toxins	Periodic α-fetoprotein measurement and liver ultrasound for patients with chronic liver disease
Immunize against infectious hepatitis	
Avoid unnecessary use of steroid hormones	

combination of 5-FU and mitomycin in addition to radiation therapy as definitive treatment [8]. Complete response in eight of nine patients with T1 and T2 disease and a median relapse-free survival of 10 months were observed. Studies such as these led the Radiation Therapy Oncology Group (RTOG), the Southwest Oncology Group (SWOG), and the North Central Cancer Treatment Group (NCCTG) to conduct a randomized trial [9] comparing a combination of fluorouracil (1000 mg/m² by continuous infusion daily for 4 d) and cisplatin (75 mg/m² on d 1) plus 5000 cGy of radiation therapy compared with 6400 cGy of radiation therapy alone in patients with epidermoid carcinoma or adenocarcinoma of the thoracic esophagus. As might be expected, severe and life-threatening side effects (predominantly mucositis and myelosuppression) were seen more frequently in patients treated with combined-modality therapy. A 5-year follow-up for all patients in this group showed a median survival of 14.1 months and overall survival of 27% in the combined treatment group, whereas the median survival duration was 9.3 months with no patient alive at 5 years in the group tested with radiation alone [10]. Control of both local and distant metastases was also superior in the combined-modality group.

Other measures sometimes employed to achieve local control include endoscopic laser therapy and endoluminal radiation. Long-term survival also has been achieved in early-stage lesions with photodynamic therapy employing systemic administration of a hematoporphyrin derivative followed by 630-µm dye laser [11]. Physical methods of maintaining esophageal patency have also improved; experience shows that expansile metal stents result in fewer complications compared with older plastic prostheses [12].

NEOADJUVANT THERAPY

An increasing amount of experience is also developing evaluating the role of combination chemotherapy with or without radiation prior to surgery. The availability of endoscopic ultrasound has been very useful in selecting patients for preoperative therapy; overall, the accuracy in identifying the correct T and N stage is 85% and 79%, respectively [13]. As with regimens used in advanced disease, cisplatin is a common denominator in neoadjuvant regimens, and the reported response rates to preoperative therapy are remarkably similar; a recent review by Philip and Ajani [14] suggests that a preoperative response rate of 50% can be achieved. Preliminary data are available from two randomized trials comparing preoperative chemotherapy with immediate surgery [15] or with radiation therapy prior to surgery [16]. In both of these trials, major objective responses (47% and 53%, respectively) were reported for preoperative chemotherapy. However, median survival did not differ significantly in the trial comparing preoperative chemotherapy with immediate surgery. Because of a crossover design in the study comparing preoperative chemotherapy with preoperative radiation therapy, it is difficult to analyze the effect of therapy on disease-free or overall survival.

Experience with the combined use of chemotherapy and radiation prior to esophagectomy is growing. Most of these studies use 5-FU as a common denominator in the induction chemotherapy as a single agent [17], in combination with cisplatin [18] or mitomycin C [19], or as a multiagent regimen [20]. Although these trials vary in their study populations with respect to the proportion of epidermoid carcinomas and adenocarcinomas and with respect to presenting stage of disease, these reports are notable for the documentation of both complete and pathologic responses in all instances. Naunheim and coworkers [21] have reported an overall median survival of 23 months; in the report by Forastiere and coworkers [20], the median survival time was 29 months, and 34% of the patients were alive at 5 years. These results appear to be better than those achieved historically. In both of the studies, the complete histologic response rate was over 20%. Because the natural history of the disease in patients with complete pathologic response to therapy is not well understood and because durable complete responses have been reported in patients who were treated with chemotherapy and radiation but without esophagectomy, the question is raised whether esophagectomy is necessary for all responding patients.

Table 8-3 TNM Staging Criteria for Esophageal Cancer

Staging	Criteria
TX	Primary tumor cannot be assessed
T0	No evidence of primary tumor
Tis	Carcinoma in situ
T1	Tumor invades lamina propria or submucosa
T2	Tumor invades muscularis propria
T3	Tumor invades adventitia
T4	Tumor invades adjacent structures
NX	Regional lymph nodes cannot be assessed
N0	No regional lymph node metastasis
N1	Regional lymph node metastasis
MX	Distant metastasis cannot be assessed
M0	No distant metastasis
M1	Distant metastasis|
Tumors of the lower thoracic esophagus:	
M1a	Metastasis in celiac lymph nodes
M1b	Other distant metastasis
Tumors of the midthoracic esophagus:	
M1a	Not applicable
M1b	Nonregional lymph nodes and/or other distant metastasis
Tumors of the upper thoracic esophagus:	
M1a	Metastasis in cervical nodes
M1b	Other distant metastasis

Stage	TNM
0	Tis, N0, M0
I	T1, N0, M0
IIA	T2, N0, M0
	T3, N0, M0
IIB	T1, N1, M0
	T2, N1, M0
III	T3, N1, M0
	T4, any N, M0
IV	Any T, any N, M1
IVA	Any T, any N, M1a
IVB	Any T, any N, M1b

Adapted from American Joint Committee on Cancer [83].

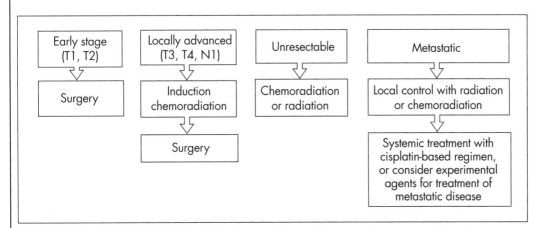

FIGURE 8-1.

Treatment strategies for esophageal and esphagogastric cancer.

In a prospective randomized trial, Walsh and coworkers [22] clearly showed the superiority of combined modality therapy (two courses of 5-FU and cisplatin with 40 cGy of radiotherapy) followed by surgery compared with surgery alone in patients with esophageal adenocarcinoma. The overall survival at 3 years was 32% and 6%, respectively. In another multicenter randomized trial in patients with squamous cell carcinoma, Bossett and coworkers [23] found improved disease-free survival and survival free of local disease but no overall survival benefit between the multimodality and the surgery-alone groups. Notably, however, cisplatin was the only chemotherapeutic agent used in the combined-treatment arm in this latter study.

All preoperative strategies are associated with a high toxicity profile, primarily from myelosuppression and esophagitis. For instance, Adelstein and coworkers [24] recently studied 5-FU and cisplatin chemotherapy in combination with accelerated fractionation radiation and found a perioperative mortality of 18%. Because of the toxicity of preoperative chemoradiotherapy, both physicians and patients should weigh the benefits and side effects when electing treatment. However, combined preoperative chemoradiotherapy should be considered in patients with clinical evidence of stage III disease (Fig. 8-1).

STOMACH CANCER

In 1998, approximately 22,400 new cases of stomach cancer will be diagnosed in United States, yet cancer of the stomach appears to be decreasing in incidence. The explanation for this perplexing change in incidence is not known; however, some have attributed the decrease to the common practice of adding ascorbic acid as a food preservative, which decreases the gastric pH and limits endogenous nitrosamine production by bacteria in the upper gastrointestinal tract. A new link between gastric cancer and *Helicobacter pylori* infections as a risk factor has now been described [25]. The overall 5-year survival rate for affected patients remains low at approximately 18%. Because the presenting symptoms of stomach cancer tend to be extremely vague, the majority of patients are diagnosed with extensive local involvement or regional lymph node metastases, which explains in part the poor 5-year survival rate following surgery (Table 8-4).

THERAPY FOR ADVANCED DISEASE

Both single-agent and combination chemotherapy have been widely tested in advanced metastatic gastric cancer. Among the most active

Table 8-4. TNM Staging Criteria for Gastric Cancer

Staging	Criteria
TX	Primary tumor cannot be assessed
T0	No evidence of primary tumor
Tis	Carcinoma in situ: intraepithelial tumor without invasion of the lamina propria
T1	Tumor invades lamina propria or submucosa
T2	Tumor invades muscularis propria or subserosa
T3	Tumor penetrates serosa (visceral peritoneum) without invasion of adjacent structures
T4	Tumor invades adjacent structures
NX	Regional lymph node(s) cannot be assessed
N0	No regional lymph node metastasis
N1	Metastasis in 1–6 regional lymph nodes
N2	Metastasis in 7–15 regional lymph nodes
N3	Metastasis in > 15 regional lymph nodes
MX	Distant metastasis cannot be assessed
M0	No distant metastasis
M1	Distant metastasis

Stage	TNM
0	Tis, N0, M0
IA	T1, N0, M0
IB	T1, N1, M0
	T2, N0, M0
II	T1, N2, M0
	T2, N1, M0
	T3, N0, M0
IIIA	T2, N2, M0
	T3, N1, M0
	T4, N0, M0
IIIB	T3, N2, M0
IV	T4, N1, M0
	T1, N3, M0
	T2, N3, M0
	T3, N3, M0
	T4, N2, M0
	T4, N3, M0
	Any T, any N, M1

Adapted from American Joint Committee on Cancer [83].

agents are 5-FU, trimetrexate, mitomycin C, hydroxyurea, epirubicin, and carmustine, which demonstrate partial response rates of 18% to 30% [26]. Combination chemotherapy with these and other marginally active agents appears to produce higher objective response rates than those with single agents. Single-institution trials have reported objective response rates of as high as 53% [27]. Recently, irinotecan in combination with cisplatin has shown an objective response of 42% with acceptable toxicity [28]. These higher objective response rates have not always held up in phase III trials, and to date, no single combination chemotherapy program tested in prospective randomized trials shows a statistically significant improvement in median survival compared with other regimens. The FAM (5-FU, doxorubicin, mitomycin C) regimen was one of the first active combination regimens described, with a partial response rate of 42% [29]. The FAM regimen has been challenged in several randomized clinical trials. An early report from the NCCTG suggested that FAM was not superior to 5-FU alone or to 5-FU plus doxorubicin in the treatment of advanced gastric cancer [30]. A more recent report from Italy [31] suggests that a combination of cisplatin, etoposide, and leucovorin preceding 5-FU produces a threefold improvement compared with FAM in objective responses but no improvement in survival. More recent modifications of the FAM regimen have included the addition of high-dose leucovorin as a biochemical modulator of 5-FU [25]. Using this approach, an objective response rate of 38% and an encouraging overall median survival of 11.5 months have been reported.

Another novel combination including etoposide, doxorubicin, and cisplatin (EAP) was first reported in 1989. An objective response rate of 64% and a complete response rate of 21% were observed in patients with advanced metastatic disease [33]. Unfortunately, severe myelosuppression was experienced in this trial, and other investigators failed to confirm these early encouraging results [34,35]. Another notable combination chemotherapy regimen includes high-dose methotrexate, 5-FU, doxorubicin, and leucovorin rescue (FAMTX). This regimen initially was shown to have an objective response rate in the range of 33% to 50%, with a 10% complete response rate [36]. A phase III trial of this regimen compared with FAM chemotherapy showed a superior objective response rate (41% vs 9%) and a significant improvement in median survival (10.5 vs 7.2 mo) [37]. Finally, the combination of etoposide, leucovorin, and 5-FU—initially chosen for expected better tolerance in elderly patients or patients with cardiac disease—has proved to be an active regimen with an objective response rate of 52% and median survival time of 11.5 months [38]. This regimen also has substantial activity in patients previously treated with carboplatin [39]. Cullinan and coworkers [40] also have evaluated whether combinations of 5-FU, doxorubicin, and methyl carmustine (with or without alternating triazinate) or 5-FU and doxorubicin are superior to 5-FU alone. These investigators identified no advantage for any of the combinations. Thus, a variety of multi-agent regimens are available with established activity against gastric cancer. Unfortunately, it is not yet clear whether any specific regimen can improve median survival compared with the best single-agent or other combination regimens. Further phase III trials are needed to clarify the role of combination chemotherapy in advanced metastatic gastric cancer.

ADJUVANT THERAPY

The higher objective response rates observed with combination chemotherapy have stimulated interest in adjuvant therapy for gastric cancer. Older studies focused primarily on postoperative chemotherapy.

The majority of these studies employed the FAM regimen or 5-FU in combination with either radiation therapy or methyl lomustine [27]. An initial encouraging report using 5-FU and methyl lomustine from the Gastrointestinal Tumor Study Group [41] was not confirmed in an identical study performed by the Eastern Cooperative Oncology Group (ECOG) [42]. A small trial evaluating the role of postoperative mitomycin C has suggested an improved median survival; confirmation of this finding awaits testing [43]. The NCCTG evaluated intensive-course 5-FU plus doxorubicin and reported no evidence of therapy benefit [44]. More recently, the British Stomach Cancer Group reported that postoperative therapy with radiation or FAM is not superior to surgery alone [45]. Finally, a recent meta-analysis involving 11 randomized trials concluded that postoperative adjuvant therapy does not appear to be a useful strategy [46].

The disappointing results with postoperative adjuvant chemotherapy have spawned attempts at improving surgical outcome with preoperative chemotherapy. Several studies are noteworthy in this regard. EAP has been tested preoperatively in patients with advanced locoregional disease (positive lymph nodes, T3 or T4 primary lesions) [47]. EAP therapy was continued until patients achieved a maximum response to therapy; resection was then attempted. The objective response rate to preoperative EAP was 70%, including a 21% complete response rate. Twenty patients subsequently underwent resection. At a median follow-up of 20 months, the relapse rate was 60% at a median survival time of 18 months. The high complete-remission rate with the EAP regimen could not be confirmed in a more recent multiinstitutional trial reported by Ajani and coworkers [48] involving early stage gastric cancers. Ajani and coworkers [49] also evaluated the preoperative response rate and resectability following administration of etoposide, 5-FU, and cisplatin. In this study, 24% of the patients had major preoperative responses to chemotherapy, including two complete responses. The resection rate was 72%, and with a median follow-up of 25 months the median survival was 15 months. Safran and coworkers [50] evaluated the combination of paclitaxel with concurrent radiation therapy for locally advanced gastric cancer and found a response rate of 70% in patients with evaluable disease; 30% of these patients subsequently underwent resection. Another approach incorporated postoperative intraperitoneal therapy with fluorouracil and cisplatin in addition to preoperative FAMTX. For patients who underwent curative resection in this study, the median survival was 31 months, and peritoneal failure with acceptable toxicity was seen in 16% of the patients [51]. These early promising reports will require confirmation in larger randomized trials before these approaches can be accepted as standard management for gastric cancer (Fig. 8-2).

PANCREATIC CANCER

ADENOCARCINOMA

Adenocarcinoma of the pancreas represents the fifth most common cause of cancer-related death in American men. Approximately 28,000 cases are expected to occur in 1998. The incidence of the disease approximately equals the age-adjusted mortality rate, underscoring the aggressive nature of this malignancy (Table 8-5). In large studies, only 5% to 22% of presenting patients have resectable tumors. Unfortunately, even successful resection is associated with a low 5-year survival rate, ranging from 3.5% to 19%. Patients with unresectable adenocarcinomas of the pancreas confined to the

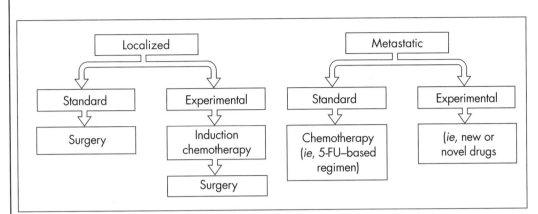

FIGURE 8-2.

Treatment strategies for gastric cancer.

pancreas often undergo palliative surgery or biliary stent placement for relief of jaundice in addition to prophylactic duodenal bypass procedures to prevent obstruction (observed in 10% of patients). Chemotherapy can add to both quantity and quality of life in advanced pancreatic cancer, although the benefit could be limited to selected patients [52].

THERAPY FOR LOCOREGIONAL DISEASE

The role of chemotherapy in the management of pancreatic carcinoma is best understood in the context of combined-modality treatment for the adjuvant therapy of pancreatic carcinoma after resection or in the management of locally unresectable lesions. The GITSG has reported a better than twofold increase in the 2-year actuarial survival (46% and 43% vs 18%) for patients treated with a combination of 5-FU and split-course radiation therapy following resection, compared with observation [53]. In addition, the GITSG has also demonstrated an almost twofold increase in median survival in patients with unresectable disease treated with 5-FU plus split-course radiation compared with high-dose radiation therapy alone [54]. Bolus 5-FU has also been studied in combination with intraoperative radiation therapy and with brachytherapy, although randomized trials are not available to determine the role of 5-FU in this clinical setting. Protracted-infusion 5-FU combined with radiation has shown similar activity to bolus 5-FU and radiotherapy but with less toxicity [55]. Taxol in combination with radiotherapy has shown some promise in preliminary trials. This combination is now under evaluation in neoadjuvant setting.

Currently, an active area of investigation involves the use of preoperative chemotherapy and radiation to improve the opportunities for complete resection. Hoffman and coworkers [56] have reported on the preoperative regimen of 5-FU, mitomycin C, and local radiation; they observed a resection rate of 32% and, with a median follow-up of 33 months, 45% of the patients had a recurrence but only one local recurrence was reported. Evans and coworkers [57] have reported a resection rate of 61% after preoperative chemoradiation but have not yet reported on long-term follow-up. It is not yet clear whether a neoadjuvant approach can alter the pattern of local and disseminated disease recurrence, but a variety of pilot trials are in progress to address these concerns. Spitz and coworkers [58] reviewed the outcome of pre- or postoperative chemoradiation and showed no difference in survival between the two groups. However, they also noted that preoperative chemoradiation could be delivered over a shorter time period and that one fourth of eligible patients were unable to receive postoperative therapy because of

prolonged recovery or perioperative complications following surgery. Thus, there may be a logistical advantage for preoperative therapy.

THERAPY FOR ADVANCED DISEASE

The use of chemotherapy for patients with widespread metastatic disease has been extremely disappointing. There appears to be no

Table 8-5. TNM Staging Criteria for Pancreatic Cancer

Staging	Criteria
TX	Primary tumor cannot be assessed
T0	No evidence of primary tumor
Tis	In situ carcinoma
T1	Tumor limited to the pancreas ≤ 2 cm or less in greatest dimension
T2	Tumor limited to the pancreas > 2 cm in greatest dimension
T3	Tumor extends directly into any of the following: duodenum, bile duct, peripancreatic tissues
T4	Tumor extends directly into any of the following: stomach, spleen, colon, adjacent large vessels
NX	Regional lymph nodes cannot be assessed
N0	No regional lymph node metastasis
N1	Regional lymph node metastasis
pN1a	Metastasis in a single regional lymph node
pN1b	Metastasis in multiple regional lymph nodes
MX	Distant metastasis cannot be assessed
M0	No distant metastasis
M1	Distant metastasis

Stage	TNM
0	Tis, N0, M0
I	T1, N0, M0
	T2, N0, M0
II	T3, N0, M0
III	T1, N1, M0
	T2, N1, M0
	T3, N1, M0
IVA	T4, any N, M0
IVB	Any T, any N, M1

Adapted from American Joint Committee on Cancer [83].

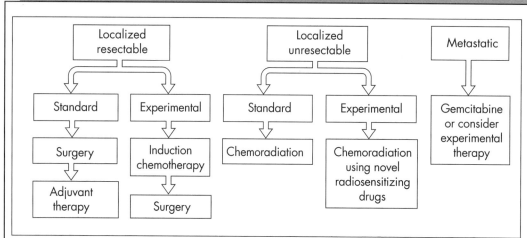

FIGURE 8-3.
Treatment strategies for pancreas cancer.

highly active single agent and virtually all approved chemotherapy drugs have now been tested. 5-FU may have activity as a single agent; for instance, a phase II trial using 5-FU and more optimal biochemical modulation with leucovorin demonstrated a modest response rate of 7% and a median survival of 6.2 months [59]. Gemcitabine has been compared to 5-FU in a phase III trial [60]. This study has demonstrated a superior median survival of 5.7 months for gemcitabine compared with 4.4 months for 5-FU; it also demonstrated improved relief of symptoms with gemcitabine. Due to its palliative potential, gemcitabine as a single agent should be considered for unresectable pancreatic adenocarcinoma [61].

Combination chemotherapy regimens have, in some cases, demonstrated improved objective response rates. However, randomized trials with popular regimens such as FAM and streptozocin, mitomycin C, and 5-FU (SMF) [60] have failed to demonstrate superiority of any single regimen. It seems clear that either new drugs or novel therapeutic approaches for pancreatic adenocarcinoma are desperately needed (Fig. 8-3).

ISLET CELL CARCINOMA

Another important subgroup of pancreatic tumors includes islet cell tumors. These include malignant insulinoma, gastrinoma, VIPoma, glucagonoma, and somatostatinoma. It is important to recognize these lesions histologically because the natural history and management of these pancreatic tumors are different.

Many of the islet cell tumors produce fascinating and distinctive syndromes related to secretory hormones produced. Although it is beyond the scope of this chapter to discuss this in detail, it is worth noting that the management of these tumors is often directed at palliation of the associated symptoms. Treatment may include surgical reduction of tumor bulk, up to and including total orthotopic liver transplantation, hepatic artery occlusion for symptomatic metastatic disease, and specific end-organ blockade of the hormonal system. Examples of the latter would include Omeprezole, an inhibitor of the parietal cell hydrogen pump, which is more effective than H-2 blockers in the management of symptomatic gastrinomas. Octreotide, a somatostatin analogue now available in a long-acting preparation, has shown beneficial effect on tumor growth with stabilization of the disease as the most favorable response [62]. Octreotide is also helpful in palliating symptoms in patients with islet cell carcinomas, depending upon the cell type.

In the past, chemotherapy was reserved for patients with these indolent tumors as a last resort. Active drugs have included streptozocin, doxorubicin, chlorozotocin, and dacarbazine. A randomized trial was conducted showing superiority of streptozocin and doxorubicin over streptozocin plus 5-FU or single-agent chlorozotocin [63]. In this trial, the combination of streptozocin and doxorubicin produced an improved response rate over the other two arms (69% vs 45% and 30%, respectively) and a significant survival advantage (median survival, 2.2 y vs 1.4 and 1.4 y, respectively). These results may justify the use of this therapy as an initial approach in some patients. Chemoembolization also appears to be an effective alternative for patients with liver metastases of neuroendocrine origin. Ruszniewski and coworkers [64] have reported that hepatic artery chemoembolization with iodized oil and doxorubicin can provide symptom control and tumor regression or stabilization in up to 80% of carcinoid tumors and gastrinomas.

HEPATOBILIARY CANCER

Together, hepatoma and biliary tract cancer will be diagnosed in more than 20,000 individuals in the United States in 1998. Worldwide, the most common risk factor for hepatoma is hepatitis B infection. In the United States, other causes of chronic liver disease, such as alcoholic cirrhosis, may be more important predisposing factors. Regardless of the etiology, the only known curative modality for hepatoma is surgical resection. Patients with unresectable disease because of severe underlying liver disease, anatomic location of tumor, or the presence of distant metastases have an extremely poor prognosis (Tables 8-6 and 8-7).

THERAPY FOR LOCOREGIONAL DISEASE

Carcinoma of the gallbladder is often an incidental finding at surgery. Nonetheless, advanced local and regional disease is usually present and the overall 5-year survival is less than 5%. The prognosis for patients with carcinoma of the distal bile duct is more optimistic, with an average 5-year survival after radical pancreaticoduodenectomy of approximately 40%. However, proximal bile duct carcinomas and hilar cholangiocarcinomas are much more difficult to treat surgically. In bile duct carcinomas, a favorable outcome is mainly determined by curative resection

Table 8-6. TNM Staging for Biliary Cancer

Staging	Criteria
TX	Primary tumor cannot be assessed
T0	No evidence of primary tumor
Tis	Carcinoma in situ
T1	Tumor invades subepithelial connective tissue or fibromuscular layer
T1a	Tumor invades subepithelial connective tissue
T1b	Tumor invades fibromuscular layer
T2	Tumor invades perifibromuscular connective tissue
T3	Tumor invades adjacent structures: liver, pancreas, duodenum, gallbladder, colon, stomach
NX	Regional lymph nodes cannot be assessed
N0	No regional lymph node metastasis
N1	Metastasis in cystic duct, pericholedochal and/or hilar lymph nodes (ie, in the hepatoduodenal ligament)
N2	Metastasis in peripancreatic (head only), periduodenal, periportal, celiac, and/or superior mesenteric and/or posterior pancreaticoduodenal lymph nodes
MX	Distant metastasis cannot be assessed
M0	No distant metastasis
M1	Distant metastasis

Stage	TNM
0	Tis, N0, M0
I	T1, N0, M0
II	T2, N0, M0
III	T1, N1, M0
	T1, N2, M0
	T2, N1, M0
	T2, N2, M0
IVA	T3, any N, M0
IVB	Any T, any N, M1

Adapted from American Joint Committee on Cancer [83].

Table 8-7. TNM Staging Criteria for Hepatocellular Carcinoma

Staging	Criteria
TX	Primary tumor cannot be assessed
T0	No evidence of primary tumor
T1	Solitary tumor ≤ 2 cm in greatest dimension without vascular invasion
T2	Solitary tumor ≤ 2 cm in greatest dimension with vascular invasion, or multiple tumors limited to one lobe, none more than 2 cm in greatest dimension without vascular invasion, or a solitary tumor > 2 cm in greatest dimension without vascular invasion.
T3	Solitary tumor > 2 cm in greatest dimension with vascular invasion, or multiple tumors limited to one lobe, none > 2 cm in greatest dimension, with vascular invasion, or multiple tumors limited to one lobe, any > 2 cm in greatest dimension, with or without vascular invasion
T4	Multiple tumors in more than one lobe or tumor(s) involve(s) a major branch of the portal or hepatic vein(s) or invasion of adjacent organs other than the gallbladder or perforation of the visceral peritoneum
NX	Regional lymph nodes cannot be assessed
N0	No regional lymph node metastasis
N1	Regional lymph node metastasis
MX	Distant metastasis cannot be assessed
M0	No distant metastasis
M1	Distant metastasis

Stage	TNM
I	T1, N0, M0
II	T2, N0, M0
IIIA	T3, N0, M0
IIIB	T1, N1, M0
	T2, N1, M0
	T3, N1, M0
IVA	T4, any N, M0
IVB	Any T, any N, M1

Adapted from American Joint Committee on Cancer [83].

in the absence of lymph nodes metastases [65]. In some cases, palliation and disease control can be achieved with brachytherapy using [192]Iridium placed through a biliary drainage catheter. Hepatic resection, when possible, is the primary curative approach for localized hepatoma. Mazzaferro and coworkers [66] have reported liver transplantation as an effective treatment for small, unresectable, hepatocellular carcinoma in patients with cirrhosis, with 4-year recurrence-free survival of 83%. Administration of an acyclic retinoid, polyprenoic acid has been shown to reduce the incidence of recurrence of new hepatomas after surgical resection or percutaneous injection of ethanol [67]. Localized but otherwise unresectable hepatobiliary tumors are sometimes managed with the orthotopic liver transplant; however, the role of liver transplantation in hepatobiliary malignancy remains undefined. The 2-year disease-free interval for incidental hepatoma identified after transplant for underlying chronic liver disease may approach 70% [68]; however, patients with known malignancy at the time of transplant fare less well. Aggressive adjuvant chemotherapy protocols aimed at improving outcome following transplantation have been designed for both cholangiocarcinoma [69] and hepatoma [70] (Figs. 8-4 and 8-5).

THERAPY FOR ADVANCED DISEASE

The use of systemic chemotherapy in the management of unresectable or metastatic hepatoma has been extremely disappointing. Although doxorubicin is often considered to be an active single agent in hepatoma, the objective response rate to this agent is low and therapy with doxorubicin probably docs not influence group survival when compared with no antitumor therapy [71]. Possible promising experimental approaches for hepatoma confined to the liver include chemoembolization [72], hepatic artery infusion chemotherapy [73], and percutaneous ethanol injection [74]. Ethanol may be a superior choice for small hepatomas unless the lesions are hypervascular [75].

Hepatoblastoma is a rare liver cancer seen primarily in children. Surgical resections can be curative, and these tumors are highly sensitive to chemotherapy. The Pediatric Oncology Group published the results of a large trial evaluating adjuvant therapy with cisplatin, vincristine, and 5-FU [76]. Patients with stage I and II disease had an actuarial survival of 90%; patients with stage III disease had a actuarial survival of 67% at 4 years. Recently, Ehrlich and coworkers [77] have shown a response rate of 91% and improved long-term survival with preoperative chemotherapy for hepatoblastoma patients using continuous infusion cisplatin and adriamycin.

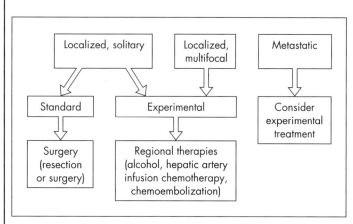

FIGURE 8-4.

Treatment strategies for hepatoma.

The role of systemic chemotherapy in unresectable metastatic biliary tract cancers also has not been well defined. Because of the low incidence of these diseases, associated medical complications,

and poor performance status of affected patients, few patients are referred for clinical trials. A recent review of the use of chemotherapy in the treatment of bile duct cancer suggests that possible active agents include 5-FU and mitomycin C either as single agents or in combination therapy with doxorubicin (FAM) [78] or a combination of 5-FU and interferon [79]. Taxol as a single agent appears to be disappointing. Combination of taxanes and other agents in combination await future testing [80]. In addition, hepatic artery infusion chemotherapy with agents such as 5-FU, fluorodeoxyuridine, and doxorubicin have been studied in small numbers in patients, and objective partial responses have been reported [81].

New techniques, such as conformal radiation (which spares uninvolved liver), have permitted studies of combined chemotherapy and radiation in hepatobiliary cancers. Robertson and coworkers [82] studied hepatic artery infusion of fluorodeoxyuridine and concurrent conformal radiation in localized hepatobiliary cancer and observed a high response to treatment, with a median survival of 19 months. Although modest progress is being made in hepatobiliary cancer, a concerted effort to better understand the role of chemotherapy in these diseases is needed.

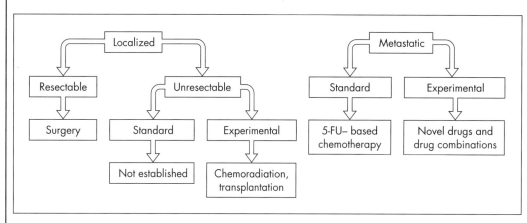

FIGURE 8-5.

Treatment strategies for gallbladder and cholangiocarcinoma.

REFERENCES

1. Farrow DC, Vaughan TL: Determinants of survival following the diagnosis of esophageal adenocarcinoma (United States). *Cancer Causes Control* 1996 7:322–327.

2. Kelsen D, Ajani J, Ilson D, *et al.*: A phase II trial of paclitaxel (taxol) in advanced esophageal cancer: preliminary report. *Semin Oncol* 1994, 21(suppl 8):44–48.

3. Kies MS, Rosen ST, Tasang TK, *et al.*: Cisplatin and 5-fluorouracil in the primary management of squamous esophageal cancer. *Cancer* 1987, 60:2156–2160.

4. Spiridonidis CH, Laufman LR, Jones JJ, *et al.*: A phase II evaluation of high dose cisplatin and etoposide in patients with advanced esophageal adenocarcinoma. *Cancer* 1996, 77:2070–2077.

5. Bamias A, Hill ME, Cunningham D, *et al.*: Epirubicin, cisplatin, and protracted venous infusion of 5-fluorouracil for esophagogastric adeno-carcinoma. *Cancer 1996*, 77:1978–1985.

6. Wadler S, Haynes H, Beitler JJ, *et al.*: Phase II clinical trial of 5-fluo-rouracil, recombinant interferon-I-2b, and cisplatin for patients with metastatic or regionally advanced carcinoma of the esophagus. *Cancer* 1996, 78:30–34.

7. Leichman L, Herskovic A, Leichman CG, *et al.*: Nonoperative therapy for squamous cell cancer of the esophagus. *J Clin Oncol* 1987, 5:365–370.

8. Coia LR, Paul AR, Engstrom PF: Combined radiation and chemotherapy as primary management of adenocarcinoma of the esophagus and gastro-esophageal junction. *Cancer* 1988, 61:643–649.

9. Herskovic A, Martz K, Al-Sarraf M, *et al.*: Combined chemotherapy and radiotherapy compared with radiotherapy alone in patients with cancer of the esophagus. *N Engl J Med* 1992, 326:1593–1598.

10. Al-Sarraf M, Martz K, Herskovic L, *et al.*: Progress report of combined chemoradiotherapy versus radiotherapy alone in patients with esophageal cancer: an intergroup study. *J Clin Oncol* 1997, 15:277–284.

11. Sibille A, Lambert R, Souquet J-C, *et al.*: Long-term survival after photodynamic therapy for esophageal cancer. *Gastroenterology* 1995, 108:337–344.

12. Knyrim K, Wagner H-J, Bethge N, *et al.*: A controlled trial of an expansile metal stent for palliation of esophageal obstruction due to inoperable cancer. *N Engl J Med* 1993, 329:1302–1307.

13. Lightdale CJ: Endoscopic ultrasound for the staging of esophageal and gastric cancer. *Principles and Practice of Oncology Update* 1995, 9:1–13.

14. Philip PA, Ajani JA: Has combined modality therapy improved the outlook in carcinoma of the esophagus? *Oncology* 1994, 8:37–52.

15. Roth JA, Pass HI, Flanagan MM, *et al.*: Randomized clinical trial of pre-operative and post-operative adjuvant chemotherapy with cisplatin, vindesine, and bleomycin for carcinoma of the esophagus. *J Thorac Cardiovasc Surg* 1988, 96:242–248.

16. Kelsen D, Bains M, Burt M, *et al.*: Randomized comparison of pre-operative (Pre-OP) chemotherapy (CT) versus radiation (RT) in epidermoid esophageal cancer (EEC). *Proc Am Soc Clin Oncol* 1988, 7(abstract):98.

17. Urba SJ, Orringer MB, Perez-Tamayo C, *et al.*: Concurrent preoperative chemotherapy and radiation therapy in localized esophageal adenocarcinoma. *Cancer* 1992, 69:285–291.

18. Lackey VL, Reagan MT, Smith RA, Anderson WJ: Neoadjuvant therapy of squamous cell carcinoma of the esophagus: role of resection and benefit in partial responders. *Ann Thorac Surg* 1989, 48:218–221.

19. Parker EF, Reed CE, Marks RD, *et al.*: Chemotherapy, radiation therapy and resection for carcinoma of the esophagus. *J Thorac Cardiovasc Surg* 1989, 98:1037–1044.

20. Forastiere AA, Orringer MB, Perez-Tamayo C, *et al.*: Preoperative chemoradiation followed by transhiatal esophagectomy for carcinoma of the esophagus: final report. *J Clin Oncol* 1993, 11:1118–1123.

21. Naunheim KS, Petruska PJ, Roy TS, *et al.*: Preoperative chemotherapy and radiotherapy for esophageal carcinoma. *J Thorac Cardiovasc Surg* 1992, 103:87–95.

22. Walsh Tn, Noonan N, Hollywood D, *et al.*: A comparison of multimodal therapy and surgery for esophageal adenocarcinoma. *N Engl J Med* 1996, 335:462–467.

23. Bosset J-F, Gignoux M, Triboulet J-P, *et al.*: Chemoradiotherapy followed by surgery compared with surgery alone in squamous-cell cancer of the esophagus. *N Engl J Med* 1997, 337:161–167.

24. Adelstein D, Rice TW, Becker M, *et al.*: Use of concurrent chemotherapy, accelerated fractionation radiation, and surgery for patients with esophageal carcinoma. Cancer 1997, 80:1011–1120.

25. Parsonnet J, Friedman GD, Vandersteen DP, *et al.*: Helicobacter pylori infection and the risk of gastric carcinoma. *N Engl J Med* 1991, 325:1127–1131.

26. Macdonald JS, Steele G Jr, Gunderson LL: Cancer of the stomach. In *Cancer Principles and Practice of Oncology*, 3rd ed. DeVita VT, Hellman S, Rosenberg SA (eds):1989, Philadelphia: JB Lippincott.

27. Kelsen D, Omar AT: Therapy of upper gastrointestinal cancer. Cancer 1991, 15:253–285.

28. Shirao K, Shimada Y, Kondo H, *et al.*: Phase I-II study of irinotecan hydrochloride combined with cisplatin in patients with advanced gastric cancer. *J Clin Oncol* 1997, 15:921–927.

29. Macdonald J, Schein P, Wooley P, *et al.*: 5-Fluorouracil, doxorubicin, and mitomycin (FAM) combination chemotherapy for advanced gastric cancer. *Ann Intern Med* 1980, 93:533–536.

30. Cullinan SA, Moertel CG, Fleming TR, *et al*: For the North Central Cancer Treatment Group: A comparison of three chemotherapeutic regimens in the treatment of advanced pancreatic and gastric carcinoma. *JAMA* 1985, 253:2061–2067.

31. Cocconi G, Bella M, Zironi S, *et al.*: Fluorouracil, doxorubicin, and mitomycin combination versus PELF chemotherapy in advanced gastric cancer: a prospective randomized trial of the Italian Oncology Group for Clinical Research. *J Clin Oncol* 1994, 12:2687–2693.

32. Arbuck SG, Silk Y, Douglass HO, *et al.*: A phase II trial of 5-fluorouracil, doxorubicin, mitomycin-C, and leucovorin in advanced gastric carcinoma. *Cancer* 1990, 65:2442–2445.

33. Preusser P, Wilke H, Achterrath W, *et al.*: Phase II study with the combination etoposide, doxorubicin, and cisplatin in advanced measurable gastric cancer. *J Clin Oncol* 1989, 7:1310–1317.

34. Kelsen D, Atiq OT, Saltz L, *et al.*: FAMTX vs. etoposide, doxorubicin, and cisplatin: a random assignment trial in gastric cancer. *J Clin Oncol* 1992, 10:541–542.

35. Lerner A, Gonin R, Steele G, and Mayer RJ: Etoposide, doxorubicin, and cisplatin chemotherapy for advanced gastric adenocarcinoma: results of a phase II trial. *J Clin Oncol* 1992, 10:536–540.

36. Wils J, Bleiberg H, Dalesio O, *et al.*: An EORTC gastrointestinal group evaluation of the combination sequential methotrexate and 5-fluorouracil combined with Adriamycin (FAMTX) in advanced measurable gastric cancer. *J Clin Oncol* 1986, 4:1799–1803.

37. Wils J, Klein H, Wagener DJ, *et al.*: Sequential high-dose methotrexate and fluorouracil combined with doxorubicin—a step ahead in the treatment of advanced gastric cancer: a trial of the European Organization of Research and Treatment of Cancer. Gastrointestinal Tract Cooperative Group. *J Clin Oncol* 1991, 9:827–831.

38. Wilke H, Preusser P, Fink U, *et al.*: High dose folinic acid/etoposide/5-fluorouracil in advanced gastric cancer—a phase II study in elderly patients or patients with cardiac arrest. *Invest New Drugs* 1990, 8:65–70.

39. Wilke H, Preusser P, Stahl M, *et al.*: Etoposide, folinic acid, and 5-fluorouracil in carboplatin-pretreated patients with advanced gastric cancer. *Cancer Chemother Pharmacol* 1991, 29:83–84.

40. Cullinan SA, Moertel CG, Wieand HS, *et al.*: For the North Central Cancer Treatment Group: controlled evaluation of three drug combination regimens versus fluorouracil alone for the therapy of advanced gastric cancer. *J Clin Oncol* 1995, 12:412–416.

41. Gastrointestinal Tumor Study Group: Control trial of adjuvant chemotherapy following curative resection for gastric cancer. *Cancer* 1982, 49:1116–1122.

42. Engstrom P, Lavin P, Douglas H, Brunner K: Post-operative adjuvant 5-fluorouracil plus methyl-CCNU therapy for gastric cancer patients. *Cancer* 1984, 55:1868–1873.

43. Estape J, Grau J, Lcobendas F, *et al.*: Mitomycin-C as an adjuvant treatment to resected gastric cancer: a 10-year follow-up. *Ann Surg* 1991, 213:219–222.

44. Crook JE, O'Connell MJ, Wieand HS, *et al.*: A prospective, randomized evaluation of intensive-course 5-fluorouracil plus doxorubicin as surgical adjuvant chemotherapy for resected gastric cancer. *Cancer* 1991, 67:2454–2458.

45. Hallissey MT, Dunn JA, Ward LC, Allum WH: The second British Stomach Cancer Group trial of adjuvant radiotherapy or chemotherapy in resectable gastric cancer: five-year follow-up. *Lancet* 1994, 343:1309–1312.

46. Herman J, Bonenkamp JJ, Boon MC, *et al.*: Adjuvant therapy after curative resection for gastric cancer: meta-analysis of randomized trials. *J Clin Oncol* 1993, 11:1441–1447.

47. Wilke H, Preusser P, Fink U, *et al.*: Preoperative chemotherapy in locally advanced and nonresectable gastric cancer: a phase II study with etoposide, doxorubicin and cisplatin. *J Clin Oncol* 1989, 7:1318–1326.

48. Ajani JA, Mayer RJ, Ota DM, *et al.*: Preoperative and postoperative combination chemotherapy for potentially resectable gastric carcinomas. *J Natl Cancer Inst* 1993, 85:1839–1844.

49. Ajani JA, Ota DM, Jessup JM, *et al.*: Resectable gastric carcinoma: an evaluation of preoperative and post operative chemotherapy. *Cancer* 1991, 68:1501–1506.

50. Safran H, King TP, Choy H, *et al.*: Paclitaxel and concurrent radiation for locally advanced pancreatic and gastric cancer: A phase I study. *J Clin Oncol* 1997, 15:901–907.

51. Kelsen D, Karpeh M, Schwartz G, *et al.*: Neoadjuvant therapy of high-risk gastric cancer: A phase II trial of preoperative FAMTX and postoperative intraperitoneal fluorouracil-cisplatin plus intravenous fluorouracil. *J Clin Oncol* 1996, 14:1818–1828.

52. Glimelius B, Hoffman K, Sjödén P-O, *et al.*: Chemotherapy improves survival and quality of life in advanced pancreatic and biliary cancer. *Ann Oncol* 1996, 7:593–600.

53. Gastrointestinal Tumor Study Group: Further evidence of effective adjuvant combined radiation and chemotherapy following curative resection of pancreatic cancer. *Cancer* 1987, 59:2006–2010.

54. Moertel CG, Fryta KS, Hahn RG, *et al.*: Therapy of locally unresectable pancreatic carcinoma: a randomized comparison of high dose (6000 rads) radiation alone, moderate dose radiation (4000 vads + 5 fluorouracil), antidose radiation + 5 fluorouracil: the Gastrointestinal Tumor Study Group. *Cancer* 1981, 48:1705–1710.

55. Ishii H, Okada S, Tokuuye K, *et al.*: Protracted 5-fluorouracil infusion with concurrent radiotherapy as a treatment for locally advanced pancreatic carcinoma. *Cancer* 1997, 79:1516–1520.

56. Hoffman JP, Weese JL, Solin LJ, *et al.*: A pilot study of preoperative chemoradiation for patients with localized adenocarcinoma of the pancreas. *Am J Surg* 1995, 169:71–77.

57. Staley CA, Lee JE, Cleary KR, *et al.*: Preoperative chemoradiation, pancreaticoduodenectomy, and intraoperative radiation therapy for adenocarcinoma of the pancreatic head. *Am J Surg* 1996, 171:118–124.

58. Spitz FR, Abbruzzese JL, Lee JE, *et al.*: Preoperative and postoperative chemoradiation strategies in patients treated with pancreaticoduodenectomy for adenocarcinoma of the pancreas. *J Clin Oncol* 1997, 15:928–937.

59. DeCaprio JA, Mayer RJ, Gonin R, Arbuck SG: Fluorouracil and high dose leucovorin in previously untreated patients with advanced adenocarcinoma of the pancreas: results of a phase 2 trial. *J Clin Oncol* 1991, 9:2128–2130. .

60. Bukowski RM, Balcerzak SP, O'Bryan RM, *et al.*: Randomized trial of 5-fluorouracil and mitomycin C with or without streptozocin for advanced pancreatic cancer: a Southwest Oncology Group Study. *Cancer* 1983, 52:1577–1582.

61. Burris HA, Moore M, Andersen J, *et al.*: Improvements in survival and clinical benefit with gemcitabine as first line therapy for patients with advanced pancreas cancer: A randomized trial. *J Clin Oncol* 1997, 15:2403–2413.

62. Arnold R, Frank M, and Kajdan U: Management of gastroenteropancreatic endocrine tumors: the place of somatostatin analogues. *Digestion* 1994, 55(suppl 3):107–113.

63. Moertel CG, Lefkopoulo M, Lipsitz S, *et al.*: Streptozocin-doxorubicin, streptozocin-fluorouracil, or chlorozotocin in the treatment of advanced islet cell carcinoma. *N Engl J Med* 1992, 326:519–523.

64. Ruszniewski P, Rougier P, Roche A, *et al.*: Hepatic arterial chemoembolization in patients with liver metastases of endocrine tumors: a prospective phase II study in 24 patients. *Cancer* 1993, 71:2624–2630.

65. Klempnauer J, Ridder GJ, von Wasielewski R, *et al.*: Resectional surgery of hilar cholangiocarcinoma: a multivariate analysis of prognostic factors. *J Clin Oncol* 1997, 15:947–954.

66. Mazzaferro V, Regalia E, Doci R, *et al.*: Liver transplantation for the treatment of small hepatocellular carcinomas in patients with cirrhosis. *N Engl J Med* 1996, 334:693–699.

67. Muto Y, Moriwaki H, Ninomiya M, *et al.*: Prevention of second primary tumors by an acyclic retinoid, polyprenoic acid, in patients with hepatocellular carcinoma. *N Engl J Med* 1996, 334:1561–1567.

68. Tan CK, Gores GJ, Steers JL, *et al.*: Orthotopic liver transplantation for preoperative early-stage hepatocellular carcinoma. *Mayo Clin Proc* 1994, 69:509–514.

69. Goldstein RM, Stone M, Tillery GW, *et al.*: Is liver transplantation indicated for cholangiocarcinoma? *Am J Surg* 1993, 166:768–771.

70. Stone MJ, Klintmalm GB, Polter D, *et al.*: Neoadjuvant chemotherapy and liver transplantation for hepatocellular carcinoma: a pilot study in 20 patients. *Gastroenterology* 1993, 104:196–202.

71. Lai CL, Wu PC, Chan GC, *et al.*: Doxorubicin vs. no antitumor therapy in an inoperable hepatocellular carcinoma: a prospective randomized trial. *Cancer* 1988, 62:479–483.

72. Venook AP, Stagg RJ, Lewis BJ, *et al.*: Chemoembolization for hepatocellular carcinoma. *J Clin Oncol* 1990, 8:1108–1114.

73. Patt YZ, Charnsangavej C, Boddie A, *et al.*: Treatment of hepatocellular carcinoma with hepatic arterial floxuridine, doxorubicin, and mitomycin C (FUDRAM) with or without hepatic artery embolization: factors associated with longer survival. *Reg Cancer Treat* 1989, 2:98–104.

74. Livraghi T, Bolondi L, Lazzaroni S, *et al.*: Percutaneous ethanol injection in the treatment of hepatocellular carcinoma and cirrhosis: a study on 207 patients. *Cancer* 1992, 69:925–929.

75. Horiguchi Y, Sekoguchi B, Imai H, *et al.*: Treatment of choice for unresectable small liver cancer: percutaneous ethanol injection therapy or transarterial chemoembolization therapy. *Cancer Chemother Pharmacol* 1994, 33:S111–114.

76. Douglass EC, Reynolds M, Finegold M, *et al.*: Cisplatin, vincristine, and fluorouracil therapy for hepatoblastoma: a Pediatric Oncology Group study. *J Clin Oncol* 1993, 11:96–99.

77. Ehrlich PF, Greenberg ML, and Filler RM: Improved long-term survival with preoperative chemotherapy for hepatoblastoma. *J Pediatr Surg* 1997, 32:999–1002–1003.

78. Oberfield RA, Rossi RL: The role of chemotherapy in the treatment of bile duct cancer. *World J Surg* 1988, 12:105–108.

79. Patt YZ, Jones Jr. DV, Hoque A, *et al.*: Phase II trial of intravenous fluorouracil and subcutaneous interferon alfa-2b for biliary tract cancer. *J Clin Oncol* 1996, 14:2311–2315.

80. Jones Jr. DV, Lozano R, Hoque A, *et al.*: Phase II study of paclitaxel therapy for unresectable biliary tree carcinomas. *J Clin Oncol* 1996, 14:2306–2310.

81. Oberfield RA, Rossi RL: The role of chemotherapy in the treatment of bile duct cancer. *World J Surg* 1988, 12:105–108.

82. Robertson JM, Lawrence TS, Dworzanin LM, *et al.*: Treatment of primary hepatobiliary cancers with conformal radiation therapy and regional chemotherapy. *J Clin Oncol* 1993, 11:1286–1293.

83. American Joint Commission on Cancer: *Manual for Staging Cancer*, edn 4. Edited by Beahrs OH, Henson DE, Hutter RVP. Philadelphia: JB Lippincott; 1992:57–66.

STREPTOZOCIN AND DOXORUBICIN

Streptozocin is a methyl nitrosourea produced by the fermentation of *Streptomyces archromogenes*. It decomposes spontaneously to generate alkylating and carbamoylating moieties, and alkylation is thought to be its principal mechanism of antitumor activity. Streptozocin is capable of transferring methyl groups to DNA but cannot form cross-links.

Doxorubicin is an antitumor antibiotic agent with an extremely wide spectrum of activity. It does not have a single mechanism of cytotoxicity but can produce cellular dysfunction and death by multiple means. Two of its most important mechanisms of cytotoxicity include intercalation among DNA base pairs and generation of toxic intracellular free radicals. These actions can cause single- and double-stranded DNA breaks, which in turn lead to inhibition of RNA and protein synthesis and defective mitoses.

DOSAGE AND SCHEDULING

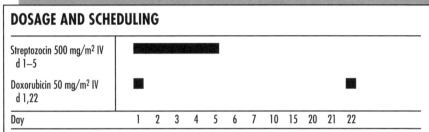

Streptozocin 500 mg/m² IV d 1–5												
Doxorubicin 50 mg/m² IV d 1,22												
Day	1	2	3	4	5	6	7	10	15	20	21	22

Cycles repeated every 6 wk.

PRIOR TO THERAPY: *CBC and platelets, liver chemistry, BUN, creatinine. Baseline estimates of cardiac ejection fraction.*

RECENT EXPERIENCE AND RESPONSE RATES

Study	Evaluable Patients, *n*	Dosage and Scheduling	Any Regression/ Complete Regression, %	Median Duration of Regression, *mo*
Moertel *et al.*, N Engl J Med 1992, 326:519–523	36	Streptozocin 500 mg/m²/d × 5 Doxorubicin 50 mg/m²/d; days 1 and 22	69/14	22
	33	Chlorozotocin, 150 mg/m² every 7 wk	30/6	21
	33	Streptozocin 500 mg/m²/d × 5 5-FU 400 mg/m²/d × 5 (repeat every 6 wk)	45/4	13

CANDIDATES FOR TREATMENT
Patients with metastatic islet cell tumors

SPECIAL PRECAUTIONS
Patients with preexisting renal or heart disease

ALTERNATIVE THERAPY
Chlorozotocin, dacarbazine

TOXICITIES
Streptozocin: renal toxicity (azotemia, anuria, hypophosphatemia, glycosuria, renal tubular acidosis), severe nausea and vomiting possible; mild-to-moderate abnormalities of glucose tolerance (hypoglycemia); hepatic toxicity and myelosuppression possible (usually mild); **Doxorubicin:** bone marrow suppression, anorexia, nausea and vomiting, alopecia, possible cardiotoxicity

DRUG INTERACTIONS
Streptozocin: none known; **Doxorubicin:** digoxin (suspected)

NURSING INTERVENTIONS
Monitor blood counts, liver function, pulmonary function, cardiac function; administer appropriate antiemetics to avoid severe nausea and vomiting; avoid extravasation; can cause severe necrosis

PATIENT INFORMATION
Myelosuppression may occur; call physician if signs and symptoms of infection develop; call physician if injection site becomes painful, red, or swollen; possible red-colored urine for 1–2 d after treatment; nausea and vomiting may occur; hair loss likely.

EAP
Etoposide, Doxorubicin, and Cisplatin

Etoposide is a semisynthetic derivative of podophyllotoxin. Its mechanism of cytotoxic action involves the inhibition of the nuclear enzyme topoisomerase II. This enzyme has the ability to disentangle topologically intertwined DNA helices, cleave double-stranded DNA, and then covalently bond to DNA to form DNA–topoisomerase II complexes. The cleaved DNA is then reunited after a second duplex DNA has passed through. Etoposide is believed to stabilize the DNA–topoisomerase II complex and prevent rejoining of the double-stranded DNA.

Doxorubicin is an antitumor antibiotic agent with an extremely wide spectrum of activity. It does not have a single mechanism of cytotoxicity but can produce cellular dysfunction and death by multiple means. Two of its most important mechanisms of cytotoxicity include intercalation among DNA base pairs and generation of toxic intracellular free radicals. These actions can cause single- and double-stranded DNA breaks, which in turn lead to inhibition of RNA and protein synthesis and defective mitoses.

Cisplatin is activated intracellularly to generate a positively charged aquated complex. This complex functions similarly to a bifunctional alkylating agent by interacting with the nucleophilic sites on DNA, RNA, and protein, producing intrastrand links and cross-links. These reactions alter the DNA template and inhibit DNA synthesis. Cisplatin lacks cell-cycle specificity.

Combination therapy with these drugs is based on in vitro and in vivo experimental data that have suggested synergistic cytotoxicity.

CANDIDATES FOR TREATMENT
Patients with advanced locoregional or metastatic gastric cancer prior to surgery

SPECIAL PRECAUTIONS
Patients with cardiac dysfunction or renal dysfunction

ALTERNATIVE THERAPIES
ELF or 5-FU, cisplatin, and etoposide for neoadjuvant therapy; FAM, FAMTX, or ELF for metastatic disease

TOXICITIES
Drug combination: severe myelosuppression (leukopenia, anemia, thrombocytopenia); **cisplatin:** renal toxicity, alopecia

DRUG INTERACTIONS
Etoposide: synergistic in vitro with cytarabine, cyclophosphamide, carmustine, vincristine, cisplatin, hydroxyurea, 5-FU, methotrexate, verapamil; **Doxorubicin:** digoxin (suspected)

NURSING INTERVENTIONS
Monitor blood counts, liver function, cardiac function, renal function, electrolytes; administer doxorubicin with caution—an extravasant; give adequate antiemetics and maintain adequate hydration; hypotension may occur with rapid administration of etoposide

PATIENT INFORMATION
Myelosuppression common; call physician if signs and symptoms of infection develop; call physician if injection site becomes painful, red, or swollen; possible red-colored urine for 1–2 d after treatment; nausea and vomiting may occur; hair loss likely.

DOSAGE AND SCHEDULING

	Day 1 2 3 4 5 6 7 8 9 10
Etoposide 120 mg/m² IV d 4,5,6	
Doxorubicin 20 mg/m² IV d 1,7	
Cisplatin 40 mg/m² IV d 2,8	

Cycles repeated every 3–4 wk

PRIOR TO THERAPY: CBC and platelets, liver chemistries, BUN, creatinine, electrolytes. Baseline estimates of cardiac ejection fraction using a gated pool scan may be useful in some patients.

RECENT EXPERIENCES AND RESPONSE RATES

Study	Evaluable Patients, n	Dosage and Scheduling	CR/PR	Median Duration of Survival, mo
Lerner et al., J Clin Oncol 1992, 10:536–540	36	Etoposide 120 mg/m²/d days 4,5,6 Doxorubicin 20 mg/m²/d days 1,7 Cisplatin 40 mg/m²/d days 2,8	3/9 (33%)	7.5
Kelsen et al., J Clin Oncol 1992, 10:541–548	30	Etoposide 120 mg/m²/d days 4,5,6 Doxorubicin 20 mg/m²/d days 1,7 Cisplatin 40 mg/m²/d days 2,8	0/6 (20%)	6.1
Preusser et al., J Clin Oncol 1989, 7:1310–1317	67	Etoposide 120 mg/m²/d days 4,5,6 Doxorubicin 20 mg/m²/d days 1,7 Cisplatin 40 mg/m²/d days 2,8	14/29 (64%)	9.0
Wilke et al., Sem Oncol 1990, 17:61–70	145	Etoposide 120 mg/m²/d days 4,5,6 Doxorubicin 20 mg/m²/d days 1,7 Cisplatin 40 mg/m²/d days 2,8	22/61 (57%)	—

FAMTX
5-Fluorouracil, Doxorubicin, Methotrexate, and Leucovorin

5-Fluorouracil (5-FU) is a fluorinated uracil analogue that is metabolized intracellularly to its active forms, fluorouridine triphosphate (FUTP) and fluorodeoxyuridine monophosphate (FdUMP). FdUMP inhibits the enzyme, thymidylate synthetase, which is necessary for DNA synthesis. Another mechanism of cytotoxicity involves the false incorporation of 5-FUTP into RNA, causing transcription errors.

Doxorubicin is an antitumor antibiotic agent with an extremely wide spectrum of activity. It does not have a single mechanism of cytotoxicity, but can produce cellular dysfunction and death by multiple means. Two of its most important mechanisms of cytotoxicity include intercalation among DNA base pairs and generation of toxic intracellular free radicals. These actions can cause single- and double-stranded DNA breaks, which in turn lead to inhibition of RNA and protein synthesis and defective mitoses.

Methotrexate is an antifolate antimetabolite that exerts its primary cytotoxic effect during the S phase. Methotrexate is actively transported across the cell membrane where it binds to its target enzyme, dihydrofolate reductase (DHFR). This enzyme is essential for regenerating the oxidized folates produced during thymidine synthesis to their active forms. In the absence of unbound DHFR, thymidylate and purine biosynthesis can no longer occur.

Leucovorin, also known as folinic acid, is the active, chemically reduced derivative of folic acid, which is involved as a cofactor for one-carbon transfer reactions in the biosynthesis of purines and pyrimidines. It is a potent antidote for the hematopoietic and reticuloendothelial effects of folic acid antagonists because it is easily converted to tetrahydrofolic acid derivatives. Leucovorin also acts as a biochemical modulator of 5-FU by enhancing the ability of 5-FU to bind and then block the action of thymidylate synthetase.

CANDIDATES FOR TREATMENT
Patients with metastatic gastric cancer

SPECIAL PRECAUTIONS
Patients with cardiac dysfunction, renal dysfunction, any third-space fluid collection or ascites, pleural effusion, seroma

ALTERNATIVE THERAPIES
EAP, FAM, ELF, 5-FU (with or without leucovorin)

TOXICITIES
Drug combination: myelosuppression, mucositis, alopecia, **5-FU:** diarrhea; **Methotrexate:** renal toxicity, pulmonary fibrosis

DRUG INTERACTIONS
5-FU: leucovorin, methotrexate, interferon α, dipyridamole, allopurinol, thymidine; **Doxorubicin:** digoxin (suspected); **Methotrexate:** salicylates, sulfonamides, tetracycline, phenylbutazone, chloramphenicol, phenytoin, probenecid, NSAIDs, L-asparaginase, vincristine, etoposide, 5-FU

NURSING INTERVENTIONS
Monitor blood counts, renal function; patient must have normal renal function, adequate hydration, and urine alkalinization prior to high-dose methotrexate administration; monitor use of all NSAIDs (can enhance methotrexate toxicity); investigate and report pulmonary symptoms (such as dry nonproductive cough); monitor for ascites or other third-space fluid collection (can enhance methotrexate toxicity); give antiemetics as necessary; monitor hepatic function; administer doxorubicin with caution—an extravasant; monitor methotrexate levels.

PATIENT INFORMATION
Myelosuppression can occur; call physician if signs and symptoms of infection develop (fever, chills, flu-like symptoms); oral mucositis and diarrhea possible; hair loss likely; call physician if injection site becomes painful, red, or swollen; possible red-colored urine for 1–2 d after treatment; maintain adequate hydration.

DOSAGE AND SCHEDULING

5-FU 1500 mg/m^2 IV d 1
Doxorubicin 30 mg/m^2 IV d 15
Methotrexate 1500 mg/m^2 IV d 1
Leucovorin 15 mg/m^2 PO every 6 h d 2,3

| Day | 1 | 2 | 3 | 4 | 5 | 6 | 7 | 8 | 9 | 10 | 11 | 12 | 13 | 14 | 15 |

Cycles repeated every 4 wk.

PRIOR TO THERAPY: *CBC and platelets, liver chemistries, BUN, creatinine. Baseline estimates of cardiac ejection fraction using a gated pool scan may be useful in some patients.*

RECENT EXPERIENCES AND RESPONSE RATES

Study	Evaluable Patients, n	Dosage and Scheduling	CR/PR	Median Duration of Survival, mo
Kelsen et al., J Clin Oncol 1992, 10:541–548	30	5-FU 1.5 g/m^2/d day 1 Doxorubicin 30 mg/m^2/d day 15 Methotrexate 1.5 g/m^2/d day 1 Leucovorin 15 mg/m^2 PO every 6 h × 3 days starting day 2	3/7 (33%)	7.3
Wils et al., J Clin Oncol 1991, 9:827–831	81	5-FU 1.5 g/m^2/d day 1 Doxorubicin 30 mg/m^2/d day 15 Methotrexate 1.5 g/m^2/d day 1 Leucovorin 15 mg/m^2 PO every 6 h × 48 h starting day 2	5/28 (41%)	10.5
Wils et al., J Clin Oncol 1986, 4:1799–1803	67	5-FU 1.5 g/m^2/d day 1 Doxorubicin 30 mg/m^2/d day 15 Methotrexate 1.5 g/m^2/d day 1 Leucovorin 15 mg/m^2 PO every 6 h × 48 h starting day 2	9/13 (33%)	6.0

ELF
Etoposide, Leucovorin, and 5-Fluorouracil

Etoposide is a semisynthetic derivative of podophyllotoxin. Its mechanism of cyto-toxic action involves the inhibition of the nuclear enzyme topoisomerase II. This enzyme has the ability to disentangle topologically intertwined DNA helices, cleave double-stranded DNA, and then covalently bond to DNA to form DNA–topoisomerase II complexes. The cleaved DNA is then reunited after a second duplex DNA has passed through. Etoposide is believed to stabilize the DNA–topoisomerase II complex and prevent rejoining of the double-stranded DNA.

Leucovorin, also known as folinic acid, is an active, chemically reduced deriva-tive of folic acid. Reduction by the enzyme dihydrofolate reductase is not required for leucovorin to participate in reactions that use folates as a source of one-carbon moieties. Leucovorin also acts as a biochemical modulator of 5-fluorouracil by enhancing the ability of 5-FU to bind and then block the action of thymidylate synthetase.

5-FU is a fluorinated uracil analogue that is metabolized intracellularly to its active forms, fluorouridine triphosphate (FUTP) and fluorodeoxyuridine monophosphate (FdUMP). FdUMP inhibits the enzyme, thymidylate synthetase, which is necessary for DNA synthesis. Another mechanism of cytotoxicity involves the false incorporation of 5-FUTP into RNA, causing transcription errors.

Etoposide and 5-fluorouracil are both active agents in gastric carcinoma. In combination, they act synergistically and are not cross-resistant in vitro or in vivo.

Leucovorin contributes to the synergism of this regimen by enhancing the cytotoxicity of 5-FU by increasing its ability to bind and then block the action of thymidylate synthetase.

CANDIDATES FOR TREATMENT
Patients with metastatic or advanced locoregional gastric cancer, especially for elderly or high-risk patients

SPECIAL PRECAUTIONS
None noteworthy

ALTERNATIVE THERAPIES
EAP, FAMTX, FAM, 5-FU (with or without leucovorin)

TOXICITIES
Myelosuppression, possible mucositis, diarrhea

DRUG INTERACTIONS:
Etoposide: synergistic in vitro with cytarabine, cyclophosphamide, carmustine, vincristine, cisplatin, hydroxyurea, 5-FU, methotrexate, verapamil; **Leucovorin:** 5-fluorouracil; **5-FU:** leucovorin, methotrexate, interferon α, dipyridamole, allopurinol, thymidine

NURSING INTERVENTIONS
Monitor blood counts; administer etoposide slowly over 45 to 60 minutes or longer (hypotension can occur if given too rapidly)

PATIENT INFORMATION
Oral mucositis may occur; skin reactions possible; call physician if diarrhea develops.

DOSAGE AND SCHEDULING

	Day 1	2	3	4	5	6	7	8	9	10	11	12	13	14	15
Etoposide 120 mg/m^2 IV d 1,2,3	▬														
Leucovorin 300 mg/m^2 IV d 1,2,3	▬														
5-FU 500 mg/m^2 IV d 1,2,3	▬														

PRIOR TO THERAPY: CBC and platelets.

RECENT EXPERIENCES AND RESPONSE RATES

Study	Evaluable Patients, n	Dosage and Scheduling	CR/PR	Median Duration of Survival, mo
Preusser et al., Sem Oncol 1990, 17:61–70	51	Etoposide 120 mg/m^2/d days 1,2,3 Leucovorin 300 mg/m^2/d days 1,2,3 5-FU 500 mg/m^2/d days 1,2,3	8/16 (53%)	11.0
Wilke et al., Invest New Drugs 1990, 8:65–70	33	Etoposide 120 mg/m^2/d days 1,2,3 Leucovorin 300 mg/m^2/d days 1,2,3 5-FU 500 mg/m^2/d days 1,2,3	4/12 (48%)	10.5

FAM
5-Fluorouracil, Doxorubicin, and Mitomycin C

5-Fluorouracil is a fluorinated uracil analogue that is metabolized intracellularly to its active forms, fluorouridine triphosphate (FUTP) and fluorodeoxyuridine monophosphate (FdUMP). FdUMP inhibits the enzyme, thymidylate synthetase, which is necessary for DNA synthesis. Another mechanism of cytotoxicity involves the false incorporation of 5-FUTP into RNA, causing transcription errors.

Doxorubicin is an antitumor antibiotic agent with an extremely wide spectrum of activity. It does not have a single mechanism of cytotoxicity but can produce cellular dysfunction and death by multiple means. Its two most important mechanisms of cytotoxicity include intercalation among DNA base pairs and generation of toxic intracellular free radicals. These actions can cause single- and double-stranded DNA breaks, which in turn lead to inhibition of RNA and protein synthesis and defective mitoses.

Mitomycin C contains both quinoline and aziridine ring structures, allowing it to exert antitumor activity by two different mechanisms. Reduction of the quinoline ring by one electron transfer allows for free radical reactions similar to those seen with the anthracyclines. The aziridine ring functions as an alkylator producing DNA cross-links.

CANDIDATES FOR TREATMENT
Patients with metastatic gastric cancer

SPECIAL PRECAUTIONS
Patients with preexisting heart disease or pulmonary dysfunction

ALTERNATIVE THERAPIES
EAP, FAMTX, ELF, 5-FU (with or without leucovorin)

TOXICITIES
Drug combination: cumulative bone marrow suppression, including enhanced leukopenia and thrombocytopenia, alopecia, anorexia, nausea and vomiting; **Doxorubicin:** congestive cardiomyopathy, **Mitomycin C:** hemolytic anemia-like syndrome, pulmonary fibrosis

DRUG INTERACTIONS
5-FU: leucovorin, methotrexate, interferon-α, dipyridamole, allopurinol, thymidine; **Doxorubicin:** digoxin (suspected); **Mitomycin C:** none

NURSING INTERVENTIONS
Monitor blood counts, liver function, pulmonary function, cardiac function; administer doxorubicin and mitomycin C with great caution—extravasation injury can be extremely severe.

PATIENT INFORMATION
Myelosuppression common; call physician if signs and symptoms of infection develop; call physician if area around site of injection becomes painful, red, or swollen; oral mucositis and diarrhea may occur; call physician if diarrhea persists; skin reactions possible; possible red-colored urine for 1–2 d after treatment.

DOSAGE AND SCHEDULING

	1	2	3	4	5	6	7	8	9	10	11	12	13	14
5-FU 600 mg/m² IV d 1 of wk 1,2,5,6	▮	▮			▮	▮								
Doxorubicin 30 mg/m² d 1 of wk 1,5	▮				▮									
Mitomycin C 10 mg/m² IV d 1 of wk 1	▮													
Week	1	2	3	4	5	6	7	8	9	10	11	12	13	14

Cycles repeated every 6 wk.

PRIOR TO THERAPY: *CBC, platelets, liver chemistries. Baseline estimates of cardiac ejection fraction using a gated pool scan may be useful in some patients. Pulmonary function tests may be useful in selected patients.*

RECENT EXPERIENCES AND RESPONSE RATES

Study	Evaluable Patients, n	Dosage and Scheduling	CR/PR	Median Duration of Response, mo
MacDonald et al., Ann Intern Med 1980, 93:533–536	62	5-FU 600 mg/m²/d days 1,8,29,36 Doxorubicin 30 mg/m²/d days 1,29 Mitomycin C 10 mg/m²/d day 1	0/26 (42%)	9
Brian et al., Oncology 1989, 46:83–87	43	5-FU 600 mg/m²/d days 1,8,29,36 Doxorubicin 30 mg/m²/d days 1,29 Mitomycin C 10 mg/m²/d day 1	0/18 (42%)	7
Arbuck et al., Cancer 1990, 65:2442–2445	26	Leucovorin 500 mg/m²/d IV over 2 h days 1,8,29,36 5-FU 600 mg/m²/d IVP 1 h after leucovorin, days 1,8,29,36 Doxorubicin 30 mg/m²/d day 1,29 Mitomycin C 10 mg/m²/d day 1	1/9 (38%)	6

5-FLUOROURACIL AND RADIATION THERAPY

5-Fluorouracil is a fluorinated uracil analogue that is metabolized intracellularly to its active forms, fluorouridine triphosphate (FUTP) and fluorodeoxyuridine monophosphate (FdUMP). FdUMP inhibits the enzyme, thymidylate synthetase, which is necessary for DNA synthesis. Another mechanism of cytotoxicity involves the false incorporation of 5-FUTP into RNA, causing transcription errors.

When 5-FU is combined with radiation, enhancement of radiation effects is observed. It is known that 5-FU can significantly affect the slope of the radiation therapy survival curve when present in cytotoxic concentrations. The mechanism of this effect is unknown but may involve incorporation into DNA or RNA and cell-cycle effects. Inhibition of sublethal damage repair does not seem to play a role.

DOSAGE AND SCHEDULING

5-FU: 500 mg/m^2/d $\times$ 3 d every 2 wk $\times$ 2, then 500 mg/m^2 every wk for a total of 2 y of therapy—weekly doses begin 1 mo after radiation therapy is complete;
Radiation: 2000 cGy over 5 d $\times$ 2 courses; 2-wk separation between doses

RECENT EXPERIENCES AND RESPONSE RATES

Study	Evaluable Patients, n	Dosage and Scheduling	Median Duration of Survival, mo	2-y Actuarial Survival, %
GI Tumor Study Group, Arch Surg 1985, 120:899–903	21	5-FU 500 mg/m^2/d x 3 days q 2 wk x 2; then 500 mg/m^2/wk starting 1 month after radiation therapy complete Plus Radiation 2000 rads/5 d x 2 (2-wk separation between doses)	21.0	43
	22	No treatment — control group	10.9	18
GI Tumor Study Group, Cancer 1987, 59:2006–2010	30	5-FU 500 mg/m^2/d x 3 days q 2 wk x 2; then 500 mg/m^2/wk starting 1 month after radiation therapy complete Plus Radiation 2000 rads/5 d x 2 (2-wk separation between doses)	18.0	46

Chemotherapy was continued on a weekly schedule for 2 y of therapy.

CANDIDATES FOR TREATMENT

Patients with locally unresectable pancreatic cancer or with pancreatic cancer causing severe back pain from retroperitoneal extension of disease

SPECIAL PRECAUTIONS

None noteworthy

ALTERNATIVE THERAPIES

Radiation therapy alone, chemotherapy

TOXICITIES

Mucositis, diarrhea, myelosuppression, anorexia, nausea, vomiting, diarrhea, skin irritation

DRUG INTERACTIONS

5-FU: leucovorin, methotrexate, interferon-α, dipyridamole, allopurinol, thymidine

NURSING INTERVENTIONS

Monitor blood counts; inform patients of possible skin reactions, diarrhea, mucositis

PATIENT INFORMATION

Possible nausea, vomiting, anorexia, oral mucositis, skin reactions, diarrhea.

CISPLATIN, 5-FLUOROURACIL, AND RADIATION THERAPY

Cisplatin is activated intracellularly to generate a positively charged aquated complex. This complex functions similarly to a bifunctional alkylating agent by interacting with the nucleophilic sites on DNA, RNA, and protein, producing intrastrand links and cross-links. These reactions alter the DNA template and inhibit DNA synthesis. Cisplatin lacks cell-cycle specificity.

5-Fluorouracil is a fluorinated uracil analogue that is metabolized intracellularly to its active forms, fluorouridine triphosphate (FUTP) and fluorode-oxyuridine monophosphate (FdUMP). FdUMP inhibits the enzyme, thymidylate synthetase, which is necessary for DNA synthesis. Another mechanism of cytotoxicity involves the false incorporation of 5-FUTP into RNA, causing transcription errors.

Both cisplatin and 5-FU, as single agents, are moderately active against esophageal carcinoma. When used in combination with radiation therapy, a radiation-enhancing effect is seen. Ideally, this multimodality approach would enhance the effects of radiation on local tumors and the systemic drug therapy would reduce the chance of distant micrometastases.

DOSAGE AND SCHEDULING

5-FU 1000 mg/m^2/d by continuous infusion every day × 5 d
Cisplatin 70–100 mg/m^2, d 1 only

PRIOR TO THERAPY: *CBC, platelets, electrolytes, BUN, creatinine.*

RECENT EXPERIENCES AND RESPONSE RATES

Study	Evaluable Patients, n	Dosage and Scheduling	Median Duration of Survival, mo	Survival Rates, % 12 mo	24 mo
Patients with Localized Disease					
Herskovic *et al.*, N Engl J Med 1992, 326:1593–1598	121	5-FU 1000 mg/m^2/d × 4 days continuous infusion Cisplatin 75 mg/m^2 day 1 only Radiation 5000 cGy/5 wk	12.5	50	38
		Radiation alone, 6400 cGy/6.4 wk	8.9	33	10
Seitz *et al.*, Cancer 1990, 66:214–219		5-FU 1000 mg/m^2/d × 5 d continuous infusion Cisplatin 70 mg/m^2/d day 2 only Radiation 20 cGy/5 d	17.0	—	41
Presurgical Chemotherapy Regimen					
Walsh *et al.*, N Engl J Med 1996, 335:462–467.	48	5-FU 15 mg/kg/d IV over 16 h daily × 5 d, wk 1 and 6 Cisplatin 75 mg/m^2 IV over 8 h ×1 dose on d 7, wk 1 and 6 Radiation 40 cGy in 15 fractions (d 1–5, 8–12, 15–19)	16.0	52	37

Study	Evaluable Patients, n	Dosage and Scheduling	CR/PR	Response Rate, %
Patients with Metastatic Disease and Control of Primary Tumor				
Debesi *et al.*, Cancer Treat Rep 1986, 70:909–910	37	5-FU 1000 mg/m^2/d × 5 d continuous infusion Cisplatin 100 mg/m^2 day 1 only Allopurinol 600 mg daily day -2 to +5	3/10	35
Kies *et al.*, Cancer 1987, 60:2156–2160	26	5-FU 1000 mg/m^2/d × 5 d continuous infusion Cisplatin 100 mg/m^2/d day 1 only	3/8	42

CANDIDATES FOR TREATMENT
Patients with esophageal carcinoma

SPECIAL PRECAUTIONS
Patients with renal dysfunction

ALTERNATIVE THERAPIES
Preoperative: 5-FU and mitomycin C; 5-FU, vinblastine, and cisplatin plus radiation; cisplatin and bleomycin with or without vindesine; cisplatin and 5-FU; etoposide, cisplatin, and 5-FU; etoposide, doxorubicin, and cisplatin; **Inoperable or metastatic disease:** cisplatin and bleomycin with or without vindesine; cisplatin, methotrexate, and bleomycin

TOXICITIES:
Cisplatin: myelosuppression, nausea, vomiting, renal dysfunction, possible ototoxicity, possible neurotoxicity; **5-FU:** myelosuppression, mucositis, diarrhea; **Chemotherapy plus radiation therapy:** enhanced myelosuppression, severe esophagitis or stomatitis, nausea, vomiting, anorexia, diarrhea, possible ototoxicity, possible neurotoxicity

DRUG INTERACTIONS
5-FU: leucovorin, methotrexate, interferon alpha, dipyridamole, allopurinol, thymidine; **Cisplatin:** none

NURSING INTERVENTIONS
Monitor blood counts, renal function, electrolytes; inform patients of possible skin reactions; give adequate amounts of antiemetics before and after cisplatin therapy; maintain adequate hydration; use diuretics as indicated

PATIENT INFORMATION
Oral mucositis and severe esophagitis may occur; myelosuppression is likely; call physician if signs of infection or diarrhea develop; call physician if hearing loss occurs; nausea and vomiting possible (possibly protracted); skin reactions possible, taste changes (metallic) possible.

5-FLUOROURACIL, RECOMBINANT INTERFERON-α-2B, AND CISPLATIN

Cisplatin is activated intracellularly to generate a positively charged aquated complex. This complex functions similarly to a bifunctional alkylating agent by interacting with the nucleophilic sites on DNA, RNA, and protein, producing intrastrand links and cross-links. These reactions alter the DNA template and inhibit DNA synthesis. Cisplatin lacks cell-cycle specificity.

5-Fluorouracil is a fluorinated uracil analogue that is metabolized intracellularly to its active forms, fluorouridine triphosphate (FUTP) and fluorodeoxyuridine monophosphate (FdUMP). FdUMP inhibits the enzyme thymidylate synthetase, which is necessary for DNA synthesis. Another mechanism of cytotoxicity involves the false incorporation of 5-FUTP into RNA, causing transcription errors.

Biochemical modulation with recombinant interferon-α (IFN-α) has been shown to augment the cytotoxicity of both 5-Fluorouracil and Cisplatin in vitro and may be a viable strategy in the treatment of esophageal carcinoma.

CANDIDATES FOR TREATMENT

Patients with regionally advanced or metastatic esophageal carcinoma

SPECIAL PRECAUTIONS

Patients with renal dysfunction

ALTERNATIVE THERAPIES

Cisplatin and bleomycin with or without vindesine, cisplatin and 5-FU, cisplatin and etoposide, methotrexate, and bleomycin

TOXICITIES

Myelosuppression, primarily thrombocytopenia, fatigue, neurologic toxicities, mucositis, diarrhea

DRUG INTERACTIONS

5-FU: leucovorin, methotrexate, dipyridamole, allopurinol, thymidine; **IFN:** cisplatin, and 5-FU (augments cytotoxicity)

NURSING INTERVENTIONS

Monitor blood counts, renal function, electrolytes; inform patients of possible skin reactions; give adequate antiemetics and maintain adequate hydration during cisplatin administration

PATIENT INFORMATION

Possible nausea, vomiting, anorexia, oral mucositis, diarrhea. Call physician if signs of infection or diarrhea develop. Possible neurologic toxicities include dizziness and gait disturbances.

DOSAGE AND SCHEDULING

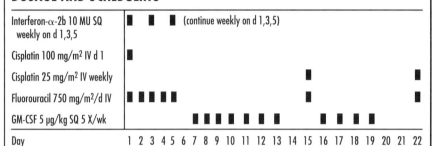

	Day 1 2 3 4 5 6 7 8 9 10 11 12 13 14 15 16 17 18 19 20 21 22
Interferon-α-2b 10 MU SQ weekly on d 1,3,5	(continue weekly on d 1,3,5)
Cisplatin 100 mg/m² IV d 1	
Cisplatin 25 mg/m² IV weekly	
Fluorouracil 750 mg/m²/d IV	
GM-CSF 5 μg/kg SQ 5 X/wk	

GM-CSF—granulocyte–macrophage colony-stimulating factor.

SEQUENCE OF ADMINISTRATION: *IFN-α → cisplatin → 5-FU with cisplatin administered immediately after IFN-α.*
5-FU is administered at 750 mg/m² daily for 5 d beginning on d 1, then at 750 mg/m² every wk beginning on d 15.
Cisplatin is administered at 100 mg/m² over 2 h on d 1, then at 25 mg/m² every wk (immediately before the 5-FU bolus) beginning on d 15.
IFN-alpha is administered at 10 MU SQ each wk on d 1 (immediately before the cisplatin), then on d 3 and 5.
GM-CSF is administered at 5 μg/kg SQ on d 7–13, then on d 2–5 each wk beginning the day after chemotherapy.

PRIOR TO THERAPY: *CBC, platelets, electrolytes, BUN, creatinine, liver function.*

RECENT EXPERIENCES AND RESPONSE RATES

Study	Evaluable Patients, *n*	Dosage and Scheduling	CR/PR	Response Rate, %
Wadler *et al.*, Cancer 1996, 78:30–34	23	5-FU 750 mg/m²/d×5 d, then 750 mg/m² q wk beginning d 15 Cisplatin 100 mg/m² IV d 1, then 25 mg/m² weekly beginning d 15 IFN-α(Intron) 10 MU SQ on d 1,3,5	1/14	65
Kelsen *et al.*, J Clin Oncol 1992, 10:269–274.	37	5-FU 750 mg/m²/d×5 d, continuous IV infusion 5-FU 750 mg/m² once weekly IVP beginning on d 12 IFN-α (Roferon-A) 9 MU SQ 3X/wk	1/9	27
Wadler *et al.*, Cancer 1993, 71:1726–1730 .	20	5-FU 750 mg/m²/d×5 d, continuous IV infusion 5-FU 750 mg/m² once weekly IVP IFN-α (Roferon-A) 9 MU SQ 3X/wk	2/3	25
Ilson *et al.*, Cancer 1995, 75:2197–2202	26	5-FU 750 mg/m²/d×5 d, continuous IV infusion q 28 d Cisplatin 100 mg/m² IV d 1, q 28 d X 3, then q 56 d IFN-α (Roferon-A) 3 MU SQ daily on d 1–28	2/13	50

HIGH-DOSE CISPLATIN AND ETOPOSIDE

Etoposide is a semisynthetic derivative of podophyllotoxin. Its mechanism of cytotoxic action involves the inhibition of the nuclear enzyme topoisomerase II. This enzyme has the ability to disentangle topologically intertwined DNA helices, cleave double-stranded DNA, and then covalently bond to DNA to form DNA–topoisomerase II complexes. The cleaved DNA is then reunited after a second duplex DNA has passed through. Etoposide is believed to stabilize the DNA–topoisomerase II complex and prevent rejoining of the double-stranded DNA.

Cisplatin is activated intracellularly to generate a positively charged aquated complex. This complex functions similarly to a bifunctional alkylating agent by interacting with the nucleophilic sites on DNA, RNA, and protein, producing intrastrand links and cross-links. These reactions alter the DNA template and inhibit DNA synthesis. Cisplatin lacks cell-cycle specificity.

Combination therapy with these drugs is based on in vitro and in vivo experimental data that have suggested synergistic cytotoxicity.

CANDIDATES FOR TREATMENT
Patients with unresectable or metastatic esophageal adenocarcinoma

SPECIAL PRECAUTIONS
Patients with renal dysfunction and patients with both renal and hepatic dysfunction

ALTERNATIVE THERAPIES
5-Fluorouracil and interferon, 5-Fluorouracil, interferon, and cisplatin

TOXICITIES
Neutropenia, thrombocytopenia, nausea and vomiting, peripheral sensory neuropathy, renal dysfunction, ototoxicity

DRUG INTERACTIONS
Cisplatin: interferon; **Etoposide:** synergistic in vitro with cytarabine, cyclophosphamide, carmustine, vincristine, cisplatin, hydroxyurea, 5-FU, methotrexate, verapamil

NURSING INTERVENTIONS
Monitor blood counts, renal function, electrolytes; give adequate amounts of antiemetics; maintain adequate hydration; use diuretics as indicated

PATIENT INFORMATION
Myelosuppression is likely; call physician if signs of infection develop. Nausea and vomiting (possibly protracted) and taste changes (metallic) may occur. Inform physician if hearing loss occurs.

DOSAGE AND SCHEDULING

Cisplatin 30 mg/m²/d days 1–5	■	■	■	■	■
Etoposide 60 mg/m²/d days 1–5	■	■	■	■	■
Day	1	2	3	4	5

Cycles repeated q 21 d for a total of 3 cycles.

DOSAGE MODIFICATIONS: Patients > 70 y of age are given reduced doses of cisplatin and etoposide. Patients with responding metastatic disease were given one additional cycle of chemotherapy. Patients with locoregional disease received radiation 1.8 Gy daily, 5 d/wk for a total dose of 41.4 Gy. 5-FU is administered by continuous infusion at 300 mg/m2/d for the duration of radiation.

PRIOR TO THERAPY: CBC, platelets, BUN, creatinine, electrolytes, liver chemistries.

RECENT EXPERIENCES AND RESPONSE RATES

Study	Evaluable Patients, n	Dosage and Scheduling	CR/PR	Response Rate, %
Spiridonidis et al., Cancer 1996, 77:2070–2077	24	Cisplatin 30 mg/m²/d × 5 d IV over 1 h Etoposide 60 mg/m²/d × 5 d IV over 2 h (3 cycles of cisplatin/etoposide followed by 5-FU and radiation in patients with locoregional disease)	5/8	54
Kelsen et al., J Clin Oncol 1992, 10:269–274	37	5-FU 750 mg/m²/d × 5 d, continuous IV infusion 5-FU 750 mg/m² once weekly IVP beginning on d 12 IFN-α (Roferon-A) 9 MU SQ 3×/wk	1/9	27
Ilson et al., Cancer 1995, 75:2197–2202	26	5-FU 750 mg/m²/d × 5 d, continuous IV infusion q 28 d Cisplatin 100 mg/m² IV d 1 q 28 d × 3, then q 56 d IFN-α (Roferon-A) 3 MU SQ daily d 1–28	2/13	50
Wadler et al., Cancer 1996, 78:30–34	23	5-FU 750 mg/m²/d × 5 d, then 750 mg/m² every wk beginning d 15 Cisplatin 100 mg/m² IV d 1, then 25 mg/m² weekly beginning d 15 IFN-α (Intron) 10 MU SQ d 1,3,5	1/14	65

COLORECTAL CANCER

Cancers of the large bowel are common and increasing in incidence. In the United States, the number of cases of colorectal carcinoma diagnosed in 1997 will exceed 131,200. Cancer deaths from colorectal malignancies number approximately 55,000 each year. The incidence for 1997 represents a downturn in newly diagnosed cases, but rates for the previous 10 to 15 years had been increasing by 2% to 3% each year as the general population aged. The number of deaths has remained fairly constant over the last 10 to 20 years. As a result, the overall death rate has declined from more than 50% of all cases to less than 40%. Earlier diagnosis and advancements in surgical and supportive care most likely account for the major portion of this improved survival rate. Advances in adjuvant therapy and progress in treatment of metastatic disease have only recently been shown to influence survival.

Three fourths of new cases originate in the colon, that is, the segment of the large bowel proximal to the peritoneal reflection. The remaining new cases arise in the rectum. A "rightward shift" of incidence has been observed over the last 25 years, with relatively fewer rectal and descending colon cases and increasing proximal colon tumors. Adenocarcinomas account for more than 90% of large bowel cancers. Carcinoid tumors account for most of the rest of malignant neoplasms arising in the colorectum. Rarely, primary lymphomas, melanomas, and sarcomas of the large bowel are reported.

ETIOLOGY AND RISK FACTORS

The average age of disease onset is 60 to 64 years, but the incidence per 100,000 patients at risk increases linearly with age from 8 per 100,000 at 40 years to 150 per 100,000 at 60 years to 500 per 100,000 at 80 years. A person's lifetime risk for developing colorectal cancer is about 1 in 10. This risk increases approximately three-fold if a first-degree relative develops a large bowel carcinoma. Several inherited syndromes are associated with an increased risk for colorectal cancer, including ulcerative colitis, Crohn's disease, familial polyposis, and hereditary nonpolyposis colon cancers such as Lynch syndromes I and II (Table 9-1) [1]. Hereditary colorectal cancers have been estimated to account for 3% to 17% of all cases with sporadic cases making up the rest. This estimate will be defined more precisely with time now that the genes associated with HNPCC on chromosomes 2 and 3 have been identified [2,3]. Cancer screening with colonoscopy or double-contrast barium enema in such settings should begin at an early age (20–35 y of age) and occur regularly. Attention should be given to screening for other tumors that can be associated with the familial Lynch syndrome II, which includes ovarian, endometrial, gastric, and urinary cancers. In asymptomatic people at normal risk, there is some controversy about the effectiveness and the appropriate frequency for colorectal cancer screening [4] (Table 9-2). However, the American Gastroenterological Association recently issued recommendations for screening in patients at low and high risk [5]. For the general population, the recommendations are on fecal blood tests beginning at age 50. Also, low-risk individuals should have a flexible sigmoidoscopy at age 50 with a complete colonoscopy if a polyp is found. Sigmoidoscopy should be performed every 3 to 5 years if the initial study is negative.

Progression of adenomatous polyps to large bowel adenocarcinoma is clearly documented, and the molecular genetic events that lead from mucosal proliferation to carcinogenesis have been well described [6]. The risk for malignant conversion of polyps is related to polyp size, number, and histology. Polyps less than 1 cm have approximately a 1% chance of containing a malignant focus. Risk increases from 5% to 10% chance for polyps 1 to 2 cm in diameter and 20% to 50% for those greater than 2 cm. In addition to the additive risk of multiple polyps (each of which has an independent chance of neoplastic transformation), a colonic epithelium in which multiple polyps develop shows increasing tendency for neoplasia with increasing numbers of polyps. Whether this tendency is due to increased exposure to environmental factors, an intrinsic genetic susceptibility, or both is unclear. The most frequently encountered adenomatous polyps (75%) are tubular adenomas. Less than 5% of these will contain foci of cancer. Tubulovillous (15% of adenomas) or villous adenomas (10% of adenomas) show malignant features in 20% and 40% of polyps, respectively.

SURGICAL CONSIDERATIONS

All polyps should be removed when detected. Even if a malignant focus is found, local removal may be curative if there is no invasion beyond the mucosa. Surgery remains the primary means for curative therapy for colorectal cancer as well. Perioperative adjuvant chemotherapy or chemoradiation therapy further decreases the risk for recurrence and improves survival rates in node-positive (stage III or Dukes' C) patients with colon or rectal primaries. A beneficial role for adjuvant therapy has also been shown for patients with rectal cancer and bowel wall penetration by tumor (stage II or Dukes' B2). There are insufficient data to confirm a benefit for similar patients with colonic (ie, nonrectal) primaries. Among patients with stage II colon cancers, a poorer prog-

Table 9-1. Risk Factors of Colorectal Cancer

Risk Factor	Lifetime Risk, %*
Individual (no predisposing history)	1–3
Individual (with one first-degree relative with colorectal cancer)	5–10
Ulcerative colitis	15–30
Crohn's disease	15
Nonpolyposis hereditary colorectal cancer (Lynch I or II)	15–20
Familial polyposis	30–100

*Risk depends on the severity and treatment of underlying disease.

Table 9-2. Prevention and Early Detection of Colorectal Cancer

Prevention*
Low fat, high fiber diet
Calcium supplements
Aspirin or nonsteroidal antiinflammatory drugs
Screening†
Age ≥ 40: digital rectal examination with fecal occult blood testing
Age ≥ 50: flexible sigmoidoscopy every 3–5 y

*None of these dietary changes or supplements has proven benefit for prevention of cancer.
†Screen earlier if family history is positive; begin at an age 5–10 years younger than the index case's age at diagnosis.

nostic group that has a higher potential to benefit from adjuvant treatment can be identified by characteristics such as bowel obstruction or perforation by tumor, direct extension of tumor to adjacent structure (T3 or Dukes' B3), or aneuploid DNA content [7].

STAGING AND PROGNOSIS

The most reproducible prognostic indicator for large bowel cancers is operative staging in one of the variations of the Dukes' system or the tumor-node metastasis (TNM) system. TNM staging is preferable to Dukes' stagings because it has been standardized by the Union Internationale Contre Cancer (UICC) and the American Joint Commission on Cancer (AJCC), and it is recognized internationally. Details of this staging may be found elsewhere [8] (Table 9-3), but stage I tumors demonstrate partial bowel invasion with extension to the muscularis propria and no lymph node involvement or distant metastatic disease (T1, T2, N0, M0, or Dukes' A and B1). Stage II tumors invade through the thickness of the bowel wall and may extend to adjacent structures but show no further tumor involvement (T3, T4, N0, M0, or Dukes' A and B1). Lymph node involvement without metastatic disease defines stage III (any T, N+, M0, or Dukes' C). The presence of distant metastases is described as stage IV (any T or N, M+, or Dukes' D).

The approximate distribution of patients at the time of diagnosis will be 15% with stage I tumor, 20% to 30% stage II, 30% to 40% stage III, and 20% to 25% stage IV. Excluding the stage IV patients, who rarely can be cured, the remaining three quarters of people have a tumor that may be approached with curative intent resection. Based on 5-year survival rates of all stages of patients with colon and rectal primaries, only about 50% of patients are cured by surgery. Patients with stage I colorectal cancer have an 85% to 90% survival rate after surgery alone. This percentage is nearly identical to that of an age-matched cohort of the general population. Sixty-five percent to 75% of stage II patients may be alive at 5 years after diagnosis. For stage III, the average 5-year survival rate is 55% for patients with colon cancer and 45% for those with rectal cancer. Patients with advanced disease (stage IV) rarely are alive five years after diagnosis (< 5%); median survival in this group ranges from 6 to 12 months (see Table 9-2).

TREATMENT STRATEGY

Follow-up after curative-intent surgery with or without adjuvant therapy includes history and physical examination, liver function tests, and chest radiograph (every 3–4 mo for the first 2 y, at 6-mo intervals for the next 3 y, and annually thereafter). Serum CEA and abdominal-pelvic CT scans are often obtained at these same intervals and when symptoms indicate a possible recurrence. Colonoscopy usually is performed annually, especially if the initial diagnosis of cancer was preceded or accompanied by the discovery of colonic polyps. The cost and intensity of follow-up must be guided by the patient's ability and willingness to undertake aggressive treatment of any recurrent disease. Anastomotic or locoregional recurrences may be completely resected and a small (5%–20%) but real cure rate can be associated with resection of isolated metastases in the liver or other sites [9].

Consideration for preoperative radiation therapy may be given to patients with resectable tumors. Proponents for this approach point out that, preoperatively, tumor tissue is well vascularized (and therefore more radiosensitive) and surgical adhesions that may retain normal loops of bowel in a radiation port have not formed. Detractors observe that without full surgical staging, 15% to 25% of patients may receive radiation therapy inappropriately for stage I or IV disease, the full extent of tumor may be best defined and marked for radiation planning at surgery, and surgical techniques for excluding the small bowel from a radiation port are effective. Several randomized clinical trials conducted over the last 25 years have compared preoperative and postoperative adjuvant therapy. Some of these studies had flawed designs, and most used radiation techniques or doses that are now considered to be outmoded. As a result, convincing data to show superiority for one of the approaches do not exist. A definitive multicenter comparison of preoperative versus postoperative adjuvant irradiation is ongoing in the Cooperative Group system, but results will not be known for at least 5 more years. Preoperative irradiation of locoregionally unresectable tumors is more generally accepted. Locally advanced tumors that cannot be resected with tumor-free margins may be reduced in size and possibly approached with curative attempt after radiation therapy [10,11].

ADJUVANT THERAPY

Standards for therapy are more clearly established for adjuvant therapy than for treatment of advanced disease. For stage III colon cancer primaries, 5-fluorouracil (5-FU) in combination with levamisole has reduced recurrence rates by 39% [12] and 5-year death rates by 31%. Mature figures from the largest clinical trial that evaluated this therapy showed overall recurrence-free rates of 47% for surgery alone and 63% for patients receiving adjuvant 5-FU and levamisole [13]. The corresponding overall survival rates were 52% and 64%. Results from large randomized studies that compare 5-FU plus levamisole with 5-FU plus leucovorin are maturing. There are already good early data that 5-FU plus leucovorin chemotherapy is an effective adjuvant treatment compared either to surgery alone [14,15] or to another 5-FU–based chemotherapy [16]. At 3 years, disease-free survival and survival for 5-FU and leucovorin–treated patients were 73% and 84% compared with corresponding survival figures of 64% and 77% for controls. A benefit from either of these chemotherapy combinations has not yet been documented by clinical trials for patients with stage II colon cancer.

For rectal cancer, studies have demonstrated an important role for 5-FU–based adjuvant chemotherapy, especially in combination with pelvic irradiation. Such therapy has reduced pelvic recurrences by 46%, systemic relapse by 37%, and has lowered death rates by 29% [17,18]. A single study that evaluated two schedules of 5-FU

Table 9-3. Staging and Prognosis of Colorectal Cancer

AJCC/UICC TNM Staging				Dukes'-MAC Staging	5-y Survival, %
Stage 0	Tis	N0	M0	—	< 95
Stage I	T1	N0	M0	A	85–90
	T2	N0	M0	B1	
Stage II	T3	N0	M0	B2	65–70
	T4	N0	M0	B3	
Stage III	Any T	N1,2,3	M0	C1–3	45–55
Stage IV	Any T	Any N	M1	D	< 5

delivery during the course of radiation therapy has shown improved tumor control with a prolonged infusion schedule compared with bolus 5-FU. Patients who received the 5 weeks of continuous infusion 5-FU had a 27% reduction in relapse rate and a 31% higher survival rate. Ongoing clinical trials are attempting to validate the apparent superiority of a prolonged infusion schedule for 5-FU. The provocative results from this report must be weighed against the costs and morbidity of the requirement for an infusion pump and a central venous device. Radiation therapy to anatomically fixed areas of the colon outside the rectum, that is, the cecum, the splenic, and the hepatic flexures, may be incorporated into a multimodality, adjuvant regimen for T4 or node positive tumors. As in the rectum, radiation with chemotherapy to these areas may reduce risk for local relapse.

THERAPY FOR ADVANCED DISEASE

Controversy exists regarding the utility of treating asymptomatic patients with metastatic disease. One view holds that there is nothing to gain from giving chemotherapy to patients with advanced disease who feel well and have good performance status. However, data from randomized prospective trials indicate that initiating chemotherapy at the time of diagnosing metastasis relieves anxiety [19], prolongs the time before symptoms appear [20], and prolongs survival by at least 6 months [20,21]. Thus, it seems that chemotherapy with a F-FU regimen is warranted and prolongs life compared with the best supportive care.

For advanced disease, 5-FU combined with leucovorin has approximately twice the response rate than that seen with 5-FU alone. A metaanalysis of randomized clinical trials comparing 5-FU with or without leucovorin revealed a collective response rate of 11% for 5-FU alone and 23% for 5-FU and leucovorin [22]. Less than 25% of the number of responses from either regimen achieved complete remission. No difference in survival of all randomized patients was seen for the two treatments, possibly because the impact of even the "best available therapy" on advanced colorectal cancer is so limited.

Several doses and schedules of 5-FU and leucovorin have been used, and none is clearly superior [23]. The two most widely used schedules are a 5-day bolus regimen repeated every 29 days and a weekly regimen administered for 6-week cycles separated by 2-week rests [24]. Stomatitis and myelosuppression are more commonly associated with the former schedule and profound diar-

rhea with the latter. A prolonged continuous infusion schedule of 5-FU also has achieved a higher response rate than that obtained with bolus therapy (30% versus 7%, respectively), but no survival difference was realized [25].

Further modulation of the effect of 5-FU with other agents, including interferon, dipyridamole, uridine, thymidine, and various combinations of these agents with or without leucovorin is the subject of ongoing clinical and preclinical research. Although reports can be found that cite provocative response rates, these combinations still should be regarded as experimental even when they employ commercially available agents. Several investigational agents, including new thymidylate synthase inhibitors and camptothecin analogues, show some activity against colorectal cancer and may be incorporated into future therapeutic regimens. High response rates have been achieved with regional therapy for liver metastases [26], but this approach has not produced improved survival and is associated with additional cost and toxicities, such as biliary sclerosis. Hepatic perfusion is an important area of clinical research, but remains experimental (Table 9-4).

Measures should be taken to reduce oral toxicity and to treat the diarrhea associated with 5-FU therapy. Because the half-life of 5-FU is short (8–12 min), stomatitis may be markedly reduced in severity with oral cryotherapy, that is, holding ice chips on or an iced slurry in the mouth before, during, and for approximately 30 minutes after bolus infusion [27]. This approach, however, is impractical with prolonged infusion schedules.

Routine antidiarrheal preparations, such as diphenoxylate hydrochloride with atropine sulfate (Lomotil) or loperamide hydrochloride (Imodium), usually are adequate to control drug-induced diarrhea. With a weekly bolus regimen of 5-FU with leucovorin, diarrhea may be cholera-like in intensity and life threatening. Patients receiving this regimen must be questioned carefully about any change in stool frequency or consistency before the administration of each week's dose, and the dose must be withheld if, compared with baseline, stools are loose or increase in number. Management of severe or greater diarrhea includes early, vigorous parenteral replacement of fluids and electrolytes. In addition, subcutaneous injections of octreotide (Sandosatin), 50 to 150 µg twice a day, may reduce or completely ablate the diarrhea within 24 to 72 hours [28].

ANAL CANCER

Anal cancer is distinct from carcinomas of the colon and the rectum. It is an uncommon tumor and one that is undergoing a demographic shift due to an association with sexually transmitted disease. The predominant squamous and transitional cell histologies differ from

Table 9-4. Standard Therapy by Stages of Colorectal Cancer

Stage	Options
I—Colon and rectum	Observation after curative-intent resection
II—Colon	Postop observation or postop adjuvant chemotherapy with 5-FU and levamisole or 5-FU and leucovorin
II—Rectum	Postop radiation + 5-FU (with or without leucovorin)
III—Colon	Postop adjuvant chemotherapy with 5-FU and levamisole or 5-FU and leucovorin
III—Rectum	Postop radiation + 5-FU (with or without leucovorin)
IV—Colon and rectum	Palliative chemotherapy with 5-FU and leucovorin or prolonged-infusion 5-FU (with local radiation if needed)

Table 9-5. Staging of Anal Cancer

AJCC/UICC	TNM Staging	Criteria
Stage 0	Tis, N0	Carcinoma in situ
Stage I	T1, N0	Tumor < 2 cm
Stage II	T2–3, N0	Tumor 2–5 cm
Stage III	T2–4, N1	Tumor any size; node involvement
Stage IV		Distant metastasis

carcinoma of the large bowel, where adenocarcinomas predominate. Most of the tumor morbidity and mortality is associated with uncontrolled locoregional disease. Nodal and distant patterns of spread tend to be systemic, beginning with inguinal nodes, rather than intra-abdominal and intrahepatic metastases, as seen with colorectal cancers. Radical surgery, which remains a mainstay of curative therapy of colorectal cancers, largely has been replaced in anal cancers with radiation or chemoradiation therapy and limited sphincter-sparing resections.

ETIOLOGY AND RISK FACTORS

In the United States, 1500 to 3000 cases of anal cancer are reported annually. The average age at diagnosis is older than 60 years. Cancers of the anal canal (from the anal verge proximal to the pectinate line) tend to occur more commonly in older females, and cancers of the anal margin (within 5 cm distal or caudal from the anal verge) occur more commonly in young men. Anal intercourse in men (but not in women) is a strong risk factor [29]. Sexually transmitted papilloma virus, development of condylomata acuminata, and other sexually transmitted diseases are probable causative agents. Immunosuppression related to organ transplant has been associated with increased incidence [30], and AIDS may have a etiologic role independent of any coexisting sexually transmitted conditions. Chronic anal fistulas, fissures, and other benign conditions have been associated with anal carcinomas, particularly adenocarcinoma.

STAGING AND PROGNOSIS

Staging based on the TNM system [7] (Table 9-5) includes stage 0 for carcinoma in situ, stage I for tumors up to 2 cm in diameter with negative nodes, and stage II for tumors 2 to 5 cm (T2) or more than 5 cm (T3) in diameter with negative nodes. Tumors of any size that extend to adjacent pelvic or peritoneal structures or have perirectal or inguinal nodes are stage III. Systemic metastases define stage IV disease. Early-stage lesions (0–I) have 5-year survival rates of 80% or greater. The presence of any nodal metastases, even with small tumors, confers approximately a 50% or worse 5-year survival rate. Locally invasive tumors, distant metastatic disease, and recurrent cancers are associated with a 7- to 12-month median survival rate. The major prognostic indicators are tumor size (< 2 cm versus all others), degree of differentiation, (well versus poorly differentiated), and site of origin (anal canal versus anal margin).

TREATMENT STRATEGY

Initial diagnostic evaluation includes anorectal digital examination and palpation of inguinal nodes as well as direct visualization with anoscopy and proctoscopy. Suspicious lesions and enlarged lymph nodes should be biopsied, but an inguinal node dissection is not useful. Concurrent benign anal pathology, such as fissures or fistulas, are commonly present. These may mask the malignant process; after a 2-week trial of appropriate analgesics and topical therapy, a malignant cause for persistent symptoms should be pursued. It is essential in the primary diagnosis and management of perianal complaints to reevaluate after no more than 2 to 4 weeks. If a presumed benign condition has not responded markedly to treatment by that time, it must be biopsied or evaluated under anesthesia.

Follow-up after treatment of the cancer includes careful examination of locoregional structures and liver function tests every 3 months for the first 2 to 3 years, then every 6 months for an additional 3 to 5 years. Radiographic imaging of the chest and abdominal–pelvic CT scan should be obtained at least at every other evaluation.

THERAPY FOR PRIMARY DISEASE

Very early lesions of the anal margin and distal anal canal may be treated with wide local resection and skin graft with cure rates of 60% to 80%. These T0 to T1 lesions are found infrequently, however, making up only about 10% of all tumors. An abdominal–perineal resection (APR) is curative in up to half of all patients but largely has been relegated to the role of salvage therapy after an initial attempt at cure with sphincter-sparing radiation or chemoradiation therapy. Radiation therapy in doses of 60 Gy may achieve cure in more than half of all cases, but subsequent APR may be required for recurrent disease or the management of radiation fibrosis and proctitis.

A chemoradiation combination of mitomycin C, 5-FU, and radiation doses to about 50 Gy produce lower long-term toxicity rates, 85% to 95% complete remission rates, and 5-year survival rate in three fourths of patients treated [31,32]. A large clinical trial designed to assess whether the dose of mitomycin C with its associated acute toxicity can be omitted has been completed but reported only in abstract form [33]. The preliminary conclusion suggests that although the toxicity is also higher with the addition of mitomycin C, disease control is substantially improved with a regimen that includes this drug. Grade 4 or 5 toxicity was 26% for the mitomycin C regimen versus 7% for radiation plus 5-FU. However, disease-free and overall survival figures were 73% and 76%, respectively, for the mitomycin C regimen compared with 51% and 67%, respectively, for radiation plus 5-FU. For patients with residual tumor at biopsy 8 to 12 weeks after initial therapy, additional chemoradiation with cisplatin, 5-FU, and RT may achieve a complete response. An abdominal–perineal resection remains a part of the therapeutic plan for patients who, after chemoradiation, do not have biopsy-proven elimination or local disease or who develop recurrent local tumor.

Most regimens that have been evaluated for treatment of anal cancer have enrolled patients who are HIV negative. Data that can serve as a basis for recommendations for therapy of the increasing number of patients with anal cancer who are HIV positive are scarce. At least one report [34] emphasizes that patients who are HIV positive suffer increased toxicity with chemoradiation treatment and require more interruptions of therapy.

THERAPY FOR ADVANCED DISEASE

Based on high rates of response in other squamous cell tumors, 5-FU and cisplatin or other cisplatin-based regimens have been suggested for metastatic or recurrent disease [35–37]. Other multidrug combinations using bleomycin, nitrosoureas, and anthracyclines are of uncertain benefit. Interstitial radiation therapy alone or with chemotherapy can be effective in controlling initial or relapsed local disease, but its success is very dependent on individual techniques and expertise.

REFERENCES

1. Lynch HT, Smyrk T, Watson P, *et al.*: Hereditary colorectal cancer. *Semin Oncol* 1991, 18:337–366.

2. Leach FS, Nicolaides NC, Papdopoulos N, *et al.*: Mutations of two PMS homologues in hereditary nonpolyposis colon cancer. *Nature* 1994, 371:75–80.

3. Nicolaides NC, Papadopoulos N, Liu B, *et al.*: Mutations of two PMS homlogues in hereditary nonpolyposis colon cancer. *Nature* 1994, 371:75–80.

4. Toribara NW, Sleisenger MH: Screening for colorectal cancer. *N Engl J Med* 1995, 332:861–867.

5. Winawer SJ, Fletcher RH, Miller L, *et al.*: Colorectal cancer screening: clinical guidelines and rationale. *Gastroneterology* 1997, 112:594–642.

6. Vogelstein B, Fearon ER, Hamilton SR, *et al.*: Genetic alterations during colorectal tumor development. *N Engl J Med* 1988, 319:525–532.

7. Moertel CG, Loprinzi CL, Witzig TE, *et al.*: The dilemma of Stage B-2 colon cancer. Is adjuvant therapy justified? A Mayo Clinic/North Central Cancer Treatment Group Study. *Proc ASCO* 1990, 9:108.

8. American Joint Committee on Cancer: Manual for Staging of Cancer, 4th ed. Philadelphia: JB Lippincott, 1992.

9. Steele G, Bleday R, Mayer RJ, *et al.*: A prospective evaluation of hepatic resection for colorectal carcinoma metastases to the liver. Gastrointestinal Tumor Study Group Protocol 6584. *J Clin Oncol* 1991, 9:1105–1112.

10. Minsky BD, Cohen AM, Enker WE, *et al.*: Combined modality therapy of rectal cancer: decreased acute toxicity with the pre-operative approach. *J Clin Oncol* 1992, 10:1218–1224.

11. Minsky BD, Cohen AM, Kemeny N, *et al.*: Enhancement of radiation induced downstaging of rectal cancer by 5-FU and high dose leucovorin chemotherapy. *J Clin Oncol* 1992, 10:79–84.

12. Moertel CG, Fleming TR, Macdonald JS, *et al.*: Levamisole and fluorouracil for adjuvant therapy of resected colon carcinoma. *N Engl J Med* 1990, 322:352–358.

13. Moertel CG, Fleming TR, Macdonald JS, *et al.*: The intergroup study of fluorouracil (5-FU) plus levamisole (Lev) and levamisole alone as adjuvant therapy for stage C colon cancer. *Proc ASCO* 1992, 11:101.

14. O'Connell MJ, Maillard J, Macdonald J, *et al.*: An intergroup trial of intensive course 5-FU and low dose leucovorin as surgical adjuvant therapy for high risk colon cancer. *Proc ASCO* 1993, 12:190.

15. Erlichman C, Marsoni S, Seitz JF, *et al.*: Event free and overall survival is increased by FUFA in resected B and C colon cancer: a prospective pooled analysis of 3 randomized clinical trials (RCTS). *Proc ASCO* 1994, 13:194.

16. Wolmark N, Rockette H, Fisher B, *et al.*: The benefit of leucovorin-modulated fluorouracil as postoperative adjuvant therapy for primary colon cancer: results from National Surgical Adjuvant Breast and Bowel Project Protocol C-03. *J Clin Oncol* 1993, 11:1879–1887.

17. Krook J, Moertel C, *et al*: Effective surgical adjuvant therapy for high risk rectal carcinoma. *N Engl J Med* 1991, 324:709–715.

18. Fisher B, Wolmark N, Rockette H, *et al.*: Postoperative adjuvant chemotherapy or radiation therapy for rectal cancer: results from NSABP R-01. *J Natl Cancer Inst* 1988, 80:21–29.

19. Earlam S, Glover L, Davies M, *et al.*: Effect of regional and systemic fluorinated pyrimidine chemotherapy on quality of life in colorectal lower metastasis patients. *J Clin Oncol* 1997, 15:2022–2029.

20. Nordic Gastrointestinal Tumor Adjuvant Therapy Group. Expectancy of primary chemotherapy in patients with advanced asymptomatic colorectal cancer: a randomized trial. *J Clin Oncol* 1992, 10:904–911.

21. Scheithauser W, Rosen H, Kornek G-V, *et al.*: Randomized comparison of combination chemotherapy plus supportive care with supportive care alone in patients with metastatic colorectal cancer. *Br Med J* 1993, 306:752–755.

22. Advanced Colorectal Cancer Meta-analysis Project: Modulation of fluorouracil by leucovorin in patients with advanced colorectal cancer: evidence in terms of response rate. *J Clin Oncol* 1992, 10:896–903.

23. Buroker TR, O'Connell MJ, Wieand HS, *et al.*: Randomized comparison of two schedules of fluorouracil and leucovorin in the treatment of advanced colorectal cancer. *J Clin Oncol* 1994, 12:14–20.

24. Peters GJ, van Groeningen CJ: Clinical relevance of biochemical modulation of 5-fluorouracil. *Ann Oncol* 1991, 2:469–480.

25. Lokich JJ, Ahlgren JD, Gullo JJ, *et al.*: A prospective randomized comparison of continuous infusion fluorouracil with conventional bolus schedule in metastatic colorectal carcinoma: a Mid-Atlantic Oncology Program Study. *J Clin Oncol* 1989, 7:425–432.

26. Wagman LD, Kemeny MM, Leong L, *et al.*: A prospective, randomized evaluation of the treatment of colorectal cancer metastatic to the liver. *J Clin Oncol* 1990, 8:1885–1893.

27. Mahood DJ, Dose AM, Loprinzi CL, *et al.*: Inhibition of fluorouracil-induced stomatitis by oral cryotherapy. *J Clin Oncol* 1991, 9:449–452.

28. Casinu S, Fedeli A, Fedeli SA, *et al.*: Control of chemotherapy-induced diarrhea with octeotide in patients receiving 5-fluorouracil. *Eur J Cancer* 1992, 28:482–483.

29. Dazing JR, Weiss NS, Hislop TG, *et al.*: Sexual practices, sexually transmitted diseases and the incidence of anal cancer. *N Engl J Med* 1987, 317:973–977.

30. Penn I: Cancer of the anogenital region in renal transplant recipient: analysis of 65 cases. *Cancer* 1986, 58:611–616.

31. Sischy B, Duggett RL, Krall JM, *et al.*: Definitive irradiation and chemotherapy for radiosensitization in management of anal carcinoma: interim report of the Radiation Therapy Oncology Group (study no. 8314). *J Nat Cancer Inst* 1989:850–856.

32. Mendenhall WM, Sombeck MD, Speer TW, *et al.*: Current management of squamous cell carcinoma of the anal canal. *Surg Oncol* 1994, 3:135–146.

33. Flam MS, John MJ, Peters T, *et al.*: Radiation and 5-fluorouracil (5-FU) vs radiation, 5-FU, and mitomycin-C (MMC) in the treatment of anal carcinoma: preliminary results of a phase III randomized RTOG/ECOG intergroup trial. *Proc ASCO* 1993, 12:192.

34. Holland JM, Swift PS: Tolerance of patients with human immue immunodeficiency virus and anal carcinoma to treatment with combined chemotherapy and radiation therapy. *Radiology* 1994, 193:251–254.

35. Majoubi M, Sadek H, Francois E, *et al.*: Epidermoid anal canal carcinoma (EACC): activity of cisplatin (P) and continuous 5-fluorouracil (5-FU) in metastatic and/or local recurrent (LR) disease. *Proc ASCO* 1990, 9:114.

36. Roca E, DeSimone G, Barugel M, *et al.*: A phase II study of alternating chemoradiotherapy including cisplatin (DDP) in anal canal carcinoma (ACC). *Proc ASCO* 1990, 9:128.

37. Rich TA, Ajani JA, Morrison WH, et al.: Chemoradiation therapy for anal cancer: radiation plus continuous infusion of 5-fluorouracil with or without cisplatin. *Radiother Oncol* 1993, 27:209–215.

5-FU AND LEVAMISOLE

5-FU is a fluorine-substituted uracil that blocks the methylation reaction of deoxyuridylic acid to thymidylic acid, interfering with DNA synthesis; it may be incorporated as a false nucleotide into DNA and RNA. The drug is most active against growing cell populations. Levamisole was introduced into clinical practice in 1973 as an antihelmintic. Early in vivo research suggested immune modulatory properties; however, its mechanism of action in adjuvant treatment remains undefined. Levamisole as a single agent is not effective for adjuvant therapy, and the combination of 5-FU and levamisole is not effective in advanced (stage IV) colon cancer.

DOSAGE AND SCHEDULING

5-FU 450 mg/m² IV bolus, daily x 5; starting d 28, weekly for 48 wk											
Levamisole 50 mg PO TID x 3 d, q other wk											
Day	1	2	3	4	5	15	16	17	29	30	31	36

5-FU 450 mg/m² IV bolus, daily x 5; starting d 28, weekly for 48 wk										
Levamisole 50 mg PO TID x 3 d, q other wk										
Day	43	44	45	50	57	58	59	64	71	72	73*

*Continue weekly 5-FU and every-other-week levamisole (x 3 d) for a total of 1 y.

RECENT EXPERIENCE AND RESPONSE RATES

Study	Evaluable Patients, n	Regimen	3.5-y Survival, %
Moertel et al., N Engl J Med 1990, 322:352–358	929	Surgery alone	55
		Levamisole	55
		5-FU/levamisole	71

CANDIDATES FOR TREATMENT
Adjuvant therapy for patients who have undergone resection for stage III (node-positive) colon cancer

SPECIAL PRECAUTIONS
Full recovery from surgery; pregnant and nursing patients

ALTERNATIVE THERAPY
5-FU and leucovorin

TOXICITIES
5-FU: loss of appetite, diarrhea, abdominal cramps, difficulty with coordination, mouth sores, dry skin or nose, splitting fingernails, metal taste in mouth, watery eyes, nausea, vomiting, temporary alopecia, leukopenia leading to an increased risk of infection, erythrocytopenia leading to anemia, photosensitivity, skin rash, hyperpigmentation, local tissue irritation if drug extravasation occurs
Levamisole: metallic taste (2%), arthralgias and myalgia (1%), mood change and dizziness (3%), exfoliative dermatitis (rare), leukoencephalopy with change in mental status (rare)
Combination: severe nausea, vomiting, diarrhea, myelosuppression (1.5%)

DRUG INTERACTIONS
5-FU: allopurinol, cimetidine, folinic acid, methotrexate, thymidine; **Levamisole:** phenytoin, warfarin, ethanol

NURSING INTERVENTIONS
Assess patient performance and mental status; monitor weight, encourage adequate fluid, caloric, and protein intake; give antiemetics, antidiarrheals, food supplements as necessary; monitor blood counts and liver function; inform patients of possible skin reactions; because of levamisole schedule, develop calendar or reminder for patient

PATIENT INFORMATION
Patient should report diarrhea > 3 × d, soreness in mouth, difficulty swallowing, rash, fever. As with all oral medications, reinforce compliance frequently.

PROLONGED CONTINUOUS IV 5-FU

5-FU is a fluorine-substituted uracil that blocks the methylation reaction of deoxyuridylic acid to thymidylic acid, interfering with DNA synthesis. Direct incorporation of fluoropyrimidine nucleotide into DNA and RNA also occurs. With continuous daily infusion, the activity and toxicity profiles are different than those seen with bolus therapy. The mechanism responsible for these differences is not completely understood.

DOSAGE AND SCHEDULING

5-FU 300 mg/m^2/24 h via ambulatory pump	███	███		
Day	1 – 7	71 – 84	85 – 155	156 – 169*

*1- to 2-wk interruptions may be required for recovery from toxicity before 10 wk of infusion; continue therapy until disease progression.

RECENT EXPERIENCES AND RESPONSE RATES

Study	Evaluable Patients, n	Regimen	Response, %
Lokich JJ et al., J Clin Oncol 1989, 7:425–432	87	5-FU bolus	7
	87	5-FU cont. IV	30

CANDIDATES FOR TREATMENT
Patients with colorectal cancer

SPECIAL PRECAUTIONS
Pregnant and nursing patients

ALTERNATIVE THERAPY
Other 5-FU-based regimens

TOXICITIES
Myelosuppression and mucositis are *less* severe, palmar planter erythrodysesthesia with peripheral neuropathy and desquamation (possibly dose-limiting); loss of appetite, diarrhea, abdominal cramps, difficulty with coordination, mouth sores, dry skin or nose, splitting fingernails, metallic taste, watery eyes, nausea, vomiting, temporary alopecia, leukopenia leading to an increased risk of infection, erythrocytopenia leading to anemia, photosensitivity, skin rash, hyperpigmentation, local tissue irritation if drug extravasation occurs

DRUG INTERACTIONS
5-FU: allopurinol, cimetidine, folinic acid, methotrexate, thymidine

NURSING INTERVENTIONS
Instruct patient in care of semipermanent IV access and ambulatory pump; assess patient performance and mental status; monitor weight, encourage adequate fluid, caloric, and protein intake; give antiemetics, antidiarrheals, food supplements as necessary; monitor blood counts and liver function

PATIENT INFORMATION
Patient should report diarrhea > 3 ×/d, soreness in mouth, difficulty swallowing, rash, fever. Patient should be informed of possible skin reactions.

INTERFERON α-2 AND 5-FU

Interferon α-2 (IFN α-2) is a biologic response modifier, that is used in a purified, recombinant form. It has demonstrated both antitumor and immunomodulatory effects.

5-Fluorouracil (5-FU) is a fluorine-substituted uracil that blocks the methylation reaction of deoxyuridylic acid to thymidylic acid, interfering with DNA synthesis. The drug is most active against growing cell populations.

Synergism of this regimen may be attributable to IFN-decreased tumor cell thymidylate synthetase production after 5-FU, protracted metabolism of 5-FU, and serum clearance of 5-FU catabolites, or to additional effects upon the 5-fluorodeoxyuridine monophosphate (FdUMP)–thymidylate synthetase complex formulation. Recombinant IFN α-2 enhances the cytotoxic effects of 5-FU against two human colon cancer cell lines in a dose- and schedule-dependent manner, demonstrating therapeutic synergism when used in a strict regimen. IFNs biochemically modulate the activity of 5-FU in vitro, enhancing intracellular levels of FdUMP and the binding of FdUMP to thymidylate synthetase, the target enzyme. Additionally, phase I clinical trials indicated decreased clearance of 5-FU with increased serum levels with IFN α-2 therapy. Finally, IFN α-2 enhances natural killer cell and macrophage activity, although it is unclear if this contributes to enhanced antitumor effects.

DOSAGE AND SCHEDULING

5-FU 750 mg/m²/d by continuous infusion (inpatient), d 1–5	████████████													
5-FU 750 mg/m² bolus (outpatient), d 8								■						
IFN 9 x 10⁶ U SC, d 1, 3, 5, 8, 10, 12	■		■		■			■		■		■		
CBC, d 1, 4, 8, 11	☐			☐				☐			☐			
LFT, ECG, d 7, 14							☐							☐
Day	1	2	3	4	5	6	7	8	9	10	11	12	13	14

RECENT EXPERIENCES AND RESPONSE RATES

Study	Evaluable Patients, n	Regimen	CR/PR (%)
Wadler et al., Cancer Res 1990, 50:2056–2059	18	5-FU: 750 mg/m²/d x 5 d (cont IV infusion); then weekly IFN α-2a: 6, 9, 12, 15, or 18 x 10⁶ U SC	1/4 (28)
Pazdur et al., J Clin Oncol 1990, 8:2027–2031	45	5-FU: 750 mg/m²/d x 5 d (cont IV infusion); then weekly IFN α-2a: 9 x 10⁶ U SC TIW	1/15 (36)
Kemeny et al., Cancer 1990, 66:2470–2475	36	5-FU: 750 mg/m²/d x 5 d (cont IV infusion); then weekly IFN α-2a: 9 x 10⁶ U SC TIW	0/9 (26)
Wadler, Wiernik, Semin Oncol 1990, 17(suppl 1):16–21, 38–41	32	5-FU: 750 mg/m²/d x 5 d (cont IV infusion); then weekly IFN α-2a: 9 x 10⁶ U SC TIW	0/20 (63)
Fornasiero et al., Tumori 1990, 76:385–388	21	5-FU: 1000 mg/wk; IFN α-2a: 6, 9, 12, 18 x 10⁶ U SC TIW (dose escalated each month)	4/5 (43)

CANDIDATES FOR TREATMENT
Patients with advanced colorectal cancers, and carcinoma of the stomach, colon, pancreas, liver, and breast

SPECIAL PRECAUTIONS
Enhanced mucositis, severe diarrhea

ALTERNATIVE THERAPIES
5-FU and leucovorin, 5-FU and levamisole

TOXICITIES
5-FU: loss of appetite, diarrhea, abdominal cramps, difficulty with coordination, mouth sores, dry skin or nose, splitting fingernails, metal taste in mouth, watery eyes, nausea, vomiting, temporary alopecia, leukopenia leading to an increased risk of infection, erythrocytopenia leading to anemia, photosensitivity, skin rash, hyperpigmentation, local tissue irritation if drug extravasation occurs; **IFN α-2:** fever, fatigue, flu-like symptoms, pancytopenia, changes in consciousness, changes in liver function tests, changes in blood pressure, numbness and tingling in fingers and toes; **less frequent:** convulsions, confusion, stupor, irregular heart beat, blood clotting abnormalities; anemia more severe than that normally seen with 5-FU alone

DRUG INTERACTIONS
IFN α-2: aspirin, NSAIDs, prostaglandin synthetase inhibitors, antihistamines, immunomodulators; **5-FU:** methotrexate, allopurinol, oxypurinol, thymidine

NURSING INTERVENTIONS
Give acetaminophen prior to IFN for flu-like symptoms and every 4 h as needed thereafter; assess patient performance and mental status; monitor weight, encourage adequate fluid, caloric, and protein intake; give antiemetics, antidiarrheals, food supplements as necessary; monitor blood counts and liver function; educate on central venous access device and pump and malfunctions

PATIENT INFORMATION
Patient may experience flu-like symptoms; fatigue likely (arrange activities in the morning and allow for frequent rest); nausea/vomiting likely; patient should report diarrhea > 3 ×/d, soreness in mouth, difficulty swallowing, rash, fever. If diarrhea develops, contact doctor (fluid replacement therapy may be necessary); possible skin reactions.

RADIATION THERAPY, 5-FU, AND MITOMYCIN C

The combination of 5-FU and mitomycin C with radiation has at the very least an additive cytotoxic effect, and it may have a synergistic "radiosensitizing" effect. 5-FU is a fluoride-substituted uracil that blocks the methylation reaction of deoxyuridylic acid to thymidylic acid, interfering with DNA synthesis; it may be incorporated as a false nucleotide into DNA and RNA. The drug is most active against growing cell populations. Mitomycin C is an antibiotic isolated from *Streptomyces caespitosus*. Its antitumor effect results from DNA cross-linking and suppression of RNA and protein synthesis.

DOSAGE AND SCHEDULING

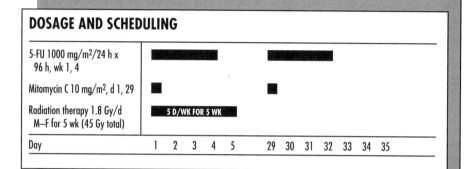

	Day
5-FU 1000 mg/m²/24 h x 96 h, wk 1, 4	
Mitomycin C 10 mg/m², d 1, 29	
Radiation therapy 1.8 Gy/d M–F for 5 wk (45 Gy total)	5 D/WK FOR 5 WK
Day	1 2 3 4 5 29 30 31 32 33 34 35

RECENT EXPERIENCES AND RESPONSE RATES

Study	Evaluable Patients, n	Regimen	Locoregional Control, %	2-y Survival, %
Sishy B *et al.*, JNCI 1989, 81:850–856	79	RT + 5-FU/MMC	90	87
Flam MS *et al.*, Proc ASCO 1993, 12:192 (#A557)	151	RT + 5-FU/MMC	92	79
	148	RT + 5-FU	86	81

CANDIDATES FOR TREATMENT

Patients with stage II or III anal carcinoma in whom sphincter preservation is option

SPECIAL PRECAUTIONS

Pregnant and nursing patients

ALTERNATIVE THERAPY

Mitomycin C may be optional component to regimen

TOXICITIES

5-FU: loss of appetite, diarrhea, abdominal cramps, difficulty with coordination, mouth sores, dry skin or nose, splitting fingernails, metal taste in mouth, watery eyes, nausea, vomiting, temporary alopecia, leukopenia leading to an increased risk of infection, erythrocytopenia leading to anemia, photosensitivity, skin rash, hyperpigmentation, local tissue irritation if drug extravasation occurs
Mitomycin C: fever, nausea, vomiting; myelosuppression, mucositis, alopecia, increased creatinine, pulmonary infiltrates and fibrosis
Chemoradiation: fatal toxicities (1%–5%)

DRUG INTERACTIONS

5-FU: Allopurinol, cimetidine, folinic acid, methotrexate, thymidine; **Mitomycin C:** vinblastine (worsened lung toxicity)

NURSING INTERVENTIONS

Moderate-to-severe pelvic/perineal skin toxicities from combined therapy; ointments and salves should not be applied to skin (mitomycin C is vesicant); good skin hygiene and Domeboro solution may provide relief

PATIENT INFORMATION

Patient should be informed about skin care. Patient should report diarrhea > 3 ×/d, soreness in mouth, difficulty swallowing, rash, fever.

ETIOLOGY AND RISK FACTORS

Cancer of the head and neck accounts for approximately 5% of malignancies in the United States [1]. Its incidence is higher in African Americans and men and is declining in white men. Tobacco and alcohol are the two major risk factors. Increasing tobacco consumption is responsible for a rising incidence of head and neck cancer in women. Tobacco chewing is a common risk factor in Asia, resulting in a higher incidence of head and neck cancer in parts of the Far East. Although alcohol and tobacco are independent risk factors, they are frequently present together, resulting in a synergistic potentiation of the carcinogenic risk [2].

Other possible risk factors include nutritional deficiencies, poor orodental care, an immunocompromised state, and a genetic predisposition (Table 10-1). Exposure to wood dust, nickel, or textile fibers is associated with adenocarcinoma of the paranasal sinuses. Nasopharyngeal carcinoma is associated with Epstein–Barr virus, and is endemic in regions of North Africa and Asia [3]. An increased incidence of oral cancer with chronic infection of herpes and papilloma viruses has been suggested. Genetic factors may account for increased susceptibility. Mutations of the *p53* tumor suppressor gene and other genes are frequent [4]. Head and neck cancer is a typical environmentally induced disease, and avoidance of the risk factors is the best prevention. Patients at risk should be followed with regular physical examinations, careful inspection of the oral cavity, questioning the patient about changes in eating habits, and early referral for laryngoscopy if hoarseness or other symptoms persist (Table 10-2).

STAGING AND PROGNOSIS

Head and neck cancer represents a heterogeneous group of cancers originating from different primary localizations. Squamous cell carcinoma is the most common histologic type in the adult. Other histologies include adenocarcinoma, adenoid cystic carcinoma, mucoepidermoid carcinoma, and undifferentiated carcinoma of the nasopharynx. Lymphoma, Hodgkin's disease, sarcoma, and melanoma may arise in the head and neck and must be distinguished. Metastases of lung cancer or gastrointestinal neoplasms may present primarily in the neck. Treatment depends on localization, resectability, and histology. For squamous cell carcinoma, local and regional extension determines the stage and prognosis.

The T staging is dependent on the exact anatomic localization of the tumor. Lesions considered to be T1 and T2 are small primary tumors, whereas T3 and T4 lesions are locally advanced, with T4 invading surrounding structures (*eg*, bone, cartilage, skin). Regional lymph nodes are staged uniformly for all anatomic sites as N1–N3 according to increasing size and number of nodes (Table 10-3). Stages I and II represent T1N0 and T2N0 lesions, respectively, whereas stages III and IV represent locally advanced disease (T3, T4) and regional involvement (N1–N3). Distant metastases are present in less than 10% of patients at diagnosis and are included in stage IV. Lungs, bones, and liver are the most commonly involved sites [5]. The majority of patients (60%) have locoregionally advanced disease (T3 and T4 or N1–N3) at presentation and die of locoregional disease, indicating the inability of currently available therapy to consistently achieve cure. Nodal involvement in the neck appears to be the most important prognostic factor (Table 10-4).

Up to 25% of patients with advanced squamous cell carcinoma will relapse with distant metastases. Autopsy series suggest that up to 40% to 50% of all patients have occult metastatic disease. Cure in locally advanced stages is less than 30% following standard therapy. In early-stage disease, cure rates are 60% to 90%. Laryngeal cancer appears to have a somewhat better prognosis than other tumor sites. Poor tissue vascularization and hoarseness as a symptom leading to early diagnosis may be contributing factors to higher cure rates in larynx cancer.

NASOPHARYNX CANCER AND EPSTEIN–BARR VIRUS

Nasopharyngeal cancer with its distinct histology must be considered separately. Surgical accessibility is difficult, and because of its hidden location the cancer causes few early symptoms. Most patients present

Table 10-1. Risk Factors

Tobacco	Smokeless tobacco (chewing)
Alcohol	Malnutrition
Poor orodental care	Mechanical irritation
Genetic susceptibility	Viruses: Epstein–Barr virus, herpes simplex
Occupational exposure: wood dust, textile fibers, nickel, cadmium, radium	virus, human papilloma virus.

Table 10-2. Prevention and Early Detection

Prevention	Early Detection (Patients at Risk)
Avoid alcohol	Yearly physical examination with special attention to the upper aerodigestive tract and neck
Avoid smoking	Digital examination of oral cavity
Avoid combination of alcohol and smoking	Refer to ear, nose, and throat specialist for unexplained symptoms lasting > 4 weeks
Discontinue risk factor exposure after diagnosis: reduction of risk of second malignancy	Leukoplakia as possible early sign of transformation: biopsy and frequent follow-up necessary
Participation in chemoprevention trials (*see* Table 10-6)	

Table 10-3. TNM-Staging and Survival

	5-y Survival	N0	N1	N2	N3
Stage I	75%–90%	T1			
Stage II	40%–70%	T2			
Stage III	20%–50%	T3			
Stage IV	<10%–30%	T4	(any M1)		

Stages I and II	Early stage	N0	no lymph node involved
T3N0, T1-2, N1	Intermediate stage	N1	single ipsilateral lymph node, <3 cm
T3, T4 and N1-3,	Locoregionally	N2	nodes > 3–6 cm
M0	advanced	N2a	single node, ipsilateral
		N2b	multiple nodes, ipsilateral
		N2c	multiple nodes, bilateral or contralateral
		N3	lymph node > 6 cm

Table 10-4. Prognostic Factors

	Comment
Nodal involvement, N-stage	Most important prognostic factor: N0 better than N+
Extracapsular spread	Tendency for recurrence in the neck and distant metastases
Tumor size	
Histological differentiation	Salivary gland cancer only
Hypopharynx	Commonly advanced with poor outcome
Larynx	Overall prognostically better, potential for organ preservation with induction chemotherapy
Nasopharynx	Chemosensitive tumor, tendency for distant metastases, median survival 4–5 y, late relapses frequent

with an advanced-stage nodal involvement and, frequently, distant metastases. Undifferentiated carcinoma of the nasopharynx is a more common tumor type, with endemic distribution in Southeast Asia. A strong etiologic association has been found for Epstein-Barr virus infection [6]. Activation of the viral genome may be caused by frequent consumption of salted fish or nitrosamines. Epstein-Barr virus genome and viral protein expression can be detected in the majority of nasopharynx tumors. Nasopharynx cancer is exquisitely sensitive to both radiation and chemotherapy, suggesting the usefulness of a combined-modality treatment approach [7]. In a randomized trial testing induction chemotherapy, Cvitkovic and coworkers [8] compared three cycles of BEC (bleomycin, epirubicin, cisplatin) followed by radiation versus radiotherapy alone. Despite an excess in toxic death in the experimental arm, which correlated with the experience of the treating center, they observed a significantly improved disease-free survival with induction chemotherapy. In a randomized

intergroup trial, concomitant chemoradiotherapy with cisplatin followed by adjuvant chemotherapy with cisplatin and 5-FU was compared to standard radiotherapy. This trial was closed early after an interim analysis showed a significantly improved outcome for the combined modality treatment (median progression-free survival: 13 mo versus 52 mo; 2-y survival: 55% versus 80%) [9].

SALIVARY GLAND CANCER

Salivary gland cancers are different from squamous carcinomas of the head and neck. Histologically these are commonly adenocarcinoma, adenoid cystic carcinoma, or mucoepidermoid carcinoma [10]. Low-grade histologic tumors tend not to recur, whereas high-grade tumors frequently invade adjacent muscle, bone, and nerves and may recur regionally or distantly. Management of these tumors, which affect primarily elderly patients, is mainly surgical; adenoid cystic carcinoma is sensitive to radiation. Chemotherapy for recurrent or metastatic disease commonly includes an anthracycline-containing regimen (*eg*, CAP: cyclophosphamide, doxorubicin, cisplatin; or FAP: 5-fluorouracil or 5-FU, doxorubicin, cisplatin).

TREATMENT STRATEGY

Stage is the main determining factor when deciding on a treatment strategy for an individual patient (Fig. 10-1). Patients are best evaluated jointly by an ENT surgeon, radiation therapist, and a medical oncologist. In addition, an experienced radiologist, an oral surgeon, a nutritionist, as well as a social worker are often very valuable resources when deciding on an overall treatment strategy.

Early stages can usually be cured with surgery, radiation therapy, or both. In the frequently locally advanced stages, a multimodality approach is necessary for optimal patient care. Local control can be

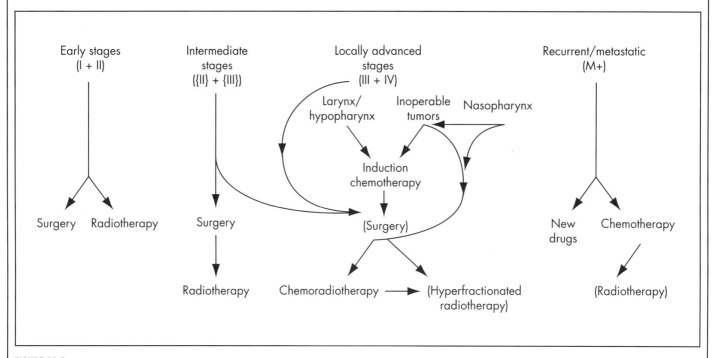

FIGURE 10-1.

Treatment strategies for head and neck cancer. (*Adapted from* Stupp and Vokes [55]; with permission.)

improved by concomitant chemoradiotherapy. Organ preservation with sequential or concomitant chemo- and radiation therapy can be an important goal for compliant patients. Surgery is then reserved for patients who fail to respond or those with recurrent disease. For patients who will not comply with a lengthy and intensive treatment and regular follow-up, radical surgery remains the treatment of choice. Patients with recurrent or metastatic disease are candidates for palliative chemotherapy [11].

Early-Stage Disease

Early-stage tumors (T1, T2) can be cured with surgery or radiotherapy alone in 60% to 90% of cases. If surgery is performed, it frequently includes an elective dissection of the regional lymph nodes. This procedure allows for more accurate pathologic staging, with important prognostic and therapeutic implications. In over 50% of cases, the pathologic stage will be higher than the clinical stage. Newer radiologic procedures (ultrasound, computed tomography, magnetic resonance imaging, positron emission tomography) also have an increasing role in the staging of this disease.

A similar outcome can be achieved in early-stage disease with radiation therapy. Primary radiotherapy may allow for organ preservation and help avoid surgery in a subgroup of patients with serious underlying morbidities (eg, chronic obstructive pulmonary disease, coronary artery disease, or liver cirrhosis). The treatment is a lengthy process over 6 to 7 weeks with mucositis, xerostomia, and loss of taste as the major secondary effects. This modality with its curative intent should only be chosen for reliable and compliant patients. For early-stage larynx cancer, radiation therapy is often the first choice. Nasopharyngeal cancer is considered unresectable and is treated with radiation.

Locally Advanced Disease

Up to 70% of patients initially present with locally advanced disease (Stage III + IV), and many patients will recur locally or regionally. In locally advanced disease, bimodal therapy with surgery followed by radiotherapy has been the standard treatment for patients who have resectable disease that is medically operable. This approach resulted in low cure rates of 20% to 30%. Depending on the extent of the tumor, surgery may lead to impaired or lost organ function, muscle atrophy, and disfigurement. New strategies have been developed to improve cure rates and overall survival. Multimodality therapy with concomitant chemoradiotherapy improve locoregional control and survival in many patients; induction chemotherapy allows for organ preservation in a majority of patients with advanced larynx and hypopharynx tumors.

Induction Chemotherapy

Rationale

The early use of chemotherapy as induction or neoadjuvant treatment has the theoretical advantage of an intact vascular bed (before surgery, with improved delivery of chemotherapy) and early control of systemic micrometastases [12]. With improvements in locoregional disease control, the latter may be important for long-term survival. Induction chemotherapy may also facilitate surgery or allow for organ preservation. Chemosensitive tumors with a better prognosis may be identified. Contrarily, the delay of surgery might result in only incomplete resectability due to tumor progression. Responding patients may subsequently refuse the planned surgery or radiation and, thus, miss the opportunity for cure. Lastly, induction

chemotherapy prolongs the overall treatment duration by another 3 months and adds toxicity and cost for no as yet proven overall survival benefit.

Induction chemotherapy with cisplatin and 5-FU results in complete response rates of 20% to 50% and an overall response rate of 80% to 90%. Responding patients survive longer. Most investigators administer three cycles of induction chemotherapy, reserving the third cycle for responding patients only. In sequential studies patients were reevaluated after two, three, and four cycles of neoadjuvant chemotherapy, and an increase in complete response rates was observed from two to three, but not from three to four, cycles [13]. A more recent trial demonstrated an increase in the complete response rate from 19% after three cycles to 31% after four cycles [14].

Randomized Trials

Although induction chemotherapy with cisplatin and 5-FU results in high response rates, this has not translated into a significant survival advantage in five conclusive randomized trials [14–19]. However, a reduction in instant metastasis was demonstrated, thus suggesting systemic activity against early micrometastatic disease [14,15,17].

Improved survival also was shown for primarily inoperable patients after induction chemotherapy followed by radiation [14]. A survival advantage also was shown by subset analysis for patients with oral cancer and N2 disease who underwent induction and adjuvant chemotherapy [20].

Organ preservation

Organ preservation has been a primary endpoint of two randomized trials [15, 19]. Patients with larynx cancer [15] and pyriform sinus cancer [19] were treated with three cycles of induction chemotherapy with cisplatin and 5-FU; responding patients then received definitive radiation. Surgery was restricted to those patients who did not respond [15], those who did not completely respond [19], and as a salvage treatment in patients with residual disease after radiation or with recurrent disease. For larynx primaries, organ preservation at 3 years was 64%; for hypopharynx primaries, the 3-year estimate of survival with a functional larynx was 42%. The feasibility of organ preservation has also been shown for nonlaryngeal sites [21]. The European Organization for Research and Treatment of Cancer (EORTC) is conducting two large randomized trials: 1) comparing alternating chemoradiotherapy with induction chemotherapy followed by radiation, and 2) standard radiotherapy versus concomitant chemoradiotherapy. Organ preservation in resectable hypopharynx and larynx cancer is the major end point.

Concomitant Chemoradiotherapy

Concepts and Rationale

High response rates and a consistently decreased incidence of distant metastases underline the efficacy of chemotherapy in the treatment of squamous cell head and neck cancer. The use of chemotherapy as a radiation sensitizer is well established. The goal of concomitant chemoradiotherapy is to administer both treatment modalities at an optimal dose and schedule simultaneously within a short time frame. Overall, three different but similar concepts have been investigated: 1) standard and uninterrupted radiation with simultaneous low-dose single-agent chemotherapy with a pure radiosensitizing objective; 2) modified radiation therapy schedule with planned treatment breaks and simultaneous, intensified (at systemically active doses), combination chemotherapy; and 3) rapidly alternating sequenced therapy with radiation and combination chemotherapy.

The rationale for concomitant chemo- and radiation therapy has been reviewed extensively [22,23]. Concomitant chemotherapy may eradicate radiation-resistant tumor cells, presumably by making the tumor cells more susceptible to radiation. Furthermore, chemotherapy may eliminate micrometastatic disease outside the radiation field (spatial cooperation). Although concomitant chemoradiotherapy enhances treatment efficacy, it also adds significant toxicity. Mucositis, neutropenia, and infections can be severe and occasionally life-threatening complications [24,25]. We consider concomitant intensive chemoradiotherapy as the treatment of choice for most patients with advanced head and neck cancer. However, because of increased acute toxicities, these treatments should be administered by an experienced and multidisciplinary team of physicians and nurses. Most patients require very close follow-up and supportive care (*eg*, percutaneous endoscopic gastrostomy).

Randomized Trials

Many well-conducted randomized trials were published in the last few years, all suggesting improved locoregional control or prolonged survival with concomitant chemoradiotherapy. 5-Fluorouracil (5-FU) has been widely used with concomitant radiation [26]. In a placebo-controlled trial 5-FU (1200 mg/m² continuous infusion, d 1–3) was added to standard radiation therapy at weeks 1 and 3. Two-year survival with 5-FU was 63% versus 50% (P=0.076) without chemotherapy [27]. There was no impact on the incidence of distant metastases. In an earlier trial, 5-FU bolus (250 mg/m2) every other day was comparable to hyperfractionated twice-daily radiotherapy (2 × 1.1 Gy) and significantly superior to standard radiotherapy alone. Median survival was 85, 84, and 38 months, respectively. Prolonged survival was also shown for cisplatin (50 mg/wk) and standard radiation versus radiotherapy alone. The corrected 2-year survival rates were 75% versus 44% (P<0.05) [28]. The combination of cisplatin (12 mg/m², d 1–5) and 5-FU (600 mg/m², d 1–5) during the first and sixth week of hyperfractionated radiotherapy was compared to twice-daily hyperfractionated (125 cGy twice daily) radiotherapy alone, suggesting an improved 3-year survival (51 versus 28%, P=0.06) and a decreased incidence of distant metastases [29].

In a large randomized multicenter trial, concomitant split-course chemoradiotherapy with cisplatin and 5-FU was compared to sequential chemotherapy (induction) followed by radiation. Locoregional control was improved in the concomitant arm; however, an excess death rate due to complications in the concomitant chemoradiotherapy arm underlined the increase in toxicity and necessity of center experience [25]. Adelstein [29a] reported on a small randomized trial of simultaneous split-course chemoradiotherapy versus sequential treatment with three cycles of chemotherapy followed by uninterrupted radiation. The survival at >30 months was 68% versus 43% (P=0.13). Vokes and coworkers [30,31] reported on their promising experience with week on/week off chemoradiotherapy with continuous infusion 5-FU, hydroxyurea [30], ± cisplatin [31, 32], or paclitaxel [33].

In a randomized trial, rapidly alternating chemoradiotherapy with cisplatin/bolus 5-FU was compared to standard radiotherapy [34]. Of 157 patients with advanced unresectable head and neck cancer, 41% of the patients treated with combined modalities survived at 3 years but only 23% survived in the radiotherapy alone treatment group (P<0.05). Recent and ongoing trials attempt to improve response and overall outcome by using hyperfractionated radiation therapy with chemotherapy [35].

Hyperfractionated Radiotherapy
Concepts and Rationale

Altered fractionation schemes have been extensively evaluated in head and neck cancer [36]. The shorter time interval between doses reduces tumor repopulation. Simple hyperfractionation (smaller dose per fraction) will lead to a better tumor control with less late toxicity, allowing for administration of higher total doses. Accelerated hyperfractionated radiation delivers higher radiation doses per treatment time. The increased treatment intensity, however, will lead to more acute toxicity.

Randomized Trials

Despite multiple randomized trials, a benefit of hyperfractionation has only been demonstrated in a few [37–39]. Possibly, the increased acute toxicity with accelerated treatment regimes leads to more treatment interruptions, thus losing the gained benefit. In a randomized trial reported by Sanchiz [39] in 1990, hyperfractionated (64 fractions of 1.1 Gy; 2 fractions/d) was equivalent to chemoradiation (30 × 2 Gy; plus 5-FU every other day), but significantly superior to conventional radiotherapy alone. Two early trials conducted by the EORTC suggest an improved local control with hyperfractionated radiation [37,38]. However, the Radiation Therapy Oncology Group (RTOG) could not demonstrate a benefit with hyperfractionation [40]. The randomized continuous hyperfractionated accelerated radiotherapy (CHART) trial giving three fractions per day (3 × 1.50 Gy) for 12 days continuously also could not confirm an earlier impression of improved locoregional control [41]. A large randomized trial by the RTOG comparing four different radiation schedules has completed accrual; a preliminary analysis is expected in the near future.

Recurrent or Metastatic Disease

Chemotherapy has a limited role within standard therapy of head and neck cancer [11]. Traditionally, it is only used in recurrent or metastatic disease [42]. In this setting, the following drugs have been found active: methotrexate, cisplatin, carboplatin, 5-FU, bleomycin, mitomycin C, cyclophosphamide, doxorubicin, hydroxyurea, and more recently, paclitaxel [43], docetaxel [44], gemcitabine [45,46], and topotecan [47,48] (Table 10-5). The response rates as single agents are 10% to 30%, with a short response duration of only 2 to 6 months. A

Table 10-5. Current Treatment Regimens

	Response Rate†
Methotrexate 40–60 mg/m² IV weekly	10%–29%
Cisplatin 100 mg/m² iv every 3–4 wk	15%–27%
Cisplatin 100 mg/m² + 5-FU 800–1000 mg/daily as continuous infusion for 4–5 d, repeat every 3–4 wk*	30%–80%
Carboplatin 300–400 mg/m² + 5-FU 800–1000 mg/m² daily as continuous infusion for 4–5 d, repeat every 3–4 wk	20%–25%
Cisplatin 100 mg/m² + 5-FU 600–800 mg/m² with leucovorin (PFL) daily as continuous infusion for 4–5 d, repeat every 3–4 wk*	15%–90%
Paclitaxel 135–175 mg/m² over 3–24 h every 3–4 wk	30%–40%
Cisplatin, 5-FU, hydroxyurea and concomitant radiation*	70%–80%

*See separate listing later in this chapter.
†Range for untreated and recurrent disease.

Table 10-6. Current Cooperative Group Trials

Group	Patient Selection	Treatment	Remarks
Intergroup	Larynx, resectable, stage III/IV (not T1 or T4)	Radiotherapy vs cisplatin/RT vs induction CT-RT	Goal: larynx preservation NCI high priority trial
Intergroup	Resectable, stage III/IV	Surgery + RT vs surgery + RT/cisplatin	
ECOG/Intergroup	Uresectable head and neck cancer	Cisplatin/RT vs PF + split course RT vs standard RT	
SAKK	Most sites, stage III/IV locoregionally advanced	Hyperfractionated RT vs hyperfract RT/cisplatin	
EORTC	Early stage oral cavity; larynx and lung cancer	Postoperative RT vs postoperative RT/cisplatin	
England	Most sites, stage III/IV locoregionally advanced	CHART vs conventional RT	
Intergroup/RTOG	T1N0, T2N0 oral cavity, pharynx, larynx	Isotretinoin vs placebo	Chemoprevention
ECOG/NCCTG	T1N0, T2N0 head and neck cancer	Isotretinoin vs placebo	Chemoprevention
SWOG	T1N0, T2N0 head and neck cancer	Beta-carotene vs placebo	Chemoprevention
Euroscan/EORTC	Early stage oral cavity; larynx and lung cancer	N-acetylcystein vs retinylpalmitat vs N-acetylc. + R.-palmitat bs observation only	Chemoprevention: accrual complete, first results expected by 1997

CHART — Continous hyperfractionated, accelerated radiation therapy; CT — Chemotherapy; ECOG — Eastern Cooperative Oncology Group; EORTC — European Organisation for Research and Treatment of Cancer; NCCTG — Northern California Cancer Treatment Group; RT — radiotherapy; RTOG — Radiation Therapy Oncology Group; SAKK — Swiss Group for Clinical Cancer Research.

combination of cisplatin and 5-FU has frequently been used for recurrent disease, with response rates of 30% to 40 %. In a randomized trial, the response rate for the combination was 32%, compared with 13% for single-agent 5-FU, and 17% for cisplatin. Despite this increased response rate, an improved survival could not been demonstrated [49]. Another randomized trial compared cisplatin/5-FU and carboplatin/5-FU with methotrexate [50]. The response rates were 32%, 21%, and 10%, respectively. Median response duration was only 4.2, 5.1, and 4.1 months, and no difference in overall survival was observed. The combination increased toxicity, causing nausea and vomiting, nephrotoxicity, and ototoxicity. Patients receiving 5-FU experienced significant mucositis. Patients with a poor performance status usually are less tolerant of chemotherapy and are more prone to complications. Because of the lack of a survival advantage, some investigators still consider single-agent methotrexate as standard chemotherapy, despite the very low response rates. Paclitaxel shows promising activity in phase II trials [43]. The EORTC is currently conducting a randomized trial comparing two schedules of paclitaxel with weekly methotrexate (Table 10-6).

CHEMOPREVENTION

Leukoplakia

Oral leukoplakia is a recognized premalignant condition that can lead to invasive squamous cell carcinoma. 13-cis-retinoic acid has been shown efficacious in reversing this precancerous condition (Table 10-7) [51]. The response rate was 67%, with a clinical complete response of 54% and a histologic one of 38%. In the high dosages used (1–2 mg/kg), the retinoic acid has significant toxicity, particularly dry and peeling skin, facial erythema, cheilitis (79%), hypertriglyceridemia (71%), and conjunctivitis (54%), as well as headaches, fatigue, anorexia, and pruritus. After discontinuation of the therapy, a high incidence of relapse is noted after a few months. Recent data suggest a maintenance therapy of 0.5 mg/kg/d, which causes only mild side effects [52]. Over 9 months only 8% of the patients receiving maintenance therapy with low-dose retinoic acid had a progression, compared with a control group treated with beta carotene, in which 55% of the patients had progression.

Second Malignancies

In the first 2 to 3 years, local recurrence is the most common type of relapse. In subsequent years, a higher percentage of patients present with secondary malignancies (eg, a second head and neck cancer, lung cancer). Regular monitoring and follow-up focusing on other potential disease sites is therefore mandatory in these patients. Instructions and support are needed to help the patient avoid further risk factor exposure (smoking, alcohol). Hong and colleagues [53] showed that the incidence of second primary tumors can be reduced markedly by daily high doses (50–100 mg/m^2) of 13-cis-retinoic acid (see Table 10-7). But this therapy does not prevent recurrence of the original tumor [53,54]. Large, long-term randomized chemoprevention trials are being conducted by several cooperative groups.

Table 10-7. Chemoprevention Trails With 13-cis Retinoic Acid

	Evaluable Patients, n	Regimen	Response Rates
Oral Leucoplakia			
Induction–3 mo	24	cis-RA 1–2 mg/kg	16 (67%)
(Hong et al. [51])	20	Placebo	2 (10%)
			(P=.0002)
			Progression
Maintenance–9 mo	26	cis-RA 0.5 mg/kg	2 (8%)
(Lippman et al. [52])	33	Beta-carotene	16 (55%)
			(P<.001)
Second Malignancies			**Second Primary**
Maintenance–12 mo	49	cis-RA 50–100 mg/m^2	2 (4%)
(Hong et al. [53])	51	Placebo	12 (24%)

REFERENCES

1. Vokes EE, Weichselbaum RR, Lippman SM, Hong WK: Medical progress: head and neck cancer. *N Engl J Med* 1993, 328:184–1894.

2. Spitz MR: Epidemiology and risk factors for head and neck cancer. *Semin Oncol* 1994, 21:281–288.

3. Fandi A, Altun M, Azli N, *et al.*: Nasopharyngeal cancer: epidemiology, staging, and treatment. *Semin Oncol* 1994, 21:382–397.

4. Li X, Lee NK, Ye YW, *et al.*: Allelic loss at chromosomes 30, 80, 13q, and 17p associated with poor prognosis in head and neck cancer. *J Natl Cancer Inst* 1994, 86:1524–1529.

5. Calhoun KH, Fulmer P, Weiss R, Hokanson JA: Distant metastases from head and neck squamous cell carcinomas. *Laryngoscope* 1994, 104:1199–1205.

6. Liebovitz D: Nasopharyngeal carcinoma: the Epstein-Barr virus association. *Semin Oncol* 1994, 21:376–381.

7. Cvitkovic E: Neoadjuvant chemotherapy with epirubicin, cisplatin, bleomycin in undifferentiated nasopharyngeal cancer: preliminary results of an international phase III trial [abstract]. *Proc Am Soc Clin Oncol* 1994, 13:283.

8. Cvitkovic E, Eschwege F, Rahal M, *et al.*: Preliminary results of a randomized trial comparing neoadjuvant chemotherapy (cisplatin, epirubicin, bleomycin) plus radiotherapy vs. radiotherapy alone in stage IV (≤ N2, M0) undifferentiated nasopharyngeal carcinoma: a positive effect on progression-free survival. *Int J Radiat Oncol Biol Phys* 1996, 35:463–469.

9. Al-Sarraf M, LeBlanc M, Giri PG, *et al.*: Superiority of chemoradiotherapy (CT-RT) vs radiotherapy (RT) in patients with locally advances nasopharyngeal cancer (NPC): preliminary results of Intergroup (0099) (SWOG 9982, RTOG 8817, ECOG 2388) randomized study [abstract]. *Proc Am Soc Clin Oncol* 1996, 15:313.

10. Kim KH, Sung MW, Chung PS, *et al.*: Adenoid cystic carcinoma of the head and neck. *Arch Otolaryngol Head Neck Surg* 1994, 120:721–762.

11. Browman GP, Cronin L: Standard chemotherapy in squamous cell head and neck cancer: what we have learned from randomized trials. *Semin Oncol* 1994, 21:311–319.

12. Forastiere AA: Randomized trials of induction chemotherapy: a critical review. *Hematol Oncol Clin North Am* 1991, 5:725–736.

13. Clark JR, Fallon BG, Dreyfuss AI, *et al.*: Chemotherapeutic strategies in the multidisciplinary treatment of head and neck cancer. *Semin Oncol* 1988, 15:35–44.

14. Paccagnella A, Orlando A, Marchiori C, *et al.*: Phase III trial of initial chemotherapy in stage III or IV head and neck cancers: a study by the Gruppo di Studio sui Tumori della Testa e del Collo. *J Natl Cancer Inst* 1994, 86:265–272.

15. The Department of Veterans Affairs Laryngeal Cancer Study Group: Induction chemotherapy plus radiation compared with surgery plus radiation in patients with advanced laryngeal cancer. *N Engl J Med* 1991, 324:1685–1690.

16. Laramore GE, Scott CB, Al Sarraf M, *et al.*: Adjuvant chemotherapy for resectable squamous cell carcinoma of the head and neck: report on intergroup study 0034. *Int J Radiat Oncol Biol Phys* 1992, 23:705–713.

17. Schuller DE, Laramore GE, Al Sarraf M, Jacobs JJ: Phase III study to determine the effect of combining chemotherapy with surgery and radiotherapy for resectable squamous cell carcinoma of the head and neck [meeting abstract]. Second International Conference on Head and Neck Cancer, 1988.

18. Head and Neck Contracts Program: Adjuvant chemotherapy for advanced head and neck squamous carcinoma: final report. *Cancer* 1987, 60:301–311.

19. Lefebvre J, Chevalier D, Luboinski B, *et al.*: Larynx preservation in pyriform sinus cancer: preliminary results of a European Organization for Research and Treatment of Cancer phase III trial. *J Natl Cancer Inst* 1996, 88:890–899.

20. Jacobs C, Makuch R: Efficacy of adjuvant chemotherapy for patients with resectable head and neck cancer: a subset analysis of the Head and Neck Contracts Program. *J Clin Oncol* 1990, 8:838–847.

21. Urba SG, Forastiere AA, Wolf GT, *et al.*: Intensive induction chemotherapy and radiation for organ preservation in patients with advanced resectable head and neck carcinoma. *J Clin Oncol* 1994, 12:946–953.

22. Stupp R, Weichselbaum RR, Vokes EE: Combined modality therapy of head and neck cancer. *Semin Oncol* 1994, 21:349–358.

23. Vokes EE, Weichselbaum RR: Concomitant chemoradiotherapy: rationale and clinical experience in patients with solid tumors. *J Clin Oncol* 1990, 8:911–934.

24. Denham JW, Abbott RL: Concurrent cisplatin, infusional fluorouracil, and conventionally fractionated radiation therapy in head and neck cancer: dose-limiting mucosal toxicity. *J Clin Oncol* 1991, 9:458–463.

25. Taylor SI, Murthy AK, Vannetzel JM, *et al.*: Randomized comparison of neoadjuvant cisplatin and fluorouracil infusion followed by radiation versus concomitant treatment in advanced head and neck cancer. *J Clin Oncol* 1994, 12:385–395.

26. Stupp R, Vokes EE: 5-FU plus radiation for head and neck cancer. *J Infusion Chemother* 1996.

27. Browman GP, Cripps C, Hodson DI, *et al.*: Placebo-controlled randomized trial of infusional fluorouracil during standard radiotherapy in locally advanced head and neck cancer. *J Clin Oncol* 1994, 12:2648–2653.

28. Bachaud JM, David JM, Boussin G, Daly N: Combined postoperative radiotherapy and weekly cisplatin infusion for locally advanced squamous cell carcinoma of the head and neck: preliminary report of a randomized trial. *Int J Radiat Oncol Biol Phys* 1991, 20:243–246.

29. Brizel D, Albers M, Fisher S, *et al.*: A phase III trial of hyperfractionated irradiation 1 concurrent chemotherapy for locally advanced carcinoma of the head and neck: superiority of combined modality treatment [abstract]. *Proc Am Soc Clin Oncol* 1997, 16:384a.

29a. Adelstein DJ, Sharan VM, Earle AS, *et al.*: Simultaneous versus sequential combined technique therapy for squamous cell head and neck cancer. *Cancer* 1990, 65:1685–1691.

30. Vokes EE, Haraf DJ, Mick R, *et al.*: Concomitant chemoradiotherapy for intermediate stage head and neck cancer (HNC) [meeting abstract]. *Proc Am Soc Clin Oncol* 1994, 13:909.

31. Vokes EE, Haraf DJ, Mick R, *et al.*: Intensified concomitant chemoradiotherapy with and without filgastrim for poor-prognosis head and neck cancer. *J Clin Oncol* 1994, 12:2351–2359.

32. Kies MS, Haraf DJ, Mittal B, *et al.*: Intensive combined therapy with C-DDP, 5-FU, hydroxyurea, and bid radiation (C-FHX) for stage IV squamous cell cancer (SCC) of the head and neck [abstract]. *Proc Am Soc Clin Oncol* 1996, 15:314.

33. Brockstein B, Haraf D, Stenson K, *et al.*: A phase I study of concomitant chemoradiotherapy with paclitaxel, 5-FU, and hydroxyurea with granulocyte colony-stimulating factor support for patients with poor prognosis cancer of the head and neck. *J Clin Oncol* 1998, 16:735–744.

34. Merlano M, Vitale V, Rosso R, *et al.*: Treatment of advanced squamous-cell carcinoma of the head and neck with alternating chemotherapy and radiotherapy. *N Engl J Med* 1992, 327:1115–1121.

35. Leyvraz S, Pasche P, Bauer J, *et al.*: Rapidly alternating chemotherapy and hyperfractionated radiotherapy in the management of locally advanced head and neck carcinoma: four-year results of a phase I/II study. *J Clin Oncol* 1994, 12:1876–1885.

36. Beck-Bronholdt HP, Dubben HH, Liertz-Petersen C, Willers H: Hyperfractionation: where do we start? *Radiother Oncol* 1997, 43:1–21.

37. Horiot JC, Bontemps P, Begg AC, *et al.*: Hyperfractionated and accelerated radiotherapy in head and neck cancer: results of the EORTC trials and impact on clinical practice. *Bull Cancer Radiother* 1996, 83:314–320.

38. Horiot JC, Le Fur R, N'Guyen T, *et al.*: Hyperfractionation versus conventional fractionation in oropharyngeal carcinoma: final analysis of a randomized trial of the EORTC cooperative group of radiotherapy. *Radiother Oncol* 1992, 25:231–241.

39. Sanchiz F, Milla A, Torner J, *et al.*: Single fraction per day versus two fractions per day versus radiochemotherapy in the treatment of head and neck cancer. *Int J Radiat Oncol Biol Phys* 1990, 19:1347–1350.

40. Marcial VA, Pajak TF, Chu C, *et al.*: Hyperfractionated photon radiation therapy in the treatment of advanced squamous cell carcinoma of the oral cavity, pharynx, larynx, and sinuses, using radiation therapy as the only planned modality: preliminary report by the Radiation Therapy Oncology Group (RTOG). *Int Radiat Oncol Biol Phys* 1987, 13:41–47.

41. Saunders MI, Disches S, Barrett A, *et al.*: Randomised multicentre trials of CHART vs conventional radiotherapy in head and neck carcinoma with distant metastases: a retrospective analysis of 44 cases treated with cisplatin-based chemotherapeutic regimens. *Anticancer Res* 1993, 13:1129–1131.

42. Gebbia V, Agostara B, Callarri A, *et al.*: Head and neck carcinoma with distant metastases: a retrospective analysis of 44 cases treated with cisplatin-based chemotherapeutic regimens. *Anticancer Res* 1993, 13:1129–1131.

43. Forastiere AA: Paclitaxel (Taxol) for the treatment of head and neck cancer. *Semin Oncol* 1994, 21:49–52.

44. Catimel G, Verweij J, Mattijssen V, *et al.*: Docetaxel (Taxotere): an active drug for the treatment of patients with advanced squamous cell carcinoma of the head and neck. *Ann Oncol* 1994, 5:533–537.

45. Catimel G, Vermorken JB, Clavel M, *et al.*: A phase II study of gemcitabine (LY 188011) in patients with advanced squamous cell carcinoma of the head and neck. *Ann Oncol* 1994, 5:543–547.

46. Couteau C, Chouaki N, Leyvraz S, *et al.*: A phase II study of docetaxel in patients with metastatic squamous cell carcinoma of the head and neck. In press.

47. Robert F, Soong SJ, Wheeler RH: A phase II study of topotecan in patients with recurrent head and neck cancer: identification of an active agent. *Am J Clin Oncol* 1997, 20:298–302.

48. Smith RE, Lew D, Rodriguez GI, *et al.*: Evaluation of topotecan in patients with recurrence for metastatic squamous cell carcinoma of the head and neck: a phase II SWOG study. *Invest New Drugs* 1996, 14:403–407.

49. Jacobs C, Lyman G, Velez Garcia E, *et al.*: A phase III randomized study comparing cisplatin and fluorouracil as single agents and in combination for advanced squamous cell carcinoma of the head and neck. *J Clin Oncol* 1992, 10:257–263.

50. Forastiere AA, Metch B, Schuller DE, *et al.*: Randomized comparison of cisplatin plus fluorouracil and carboplatin plus fluorouracil versus methotrexate in advanced squamous-cell carcinoma of the head and neck: a Southwest Oncology Group study. *J Clin Oncol* 1992, 10:1245–1251.

51. Hong WK, Endicott J, Itri LM, *et al.*: 13-cis-Retinoic acid in the treatment of oral leukoplakia. *N Engl J Med* 1986, 315:1501–1505.

52. Lippman SM, Batsakis JG, Toth BB, *et al.*: Comparison of low-dose isotretinoin with beta carotene to prevent oral carcinogenesis. *N Engl J Med* 1993, 328:15–20.

53. Hong WK, Lippman SM, Itri LM, *et al.*: Prevention of secondary primary tumors with isotretinoin in squamous-cell carcinoma of the head and neck. *N Engl J Med* 1990, 323:795–801.

54. Papadimitrakopoulou VA, Hong WK, Lee JS, *et al.*: Low-dose isotretinoin versus beta carotene to prevent oral carcinogenesis: long-term follow-up. *J Natl Cancer Inst* 1997, 89:257–258.

55. Stupp R, Vokes EE: *Therapiekonzepte Onkologie*, ed 3. Heidelberg: Springer Verlag; 1998.

The information here is provided as guidance only. Prescribers should always consult the manufacturer's current prescribing information.

171

CISPLATIN AND 5-FLUOROURACIL

Platinum compounds are complex molecules that covalently bind to DNA and also interact with proteins. The two available agents in this class, cisplatin and carboplatin, have a different toxicity profile. Carboplatin has less renal toxicity, but myelo-suppression and mainly thrombocytopenia can be pronounced. Response rates for single-agent use are ~30% for cisplatin and 20% for carboplatin.

The antimetabolite 5-FU is commonly used in many combination regimens and as a single agent. This pyrimidine analogue interferes with DNA and RNA synthesis by binding to thymidylate synthase, or it can be incorporated into RNA as a false messenger. In head and neck cancer, 5-FU alone has not commonly been used, but a single-agent response rate of 15% has been reported. The response rate depends on the dose and schedule. A randomized trial has suggested that continuous infusion therapy over 4–5 d is superior to IV bolus administration (when 5-FU is given in combination with cisplatin) in recurrent disease.

The combination of the two agents can significantly improve the overall response rate. Several trials using this combination showed an overall response rate of 25%–40%, with 15% complete responders in the recurrent disease groups. However, randomized trials have failed to demonstrate improved survival using this combination compared with single-agent chemotherapy.

CANDIDATES FOR TREATMENT

Recurrent or metastatic disease; locally advanced advanced larynx and hypopharynx cancer for organ preservation

SPECIAL PRECAUTIONS

Hydration for 6–12 h before and after cisplatin administration; antiemetic prophylaxis during initial 48 h after cisplatin administration

ALTERNATIVE THERAPIES

Methotrexate, carboplatin and 5-FU, cisplatin or 5-FU (single agent), paclitaxel

TOXICITIES

Cisplatin: highly emetogenic, nephrotoxicity, cumulative ototoxicity, metallic taste in mouth; late chronic neuropathy (up to 40% of patients); myelosuppression (nadir after approx 10 d); electrolyte wasting (K, Mg); **5-FU:** mucositis, diarrhea, increased liver enzymes

DRUG INTERACTIONS

Cisplatin: antimetabolites, nephrotoxic agents (*eg*, aminoglycoside); **5-FU:** leucovorin, interferon, dipyridamole

RECENT EXPERIENCE AND RESPONSE RATES

Study	Evaluable Patients, *n*	Regimen	Response Rates/Survival
Recurrent disease			
Clavel *et al.*/EORTC Ann Oncol 1994, 5:521–526	116	cDDP 100 mg/m2 x 1 + 5-FU 1000 mg/m² x 4 d ci	CR=1.7%, RR=31%; TTP 17 wk,
	127	cDDP 50 mg/m², d 4; methotrexate 40 mg/m², d 1, 8; bleomycin 10 mg + vincristine 2 mg, d 1, 8, 15	CR=9.5%, RR=34%; TTP 19 wk, median survival for all 365 patients: 29 wk
	122; mainly recurrent, no prior chemotherapy	cDDP 50 mg/m2, d 1, 8	CR=2.5%, RR=15%; TTP 12 wk
Jacobs *et al.* J Clin Oncol 1992, 10:257–263	79, eval. 63	cDDP 100 mg/m2 x 1 + 5-FU 1000 mg/m2 x 4 d ci	CR=5, PR=20; RR=32%; surv. > 9 mo: 40
	83, eval. 80	cDDP 100 mg/m2 x 1	CR=3, PR=11; RR=17%; surv. > 9 mo: 24
	83, eval. 75; recurrent or metastatic	5-FU 1000 mg/m2 x 4 d	CR=2, PR=9; RR=13%; surv. > 9 mo: 27
Forastiere *et al.* (SWOG), J Clin Oncol 1992, 10:1245–1251	87; randomized	CDDP 100 mg/m² + 5-FU 1000 mg/m² x 4 d ci	RR=32%; surv. 6.6 mo
	86	Carboplatin 300 mg/m² + 5-FU 1000 mg/m² x 4 d ci	RR=21% (ns); surv. 5.0 mo
	88; recurrent or metastatic	MTX 40 mg/m2 IV every week	RR=10%; surv. 5.6 mo
Kish *et al.* Cancer 1985 56:2740–2744	18; randomized	cDDP 100 mg/m² + 5-FU 600 mg/m² bolus d 1 + 8	CR=2, PR=2; RR=20%
	20; locally adv. + recurrent	cDDP 100 mg/m² + 5-FU 1000 mg/m² x 4 d ci	CR=4, PR=9; RR=72%

Continued

CISPLATIN AND 5-FLUOROURACIL (Continued)

RECENT EXPERIENCE AND RESPONSE RATES Continued

Study	Evaluable Patients, n	Regimen	Response Rates/Survival
No prior therapy/induction chemotherapy			
Paccanella et al. J Natl Cancer Inst 1994, 86:265–272	118	cDDP 100 mg/m² x 1 + 5-FU 1000mg/m², d 1–5 ci x 4 cycles, followed by (surgery) + XRT 200 cGy/1 x d versus	CR=31, PR=55, RR=80%; 2-y survival: 37; inop. pts, 2-y survival: 30; distant mets: 9 at 2 y
	119; locally advanced	(Surgery) + XRT 200 cGy/1 x d	CR=67 (56%); 2 y survival: 29; inop. pts, 2-y survival: 19; distant mets: 32 at 2 y
Veterans Affairs Larynx Cancer Study Group. N Engl J Med 1991,	166	cDDP 100 mg/m² x 1 + 5-FU 1000mg/m², d 1–5 ci, x 3 cycles, followed by XRT 200 cGy/1 x d ± salvage surgery versus	CR=31, RR=54%; distant mets: 11%
	166	surgery + XRT 200 cGy/1 x d	larynx preservation: 64%; distant mets: 17%
Vokes et al. J Clin Oncol 1991, 9:1376–1384	advanced larynx; 51, neoadjuvant and adjuvant	cDDP 100 mg/m² x 1, 5-FU 1000 mg/m² x 5 d ci	CR=22 (43%); pCR=24%; PR=24 (47%); RR=90%

NURSING INTERVENTIONS

Agents can be administered by a peripheral venous access. Extravasation causes local irritation; monitor fluid status; watch for dehydration and overhydration; do not administer cisplatin if urine output <100 mL/h over the last 4 h prior to start; monitor electrolytes including magnesium and start supplements early

PATIENT INFORMATION

Patient may experience delayed nausea/vomiting with cisplatin; antiemetic must be available at all times; contact physician immediately for fevers (neutropenia possible), bleeding (thrombocytopenia rare), and diarrhea (electrolyte wasting, dehydration).

DOSAGE AND SCHEDULING

Cisplatin 100 mg/m² IV over 2–6 h: d l	■									
5-FU 1000 mg/m²/d IV continuous infusion for 4–5 d	▬▬▬▬▬									
CBC, platelets: d 1, 5, 10	☐				☐					
Na, K, Mg, BUN, Crea: d 1, 3, 5, 10	☐		☐		☐					☐
SGOT, SGPT, alk. Phos, Albumin: d 1	☐									
Day	1	2	3	4	5	6	7	8	9	10

Repeat every 3–4 wk.
CR—complete response; pCR—pathologic complete response; PR—partial response.
Dosage Modifications: For impaired renal function, reduce cDDP to 75% for creatinine clearance of 50–75 mL/min, to < 50% for clearance of 25–50 mL\min. Do not administer if clearance < 25 mL/min. For grade III mucositis decrease 5-FU to 80% (eg, administer 4 d only).

CONCOMITANT CHEMORADIOTHERAPY WITH SINGLE-AGENT 5-FLUOROURACIL OR CISPLATIN

Cisplatin and 5-fluorouracil (5-FU) are known for their radiosensitizing effects. The mechanism of this interaction is not completely known. Theoretically, several mechanisms have been postulated. Ideally both, the chemotherapeutic agent and the radiation must have independent antitumor activity. Acting against different sites of the tumor cell, they enhance each other by inhibiting tumor cell recovery from sublethal damage. They have additive cytotoxicity and prevent tumor resistance. Because radiation therapy is cell-cycle specific, the chemotherapy may synchronize and block the tumor cells in S phase and, thus, make them more radiosensitive. Decreased tumor bulk may improve drug delivery to the remaining tumor cells.

Cisplatin causes direct DNA damage by intrastrand crosslinks and breaks. It acts mainly with synergistic cytotoxicity by inhibiting DNA repair from sublethal cell damage.

5-FU is either incorporated into RNA or binds to thymidylate synthase and, thus, inhibits DNA synthesis. Synergy with radiation has been shown in several in vitro studies in which subtherapeutic doses of radiation or 5-FU were not able to induce cell death, but the combination showed increased cytotoxicity. The mechanism of this interaction remains unclear; possibly the cells become more sensitive to the radiation by modification of the cell kinetics.

CANDIDATES FOR TREATMENT
Patients with locally advanced squamous cell carcinoma of the head and neck, recurrent unresectable disease for locoregional control; patients who are candidates for postoperative radiotherapy

TOXICITIES
Mucositis, weight loss, myelosuppression, renal insufficiency (with cisplatin)

NURSING INTERVENTIONS
Good oral hygiene with nonalcoholic antiseptic mouthwashes (4 x d); fungal prophylaxis with nystatin mouthwash or clotrimazole troches; watch nutritional status (if insufficient, suggest feeding tube)

PATIENT INFORMATION
Patient should be aware of mucositis potential; mouth care needs to be emphasized; encourage good and regular nutrition and fluid intake.

RECENT EXPERIENCES AND RESPONSE RATES

Study	Evaluable Patients, n	Regimen	Response Rates	Survival
Browman et al.: J Clin Oncol 1994, 12: 2648–2653	87	Placebo infusion + XRT 200 cGy/d	CR 49 (56%)	24 mo: 50%
		vs.		
	88	5-FU 1200 mg/m^2/d × 3 d ci, wk 1 & 3, + concomitant XRT 200 cGy/d	CR 60 (68%)	24 mo: 63%
Sanchiz et al.: Int J Radiat Oncol Biol Phys 1990, 19:1347–1350	306	5-FU 250 mg/m^2 qod + RT 2.0 Gy qd	CR 96%	Median: 85 mo
		vs.		
	292	RT 1.1 Gy bid	CR 90%	Median: 84 mo
		vs.		
	294	RT 2.0 Gy qd	CR 68%	Median: 38 mo
Bachaud et al.: Int J Radiat Oncol Biol Phys 1991, 20:243–246	39	Cisplatin 50 mg/wk + RT qd	postoperative RT	2-y: 75%
		vs.		
	44	RT qd		2-y: 44% ($P < 0.05$)
Glicksman et al.: Int J Radiat Oncol Biol Phys 1994, 30:1043–1050	101	Cisplatin 20 mg/m^2, d1-4, wk 1 & 3 + RT qd	pathologic CR of operated patients: 82%	3-y: 78% (other causes of death excluded) actuarial 9-y: 49%
Al-Sarraf (RTOG 88-24): Int J Radiat Oncol Biol Phys 1997, 37:777–782	52	Cisplatin 100 mg/m^2; d 1, 23, 43; + RT qd (30 X 2 Gy)	postoperative RT	3-y: 48% (actuarial)
Jeremic et al.: Radiother Oncol 1997, 43:29–37	53	Carboplatin 25 mg/m^2 qd + RT qd (35 × 2 Gy)	CR 68%, PR 17%	Median: 30 mo, 2 y: 55%
		vs.		
	53	Cisplatin 6 mg/m^2 qd + RT qd (35 × 2 Gy)	CR 72%, PR 9%	Median: 32 mo, 2 y: 58%
		vs.		
	53	RT qd (35 × 2 Gy)	CR 38%, PR 21%	Median: 16 mo, 2 y: 35%

CONCOMITANT CHEMORADIOTHERAPY WITH SINGLE-AGENT 5-FLUOROURACIL OR CISPLATIN (Continued)

DOSAGE AND SCHEDULING

	Week 1	2	3	4	5	6	7	8	9	10
Cisplatin 100 mg/m² iv over 1–6 h: d 1	■			■			■			
or										
5-FU 1200 mg/m² continual infusion over 24 h: d 1–3	■			■			■			
Radiotherapy 200 cGy qd: d 1–5	□	□	□	□	□	□	□	□	□	
CBC, platelets: weekly	▭▭▭▭▭▭▭▭▭▭ (continuous)									
Na, K, Mg, BUN, Creatinine: d 1, 3, 5	□□□			□□□			□□□			□□□
SGOT, SGPT, alk.Phos, Albumin: d 1	□			□			□			□

Repeat every 3–4 wk; cisplatin every other cycle.

Dosage Modifications: For impaired renal function, reduce cisplatin to 75% for creatinine clearance of 50–75 mL/min and then to 50% of clearance of 25–50 min. Do not administer if clearance < 25 mL/min. Avoid cisplatin in patients who are hearing impaired. For grad III mucositis, decrease 5-FU to 80%.

CONCOMITANT SPLIT-COURSE CHEMORADIOTHERAPY (WEEK ON/WEEK OFF)
5-Fluorouracil, Hydroxyurea ± Cisplatin

Cisplatin, 5-FU, and hydroxyurea have long been known for their radiosensitizing effects. The mechanism of this interaction is not completely known. Several mechanisms have been postulated. Ideally both the chemotherapeutic agent and the radiation must have independent antitumor activity. Acting against different sites of the tumor cell, they enhance each other by inhibiting tumor cell recovery from sublethal damage. They have additive cytotoxicity and prevent tumor resistance. As radiation therapy is cell-cycle specific, the chemotherapy may synchronize and block the tumor cells in S phase and thus make them more radiosensitive. Decreased tumor bulk may improve drug delivery to the remaining tumor cells. These drugs have been used as single agents with simultaneous radiation therapy in a variety of malignant diseases.

Concomitant radiation therapy with full-dose chemotherapy significantly increase toxicities. Severe mucositis is very common, and the majority of patients require placement of a feeding tube. For regeneration of the normal tissues, this approach requires scheduled rest periods.

Cisplatin causes direct DNA damage by intrastrand cross-links and breaks. It acts mainly with synergistic cytotoxicity by inhibiting DNA repair from sublethal cell damage.

5-Fluorouracil is either incorporated into RNA or binds to thymidylate synthase and thus inhibits DNA synthesis. Synergy with radiation has been shown in several in vitro studies, where subtherapeutic doses of radiation or 5-FU were not able to induce cell death, but the combination showed increased cytotoxicity. The mechanisms of this interaction remains unclear. Possibly the cells become more sensitive to the radiation by modification of the cell kinetics.

Hydroxyurea inhibits ribonucleotide reductase specifically in the S phase. It alters the cell kinetics by inhibiting entry into the radioresistant S phase. As an antimetabolite hydroxyurea inhibits DNA synthesis or repair. Although it has single-agent activity in head and neck cancer, it is rarely used other than as a radiosensitizer.

Paclitaxel stabilizes the mitotic spindle tubules, causing cell cycle arrest in the radiation sensitive G_2/M-phase of the cell cycle. Prolonged exposure appears to increase radiosensitizing properties. Paclitaxel has single-agent activity against head and neck cancer.

CANDIDATES FOR TREATMENT
Patients with locally advanced and recurrent squamous cell carcinoma of the head and neck

TOXICITIES
Severe mucositis, weight loss (forced feeding commonly necessary)

NURSING INTERVENTIONS
Good oral hygiene with nonalcoholic antiseptic mouthwashes (4 ×/d); fungal prophylaxis with nystatin mouthwash or clotrimazole troches; insufficient food and fluid intake commonly requires feeding tube

PATIENT INFORMATION
Patient should be aware of mucositis potential; mouth care needs to be emphasized.

CONCOMITANT SPLIT-COURSE CHEMORADIO-THERAPY (WEEK ON/WEEK OFF) (Continued)
5-Fluorouracil, Hydroxyurea ± Cisplatin

RECENT EXPERIENCES AND RESPONSE RATES

Study	Evaluable Patients, n	Regimen	Response Rates	Survival/Remarks, %
Vokes et al. J Clin Oncol 1994, 12:2351–2359	17 (recurrent)	CDDP 100 mg/m^2, d 1 + 5-FU 800 mg/m^2, d 1–5 + HU 1000 mg bid plus concomitant XRT 200 cGy/1 × d ± G-CSF	CR=11 (64%) RR=76%	Median survival: 12 mo Median TTF: 8 mo
	28 (no prior therapy)		CR=21 (75%) RR=89%	Median survival: 12 mo Median TTF: not reached
Taylor et al. J Clin Oncol 1994, 12:385–395	107 vs.	CDDP 100 mg/m^2, d 1 + 5-FU 1000 mg/m^2/d, d 1-5 ci × 3 cycles followed by XRT (seq)	CR=50 (47%) PR=28 (26%) RR=73%	Marked differences in response rates depending on treatment institution; significantly improved local control with concomitant therapy
	107 (locally advanced)	CDDP 60 mg/m^2, d1 +5-FU 800 mg/m^2/d, d 1–5 ci plus concomitant XRT 200 cGy/1× d, every other week	CR=52 (49%) PR=41 (38%) RR=87	
Adelstein et al./ECOG J Clin Oncol 1993, 11:2136–2142	52 (locally advanced)	CDDP 75 mg/m^2 × 1 + 5-FU 1000 mg/m^2 × 4 d ci plus concomitant XRT 200 cGy qd × 15 (3000 cGy total), followed by chemotherapy only × 1 cycle and subsequently the same chemoradiotherapy	CR=77%	4-y survival: 49%
Adelstein et al. Cancer 1990, 65:1685–1691	24 (simultaneous therapy) vs.	CDDP 75 mg/m^2 × 1 + 5-FU 1000 mg/m^2 × 4 d ci (repeat chemo on d 28) plus concomitant XRT 200 cGy qd × 15 (3000 cGy total), possibly surgery and repeat above	CR=16, PR=8 RR=100%	Neutropenia grade IV: 10 (42%), one toxic death; trend for improved overall survival with simultaneous therapy
	24 (sequential therapy)	CDDP 100 mg/m^2 × 1 + 5-FU 1000 mg/m^2 × 5 d ci × 3 cycles, followed by possible surgery and RT 6000 cGy total	CR=7, PR=13 RR=83%	Neutropenia grade IV: 14 (58%), two toxic deaths
Weppelmann et al. Int J Radiat Oncol Bio Phys 1992, 22:1051–1056	21 (evaluated 20) Recurrent or metastatic, after previous surgery and radiation	5-FU 300 mg/m^2 × 5 d ci + HU > 1500 mg/m^2 qd × 5 d + XRT 200 cGy qd × 5 d every other week	CR=9, PR=6, RR=75%	1-y survival: 56%
Wendt et al. J Clin Oncol 1989, 7:471–476	59 (locally advanced)	CDDP 60 mg/m^2 × 1 + 5-FU 350 mg/m^2 × 4 d ci + LV 50 mg/m^2 × 4 d ci plus concomitant XRT 180 cGy qd × 11 d	CR=48 (81%) PR=11 (19%) RR=100%	
Brockstein et al.: J Clin Oncol 1998, 16:735–744	55 (mainly recurrent) phase II:20	Paclitaxel 5–20 mg/m^2, d 1-5 ci + 5-FU 600 mg/m2, d 1-5 ci + HU 500 mg bid plus concomitant XRT 200 cGy/once daily or 150 cGy/twice daily	CR 65%, PR 10%	Phase I/II dose finding study

CDDP—cisplatin; ci—continuous infusion; CR—complete response rate; 5-FU—5-Fluorouracil; HU—hydroxyurea; PR—partial response rate; RR—overall response rate; XRT—external radiation therapy.

DOSAGE AND SCHEDULING

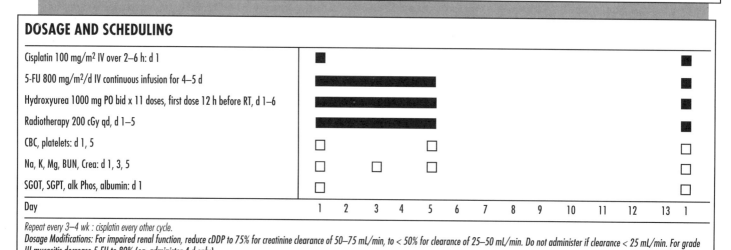

	1	2	3	4	5	6	7	8	9	10	11	12	13	1

Cisplatin 100 mg/m^2 IV over 2–6 h: d 1
5-FU 800 mg/m^2/d IV continuous infusion for 4–5 d
Hydroxyurea 1000 mg PO bid x 11 doses, first dose 12 h before RT, d 1–6
Radiotherapy 200 cGy qd, d 1–5
CBC, platelets: d 1, 5
Na, K, Mg, BUN, Crea: d 1, 3, 5
SGOT, SGPT, alk Phos, albumin: d 1
Day

Repeat every 3–4 wk : cisplatin every other cycle.
Dosage Modifications: For impaired renal function, reduce cDDP to 75% for creatinine clearance of 50–75 mL/min, to < 50% for clearance of 25–50 mL/min. Do not administer if clearance < 25 mL/min. For grade III mucositis decrease 5-FU to 80% (eg, administer 4 d only).

Lung cancer is the leading cause of cancer mortality in both men and women in the Unites States, accounting for more than 29% of all cancer deaths in 1997. The estimated number of new cases of lung cancer in 1997 is 178,000, with an estimated 160,400 lung cancer deaths [1]. Lung cancer is the third most common cancer in the U.S. behind prostate and breast cancer, but more Americans will die from this dreaded disease than from breast cancer, prostate cancer, and colorectal cancer combined because of the low 14% cure rate [1]. This low rate can be ascribed almost exclusively to the high propensity for metastatic spread, the lack of effective screening measures, and the inability of systemic therapy to cure metastatic disease. The majority of patients present with inoperable stage III disease or with metastasis to distant organs (stage IV) [2]. Patients with stage IV disease are rarely cured with previous chemotherapeutic approaches [2]. A small minority of patients (approximately 10%–15%) with advanced regional stage III disease with either small cell lung cancer (SCLC) or non–small cell lung cancer (NSCLC) may be cured with intensive combined modality approaches. Surgery cures 20% to 60% of operable cases depending on stage [2]. Because most patients develop systemic disease, chemotherapy will be indicated for a high percentage of patients. Chemotherapeutic options have improved considerably in recent years, with more effective and less toxic regimens now available. Chemotherapy improves symptoms, quality of life, and survival of lung cancer patients.

ETIOLOGY AND RISK FACTORS

The majority of lung cancers are caused by carcinogens and tumor promoters ingested via cigarette smoking (Table 11-1). Overall, the relative risk of developing lung cancer is increased approximately 13-fold by active smoking and approximately 1.5-fold by long-term passive exposure to cigarette smoke [2]. There appears to be a dose-response relationship between the lung cancer death rate and the total amount of cigarette smoke (often expressed in "cigarette-pack years"), such that the risk increases 60- to 70-fold for a man or woman smoking two packs per day for 20 years compared with a nonsmoker. Conversely, the chance of developing lung cancer decreases with cessation of smoking but never returns to the level of the nonsmoker. For this reason, more than half of all lung cancer diagnosis is the United States are now in former smokers [3,4].

Cigarette smoking is more common in blacks than whites. In 1993, 32% of American blacks and 27% of whites were smokers, although whites smoked more cigarettes per day. The largest differences in smoking was seen between educational groups with a 36% incidence in those with less than a high school education compared with 14% among college graduates [5]. Many countries have launched programs to decrease tobacco use and to educate the public. These programs include legislative activity (eg, smoke-free areas and the banning of tobacco advertisements), educational activities (through mass media and schools), and interventional approaches targeted to groups at highest risk for developing tobacco-related cancer. The greatest impact on decreased smoking habits appears to be the stigma placed on smokers by society. These activities have reduced the percentage of the U.S. population who smoke from a high of approximately 50% to approximately 25%. The linkage of cigarette smoking to lung cancer and other diseases has resulted in a decrease in tobacco use among men. As a result, there has been a modest decrease in the death rate due to lung cancer among American men. Unfortunately, the rate of lung cancer among American women continues to rise largely due to their continued use of cigarettes. Young women continue to take up the habit of cigarette smoking more rapidly than their male counterparts. This observation suggests that the death rate due to lung cancer will continue to increase in American women for many years to come.

A small minority of lung cancer cases may be caused by exposure to other carcinogens [2]. Increases in lung cancer risk accompany exposure to carcinogens such as asbestos, radon, bis (chloromethyl) ether, polycyclic aromatic hydrocarbons, chromium, nickel, and inorganic arsenic compounds. The association with occupational exposure to these agents appear to be independent of cigarette smoking [6]. However, exposure to both increases the risk of lung cancer in an exponential manner.

PATHOLOGY

Four major cell types make up 95% of all primary lung neoplasms [7,8]. These are SCLC, squamous (epidermoid) carcinoma, adenocarcinoma (including bronchoalveolar) and large-cell (undifferentiated) carcinoma (Table 11-2). The latter three cell types are often lumped together and referred to as NSCLC. The remaining 5%

Table 11-1. Lung Cancer Etiology*

Cause	Percentage, %
Active tobacco smoking	85
Current smoking	35
Former smoking	50
Passive tobacco exposure	3
Radon	3
Other environmental factors (eg, asbestos, arsenic, chloromethyl ether)	0.1–3.0

*Data from Schottenfeld [6] and Fraumeni et al. [7].

Table 11-2. Lung Cancer Pathology*

Cell type	Frequency, %	Features
Non–small cell lung cancer Squamous	35	Central location; more common in males; less metastases; associated with hypercalcemia, clubbing, hypertrophic pulmonary osteoarthropathy
Adenocarcinoma (includes bronchalveolar)	35	Peripheral in location; equal frequency in both sexes; associated with scars; metastatic potential common; most common type in nonsmokers; hypercoagulable states; associated with filtered cigarettes
Large cell	10	Peripheral in location; equal frequency in both sexes; anaplastic; undifferentiated metastatic potential
Small cell lung cancer	20	Central location; strong relationship with smoking; associated with neuroendocrine features, paraneoplastic syndromes; metastasizes widely; most sensitive to chemotherapy and radiotherapy

*Data from Travis et al. [8].

include carcinoids, bronchial gland tumors, and mesotheliomas. The various cell types have different natural histories and responses to therapy, and thus, a correct histologic diagnosis by an experienced pathologist is the first step to correct treatment. Major treatment decisions are made on the basis of the crucial distinction between histologic classification of a tumor as SCLC or NSCLC. Therapy shall be discussed separately for SCLC and NSCLC. With regards to chemotherapy, all NSCLC cases are considered together because there is no evidence that there are response differences for specific therapies based on cell type.

Squamous cell carcinoma, at one time, was the most frequent of all lung cancers. Squamous cell carcinoma arises most frequently in proximal segmental bronchi and is preceded by squamous metaplasia. Because of its central location and ability to exfoliate, squamous cancers can be detected by cytologic examination in an early stage. With further growth, squamous cancers invade the basement membrane and extend into the bronchial lumen, producing obstruction with resultant atelectasis or pneumonia. These tumors tend to be slow growing, and it is estimated that up to 3 or 4 years are required for an in situ carcinoma to advance to a clinically apparent tumor. Histologically, the squamous cell tumor is composed of sheets of epithelial cells that may be well or poorly differentiated. Most well-differentiated tumors demonstrate keratin pearls.

Adenocarcinoma has become the most frequent lung cancer histology in North America, accounting for approximately 35% to 40% of all cases of lung cancer. Most of these tumors are peripheral in origin, arising from alveolar surface epithelium or bronchial mucosal glands. They also can arise from peripheral scar tumors. Adenocarcinoma appears to have a worse prognosis for operable stages than squamous cell carcinoma because of its propensity for early metastases. Histologically, these tumors form glands and produce mucin. Bronchoalveolar carcinoma is a distinct clinicopathologic type of adenocarcinoma. This tumor appears to arise from type II pneumocytes, growing along alveolar septa by lepidic growth, and showing little if any desmoplastic or glandular change. They can present in three different fashions: a solitary peripheral nodule, multifocal disease, or a rapidly progressive pneumonic form that appears to spread from lobe to lobe and ultimately encompasses both lungs.

Large cell carcinoma is the least common of all NSCLC tumors, accounting for approximately 15% of all lung cancers. Most are located peripherally and are similar to adenocarcinomas in prognosis.

Small cell lung cancers have both biologic and clinical differences from NSCLC tumors. Biologically, SCLCs have neuroendocrine features. These features lead to frequent endocrine and neurologic paraneoplastic syndromes. SCLCs also have more rapid growth and a greater propensity for early metastatic spread [9]. More than 90% of patients with SCLC have mediastinal lymph node metastases, and more than two third of cases have distant organ metastases at the time of diagnosis. SCLC has the most aggressive clinical course of any type of pulmonary tumor, with median survival from diagnosis of only 2 to 4 months without treatment. Because of its propensity for distant metastases, localized forms of treatment, such as radiotherapy or surgical resection, rarely produce long-term survival [9]. SCLCs are more sensitive to chemotherapy than NSCLCs, and chemotherapy represents the cornerstone of therapy.

EARLY DETECTION AND SCREENING

No method has been established as effective in the early detection or screening for lung cancer [10]. Annual chest radiographs, routine sputum cytology examinations, or both were studied in large-scale trials because they were thought to be useful as screening/early detection strategies to reduce lung cancer mortality [11–15]. No decreased lung cancer mortality rate was observed in any of these studies. These trials, therefore, did not prove a screening role for either sputum or chest radiographs. Subsequently, the American Cancer Society, the National Cancer Institute, and other organizations resolved that large-scale radiologic and cytologic screening for lung cancer could not be justified [16]. These studies lacked the power to exclude a useful role for chest radiographs, and thus, the PLCO (prostate, lung, colorectal and ovarian cancer) study is currently examining the role of annual chest radiographs. Although standard sputum cytology may not be sufficiently sensitive for a routine screening examination, it remains as an excellent diagnostic test for smokers with symptoms.

PREVENTION OF LUNG CANCER

The fact that 85%–87% of lung cancer is caused by active tobacco smoking makes primary prevention an essential element of any prevention strategy. Worldwide efforts to limit tobacco use have been relatively ineffective. In the United States, the fraction of adult smokers declined progressively from the time of the Surgeon General's report on the association between tobacco smoke and lung cancer in 1964 until the early 1990s when approximately 25% of the population were active smokers [17]. Unfortunately, over the past several years, the fraction of smokers has ceased declining and may even have increased slightly. Education and public awareness can aid in preventing individuals from starting smoking and becoming addicted to nicotine. Other efforts are aimed at helping smokers quit. Effort to get people to cease smoking (including physician and nurse advice and nicotine replacement therapy) can increase the rate of successful quitting. Although the minority of smokers (< 10%) are able to successfully stop smoking for a year or more in their first attempt, more than half have been able to stop with the assistance of health professionals [18].

The risk of lung cancer declines within one or two years after the cessation of smoking and continues to decline through at least 15 years but never reaches that of a nonsmoker [19]. Consequently, approximately 50% of the lung cancers now diagnosed in the United States are in former smokers [3,4]. Thus, secondary preventive measures (eg, chemoprevention) must be considered as well. Epidemiologic evidence has supported a protective association between the consumption of large amounts of carrots and yellow and green leafy vegetables (all rich in vitamin A and beta carotene) and the risk of lung cancer [20]. These compounds have relatively little toxicity when given in therapeutic doses and have been the first agents studied for the secondary prevention of lung cancer.

Two prevention studies were initiated, the alpha-tocopherol–beta carotene study (ATBC) in Finland and the beta carotene–retinol efficacy trial (CARET) in the United States. Surprisingly, both studies confirmed the increased risk of lung cancer in the group taking beta carotene [21,22]. A more recent strategy has been to study chemoprevention agents in patients with early-stage aerodigestive cancers treated for cure. This represents a group with the highest risk of developing new primary lung cancers. The European Oncology Research Treatment Center (EORTC) study randomized patients with completely resected stage I and II NSCLC to receive retinyl palmitate (vitamin A) or placebo [23]. The occurrence of a new primary aerodigestive cancer significantly decreased in the group receiving vitamin A compared with the placebo group.

In another study performed at MD Anderson Cancer Center, patients with completely resected head and neck cancers were randomized to receive high-dose 13-*cis*-retinoic acid (a vitamin A derivative) or placebo for 12 months [24]. There was no difference in the rate of recurrence of the primary tumor, but the rate of developing secondary primary tumors was significantly lowered in the 13-*cis*-retinoic acid treatment group. A U.S. intergroup study randomizing patients with completely resected stage I lung cancer to low-dose 13-*cis*-retinoic acid or placebo for 3 years recently completed accrual, and the results will be available in a few years. A European study randomizing patients with resected early-stage lung and head and neck cancer to placebo, retinyl palmitate, N-acetyl cysteine, or both agents for 2 years has also completed accrual ,and results will be available in a few years. Selenium, nonsteroidal anti-inflammatory agents and diets high in fresh fruits and vegetables are also under study.

STAGING AND PROGNOSIS

The most important prognostic factors for lung cancer are the stage, the patient's performance status, and the amount of weight loss prior to the diagnosis of lung cancer. The staging classification for NSCLC was recently modified, and the current classification is shown in Table 11-3 [25]. The primary tumor is indicated by the T-stage, which goes from the smallest lesion (< 3 cm) T1 to the most extensive lesion with invasion of the mediastinum and great vessels, extensive pleural involvement with pleural effusion, or satellite lesions within the same lobe of the lung (T4). Regional lymph node metastases may be uninvolved (N0); involve hilar or peribronchial nodes (N1); ipsilateral mediastinal nodes (N2); or may be extensively involved and include high paratracheal, supraclavicular, or contralateral nodes (N3). Distant spread to other organs indicates metastatic involvement (M1). The T, N, and M designations are then used to divide patients into stages. As shown in Table 11-3, the survival rates

Table 11-3. Staging Classification of Lung Cancer

Primary tumor (T)

TX: primary tumor cannot be assessed, or tumor is proven by the presence of malignant cells in sputum or bronchial washings but not visualized by imaging or bronchoscopy

T0: No evidence of primary tumor

Tis: Carcinoma in situ

T1: Tumor that is ≤ 3.0 cm in greatest diameter and surrounded by lung or visceral pleura, without evidence of invasion more proximal than the lobar bronchus (*ie*, not in the main bronchus)

T2: Tumor with any of the following features of size or extent:
> 3.0 cm in greatest dimension
Involving the main bronchus, > 2.0 cm or more distal to the carina
Invading the visceral pleura
Associated with atelectasis or obstructive pneumonitis that extends to the hilar region but does not involve the entire lung

T3: Tumor of any size with direct extension to the chest wall (including superior sulcus tumors), diaphragm, mediastinal pleura, parietal pericardium; tumor in the main bronchus < 2.0 cm distal to the carina but without involvement of the carina; associated atelectasis or obstructive pneumonitis of the entire lung

T4: Tumor of any size that invades any of the following: mediastinum, heart, great vessels, trachea, esophagus, vertebral body, carina; or tumor with a malignant pleural or pericardial effusion or with satellite tumor nodule(s) within the ipsilateral primary-tumor lobe of the lung

Nodal involvement (N)

NX: Regional lymph nodes cannot be assessed

N0: No regional lymph node metastasis

N1: Metastasis in ipsilateral peribronchial and/or ipsilateral hilar lymph nodes, including direct extension

N2: Metastasis in ipsilateral mediastinal and/or subcarinal lymph nodes

N3: Metastasis in contralateral mediastinal, contralateral hilar, ipsilateral or contralateral scalene, or supraclavicular lymph nodes

Distant metastasis (M)

MX: Presence of distant metastasis cannot be assessed

M0: No distant metastasis

M1: Distant metastasis (beyond the ipsilateral supraclavicular nodes)

Staging	TNM	5-y Survival, %
Stage 0	Tis, N0, M0	0
StageIA	T1, N0, M0	67
Stage IB	T2, N0, M0	57
Stage IIA	T1, N1, M0	34
Stage IIB	T2, N1, M0	24
Stage IIB	T3, N0, M0	22
Stage IIIA	T3, N1, M0	9
Stage IIIA	T1–3, N2, M0	13
Stage IIIB	T4, any N, M0	7
Stage IIIB	any T, N3, M0	3
Stage IV	any T, any N, M1	< 1

decline as the stage increases, with a 5-year survival rate of approximately 67% for stage I compared with 1% for stage IV disease.

The stage of disease is based on a combination of clinical (physical examination and radiologic and laboratory studies) and pathologic (biopsy of lymph nodes, bronchoscopy, mediastinoscopy, or other type of thoracotomy) studies. For asymptomatic patients, a complete history and physical examination, a chest radiograph, a computer tomography (CT) scan of the chest and upper abdomen to include the liver and adrenals, a complete blood count (CBC), and blood chemistry usually are all that is required to determine the clinical stage. Additional studies, such as magnetic resonance imaging (MRI) scans of the brain or bone scans, are only indicated if there is a question of metastatic spread based on patient's symptoms, signs, or laboratory data. Evaluation should include questions regarding weight loss, focal skeletal pain, chest pain, seizures, syncope, extensive weakness, headache, and mental status changes. CT scans of the chest can provide an accurate assessment of the size of lymph nodes in the mediastinum, but lymph node size is a poor predictor of cancer involvement. Thus, mediastinoscopy with biopsy of these nodes is indicated in most cases for adequate staging of nodal status.

Small cell lung cancer is classified as either being limited or extensive stage [9]. Limited-stage disease is confined to the hemithorax of origin, the mediastinum, or the supraclavicular lymph nodes, all of which are able to be encompassed within a "tolerable" radiotherapy port. Radiation therapy cannot be delivered to an entire hemithorax; therefore, patients with malignant pleural effusions as well as distant metastases are included in extensive-stage disease.

Performance status describes the functional ability of patients to carry out their usual daily activity. It is usually scored from 0 to 4 (Eastern Cooperative Oncology Group [ECOG] scale) or from 0% to 100% (Karnofsky scale). Patients with decreased activity have a poor prognosis and more toxicity after therapy [26]. Similarly, the degree of weight loss also correlates with a shorter survival [27]. In SCLC, other prognostic factors in addition to stage and performance status include the amount of lactate dehydrogenase and gender. Patients with performance status of 0 or 1, a normal amount of lactate dehydrogenase, and female gender have a better prognosis.

THERAPY FOR SMALL CELL LUNG CANCER

Small cell lung cancer has a high tendency for early metastatic spread [9]. At the time of diagnosis, more than 90% of patients with SCLC have mediastinal lymph node metastases, and more than two thirds of cases have distant organ metastases. The median survival from diagnosis is only 2 to 4 months without treatment. Because of its propensity for distant metastases, localized forms of treatment, such as radiotherapy or surgical resection, rarely produce long-term survival. The tumor cells are highly sensitive to chemotherapy. Active single-agent therapy has shown to produce responses in the 20%–70% range and to prolong survival [9]. With first-line multiagent chemotherapy, response rates approximate 80% to 90%, with complete response in 10% to 50% of patients, depending on disease stage. Survival is improved to a median of 8 to 12 months for extensive stage and 14 to 20 months for limited stage. Thus, combination chemotherapy is the cornerstone of treatment.

Treatment for Limited-Stage Small Cell Lung Cancer

The vast majority of patients with limited-stage SCLC are currently treated with chemotherapy and chest irradiation. This bimodality therapy was shown to be superior to either modality alone, resulting in increased complete response rate, decreased local recurrence, and improved survival [28]. A recent meta-analysis of 13 randomized trials showed a modest but significant 14% reduction in the relative mortality rate for patients receiving combined-modality therapy, with 14% of patients alive after 3 years compared with 9% in the chemotherapy-only group [29]. Patients receiving chemotherapy and chest irradiation had more toxicity, but the gain in response and survival is thought to outweigh the increased toxicity in most instances.

The optimal chemotherapy regimen for combined modality approaches has not been defined. The current, most widely used regimen is cisplatin and etoposide (Table 11-4) [30–34]. It has largely replaced the CAV regimen (cyclophosphamide, doxorubicin, vincristine) of the 1970s and the CAE regimen (cyclophosphamide, doxorubicin, etoposide) of the early 1980s because it appears to be less toxic and more effective [35]. New chemotherapy combinations, such as carboplatin and paclitaxel, are under evaluation.

The optimal means of combining chemotherapy and radiotherapy remains undefined. It can either be given in a sequential, concurrent, or alternating manner. Several randomized trials, confounded by differences in chemotherapeutic regimen and dose modification, demonstrated conflicting results [36,37]. For example, in six consecutive Southwest Oncology Group (SWOG) studies, the best 5-year survival rate of 25% was obtained in the trial in which etoposide, cisplatin, and vincristine were given concurrently with chest irradiation as the initial therapy [35,38]. It must be mentioned, however, that the other five protocols, (which gave the modalities in sequence and resulted in a 5-y survival of 5%–10%) used the combination of cyclophosphamide, doxorubicin, and vincristine. A recent meta-analysis supports the evidence that starting radiotherapy concurrent and early in the course of chemotherapy is most beneficial for long-term survival [39].

Increasing the frequency of delivery of the radiotherapy by giving it twice daily in fractions that are one half (hyperfractionated) or more than the usual daily dose (accelerated hyperfractionated) has also been evaluated. A randomized trial of ECOG showed that this approach produced a significant improvement in local control, a small improvement in survival, but also increased toxicity [34]. Thus, these approaches remain experimental. More recent studies have altered the radiotherapy by reducing volumes using ports designed by CT scans and by using postchemotherapy volumes or shrinking fields. These studies suggest volume reductions have reduced toxicity but have not adversely affected outcome. Unfortunately, patients with limited-stage SCLC who receive combined modality therapy still have a high relapse rate at both local and distant sites.

For the rare stage I patient without nodal involvement or distant metastases (T1,N0; T2,N0), surgery followed by chemotherapy (and radiotherapy) appears to be a reasonable treatment option [9,40]. Cure rates exceeding 60% are reported in these instances. For stage II and III disease, surgery in addition to chemotherapy and radiotherapy failed to improve outcome [41].

Treatment for Extensive-Stage Small Cell Lung Cancer

During the 1970s, the three-drug CAV regimen became one of the most commonly used regimens in both limited- and extensive-stage disease. This regimen produced responses in 80% to 90% of patients and markedly prolonged survival with a median of 8 to 14 months compared with no treatment or single-agent chemotherapy [9]. A small fraction of patients were long-term survivors (2%–10%); however, a relatively high rate of grade 4 myelosuppression, pulmonary toxicity, and neuropathy was noted. After failure on

Table 11-4. Combined Chemotherapy With Cisplatin and Etoposide Plus Thoracic Radiotherapy in Limited-Stage Small Cell Lung Cancer

Study	Patients, n	Chemotherapy Dosage Schedule	Chest Radiopathy	CR, %	PR, %	MS, mo	2-y Survival, %	Comments
McCracken [30]	154	CDDP: 50 mg/m² IV; d 1–8, 29–36, 57–64 E: 50 mg/m² IV; d 1–5, 29–33, 57–61 V: 1–4 mg/m² IV; d 15, 22, 43, 50	45 Gy concurrent, 180 cGy/fr qd × 25 fr, d 1–25	56.0	27.0	17.5	45.0	Every 4 wk × 3 cycles; PCI 30 Gy; consolidation with V, M & E alternating with A & Cy
Turrisi [31]	40	CDDP: 60 mg/m² IV; d 1 E: 120 mg/m² IV; d 4, 6, 8	45 Gy concurrent, 150 cGy/fr bid × 30 fr, d 1–21	78.0	18.0	20.0	36.0	Every 3 wk × 2 cycles; PCI 30 Gy; consolidation with P & E alternating C, A & V × 6 cycles
Johnson DH [32]	34	CDDP: 30 mg/m² IV, d 1–3 E: 120 mg/m² IV, d 1–3	45 Gy alternating, 150 cGy/fr bid × 30 fr, d 8–12, 29–33, 50–54	59.0	38.0	18.0	44.0	Every 3 wk × 4 cycles; PCI optional; consolidation with Cy & E
Johnson BE [33]	54	CDDP: 80 mg/m² IV, d 1 E: 80 mg/m² IV, d 1–3	45 Gy concurrent, 150 cGy/fr bid × 30 fr, d 6–24	74.0	22.0	21.3	43.0	Every 4 wk × 4 cycles; PCI optional; consolidation with C, A & V × 4 cycles or individualized chemotherapy
Johnson DH [34]	182	CDDP: 60 mg/m² IV, d 1 E: 120 mg/m² IV, d 1–3	45 Gy, concurrent 180 cGy/fr qd × 30 fr, d 1–41	46.0	35.2	18.6	41.7	Every 3 wk × 4 cycles, PCI for patients with CR
	176	CDDP: 60 mg/m² IV, d 1 E: 120 mg/m² IV, d 1–3	45 Gy, concurrent 150 cGy/fr bid × 30fr, d 1–20	52.7	29.1	20.3	44.3	

A—doxorubicin; C—cyclophosphamide; CDDP—cisplatin; CR—complete response; Cy—cyclophosphamide; E—etoposide; fr—fraction; LD—limited stage disease; M—metothrexate; P—paclitaxel; PCI—prophylactic cranial irradiation; PR—partial response; V—vincristine.

CAV, the response rate to second-line chemotherapy was less than 10% with a dismal survival of 8 to 12 weeks.

During the late 1970s, cisplatin and etoposide (VP-16) were shown to be active in SCLC. The combination of cisplatin and etoposide (PE) produced response rates in 90% of patients with complete responses in up to 50% [42]. This combination was also active in patients who failed CAV therapy, producing responses in up to 50% of such patients [43]. The PE regimen's toxicity consisted primarily of myelosuppression, nephrotoxicity, ototoxicity, and peripheral neuropathy. The incidence of neuropathy was similar to CAV, but myelosuppression was less severe. In order to overcome the high relapse rate due to acquired drug resistance the PE regimen was combined with CAV in an alternating manner. Two large randomized studies, however, showed no significant difference in the response rates; complete response rates; or survival in patients given continuous PE, continuous CAV, or alternation of the two regimens (Table 11-5) [44,45]. In the study conducted by Roth and coworkers [45], the PE arm was associated with the least myelosuppression and was only given for 4 cycles as compared with 6 cycles of CAV or alternating CAV/EP. Thus, PE given for 4 to 6 cycles compares favorably in terms of efficacy and toxicity compared with other regimens.

Attempts to enhance the efficacy of the CAV or EP regimens by increasing the dose or increasing the frequency of drug delivery have largely been unsuccessful. Individual randomized trials comparing standard-dose CAV to dose-intensified CAV and comparing standard-dose PE to dose-intensified PE revealed enhanced toxicity without improving survival [46,47]. In another randomized trial, G-CSF has been used to increase the dose of the standard three-drug

CAE regimen [48]. Despite improved dose intensity, the study failed to demonstrate improvement in response rate or survival. The use of G-CSF reduced the myelosuppression associated with intensified dose. It is interesting to note that these growth factors should not be given in limited-stage disease patients with concurrent radiotherapy because they produce a significant increase in thrombocytopenia, other toxicities, and cost [9].

Increasing dose intensity by increasing the frequency of drug delivery led to the testing of weekly regimens. Randomized trials reported to date have failed to show an advantage compared with standard regimens, and toxicity has been greater on the weekly regimens. A number of trials attempted to improve results by using high-dose chemotherapy that required autologous bone marrow rescue. In general, these studies showed marked increases in toxicity without improvement in survival compared with the standard approaches [9]. Thus, an international consensus panel concluded that this approach remains experimental [49].

There has been some debate over the optimal number of chemotherapy cycles and the role of maintenance therapy. Three large randomized trials showed that the time to progression was longer in the groups receiving maintenance chemotherapy, but there were no difference in survival [50–52]. Toxicity was greater in patients receiving the maintenance therapy. At present, both continued exposure to the toxic chemotherapy and the fact that patients who progress under maintenance chemotherapy tend to do poorly under salvage treatment make the discontinuation of chemotherapy after 4 to 6 cycles a preferred approach. Randomized trials using interferons as maintenance therapy showed an increase in cost and toxicity without an effect on survival [53].

Table 11-5. Randomized Trials: PE versus CAV versus CAV Alternating With PE

Study	Patients, n	Treatment	Complete Response, %	Partial Response, %	Median Survival, mo	Comments
Fukuoka et al. [44]	97	CAV	15	40	9.9	Slightly significant survival advantage in favor of CAV/PE
	97	PE*	14	64	9.9	
	92	CAV/PE	16	60	11.8	
Roth et al. [45]	140	CAV	7	44	8.3	No significant survival difference among the three regimens
	140	PE†	10	51	8.6	
	138	CAV/PE	7	52	8.1	

* CDDP 80 mg/m^2 IV, d 1; VP-16 100 mg/m^2 IV, d 1, 3, 5 every 3–4 wk.
† CDDP 20 mg/m^2 iv, d 1–5; VP-16 80 mg/m^2 IV, d 1–5.
CAV—cyclophosphamide, doxorubicin, and vincristine; CDDP—cisplatin; PE—cisplatin and etoposide; VP-16—etoposide.

There are many elderly and unfit patients with SCLC who often have other comorbid diseases, especially because of their smoking histories. Several studies showed that single-agent oral VP-16 was tolerated by this patient group and that response rates and survival were similar to those reported in younger and more fit patients. However, randomized trials comparing oral VP-16 to standard combinations showed that standard combination regimens produced better quality of life and longer survival without an increase in toxicity and, therefore, were the preferred treatment for this poor prognostic group [54,55].

The activity of carboplatin in SCLC was recognized some time after cisplatin had become a standard agent. Carboplatin has the advantage of producing less renal toxicity, ototoxicity, neuropathy, nausea, vomiting, and it is easier to administer. Two randomized trials showed carboplatin to be equivalent in efficacy and less toxic compared with cisplatin [56,57]. Thus, the etoposide-carboplatin regimen is often used in the today.

Unfortunately, the vast majority of SCLC patients relapse and die from progressive disease. Extensive stage SCLC patients who receive chemotherapy have a 5-year survival rate of only 1%. Thus, it was reasonable to study new agents in untreated extensive stage patients. In some trials in which ineffective agents were studied in untreated patients, the patients receiving the ineffective agent had a worse outcome than patients receiving standard therapy. In other instances, patients were crossed over rapidly to standard PE regimens if there was no response to the new agent; no negative impact from the study of the new agent was found in these untreated patients [49]. Thus, it is reasonable to study new agents in either setting if attention to study crossover is built into studies of untreated patients.

Several new agents with novel mechanisms of action have been studied in SCLC. These include the taxanes, paclitaxel, and docetaxel, the topoisomerase I inhibitors, irinotecan (CPT-11), topotecan (another vinca alkaloid), vinorelbine, and gemcitabine (an antimetabolite) [58].

Paclitaxel, unlike the vinca alkaloids, which prevent microtubule assembly, stabilizes microtubules against depolymerization. Paclitaxel inhibits proliferation of cells by inducing a sustained mitotic block at the metaphase/anaphase boundary. Two phase II trials of paclitaxel given as a 24-hour continuous infusion at a dose of 250 mg/m^2 every 3 weeks with G-CSF support showed response rates of approximately 60%. The first study conducted by ECOG showed a confirmed response rate of 34%, but the confirmed plus unconfirmed rate, which most likely represents the true response rate, was 53% [59]. The other trial by the North Central Cancer Treatment Group treated 37 patients with an overall response rate of 68% [60]. When

the studies were combined, there were 42 responses among 71 evaluable patients (59%). In an European Organization for Research and Treatment of Cancer (EORTC) study, docetaxel (another taxane) at a dose of 100 mg/m^2 resulted in an objective response rate of 25% among 28 patients, most of whom had received prior therapy. Ninety percent of the patients, however, developed grade 4 neutropenia, and a significant minority of patients developed clinically significant effusions, ascites, and edema [58].

The topoisomerases, CPT-11 and topotecan, also appear to have considerable activity in SCLC. Two studies from Japan using CPT-11 showed an objective response of 40% in previously treated patients (5% complete response [CR] and 35% partial response [PR]). In contrast, a French phase II study reported only a 16% response rate in patients who had progressed on a cisplatin–etoposide regimen [61]. Topotecan showed considerable activity in both previously treated (35%) and untreated (39%) patients [58]. A randomized study of topotecan versus the CAV combination in "sensitive relapse" patients who progressed more than 10 weeks after etoposide-based therapy showed a higher response rate in the topotecan-treated patients (25% vs 15%) [62]. Survival and toxicity were similar in the two arms.

Vinorelbine (a vinca alkaloid) was reported to have a response rate of 13% in pretreated SCLC patients. Because of its myelosuppressive properties, its ability to be combined with other myelosuppressive agents is limited. Gemcitabine was reported to have a response rate of 36% in 26 untreated patients with extensive-stage SCLC [58]. These agents need additional evaluation in combination studies.

Combinations of these new agents with established agents, such as cisplatin, carboplatin and etoposide, in SCLC are just being reported. Five phase II studies have evaluated the addition of paclitaxel to cisplatin or carboplatin and etoposide. Bunn and Kelly [63], using a combination of cisplatin, etoposide, and paclitaxel reported an overall response rate of 94% (22% CR, 72% PR). The group from the Sarah Cannon Cancer Center used a combination of paclitaxel, carboplatin, and extended-schedule etoposide showed a 76% response rate (26% CR, 50% PR) with a complete response of 17% for extensive disease and 40% for limited disease [64]. When the dose of carboplatin was increased to an area under the curve (AUC) of 6 and paclitaxel to 200 mg/m^2 as a 1-hour infusion, the latter investigators showed a 91% response rate (47% CR, 44% PR) with a 71% CR for limited disease and an overall response rate for extensive disease of 84% [65]. Gatzemeier and coworkers [66] evaluated paclitaxel, carboplatin, and oral etoposide in limited-stage SCLC. They reported an overall response rate of 88% (37% CR, 51% PR). A similar study at MD Anderson Cancer Center showed an overall

LUNG CANCER

response rate of 96% (19% CR, 77% PR) [67]. These five studies showed an overall response rate of approximately 88% using the three-drug combination of paclitaxel, a platinum agent, and etoposide. Randomized trials are now clearly indicated to determine whether these new combinations are superior to older combinations.

Because of the high frequency of development of brain metastases in SCLC, prophylactic cranial irradiation (PCI) was evaluated as a means to reduce metastases of the central nervous system (CNS) and to prolong survival [9]. Prospective randomized studies showed that PCI reduced the frequency of clinically detected brain metastases, particularly in patients with a complete response to therapy, but have not shown improvement in overall survival. There are reports of significant neurologic, mental, and psychometric deficits in long-term survivors treated with PCI. A review of 7 studies in which PCI was employed revealed that in 96 long-term survivors, neuropsychologic impairment was noted in 76% of examined patients as compared with 15% in a group of 20 long-term survivors not treated with PCI [9]. Other studies have shown little difference in long-term neurologic function between those receiving and those not receiving PCI. Most likely, the explanation for the failure to affect survival is the fact that brain metastases are rarely the sole site of metastatic spread. Thus, the major issue is whether a delay and reduction in brain metastases by PCI in a small fraction of patients is justified by the toxicity and the treatment of patients.

THERAPY OF NON–SMALL CELL LUNG CANCER
Treatment of Stage I–II Non–Small Cell Lung Cancer

Surgery is the primary therapy for patients with stage I and II NSCLC, the goal being to remove the entire tumor en bloc. Assessment of lung function by simple spirometry remains one of the most important determinants of operability. In general, an forced expiratory volume of 1 second (FEV$_1$) ≥ 2.0 L (> 60% of predicted value), a maximum voluntary ventilatory capacity > 50%, or a diffusing capacity of carbon monoxide (CO) > 60% means that a patient likely has the pulmonary reserve to tolerate a pneumonectomy or lesser resection.

For those patients who do not meet these criteria, smoking cessation, pulmonary rehabilitation, and intensive preoperative respiratory therapies can help. Patients continuing to have poor pulmonary function tests after these measures can still undergo resection if a post operative predictive FEV$_1$ > 40% (or 800 mL) is obtained. Most often this requires a lobectomy or a pneumonectomy (the latter is required only in a minority of cases; when the tumor is central in location or extends into several lobes, it can only be removed in its entirety with a pneumonectomy). Lesser resection (eg, wedge resection, segmental resection, or sleeve lobectomy) should be reserved for patients with compromised pulmonary function who could not tolerate a lobectomy. This was shown in an Lung Cancer Study Group study in T1,N0 NSCLC, comparing limited resection with lobectomy. In this study, a higher local recurrence rate was noted in the limited resection group [68]. Chest wall resection and sleeve resection may be performed for T3 lesions. Sleeve resections are performed for tumors near the carina where a distal bronchus from an uninvolved lobe is sewn into the carina after resection.

Surgical therapy provides excellent results with cure rates exceeding 70% for only stage IA (T1,N0,M0) NSCLC. There is no evidence that any adjuvant therapy (including immunotherapy, radiotherapy, or chemotherapy) improves survival for these patients. Because the majority of these patients are cured by surgery, it is probably best to reserve further study of adjuvant chemotherapy until such adjuvant therapy shows value in NSCLC patients at higher risk of relapse. However, stage I lung cancer patients resected for cure have a high risk of developing second primary tumors, which exceeds the risk of disease recurrence. Because of this, patients should be encouraged to stop smoking. These patients also serve as excellent subjects for chemoprevention studies.

The majority of patients with stage IB-IIIA NSCLC will recur after surgical therapy, and the majority of these recurrences are in distant sites [69]. Postoperative radiation therapy in stage IB-IIIA NSCLC has been found to reduce the rate of local recurrence but has no benefit in overall survival [69]. A randomized trial by the Lung Cancer Study Group (which was investigating the efficacy of postoperative mediastinal irradiation in completely resected squamous cell carcinoma of the lung) demonstrated a reduction in local recurrence (from 41% to 3%), but this improvement did not translate into a survival benefit because most of the failures were distant [70]. Meta-analysis of all randomized trials of postoperative radiotherapy also showed no improvement in survival, although local relapses were reduced significantly.

The earliest studies of postoperative adjuvant chemotherapy used alkylating agents alone or in combination [71]. These studies showed no benefit for the postoperative chemotherapy, and in several studies, survival was actually shortened. A meta-analysis of all postoperative adjuvant studies with alkylating-agent–based therapy confirmed an increased hazard ratio for death and a shortened survival [71]. These therapies were also relatively toxic, all of which led to considerable pessimism for the role of adjuvant chemotherapy.

After cisplatin-based chemotherapy was shown to have activity in advanced NSCLC, it was evaluated as postoperative therapy in resected patients [69]. Many trials used the CAP regimen (cyclophosphamide, adriamycin, and low-dose cisplatin [40 mg/m^2]). Compliance in the postoperative setting was often poor. Some of these studies showed survival advantages for the chemotherapy, whereas others did not. A meta-analysis was therefore performed, showing that the cisplatin therapy was associated with an absolute increase of 5% in the 5-year survival rate—a 13% reduction in the hazard rate of death [71]. Given the small number of patients in these studies, this survival increase was of borderline statistical significance. Physicians in the United Kingdom were surveyed after being shown these data, and < 5% indicated that they would recommend chemotherapy for their patients. In contrast, when such data were explained to patients, more than 90% wished to be offered chemotherapy, and more than 50% wanted chemotherapy if it would improve the cure rate by 1%. Fortunately, chemotherapy today is far superior with lower toxicity. Randomized trials using these new agents in a neoadjuvant or adjuvant manner are required to determine if they should be used routinely.

Treatment of Stage IIIA-N2 Non–Small Cell Lung Cancer

The 5-year survival rates for patients with clinical stage IIIA-N2 NSCLC treated with surgery alone is poor (10%–20%). Postoperative radiotherapy improves local control but fails to improve survival [69]. The poor survival and high rate of distant relapse made studies of preoperative chemotherapy logical. Phase II studies of such an approach provided encouraging results. Typical results from some studies are summarized in Table 11-6. The Memorial Sloan-Kettering Cancer Center evaluated 2 or 3 cycles of neoadjuvant mitomycin, vinblastine, and cisplatin chemotherapy [72]. The objective response rate to chemotherapy was 77%, the

Table 11-6. Selected Phase II Neoadjuvant Results in Stage IIIA Non–Small Cell Lung Cancer

Study group	Treatment	Patients, n	Response Rates, %	Median Survival, mo	Overall Survival, %*
MKSCC (Martini et al. [72])	MVP	136	77	19.0	17 (5)
Toronto (Burkes et al. [73])	MVP	55	71	21.0	20 (5)
CALGB (Sugarbaker et al. [74])	VP	74	88†	20.9	33 (3)
SWOG (Albain et al. [75])	EP + RT	75	88†	13.0	27 (3)

Percent of patients alive at 1 y is indicated in parenthesis.
† Includes stable disease and responders.
CALGB—Cancer and Leukemia Group B; EP—etoposide and cisplatin; MSKCC—Memorial Sloan-Kettering Cancer Center; MVP—mitomycin, vinblastine, and cisplatin; RT—radiation therapy; SWOG—Southwest Oncology Group; VP—vinblastine and cisplatin.

complete resection rate was 78%, the pathologic complete response rate was 14%, and for all the patients, the 5-year survival rate was 17%. Nearly all the 5-year survivors were in the subgroup of patients undergoing complete resection. This subset had a 5-year survival of 26%. The group in Toronto using the same chemotherapy regimen reported a 71% response rate and a 51% complete resection rate [73]. The median survival was 21.3 months. The 5-year survival rates were encouraging (> 20%).

A large phase II trial by the Cancer and Leukemia Group B (CALGB) evaluated 74 patients with stage IIIA NSCLC who were treated with two cycles of vinblastine/cisplatin prior to complete resection, followed by chest irradiation in patients who had incomplete resection or no response to chemotherapy Table 11-6 [74]. The objective response plus stable disease rate was 88%. Eighty-six percent of patients were treated with surgery and 36% had complete resection. The 3-year overall survival rate was 23%, with median survivals of 20.9 months in patients undergoing complete resection, 17.8 months in those with incomplete resection, and only 8.5 months in patients who were not resected. A SWOG phase II study was performed to assess the feasibility of concurrent chemotherapy and irradiation followed by surgery in locally advanced NSCLC [75]. This study reported an 85% resectability for the stage IIIA-N2 group and an 80% resectability for the IIIB group. Two- and 3-year survival rates were 37% and 27%, respectively.

The encouraging results in these phase II neoadjuvant studies led to two prospective phase III randomized trials using neoadjuvant cisplatin based chemotherapy. The Spanish trial compared cisplatin, ifosfamide, and mitomycin C for 3 cycles followed by surgery with surgery alone [76]. The median (26 mo vs 8 mo) and the 3-year survival (25% vs 0%) favored the chemotherapy. In the study from the MD Anderson Cancer Center, the preoperative chemotherapy consisted of cisplatin, cyclophosphamide, and etoposide for three cycles before surgery or surgery alone [77]. Postoperative chemotherapy was also administered and postoperative radiotherapy was allowed at the discretion of the physician. Survival results again favored the chemotherapy with improved median (64 mo vs 11 mo) and 3-year survival (56% vs 15%). Both of these studies had a very small number of patients (60 in each study) because the statisticians closed the studies at an early-stopping rule due to the highly statistically significant improvement in survival. Many physicians concluded that these studies showed that single-modality surgical therapy for preoperatively defined N2 disease could no longer be justified.

The optimal combined therapy approach remains undefined. Excellent results have been achieved with chemotherapy plus surgery, with chemotherapy plus radiotherapy, and with all three modalities.

Future randomized trials will be necessary to clarify the optimal approach. An intergroup study is currently in progress to determine whether all three modalities are better than combined modality with chemotherapy plus radiotherapy. Future trials should also address whether chemotherapy plus radiotherapy or chemotherapy plus surgery is preferred for stage IIIA-N2 NSCLC patients.

Treatment of Stage IIIB Non–Small Cell Lung Cancer

Radiotherapy was the primary therapy for stage IIIB NSCLC for many years because it alleviated symptoms and because approximately 5% to 10 % of patients experienced 5-year survival [2]. Survival of patients with locally advanced, unresectable NSCLC treated with radiotherapy is poor with a median survival of only 9 to 10 months. The addition of chemotherapy was tested to evaluate its ability to improve local control and eliminate or delay the emergence of metastatic disease. Multiple randomized trials of radiotherapy alone versus radiotherapy plus chemotherapy have been completed; most of the trials showed a survival advantage for the combined approach (Table 11-7).

The CALGB, using sequential radiotherapy plus chemotherapy, compared two cycles of cisplatin- and vinblastine-induction chemotherapy followed by definitive chest irradiation with the same radiotherapy alone in 155 patients with stage III NSCLC (see Table 11-7) [78]. The median duration of survival was 13.8 months for the combined modality group and 9.7 months for the radiotherapy group alone (P=0.0066). Survival rates at 2 and 3 years were 24% and 23%, respectively, for the combined modality group compared with 14% and 11%, respectively, for the radiotherapy group alone. After more than 7 years of follow-up, long-term survival remained greater for the radiotherapy–chemotherapy group (5-y survival rate of 17% vs 6%) [79]. The superiority of this combined regimen was confirmed by the Radiation Therapy Oncology Group study that compared standard radiation therapy with induction chemotherapy of cisplatin and vinblastine followed by radiation therapy with twice-daily radiation therapy in unresectable NSCLC patients [80]. The combined-modality arm was statistically superior to the other two treatment arms (median and 1-y survival of 13.8 mo and 60% compared with 11.4 mo and 46% in the standard arm, and 12.3 mo and 51% in the hyperfractionated arm).

A French group compared chemotherapy and radiotherapy with thoracic irradiation alone (65 Gy) (see Table 11-7) [81]. Chemotherapy consisted of three monthly cycles of vindesine, cyclophosphamide, cisplatin, and lomustine. In the radiotherapy group, 20% of patients achieved complete remission as did 16% in the combined-modality group. The rate of distant metastases at 2 years was 64% in the radiotherapy group compared with 43% in the

Table 11-7. Randomized Trials of Sequential or Concurrent Chemotherapy and Radiation Therapy

Study Group	Patients, n	Type	CT+RT Schedule	Median Survival, mo CT+RT	Median Survival, mo RT Alone	2-y Survival, % CT+RT	2-y Survival, % RT Alone
Dillman et al. [78,79]	155	Sequential	P/Vb × 2 + 60 Gy for 6 wk	13.8	9.7	26	13
Sause et al. [80]	452	Sequential	P/Vb × 2 + 60 Gy for 6 wk	13.8	11.4	30	19
LeChevalier et al. [81]	353	Sequential	VCPC × 3 + 65 Gy for 5.5 wk + VCPC × 3	12.0	10.0	21	14
Schaake-Koning et al. [82]	308	Concurrent	P + 30 Gy for 2 wk +25 Gy for 2 wk (split)	13.0	12.0	26	13
Jeremic et al. [84]	131	Concurrent	CBDCA/VP-16 + 69.9 Gy/1.2 Gy twice daily for 5 wk	22.0	14.0	23	9 (4-y)
Takada et al. [87]	314	Concurrent	MVP + 28 Gy for 3 wk + 28 Gy for 3 wk	16.5	—	37	—
		Sequential	MVP + 56 Gy	13.3	—	25.6	—

CBDCA/VP-16—carboplatin (50 mg/m²) and etoposide (50 mg daily); MVP—mitomycin (8 mg/m² d 1, 29), vinblastine (3 mg/m² d 1, 8, 29, 36), and cisplatin (80 mg/m² d 1, 29); P/Vb—cisplatin (100 mg/m²) and vinblastine (5 mg/m²); VCPC—vindesine (1.5 mg/m² d 1,2), lomustine (50 mg/m² d 2 and 25 mg/m², d 3), and cyclophosphamide (200 mg/m² d 2, 4); P—cisplatin (30 mg/m² every wk × 4 or 6 mg/m² every d × 20).

combined-modality group (P < 0.001). Combined-modality therapy was associated with significant improvement in length of survival (median survival, 12 mo vs 10 mo) and reduced incidence of distant disease.

A concurrent combined-modality approach was evaluated in an EORTC phase III trial in inoperable, non-metastatic NSCLC. This study compared split-course radiation therapy alone with split-course radiation therapy combined with cisplatin (given either weekly or daily) (see Table 11-7) [82]. Survival was significantly improved in the combination group compared with the radiotherapy group only (P=0.009). Also noted was improved local control in the daily cisplatin–radiotherapy group (P=0.003), suggesting that this schedule results in maximal radiation enhancement.

A randomized study of hyperfractionated radiation therapy with or without concurrent chemotherapy of carboplatin and etoposide in stage III NSCLC was conducted by Jeremic and coworkers [83]. The median and 3-year survival was substantially greater for the chemotherapy groups (13 mo and 16% in the high-dose carboplatin arm, 18 mo and 23% in the low-dose carboplatin arm, and 8 mos and 6.6% in the radiation arm alone). There was a higher incidence of acute and/or late high-grade toxicity in the combined groups, but no patient died of treatment-related toxicity. A subsequent study was performed comparing hyperfractionated radiation therapy with or without concurrent low-dose daily carboplatin (50 mg) and etoposide (50 mg). A significantly longer survival time was found in the group receiving both radiation and chemotherapy (median survival of 22 mo vs 14 mo and 4-y survival rates of 23% vs 9%) [84].

A meta-analysis of 14 randomized trials of combination therapy and radiotherapy alone in locally advanced, unresectable NSCLC was subsequently performed [85]. Compared with radiotherapy, the combination of chemotherapy and radiotherapy reduced the risk for death by 12% at 1 year, 13% at 2 years, and 17% at 3 years. This corresponds to a mean gain in life expectancy of approximately 2 months from 10.3 months to 12.0 months by the end of 3 years. When considered separately, trials of concurrent and sequential chemotherapy yielded similar treatment effects. The addition of chemotherapy to radiotherapy was associated with a 10% to 20% decrease in the risk for death. When the analysis was restricted to only trials in which cisplatin was used as part of the chemotherapy regimen, the results were similar. The absolute benefit is relatively small, however, and should be balanced against the increased toxicity associated with the addition of chemotherapy. A United Kingdom study showed an improved quality of life when chemotherapy was added to radiation therapy in patients with localized disease [86]. The meta-analysis showed that the combination of chemotherapy and radiotherapy, either concurrently or sequentially, had a positive effect on survival and quality of life. The optimum approach, however, needs to be sorted out.

Takada and coworkers [87] compared concurrent versus sequential thoracic radiotherapy in combination with mitomycin, vindesine, and cisplatin in unresectable stage III NSCLC (see Table 11-7) [87]. Preliminary analysis showed a significantly better response and survival in the concurrent chemoradiotherapy arm compared with the sequential arm (84% overall response, 16.5 mo median survival, and 27% 3-y survival compared with 66.4%, 13.3 mo, and 12.5%, respectively).

Treatment of Stage IV Non–Small Cell Lung Cancer

Until the past several years, there was considerable pessimism about the role of chemotherapy in advanced NSCLC. No agent consistently produced objective responses in more than 20% of patients, and no evidence showed that chemotherapy prolonged the survival of these patients. During the 1980s, a number of randomized trials compared cisplatin-based chemotherapy combinations with best supportive care. All of the studies showed superior survival results with the cisplatin therapy, but this difference was not always statistically significant. A meta-analysis was performed and showed a highly statistically significant survival advantage for patients receiving cisplatin-based therapy. However, the survival advantage was modest [71]. A randomized study by the Canadian National Cancer Institute showed a median survival of 33 weeks in patients treated with chemotherapy compared with 17 weeks in patients treated with best supportive care [88]. The 1-year survival was more than doubled from 10% to 20%, and symptoms improved in responding patients. In the meta-analysis, cisplatin-based combinations significantly improved median survival by approximately 2 months with a 10% increase (from 10% to 20%) in the percent of patients alive at 1 year [71]. Combination chemotherapy also improved quality of life and palliated symptoms. A United Kingdom study showed that chemotherapy (mitomycin, ifosfamide, and cisplatin), significantly improved quality of life in addition to survival compared with standard treatment in inoperable NSCLC of stages III and IV [86].

Five new chemotherapeutic agents, including the two taxanes (paclitaxel and docetaxel), a topoisomerase I inhibitor (CPT-11), a novel antimetabolite (gemcitabine), and a novel vinca alkaloid (vinorelbine) have shown better activity than any agent previously available and have improved the survival and quality of life of NSCLC patients.

Table 11-8. Randomized Trials of New Drug Combinations

Study Group	Treatment	Patients, n	Response Rates, %	Median Survival, wk	1-y Survival, %
SWOG (Wozniak et al. [107])	CDDP 100 mg/m² every 3 wk V 25 mg/m² weekly × 3	214	25	30.0	33
	CDDP 100 mg/m² every 4 wk	218	10	26.0	12
IGR (LeChavalier et al. [101])	V 30 mg/m² weekly	206	14	31.0	30
	CDDP 120 mg/m2 d 1, 29 V 30 mg/m² weekly	206	30	40.0	35
ECOG (Bonomi et al. [104])	P 135 mg/m² IV over 24 h CDDP 75 mg/m² d 1	201	27	41.0	37
	P 250 mg/m² IV over 24 h + GCSF CDDP 75 mg/m² d 1	196	32	43.0	40
	E 100 mg/m² IV d 1-3 CDDP 75 mg/m² d 1	200	12	32.0	31
EORTC (Giaccone et al. [105])	P 175 mg/m² IV over 3 h CDDP 80 mg/m² d 1	155	41	38.8	43
	T 100 mg/m² d 1, 3, 5 C 80 mg/m² d 1	162	28	39.6	41
Spain (Lopez et al. [110])	G 1250 mg/m² d 1, 8 CDDP 100 mg/m² d 1	69	41	35.0	30
	E 100 mg/m² IV d 1–3 CDDP 100 mg/m²	64	21	29.0	24

CDDP—cisplatin; E—etoposide; ECOG—Eastern Cooperative Oncology Group; EORTC—European Organization for Research and Treatment of Cancer; G—gemcitabine; IGR—Institute Goustave Roussy; P—paclitaxel; SWOG—Southwestern Oncology Group; T—tenoposide; V—vinorelbine.

Two initial phase II studies of paclitaxel as 24-hour infusions of a high dose (200–250 mg/m²) showed a response rate of 22% among the 49 patients [89]. Subsequent studies of short infusion paclitaxel given in 1 hour or 3 hours showed a response rate of 21% among the 105 patients in these trials [89]. The survival rates were even more impressive than the response rates. In the 24-hour infusion studies, the 1-year survival rates were 40% and the 2-year survival rates were approximately 20%.

Docetaxel produced response rates of 18% to 38%, with an average of 25% in five studies [90–94]. In previously treated patients, docetaxel was nearly as active with a response rate of 33% with an estimated 1-year survival rate of 45% in one study [94]. The topoisomerase I inhibitors have also been shown to be effective. Three phase II studies of CPT-11 in advanced untreated NSCLC patients reported response rates of 32% to 41%, with an average of 34% among 161 patients [95–97]. Gemcitabine had an overall response rate of 20% among 332 patients in several phase II trials [98]. In one study, gemcitabine was shown to have equivalent efficacy with less toxicity than the two-drug combination of etoposide and cisplatin [99].

Vinorelbine, a novel vinca alkaloid, produced response rates ranging from 14% to 29%, with median survival time of approximately 32 weeks [100]. In a large European study, vinorelbine alone was shown to have similar median survival times to the combination of vindesine and cisplatin (32 wk vs 31 wk), with substantially less toxicity [101]. A U.S. study showed single-agent vinorelbine was superior to the combination of 5-fluorouracil plus leucovorin with a median survival of 29 weeks and with 25% of patients alive at 1 year [102].

Because of the impressive results of these new single agents, attempts were made to combine these drugs with older agents, including cisplatin and carboplatin. In studies using paclitaxel and cisplatin, the overall response rate varied from 27% to 63%, with an

average of 48% [89]. There was a suggestion of a dose-response effect with a response rate of 24% at 135 mg/m², 42% at 175 mg/m², and 63% at 200 to 215 mg/m². Survival was also impressively long with a median exceeding 52 weeks in the largest study [103]. In studies of paclitaxel combined with carboplatin without G-CSF support, response rates varied from 33% to 47% with an average of 41% [89]. There was suggestion of a dose response with a response rate of 17% at paclitaxel doses of 135 mg/m² and 150 mg/m² and 41% at doses of ≥ 175 mg/m² [89]. The recommended dose appears to be 225 mg/m² of paclitaxel and an AUC of 6 of carboplatin. This combination is being compared with the cisplatin–vinorelbine combination in ongoing SWOG, ECOG, and CALGB studies.

There is evidence that the combination of paclitaxel with a platinum agent is superior to prior cisplatin combinations. Several randomized trials of these new agents with cisplatin are summarized in Table 11-8. The ECOG completed a randomized study comparing their standard etoposide–cisplatin combination to the paclitaxel–cisplatin combination with paclitaxel over 24 hours at 135 mg/m² without G-CSF support or 250 mg/m² with G-CSF support [104]. Both of the paclitaxel arms were superior to the etoposide–cisplatin arm with respect to response (30% vs 12%) and survival (1-y survival of 38.5% vs 31.6%). The EORTC compared a short (3-hour) infusion of paclitaxel and cisplatin with teniposide and cisplatin [105]. The paclitaxel arm was superior with respect to response rate, toxicity, and quality of life. In both of these randomized studies, 37% to 40% of patients on the paclitaxel arms were alive at 1 year. This compares with 10% alive at 1 year in studies of best supportive care.

Docetaxel was also combined with cisplatin in many phase II studies in advanced NSCLC. Among 255 patients reported in these studies, the response rate was 35%, and the average median survival was 39 weeks [106]. The ECOG is conducting a 4-arm randomized study comparing docetaxel and cisplatin with paclitaxel and cisplatin, paclitaxel and carboplatin, and gemcitabine and cisplatin.

A SWOG phase III trial comparing the combination of vinorelbine and cisplatin to cisplatin alone showed the combination of vinorelbine and cisplatin to be superior to cisplatin or vinorelbine alone [107]. A large European study reported a 30% response rate for the combination, with a median survival of 40 weeks [101]. A significantly higher rate of neutropenia, however, was noted. A randomized study comparing a three-drug regimen of cisplatin, mitomycin, and vindesine versus cisplatin, mitomycin, and vinorelbine reported a 25% response rate for the vinorelbine arm and an overall median survival time of 33 weeks. For stage IIIB patients, median survival rates were 46 weeks in the vinorelbine arm with a 1-year survival rate of 40% [108].

Several phase II studies of gemcitabine and cisplatin have reported an overall response rate of 47%, higher than the 35-46% response rate reported with paclitaxel or docetaxel and cisplatin or carboplatin [109]. The average median survival was 48 weeks, and an average 1-year survival rate was 48%. A Spanish trial comparing the combination of gemcitabine and cisplatin to etoposide and cisplatin showed a higher objective response in the gemcitabine arm (41%) compared with the etoposide arm (21%) [110]. A large multicenter study comparing gemcitabine and cisplatin with cisplatin alone showed an overall response rate of 31% versus 9%. Thus, the combination of cisplatin and etoposide can no longer be considered standard therapy because randomized studies have shown the combinations of paclitaxel and cisplatin, Navelbine and cisplatin, and gemcitabine and cisplatin to be superior.

Compared with the 16- or 17-week median survival of patients who received best supportive care, patients treated with new agents alone or in combination have median survival of approximately 39 to 48 weeks, a gain of approximately 26 weeks. Chemotherapy, especially new agents, is expensive. Because they prolong survival, the costs per year of life gained can be determined and compared with other medical therapies. In a Canadian study, the survival benefit of 8 weeks in favor of patients receiving CAP chemotherapy was associated with an economic saving of $949.49 (in Canadian dollars), when compared with best supportive care [111]. This translated into a savings of $6171 per year of life gained. The VP-16 arm (etoposide and high-dose inpatient cisplatin) resulted in a mean survival benefit of 12.8 weeks and an increased cost of $3637 per patient, translating to $14,777 per added year of life. The VP-16 arm resulted in both increased costs and increased survival when compared with BSC. It was, therefore, less economically favorable than CAP, but the costs associated with its use are still acceptable when compared with the benefits. Evans [112], using a model of lung cancer diagnosis and treatment by disease stage and cell type, examined the cost effectiveness of common chemotherapy regimens compared with BSC. Cisplatin and etoposide saved $1461 per case relative to supportive care. Newer chemotherapeutic regimens were compared with etoposide and cisplatin as the standard regimen. Cisplatin and vinorelbine

cost $8,566 per year of life saved, gemcitabine and cisplatin cost $10,963, and paclitaxel and cisplatin cost $12,116. Thus, the cost of chemotherapy for advanced NSCLC, though expensive, is well within the range of other accepted medical therapies and will be lowered considerably when generic agents become available.

SUMMARY

Chemotherapy is a major component of treatment for both SCLC and NSCLC patients. Completely resected stage I NSCLC patients have a high risk of developing second primary tumors and should be encouraged to stop smoking and be considered for screening and chemoprevention studies. For resectable NSCLC patients with stage IB, IIA, and IIB disease, postoperative radiotherapy reduces local failures that occur in approximately 20% of patients but does not improve overall survival. Old randomized studies with low-dose cisplatin (40 mg/m^2) based postoperative chemotherapy showed a 13% reduction in the hazard rate of death, which translated into a 5% absolute increase in 5-year survival. However, because modern chemotherapy regimens are markedly superior to both low-dose and high-dose cisplatin combinations, it is likely they will further increase the cure rate when given preoperatively in these NSCLC patients.

For patients with stage III disease, chemotherapy improves survival in stage IIIB (when added to radiotherapy) and stage IIIA (when added to surgery) patients. In stage IIIA-N2, one treatment modality is not sufficient. Randomized trials have shown that combined chemotherapy and radiotherapy is superior to either modality alone in both SCLC and NSCLC. Combined chemotherapy and surgery has also been shown to be superior to surgery alone in stage IIIA NSCLC. It remains unclear which combination is better—chemotherapy and radiotherapy or chemotherapy and surgery. Would combining all three regimens be more effective? In stage III SCLC, the combination of chemotherapy, radiotherapy, and surgery was not found to be superior to chemotherapy and radiotherapy. In stage III NSCLC, this question is currently being addressed in a randomized intergroup study. For stage IIIB NSCLC patients, the combined chemotherapy and radiotherapy approach is favored over either modality alone, with median survivals of 14 to 16 months and 5-year survival rates of 15% to 20%.

Meta-analyses of randomized trials show that chemotherapy prolongs the survival of patients with stage III and stage IV SCLC and NSCLC. In extensive stage SCLC, chemotherapy improves median survival from 2 months to 9 to 10 months. In NSCLC, chemotherapy based on newer agents improves survival from 4 months to approximately 10 months and improves one-year survival from 10% to 40% or 50%. These therapies also improve one's quality of life, and their cost is similar to that of other accepted medical therapies. The guidelines of lung cancer therapy of the American Society of Clinical Oncology reflect the contribution of chemotherapy to prolonging the survival of these patients [113]. Thus, it is reasonable to offer chemotherapy to advanced NSCLC patients with good performance status.

REFERENCES

1. Parker SL, Tong T, Bolden S, Wingo PA: Cancer statistics, 1997. *Cancer J Clin* 1997, 47:5–27
2. Ginsberg RJ, Vokes EE, Raben A: Non-small cell lung cancer in cancer. *Principles and Practice of Oncology*, ed 5. Edited by DeVita VT, Hellman S, Rosenberg SA. Philadelphia: Lippincott-Raven; 1997:858–911
3. Strauss G, DeCamp M, Dibiccaro E, *et al.*: Lung cancer diagnosis is being made with increasing frequency in former cigarette smokers [abstract]. *Proc Am Soc Clin Oncol* 1995, 14:A1106.
4. Okene JK, Kuller LH, Svendsen KH, *et al.*: The relationship of smoking cessation to coronary artery disease and lung cancer in the multiple risk-factor intervention trial (MRFIT). *Am J Public Health* 1990, 80:954–958.

5. *Cancer facts and figures.* American Cancer Society; 1996.

6. Schottenfeld D. Epidemiology of lung cancer. In *Lung Cancer: Principles and Practice.* Edited by Pass HI, Mitchell JB, Johnson DH, and Turrisi AT. Philadelphia: Lippincott-Raven; 1996:305–321.

7. Fraumeni JF: Lung and pleura. In *Cancer Epidemiology and Prevention.* Edited by Schottenfeld D, Fraumeni JF. Philadelphia: WB Saunders; 1982:564–670.

8. Travis WD, James L, Mackey B: Classification, histology, cytology and electron microscopy. In *Lung Cancer: Principles and Practice.* Edited by Pass HI, Mitchell JB, Johnson DH, Turrisi AT. Philadelphia: Lippincott-Raven; 1996:361–395.

9. Cook R, Miller Y, Bunn PA: Small cell lung cancer: tiology, biology, clinical features, staging and treatment. *Curr Probl Cancer* 1993, 17:69–144.

10. Berlin NI, Buncher CR, Fontana RS, *et al.*: National Cancer Institute Cooperative Lung Cancer Detection Program: results of initial screen (prevalence) early lung cancer detection (introduction). *Am Rev Resp Dis* 1984, 130:545–549.

11. Shaw GL: Screening for lung cancer. In *Lung Cancer.* Edited by Johnson BE, Johnson DH. New York: Wiley-Liss; 1995:55–72.

12. Early Lung Cancer Cooperative Study Group: Early lung cancer detection: summary and conclusions. *Am Rev Respir Dis* 1984, 130:565–570.

13. Flehinger BJ, Melamed MR, Zaman MB, *et al.*: Early lung cancer detection: results of the initial (prevalence) radiologic and cytologic screening in the Memorial Sloan-Kettering Study. *Am Rev Respir Dis* 1984, 130:555–560.

14. Fontana RS, Sanderson DR, Taylor WF, *et al.*: Early lung cancer detection: results of the initial (prevalence) radiologic and cytologic screening in the Mayo Clinic Study. *Am Rev Respir Dis* 1984, 130:561–565.

15. Frost JK, Ball WC Jr, Levin ML, *et al.*: Early lung cancer detection: results of the initial (prevalence) radiologic and cytologic screening in the Johns Hopkins Study. *Am Rev Respir Dis* 1984, 130:549–554.

16. Eddy, DM. Screening for lung cancer. *Ann Int Med* 1989, 111:232–237.

17. Centers for Disease Control, USA: Cigarette smoking among adults: United States, 1993. *MMWR* 1994, 43:925–930.

18. Hunt RD, Dale LC, Frederickson PA, *et al.*: Nicotine patch therapy for smoking cessation combined with physician advice and nurse followup. *JAMA* 1994, 27:595–600.

19. Ockene JK, Kuller LH, Svendsen KH, *et al.*: The relationship of smoking cessation to coronary heart disease and lung cancer in the multiple risk factor intervention trial (MRFIT). *Am J Public Health* 1990, 80:954–958.

20. Kvale G, Bjelke E, Gart JJ: Dietary habits and lung cancer risk. *Int J Cancer* 1983, 31:397–405.

21. The Alpha-Tocopherol, Beta Carotene Cancer Prevention Study Group: The effect of vitamin E and beta carotene on the incidence of lung cancer and other cancers in male smokers. *N Engl J Med* 1994, 330:1029–1035.

22. Omenn GS, Goodman GE, Thornquist MD, *et al.*: Risk factors for lung cancer and for intervention effects in CARET, the Beta Carotene and Retinol Efficacy Trial. *J Nat Cancer Inst* 1996, 88:1550–1559.

23. Pastorino U, Infante M, Maioli M, *et al.*: Adjuvant treatment of stage I lung cancer with high-dose vitamin A. *J Clin Oncol* 1993, 11:1216–1222.

24. Hong, WK, Lippman SM, Itri LM, *et al.*: Prevention of second primary tumors with isotretinoin in squamous cell carcinoma of the head and neck. *N Engl J Med* 1990, 323:795–801.

25. Mountain CF. Revisions in the international system for staging lung cancer. *Chest* 1997, 111:1710–1717.

26. O'Connell JP, Kris MG, Gralla RJ, *et al.*: Frequency and prognostic importance of pretreatment clinical characteristics in patients with advanced non-small cell lung cancer treated with combination chemotherapy. *J Clin Oncol* 1986, 4:1604–1614.

27. DeWys WD, Begg C, Lavin PT, *et al.*: Prognostic effect of weight loss prior to chemotherapy in cancer patients. *Am J Med* 1980, 69:491–497.

28. Warde P, Payne D: Does thoracic irradiation improve survival and local control in limited-stage small-cell carcinoma of the lung?: a meta-analysis. *J Clin Oncol* 1992, 10:890–895.

29. Pignon JP, Arriagada R, Ihde CE, *et al.*: A meta-analysis of thoracic irradiation for small cell lung cancer. *N Eng J Med* 1992, 327:1618–1624.

30. McCracken JD, Janaki LM, Crowley JJ, *et al.*: Concurrent chemotherapy/radiotherapy for limited small-cell lung carcinoma: a Southwest Oncology Group Study. *J Clin Oncol* 19908:892–898.

31. Turrisi AT, Wagner H, Glover B, *et al.*: Limited small cell lung cancer (LSCLC): concurrent BID thoracic radiotherapy (TRT) with platinum-etoposide (PE): an ECOG study [abstract]. *Proc Am Soc Clin Oncol* 1990, 9:A887.

32. Johnson DH, Turrisi AT, Chang AY, *et al.*: Alternating chemotherapy ad twice-daily thoracic radiotherapy in limited-stage small-cell lung cancer: a pilot study of the Eastern Cooperative Oncology Group. *J Clin Oncol* 1993, 11:879–884.

33. Johnson BE, Bridges JD, Sobczeck M, *et al.*: Patients with limited-stage small-cell lung cancer treated with concurrent twice-daily chest radiotherapy and etoposide/cisplatin followed by cyclophosphamide, doxorubicin, and vincristine. *J Clin Oncol* 1996, 14:806–813.

34. Johnson DH, Kim K, Turrisi AT, *et al.*: Cisplatin and etoposide plus concurrent thoracic radiotherapy administered once versus twice daily for limited-stage small cell lung cancer: Preliminary results of an Intergroup trial [abstract]. *Proc Am Soc Clin Oncol* 1994, 13:A1105.

35. Albain KS, Crowley JJ, Le Blanc M, *et al.*: Determinants of improved outcome in small-cell lung cancer: an analysis of 2850 patient Southwest Oncology Group data base. *J Clin Oncol* 1990, 8:1563–1547.

36. Perry MC, Eaton WL, Propert KJ, *et al.*: Chemotherapy with or without radiation therapy in limited small-cell carcinoma of the lung. *N Engl J Med* 1987, 316:912–918.

37. Murray N, Coy P, Pater JL, *et al.*: Importance of timing for thoracic irradiation in the combined modality treatment of limited-stage small-cell lung cancer. *J Clin Oncol* 1993, 11:336–344.

38. Janaki L, Rector D, Turrisi AT, *et al.*: Patterns of failure and second malignancies from SWOG 8269: concurrent cisplatin, etoposide, vincristine, and once daily radiotherapy for the treatment of limited small-cell lung cancer [abstract]. *Proc Am Soc Clin Oncol* 1994, 13:A1096.

39. Murray N, Coldman C: The relationship between thoracic irradiation timing and the long-term survival in combined modality therapy of limited stage small-cell lung cancer [abstract]. *Proc Am Soc Clin Oncol* 1995, 14:A1099, 1995.

40. Shepherd FA, Ginsberg RJ, Evans WK, *et al.*: Surgical treatment for limited small-cell lung cancer. *J Thorac Cardiovasc Surg* 1991, 101:385–393.

41. Lad T, Piantandosi S, Thomas P, *et al.*: A prospective randomized trial to determine the benefit of surgical resection of residual disease following response of small-cell lung cancer to combination therapy. *Chest* 1994, 106(suppl):S320–S323.

42. Einhorn LH. Initial therapy with cisplatin plus VP-16 in small cell lung cancer. *Semin Oncol* 1986, 13:5–9.

43. Evans WK, Osoba D, Feld R, *et al.*: Etoposide (VP-16) and cisplatin: an effective treatment for relapse in small-cell lung cancer. *J Clin Oncol* 1985, 3:65–71.

44. Fukuoka M, Furese K, Saijo N, *et al.*: Randomized trial of cyclophosphamide, doxorubicin, and vincristine versus cisplatin and etoposide versus alternation of these regimens in small cell lung cancer. *J Natl Cancer Inst* 1991, 83:855–861.

45. Roth BJ, Johnson DH, Einhorn LH, *et al.*: Randomized study of cyclophosphamide, doxorubicin, and vincristine versus cisplatin and etoposide versus alternation of these regimens in small cell lung cancer: a phase III trial of the Southeastern Cancer Study Group. *J Clin Oncol* 1992, 10:282–291.

46. Johnson DH, Einhorn LH, Birch R, *et al.*: A randomized comparison of high-dose versus conventional dose cyclophosphamide, doxorubicin and vincristine for extensive-stage small cell lung cancer: a phase III trial of the Southeastern Cancer Study Group. *J Clin Oncol* 1987, 5:1731–1738.

47. Ihde DC, Johnson BE, Mulshine JL, *et al.*: Randomized trial of high dose versus standard dose etoposide and cisplatin in extensive stage small cell lung cancer. *J Clin Oncol* 1994, 12:2022–2034.

48. Crawford J, Ozer H, Stoller R, *et al.*: Reduction by granulocyte colony-stimulating factor of fever and neutropenia induced by chemotherapy in patients with small cell lung cancer. *N Engl J Med* 1991, 235:164–170.

49. Bunn PA, Cullen M, Fukuola M, *et al.*: Chemotherapy in small cell lung cancer: a consensus report of the International Association for the Study of Lung Cancer Workshop. *Lung Cancer* 1989, 5:127–134.

50. Giaccone G, Dalesio O, McVie GJ, *et al.*: Maintenance Chemotherapy in small cell lung cancer: long-term results of a randomized trial. *J Clin Oncol* 1993, 11:1230–1240.

51. Spiro SG, Souhami RL, Geddes DM, *et al.*: Duration of chemotherapy in small cell lung cancer: a Cancer Research Campaign trial. *Br J Cancer* 1989, 58:578–583.

52. Bleehan NM, Fayers PM, Girling DJ, *et al.*: Controlled trials of twelve versus six courses of chemotherapy in small cell lung cancer. *Br J Cancer* 1989, 59:584–590.

53. Kelly K, Crowley JJ, Bunn PA, *et al.*: Role of recombinant interferon alpha-2a maintenance in patients with limited-stage small-cell lung cancer responding to concurrent chemoradiation: a Southwest Oncology Group study. *J Clin Oncol* 1995, 13:2924–2930.

54. Souhami RL, Spiro SG, Rudd RM, *et al.*: Five-day oral etoposide treatment for advanced small cell lung cancer: randomized comparison with intravenous chemotherapy. *J Natl Cancer Inst* 1997, 89:577–580.

55. Clark PI, Thatcher N, Lallenand G, *et al.*: Updated results of a randomized trial confirm that oral etoposide alone is inadequate palliative chemotherapy for small cell lung cancer (SCLC). *Lancet* 1996, 3–566.

56. Wolf M, Drings P, Hans K, *et al.*: Alternating chemotherapy with adriamycin/ifosfamid/ vincristine (AIO) and either cisplatin/etoposide (PE) or carboplatin/etoposide (JE) in small cell lung cancer (SCLC) [abstract]. *Lung Cancer* 1991, 7(suppl):A527.

57. Skarlos DV, Samantas E, Kosmidis P, *et al.*: Randomized comparisons of etoposide-cisplatin versus etoposide-carboplatin and irradiation in small cell lung cancer: a Hellenic Co-operative Oncology Group Study. *Ann Oncol* 1994, 5:601–607.

58. Bunn PA Jr: Future directions in therapeutic approaches for small cell lung cancer. *Semin Oncol* 1996, 23(suppl 16):136–138.

59. Chang AY, Kim K, Glick J, *et al.*: Phase II study of taxol, merbarone and piroxantrone in stage IV non-small cell lung cancer: The Eastern Cooperative Group results. *J Natl Cancer Inst* 1993, 85:388–394.

60. Murphy WK, Fossella FV, Winn RJ, *et al.*: Phase II study of Taxol in patients with untreated advanced non-small cell lung cancer. *J Natl Cancer Inst* 1993, 85:384–388.

61. Le Chevalier T, Ibrahim N, Chomy N, *et al.*: A phase II study of irinotecan (CPT-11) in patients with small cell lung cancer progressing after initial response to first line chemotherapy [abstract]. *Proc Am Soc Clin Oncol* 1997, 16:A1617.

62. Schiller JH, von Pawel J, Clarke P, *et al.*: Preliminary results of a randomized comparative phase III trial of topotecan (T) versus CAV as second-line therapy of small cell lung cancer (SCLC) [abstract]. *Lung Cancer* 1997, 18(suppl 1):A41.

63. Bunn PA, Kelly K. A phase I study of cisplatin, etoposide, and paclitaxel in small cell lung cancer: a University of Colorado Cancer Center Study. *Semin Oncol* 1997, 24(suppl 12):144–148.

64. Hainsworth JD, Strupp SL, Greco FA: Paclitaxel, carboplatin and extended schedule etoposide in the treatment of small cell lung cancer. *Cancer* 1996, 77:2458–2463.

65. Hainsworth JD, Gray JR, Hopkins LG, *et al.*: Paclitaxel (1 hour infusion), carboplatin and extended schedule etoposide in small cell lung cancer (SCLC) [abstract]. *Proc Am Soc Clin Oncol* 1997, 16:A1623.

66. Gatzemeier U, Jagos U, Kaukel E, *et al.*: Paclitaxel, carboplatin and oral etoposide: a phase ii trial in limited stage small cell lung cancer. *Semin Oncol* 1997, 24(suppl 12):149–152.

67. Glisson BS, Kurie JM, Fox NJ, *et al.*: Phase I-II study of cisplatin,etoposide and paclitaxel (PET) in patients with extensive small cell lung cancer (ESCLC) [abstract]. *Proc Am Soc Clin Oncol* 1997, 16:A1635.

68. Ginsberg RJ, Rubinstein L: The comparison of limited resection to lobectomy for T1N0 non-small cell lung cancer. *Chest* 1994, 106:318S–319S.

69. Bunn PA Jr: The treatment of non-small cell lung cancer: current perspectives and controversies, future directions. *Semin Oncol* 1994, 21(suppl 6):49–59.

70. Weisenburger JH, Lung Cancer Study Group. Effects of postoperative mediastinal radiation on completely resected stage II and stage III epidermoid carcinoma of the lung. *N Engl J Med* 1986, 315:1377–1381.

71. Non-small Cell Lung Cancer Collaborative Group: chemotherapy in non-small cell lung cancer: a meta-analysis using updated data on individual patients from 52 randomized clinical trials. *Br Med J* 1995, 311:899–909.

72. Martini N, Kris M, Flehinger B, *et al.*: Preoperative chemotherapy for stage IIIA (N2) lung cancer: the Sloan Kettering experience with 136 patients. *Ann Thorac Surg* 1993, 55:1365–1374.

73. Burkes R, Ginsberg, Shepherd F, *et al.*: Induction chemotherapy with mitomycin C, vindesine and cisplatin for stage III unresectable non-small cell lung cancer: results of the Toronto phase II trial. *J Clin Oncol* 1992, 10:580–586.

74. Sugarbaker DJ, Herndon J, Kohman LJ, *et al.*: Results of Cancer and Leukemia Group B protocol 8935: multi-institutional phase II trimodality trial for stage IIIA (N2) NSCLC. *J Thorac Cardiovasc Surg* 1995, 109:473–485.

75. Albain KS, Rusch V, Crowley J, *et al.*: Concurrent cisplatin/etoposide plus chest radiotherapy followed by surgery for stages IIIA and IIIB non-small cell lung cancer: mature results of Southwest Oncology Group phase II study 8805. *J Clin Oncol* 1995, 13:1880–1892.

76. Rosell R, Gomez-Codina J, Camps C, *et al.*: A randomized trial comparing preoperative chemotherapy plus surgery with surgery alone in patients with non-small cell lung cancer. *N Engl J Med* 1994, 330:153–158.

77. Roth JAB, Fossella F, Komaki R, *et al.*: A randomized trial comparing perioperative chemotherapy and surgery with surgery alone in resectable stage IIIA non-small cell lung cancer. *J Natl Cancer Inst* 1992, 86:673–680.

78. Dillman RO, Seagren SL, Herndon J, *et al.*: A randomized trial of induction chemotherapy plus high-dose radiation versus radiation alone in stage III non-small cell lung cancer. *N Engl J Med* 1990, 323:940–945.

79. Dillman RO, Herndin J, Seagren SL, *et al.*: Improved survival in stage III non-small cell lung cancer: seven year follow-up of cancer and leukemia group B (CALGB) 8433 trial. *J Natl Cancer Inst* 1996, 88:1210–1215.

80. Sause WT, Scott C, Taylor S, *et al.*: Radiation Therapy Oncology Group (RTOG) 88-08 and Eastern Cooperative Oncology Group (ECOG) 4588: preliminary results of a phase III trial in regionally advanced, unresectable non-small cell lung cancer. *J Natl Cancer Inst* 1995, 87:198–205.

81. Le Chevalier T, Arrigada R, Quiox E, *et al.*: Radiotherapy alone versus combined chemotherapy and radiotherapy in nonresectable non-small cell lung cancer: first analysis of a randomized trial in 353 patients. *J Natl Cancer Inst* 1991, 83:417–423.

82. Schaake-Koning C, Van Den Bogert W, Dalesio O, *et al.*: Effects of concomitant cisplatin and radiotherapy in inoperable non-small cell lung cancer. *N Engl J Med* 1992, 326:524–530.

83. Jeremic B, Shibamoto Y, Acinovic L, *et al.*. Randomized trial of hyperfractionated radiation therapy with or without concurrent chemotherapy for stage III non-small cell lung cancer. *J Clin Oncol* 1995, 13:452–458.

84. Jeremic B, Shibamoto Y, Acinovic L, et al.: Hyperfractionated radiation therapy with or without concurrent low dose daily carboplatin/etoposide for stage III non-small cell lung cancer: a randomized study. J Clin Oncol 1996, 14:1065–1070.

85. Pritchard RS, Anthony SP: Chemotherapy plus radiotherapy compared with radiotherapy alone in the treatment of locally advanced, unresectable, NSCLC: a meta-analysis. Ann Intern Med 1996, 125:723–729.

86. Billingham LJ, Cullen J, Woods AD, et al.: Mitomycin, ifosfamide and cisplatin (MIC) in non-small cell lung cancer (NSCLC): 3 results of a randomised trial evaluating palliation & quality of life [abstract]. Lung Cancer 1997, 18(suppl 1):A26.

87. Takada Y, Furuse K, Fukuoka YH, et al.: A randomized phase III study of concurrent versus sequential thoracic radiotherapy (TRT) in combination with mitomycin, vindesine, and cisplatin in unresectable stage III non-small cell lung cancer (NSCLC) [abstract]. Lung Cancer 1997, 18(suppl 1):A294.

88. Rapp E, Pater JL, Willan A, et al.: Chemotherapy can prolong survival in patients with advanced non-small cell lung cancer: report of a Canadian multi-center randomized trial. J Clin Oncol 1988, 6:663–641.

89. Bunn PA Jr: The North American experience with paclitaxel combined with cisplatin or carboplatin in lung cancer. Semin Oncol 1996, 23(suppl 16):18–25.

90. Cerny T, Kaplan S, Pavlidis N, et al.; Docetaxel (Taxotere) is active in non-small cell lung cancer: a phase II trial of the EORTC early clinical trials group (LCTG). Br J Cancer 1994, 70:384–387.

91. Francis PA, Rigas JR, Kris MG, et al.: Phase II trial of docetaxel in patients with stage III and IV non-small cell lung cancer. J Clin Oncol 1994, 12:1232–1237.

92. Burris H, Eckardt J, Fields S, et al.: Phase II trials of taxotere in patients with non-small cell lung cancer [abstract]. Proc Am Soc Clin Oncol 1993, 12:A335.

93. Fosella FV, Lee JS, Murphy WK, et al.: Phase II study of docetaxel for recurrent or metastatic non-small cell lung cancer. J Clin Oncol 1994, 12:1238–1244.

94. Fosella FV, Lee JS, Shin DM, et al.: Phase II study of docetaxel for advanced or metastatic platinum-refractory non-small cell lung cancer. J Clin Oncol 1995, 13:645–651.

95. Fukuoka M, Nutani H, Suzuki A, et al.. A phase II study of CPT-11, a new derivative of camptothecin, for previously untreated non-small cell lung cancer. J Clin Oncol 1992, 10:16–20.

96. Ogawa M, Tauchi T: Clinical studies with CPT-11: the Japanese experience [abstract]. Ann Oncol 1992, 3(suppl 1):118.

97. Negoro S, Fukuoka M, Masuda N, et al.: Phase I study of weekly intravenous infusions of CPT-11: a new derivative of camptothecin in the treatment of advanced non-small cell lung cancer. J Natl Cancer Inst 1991, 83:1164–1168.

98. Anderson H, Thatcher N, Walling J, et al.: Gemcitabine and palliation of symptoms in non-small cell lung cancer [abstract]. Proc Am Soc Clin Oncol 1995, 13:A367.

99. Manegold C, Stahel R, Mattson K, et al.: Single-agent Gemzar (gemcitabine) versus cisplatin plus etoposide (C/E): a randomized phase II study in patients with locally advanced or metastatic non-small cell lung cancer (NSCLC) [abstract]. Lung Cancer 1997 18(suppl 1):A32, 1997.

100. Vokes EE: Integration of vinorelbine into chemotherapy strategies for non-small cell lung cancer. Oncology 1995, 9:565–575.

101. LeChevalier T, Pujol JL, Douillard JY, et al.: A three arm trial of vinorelbine (Navelbine) plus cisplatin, vindesine plus cisplatin, and single agent vinorelbine in the treatment of non-small cell lung cancer: an expanded analysis. Semin Oncol 1994, 21:28–33.

102. Crawford J, O'Rourke M, Schiller J, et al.: Randomized trial of vinorelbine compared with flourouracil plus leucovorin in patients with stage IV non-small cell lung cancer. J Clin Oncol 1996, 14:2777–2784.

103. Langer CJ, Leighton JC, Comis RL, et al.: Paclitaxel and carboplatin in combination in the treatment of advanced NSCLC: a phase II toxicity, response and survival analysis. J Clin Oncol 1995, 13:1860–1870.

104. Bonomi P, Kim K, Kugler K, et al.: Results of a phase III trial comparing taxol-cisplatin (TC) regimens to etoposide-cisplatin (EC) in non-small cell lung cancer (NSCLC) [abstract]. Lung Cancer 1997, 18(suppl 1):A28.

105. Giaccone P, Splinter TA, Debruyne C, et al.: A randomized study of paclitaxel-cisplatin versus cisplatin-teniposide in patients with advanced non-small cell lung cancer. J Clin Oncol 1998: in press.

106. Berille J, LeChavelier T, Zalcberg JR, et al.: Overview of taxotere-cisplatin combination in non-small cell lung cancer [abstract]. Ann Oncol 1996, 7(suppl 5):90.

107. Wozniak AJ, Crowley JJ, Balcerzak SP, et al.: Randomized phase III trial of cisplatin (CDDP) vs CDDP plus navelbine (NVB) in treatment of advanced non-small cell lung cancer (NSCLC): report of a Southwest Oncology Group Study (SWOG-9308) [abstract]. Proc Am Soc Clin Oncol 1996, 15:A1110.

108. Perol M, Guerin JC, Thomas P, et al.: Multicenter randomized trial comparing cisplatin-mitomycin-vinorelbine versus cisplatin-mitomycin-vindesine in advanced non-small cell lung cancer: Groupe Francais de Pneumo-cancerologie. Lung Cancer 1996, 14:119–134.

109. Bunn PA, Kelly K. New chemotherapeutic agents are as useful in non-small cell lung cancer as older chemotherapeutic agents in small cell lung cancer and breast cancer and may increase the cure rate. Clin Cancer Res 1998: in press.

110. Lopez Cabrerizo MP, Cardenal F, Artal A, et al.. Gemcitabine plus cisplatin versus etoposide plus cisplatin in advanced non-small cell lung cancer: A randomized trial by the Spanish Lung Cancer Group [abstract]. Lung Cancer 1997, 18(suppl 1):A27.

111. Jaakkimainen L, Goodwin PJ, Pater J, et al.: Counting the costs of chemotherapy in a National Cancer Institute of Canada randomized trial in nonsmall-cell lung cancer. J Clin Oncol 1990, 8:1301–1309.

112. Evans, WK. Treatment of NSCLC with chemotherapy is controversial because of low response and high cost. Lung Cancer 1997, 18(suppl2):117–118.

113. Clinical practice guidelines for the treatment of unresectable non-small cell lung cancer. J Clin Oncol 1997, 15:2996–3018.

114. Livingston RB, Moore TN, Heilburn L, et al.: Small-cell carcinoma of the lung: combined chemotherapy and radiation. Ann Int Med 1978, 88:194–199.

115. Feld R, Evans WK, DeBoer G et al.: Combined modality induction therapy without maintenance chemotherapy for small cell carcinoma of the lung. J Clin Oncol 1984, 2:294–304.

116. Ettinger DS, Finkelstein DM, Abeloff MD, et al.: A randomized comparison of standard chemotherapy versus alternating chemotherapy and maintenance versus no maintenance therapy for extensive-stage small cell lung cancer: a phase III study of the Eastern Cooperative Oncology Group. J Clin Oncol 1990, 8:230–240.

117. Jett JR, Everson L, Therneau TM, et al.: Treatment of limited-stage small-cell lung cancer with cyclophosphamide, doxorubicin, and vincristine with or without etoposide: a randomized trial of the North Central Cancer Treatment Group. J Clin Oncol 1990, 8:33–39.

118. Smith JE, Evans BD, Gore ME, et al.: Carboplatin (Paraplatin; JM8) and etoposide (VP-16) as first-line combination therapy for small-cell lung cancer. J Clin Oncol 1987 5:185–189.

119. Evans WK, Radwi A, Tomiak E, et al.: Oral etoposide and carboplatin: effective therapy for elderly patients with small cell lung cancer. Am J Clin Oncol 1995, 18:149–155.

120. Pfeiffer P, Sorensen P, Rose C: Is carboplatin and oral etoposide an effective and feasible regimen in patients with small cell lung cancer? Eur J Cancer 1995, 31A:64–69.

121. Carney DN: Carboplatin/etoposide combination chemotherapy in the treatment of poor prognosis patients with small cell lung cancer. *Lung Cancer* 1995, 12(suppl 3):77–83.

122. Klastersky J, Sculier JP: Dose-finding study of paclitaxel (Taxol) plus cisplatin in patients with NSCLC: European Lung Cancer Working Party. *Lung Cancer* 1995, 12(suppl 2):117–125.

123. Pirker R, Krajnik G, Zochbauer S, *et al.*: Paclitaxel and cisplatin in advanced NSCLC. *Ann Oncol* 1995, 6:833–835.

124. Belli L, LeChevalier T, Gottried M, *et al.*: Phase I-II trial of paclitaxel (Taxol) and cisplatin in previously untreated advanced NSCLC [abstract]. *Pro Am Soc Clin Oncol* 1995, 14:A1058.

125. Niederle N, Heider A, Von Pawel J, *et al.*: Phase II study of paclitaxel and cisplatin in patients with NSCLC [abstract]. *Proc Am Soc Clin Oncol* 1997, 16:A1716.

126. Belani CP, Aisner J, Hiponia D, *et al.*: Paclitaxel and carboplatin in metastatic NSCLC: preliminary results of a phase I study. *Semin Oncol* 1996, 23(supp 12):19–21.

127. Johnson DH, Paul DM, Hande KR, *et al.*: Paclitaxel plus carboplatin in advanced NSCLC: a phase II trial. *J Clin Oncol* 1996, 14:2054–2060.

128. Muggia FM, Vafai D, Natale R, *et al.*: Paclitaxel 3 hour infusion given alone and in combination with carboplatin: preliminary results of dose escalation trials. *Semin Oncol* 1995, 22(suppl 9):63–66.

129. Kelly K, Zhaoxing Pan, Murphy J, *et al.*: A phase I trial of paclitaxel plus carboplatin in untreated patients with advanced non-small cell lung cancer. *Clin Cancer Res* 1997, 3:1117–1123.

130. Huizing MT, Giaccone G, van Warmerdan LJ: Pharmacokinetics of paclitaxel and carboplatin in a dose-escalating and dose-sequencing study in patients with NSCLC: the European Cancer Centre. *J Clin Oncol* 1997, 15:317–329.

131. Schutte W, Bork I, Sucker S: Phase II trial of paclitaxel and carboplatin as front line treatment in advanced NSCLC [abstract]. *Proc Am Soc Clin Oncol* 1996, 15:A1208.

132. Depierre A, Chastang C, Quiox *et al.*: Vinorelbine plus cisplatin in advanced non-small cell lung cancer: a randomized trial. *Ann Oncol* 1994, 5:37–42.

133. Berthaud P, LeChevalier T, Ruffie P, *et al.*: Phase I-II study of vinorelbine (Navelbine) plus cisplatin in advanced non-small cell lung cancer. *Eur J Cancer* 1992 28A(11):1863–1865.

134. Frontini L, Candido P, Cattaneo MT, *et al.*: Cisplatin-vinorelbine combination chemotherapy in locally advanced non-small cell lung cancer. *Tumor* 1996, 82:57–60.

135. Manegold C, Stahel R, Mattson K, *et al.*: A randomized phase II study of gemcitabine monotherapy versus cisplatin plus etoposide in patients with locally advanced or metastatic NSCLC [abstract]. *J Clin Oncol* 1997, 16:A1651.

136. Perng RP, Chen YM, Ming-Liu J, *et al.*: Gemcitabine versus the combination of cisplatin and etoposide in patient with inoperable non-small cell lung cancer in a phase II randomized study. *J Clin Oncol* 1997, 15:2097–2102.

137. Einhorn LH. Phase II trial of gemcitabine plus cisplatin in NSCLC: a Hoosier Oncology Group study. *Semin Oncol* 1997, 24(suppl 8):24–26.

138. Abratt RP, Hacking DJ, Goedhals L, *et al.*: Weekly gemcitabine and monthly cisplatin for advanced non-small cell lung cancer. *Semin Oncol* 1997, 24(suppl 8):18–23.

139. Anton A, Artal A, Carrato A, *et al.*: Gemcitabine plus cisplatin in advanced NSCLC: final phase II results [abstract]. *Proc Am Soc Clin Oncol* 1997, 16:A1656.

140. Shepherd FA, Cormier Y, Burkes R, *et al.*: Phase II trial of gemcitabine and weekly cisplatin for advanced non-small cell lung cancer. *Semin Oncol* 1997, 23(suppl 8):27–30.

141. Gonzales-Baron M, Ordonez A, Gracia M, *et al.*: Gemcitabine and cispaltin in advanced NSCLC: results of a phase II study [abstract]. *Proc Am Soc Clin Oncol* 1997, 16:A1687.

CYCLOPHOSPHAMIDE, DOXORUBICIN, AND VINCRISTINE IN SMALL CELL LUNG CANCER

During the 1970s, it was demonstrated that combination chemotherapy with three or four active drugs improved response rates and survival in small cell lung cancer compared with single-agent chemotherapy or two-drug combinations [114–117]. The three-drug combination of cyclophosphamide, doxorubicin, and vincristine (CAV) produced objective responses in ~80%–90% of patients, with complete responses up to 40%. The median survival was ~8–14 mo. Occasionally, long-term survivors were seen (2%–10%). However, large randomized trials in the late 1980s confirmed that cisplatin and etoposide given for 4–6 cycles was as active as CAV or alternating CAV with cisplatin and etoposide [44,45]. In patients who failed CAV, the cisplatin and etoposide regimen produced responses in up to 50% of patients with increased survival up to 6 mo [43]. Today, CAV (like many other regimens) still offers a reasonable approach in extensive-stage disease. In limited-stage disease, CAV is not preferentially used in combination with concurrent radiotherapy due to its enhanced lung toxicity.

RECENT EXPERIENCES AND RESPONSE RATES

Study	Patients, n	Dosage Schedule, mg/m^2	CR, % LD	CR, % ED	PR, % LD	PR, % ED	Median Survival, wk LD	Median Survival, wk ED	Comments
Livingston et al. [114]	403	Cy: 750 IV; d 1 A: 50 IV; d 1 V: 1 IV; weekly (total 12 mg)	41	14	34	42	52.0	25.0	Repeat every 3 wk; chest-RT and PCI for LD and ED patients
Feld et al. [115]	370	Cy: 900 IV; d 1 A: 45 IV; d 1 V: 2 (total) IV; d 1	52	10	32	63	49.0	34.0	Repeat every 3 wk; chest-RT and PCI for LD and ED patients
Ettinger et al. [116]	294	Cy: 1000 IV; d 1 A: 50 IV; d 1 V: 1,2 IV; d 1	16	—	45	—	42.7	—	Repeat every 3 wk; ED patients only
Jett et al. [117]	113	Cy: 750 IV; d 1 A: 40 IV; d 1 V: 1,4 IV; d 1	57	—	8	—	50.0	—	Repeat every 4 wk; LD patients only; chest-RT and PCI for all patients

A—doxorubicin (adriamycin); chest-RT—chest-radiotherapy; CR—complete response; Cy—cyclophosphamide; ED—extensive-stage disease; LD—limited-stage disease; PCI—prophylactic cranial irradiation; PR—partial response; V—vincristine.

CANDIDATES FOR TREATMENT
Small cell lung cancer: extensive- and limited-stage disease; first- and second-line treatment.

SPECIAL PRECAUTIONS
Obtain electrocardiogram and consider baseline cardiac ejection fraction in high-risk patients before starting doxorubicin therapy; perform dose modification for doxorubicin and vincristine in patients with hepatic dysfunction

ALTERNATIVES THERAPIES
Cisplatin and etoposide; cyclophosphamide and etoposide; cyclophosphamide, doxorubicin, and etoposide; new drugs such as taxanes, topotecan, and gemcitabine in combination with standard chemotherapy (experimental)

TOXICITIES
Myelosuppression, nausea, vomiting, alopecia, cardiotoxicity (acute arrhythmias, delayed congestive heart failure), neurotoxicity (peripheral neuropathy, cranial nerve paralysis, autonomic effects, central nervous system effects) hemorrhagic cystitis, nephrotoxicity, mucositis, diarrhea, local extravasation (necrosis)

DRUG INTERACTIONS
Cyclophosphamide: may interfere with microsomal enzyme activity in liver (eg, cimetidine); Vincristine: digoxin

NURSING INTERVENTIONS
Myelosuppression: monitor blood counts; inquire about symptoms of infection, bleeding, and anemia; Neurotoxicity: assess for weakness and numbness of arms, hand, legs, and feet; assess for jaw pain, foot drop, loss of deep tendon reflexes; Constipation: assess bowel habits and nutritional pattern; encourage a high-fiber diet and fluid intake; Cardiac toxicity: note patient's cumulative dose (maximum 450 mg/m^2); high-risk patients include those receiving concurrent cyclophosphamide therapy and radiation; monitor signs and symptoms of congestive heart failure; Local: doxorubicin and vincristine are vesicants, so check for good blood return before and during administration; monitor for clinical signs of extravasation (pain, burning, swelling, erythema, absence of blood return); be prepared for emergency procedures for extravasation

PATIENT INFORMATION
Report immediately signs of heart burn, chest pain, breathing problems, irregular heart beat; report immediately symptoms of infection (fever, chills, sore throat) and unusual bleeding or bruising; report upset stomach, numbness, tingling; maintain good nutrition and exercise.

CISPLATIN AND ETOPOSIDE IN SMALL CELL LUNG CANCER

Cisplatin, a platinum analogue, is one of the most active antineoplastic agents for lung cancer. It inhibits DNA synthesis by producing intrastrand and interstrand crosslinks, similar to bifunctional alkylating agents. Etoposide exerts its effect on DNA by forming a complex with DNA and the DNA-unwinding enzyme topoisomerase II, which causes strand breakage. The combination of cisplatin and etoposide (PE) is currently considered to be one of the most active drug combinations for small cell lung cancer, reaching response rates up to 90% of patients with complete remissions in up to 50% [42]. In limited-stage disease, PE combined with chest irradiation has been shown to improve local control and median survival. In fact, a concurrent application of chemotherapy and radiotherapy is preferred by most centers (see Table 11-4) [30-34]. Although the PE regimen produces considerable nausea and vomiting, it generally causes less myelosuppression, cardiac toxicity, and neurotoxicity than the older CAV regimen (cyclophosphamide, doxorubicin, vincristine).

CANDIDATES FOR TREATMENT

Small cell lung cancer: limited-stage disease concurrent with, alternated with, or followed by chest irradiation; extensive-stage disease

SPECIAL PRECAUTIONS

Patients with renal dysfunction and impaired hearing function

ALTERNATIVE THERAPIES

Carboplatin and etoposide; cyclophosphamide, doxorubicin, and etoposide; cyclophosphamide, doxorubicin, and vincristine; new drugs such as taxanes, topotecan, and gemcitabine as a single-agent or in combination with a platinum compound (experimental)

TOXICITIES

Myelosuppression, nausea, vomiting, nephrotoxicity with electrolyte wasting, neurotoxicity (peripheral neuropathy), auditory impairment, hypotension, and hypersensitivity (including anaphylactic reactions), mucositis, diarrhea, alopecia, asthenia

DRUG INTERACTIONS

Cisplatin: other nephro- and ototoxic drugs (eg, aminoglycosides, furosemide); **Etoposide:** not known

NURSING INTERVENTIONS

Hypersensitivity: anaphylactic reactions have been documented with both agents; benedryl and epinephrine should be readily available as well as a crash cart; **Myelosuppression:** monitor blood counts; inquire about symptoms of infection, bleeding, and anemia; **Nausea and vomiting:** give antiemetics before chemotherapy and as needed; **Nephrotoxicity:** monitor renal function indices (serum creatinine, blood urea nitrogen, creatinine clearance) and electrolytes (especially magnesium and calcium); encourage adequate oral and intravenous hydration as well as high urine flow during therapy; **Neurotoxicity:** assess for weakness and numbness of legs, feet, arms, and hands; **Hypotension:** usually attributed to fast infusion rate of etoposide (due to vehicle); stop infusion and give supportive care; restart infusion at slower rate or consider change to etoposide phosphate; **Local:** venous spasm and occasionally phlebitis

PATIENT INFORMATION

Drink plenty of fluids and urinate frequently; report immediately symptoms of infection (fever, chills, sore throat), unusual bleeding, bruising, breathing problems, upset stomach, numbness, and tingling; maintain good nutrition and exercise.

The information here is provided as guidance only. Prescribers should always consult the manufacturer's current prescribing information.

CARBOPLATIN AND ETOPOSIDE IN SMALL CELL LUNG CANCER

Carboplatin, a platinum analogue like cisplatin, inhibits DNA synthesis by causing irreversible intra- and interstrand crosslinks. Carboplatin is highly effective in small cell lung cancer as a single agent. Etoposide, a topoisomerase II inhibitor produces irreversible strand breakage. In two randomized studies, the combination of carboplatin and etoposide was shown to be as active but less toxic than the combination of cisplatin and etoposide in patients with limited- and extensive-stage disease [56,57]. The nonhematologic toxicity (*eg*, neuropathy, renal toxicity, asthenia, nausea, and vomiting) compares favorably with the cisplatin–etoposide regimen. Therefore, the combination of carboplatin and etoposide (intravenous or perioral) is frequently used in elderly patients with poor performance status and extensive-stage disease, showing a remarkable response and survival rates [118–121].

RECENT EXPERIENCES AND RESPONSE RATES

RANDOMIZED TRIALS COMPARING CARBOPLATIN AND ETOPOSIDE WITH CISPLATIN- CONTAINING REGIMENS IN LIMITED AND EXTENSIVE-STAGE SMALL CELL LUNG CANCER

Study	Patients, n	Dosage Schedule, mg/m^2	CR, % LD	CR, % ED	PR, % LD	PR, % ED	Median Survival, mo LD	Median Survival, mo ED	Comments
Wolf et al. [56]	129	A, I, and V alternating with C: 300 IV, d 1 E: 120 IV, d 1, 2, 3	20	17	53	34	12.0	9.3 / 9.3	Every 4 wk × 4 cycles; chest RT for LD
		vs.							
	133	A, I, and V alternating with CDDP: 90 IV, d 1 E: 150 IV, d 1–3	22	14	56	36	14.3		
Skarlos et al. [57]	72	C: 300 IV, d 1 E: 100 IV, d 1, 2, 3	37	19	49	48	11.8 (LD & ED)		Every 3 wk × 6; chest RT for LD; PCI if complete remission
		vs.							
	71	CDDP: 50 IV, d 1, 2 E: 100 IV, d 1, 2, 3	44	10	29	40	12.5 (LD & ED)		

A—doxorubicin (adriamycin); C—carboplatin; CDDP—cisplatin; chest RT—chest radiotherapy; CR—complete response; E—etoposide; ED—extensive-stage disease; I—ifosfamide; LD—limited-stage disease; PCI—prophylactic cranial irradiation; PR—partial response; V—vincristine.

CANDIDATES FOR TREATMENT

Small cell lung cancer: limited-stage disease with chest irradiation and extensive-stage disease; elderly patients

SPECIAL PRECAUTIONS

Treatment delay and transfusions may be mandatory due to myelosuppression. In case of impaired renal function, consult drug instruction form or consider use of Calvert formula (in which the total dose is in mg, area under the curve [AUC] = 4–5, and GFR is the glomerular filtration rate [use creatinine clearance]):

Total Dose = AUC × (GFR + 25)

ALTERNATIVE THERAPIES

Carboplatin and etoposide; cyclophosphamide, doxorubicin, and etoposide; cyclophosphamide, doxorubicin, and vincristine; new drugs such as taxanes, topotecan, and gemcitabine in combination with standard regimens (experimental)

TOXICITIES

Myelosuppression, nausea, vomiting, alopecia, mucositis, infection, peripheral neuropathy, hypotension, hypersensitivity (including anaphylactic reactions), anorexia, mild renal toxicity

DRUG INTERACTIONS

Other nephro- or ototoxic drugs (*eg*, aminoglycosides, furosemide)

NURSING INTERVENTIONS

Hypersensitivity: anaphylactic reactions have been documented with both agents; benedryl and epinephrine should be readily available as well as crash cart; **Myelosuppression:** monitor blood counts; inquire about symptoms of infection, bleeding, and anemia; **Nausea, vomiting:** give antiemetics before chemotherapy and as needed; **Nephrotoxicity:** monitor renal function indices (serum creatinine, blood urea nitrogen) and magnesium; **Neurotoxicity:** assess for weakness and numbness of legs, feet, arms, and hands; **Hypotension:** usually attributed to fast infusion rate of etoposide (due to vehicle); stop infusion and give supportive care; restart infusion at slower rate or consider change to etoposide phosphate; **Local:** venous spasm and occasionally phlebitis

CARBOPLATIN AND ETOPOSIDE IN SMALL CELL LUNG CANCER (Continued)

NON-RANDOMIZED CARBOPLATIN AND ETOPOSIDE TRIALS IN LIMITED- AND EXTENSIVE-STAGE SMALL CELL LUNG CANCER

Study	Patients, n	Dosage Schedule, mg/m²	CR, %		PR,%		Median Survival		Comments
			LD	ED	LD	ED	LD	ED	
Smith *et al.* [118]	52	C: 300 IV, d 1 E: 100 IV, d 1, 2, 3	29	13	53	75	9.5 mo	9.5 mo	Every 4 wk
Evans *et al.* [119]	47	C: 150 IV, d 1 E: 100 PO, d 1–7	50	23	38	67	59.0 wk	45.0 wk	Elderly, unfit patients; every 3–4 wk
Pfeiffer *et al.* [120]	106	C: 300 IV, d 1 E: 240 PO, d 1, 2, 3	41	8	48	45	15.0 mo	8.5 mo	Every 4 wk
Carney *et al.* [121]	83	C: 300 IV, d 1 E: 200 PO, (total) d 1–5	53	26	45	—	43.0 wk (LD & ED)		Elderly patients; every 4 wk; PS ≥ 3

C—carboplatin; CR—complete response; E—etoposide; ED—extensive stage disease; LD—limited stage disease; PR—partial response; PS—performance status.

PATIENT INFORMATION

Report immediately symptoms of infections (fever, chills, sore throat) and unusual bleeding or bruising; report upset stomach, numbness, tingling; maintain good nutrition, fluid intake, and exercise.

PACLITAXEL AND CISPLATIN IN NON-SMALL CELL LUNG CANCER

Paclitaxel is a unique diterpene anticancer agent derived from the bark of the *Taxus brevifola* tree . It exerts its antitumor effect by stabilizing microtubules, rendering them resistant to disassembly. This differs from the other antimicrotubule agents like the vinca alkaloids, which induce microtubule disassembly. Two initial phase II studies of paclitaxel as 24-h infusions showed a response rate of 22% among the 49 patients with an improved median survival of ~40 wk [89]. Subsequent studies in combination with cisplatin ensued. The Eastern Cooperative Oncology Group did a randomized study comparing low and high-dose paclitaxel with cisplatin to the standard regimen of cisplatin and etoposide [104]. Both the paclitaxel arms showed a higher response rate (26.5% and 32.1% vs. 12.0%) and better 1-y survival rates. The European Organization for Research in Cancer Therapy did a randomized study using a short infusion of paclitaxel and cisplatin compared with teniposide and cisplatin [105]. This study showed a higher response rate (44% vs. 30%), reduced toxicity, and improved quality of life in patients receiving paclitaxel. Survival was similar in both treatment groups.

RECENT EXPERIENCES AND RESPONSE RATES

Study	Patients, n	Chemotherapy Dosage Schedule, mg/m²	Response Rate, %	Median Survival, wk	1-y Survival, %	Comments
Bonomi *et al.* [104]	201	P: 135 IV over 24 h, d 1 CDDP:75 d 1	27	41	37	Phase III study every 3 wk
		or				
	196	P: 250 IV over 24 h, d 1 + GCSF 5 μg/kg SQ d 3–10 CDDP: 75 D1	32	43	40	
Giaccone *et al.* [105]	154	P: 175 IV over 3 h, d 1 CDDP: 80 IV, d 1	44	39	NR	Phase III study every 3 wk
Klastersky *et al.* [122]	17	P: 135-200 IV over 3 h CDDP: 100 IV, d 1	47	NR	NR	Phase I study every 3 wk; severe polyneuropathy with > 3 cycles
Pirker *et al.* [123]	20	P: 175 IV over 3 h, d 1 CDDP: 100 IV, d 1	35	10	35	Phase II study every 3 wk; neurotoxicity dose limiting
Belli *et al.* [124]	29	P: 135-225 IV over 3 h CDDP 100-200 IV, d 1	38	NR	NR	Phase I/II study every 3 wk; efficacy of taxol superior at 200 mg/m²
Niederle *et al.* [125]	67	P: 175 IV over 3 h, d 1 CDDP: 75 IV, d 1	43	43	33	Phase II study every 3 wk

CDDP—cisplatin; NR—not reported; P—paclitaxel.

CANDIDATES FOR TREATMENT

Patients with stage III and stage IV disease as well as preoperatively in resectable early-stage disease

SPECIAL PRECAUTIONS

Patients with renal dysfunction; a history of cardiac toxicity should caution the caregiver

ALTERNATIVE THERAPIES

Etoposide and paclitaxel, etoposide and carboplatin, carboplatin and paclitaxel, cisplatin and vinorelbine, cisplatin and gemcitabine, vinorelbine alone, or gemcitabine alone

TOXICITIES

Paclitaxel: myelosuppression (almost exclusively neutropenia; thrombocytopenia is rare), neurotoxicity (peripheral neuropathy, seizures), gastrointestinal (nausea, vomiting, diarrhea, mucositis, neutropenic enterocolitis), cardiac (arrhythmia, ventricular tachycardia, myocardial infarction, bradycardia), anaphylactic and urticarial reactions, and alopecia and radiation pneumonitis (when administered concomitantly with radiation); **Cisplatin:** gastrointestinal (nausea, vomiting, anorexia), renal toxicity (with an elevation of blood urea nitrogen, creatinine, serum uric acid, impairment of endogenous creatinine clearance, and renal tubular damage), ototoxicity (with hearing loss that initially is in the high-frequency range and tinnitus), peripheral neuropathy, and hyperuricemia; anaphylactic-like reactions (*eg*, facial edema, bronchoconstriction, tachycardia, and hypotension) may occur; myelosuppression often with delayed erythrosuppression is expected; electrolyte disturbances (*eg*, hypomagnesemia and/or hypocalcemia) can occur, resulting in tetany or seizures; subsequent courses should not be given until serum creatinine returns to normal if elevated

DRUG INTERACTION

Agents that are nephrotoxic should be given with caution

NURSING INTERVENTIONS

Hypersensitivity: give premedications for prevention of allergic reactions to paclitaxel (dexamethasone, diphenhydramine, and cimetidine); **Myelosuppression:** monitor blood counts; inquire about symptoms of infection, bleeding, and anemia; **Nausea, vomiting:** give antiemetics before chemotherapy and as needed; **Nephrotoxicity:** monitor renal function indices (serum creatinine, blood urea nitrogen), monitor magnesium, give adequate hydration; **Neurotoxicity:** assess for weakness and numbness of legs, feet, arms, and hands

PATIENT INFORMATION

Patient should drink plenty of fluids and urinate frequently; report prolonged upset stomach and symptoms of infection (fever, chills, sore throat) or neurotoxicity (numbness and tingling sensation of hands or toes).

PACLITAXEL AND CARBOPLATIN IN NON–SMALL CELL LUNG CANCER

Due to a higher incidence of peripheral neuropathy associated with the cisplatin–paclitaxel combination, several trials combining carboplatin with paclitaxel (either as a 24-h or 3-h infusion) have been initiated. It appears that short infusion schedules of paclitaxel have similar degrees of efficacy as compared with 24-h infusion schedules. Shorter infusion schedules result in less myelosuppression, and neuropathy becomes dose limiting. The Southwest Oncology Group is currently doing a study comparing carboplatin and paclitaxel versus cisplatin and vinorelbine, and the European Eastern Cooperative Oncology Group is conducting a 4-arm study comparing docetaxel and cisplatin versus paclitaxel and cisplatin versus paclitaxel and carboplatin versus gemcitabine and cisplatin.

RECENT EXPERIENCES AND RESPONSE RATES

Study	Patients, n	Chemotherapy Dosage Schedule	Response Rate, %	Median Survival, wk	1-y Survival, wk	Comments
Langer et al. [103]	53	P: 135–215 mg/m² IV over 24 h; C: AUC 7.5	62	53	54	Phase I/II study every 3 wk
Belani et al. [126]	30	P: 135–225 mg/m² IV over 24 h; C: AUC 5–11	50	NR	NR	Phase I study every 3 wk
Johnson DH et al. [127]	51	P: 135–175 mg/m² IV over 24 h; C: 300 mg/m² or AUC 6	27	38	32	Phase I/II study every 4 wk × 6 cycles
Muggia et al. [128]	44	P: 150–250 mg/m² IV over 3 h; C: AUC 6	48	NR	NR	Phase I/II study every 3 wk
Kelly et al. [129]	50	P: 135–250 mg/m² IV over 3 h; C: 250–400 mg/m²	26	31	28	Phase I study every 3 wk
Huizing et al. [130]	45	P: 100–250 mg/m² IV over 3 h; C: 300–400 mg/m²	12	NR	NR	Phase I study every 4 wk
Schutte et al. [131]	25	P: 200 mg/m2 IV over 3 h; C: AUC 5	52	NR	NR	Phase II study every 3 wk

AUC—area under the curve; C—carboplatin; NR—not reported; P—paclitaxel.

CANDIDATES FOR TREATMENT
Patients with stage III and IV disease who have been untreated or refractory to other regimens

SPECIAL PRECAUTIONS
Patients with renal dysfunction; a history of cardiac toxicity should caution the caregiver

ALTERNATIVE THERAPIES
Etoposide and paclitaxel, etoposide and carboplatin, cisplatin and paclitaxel, cisplatin and vinorelbine, cisplatin and gemcitabine, vinorelbine alone, or gemcitabine alone

TOXICITIES
Carboplatin: myelosuppression, nausea, vomiting, and loss of appetite are common; rare toxicities include gross hematuria, hyponatremia, ageusia, allergic reaction, peripheral neuropathy, venoocclusive disease, liver and kidney damage, hearing loss, dizziness, and blurred vision; **Paclitaxel:** myelosuppression (almost exclusively neutropenia; thrombocytopenia is rare), neurotoxicity (peripheral neuropathy, seizures), gastrointestinal (nausea, vomiting, diarrhea, mucositis, neutropenic enterocolitis), cardiac (arrhythmia, ventricular tachycardia, myocardial infarction, bradycardia), anaphylactic and urticarial reactions, and alopecia and radiation pneumonitis (when administered concomitantly with radiation)

DRUG INTERACTIONS
None known

NURSING INTERVENTION
Hypersensitivity: give premedications for prevention of allergic reactions to paclitaxel (dexamethasone, diphenhydramine, and cimetidine); **Myelosuppression:** monitor blood counts; inquire about symptoms of infection, bleeding, and anemia; **Nausea, vomiting:** give antiemetics before chemotherapy and as needed; **Nephrotoxicity:** monitor renal function indices (serum creatinine, blood urea nitrogen) and magnesium; give adequate hydration; **Neurotoxicity:** assess for weakness and numbness of legs, feet, arms, and hands

PATIENT INFORMATION
Patient should drink plenty of fluids and urinate frequently; report prolonged upset stomach and irregularities in heart rhythm, and symptoms of infection (fever, chills, sore throat) or neurotoxicity (tingling or numbness of hands and toes).

VINORELBINE AND CISPLATIN IN NON–SMALL CELL LUNG CANCER

Vinorelbine is a unique semisynthetic vinca alkaloid. Its mechanism of action is similar to the other vinca alkaloids in that it is an inhibitor of microtubule assembly. It binds to tubulin, resulting in disruption of the mitotic spindle apparatus during metaphase. Vinorelbine has a lesser effect on axonal microtubules, and because neurotoxicity of vinca alkaloids is postulated to derive from damage to axonal microtubules, a more favorable therapeutic index of vinorelbine has been postulated. Preclinical studies with vinorelbine indicate activity against several tumor cell lines representing leukemia, small and non–small cell lung cancer, breast and colon cancer, and melanoma. Depierre and coworkers [132] demonstrated significant activity of vinorelbine in previously untreated patients with non–small cell lung cancer. Of 78 eligible patients, the objective response rate was 29%, median survival was 34 wk, and 1-y survival rate was ~30%. Crawford and coworkers [102], in a randomized study comparing vinorelbine with 5-fluorouracil and leucovorin showed superior activity in the vinorelbine arm. Subsequent studies combining vinorelbine with cisplatin have been performed.

CANDIDATES FOR TREATMENT
Preoperative resectable stage II–IIIA as well as stage IIIB and IV disease

SPECIAL PRECAUTIONS
Patients with renal dysfunction; a history of peripheral neuropathy should caution the caregiver

ALTERNATIVE THERAPIES
Etoposide and paclitaxel, etoposide and carboplatin, carboplatin and taxol, cisplatin and gemcitabine, or phase II agents

TOXICITIES
Vinorelbine: myelosuppression with neutropenia and leukopenia are the most frequent dose-limiting toxicities (thrombocytopenia is rare; however, thrombocytosis is fairly common); mild to moderate constipation and decreased deep tendon reflexes are the most frequent occurring neurotoxicities; paresthesias occur infrequently; foot drop, peripheral neuropathy, and paralytic ileus have also been observed; mild to moderate nausea and vomiting occur in ~50% of patients; phlebitis characterized by erythema and tenderness extending over the palpable length of the infused vein has been associated with intravenous vinorelbine; mild to moderate alopecia has occurred and is related to duration of treatment; allergic reactions, fatigue, inappropriate antidiuretic hormone syndrome, hemorrhagic cystis, and insomnia have been reported

DRUG INTERACTIONS
None known

NURSING INTERVENTIONS
Myelosuppression: monitor blood counts; ask for symptoms of infection, bleeding, and anemia; **Nausea, vomiting:** give antiemetics before chemotherapy and as needed; **Nephrotoxicity:** monitor renal function indices (serum creatinine, blood urea nitrogen) and magnesium; give adequate hydration; **Neurotoxicity:** assess for weakness and numbness of legs, feet, arms, and hands.

RECENT EXPERIENCES AND RESPONSE RATES

Study group	Patients, n	Chemotherapy Dosage Schedule, mg/m²	Response Rate, %	Median Survival, wk	1-y Survival, %	Comments
Depierre [132]	116	CDDP: 80 IV every 3 wk V: 30 weekly	43.0	32	NR	Phase III study with patients treated a minimum of 6 wk
Berthaud [133]	32	CDDP: 120 IV every 4–6 wk V: 30 weekly	33.0	44	NR	Phase I–II study
Frontini [134]	74	CDDP: 80 IV d 1 V: 25 IV d 1, 8	56.7	52	NR	Phase II study with regimen every 3 wk for 3 cycles
Wozniak [107]	195	CDDP: 100 IV every 3 wk V: 25 mg/m2/wk × 3	25.0	28	33	Phase III study that showed a better 1-y survival rate of this combination compared with CDDP alone
LeChevalier [101]	206	CDDP: 120 mg/m2 IV d 1, 28 then every 6 wk V: 30 mg/m2/wk × 6 then every 2 wk	30.0	40	35	Phase III study comparing this regimen with vinorelbine alone and with cisplatin and vindesine; it showed higher response and 1-y survival rates with a major difference in survival in stage IV patients

CDDP—cisplatin; V—vinorelbine.

GEMCITABINE AND CISPLATIN IN NON–SMALL CELL LUNG CANCER

Gemcitabine is a new deoxycytidine analog related to cytosine arabinoside and has been found to have considerable activity in non–small cell lung cancer (NSCLC). Several phase II trials using gemcitabine in advanced, untreated NSCLC patients showed an overall response rate of 20% among 332 patients. In a randomized study, Manegold and coworkers [135] showed that gemcitabine was equally efficacious with less toxicity compared with the two-drug combination of cisplatin and etoposide. The impressive low toxicity profile of gemcitabine adds to its appeal in combining it with other active agents such as cisplatin. Several phase II studies in combination with cisplatin have reported an overall response rate of 47%, an average median survival of 48 weeks, and a 1-y survival rate of 48%. A randomized study in Spain comparing gemcitabine and cisplatin with etoposide and cisplatin showed a higher objective response in the gemcitabine arm (49% vs. 28%) [110].

RECENT EXPERIENCES AND RESPONSE RATES

Study	Patients, n	Chemotherapy Dosage Schedule	Response Rate, %	Median Survival, wk	1-y Overall Survival, %	Comments
Manegold et al. [135]	66	G: 1000 mg/m²/wk × 3 wk	18.2	15.3	29	Phase III study every 4 wk for a minimum of 6 cycles
Perng et al. [136]	26	G: 1250 mg/m²/wk × 3 wk	19.2	37.0	38	Phase III study every 4 wk
Einhorn et al. [137]	27	G: 1000 mg/m²/wk × 3 wk CDDP: 100 mg/m² d 1	37.0	33.6	37	Every 4 wk
Abratt et al. [138]	50	G: 1000 mg/m²/wk × 3 wk CDDP: 100 mg/m² d 15	52.0	42.0	61	Every 4 wk
Anton et al. [139]	40	G: 1250 mg/m²/wk × 3 wk CDDP: 100 mg/m² d 15	47.5	10.4	35	Every 4 wk
Shepherd et al. [140]	39	G: 1250 mg/m²/wk × 3 wk CDDP: 30 mg/m² weekly × 3 wk	26.0	26.0	NR	Every 4 wk
Lopez-Cabrezio et al. [110]	65	G: 1250 mg/m² d 1, 8 CDDP: 100 mg/m² d 1	49.0	NR	NR	Every 4 wk; a higher response rate compared with EP
Gonzalez-Baron et al. [141]	51	G: 1200 mg/m²/wk × 3 wk CDDP: 100 mg/m² d 1	43.0	NR	NR	Every 4 wk

CDDP—cisplatin; EP—etoposide and cisplatin; G—gemcitabine; NR—not reported.

CANDIDATES FOR TREATMENT
Patients refractory to standard chemotherapy; patients with stage III and stage IV NSCLC

SPECIAL PRECAUTIONS
Patients with renal dysfunction and impaired liver function

ALTERNATIVE THERAPIES
Etoposide and paclitaxel, etoposide and carboplatin, carboplatin and paclitaxel, cisplatin and vinorelbine, vinorelbine alone, or gemcitabine alone

TOXICITIES
Gemcitabine: myelosuppression is the dose-limiting toxicity; thrombocytopenia occurs occasionally, but thrombocytosis is also reported; abnormalities in liver transaminase enzymes can occur; nausea and vomiting occurs in two thirds of patients; mild proteinuria and hematuria can be present but is not associated with any change in serum creatinine or blood urea nitrogen; a rash is seen in 25% of patients and is associated with pruritus in ~10% of patients; other reported toxicities include a flu-like syndrome, mild to moderate peripheral edema, pulmonary edema, and rarely facial edema.

DRUG INTERACTION
Cisplatin with other nephro- or ototoxic drugs

NURSING INTERVENTIONS
Myelosuppression: monitor blood counts; inquire about symptoms of infection, bleeding, and anemia; **Nausea, vomiting:** give antiemetics before chemotherapy and as needed; **Nephrotoxicity:** monitor renal function indices (serum creatinine, blood urea nitrogen) and magnesium; give adequate hydration; **Neurotoxicity:** assess for weakness and numbness of legs, feet, arms, and hands

PATIENT INFORMATION
Patients should drink plenty of fluids and urinate frequently; report prolonged upset stomach, symptoms of infection (fever, chills, sore throat), and unusual bleeding or bruising.

CHAPTER 12: MELANOMA AND OTHER TUMORS OF THE SKIN

John M. Kirkwood, Michael T. Lotze

The most frequent human neoplasms are those of the skin. The nonmelanoma neoplasms are chiefly squamous and basal cell carcinomas that evolve slowly, generally permitting early recognition and cure by local measures. Less often, radiation and topical chemotherapeutic approaches are used. Melanoma is a less common but more aggressive cutaneous neoplasm that has a considerable lethal potential following progression to involve regional and distant sites. More than 15% of patients developing cutaneous melanoma will succumb to this disease, and major research efforts have recently yielded new immunologic therapies capable of preventing relapse after surgery. Melanoma also occurs in a variety of noncutaneous sites, such as the mucosae and subungual areas of the toes and fingers and the uveal tract of the eye (where it is the most lethal tumor of the eye in adults). The incidence of melanoma has risen more rapidly than other solid tumor. Currently, approximately 40,000 patients develop melanoma annually, with one in 75 white patients expected to be at risk by the year 2000 [1]. The following discussion will deal predominantly with cutaneous melanoma and basal and squamous cell carcinoma as the leading skin cancers that confront the clinician.

MELANOMA

Melanoma is a fascinating tumor with well-described patterns of genetic predisposition in 10% of cases, a clear association with episodic ultraviolet exposure, and strong evidence of host immunologic response that has recently been brought to bear on the disease in terms of its therapy. Spontaneous regression is observed in < 1% of patients, and as many as 10% of patients may develop metastases without a known primary. Although the incidence of melanoma increases with age, young adults and even children develop this tumor. Surgical excision of the primary lesion remains the mainstay of treatment for localized melanoma. New techniques of isotopic and dye localization of lymphatic drainage suggest the potential to perform selective lymph node dissection for prognostic and/or therapeutic gain. Biologic therapy of patients with regional metastatic spread has recently shown the possibility of prolonging life and increasing the cure rate of this disease for the first time.

Etiology and Risk Factors

Evidence for an inherited predisposition to melanoma comes from observations that defined family history is a risk factor for melanoma, especially in association with a characteristic precursor lesion termed the dysplastic nevus. Genes localized on chromosomes (including 1, 6, 7 and 10) appear to be important. The genetic predisposition of a subset of patients has recently been linked with mutations in p16, a gene encoding a cell cycle regulatory protein that also enhances the risk for pancreatic cancer [2–4]. Ten percent of all melanoma is associated with a family history, and in this setting, the role of the dysplastic nevus syndrome was first established as a precursor lesion. With dysplastic nevi and two cases of melanoma in a family, the risk of developing melanoma approaches 100% at 70 years of age [5]. Dysplastic nevi are suspected precursors in 25% to 40% of sporadic cases, but the molecular and immunologic features of progression from normal nevi to atypical and frankly malignant melanocytic lesions are still unclear. Early evidence suggests that alterations in growth factors and their receptors, as well as vascularization and the presence of integrins and adhesion molecules, are important [6]. Congenital melanocytic nevi are precursors related to a small subset of melanoma in the population at large. Apart from the presence of

dysplastic nevi, the risk for primary melanoma is directly related to the total number of all moles. With a personal history of melanoma, the presence of atypical nevi increases eight-fold the risk of a second primary [7].

Ultraviolet exposure clearly plays a role in development of melanoma [8]. Evidence to support this notion is found in the topographic distribution of melanoma in the body, which is directly related to sun exposure. The incidence of melanoma is associated with latitude and the intensity of solar exposure among susceptible populations. Fair-skinned individuals who have migrated to Australia and New Zealand are at particularly high-risk because of the high degree of solar radiation and the constitutional susceptibility of this population. In melanoma found to arise in the background of an atypical/dysplastic nevus, the neoplastic component most frequently arises in the junctional rather than the dermis component. Educational programs designed to modify the population's behavior in relation to sun exposure are needed [9].

The evidence for host immune reactivity to melanoma includes the frequent observation of regression in both acquired nevi and, on rare occasion, melanoma. Aside from the aforementioned risk factors, a variety of conditions associated with immunodeficiency are also associated with increased risk of melanoma and include ataxia telangiectasia, chronic lymphocytic leukemia, Hodgkin's disease, immunosuppression for organ transplantation, and AIDS (Table 12-1) [10]. Histologic evidence supporting a role of the immune response in melanoma includes the frequent finding of lymphocytic infiltrates in primary lesions and dysplastic nevi, which are diminished (if present at all) in metastatic lesions. Melanoma is responsive to many immunologic therapies, including interferon (IFN) α and interleukin (IL)-2 (*see* Treatment section) . Serologic and/or cellular

Table 12-1. Risk factors of melanoma and nonmelanoma skin cancers

Risk factor	Lifetime risk	Cancer type
Sun exposure	1%–2% (in whites)	Melanoma & SCC/BCC
Light complexion (skin that tans poorly or burns easily)	1%–2%	Melanoma & SCC/BCC
Cigarette smoking	1%–2%	SCC
Human papillomavirus (HPV 16, 18)	ND	SCC/BCC
Arsenic	ND	SCC/BCC
Polycyclic aromatic hydrocarbons	ND	SCC/BCC
Xeroderma pigmentosum (autosomal recessive)	2%–100%	Melanoma & SCC/BCC
Basal-cell nevus syndrome (autosomal dominant)	1%–5%	SCC/BCC
Albinism (autosomal recessive)	1%–5%	SCC/BCC
Epidermodysplasia verruciformis (autosomal recessive)	1%–5%	SCC/BCC
Acquired immunodeficiency syndrome	5%	Melanoma & SCC/BCC
Chronic wounds and scars	ND	SCC/BCC
Chronic immunosuppression	5%	SCC
Familial Syndromes (including atypical nevi) — p16 and p53 mutations	2%–5%	Melanoma & SCC/BCC
Multiple nevi (especially > 50 y of age)	2–12 times	Melanoma

BCC — basal cell carcinoma; ND — not determined; SCC — squamous cell carcinoma

reactivity to melanoma has been detected in a significant fraction of patients. An enlarging array of protein peptide antigens recognized by cloned T cells [11-13] and ganglioside tumor antigens identified serologic expression will enable measurement of host response to these tumor antigens in relation to vaccination and other therapies and will allow their therapeutic roles to be established (Table 12-2).

Clinical and Pathologic Appearance

The clinical characteristics of melanoma have been well described. These include the "ABCDE" criteria of asymmetry, border variation, color variation, diameter greater than 4 mm, and evolution or change noted by the patient or by a friend or family member. Bleeding and ulceration are findings that clinically suggest a poor prognosis. Evolution in the characteristics of a lesion should prompt investigation and possible biopsy. The various gradations of progression in human melanoma appear to involve a series of stages of morphologic and histopathologic steps: 1) an acquired melanocytic nevus, 2) melanocytic nevus with various degrees of architectural and cytologic atypia (dysplasia), 3) radial growth phase primary melanoma, 4) vertical growth phase primary, 5) regional lymph node metastatic melanoma, and 6) distant hematogenous metastatic melanoma. Often a patient can give a clear-cut history of progression from a pigmented lesion appearing as a nevus to the appearance of surface irregularity or ulceration associated with a vertical growth phase. A variety of different morphologic types of melanoma have been identified: 1) superficial spreading (flat) melanoma, 2) nodular melanoma, 3) lentigo maligna melanoma, 4) acral lentiginous (including subungual) melanoma, and 5) ocular melanoma. However, with the availability of microstaging for tumor depth in the past 25 years, their prognostic importance is no longer as great.

Diagnosis, Prognosis, and Staging

The treatment of melanoma varies according to disease stage as defined by the American Joint Commission on Cancer (AJCC) staging system (Table 12-3). Previously, melanoma was simply divided into three general prognostic subgroups: 1) local disease, for which surgical therapy is the predominant therapy; 2) regional disease, for which adjuvant IFNα therapy has recently entered standard practice, and selective lymph node surgery is in current evolution; and 3) systemic disease, for which a variety of experimental chemotherapeutic and immunologic approaches exist, but none have been proven to prolong survival. In the AJCC staging system, stage I and II encompass localized disease of low- and intermediate/high-recurrence risk, stage III encompasses lymph nodal disease, and stage IV represents distant metastatic disease. In stage III, the most important factors relating to local- and distant-recurrence risk are the presence or absence of extranodal/extracapsular extension and the number of

lymph nodes involved. The AJCC staging system is currently the standard for melanoma staging, although revisions have been suggested that would incorporate such factors as ulceration in the primary and node number involved for regional disease. These are widely accepted prognostic factors not formally included in the current AJCC classification [14].

A workup for primary melanoma includes a physical examination with attention to skin pigmentation, including the presence of hypopigmentation, which may reflect obliterated primary site or paraneoplastic vitiligo-like destruction of the normal pigment cells in the skin. If a patient presents with nodal or metastatic disease in the absence of an obvious primary, it is important to examine the less obvious potential noncutaneous sites of melanoma, including mucosal surfaces and the uveal tract of the eye. A chest radiograph and liver function test for the lactate dehydrogenase enzyme are performed to detect signs of occult metastatic disease in these two major organs, although neither is highly sensitive. More intensive protocols may specify computer tomography or magnetic resonance imaging to evaluate the head, chest, and abdomen to identify with greater sensitivity (although with less specificity) the potential site of metastasis.

The recognition of primary melanoma and its precursor lesions (including dysplastic nevi) depends on awareness of change in pigmented lesions. Photographic evaluation is useful in providing a reference frame for the follow-up of skin lesions in patients with particularly numerous or varied lesions. Excisional surgical or punch biopsy is required to evaluate lesions suspected of being melanoma. Patients with regional lymphadenopathy in the absence of evidence of systemic spread are best treated with regional lymphadenectomy. Patients without regional lymphadenopathy who have primary tumors of intermediate-risk (AJCC stage II) are potential candidates for the evaluation of regional lymph nodes if they would be considered for further systemic adjuvant therapy, as follows. Previously, lymphadenectomy was performed electively for the drainage basin at greatest risk defined according to the anatomic location of the primary. However, this method of determination has been found to be erroneous in up to 30% of cases. Scintigraphic and dye methods have been developed to more precisely ascertain the exact drainage of melanoma and other tumors, allowing sentinel node

Table 12-2. Antigens of human melanoma defined by T cell and antibody response

Cancer–testis antigens	Differentiation antigens
MAGE 1, 3	Tyrosinase (internal, leader)
BAGE, GAGE, RAGE	gp100 (HMB-45) (multiple, both mutated and native)
NY ESO-1	Melan-A/MART-1 (multiple)
	TP1/gp75
	TRP2/dopachrome tautomerase

Table 12-3. Staging and prognosis of melanoma

Stage	TNM	Criteria	5-y survival, %
IA	T1	Breslow ≤ 0.75 mm (Clark II)	95
IB	T2	Breslow 0.76–1.50 mm (Clark III)	90
IIA	T3	Breslow 1.51–4.00 mm (Clark IV)	80
IIB	T4	Breslow ≥ 4.10 mm (Clark V) or satellites (within 2 cm)	70
III	Any T, N1	One regional node station, node(s) mobile, diameter ≤ 5 cm < 5 in-transit metastases	25–35
IIIB	Any T, N2	≥ 1 lymph node or lymph node > 3 cm or fixed or ≥ 5 in-transit metastases	10–20
IVA	Any T, any N, M1	Involvement of skin or subcutaneous tissue beyond site of primary tumor and its drainage	10
IVB	Any T, any N, M2	Visceral metastasis	< 5%

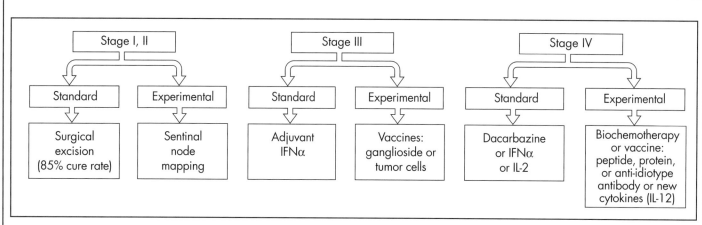

FIGURE 12-1.

Algorithm for melanoma therapy by stage. This approach to patients with melanoma includes both standard and experimental strategies. This schematic represents the current approach to patients at the University of Pittsburgh Medical Center. IFNα — interferon α; IL-2 — interleukin-2; IL-12 — interleukin-12.

biopsy and selective lymphadenectomy for diagnostic and potential therapeutic purposes [15].

Elective lymphadenectomy has shown no survival benefit in any of several large randomized controlled trials, and the therapeutic value of selective lymph node dissection is currently under study. Selective lymphadenectomy offers greater precision and lower morbidity for staging of regional lymph nodes than elective full regional lymphadenectomy. This procedure, coupled with the more effective adjuvant IFN therapy now available (see Treatment section), is becoming more widely adopted in the treatment of melanoma. The presence of distant metastasis has a radical impact on the therapeutic options and likely outcome for patients, and suspected metastatic sites of tumor are reasonable to document by needle biopsy or by serial radiological follow-up when a change of therapy is not at issue.

Prognostic factors for survival include microstage of disease as defined by tumor thickness (Breslow depth) and, previously, skin layer penetration (Clark level) (see Table 12-3). Mitotic rate, ulceration, and the presence of satellites are prognostically important histologic factors (Table 12-4). Younger patients, females, and patients with extremity lesions fare better than older males and those with truncal tumors. Although T-cell infiltrate is a factor associated with improved prognosis, expression of the class II MHC molecules, (DR, DP, DQ) has been associated with poorer prognosis. The loss of class I MHC expression is recognized as a factor relevant to the evasion of immune recognition, but further study is required.

Treatment

The surgical treatment for primary melanoma has been studied for many years now. Consensus from a number of published studies indicates that a wide local excision should be performed for lesions deeper than 1.0 mm; 2-cm margins have recently been demonstrated to be equivalent to 4-cm margins in a prospective randomized trial for primary tumors of 1–4 mm Breslow depth [16]. Therapeutic lymphadenectomy is indicated for manifest, regional lymph node metastases in the absence of distant disease. Prophylactic regional lymph node dissection has not been demonstrated to be of value in prolonging survival or time to relapse in any of a number of large, randomized controlled studies. Selective regional lymphadenectomy performed after scintigraphic and dye-lymphographic identification of the sentinel draining lymph

node(s) offers improved prognostic precision as noted above, and its therapeutic role is currently under study in the Multicenter Selective Lymphadenectomy Trial. Limited cutaneous or nodal tumor resection has a role in palliation of symptomatic mass lesions without any demonstrable impact on survival. Patients with isolated visceral metastatic brain disease or with gastrointestinal tract tumors may obtain significant benefit from resection of limited metastatic disease, especially following long disease-free intervals or with disease that has a long doubling time on serial radiologic follow up. In general, resection of metastases of lung, liver, and other abdominal viscera has shown little advantage [17,18].

Radiation therapy is an alternative palliative modality for inoperable visceral metastases sites, particularly in bone and in the brain. In high-dose fractions given for metastatic brain disease, steroid premedication should be used to prevent edema, which may exacerbate symptoms or provoke hemorrhage. Bleeding into brain metastases is particularly frequent in patients with melanoma. Intensive local irradiation using a stereotactic delivery in special multibeam units (gamma-knife therapy) appears to be useful for treatment of patients with unresectable, isolated, or a limited number of small (< 2.5 cm) lesions [19]. Whole-brain radiotherapy has been used to reduce the size and risk of bleeding from brain metastases, although studies to evaluate its role in conjunction with stereotactic radiation therapy are incomplete.

Table 12-4. Adverse prognostic factors

Histoligic
Increased tumor thickness (Breslow depth) or skin layer penetration (Clark level), increased mitotic rate, presence of ulceration or satellites

Clinical
Advanced age, male gender, trunk or head and neck as site of origin, mucosal melanoma, morphology of the primary tumor (nodular as opposed to superficial spreading)

Immunologic
Lack of lymphoid inflammatory infiltrate within the primary lesion, HLA-antigen expression decreased or absent, serum antibody to melanoma absent, lack of delayed type hypersensitivity response to tumor

Table 12-5. Prevention and early detection.

Sunscreens, limit exposure to midday sun, sunglasses, hats
Regular examination of skin particularly in light-skinned, fair-haired individuals
Wood's lamp examination of skin; epiluminescence
Topical retinoids (under investigation)

Table 12-6. Current noninvestigational regimens for melanoma

Regimen	Response rates
IFNα-2	15%–20% in established disease, in which durable complete responses noted in one-third improvement in disease-free and overall survival as adjuvant
Dacarbazine Temuzolomide	15%; randomized studies combined ± IFN ± tamoxifen (E3690) not demonstrably better.
Melphalan	80%–100%; combination therapy with TNFα and IFNγ under study in perfusion patients with in-transit metastases
Interleukin-2	15%–25% in established disease; complete responses (10%) durable up to 10 y; partial responses (10%) of 18–24 mo median duration; response improved at highest doses tested

Dacarbazine (dimethyl triazeno imidazole carboxamide or DTIC) is the only FDA-approved chemotherapeutic agent for treatment of metastatic melanoma in the United States. Complete and partial responses with dacarbazine alone or combined with cisplatin and biologic agents occur in approximately 20% of patients, with a mean duration of response that is 5 to 7 months [20–22]. Response to this agent has been correlated with disease limited to soft tissues and female gender. Dacarbazine requires hepatic transformation to its active intermediate, whereas temozolomide, a newer fully-absorbed oral prodrug, shows a wider distribution in the body (including central nervous system) and spontaneously transforms into the same active intermediate as for dacarbazine. To date, no benefit has been demonstrated for adjuvant chemotherapy with dacarbazine alone or in combination with other chemotherapeutic and hormonal agents. No other single agent has shown results, suggesting a true response rate in patients with metastatic disease greater than or equal to 20%.

Patients presenting with asymptomatic or minimally symptomatic metastatic melanoma can reasonably be offered a variety of investigational treatment programs. Combination chemotherapy historically has been associated with increased toxicity that outweighs the minimal gains in response rate obtained using a variety of different protocols. Early studies of dacarbazine with tamoxifen appeared to have been of benefit for subjects in one randomized trial, whereas dacarbazine and IFN showed benefit in another. Unfortunately, larger multicenter studies of these two combinations conducted in the Eastern Cooperative Oncology Group (ECOG) (E3690) have shown no survival benefit for either combination or for all three agents together over dacarbazine alone [23]. A considerable degree of interest and enthusiasm has been raised in a series of reports of uncontrolled trials using the four-agent combination of dacarbazine, bischlorethylnitrosourea (BCNU), cisplatin, and tamoxifen, which is known as the Dartmouth regimen [24]. Careful controlled studies of the National Cancer Institute–Canada have dismissed the previous suggestion of benefit from tamoxifen in this combination [22], and a recently concluded trial of the ECOG and Memorial-Sloan Kettering Cancer Center (MSKCC) (M91-140) will complete the evaluation of this Dartmouth combination against dacarbazine. High-dose chemotherapy with bone marrow rescue using melphalan, thiotepa, or BCNU have achieved improved short-term responses but not durable complete remissions or overall survival benefit.

IFNα treatment is associated with response in 16% to 22% of a collected series of patients with metastatic melanoma [25]. Treatment has been reported to achieve durable complete remissions in one third of responders. Response is associated with soft tissue or pulmonary sites and is higher in smaller-bulk disease. A variety of combinations with chemotherapy have been investigated with contradictory results, which may be due to the dose and sequence of agents used [26].

IL-2 (a T-cell growth factor employed since 1984 in the treatment of patients with melanoma [27-30]) has achieved a response rate of 20% to 25% with a subset of patients who experience durable complete response. Treatment with IL-2 (recently approved by the FDA for treatment of metastatic renal cell cancer) requires very high doses for induction of response. Associated vascular leak syndrome, hypotension, myocardial infarction, and renal failure has tempered the application of this modality.

Other cytokines (including IL-4, IL-12, tumor necrosis factor [TNF], and IL-1) have attractive rationale but as yet have no clinical substantiation for the treatment of melanoma. Significant interest in vaccines has existed in the field of melanoma for many years, and a variety of vaccines have been tested, but none has yet shown evidence of an increase in survival in properly controlled trials [15,31]. Adoptive immunotherapy with transfer of cellular reagents (including tumor infiltrating lymphocytes or lymphokine-activated killer cells with IL-2) have been shown to induce response rates of 30% to 50% in limited series, although their role beyond that associated with IL-2 alone has been difficult to prove. Gene therapy that introduces cytokine genes or costimulatory molecules such as CD80 (B7.1) into tumors are currently undergoing evaluation at a number of centers [32].

Isolated limb perfusion using melphalan has been applied for many years and has gone through a resurgence of interest in combination with TNFα administered by perfusion and with IFNγ administered systemically [33,34]. Recent results from a randomized study comparing melphalan alone with the combination performed at the NCI have not shown improved outcome with the combination overall, although there is a suggestion that it may be superior for patients with extensive disease (> 10 lesions).

The risk factors predicting outcome in the setting of metastatic disease have recently been analyzed [14,35–37], with three independent variables predicting survival: 1) initial site of the metastases (patients with distant cutaneous, nodal, and gastrointestinal disease fare better than those presenting with lung disease, which is better than other visceral sites), 2) disease-free interval prior to distant metastases, and 3) stage of disease preceding distant metastases. In long-term survivors, younger age and female gender tended to be correlated with improved survival, but the only significant difference was the ability of the long-term surviving patients to have all metastatic disease resected or a complete or partial response with initial chemotherapy or immunotherapy. Multivariate analysis of a recent series of patients with metastatic disease has shown independent prognostic roles for blood lactic dehydrogenase and albumin levels. These factors should be considered in the design of future trials in the setting of metastatic disease.

Table 12-7. Current and planned cooperative group adjuvant trials for treatment of melanoma

Group No.	Regimen	Principle investigators
E1694	Phase III study of adjuvant ganglioside vaccination therapy for high-risk melanoma (T4 > 4 mm primary or N1 [regional lymph node metastasis AJCC stages IIB/III]) compared with interferon α-2b	Kirkwood J, Lawson D
E1697	Phase III study of 1 mo of adjuvant high-dose interferon α-2b in patients with resected stage IIA melanoma	Agarwala S, Kirkwood J (ECOG), Isacove N (NCI-C)
E3697	Phase III clinical trial evaluating the use of postoperative adjuvant radiotherapy in the treatment of patients with extranodal extension of melanoma	Wazer D
E2696	Phase II trial of GMK vaccine in combination with interferon α-2b vs GMK vaccine alone in high-risk resectable melanoma	Kirkwood J, Chapman P
E3695	Phase III randomized intergroup trial of concurrent biochemotherapy with cisplatin, dacarbazine, vinblastine, interleukin-2, and interferon α-2b versus dacarbazine alone in patients with metastatic malignant melanoma	Atkins M (ECOG) Flaherty L (SWOG)

AJCC—American Joint Commission on Cancer; ECOG—Eastern Cooperative Oncology Group; NCI-C—National Cancer Institute–Canada; SWOG—Southwestern Oncology Group.

Adjuvant Therapy

The staging of melanoma by classical tumor-node-metastasis (TNM) and AJCC systems is detailed in Table 12-3. In AJCC staging (the current standard), primary melanomas deeper than 0.76 mm (T2) without associated metastatic involvement of regional lymph nodes (N0) are defined as stage IB, whereas melanomas deeper than 1.50 mm (T3) in the absence of lymphadenopathy are defined as stage IIA. Those deeper than 4.0 mm (T4) and free of clinically apparent regional nodal involvement or other signs of metastasis are defined as stage IIB, with a risk that approaches that of patients with clinical manifestations of regional lymph node metastasis, which is defined as stage IIIA (N1). The prognostic subclassification of nodal involvement is formally defined by node size (> 3 cm), but it is widely recognized that the prognosis for node-positive patients is better quantified by the number of tumor-involved lymph nodes. Patients with distant metastasis beyond the regional draining nodal group (M1) are defined as stage IV. These disease groupings contrast to the three classical staging groups of primary disease (old stage I), regional nodal involvement (old stage II), and distant metastases (old stage III). Newer systems, incorporating the presence of ulceration and satellite involvement in the prognostication of localized disease and the number of involved nodes for patients in stage III, have been proposed and are expected to be assimilated into the AJCC system [14].

High risk of relapse, generally exceeding 50% in the first 2 years of follow-up, is associated with AJCC stage III melanoma and the presence of regional lymph node metastasis (stage IIB disease with deep invasion at the site of the primary lesion > 4 mm). These have ominous prognostic significance. For this reason, patients in these prognostic groups have been widely considered for new therapies (ranging from chemotherapy to biologicals), including interferons, cytokines, antibodies, and tumor vaccines.

Extensive literature has been published detailing the results of multiple randomized controlled trials of chemotherapy and chemotherapy with older biologicals (*eg*, the crude microbial immunostimulants bacille Calmette–Guérin [BCG], *Corynebacterium parvum*, and OK 432 [38]. These studies failed to yield consistent beneficial evidence to support further investigation of these regimens (based largely on the drug dacarbazine). Chemical immunomodulators and the antihelminthic agent levamisole have also been intensively investigated, with controversial results that have not led to regulatory approval or clinical use of levamisole as adjuvant therapy outside Canada [39,40].

The largest and most positive literature for adjuvant therapy surrounds IFNα-2, which has been tested in high-risk groups of patients with resected stage III and IIB melanoma [41]. This study shows the first significant benefit of adjuvant therapy, both in terms of survival rate and relapse-free interval. The ECOG high-dose regimen, which employed intravenous office therapy (20 MU/m^2/d, 5 d/wk for 4 wk) followed by subcutaneous patient-administered therapy (10 MU/m^2/d three times weekly for 11 mo) with IFNα-2b, has significantly prolonged relapse-free survival (p_1 = 0.002) and overall survival (p_1 = 0.023) of patients treated within 56 days of surgery. This agent has been approved by the FDA as the first and only agent capable of preventing relapse and death in high-risk melanoma. The toxicity of treatment at the maximally tolerable dosages employed in the study were significant, and severe toxicity was noted in a majority of patients at one or more times during therapy. However, the regimen was given entirely in the outpatient setting, and (with dose modification for these dose-limiting constitutional [50%], hematologic [24%], or hepatic [15%] toxicities) 74% of patients without relapse continued on treatment through the full year [41].

The quality of life during and following this therapy has been evaluated since 1984 in the ECOG. Adjuvant therapy for resected stage IIB–III AJCC disease using the foregoing intravenous and subcutaneous high-dose regimen showed benefit (even accounting for toxicity), significantly prolonged survival (2.8–3.8 y), and improved by 40% the fraction of patients who never relapsed at a mature median follow-up of 7 years. This adjuvant regimen approved by the FDA for use in high-risk postoperative patients has been assessed for cost efficacy and shows figures comparable with accepted adjuvant chemotherapy in breast and colorectal cancer [41–43].

A variety of programs of IFN therapy seeking to obtain similar benefit with lower dosages or shorter intervals of treatment have been pursued. None of these has yet shown a significant impact on relapse-free and overall survival rates; negative results have been reported with lower dosages of subcutaneous IFNα-2a given for 3 years in the World Health Organization Melanoma Programme trial #16 [44], as well as shorter intramuscular regimens given for 3 months at 20 MU/m^2. Adjuvant radiation therapy to the area of potential nodal disease may provide local benefit [45] and will be tested in a prospective trial through the ECOG for patients with increased regional relapse risk on the basis of extracapsular extension of tumor.

A variety of vaccines have been developed and tested for melanoma, ranging from the whole-cell vaccines administered with either the immunostimulant BCG, or a detoxified Lipid A derivative (Detox Ribi Immunochemicals, Inc.). The results obtained by these investigators in uncontrolled trials have led to the development of a randomized controlled trial performed by the Southwestern Oncology Group (S9035). This trial tested the efficacy of a commercially produced allogeneic tumor cell vaccine (Melacine; Ribi Immunochemicals, Inc.) in more than 600 patients accrued over the past 7 years with resected stage II primary melanoma. The results of this trial are not anticipated for several years. A larger multicenter trial of Newcastle disease virus in viral melanoma oncolysate is the only published multicenter controlled trial of vaccine therapy in the literature, and it is negative [46].

Vaccine therapies designed to induce antibody reactive with the gangliosides of melanoma (GM2, GD2) have been tested in controlled phase II–III single-institution trials at MSKCC. Initial vaccines employed the older immunostimulant BCG; prolonged relapse-free survival was observed among vaccinated patients with high titers of antibody against GM2 (IgM). The unbalanced presence of native antibody in the unvaccinated control population (9%), and the limited size of this phase III trial (122 patients) resulted in findings that are not significant, despite a trend to benefit from this GM2/BCG vaccine. Recently, a modified commercial vaccine composed of GM2 coupled to keyhole-limpet hemocyanin administered with the potent immunologic adjuvant QS-21 has given higher and more durable titers of antibodies IgM and IgG against GM2 (GMK, Progenics Inc., Tarrytown, NJ). This agent is under evaluation in an intergroup phase III trial (E1694) that commenced in 1996 and will accrue subjects through 1999. Although this phase III trial asks whether GM2 vaccine is more effective than the current standard E1684 regimen of IFN, further questions relate to the potential for synergistic and additive (or, on the other hand, antagonistic) effects of IFN given concurrently with or directly following the initiation of this vaccine. To test this question, the ECOG has conducted a study of GM2 vaccination versus GM2 with IFN (or GM2 followed after a month of vaccination by IFN). This trial (E2696) will provide evidence that may permit the rational selection of combined modality approaches in the next year.

Cellular Immunity

During the past several years, a number of studies have been conducted on the autologous CD4 and CD8 T-cell–mediated response to human melanoma [13,47–50]. The emerging picture indicates that melanomas express multiple T-cell–defined epitopes, some of which are unique to a given tumor and reflect mutations, whereas others are shared by allogeneic melanomas of patients who are of similar HLA type. These epitopes represent short (9–10) amino acid peptides derived from tumor-associated antigens that are recognized by the CD8+ T cells in the context of major histocompatibility complex (MHC) class I antigens of the host antigen-presenting cell. A classification of antigens defined by T-cell recognition in human cancers includes three categories: 1) differentiation or lineage antigens (chiefly associated with the process of melanization and pigment formation in melanoma); 2) cancer–testis antigens, referring to a series of melanoma antigens (MAGE 1,2,3; NY-ESO-1; and HO-MEL-40) specified by X-linked genes and expressed only in cancers of a range of organs as well as normal testis (and ovary); and 3) a group of antigens found to result from mutation of normal gene products [51]. Clinical trials evaluating representa-

tives of these peptide vaccines are underway at many centers in the U.S. and Europe with surprising early successes.

The most exciting new prospect for the specific vaccine therapy of melanoma may lie in the use of the peptide epitopes or whole protein recognized by the host T cell. T-cell recognition occurs in conjunction with the presenting MHC molecules of the host, with restrictions that to date have limited the application of these vaccine approaches. The genes encoding these targets have been cloned by investigators in the U.S. and Europe over the past several years [46], and alternative strategies using the whole proteins (or DNA encoding these antigens) may obviate the difficulties associated with MHC-restricted recognition of peptide antigens. These peptides, proteins, and complimentary DNA vaccines are currently undergoing testing in clinical trials.

Ocular Melanoma

Arising from the pigmented epithelium of the choroid, ocular melanoma is associated with visual disturbances at presentation and rarely with metastatic disease. The usual clinical treatment is either enucleation or radiotherapy, which are being evaluated against one another in a formal trial by the collaborators of the Ocular Melanoma Study Committee with the support of the National Eye Institute and the NCI. Photodynamic therapy has been tested with an apparent improved response rate [52]. The risk of metastasis varies with the histologic type and size of these tumors as well as their location in the eye. Historically, metastases occur most frequently in the liver but have been well documented in bone, skin, lung, and a variety of other tissues. Hepatic metastases from ocular melanoma are unusually resistant to systemic chemotherapy or immunotherapy. Remarkably, even the 10% to 20% response rate observed with cutaneous melanoma is not observed, and current trials are evaluating regional intra-arterial chemotherapy.

NONMELANOMA SKIN CANCERS

The most frequent tumors in the white population are nonmelanoma skin tumors [53]. More than 500,000 new cases of basal cell carcinoma and 100,000 cases of squamous cell carcinomas occur each year. The incidence has increased by 65% since 1980, probably due to increased sun exposure [1]. Most of the tumors occur on skin exposed to the sun, and there is clearly a relationship between latitude and cumulative solar exposure and incidence of these tumors. Deaths due to these tumors are extremely infrequent, allowing most cancer protocols treating tumors at other sites to permit these as preceding malignancies. Approximately 1500 deaths occur each year due largely to squamous cell carcinoma (~1:500 patients). This death rate is approximately one fourth of that due to melanoma.

There are multiple risk factors associated with these nonmelanoma skin cancers (*see* Table 12-1). Clearly, efforts are needed to decrease exposure to the sun and other carcinogenic factors associated with a concomitant decrease in skin tumors. The most common sites of metastases (which occur infrequently) are regional lymph nodes. Rarely, liver, lung, bone, and brain metastases are found. The primary treatment for skin tumors is local ablative therapy. This may consist of simple excisional procedures, excision and grafting or flap rotation, electrodesiccation and curettage, cryosurgery, Mohs' surgery, or radiation therapy. Each procedure is designed to ablate the tumor. Because local recurrence is the major risk—and the margin of excision needed to control these tumors may be less than for tumors like melanoma with discontinuous local extension—a variety of procedures have been developed to try to encompass the tumor while preserving normal skin, especially in cosmetically sensitive areas. One such technique, known after its originator as Mohs' surgery, attempts to remove successive shells of tissue so as to take the minimal amount of tissue while completely excising the tumor. This is a time-consuming and costly procedure.

Radiation therapy is perhaps best used in older patients who may not tolerate the necessary surgery. Topical fluorouracil can be used to treat multiple basal cell carcinomas or actinic keratosis, in which the multiplicity of established or emerging new tumors in some patients makes surgical removal problematic [54,55]. Beta carotene and isotretinoin have shown benefit in clinical trials and await definitive evaluation in this context.

REFERENCES

1. Rigel DS: Epidemiology and prognostic factors in malignant melanoma. *Ann Plast Surg* 1992, 28:7–8.

2. Skolnick, MH, Cannon-Albright LA, Kamb A: Genetic predisposition to melanoma. *Eur J Cancer* 1994, 30A:1991–1995.

3. Whelan AJ, Bartsch D, Goodfellow PJ: A familial syndrome of pancreatic cancer and melanoma with a mutation in the CDKN2 tumor-suppressor gene. *N Engl J Med* 1995, 333:970–974.

4. Goldstein AM, Fraser MC, Struewing JP, *et al.*: Increased risk of pancreatic cancer in melanoma-prone kindreds with p16INC4 mutations. *N Engl J Med* 1995, 333:970–974.

5. Greene MH, Clark WJ Jr, Tucker MA, *et al.*: High risk of malignant melanoma in melanoma-prone families with dysplastic nevi. *Ann Intern Med* 1985, 102:458–465.

6. Wang Y, Rao U, Mascari R, Richards TJ, *et al.*: Molecular analysis of melanoma precursor lesions. *Cell Growth Differ* 1996, 7:1733–1740.

7. Titus-Ernstoff L, Duray PH, Ernstoff MS, *et al.*: Dysplastic nevi in association with multiple primary melanoma. *Cancer Res* 1998, 48:1016–1018.

8. Ziegler A, Jonason AS, Leffel DJ, *et al.*: Sunburn and p53 in the onset of skin cancer. *Nature* 1994, 372:773–776.

9. Rhodes AR: Public education and cancer of the skin. *Cancer* 1995, 75:613–636.

10. Wang C, Brodland DG, Su WPD: Skin cancers associated with acquired immunodeficiency syndrome [abstract]. *Mayo Clin Proc* 1995, 70:766–772.

11. Boon T: Toward a genetic analysis of tumor rejection antigens. *Adv Cancer Res* 1992, 58:177–210.

12. Sahin U, Tureci O, Schmitt H, *et al.*: Human neoplasms elicit multiple specific immune response in the autologous host. *Proc Natl Acad Sci U S A* 1995, 92:11810–11813.

13. Maeurer MJ, Storkus WJ, Kirkwood JM, Lotze MT: New treatment option for patient with melanoma: review of melanoma-derived T-cell epitope-based peptide vaccines. *Melanoma Res* 1996, 6:11–24.

14. Ross MI, Balch CM, Soong S, *et al.*: Critical analysis of the current american joint committee on cancer staging system for cutaneous melanoma and proposal of a new staging system. *J Clin Oncol* 1997, 15:1039–1051.

15. Morton DL, Foshag LJ, Hoon DS, *et al.*: Prolongation of survival in metastatic melanoma after active specific immunotherapy with a new polyvalent melanoma vaccine. *Ann Surg* 1992, 216:463–482.

16. Balch, CM, Urist MM, Karakousis CP, *et al.*: Efficacy of 2-cm surgical margins for intermediate-thickness melanomas (1–4 mm): results of a multi-institutional randomized surgical trial. *Ann Surg* 1993, 218:262–269.

17. Karakousis, CP, Velez A, Driscoll DL, Takita H: Metastasectomy in malignant melanoma. *Surgery* 1994, 115:295–302.

18. Karp NS, Boyd A, DePan HJ, *et al.*: Thoracotomy for metastatic malignant melanoma of the lung. *Surgery* 1990, 107:256–261.

19. Loffler JS, Larson DA, Shrieve DC, Flickinger JC: Radiosurgery for the treatment of intracranial lesions. In *Important Advances in Oncology*.

Edited by DeVita V, Hellman S, Rosenberg S. Philadelphia; Lippincott; 1995:141–156.

20. Falkson CI, Falkson G, Falkson HC. Improved results with the addition of interferon alfa-2b to dacarbazine in the treatment of patients with metastatic malignant melanoma. *J Clin Oncol* 1991, 9:1403–1408.

21. Bleehan NM, Newlands ES, Lee SM, *et al.*: Cancer research campaign phase II trial of temozolomide in metastatic melanoma. *J Clin Oncol* 1995, 13:910–913.

22. Rustoven JJ, Quirt IC, Iscoe NA, *et al.*: Randomized, double-blind, placebo-controlled trial comparing the response rates of carmustine, dacarbazine, and cisplatin with and without tamoxifen in patients with metastatic melanoma. *J Clin Oncol* 1996, 14:2083–2090.

23. Falkson CI, Ibrahim J, Kirkwood JM, *et al.*: A phase III trial of dacarbazine versus dacarbazine with interferon alpha-2b versus dacarbazine with tamoxifen (TMX) versus dacarbazine with interferon alpha-2b and tamoxifen in patients with metastatic malignant melanoma: an Eastern Cooperative Oncology Group Study (E3690). *J Clin Oncol* 1998, in press.

24. Del Prete SA, Maurer LH, O'Donnell J, *et al.*: Combination chemotherapy with cisplatin, carmustine, dacarbazine and tamoxifen in malignant melanoma. *Cancer Treat Rep* 1984, 68:1403–1405.

25. Kirkwood JM: Biologic therapy with interferon a and b: clinical applications—melanoma. In *Biologic Therapy of Cancer: Principles and Practice*. Edited by DeVita VT Jr, Hellman S, Rosenberg SA. Philadelphia: JB Lippincott; 1995:388–411.

26. Atkins MB: The role of cytotoxic chemotherapeutic agents either alone or in combination with biological response modifiers. In *Molecular Diagnosis and Treatment of Melanoma*. Edited by Kirkwood JM. New York:Marcel Dekker, Inc.; 1998.

27. Lotze MT: Biologic therapy with interleukin-2: preclinical studies. In *Biologic Therapy of Cancer: Principles and Practice*. Edited by DeVita VT Jr, Hellman S, Rosenberg SA. Philadelphia: JB Lippincott; 1995:207–233.

28. Royal RE, Steinberg SM, Krouse RS, *et al.*: Correlates of response to IL-2 therapy in patients treated for metastatic renal cancer and melanoma. *Sci Am* 1996, 2:91–98.

29. Keilholz U, Scheibenbogen C, Tilgen W, *et al.*: Interferon-a and interleukin-2 in the treatment of metastatic melanoma: comparison of two phase II trials. *Cancer* 1993, 72:607–614.

30. Rosenberg SA, Yang JC, Topalian SL: The treatment of 283 consecutive patients with metastatic melanoma or renal cell cancer using high-dose bolus interleukin-2. *JAMA* 1994, 271:907–913.

31. Hoon DS, Yuzuki D, Hayashida M, *et al.*: Melanoma patients immunized with melanoma cell vaccine induce antibody responses to recombinant MAGE-1 antigen. *J Immunol* 1995, 154:730–737.

32. Lotze MT: A new perspective: cytokine gene therapy of cancer. *Cancer J Sci Am* 1996, 2:63–72.

33. Lienard D, Ewalenko P, Delmotte JJ, *et al.*: High-dose recombinant tumor necrosis factor alpha in combination with interferon gamma and melphalan in isolation perfusion of the limbs for melanoma and sarcoma. *J Clin Oncol* 1992, 10:52–60.

34. Thom AK, Alexander HR, Andrich MP, *et al.:* Cytokine levels and systemic toxicity in patients undergoing isolated likb perfusion with high-dose tumor necrosis factor, interferon gamma, and melphalan. *J Clin Oncol* 1995, 13:264–273.

35. Barth A, Wanke LA, Morton DL: Analysis of prognostic factors in 1521 patients with metastatic melanoma [abstract]. *Proc ASCO* 1995, 14:410.

36. Flaherty LE, Robinson W, Redman BG, *et al.:* A phase II study of dacarbazine and cisplatin in combination with outpatient administered interleukin-2 in metastatic malignant melanoma. *Cancer* 1993, 71:3520–3525.

37. Sirott MN, Bajorin DF, Wong GY, *et al.:* Prognostic factors in patients with metastatic malignang melanoma: a multivariate analysis. *Cancer* 1993, 72:3091–3098.

38. Kirkwood JM, Wilson J, Whiteside TL, *et al.:* Phase IB trial of picibanil (OK-432) as an immunomodulator in patients with resected high-risk melanoma. *Cancer Immunol Immunother* 1997, 44:137–149.

39. Lear JT, Strange RC, Fryer AA: Relationship between sunlight exposure and a key genetic alteration in basal cell carcinoma. *J Natl Cancer Inst* 1997, 89:454–455.

40. Spitler, LE: A randomized trial of levamisole versus placebo as adjuvant therapy in malignant melanoma. *J Clin Oncol* 1991, 9:736–740.

41. Kirkwood, JM, Strawderman MH, Ernstoff MS, *et al.:* Interferon alfa-2b adjuvant therapy of high-risk resected cutaneous melanoma: the Eastern Cooperative Oncology Group Trial EST1684. *J Clin Oncol* 1996, 14:7–17.

42. Cole BF, Gelber RD, Kirkwood JM, *et al.:* A quality-of-life-adjusted survival anaysis of interferon alfa-2b adjuvant treatment for high-risk resected cutaneous melanoma: an Eastern Cooperative Oncology Group Study (E1684). *J Clin Oncol* 1996, 14:2666–2673.

43. Hillner BE, Kirkwood JM, Atkins MB, *et al.:* Economic analysis of adjuvant interferon alfa-2b in high-risk melanoma based on projections from ECOG 1684. *J Clin Oncol* 1997, 15:2351–2358.

44. Cascinelli N: Evaluation of efficacy of adjuvant rIFN alpha-2a in melanoma patients with regional node metastases [abstract]. *Proc ASCO* 1995, 14:A1296.

45. Strom EA, Ross MI: Adjuvant ratiation therapy after axillary lymphadenectomy for metastatic melanoma: toxicity and local control. *Ann Surg Onc* 1995, 2:445–449.

46. Wallack MK, Sivanandham M, Balch CM, *et al.*: 1995. A phase III randomized, double-blind, multiinstitutional trial of vaccinia melanoma oncolysate-active specific immunotherapy for patients with stage II melanoma. Cancer 75:34–42.

47. Maeurer MJ, Hurd S, Martin DS, *et al.*: Cytolytic T cell clones define HLA-A2 restricted human cutaneous melanoma peptide epitopes: correlation with T cell receptor usage. *Cancer* 1995, 1:162–170.

48. van der Bruggen P, Traversari C, Chomez P, *et al.*: A gene encoding an antigen recognized by cytolytic T lymphocytes on a human melanoma. *Science* 1991, 254:1643–1647.

49. Marincola FM, Shamamian P, Alexander RB, *et al.*: Loss of HLA haplotype and B locus down-regulation in melanoma cell lines. *J Immunol* 1994, 153:1225–1237.

50. Topalian SL, Rivoltini L, Mancini M, *et al.*: Human CD4+ T cells specifically recognize a shared melanoma-associated antigen encoded by the tyrosinase gene. *Proc Natl Acad Sci U S A* 1994, 91:9461–9465.

51. Wolfel T, Hauer M, Schneider J, *et al.*: A p161NK4a-insensitive CDK4 mutant targeted by cytolytic T lymphocytes in a human melanoma. *Science* 1995, 269:1281–1284.

52. Favilla I, Favilla ML, Gosbell AD, *et al.*: Photodynamic therapy: a 5-year study of its effectiveness in the treatment of posterior uveal melanoma, and evaluation of haematoporphyrin uptake and photocytotoxicity of melanoma cells in tissue culture. *Melanoma Res* 1995, 5:355–364.

53. Preston DS, Stern RS: Nonmelanoma cancers of the skin. *N Engl J Med* 1992, 327:1649–1662.

54. Cullen SI: Topical fluorouracil therapy for precancer and cancers of the skin. *J Am Geratr Soc* 1997, 27:529–535.

55. Ashton H, Beveridge GW, Stevenson CJ: Topical treatment of skin tumors with 5-flourouracil. *Br J Dermatol* 1970, 82:207–209.

INTERFERON α-2

Interferon α-2 has shown modest levels of antitumor activity as a single agent in patients with metastatic melanoma, ranging from 15% to 20% in multiple trials. The highest response rates with IFN α-2 were noted in patients with the smallest bulk of disease. Immune mechanisms of antitumor response have their greatest impact in microscopic (or adjuvant) therapy rather than the advanced disease [30].

DOSAGE AND SCHEDULING

Arm A: high-dose IFN α-2b for 1 y
Induction therapy: 20 MU/m² QID IV for 5 d × 4 wk
Maintenance: 10 MU/m²/d 3 × weekly SC × 48 wk
Arm B: chronic low-dose IFN α-2b for 2 y
        3 MU/m²/d 3 × weekly SC
Arm C: Observation: studies at serial intervals (control)

DOSAGE MODIFICATION: *Reduce dose if bilirubin is elevated (2.6–5 × ULN) or SGOT, alkaline phosphatase is elevated (2.6–5 × ULN).*

CANDIDATES FOR TREATMENT

High-risk patients with deep primary melanoma (> 4 mm Breslow depth) with or without lymph node involvement (T4, NO, MO)

TOXICITIES

Fever, chill, myalgia and arthralgia, fatigue, headache; neutropenia, anemia, thrombocytopenia (not dose limiting unless severe); hepatotoxicity (at high doses), hyperbilirubinemia, apparent hepatic necrosis (rare); proteinuria, elevated creatinine or BUN (at high doses)

ALTERNATIVE THERAPIES

Vaccination with cultured irradiated lines of tumor cells or partially purified proteins, whole tumor cells, partially purified proteins shed from cultured tumor cells, virus-modified tumor cell vaccine, defined gangliosides for immunization against melanoma, defined peptides and proteins for immunization against melanoma, antiidiotype antibodies as vaccine

ENTRY TO THE INTERGROUP STUDY

Patients may be formally entered into study by investigators in the Eastern Cooperative Oncology Group, Cancer and Leukemia Group B, and Southwest Oncology Group or at the MD Anderson and Memorial Sloan-Kettering Cancer Centers

DRUG INTERACTIONS

Aspirin, prostaglandin synthetase inhibitors, antihistamines, other immunomodulators, NSAIDs

DACARBAZINE, ALONE OR IN COMBINATION

The ECOG study group is conducting a phase III trial of dacarbazine alone versus pairwise combinations with interferon treatment-2, tamoxifen, or a combination of these agents for surgically incurable metastatic melanoma. This trial is designed to confirm or refute initial reports using dacarbazine combined with IFN α-2 in South Africa and with tamoxifen in Italy to a reasonably high level of confidence.

Dacarbazine is the only single agent that is FDA-approved for the indication of palliative therapy of metastatic melanoma. Combined chemotherapy for melanoma has not previously induced remissions significantly more frequently (> 15%) than dacarbazine nor prolonged survival of tested patients. However, two approaches have suggested prolonged survival of patients with metastatic melanoma through combined-modality treatment: tamoxifen plus dacarbazine [15,29] and IFN α-2 plus dacarbazine.

TRIAL DESIGN

Phase III comparison of dacarbazine or dacarbazine combined with either IFN α-2, tamoxifen, or both: dacarbazine alone, dacarbazine plus tamoxifen, dacarbazine plus IFN α-2, or dacarbazine plus IFN α-2 plus tamoxifen

This efficient trial design will allow analysis of groups separately and collapsed into larger groups with or without tamoxifen and with or without IFN.

CANDIDATES FOR TREATMENT

Histologically confirmed surgically incurable metastatic melanoma; measurable disease; performance status of 0–2; normal hematologic and biochemical values; SGOT < 3 times the upper limit of normal (unless deviation due to metastases); no prior chemotherapy; no prior radiotherapy to measurable disease; and no brain metastases
Exclusion criteria: ocular melanoma; angina pectoris; ventricular arrhythmias or myocardial infarction within 6 mo; prior malignancy; history of clinical depression

TOXICITIES

Flu-like syndrome (anorexia, fatigue and malaise, chills or rigors, myalgias and arthralgias); hematologic, renal, hepatic, CNS, and GI toxicities; weight gain (fluid retention) or loss (anorexia)

ALTERNATIVE THERAPIES

Three-drug regimen of cisplatin, vinblastine, decarbazine, with response rates of 50%, four-drug regimen of cisplatin, BCNU, tamoxifen, and dacarbazine with response rates of 50%; six-drug regimen with IFN α-2 and IL-2 added to the 4-day combination: response rates of up to 57%

HYPERTHERMIC PERFUSION WITH MELPHALAN

Locoregional spread of melanoma of the extremity is a problem for a subset of approximately 10% of patients. In spite of the lack of systemic spread, many patients develop local complications related to in-transit spread that are difficult to manage. Creech developed a method to apply locoregional perfusion using cytotoxic agents. The application of chemotherapy, heat, and/or immunotherapy using this method has been used by a variety of surgeons. One prospective randomized study showing benefit was carried out by Ghussen and colleagues from 1980 to 1983. In a control group (n = 54) the tumors were widely excised and the regional lymph nodes removed. The perfusion group received this treatment, as well as hyperthermic (42°C) perfusion with melphalan. After a median observation time of 5 years, 11 months, 26 recurrences were diagnosed in the control group and 6 noted in the perfusion group (*P* < .001). A survival advantage was also noted for the perfusion group (*P* < .01). Other studies have not shown a significant advantage, however. Recent variations that have used this approach have included coadministration of TNF and interferon γ [26,27].

Hyperthermic perfusion alone has been used with apparent antitumor effects. Subsequently, Stehlin reported that the antitumor effect could be increased by adding chemotherapy. Melphalan (L-phenylalanine mustard) is used most frequently in perfusates. Recently cisplatin has also been tested in some protocols. The maximally tolerated dose used in the randomized study was 1 mg/kg for the upper extremity and 1.5 mg/kg for the lower extremity. Morbidity and mortality for the isolation limb perfusion have been reported. A 6% to 39% morbidity, including requirement for major skin grafting and limb loss due to a compartment syndrome, has been reported in various series. Mortality is unusual but has been reported up to 3% in some series.

DOSAGE AND SCHEDULING

Upper extremity (UE): The axillary vein and artery are exposed through an incision from the clavicle to the anterior axillary line. The patient is heparinized systemically (100 U/kg), and the vessels are occluded and catheters inserted. The initial perfusate is whole blood using an extracorporeal heater/bubble oxygenator/low flow pump. Flow rates range from 250 to 400 mL/min.

Lower extremity (LE): The femoral vessels are exposed through an incision from a point medial to the anterosuperior iliac spine to the femoral triangle. The inferior epigastric and circumflex iliac vessels are temporarily occluded and catheters inserted into the external iliac vessels so that the catheters are lying in the proximal femoral vessels. An Esmarch is applied around the root of the limb to prevent circulation through cutaneous or subcutaneous blood vessels. Leakage is measured using dye dilution techniques.

The perfusate temperature is maintained at 42.5°C, monitored by thermistor probes between the muscles and in the subcutaneous tissues of the thigh and calf. Melphalan is given in the UE (1.0 mg/kg) and in the LE (1.5 mg/kg). The first half of the dose is administered when the limb has reached 40°C, and the balance is injected in 3 equal aliquots at 15, 30, and 45 minutes, the entire procedure taking place over 1 hour.

CANDIDATES FOR TREATMENT

Patients with deep primary melanoma of the extremity, or in transit, advanced locoregional melanoma; other advanced locoregional diseases confined to the extremity (squamous carcinomas, sarcomas)—currently under investigation.

DRUG INTERACTIONS

TNFα and IFNγ (septic shock-like syndrome and death in some instances [5]) appear to enhance melphalan activity

TOXICITIES

Wound healing (5.7%), lymphatic fistulas (7.5%), low-grade fever, mild pain and erythema of the extremity, compartment syndrome (approximately 10%, amputation possibly required)

Give acetaminophen and/or indomethacin in the first 24–48 h to control fever and chills; observe perfusion of the extremities to assess circulation, swelling, and presence of pulse (using handheld Doppler device); monitor vital signs every 4 h during immediate postoperative period; refrain from movement of the extremity until drains are removed.

PATIENT INFORMATION

Patient should be informed of benefits and side effects. Possible injury to the skin or other structures in the extremity may require additional operations and even amputation. The procedure is done under anesthesia and a hospital stay of approximately 1–2 wk is required.

TOPICAL APPLICATIONS OF 5-FU

Patients with multiple actinic solar keratoses are at risk for development of nonmelanoma skin cancers. In addition, patients with established basal cell carcinomas or multiple basal cell carcinomas may be treated with a 5% fluorouracil cream.

Fluorouracil blocks the methylation reaction of deoxyuridylic acid to thymidylic acid. It inhibits the synthesis of DNA and, to a lesser extent, RNA. The primary effect of 5-FU is on rapidly growing cells, and topical application has been shown to lead to insignificant absorption and primarily local antitumor effects.

DOSAGE AND SCHEDULING

When Efudex is applied to a tumor, local inflammation occurs associated with erythema, blister formation, ulceration, local necrosis and ultimately reepitheliazation [43]. 5-FU cream or solution is applied twice daily in an amount sufficient to cover lesions [44]. The treatment is continued until inflammation resolves, usually for a period of 2 to 4 weeks. For treatment of basal cell carcinomas, applications for as long as 12 weeks may be required. A patient should be followed to determine the antitumor effects.

CANDIDATES FOR TREATMENT
Patients with Bowen's disease, actinic keratosis, or multiple basal cell carcinomas

SPECIAL PRECAUTIONS
Patients must not have a known hypersensitivity to any components of the drug

DRUG INTERACTIONS
None

TOXICITIES
Local reactions: pain, pyrites, hyperpigmentation, burning at the site of application; other reactions: contact dermatitis, scarring, tenderness, local infection, swelling

NURSING INTERVENTIONS
Instruct the patient in the expected side effects and to keep the area clean, dry, and potentially bandaged to prevent exposure to exogenous pathogens

PATIENT INFORMATION
This treatment is useful for patients thought to be at high risk for development of tumors of the skin or those who have had multiple previous tumors of the skin. In addition, some people with very early tumors, such as Bowen's disease or some basal cell carcinomas, will benefit from application of the cream. The cream should be applied in amounts sufficient to cover the lesions and the area lightly bandaged. Treatment may continue as long as 10 to 12 wk and will cause redness, swelling, some pain, and itching. The patient should be followed closely by the physician during the course of treatment and thereafter to insure that tumor eradication has occurred.

Herbert J. Zeh, David L. Bartlett

Sarcomas are a histologically diverse group of tumors that arise most often from tissues of mesodermal origin. Despite the fact that approximately 75% of the body is derived from mesoderm, sarcomas are relatively rare, representing only 1% of all adult tumors and 15% of pediatric neoplasms. Approximately 5000 to 6000 new cases of sarcoma are diagnosed each year, and half of these patients will eventually succumb to their disease. Sarcomas may arise in any anatomic location, but are most commonly found in the extremities. This chapter will focus on the current management of sarcomas arising in the soft tissue and bone in the adult population.

ETIOLOGY AND RISK FACTORS

The majority of patients presenting with soft tissue sarcomas have no identifiable risk factors. However, several genetic and environmental conditions have been described that clearly increase the risk of developing these tumors (Table 13-1). Individuals with germline mutations in the regulatory genes p53 (Li-Fraumeni syndrome), familial retinoblastoma, or neurofibromatosis have increased the incidence of a variety of tumors, including sarcomas of bone and soft tissue [1–3]. Several other genetic syndromes (including familial adenomatous polyposis and Gardener's syndrome) have been implicated as well [1].

In addition to hereditary predisposition, exposure to ionizing radiation also increases the risk of developing bone and soft tissue sarcomas. Radiation-induced sarcomas have been reported with increasing incidence after therapy for a variety of common malignancies, especially breast cancer and Hodgkin's disease [4–6]. These secondary neoplasms are most often osteosarcomas (35%) or malignant fibrous histiocytomas (22%) and have been reported after doses as low as 800 cGy [5].

Increased incidence of sarcomas have also been reported following exposure to a variety of chemical agents. Exposure to throrotrast and vinyl chloride have been firmly linked to the development of hepatic angiosarcomas [7]. Several conflicting reports have attempted to link phenoxy herbicide and agent orange exposure to the subsequent development of soft tissue sarcomas. More recently, treatment with several common chemotherapeutic agents have been linked to an increased risk of osteosarcoma in children [1]. Trauma, infection, and chronic lymphedema have also been implicated in the development of soft tissue sarcomas [1,8].

Table 13-1. Sarcoma Risk Factors and Predominate Histology

Risk Factors	Predominate Histology
Genetic syndromes	
Li-Fraumeni (p53)	Osteosarcoma, STS
Familial retinoblastoma (Rb)	Osteosarcoma, STS
Neurofibromatosis (NF-1)	Osteosarcoma, STS
Radiation therapy	Osteosarcoma, malignant fibrous histiocytoma
Chemical agents	
Alkylating agents	Hepatic angiosarcoma
Polyvinyl chloride	Hepatic angiosarcoma
Thorium	Hepatic angiosarcoma
Chronic lymphedema	
After mastectomy	Angiosarcoma
Congenital	Angiosarcoma

STS—soft tissue sarcoma.

ADULT SOFT TISSUE SARCOMAS

PATHOLOGIC CLASSIFICATION, GRADE, AND STAGING

Sarcomas are classified according to the differentiated tissue they most resemble histologically (Table 13-2). Although each subtype has distinct histologic features, tumor grade is the best predictor of the biologic aggressiveness for soft tissue sarcomas [9]. The major exceptions to this point are the pediatric sarcomas (rhabdomyosarcoma, Ewing's sarcoma, and peripheral neuroectodermal tumors) whose prognosis and treatment strategies differ based on the histologic subtype. Unfortunately, the criteria for grading soft tissue sarcomas is not standardized. Currently there exist three dominant systems for grading soft tissue sarcomas [10–12]: a four-grade system as proposed by Broders and coworkers [11], a three-grade system based on the American Joint Commission on Cancer (AJCC), and a binary system as used at Memorial Sloan-Kettering Cancer Center (MSKCC). Despite the lack of a standardized grading system, pathologists agree that cellularity, mitotic activity, nuclear atypia, and degree of necrosis are the most important histopathologic correlates of tumor grade.

Staging of soft tissue sarcomas is based on histologic grade, size of primary tumor, and presence or absence of distant metastases.

Table 13-2. Common Histologic Subtypes of Soft Tissue Sarcomas

Histology	Cell Type	Frequency, %	Comments
Malignant fibrous histiocytoma	Fibroblast	22	Most common subtype; peak incidence 7th decade
Liposarcoma	Adipocyte	17	Occur commonly on thigh or retroperitoneum
Fibrosarcoma	Fibroblast	10	Peak incidence in 3rd to 5th decade
Synovial cell sarcoma	Synovial cells	7	Commonly occurs in young adults around knee
Leiomyosarcoma	Smooth muscle	19	Most common in viscera or retroperitoneum; surgery is primary treatment
Embryonal/rhabdomyosarcoma	Smooth muscle/mesoderm	4	Occur in young adults; treated primarily with chemoradiotherapy
Malignant peripheral nerve sheath (malignant Schwannoma)	Schwann cell	5	Arise from nerve sheath; appearance in lower extremity or retroperitoneum common
Angiosarcoma	Mesoderm	1	Arise in chronic lymphedema, postirradiation, on scalp of elderly men, or in breast tissue

Table 13-3. American Joint Committee on Cancer's Staging System for Soft Tissue Sarcomas

TNM Classification	Characteristics
Histologic Grade	
G1	Low grade, well differentiated
G2	Intermediate grade, moderately differentiated
G3	High grade, poorly differentiated
G4	High grade, undifferentiated
Primary Tumor	
T1	Tumor < 5 cm
a	Superficial tumor
b	Deep tumor
T2	Tumor > 5 cm
a	Superficial tumor
b	Deep tumor
Regional Nodes	
N0	No histologically verified lymph node metastases
N1	Histologically verified lymph node metastases
Distant Metastases	
M0	No distant metastases
M1	Distant metastases

Stage Group	5-y Survival, %
IA (G1–2,T1a–T1b,N0, M0)	98
IB (G1–2,T2a,N0,M0)	
IIA (G1–2,T2b,N0,M0)	81
IIB (G3–4,T1a–T1b,N0,M0)	
IIC (G3–4,T2a,N0,M0)	
III (G3–4,T2b,N0,M0)	51
IV (Any G,any T,N0,M0)	18

Table 13-3 shows the current AJCC staging system [12]. Historically, staging has been predominately based on histologic grade of the primary tumor. Low-grade lesions carry a low risk for developing distant metastases (< 15%) and an excellent survival rate, whereas high-grade lesions are associated with greater than 50% risk for developing distant metastases. Recent experience suggests that small superficial lesions (< 5 cm) regardless of histopathologic grade may best be categorized into stage II lesions, because these patients have a greater than 80% chance of long-term event-free survival when treated with current standards [12]. The strong influence of tumor grade on prognosis, staging, and therapy of patients with soft tissue sarcomas combined with the lack of a uniform grading scheme underscores the importance of having all sarcoma specimens reviewed by a skilled pathologist experienced in sarcomas.

PRESENTATION AND DIAGNOSIS

Fifty percent of all soft tissue sarcomas arise in the extremities, with retroperitoneal (14%), visceral (15%), and truncal (10%) lesions accounting for the majority of other sites. These tumors typically present as a painless enlarging mass. Any enlarging or persistent (> 4 wk) soft tissue mass or any mass larger than 5 cm, should be biopsied. The choice of biopsy technique is critical and should provide maximal histopathologic information while not jeopardizing subsequent surgical procedures. Historically, incisional biopsy has been the preferred technique for lesions greater than 5 cm, but the complication rate and chance of spreading tumor cells through uncontaminated tissue planes is significant.

Recently, the accuracy of core needle biopsy in the diagnosis of soft tissue masses has been addressed by several investigators [13–15]. Barth and coworkers [13] at the National Cancer Institute (NCI) correlated the results of 27 core needle biopsies to the final resected specimen. Core needle biopsy correctly identified 16 of 16 malignant lesions and 10 of 11 benign lesions. In each of the malignant lesions, tumor grade was correctly identified by core needle biopsy. More recently, Heslin and coworkers [15] reviewed 60 core needle biopsies performed at MSKCC. In this series, the results of core needle biopsy correlated with final pathology 95% of the time with respect to malignancy and 88% of the time with respect to tumor grade. The high specificity and sensitivity, coupled with the lower morbidity and cost of core needle biopsy, should make it the preferred technique when feasible. For lesions less than 5 cm, an excisional biopsy is adequate. Excisional biopsies should be performed with the intent to obtain negative margins. This will avoid an unsatisfactory re-resection of the surgical bed. Fine needle aspiration does not provide adequate sample to determine tumor grade and should not be routinely used in the initial diagnosis of soft tissue masses [13].

THERAPY

Surgery is the most effective modality in the treatment of localized soft tissue sarcomas. The goal of surgical excision should be complete removal of the tumor with a margin of normal tissue. In cases where the tumor abuts major neurovascular structures, every attempt at conservation should be made. Local control rates with limited wide local excision (limb-sparing surgery [LSS]) and adjuvant radiotherapy now approach those obtained historically with amputation [16]. Amputation, once the standard for surgical control of extremity soft tissue sarcomas, should only be applied in select cases of advanced or recurrent local regional disease. Currently, greater than 95% of all patients with extremity sarcomas are managed without amputation. For patients with stage I or II disease, surgery with adjuvant radiotherapy results in 5-year disease-free survival rates of 60% to 80% and overall survival rates of 80% to 98%.

Despite the wide acceptance of LSS in extremity soft tissue sarcomas, its impact on long-term survival has only been addressed in a single randomized trial [17]. In this study at the NCI, patients with extremity sarcoma were randomized to amputation or to wide local excision of the tumor with adjuvant radiotherapy (both arms received adjuvant chemotherapy). With follow-up greater than 10 years, five of the 27 patients in the LSS arm had a local recurrence versus one of 17 patients in the amputation arm (P = 0.22). Despite this slightly higher rate of local recurrence in the LSS arm, overall survival was not different (70% in the LSS arm and 71% in the amputation group; P = 0.97). The link between local recurrence and the development of distant metastases is unclear and complex. Retrospective data correlates local recurrence with increased risk of developing distant metastases and decreased overall survival [18,19]. Yet in two prospective randomized trials, better local control rates did not translate into improved survival. In the NCI trial, local recurrence in the LSS arm was higher than with amputation, whereas overall survival did not differ between arms. Similarly, in the adjuvant brachytherapy trial from MSKCC improved local control in the adjuvant radiotherapy group did not result in improved overall survival. It appears that survival is dictated by the biologic aggressiveness of the tumor and the presence of microscopic metastatic disease at the time of diagnosis. Local recurrence in patients with adequately treated primary tumors probably represents aggressive tumor biology, a harbinger for the development of distant disease.

Adjuvant radiotherapy combined with surgical resection results in improved local control over surgery alone for patients with soft tissue sarcoma of the extremities [16,20–23]. Postoperative adjuvant radiotherapy for high-grade lesions may be delivered in the form of external beam or brachytherapy. Brachytherapy delivers radiation to the tumor bed by way of interstitial catheters placed at the time of resection. This has several potential benefits over traditional external-beam radiotherapy, including shorter length of treatment, lower cost, and greater sparing of normal tissues [10,24]. In a prospective randomized trial of 164 patients from MSKCC, patients treated with surgery plus adjuvant brachytherapy had better local control rates when compared to surgery alone (82% vs 69%; $P = 0.04$) [24]. Subset analysis revealed that patients with high-grade lesions benefited from adjuvant brachytherapy, whereas no improvement in local control rate was observed for patients with low-grade sarcomas.

The effectiveness of adjuvant external-beam radiotherapy in the treatment of soft tissue sarcomas of the extremities has recently been addressed in a randomized trial [25]. In an ongoing study at the NCI, 91 patients with high-grade and 50 patients with low-grade soft tissue sarcomas of the extremity have been randomized to surgery alone or surgery plus adjuvant external-beam radiotherapy (6300 cGy). With a median follow up at 9.9 years, a statistically significant decrease in local recurrence has been seen in both the high-grade ($P = 0.0028$) and low-grade tumors ($P = 0.0160$) after adjuvant external-beam radiotherapy.

Several centers have reported on the use of preoperative adjuvant radiotherapy [26–29]. Local control rates for small (T1 and T2)

lesions have been reported to be similar to those obtained with postoperative treatment. No randomized trial as addressed whether preoperative or postoperative radiotherapy is superior. Furthermore, given the excellent local control rates with small lesions, it is unlikely that a randomized trial could accrue enough patients to definitively answer this question. Studies are ongoing to explore the effectiveness of preoperative radiotherapy in the treatment of advanced local disease (large primary tumores 710 cm). Theoretically, the application of preoperative radiotherapy in this setting will allow for more limb-sparing resections.

Patients with low-grade soft tissue sarcoma should not be candidates for adjuvant chemotherapy, given their extremely low risk of metastatic disease and excellent overall survival. However, greater than 50% of patients with high-grade sarcomas will eventually develop distant metastases and succumb to their disease. The goal of adjuvant chemotherapy is to improve survival by early elimination of microscopic hematogenous metastases. Successful adjuvant chemotherapy has been defined for a number of other cancers, including colon and breast cancer and osteosarcoma. However, adjuvant chemotherapy for patients with high-grade soft tissue sarcomas remains controversial. Table 13-4 summarizes several of the largest randomized trials examining adjuvant chemotherapy for this disease [30–43]. The two largest trials (European Organization for Research in Cancer Therapy [EORTC] and Scandanavian Sarcoma Group) do not support the use of adjuvant chemotherapy because neither showed a statistically significant improvement in overall survival [33,40]. Several smaller trials (Rizzoli, Bergonie) have shown some survival advantage to adjuvant therapy; however, these studies have been extensively criticized for inadequate randomization, small size, and poor design [44,45].

The low incidence of sarcoma and the diversity of this disease has made it difficult for many of these trials to accrue sufficient patients for meaningful randomization and statistical evaluation. In an

Table 13-4. Adjuvant Chemotherapy for Soft Tissue Sarcomas

Study	Regimen	Disease Sites	Patients, n	Improved Disease Free Survival?	Improved Overall Survival?
GOG [30]	Doxorubicin	Uterus	225	No	No
DFCI [31]	Doxorubicin	Extremities, trunk, head and neck, retroperitoneum	42	No	No
ECOG [32]	Doxorubicin	Extremities, trunk, head and neck, retroperitoneum	47	No	No
SSG [33]	Doxorubicin	Extremities, trunk, head and neck, breast, chest	240	No	No
Rizzoli [34]	Doxorubicin	Extremities	77	Yes	Yes
ISSG [35]	Doxorubicin	Extremities, trunk, head and neck, retroperitoneum	92	No	No
UCLA [37]	Doxorubicin	Extremities	119	No	No
MD Anderson [36]	Doxorubicin, cyclophosphamide, actinomycin-D, vincristine	Extremities, trunk	43	Yes	No
Mayo Clinic [38]	Doxorubicin, vincristine, dacarbazine, vincristine, actinomycin-D, cyclophosphamide	Extremities, trunk	74	No	No
				No	No
NCI [39,42]	Doxorubicin, cyclophosphamide, methotrexate	Extremities	65	Yes	No
NCI [41]	Doxorubicin, cyclophosphamide, methotrexate	Trunk, breast, head and neck	57	No	No
EORTC [40]	Doxorubicin, cyclophosphamide, vincristine, dacarbazine	Extremities, trunk, head and neck	468	Yes*	No
Bergonie [43]	Doxorubicin, cyclophosphamide, vincristine, dacarbazine	Extremities, trunk, head and neck, retroperitoneum	65	Yes	Yes

* Limited to patients with head and neck or trunk lesions.
DFCI—Dana Farber Cancer Institute; ECOG—Eastern Cooperative Oncology Group; EORTC—European Organization for Research in Cancer Therapy; GOG—Gynecologic Oncology Group; ISSG—Intergroup Sarcoma Study Group; NCI—National Cancer Institute; SSG—Scandinavian Sarcoma Group; UCLA—University of California, Los Angeles.

attempt to integrate the data from many of these trials, several meta-analyses have been performed [46–48]. These have suggested a small advantage in recurrence of free survival and overall survival to doxorubicin-based adjuvant chemotherapy. However, these studies should be interpreted with caution because they are subject to selection bias (exclusion of unpublished negative trials). Furthermore, the large heterogeneity in design and methods of assessing outcome among the various trials makes synthesis of the data complex and potentially unreliable. Recently, a meta-analysis encompassing individual patient data from a number of large published and unpublished trials was performed [49]. Theoretically, this method of meta-analysis is more reliable because it combines the individual patient's data into a single time-to-event analysis. With a median follow-up of 9.4 years, this study showed a statistically significant advantage in disease-free survival to doxorubicin-based adjuvant chemotherapy. A statistically nonsignificant trend towards better overall survival was also observed. Subgroup analysis in this study demonstrated that patients with high-grade extremity lesions received the most benefit from adjuvant chemotherapy.

Neoadjuvant chemotherapy has several theoretical advantages, including the early treatment of microscopic metastatic disease, ability to monitor the primary tumor to gauge responsiveness to particular agents, and shrinkage of advanced local tumors that may allow limb salvage. A retrospective analysis of 46 patients from MD Anderson Cancer Center who received doxorubicin-based neoadjuvant chemotherapy found significantly improved disease free and overall survival in those patients whose primary tumors responded [50]. However, prospective trial at MSKCC of 29 patients with large (> 10 cm) high-grade extremity sarcomas failed to demonstrate improved survival compared to historical controls [51]. Studies are ongoing to evaluate the efficacy of preoperative chemotherapy, especially in patients with large high-grade lesions.

In summary, the sum total experience with doxorubicin-based adjuvant chemotherapy suggests that it may provide a small advantage in disease-free survival . Nevertheless, its application outside of well-constructed clinical trials cannot be advocated at this time. The rarity and complexity of soft tissue sarcomas continues to confound efforts to construct clinical trials with sufficient power to demonstrate a definitive survival benefit to these potentially toxic therapies. The experience to date underscores the importance of enrolling all eligible patients in clinical trials if progress is to be made. Future trials will focus on preoperative or postoperative adjuvant therapy in high-risk patients (those with large high-grade tumors) with dose intensification of chemotherapeutic regimens.

Unresectable and Recurrent Tumors

Despite adequate treatment of their primary tumors, 8% to 20% of patients with high-grade extremity sarcomas will recur locally. The vast majority of these patients may be managed with re-resection and additional adjuvant radiotherapy [18,52]. In cases of multifocal recurrence or previous maximum radiotherapy, amputation may be necessary. In select patients with advanced unresectable or recurrent local disease, administration of chemotherapeutic drugs via direct arterial infusion or in the setting of isolated limb perfusion has been evaluated in an attempt to improve the rate of limb salvage. A recent review of 186 patients enrolled in an ongoing multicenter trials in Europe showed an 82% major response rate using a regimen of tumor necrosis factor and melphalan [53]. Eighty-two percent of these initially unresectable patients were able to undergo limb salvage surgery. In 21 patients with unresectable or recurrent extremity sarcoma using

isolated limb perfusion with TNF and melphalan, the authors saw a 65% objective response rate and 48% limb salvage rate (Unpublished data, Alexander HR and Bartlett RL).

Figure 13-1 summarizes an algorithm for the approach to soft tissue sarcomas. In brief, current standards entail complete surgical excision of the tumor with a negative margin, followed by adjuvant radiotherapy when necessary to decrease the rate of local recurrence. Adjuvant chemotherapy should only be administered in the setting of clinical trials. Clinical trials of preoperative chemoradiotherapy should be considered in patients presenting with advanced local disease.

MANAGEMENT OF METASTATIC DISEASE.

Approximately one half of all patients with high-grade soft tissue sarcomas will eventually develop distant metastases. The site of recurrence depends on the location of the primary tumor . For patients with extremity and truncal sarcomas, by far the most common site is the lung. Surgery is the treatment of choice for patients with isolated pulmonary metastases. In several large retrospective series examining pulmonary metastasectomy, the average 3-year survival rate was reported to be between 23% and 42% [54–61]. Important independent prognostic factors in survival after metastasectomy include disease-free interval, metastases doubling time of 40 days or greater, unilateral disease, three or fewer nodules on preoperative computed tomography scan of the chest, and two or less nodules found at time of resection [62]. Long-term disease-free survival has been reported after repeat thoracotomy and metastasectomy [61].

Soft tissue sarcomas are among the most chemoresistant of all malignancies. Currently, there are only two agents that reproducibly demonstrate greater than 20% response rate in metastatic sarcoma—doxorubicin and ifosfamide. Doxorubicin is the single most effective agent against soft tissue sarcoma with response rates reported from 9% to 70% [63–66]. Response to doxorubicin is dose related. Unfortunately increasing the dose of doxorubicin is associated with severe myelosuppression and cardiotoxicity. Several anthracycline derivatives have been examined in an attempt to find agents with similar efficacy and less toxic profiles.

Epirubicin, an anthracycline derivative, has been recently examined for its activity in soft tissue sarcomas. A large randomized trial by the EORTC comparing doxorubicin with epirubicin showed similar overall response rates (18%) with no significant difference in toxicity profiles [67]. Ifosfamide, an analogue of the alkylating agent cyclophosphamide, also has activity as a single agent in the treatment of soft tissue sarcomas [68,69]. Ifosfamide has been shown to be superior to cyclophosphamide in a randomized trial conducted by the EORTC [70]. Ifosfamide is active in patients who have failed doxorubicin-based therapy [71]. The severe hemorrhagic cystitis associated with the use of ifosfamide has been greatly reduced by the introduction of the uroprotective agent mesna [72]. Dacarbazine (DTIC) is another agent frequently used in combination regimens for the treatment of soft tissue sarcomas. Its effectiveness as a single agent in phase II trials was limited with response rates of approximately 18% [73]. Toxicity to DTIC is severe and includes significant nausea , vomiting, and myelosuppression.

In an attempt to improve upon the response rates seen with single agent therapies, several important randomized trials of combination chemotherapy have been conducted by the large cooperative groups (Table 13-5) [63,65,74–78]. The Eastern Cooperative Oncology Group (ECOG) conducted a series of randomized trails comparing single-agent doxorubicin to combination regimens. Higher response rates were observed for regimens combining doxorubicin with ifosfamide and doxorubicin with DTIC. However, the combination therapies offered no survival advantage and were associated with significantly higher toxicity [65,76]. The CyVADIC regimen (cyclophosphamide, vincristine, doxorubicin, DTIC) has been extensively studied by the Southwestern Oncology Group (SWOG). Several large randomized trials have demonstrated response rates ranging from 38% to 71% [77,79].

However, a recent study by the EORTC, comparing doxorubicin alone (75 mg/m^2 every 3 wk) or doxorubicin (50 mg/m^2) plus ifosfamide (5 g/m^2) to the CyVADIC regimen, showed no advantage to combination regimens over single-agent doxorubicin. Response rates were 23%, 28% and 28% respectively with a median survival of 52, 51, and 55 weeks, respectively [78]. In a large randomized intergroup trial, the MAID (mesna, doxorubicin, ifosfamide, DTIC) regimen was shown to have higher response rates than combination regimens of doxorubicin and DTIC (32% vs 17%) [74]. The overall survival advantage for the three-drug regimen was not significantly different (12 vs 13 mo). Moreover, toxicity was significantly greater in the MAID arm of this study, which resulted in significantly lower doses of doxorubicin

delivered. Because the dose of doxorubicin is thought to be critical in soft tissue sarcoma, recent studies have focused on dose intensification of doxorubicin with hematopoietic stem cell support [80–84].

A recent EORTC trial evaluated doxorubicin (75 mg/m^2) and ifosfamide (5 g/m^2) with granulocyte–macrophage colony-stimulating factor (GM-CSF) (250 mug/m^2) support [82,84]. In 104 evaluable patients, an overall response rate of 45% was seen with a 10% complete response rate. A randomized trial comparing doxorubicin and GM-CSF to ifosfamide and doxorubicin is currently being conducted by this group. The SWOG has recently reported the results of a phase I trial of dose-intensified doxorubicin within the MAID regimen. In this trial of 13 patients, the addition of GM-CSF did not allow for significant dose intensification of doxorubicin [83]. To date, very little information regarding the value of high dose myeloablative therapy with bone marrow support exists.

In summary, treatment of widely metastatic soft tissue sarcoma is difficult. Single-agent doxorubicin remains the standard for treatment of this disease. Combination regimens, including doxorubicin and ifosfamide or DTIC demonstrate higher response rates at the cost of increased toxicity. Moreover, they have failed to significantly improve

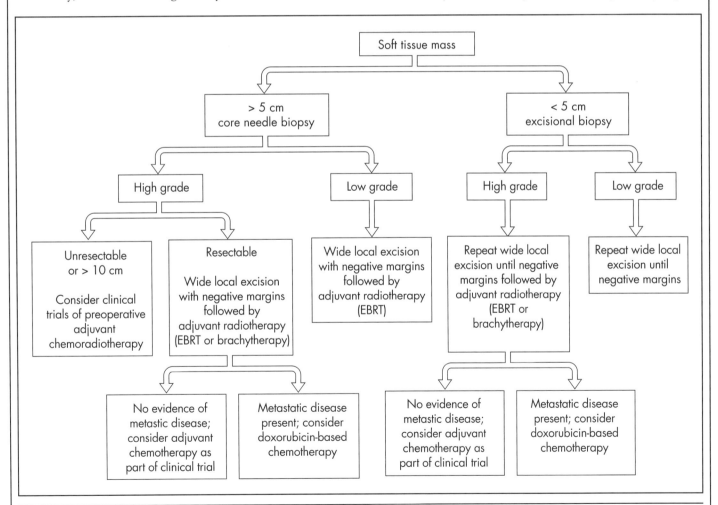

FIGURE 13-1.

Algorithm for management of primary soft tissue sarcoma. EBRT—external-beam radiotherapy.

overall survival. Dose intensification of doxorubicin within these combination regimens may offer promise for increasing their effectiveness.

FEATURES OF NONEXTREMITY AND ATYPICAL SOFT TISSUE SARCOMAS

Retroperitoneal Sarcomas

Retroperitoneal sarcomas are relatively rare, accounting for approximately 15% of all sarcomas. Because of the large permissive nature of the retroperitoneal space, these patients will often present with large bulky tumors late in the course of their disease. The differential diagnosis of retroperitoneal masses should include lymphoma, sarcoma, and metastatic testicular cancer. Every attempt to completely resect the tumor with negative margins at initial exploration should be made because this is the only potentially curative therapy. Unlike with extremity tumors, survival from retroperitoneal sarcomas is most dependent on locoregional control. Whenever necessary, adjacent viscera involved with the tumor should be removed en bloc with the specimen. Resectability of retroperitoneal sarcomas has been reported to be between 50% and 80% [85–87]. The 5-year actuarial survival for patients completely resected is 30% to 40% [87–88]. Despite complete resection, local recurrence will develop in 40% to 50 % of patients [85–87]. Local recurrences are managed by successive surgical resections that can go on for many years, increasing in frequency over time. Unfortunately, efforts to improve local control with adjuvant radiotherapy are limited by the radiosensitivity of overlying viscera. Attempts to minimize the

dose of radiotherapy to normal tissue by means of intraoperative delivery of radiotherapy (IORT) have been successful in decreasing local failure rates but do not appear to improve survival [89]. Current studies are ongoing to evaluate methods to improve local control in these patients.

Sarcomas Arising in the Head and Neck or Trunk

Sarcomas arising in the head and neck region are uncommon, representing less than 5% of all sarcomas. The most common histologic subtypes in this region are fibrosarcoma, malignant schwannoma, and rhabdomyosarcoma. Treatment of these lesions is similar to sarcomas in other locations. Local failure is a significant problem for head and neck sarcomas. Surgical excision of the primary tumor with negative margins is more difficult, given the complex nature of this area. Adjuvant radiotherapy may play a role in preventing local recurrence. Successful treatment is predicted by the grade and size of the primary tumor, status of the surgical margins, and presence or absence of bony invasion [90]. Lymph node metastases, as with other sarcomas, are rare and routine; lymphadenectomy is not recommended. Five-year survival has been reported to vary from 20% to 68%. Sarcomas arising on the trunk or chest are managed primarily with surgery and adjuvant radiotherapy. As with other nonextremity sarcomas, local control is a significant problem with these lesions. Unlike extremity soft tissue sarcomas, survival correlates with the ability to locally control the primary tumor.

Rhabdomyosarcoma

Rhabdomyosarcoma is an uncommon histologic subtype of soft tissue sarcomas, occurring most commonly in childhood or adoles-

Table 13-5. Randomized Trials Comparing Efficacy of Combination Chemotherapy Regimens for Soft Tissue Sarcomas

Study	Agents	Number of Patients	Response Rate, %	Improvement in response rate?*	Improvement in overall survival?*
ECOG [75]	Doxorubicin	200	27	—	—
	Doxorubicin/vincristine		19	No	No
	Cyclophosphamide, actinomycin-D, vincristine/cyclophosphamide		11	No	No
ECOG [76]	Doxorubicin (70 mg/m^2)	275	18	—	—
	Doxorubicin (45 mg/m^2)		16	No	No
	Doxorubicin/dacarbazine		30	Yes	No
ECOG [63]	Doxorubicin	298	17	—	—
	Doxorubicin/vindesine		18	No	No
ECOG [65]	Doxorubicin	262	20	—	—
	Doxorubicin/ifosfamide		34	Yes	No
	Mitomycin/doxorubicin, cisplatin		32	Yes	No
SWOG [77]	Doxorubicin/dacarbazine	276	33	—	—
	Doxorubicin/dacarbazine/cyclophosphamide		34	No	No
	Doxorubicin/dacarbazine/actinomycin-D		24	No	No
EORTC [78]	Doxorubicin	663	23	—	—
	Doxorubicin/ifosfamide		28	No	No
	Doxorubicin/vincristine/cyclophosphamide/actinomycin-D		28	No	No
ISSG [74]	Doxorubicin/dacarbazine	340	17	—	—
	Doxorubicin/ifosfamide/dacarbazine/mesna		32	Yes	No

*As compared with single-agent doxorubicin or control indicated by a dash.
ECOG—Eastern Cooperative Oncology Group; EORTC—European Organization for Research in Cancer Therapy; ISSG—Intergroup Sarcoma Study Group; SWOG—Southwestern Oncology Group.

cence. These tumors are more chemoradiosensitive than other soft tissue sarcomas. The treatment of rhabdomyosarcomas is primarily nonsurgical, involving early and aggressive chemoradiation therapy.

Kaposi's Sarcoma

Kaposi's sarcoma is an unusual vascular sarcoma that occurs in the skin of elderly men or in the setting of AIDS. The staging , prognosis, and therapy for Kaposi's sarcoma is completely different from that of other soft tissue sarcomas. Treatment strategies vary depending on the clinical scenario in which the tumor arises, but in general, systemic chemotherapy is the treatment of choice and excellent responses have been noted with single-agent vincristine, doxorubicin, vinblastine, or etoposide.

SARCOMAS OF THE BONE

PATHOLOGIC CLASSIFICATION, GRADING, AND STAGING

Sarcomas may arise form any of the four tissues that comprise mature bone—cartilage, bone, fibrous tissue, and marrow. As with soft tissue sarcomas, sarcomas of the bone are staged primarily on the grade. This is reflected in the staging system adopted by the Musculoskeletal Tumor Society (MSTS). Size of primary tumor and presence of distant metastases are also important prognostic factors.

PRESENTATION AND DIAGNOSIS

The two most common histologic subtypes of bone sarcomas (osteosarcoma and Ewing's sarcoma) are most common in childhood or adolescence (Table 13-6). These tumors typically present as a painless mass firmly fixed to underlying bone. Radiographic evaluation is usually quite characteristic with a pattern of permeative cortical destruction, periosteal elevation, and soft tissue ossification. The biopsy of sarcomas arising in the bone must be performed with consideration for the definitive procedure. Poorly placed biopsies will often limit limb-sparing options later. In general, core needle biopsy is the preferred technique and will yield adequate specimen for diagnosis in the majority of cases [91].

THERAPY

Surgery plus adjuvant chemotherapy is standard treatment of sarcomas arising from the bone. Prior to the 1980s, amputation one joint above the lesion was the standard of care for all osteosarcomas [92]. Developments in reconstructive techniques and chemotherapy have made limb-sparing options more prevalent. As with soft tissue sarcoma, limited resections do not appear to affect survival. With current techniques, 50% to 80% of all osteosarcomas may be managed without amputation [92]. Contraindications to the use of limb-sparing surgery include major neurovascular involvement, pathologic fractures, inappropriate biopsy site, infections, and skeletal immaturity.

Unlike soft tissue sarcomas, adjuvant chemotherapy effectively prolongs disease-free and overall survival in patients with osteosar-

Table 13-6. Common Histologic Types of Sarcomas Arising in Bone

Histologic Type	Comments
Osteosarcoma	Most common subtype; treated with adjuvant chemotherapy and surgery
Chondrosarcoma	Second most common sarcoma of bone; slow growing; low grade; treated primarily with surgery
Ewing's sarcoma	Small cell sarcoma; best treated with combination chemotherapy and radiation; surgery reserved for select cases

coma [93,94]. Currently, a majority of the regimens incorporate adriamycin and cisplatin with or without high dose methotrexate [92]. Other regimens used include bleomycin, cyclophosphamide, and dactinomycin [95]. Relapse-free survival rates between 40% and 60% have been reported using these regimens [95]. A major area of study in the treatment of osteosarcoma is the preoperative administration of adjuvant chemotherapy. Several early retrospective trials from MSKCC suggested that this approach may be better than traditional postsurgical adjuvant therapy [96–98]. However, preliminary results from a randomized trial by the Pediatric Oncology Group has failed to demonstrate a significant disease free survival advantage to preoperative chemotherapy versus traditional postsurgical adjuvant therapy [99]. Nevertheless, the response to preoperative chemotherapy remains the best predictor of future performance for patients with osteosarcoma.

Patients whose primary tumors demonstrate significant histologic response are less likely to develop distant metastases and have better overall survival. This finding led to "custom tailoring" therapy, where postsurgical adjuvant therapy is modified according to the response of the primary tumor to preoperative therapy. Early results from the T10 protocol conducted at MSKCC showed 70% to 90% long-term disease-free survival using this approach [100,101]. Subsequent multicenter trials have failed to reproduce these numbers [102,103]. It appears that poor responders will relapse and modifications of postsurgical chemotherapy do not significantly improve their survival. Current trials are evaluating dose intensification of preoperative chemotherapy in an attempt to increase the number of initial responders.

TREATMENT OF METASTATIC DISEASE

Like with soft tissue sarcomas, the most common site of metastatic disease in osteosarcoma is the lung. The single most effective treatment for patients with isolated pulmonary metastases remains surgery. Long-term survival after pulmonary metastasectomy has been reported to vary from 15% to 30% [104–108]. Adjuvant therapy after metastasectomy has not been well studied, but some have suggested that it may be of use in select cases [95]. Despite the effectiveness of adjuvant chemotherapy for osteosarcoma, treatment of established metastatic disease is difficult and associated with poor response rates.

REFERENCES

1. McClay E: Epidemiology of bone and soft tissue sarcomas. *Sem Oncol* 1989, 16:264–272.

2. Roos K, Dunn D: Neurofibromatosis. *CA Cancer J Clin* 1992, 42:241–254.

3. Birch JM: Li-Fraumeni Syndrome. *Eur J Cancer* 1994, 30A:1935–1941.

4. Robinson E, Neugut A, Wylie P: Clinical aspects of post irradiation sarcoma. *J Natl Cancer Inst* 1988, 19:230–240.

5. Nanus D, Kelsen D, Clarck D: Radiation induced angiosarcoma. *Cancer* 1987, 60:777–779.

6. Davidson T, Westbury G, Harmer C: Radiation-induced soft tissue sarcoma. *Br J Surg* 1986, 73:308–309.

7. Falk H, Herbert J, Crowley S, *et al.*: Epidemiology of hepatic angiosarcoma in the United States: 1964-1974. *Environ Health Perspect* 1981, 41:107–113.

8. Hayman J, Huygen H: Angiosarcoma developing around a foreign body. *J Clin Pathol* 1983, 36:515–518.

9. Gaynor J, Tan C, Casper E, *et al.*: Refinement of clinicopathological staging for localized soft tissue sarcoma of the extremity: a study of 423 adults. *J Clin Oncol* 1992, 10:1317–1325.

10. Brennan MF, Casper ES, Harrison LB: Soft tissue sarcoma. In *Principles and Practice of Oncology* ed 5. Edited by Rosenberg S, Devita V, Hellman S. Philadelphia: Lippincott-Raven; 1997:1738–1787.

11. Broders O, Hargrave R, Meyerding H: Pathological features of soft tissue fibrosarcomas with special reference to the grading of its malignancy. *Surg Gyencol Obstet* 1939, 69:237–241.

12. American Joint Committee on Cancer: *AJCC Cancer Staging Manual*, ed 5. Edited by Fleming I, Cooper J, Heuson D, *et al.* Philadelphia: Lippincott-Raven Publishers; 1997.

13. Barth R, Merino M, Solomon D, *et al.*: A prospective study of the value of core needle biopsy and fine needle aspiration in the diagnosis of soft tissue masses. *Surgery* 1992, 112:536–543.

14. Ball A, Fisher C, Pittan M, *et al.*: Diagnosis of soft tissues tumor by tru-cut biopsy. *Br J Surg* 1990, 77:756–760.

15. Heslin MJ, Lewis JJ, Woodruff JM, Brennan MF: Core needle biopsy for diagnosis of extremity soft tissue sarcoma. *Ann Surg Oncol* 1997, 4:425–431.

16. Spiro IJ, Rosenberg AE, Springfield D, Suit H: Combined surgery and radiation therapy for limb preservation in soft tissue sarcoma of the extremity: the Massachusetts General Hospital experience. *Cancer Invest* 1995, 13:86–95.

17. Rosenberg SA, Tepper J, Glatstein E: The treatment of soft tissue sarcomas of the extremities: prospective randomized evaluations of limb sparing surgery plus radiation therapy compared with amputation and the role of adjuvant chemotherapy. *Ann Surg* 1982, 196:305–315.

18. Brennan MF: The enigma of local recurrence: the Society of Surgical Oncology. *Ann Surg Oncol* 1997, 4:1–12.

19. Lewis JJ, Leung D, Heslin M, *et al.*: Association of local recurrence with subsequent survival in extremity soft tissue sarcoma. *J Clin Oncol* 1997, 15:646–652.

20. Lindberg RD, Martin RG, Romsdahl MM, Barkley HT Jr: Conservative surgery and postoperative radiotherapy in 300 adults with soft-tissue sarcomas. *Cancer* 1981, 47:2391–2397.

21. Abbatucci JS, Boulier N, de Ranieri J, *et al.*: Local control and survival in soft tissue sarcomas of the limbs, trunk walls and head and neck: a study of 113 cases. *Int J Radiat Oncol Biol Phys* 1986, 12:579–586.

22. Karakousis CP, Emrich LJ, Rao U, Krishnamsetty RM: Feasibility of limb salvage and survival in soft tissue sarcomas. *Cancer* 1986, 57:484–491.

23. Potter DA, Kinsella T, Glatstein E, *et al.*: High-grade soft tissue sarcomas of the extremities. *Cancer* 1986, 58:190–205.

24. Pisters PW, Harrison LB, Leung DH, *et al.*: Long-term results of a prospective randomized trial of adjuvant brachytherapy in soft tissue sarcoma. *J Clin Oncol* 1998, 14:859–868.

25. Yang J, Chang A, Baker A, *et al.*: A randomized prospective study of the benefit of adjuvant radiation therapy in the treatment of soft tissue sarcomas of the extremity. *J Clin Oncol* 1998, 16:197–203.

26. Spiro IJ, Gebhardt MC, Jennings LC, *et al.*: Prognostic factors for local control of sarcomas of the soft tissues managed by radiation and surgery. *Semin Oncol* 1997, 24:540–546.

27. Suit HD, Willett CG: Radiation therapy of sarcomas of the soft tissues. *Cancer Treat Res* 1991, 56:61–74.

28. Suit HD, Mankin HJ, Wood WC, Proppe KH: Preoperative, intraoperative, and postoperative radiation in the treatment of primary soft tissue sarcoma. *Cancer* 1985, 55:2659–2667.

29. Suit HD, Proppe KH, Mankin HJ, Wood WC: Preoperative radiation therapy for sarcoma of soft tissue. *Cancer* 1981, 47:2269–2274.

30. Omura A, Blessinf J, Major F, *et al.*: A randomized trial of adjuvant adriamycin in uterine sarcomas: a Gynecologic Oncology Group study. *J Clin Oncol* 1985, 3:1240–1245.

31. Antman K, Suit H, Amato D, *et al.*: Preliminary results of a randomized trial of adjuvant doxorubicin for sarcomas: lack of apparent difference between treatment groups. *J Clin Oncol* 1984, 2:601–608.

32. Lerner H, Amato D, Savlov E, *et al.*: Eastern Oncology Cooperative Group: a comparison of adjuvant doxorubicin and observation for patients with localized soft tissue sarcoma. *J Clin Oncol* 1987, 5:613–617.

33. Alvegard T, Sigurdsson H, Mouridsen H, *et al.*: Adjuvant chemotherapy with doxorubicin in high-grade soft tissue sarcoma: a randomized trial of the Scandinavian Sarcoma Group. *J Clin Oncol* 1989, 7:1504–1513.

34. Gherlinzoni F, Bacci G, Picci P, *et al.*: A randomized trial for the treatment of high-grade soft-tissue sarcomas of the extremities: preliminary observations. *J Clin Oncol* 1986, 4:552–558.

35. Antman KH, Ryan LM, Borden EC, *et al.*: Pooled results from three randomized adjuvant studies of doxorubicin versus observation in soft tissue sarcoma: 10-year results and review of the literature. In *Adjuvant Therapy of Cancer VI*. Edited by Salmon SE. Philadelphia: WB Saunders; 1990:529–543.

36. Benjamin RS, Terjanian TO, Fenoglio CJ, *et al.*: The importance of combination chemotherapy for adjuvant treatment of high risk patients with soft tissue sarcomas of the extremities. In *Adjuvant Therapy of Cancer V*. Edited by Salmon S. Orlando, FL: Grune and Stratton; 1987:735–744.

37. Eilber FR, Giuliano AE, Huth JF, Morton DL: Post operative adjuvant chemotherapy (adriamycin) in high grade extremity soft tissue sarcoma: a randomized prospective trial. In *Adjuvant Therapy of Cancer V*. Edited by Salmon S. Orlando, FL: Grune and Stratton; 1987:719–726.

38. Edmonson JH, Fleming TR, Ivins JC, *et al.*. Randomized study of systemic chemotherapy following complete excision of nonosseous sarcomas. *J Clin Oncol* 1984, 2:1390–1406.

39. Rosenberg SA, Tepper J, Glatstein E, *et al.*: Prospective randomized evaluation of adjuvant chemotherapy in adults with soft tissue sarcomas of the extremities. *Cancer* 1983, 52:424–434.

40. Bramwell VH, Rousse J, Steward WP, *et al.*: Adjuvant CYVADIC chemotherapy for adult soft tissue sarcoma-reduced local recurrence but no improvement in survival: a study of the European Organization for research and treatment of cancer, soft tissue and bone sarcoma group. *J Clin Oncol* 1994, 12:1137–1149.

41. Glenn J, Kinsella T, Glatstein E, *et al.*: A randomized, prospective trial of adjuvant chemotherapy in adults with soft tissue sarcomas of the head and neck, breast, and trunk. *Cancer* 1985, 55:1206–1214.

42. Chang AE, Kinsella T, Glatstein E, *et al.*: Adjuvant chemotherapy for patients with high-grade soft-tissue sarcomas of the extremity. *J Clin Oncol* 1988, 6:1491–1500.

43. Ravaud A, Bui NB, Coindre JM, *et al.*: Adjuvant chemotherapy with Cyvadic in high risk soft tissue sarcoma: a randomized prospective trial. In *Adjuvant Therapy of Cancer*. Edited by Salmon S. Philadelphia: WB Saunders; 1990:556–566.

44. Steward WP: Chemotherapy for metastatic soft tissue sarcomas. *Cancer Treat Res* 1997, 91:157–172.

45. Phillips KA, Toner GC: Chemotherapy for soft tissue sarcomas. *Acta Orthop Scand* 1997, 68:133–138.

46. Zalupski M, Ryan JR, Hussein ME, Baker LH: Systemic adjuvant chemotherapy for soft tissue sarcomas of the extremities. *Surg Oncol Clin North Am* 1993, 2:621–636.

47. Jones GW, Chouinard E, Patel M: Adjuvant adriamycin (doxorubicin) in adult patients with soft tissue sarcomas: a systematic overview and quantitative meta-analysis [abstract]. *Clinical Ivest Med* 1991, 14:A772.

48. Zalupski M, Ryan JR, Hussein ME: Defining the role of adjuvant chemotherapy for patients with soft tissue sarcoma of the extremities. In *Adjuvant Therapy of Cancer VII*. Edited by Salmon SE. Philadelphia: JB Lippincott; 1993:385–392.

49. Tierney JF: Adjuvant chemotherapy for localized resectable soft tissue sarcoma of adults: a meta-analysis of individual patient data. *J Clin Oncol* 1998, in press.

50. Pezzi CM, Pollock RE, Evans HL, *et al.*: Preoperative chemotherapy for soft-tissue sarcomas of the extremities *Ann Surg* 1990, 211:476–481.

51. Casper ES, Gaynor JJ, Panicek DM, Harrison LB: Preoperative and Postoperative adjuvant chemotherapy for adults with high grade soft tissue sarcoma. *Cancer* 1994, 73:1644–1650.

52. Singer S, Antman K, Corson J, Eberlein TJ: Long-Term salvagability for patients with locally recurrent soft-tissue sarcomas. *Arch Surg* 1992, 127:548–554.

53. Eggermont AM, Schraffordt-Koops H, Klausner JM, *et al.*: Isolated limb perfusion with tumor necrosis factor and melphalan for limb salvage in 186 patients with locally advanced soft tissue extremity sarcomas: the cumulative multi-center European experience. *Ann Surg* 1996, 224:756–764 (discussion 764–765).

54. Maruyama R, Mitsudomi T, Ishida T, *et al.*: Aggressive pulmonary metastasectomies for synovial sarcoma. *Respiration* 1997, 64:316–318.

55. Choong PF, Pritchard DJ, Rock MG, *et al.*: Survival after pulmonary metastasectomy in soft tissue sarcoma. Prognostic factors in 214 patients. *Acta Orthop Scand* 1995, 66:561–568.

56. Putnam JB Jr, Roth JA: Surgical treatment for pulmonary metastases from sarcoma. *Hematol Oncol Clin North Am* 1995, 9:869–887.

57. Schirren J, Krysa S, Bulzebruck H, *et al.*: Results of surgical treatment of pulmonary metastases from soft tissue sarcomas. *Recent Results Cancer Res* 1995, 138:123–138.

58. Shimizu J, Oda M, Hayashi Y, *et al.*: Results of surgical treatment of pulmonary metastases. *J Surg Oncol* 1995, 58:57–62.

59. Casson AG, Putnam JB, Natarajan G, *et al.*: Efficacy of pulmonary metastasectomy for recurrent soft tissue sarcoma. *J Surg Oncol* 1991, 47:1–4.

60. Jablons D, Steinberg SM, Roth J, *et al.*: Metastasectomy for soft tissue sarcoma: further evidence for efficacy and prognostic indicators. *J Thorac Cardiovasc Surg* 1989, 97:695–705.

61. Pogrebniak HW, Roth JA, Steinberg SM, *et al.*: Reoperative pulmonary resection in patients with metastatic soft tissue sarcoma. *Ann Thorac Surg* 1991, 52:197–203.

62. Casson AG, Putnam JB, Natarajan G, *et al.*: Five-year survival after pulmonary metastasectomy for adult soft tissue sarcoma. *Cancer* 1992, 69:662–668.

63. Borden EC, Amato DA, Edmonson JH, *et al.*: Randomized comparison of doxorubicin and vindesine to doxorubicin for patients with metastatic soft-tissue sarcomas. *Cancer* 1990, 66:862–867.

64. Casper ES, Gaynor JJ, Hajdu SI, *et al.*: A prospective randomized trial of adjuvant chemotherapy with bolus versus continuous infusion of doxorubicin in patients with high-grade extremity soft tissue sarcoma and an analysis of prognostic factors. *Cancer* 1991, 68:1221–1229.

65. Edmonson JH, Ryan LM, Blum RH, *et al.*: Randomized comparsion of doxorubicin alone versus ifosfamide plus doxorubicin or mitomycin ,doxorubicin and cisplatin against advanced soft tissue sarcomas. *J Clin Oncol* 1993, 11:1269–1275.

66. Verweij J, van Oosterom AT, Somers R, *et al.*: Chemotherapy in the multidisciplinary approach to soft tissue sarcomas: EORTC Soft Tissue and Bone Sarcoma Group studies in perspective. *Ann Oncol* 1992, 3(suppl 2):S75–S80.

67. Mouridsen HT, Bastholt L, Somers R, *et al.*: Adriamycin versus epirubicin in advanced soft tissue sarcomas: a randomized phase II/phase III study of the EORTC Soft Tissue and Bone Sarcoma Group. *Eur J Cancer Clin Oncol* 1987, 23:1477–1483.

68. Stuart-Harris RC, Harper PG, Parsons CA, *et al.*: High-dose alkylation therapy using ifosfamide infusion with mesna in the treatment of adult advanced soft-tissue sarcoma. *Cancer Chemother Pharmacol* 1983, 11:69–72.

69. Stuart-Harris R, Harper PG, Kaye SB, Wiltshaw E: High-dose ifosfamide by infusion with mesna in advanced soft tissue sarcoma. *Cancer Treat Rev* 1983, 10(suppl A):163–164.

70. Bramwell VH, Mouridsen HT, Santoro A, *et al.*: Cyclophosphamide versus ifosfamide: final report of a randomized phase II trial in adult soft tissue sarcomas. *Eur J Cancer Clin Oncol* 1987, 23:311–321.

71. Antman KH, Elias AD: Dana-Farber Cancer Institute studies in advanced sarcoma. *Semin Oncol* 1990, 17:7–15.

72. Elias AD, Eder JP, Shea T, *et al.*: High-dose ifosfamide with mesna uroprotection: a phase I study. *J Clin Oncol* 1990, 8:170–178.

73. Buesa JM, Mouridsen HT, van Oosterom AT, *et al.*: High-dose DTIC in advanced soft-tissue sarcomas in the adult: a phase II study of the EORTC Soft Tissue and Bone Sarcoma Group. *Ann Oncol* 1991, 2:307–309.

74. Antman KH, Crowley J, Balcerzak S, *et al.*: An Intergroup phase III randomized study of doxorubicin and dacarbazine with or without ifosfamide and mesna in advanced soft tissue and bone sarcomas. *J Clin Oncol* 1993, 11:1276–1285.

75. Schoenfeld DA, Rosenbaum C, Horton J, *et al.*: A comparison of adriamycin versus vincristine and adriamycin, and cyclophosphamide versus vincristine, actinomycin-D, and cyclophosphamide for advanced sarcoma. *Cancer* 1982, 50:2757–2762.

76. Borden EC, Amato DA, Rosenbaum C, *et al.*: Randomized comparison of three adriamycin regimens for metastatic soft tissue sarcomas. *J Clin Oncol* 1987, 5:840–850.

77. Baker LH, Frank J, Fine G, *et al.*: Combination chemotherapy using adriamycin, DTIC, cyclophosphamide, and actinomycin D for advanced soft tissue sarcomas: a randomized comparative trial: a phase III Southwest Oncology Group Study (7613). *J Clin Oncol* 1987, 5:851–861.

78. Santoro A, Tursz T, Mouridsen H, *et al.*: Doxorubicin versus CYVADIC versus doxorubicin plus ifosfamide in first-line treatment of advanced soft tissue sarcomas: a randomized study of the EORTC Soft Tissue and Bone Sarcoma Group. *J Clin Oncol* 1995, 13:1537–1545.

79. Pinedo HM, Bramwell VH, Mouridsen HT, *et al.*: Cyvadic in advanced soft tissue sarcoma: a randomized study comparing two schedules: a study of the EORTC Soft Tissue and Bone Sarcoma Group. *Cancer* 1984, 53:1825–1832.

80. Edmonson JH, Long HJ, Kvols LK, *et al.*: Can molgramostim enhance the antitumor effects of cytotoxic drugs in patients with advanced sarcomas? *Ann Oncol* 1997, 8:637–641.

81. Bokemeyer C, Franzke A, Hartmann JT, *et al.*: A phase I/II study of sequential, dose-escalated, high dose ifosfamide plus doxorubicin with peripheral blood stem cell support for the treatment of patients with advanced soft tissue sarcomas. *Cancer* 1997, 80:1221–1227.

82. Steward WP, Verweij J, Somers R, *et al.*: Doxorubicin plus ifosfamide with rhGM-CSF in the treatment of advanced adult soft-tissue sarcomas: preliminary results of a phase II study from the EORTC Soft-Tissue and Bone Sarcoma Group. *J Cancer Res Clin Oncol* 1991, 117(suppl 4):S193–S197.

83. Hicks LG, Balcerzak SP, Zalupski M: GM-CSF did not allow doxorubicin dose escalation in the MAID regimen: a phase I trial: a Southwest Oncology Group study. *Cancer Invest* 1996, 14:507–512.

84. Steward WP, Verweij J, Somers R, *et al.*: Granulocyte-Macrophage Colony Stimulating factor allows safe escalation of dose -intensity of chemotherapy in metastatic adult soft tissue sarcomas: a study of the EORTC Soft Tissue and Bone Sarcoma Group. *J Clin Oncol* 1993, 11:15–21.

85. Jaques DP, Coit DG, Hajdu SI, Brennan MF: Management of primary and recurrent soft-tissue sarcoma of the retroperitoneum. *Ann Surg* 1990, 212:51–59.

86. Kilkenny JW III, Bland KI, Copeland EM III. Retroperitoneal sarcoma: the University of Florida experience. *J Am Coll Surg* 1996, 182:329–339.

87. Dalton RR, Donohue JH, Mucha P Jr, *et al.*: Management of retroperitoneal sarcomas. *Surgery* 1989, 106:725–732 (discussion 732–733).

88. Heslin MJ, Lewis JJ, Nadler E, *et al.*: Prognostic factors associated with long-term survival for retroperitoneal sarcoma: implications for management. *J Clin Oncol* 1997, 15:2832–2839.

89. Kinsella TJ, Sindelar WF, Lack E, *et al.*: Preliminary results of a randomized study of adjuvant radiation therapy in resectable adult retroperitoneal soft tissue sarcomas. *J Clin Oncol* 1988, 6:18–25.

90. Farhood A, Hajdu S, Shiu M, Strong E: Soft tissue sarcomas of the head and neck in adults. *Am J Surg* 1990, 160:365–369.

91. Mankin HJ, Lange TA, Spanier SS: The hazards of biopsy in patients with malignant primary bone and soft-tissue tumors. *J Bone Joint Surg Am* 1982, 64:1121–1127.

92. Malawer M, Link MP, Donaldson SS: Sarcomas of bone. In *Principles and Practice of Oncology*, ed 5. Edited by Rosenberg S, Devita V, Hellman S. Philadelphia: Lippincott-Raven; 1997:1789–1852.

93. Link MP, Goorin AM, Miser AW, *et al.*: The effect of adjuvant chemotherapy on relapse-free survival in patients with osteosarcoma of the extremity. *N Engl J Med* 1986, 314:1600–1606.

94. Eilber F, Giuliano A, Eckardt J, *et al.*: Adjuvant chemotherapy for osteosarcoma: a randomized prospective trial. *J Clin Oncol* 1987, 5:21–26.

95. Mosende C, Gutierrez M, Caparros B, Rosen G: Combination chemotherapy with bleomycin, cyclophosphamide and dactinomycin for the treatment of osteogenic sarcoma. *Cancer* 1977, 40:2779–2786.

96. Rosen G, Marcove RC, Huvos AG, *et al.*: Primary osteogenic sarcoma: eight-year experience with adjuvant chemotherapy. *J Cancer Res Clin Oncol* 1983, 106(suppl):55–67.

97. Rosen G, Nirenberg A: Neoadjuvant chemotherapy for osteogenic sarcoma: a five year follow-up (T-10) and preliminary report of new studies (T-12). *Prog Clin Biol Res* 1985, 201:39–51.

98. Rosen G: Preoperative (neoadjuvant) chemotherapy for osteogenic sarcoma: a ten year experience. *Orthopedics* 1985, 8:659–664.

99. Goorin A, Baker A, Gieser P, Ayala A, *et al.*: No evidence for improved event free survival (EFS) with presurgical chemotherapy (PRE) for nonmetastatic extremity osteogenic sarcoma (OGS): preliminary results of randomized Pediatric Oncology Group (POG) trial [abstract]. *Proc Am Soc Clin Oncol* 1995, 14:444.

100. Meyers PA, Heller G, Healey J, *et al.*: Chemotherapy for nonmetastatic osteogenic sarcoma: the Memorial Sloan-Kettering experience. *J Clin Oncol* 1992, 10:5–15.

101. Glasser DB, Lane JM, Huvos AG, *et al.*: Survival, prognosis, and therapeutic response in osteogenic sarcoma: the Memorial Hospital experience. *Cancer* 1992, 69:698–708.

102. Provisor AJ, Ettinger LJ, Nachman JB, *et al.*: Treatment of nonmetastatic osteosarcoma of the extremity with preoperative and postoperative chemotherapy: a report from the Children's Cancer Group. *J Clin Oncol* 1997, 15:76–84.

103. Winkler K, Beron G, Delling G, *et al.*: Neoadjuvant chemotherapy of osteosarcoma: results of a randomized cooperative trial (COSS-82) with salvage chemotherapy based on histological tumor response. *J Clin Oncol* 1988, 6:329–337.

104. Beattie EJ, Harvey JC, Marcove R, Martini N: Results of multiple pulmonary resections for metastatic osteogenic sarcoma after two decades. *J Surg Oncol* 1991, 46:154–155.

105. Burk CD, Belasco JB, O'Neill JA Jr, Lange B: Pulmonary metastases and bone sarcomas: surgical removal of lesions appearing after adjuvant chemotherapy. *Clin Orthop* 1991, 88–92.

106. Goorin AM, Delorey MJ, Lack EE, *et al.*: Prognostic significance of complete surgical resection of pulmonary metastases in patients with osteogenic sarcoma: analysis of 32 patients. *J Clin Oncol* 1984, 2:425–431.

107. Flye MW, Woltering G, Rosenberg SA: Aggressive pulmonary resection for metastatic osteogenic and soft tissue sarcomas. *Ann Thorac Surg* 1984, 37:123–127.

108. Putnam JB Jr, Roth JA, Wesley MN, *et al.*: Survival following aggressive resection of pulmonary metastases from osteogenic sarcoma: analysis of prognostic factors. *Ann Thorac Surg* 1983, 36:516–523.

MAID FOR THE TREATMENT OF ADVANCED SOFT TISSUE SARCOMA
Mesna, Doxorubicin, Ifosfamide, and Dacarbazine

Doxorubicin is the most effective single agent in the treatment of soft tissue sarcomas in the adult. Ifosfamide has been shown to also have good activity as a single agent. The combination regimen of doxorubicin and ifosfamide with or without dacarbazine (DTIC) has been shown to have higher response rates than treatment with single agents. Unfortunately, overall survival has not been shown to be improved by combination regimens. Moreover, toxicity is significantly greater. Efforts to limit myelosuppressive toxicity and increase the dose of doxorubicin in these regimens is currently being investigated.

RECENT EXPERIENCE AND RESPONSE RATES

Group	Regimen	Dose of A	Patients, n	RR, %	CR, %
DFCI [71]	MAID	60 mg/m²/course	108	47	10
SWOG [83]	MAID + GM-CSF	75 mg/m²/course	13	—	—
EORTC [84]	A + I + GM-CSF	60 mg/m²/course	145	45	10

A—doxorubicin; CR—complete response rate; DFCI—Dana-Farber Cancer Institute; EORTC—European Organization for Research in Cancer Therapy; GM-CSF—granulocyte–macrophage colony-stimulating factor; I—ifosfamide; MAID—mesna, doxorubicin, ifosfamide, and dacarbazine; RR—response rate; SWOG—Southwestern Oncology Group.

INDICATIONS
Doxorubicin is the only drug with labeled indication for the treatment of soft tissue sarcomas; combination regimens incorporating ifosfamide with mesna and or dacarbazine have been shown in randomized trials to improve response rates in soft tissue sarcoma; currently little data exists to support the use of these drugs in the adjuvant setting outside of clinical trials; for patients with advanced disease, single agent doxorubicin may provide palliative benefit; the greater response rates with combination regimens should be balanced against the increased toxicity

CANDIDATES FOR TREATMENT
Patients with advanced soft tissue sarcomas who have normal renal and cardiac function

TOXICITY
Enhanced myelosuppression with combination regimen: administration of hematopoietic growth factors may blunt severe neutropenia; severe nausea and emesis is common; alopecia is to be expected; **Doxorubicin:** cardiac toxicity is the single most important concern with doses exceeding 400 mg/m²; may also tinge urine red-orange; hyperpigmentation and creasing of nail beds may occur; should be administered through central venous line because local extravasation will result in severe cellulitis, vesication, and tissue necrosis; **Ifosfamide** severe hemorrhaged cystitis; should only be administered with vigorous hydration in combination with uroprotective agent mesna; neurological manifestations (*eg*, somnolence, confusion, and hallucinations); **Dacarbazine:** severe nausea and vomiting are the most common toxicities

DRUG INTERACTIONS
Administration of live vaccines should be avoided in all patients receiving myelosuppressive chemotherapy; **Doxorubicin:** cyclosporine may induce coma and/or seizures; phenobarbitol increases elimination of doxorubicin; phenytoin levels may be decreased by concomitant administration of doxorubicin; **Ifosfamide and DTIC:** no specific interactions cited in literature; physician should be alert to possible combined drug interactions

NURSING INTERVENTIONS
Strict sterile technique when accessing central venous devices should be practiced; general supportive measures, including prophylactic antiemetics and mouth care to minimize symptoms from stomatitis; vigorous hydration with administration of ifosfamide; immediately report any symptoms of infection, bleeding, or shortness of breath

PATIENT INFORMATION
Common side effects from administration of these agents include nausea, vomiting, and stomatitis; in addition, doxorubicin may have direct cardiac toxicity manifested by acute left ventricular failure; immunosuppression is expected and occurs at a maximum of 10–14 d after therapy; patients should notify their physician immediately if they develop a fever, abnormal bleeding, or shortness of breath

ADMINISTRATION NOTES
Doxorubicin: (Rubex, Bristol-Meyers Squibb, Princeton, NJ) supplied as 10-mg, 50-mg, and 100-mg vials. Reconstitute with sterile sodium chloride (0.9%) to final concentration of 2 mg/mL. Reconstituted solution is stable up to 24 h at room temperature and 48 h under refrigeration (2°C–8°C)
Ifosfamide: (Ifex, Bristol-Meyers Squibb, Princeton, NJ) supplied as 1-gm or 3-gm single- or multiple-dose vials in combination packages with mesna. Should be reconstituted in sterile water to final concentration of 50 mg/mL. Should be refrigerated and used within 24 h of reconstitution
Dacarbazine: (multiple manufactures) supplied as 100-mg or 200-mg vials. May be reconstituted and mixed with doxorubicin for injection.

MABCDP FOR TREATMENT OF OSTEOSARCOMA
Methotrexate, Doxorubicin, Bleomycin, Cyclophosphamide, Dactinomycin, and Cisplatin

Chemotherapy for osteosarcoma is most often given in the setting of adjuvant therapy. The development of effective regimens for these tumors has been largely empirical given the extremely poor response rates in macroscopic disease. Currently, the area under study is whether there is an advantage to early preoperative treatment versus traditional postoperative adjuvant therapy. Additionally, the value of modifying postoperative regimens in patients who respond poorly to preoperative therapy is being studied. The majority of randomized trials incorporate chemotherapy regimens based on doxorubicin and cisplatin. Other agents, such as high-dose methotrexate and the BCD (bleomycin, cyclophosphamide, dactinomycin) combination, are controversial.

INDICATIONS

FDA-approved: only doxorubicin has a labeled indication for the treatment of bone sarcomas; methotrexate, bleomycin, cyclophosphamide, dactinomycin, and cisplatin are all FDA-approved for the treatment of cancer and have shown effectiveness in various randomized trials against osteosarcoma

CANDIDATES FOR TREATMENT

Patients with osteosarcoma who have normal renal, cardiac, and pulmonary function

TOXICITIES AND ADVERSE REACTIONS

Enhanced myelosuppression with combination regimen: administration of hematopoietic growth factors may blunt severe neutropenia; severe nausea and emesis is common; alopecia is to be expected; **Doxorubicin:** cardiac toxicity is the single most important concern with doses exceeding 400 mg/m^2; may also tinge urine red-orange; hyperpigmentation and creasing of nail beds may occur; should be administered through central venous line because local extravasation will result in severe cellulitis, vesication, and tissue necrosis; **Methotrexate:** may result in renal failure or death if not given with appropriate support; cumulative toxicity includes hepatic fibrosis, osteoporosis, and pulmonary dysfunction; **Bleomycin:** severe idiosyncratic, anaphylactic reactions have been reported; pulmonary fibrosis that begins as pneumonitis is the most serious side effect, arising in 10% of patients treated; **Cyclophosphamide:** hemorrhagic cystitis; should be given with vigorous hydration; **Dactinomycin:** GI toxicity most predominate; locally irritating if extravasated

DRUG INTERACTIONS

Administration of live vaccines should be avoided in all patients receiving myelosuppressive chemotherapy; **Doxorubicin:** cyclosporine may induce coma and/or seizures; phenobarbitol increases elimination of doxorubicin; **Methotrexate:** nonsteroidal anti-inflammatories, ethanol, 5-fluorouracil, and salicylates. **Bleomycin:** granulocyte colony-stimulating factor may increase risk of pulmonary fibrosis

NURSING INTERVENTIONS

Strict sterile technique when accessing central venous devices should be practiced; general supportive measures, including prophylactic antiemetics and mouth care to minimize symptoms from stomatitis; vigorous hydration with administration of cyclophosphamide; immediately report any symptoms of infection, bleeding, pulmonary dysfunction, or symptoms of congestive heart failure

MABCDP FOR TREATMENT OF OSTEOSARCOMA (Continued)
Methotrexate, Doxorubicin, Bleomycin, Cyclophosphamide, Dactinomycin, and Cisplatin

RECENT EXPERIENCES AND RESPONSE RATES

Group	Preoperative regimen	Preoperative regimen	Patients, n	Disease-free survival, %	Overall survival, %
POG [99]	None or methotrexate, doxorubicin, and cisplatin	None or methotrexate, doxorubicin, and cisplatin	106	70.0 (preoperative) 72.8 (postoperative)	—
CCG [99]	Methotrexate and BCD	methotrexate, doxorubicin, cisplatin and BCD	231	53.0	60

BCD—bleomycin, cyclophosphamide, and dactinomycin; CCG—Children's Cancer Group; POG—Pediatric Oncology Group.

PATIENT INFORMATION

Common side effects from administration of these agents include nausea, vomiting, and stomatitis; in addition, doxorubicin may have direct cardiac toxicity manifested by acute left ventricular failure; bleomycin may result in severe pulmonary fibrosis; immunosuppression is expected and occurs at a maximum of 10–14 d after therapy; patients should notify their physician immediately if they develop a fever, abnormal bleeding or swelling, or shortness of breath

ADMINISTRATION NOTES

Doxorubicin: (Rubex, Bristol Meyers Squibb) supplied as 10-mg, 50-mg, and 100-mg vials. Reconstitute with sterile sodium chloride (0.9%) to final concentration of 2 mg/ml. Reconstituted solution is stable up to 24 h at room temperature and 48 h under refrigeration (2°C–8°C)

Cisplatin: (Bristol Meyers Squibb) supplied as 10 mg or 50 mg of powder to be resuspended into solution at 50 mg/mL

Methotrexate: (multiple suppliers) supplied as 1-g vial lyophilized powder

Bleomycin: (Bristol Meyers Squibb) supplied as 15-U vial

Cyclophosphamide: (Bristol Meyers Squibb) supplied as 100-mg to 2-g vials

Dactinomycin: (Merck, Sharp and Dohme) supplied as 0.5-mg/mL vial

Leucovorin calcium: (multiple suppliers) 5–25-mg tablets; 3-mg/mL injection and 50–350-mg vial of powder for injection.

Although tremendous strides have been made in the treatment of genitourinary malignancies in the past 10 to 15 years, the explosion of new findings in cell biology, physiology, biochemistry, pharmacology, immunology, and radiobiology has broadened and deepened our understanding of biology and treatment for the 1990s. This chapter summarizes present medical and surgical therapies employed for prostate, urinary bladder, testicular, and renal cancers. We highlight salient basic and clinical observations that have formed the foundation of our current therapeutic strategies in genitourinary cancers.

TESTICULAR CANCER

ETIOLOGY AND RISK FACTORS

Germ cell cancers arise from pleuripotent cells capable of differentiating along five different embryonic lines. These tumors are commonly grouped into seminoma and nonseminoma. Seminoma tumors arise from the spermatocyte, the earliest cell with the greatest ability to differentiate into embryonic or placental tissue. Nonseminoma tumors often are mixed and contain elements of embryonal cells, teratoma, yolk sac, and choriocarcinoma.

Germ cell tumors are rare, and if treatment for a suspicious testicular mass is approached promptly, the clinical outcome for the overwhelming majority of patients is cure. It is of no surprise that screening for early-stage testicular malignancies has not proved to be beneficial [1]. Etiology and risk factors are described in Table 14-1.

STAGING AND PROGNOSIS

The diagnosis and therapeutic approaches to germ cell tumor of the testis must consider the anatomy of lymphatic drainage and course of the neurovascular bundles, stage, histologic type, and the presence of vessel invasion (Table 14-2). In addition, the relative sensitivity to chemotherapy or radiation therapy may dictate choice of treatment for these tumors. When testicular malignancy is suspected, a routine battery of laboratory and radiologic evaluations should be performed, including a complete blood count, lactate dehydrogenase, β-human chorionic gonadotropin (βhCG), α-fetoprotein, urine analysis, and computed tomography of the chest and abdomen. Magnetic resonance imaging and new modalities, such as positron emission tomography, may improve our ability to detect metastatic disease but await further study. Other tests that may prove useful for the diagnosis and management of testicular tumors include testicular ultrasound and IV pyelography.

We are fortunate to have accurate tumor markers for assessment of germ cell cancers, and these markers have become essential for the correct management of these malignancies (Table 14-3). Elevation of α-fetoprotein, βhCG, or both is found in 85% of nonseminomatous germ cell cancer, whereas only 10% of seminomas show mild elevation in βhCG. False elevations in serum markers are rare but should be recognized because treatment decisions are based, in part, on these measurements. Although lactate dehydrogenase is a nonspecific marker, it is helpful in suggesting bulky lymph node involvement.

For patients with metastatic disease a number of prognostic factors have been used in devising staging systems. Commonly used are the M.D. Anderson Classification, the Memorial Sloan-Kettering Cancer Institute Classification, and the Indiana Classification. These systems attempt to estimate the bulk of disease

Table 14-2. Staging of Testicular Cancers

Stage*		TNM Staging	Criteria
0		Tis N0 M0	Intratubular, preinvasive tumor
I (A)		T1 T2 N0 M0	Tumor limited to testes and/or rete testis Invasion beyond tunica albuginea or into epididymis
II (A)		T3 T4 N0 M0	Invasion of spermatic cord Invasion of scrotum Invasion of scrotum
III (B1)		Any T N1 M0	Metastasis to one lymph node ≤ 2 cm in dimension
IV (B2)		Any T N2	Metastasis to one lymph node 2–5 cm in size or multiple lymph nodes < 5 cm
(B3)		N3 M0	Metastasis to lymph node ≥ 5 cm in diameter
(C)	or	Any T Any N M1	Distant metastases

*American Urological Association staging in parentheses.

Table 14-1. Risk Factors for Testicular Cancers

Genetic Factors
Association of Lewis antigen Le(a-b-) with germ cell tumors [2]
Association of HLABw41 with seminoma [2]

Acquired Factors
Cryptorchidism (relative risk of 7.4) [3]
Exposure to diethylstilbesterol in utero (relative risk 9.8) [4]
Decreased risk with birth order (for fourth or later child compared to first-born a relative risk of 0.3) [5]
Occupational exposure to extreme temperature (odds ratio 1.7) [6]

Table 14-3 Prognostic Factors for Patients with Stage I Testicular Cancers

Preoperative α-fetoprotein
Vascular invasion
Absence of teratoma

From Klepp et al. [7]; with permission.

and do so relatively well. We use the Indiana system, which classifies patients with testicular cancer into three categories (Table 14-4).

Clinical outcome for minimal and moderate-stage metastatic germ cell cancer remains excellent with 3-year survival rates of approximately 98% and 92%, respectively. A high percentage (approximately 90%) of advanced-stage metastatic cancers enter complete remission, with approximately 85% of patients remaining disease free at 2 years.

PRIMARY DISEASE THERAPY

There is no controversy over the appropriate initial diagnostic and therapeutic approach to suspected testicular malignancies (Table 14-5). An inguinal orchiectomy allows for control of blood and lymphatic vessels and en bloc removal of the affected testicle. Transscrotal biopsies or orchiectomy may lead to locoregional recurrences in as many as one quarter of patients and are discouraged. Lymphatic pathways from the testicle pass first to the periaortic and preaortic lymph nodes on the left and interaortocaval, preaortic, and precaval lymph nodes on the right. Identification of the sympathetic nerves that supply the ejaculatory muscles and understanding of which nodal groups are likely to be involved with tumor have allowed for an effective and more limited retroperitoneal lymph node dissection (RPLND), a procedure that preserves fertility. Laparoscopic technique for lymph node dissections has become available. As this technique becomes more popular, its role in evaluation of nodal status must be assessed.

ADJUVANT THERAPY FOR REGIONAL DISEASE

The success of platinum-based multichemotherapy for the treatment of nonseminomatous testicular cancers has provided the foundation for the treatment of early-stage disease as well. The question in stage I nonseminomatous disease following an inguinal orchiectomy and demonstration of no other metastases by serologic, radiologic, and physical examination is whether to do an elective RPLND or recommend surveillance. Studies of surveillance suggest that disease progression occurs in approximately 30% of patients and frequently presents with bulkier disease. Embryonal, yolk sac, and choriocarcinoma histologic elements are highly prone to metastatic spread. Venous or lymphatic invasion and tumor outside the tunica albuginea or involving the epididymis (T2) suggest a tumor with the ability to metastasize. Vessel invasion was the single most important histologic risk factor in a report by the Testicular Cancer Intergroup Study. People with these findings are poor candidates for surveillance [10].

Approximately 25% of patients who undergo RPLND for clinical stage I disease have evidence of microscopic metastases. Approximately 10% to 15% of patients undergoing RPLND relapse with cancer, usually outside the operative field. Randomized studies have shown that two cycles of cisplatin, vinblastine, and bleomycin chemotherapy following RPLND for stage II disease yield a cure in approximately 98% of patients. The management of low-volume stage II disease (stage IIa, stage IIb, and patients with persistent marker elevation after orchiectomy) continued to generate considerable controversy. Lack of randomized, well-conducted studies and small sizes of prospective analyses have not clarified the controversies. One area of consensus is to reduce the type and number of therapies to minimize toxicity and cost.

Identification of factors that would predict benefit of combined RPLND and drug therapy could reduce the use of combined therapy by as much as 68% to 71% [11,12]. Baniel and coworkers [13] compared the direct costs, toxicity, and quality of life for nonseminomatous stage IIa/IIb cancers treated with primary RPLND plus adjuvant chemotherapy or cisplatin-based chemotherapy along. They found that primary RPLND plus chemotherapy is equivalent to chemotherapy in producing 5-year disease-free status but is associated with less overall morbidity, mortality, and lost weeks of work and better fertility. If needed, postchemotherapy nerve-sparing RPLND is considerably more difficult and is associated with a decrease in the likelihood of the preservation of ejaculatory function.

We recommend that primary RPLND should be considered for patients with clinical stage IIa or IIb nonseminomatous germ cell

Table 14-4. Indiana Staging System for Metastatic Testicular Malignancies

Minimal disease

Elevated βhCG and or α-fetoprotein

Palpable cervical nodes with or without nonpalpable retroperitoneal nodes

Unresectable, but nonpalpable, retroperitoneal nodes

Less than five metastatic lesions per lung field with none > 2 cm in largest diameter, with or without nonpalpable retroperitoneal nodes

Moderate disease

Palpable abdominal mass as only anatomical disease

Five to ten pulmonary metastases per lung field < 3 cm in largest diameter, or a mediastinal mass < 50% of the intrathoracic diameter, or a solitary pulmonary metastasis > 2 cm in largest diameter with or without nonpalpable retroperitoneal nodes

Advanced disease

Mediastinal mass > 50% of the intrathoracic diameter, or > 10 pulmonary nodules per lung field, or multiple pulmonary metastases > 3 cm with or without nonpalpable retroperitoneal nodes

A palpable abdominal mass with any pulmonary or intrathoracic metastases

Liver, bone, or CNS metastases

Other factors identified with poor outcome [6]

α-Fetoprotein > 500 IU/L

βhCG > 1000 IU/L

Age > 35 y

Factors associated with poor outcome in patients with low-volume disease (ie, minimal disease)

α-Fetoprotein > 1000 IU/L

βhCG > 10,000 IU/L

Adapted from Birch et al. [8] and Aass et al. [9]; with permission.

Table 14-5. Management of Early-Stage Primary Testicular Disease

Inguinal orchiectomy

Surveillance for good candidates

RPLND for nonseminomatous tumors to determine adjuvant chemotherapy

For seminoma, radiotherapy to nodal groups at risk

RPLND—retroperitoneal lymph node dissection.

tumors of the testes, except in cases of large retroperitoneal masses (> 5 cm), in high percentage of embryonal carcinoma or vascular invasion in primary tumor, or in multiple large lymph nodes. Two cycles of cisplatin-based adjuvant chemotherapy are employed if tumor markers drop to normal levels.

Finally, patients with persistent elevation of tumor markers postorchiectomy in what otherwise appears to be stage I disease (so-called "IIm") should be considered for primary chemotherapy because this may represent systemic rather than nodal metastases [14]. Newer markers and histopathologic factors may identify high-risk patients in this category, which allow for a more selective approach to adjuvant therapy.

ACTIVE AGENTS FOR ADVANCED DISEASE

Modern multiagent chemotherapy has had a significant impact on the treatment of testicular tumors. In the early 1970s, investigators at Memorial Sloan-Kettering Cancer Center began to evaluate the combination called VAB-I (vinblastine, dactinomycin, and bleomycin) in patients with metastatic nonseminomatous cancers and demonstrated a 36% objective response rate (14% complete response rate, or CR). The addition of cyclophosphamide and cisplatin to this regimen (VAB-VI) improved the CR rate to 78%. Concomitantly, the group at Indiana University began using the combination called PVB (cisplatin, vinblastine, and bleomycin) and demonstrated a 70% CR rate and a 60% 10-year survival. Toxicity of PVB chemotherapy principally was due to the high dose of vinblastine (0.4 mg/kg). Subsequent trials evaluated lower doses of vinblastine and led to a comparative randomized study of PVB chemotherapy versus PEB (cisplatin, etoposide, and bleomycin). This study demonstrated a significant reduction of toxicity for the PEB arm with equal or better response and survival rates (83% CR for PEB vs 71% CR for PVB). More recent studies have continued to focus on diminishing toxicity. A recent multicenter, randomized trial compared the efficacy and toxicity of four cycles of carboplatin and etoposide versus cisplatin and etoposide in 270 patients with good-risk metastatic germ cell tumor [15]. Carboplatin doses ranged from 350 mg/m^2 to 500 mg/m^2. The carboplatin regimen was associated with more hematologic toxicity, more relapses from CR, and lower event-free survival compared with the cisplatin-based therapy.

The feasibility of removing bleomycin from PEB chemotherapy was tested in a randomized study. The initial study evaluating PEB versus PE (cisplatin and etoposide), performed through the Eastern Cooperative Oncology Group (ECOG) in good-prognosis metastatic nonseminomatous cancers (Indiana stage minimal disease), was discontinued after investigators noted that response rates were lower in the PE arm. A subsequent ECOG trial reported the relative efficacy and toxicity of three cycles of PEB (bleomycin 30 IU/wk for 9 wk) versus three cycles of EP [16]. Once again, relapse rates (23% vs 10%) and 3-year disease-free survival favored the PEB arm, and there were no cases of significant pulmonary toxicity in either arm. The Australian Germ Cell Trial Group compared PVB with cisplatin and vinblastine (PV) in 222 patients with inoperable gonadal cancer. Patients were matched on prognostic risk factors. Minimum duration of follow-up was 4 years. Although relapse rates (7% for PV and 5% for PVB) and overall survival were not different for the two groups, tumor-related deaths occurred in 16 patients (15%) in the PV group and 6 patients (5%) in the PVB arm (P=0.02). Although toxicity was greater in the PVB arm, it was concluded that bleomycin significantly enhanced the therapeutic

benefit of cisplatin and vinblastine [17]. Thus, the weight of the evidence at this time favors the continued inclusion of bleomycin in the treatment of good-risk metastatic germ cell tumors.

Response rates in metastatic seminoma to platinum-based combination chemotherapy regimens have proved to be as good as response rates in nonseminomatous cancers, with better than 80% cure rates. This has led to a rethinking of recommendations for radiotherapy, which was previously employed for the treatment of early-stage seminoma. Initial treatment of stage I and II disease has consisted of involved- and extended-field radiation therapy. Trials of radiation therapy for stage II disease reveal a 70% to 90% 5-year survival. In stage II disease, approximately 30% of patients have failures outside the radiation ports. Salvage of treatment failures with combination chemotherapy may be compromised by radiation damage to the bone marrow. We suggest treating stage II seminoma patients with evidence of residual cancer with up-front chemotherapy followed by radiation therapy. Treatment strategies for stage I seminoma are more controversial. It appears that prophylactic radiation of the mediastinum does not provide survival advantage and adds to morbidity and late toxicity, as well as causing difficulty in administering chemotherapy at a later time if needed. Inguinal orchiectomy and postsurgery radiation therapy to abdominal lymph nodes are associated with 5-year survival of better than 98%. Chemotherapy is reserved for the few patients who have relapses.

With the use of platinum-based multiagent chemotherapy, extragonadal testicular tumors are treated with equal success, stage for stage, to primary gonadal tumors that have metastasized [18].

Options do exist for metastatic germ cell tumors of the testis that are refractory to or recur after cisplatin-based chemotherapy. Salvage chemotherapy (consisting of ifosfamide, cisplatin, and either vinblastine or etoposide) can cure up to 25% of patients [19]. A recent phase II trial examined the use of two cycles of high-dose carboplatin and taxol with stem cell rescue following one to two cycles of cisplatin-based salvage chemotherapy in patients with refractory or recurrent disease [20]. Out of 25 patients with a median follow-up, 56% were free of disease. Thus, high-dose chemotherapy with stem cell rescue is a viable option for refractory or recurrent malignancy but should be carried out in an experienced center.

Long-term follow-up for patients with testicular cancers should include evaluation for secondary leukemia in patients treated with chemotherapy, and solid organ malignancies, such as gastric carcinoma in patients who received abdominal radiation therapy.

PROSTATE CANCER

ETIOLOGY AND RISK FACTORS

Therapy for prostate cancer continues to generate controversy. A significant number of men are diagnosed with this cancer and die from their illness each year. In the United States, 209,000 men with prostate cancer will be diagnosed in 1997, and 41,800 deaths will be attributed to this disease. In autopsy studies, 30% of men between the ages of 50 and 70 years with no overt evidence of prostate cancer before death had evidence of prostate carcinoma. Prostate cancer risk factors (Table 14-6) include first-degree relatives with prostate cancer, race (in the United States), testosterone level, vasectomy, monosaturated fat intake, and other dietary factors.

For the most part, prostate cancers are slow growing and metasta-

Table 14-6. Etiology and Risk Factors for Prostate Cancer

Age [21]
Race [21]
Family history [21]

Suspected but not yet fully accepted risk factors
Vasectomy (methodologic issues remain in the major studies evaluating vasectomy and
   prostate cancer) [22]
Dietary fat [23]
5-α reductase activity [24]
Socioeconomic status [25]
Cadmium [26]

Table 14-7. Staging of Prostate Cancer

Stage*	TNM Staging	Criteria
0 (A1)	T1a	Tumor is incidental histologic finding in < 3 microscopic foci
(B1)	T2a	Tumor ≤ 1.5 cm with normal tissue on at least three sides in one lobe of the prostate gland
	N0	
	M0	
	G1	Well-differentiated cancer
I (A1)	T1a	
(B1)	or T2a	
	N0	
	M0	
	G2,G3–4	Moderately differentiated or poorly differentiated, respectively
II (A2)	T1b	Tumor is incidental histologic finding in > 3 microscopic foci
(B2)	or T2b	Tumor > 1.5 cm or in > 1 lobe
	N0	
	M0	
	Any G	
III (C1 or C2)	T3	Invasion of prostatic apex, or into or beyond prostatic capsule, bladder neck, or seminal vesicle, but not fixed
	N0	
	M0	
	Any G	
IV (C2)	T4	Tumor is fixed or invades adjacent structure other than those for T3
	N0	
	M0	
	Any G	
(D)	Any T	
	N1	Single lymph node, ≤ 2 cm involved with cancer
	N2	Metastasis in a single lymph node 2–5 cm in diameter or multiple lymph nodes < 5 cm
	N3	Metastasis to lymph node > 5 cm
	M0	
	Any G	
(D)	Any T	
	Any N	
	M1	Distant metastases
	Any G	

American Urological Association staging in parentheses.

size late in their natural history. This presents to the treating clinician a therapeutic dilemma in patients with early-stage disease: which patients will have aggressive cancers needing treatment, and which will have indolent disease requiring no further therapy? Furthermore, if treatment is chosen, which treatment will provide the best outcome with the least morbidity? Although radical prostatectomy and radiotherapy have remained the keystones for initial therapy for early-stage prostate cancers (A and B), recent outcome analyses have questioned these approaches, raising more questions than answers [27,28]. The controversies over treatment for early-stage prostate cancer will continue; treatment for metastatic disease remains palliative, but the issue of when to begin therapy is unresolved.

SCREENING

Early diagnosis of prostate cancer is the focus of numerous screening modalities, including digital rectal examination, transrectal ultrasound, and serum prostate-specific antigen. No study has documented that screening affects overall survival from prostate cancer [29]. Furthermore, the controversy over treatment requirements for early-stage disease causes increasing difficulty in assessing the role of screening. The American Cancer Society recommends screening for prostate cancer with digital rectal examinations beginning at age 40. Assessment of PSA levels using 4 ng\mL as the upper limits of normal has been shown to improve prostate cancer detection [30]. Free prostate-specific antigen and other members of the human kallikrein gene family are also useful in the diagnosis of prostate cancer [31]. A survey of 4.7% practicing urologists who are members of the American Urological Association (AUA) found that screening for prostate cancer was recommended for men between the ages of 50 and 80 years [32].

STAGING AND PROGNOSIS

With early diagnosis comes the dilemma of identifying clinically aggressive cancer that causes significant morbidity by metastasizing or premature death. Except for invasion outside the capsule of the gland (T3, stage C) and histologic grade, which portend a bad prognosis, other factors have failed to further delineate aggressive from indolent disease, causing considerable difficulty in interpreting screening results and confounding treatment decision (Tables 14-7 and 14-8).

Evaluation of prostate cancer should consist of technetium pyrophosphate bone scan for patients with prostate-specific antigen above 10, chest radiography, computed tomography or magnetic resonance imaging of the prostate and evaluation of blood work, including complete blood cell counts, coagulation profile measurement of tumor markers including prostate-specific antigen and lactate dehydrogenase. Usually, prostate-specific antigen alone, if elevated, is used in following patients with prostate cancer. Approximately 90% of nodal tissue can be examined using peritoneoscopy. The best clinical setting for the use of laparoscopic node dissection still needs to be determined. Another modality being tested for staging purposes is radiolabeled murine monoclonal antibodies. Small published series employing CYT-356 antibody

Table 14-8. Test for Evaluation of Prostate Cancer

Serum prostate-specific antigen

Chest radiograph

Bone scan

Computed tomography or magnetic resonance imaging of the pelvis and prostate

Coagulation Profile

Lactate dehydrogenase

(Prostascint; Cytogen, Princeton, NJ) suggest the use of this agent in detecting small microscopic foci. (The FDA has approved the use of Prostascint for the detection of microscopic disease.

A new technique using reverse transcriptase polymerase chain reaction (RT-PCR) allows the detection of circulating prostate cancer cells in the peripheral blood. RNA is extracted from 5 mL of circulating nucleated cells and, using primers for PSA, prostate cancer cells can be detected. This technique appears to be able to predict for capsular penetration with a sensitivity of approximately 67% and for detecting positive surgical margins with a sensitivity of approximately 87% [33]. A positive RT-PCR test was found in 16 of 18 patients with metastatic disease.

Patients with early-stage prostate cancers (A or B) and well- or moderately differentiated tumors have a 10-year survival of approximately 60% to 75%, whereas 20% to 40% of patients with poorly differentiated tumors may survive a decade. Less than half of patients with stage C disease may be expected to live 10 years or more. Gleason grade alone predicted for distant metastases in patients with D1 disease [34]. Gleason grades 8 to 10 correlated with rapid progression to distant metastases (85% at 5 y), whereas patients with a well- or moderately differentiated tumor had a 41% chance of distant metastases at 5 years.

TREATMENT OF EARLY STAGE PROSTATE CANCER

Initial treatment recommendations depend on clinical staging, radiographic findings, level of serum tumor markers, and histology. Assessment of clinical stage prostate-specific antigen level and histologic grade can be used to determine the likelihood of invasion outside the confines of the prostate gland or for metastatic spread. Survival for men with stage A1 (T1a) disease appears about the same as for age-matched controls and is followed with close observation and repeat biopsies of the prostate when clinically indicated. A mathematical model of patients with localized prostate cancer (A2, B1, B2 or T1b, T2a, T2b) suggests a benefit for therapeutic intervention (surgery or radiotherapy) for men younger than 65 years only. The model is provocative and suggests that a clinical trial should be performed to confirm these predictions. The Prostate Intervention versus Observation Trial (PIVOT) for early-stage prostate cancer is being conducted at an intergroup study to address this question. The best initial treatment of stage A2 and B disease continues to be hotly debated between surgeons and radiotherapists. The only randomized study between radiation therapy and radical prostatectomy in patients with A2 and B disease was reported by Paulson [35] in 1982 but remains controversial owing to methodologic issues. Although the study suggests a survival advantage to surgery, the radiotherapy-treated patients appear to have a worse outcome than other reported by other radiotherapy programs. The Veterans Administration Cooperative Urologic Research Group (VACURG) reported a small study of stage A and B patients randomly assigned to radical prostatectomy plus placebo versus placebo alone. Although there appeared to be a survival advantage for the patients treated in the placebo-alone arm, the study is flawed by its small patient sample and high percentage of poorly differentiated tumors in the surgery arm (there were none in the placebo arm). It is unlikely that an answer to this time-worn question is forthcoming in the foreseeable future.

Both surgical and radiation techniques continue to improve for the treatment of early-stage disease. One technique that most likely will yield a lower morbidity and higher dose of radiation is three-dimensional conformal radiotherapy, which allows specifically for more accurate delivery of the radiation dose. Recent attention has focused on the timing of adjuvant hormonal intervention.

ADJUVANT THERAPY FOR REGIONAL DISEASE

Regional disease, defined as penetration through the capsule of the prostate gland (T3) with or without spread to neighboring organs (T4) or first-tier pelvic lymph nodes (N1), is incurable with surgical or radiotherapy techniques. Treatment choices must again reflect the natural history of the disease and development of symptoms. There have been a number of recent randomized studies exploring different schedules of adjuvant hormonal therapy with radiation treatment for patients with local advanced prostate cancer [36]. Goserelin (Zoladex; Zeneca Pharmaeuticals, Wilmington, DE) 3.6 mg every 4 weeks for 3 years given in combination with 5 weeks of pelvic radiation (50 Gy with a 2-wk boost of 20 Gy) and cyproterone acetate 150 mg for 1 month improved 5-year overall survival by 17% compared with radiation therapy alone. Even more striking was an 85% disease-free survival for the adjuvant hormone group compared with 48% in the radiotherapy group. The choice of adjuvant/normal therapy and the length of treatment has not yet been optimally defined.

ACTIVE SINGLE AGENTS FOR ADVANCED DISEASE

Hormone therapy using castration or estrogens has been considered standard therapy for D2 disease since the observations in the 1940s by Huggins and Hodges that hormonal intervention causes improvement in symptoms from bone metastases and decrease in alkaline phosphatase. With the advent of newer hormonal agents, the question of the optimal hormonal therapy must be addressed. Historically, the VACURG series of randomized studies provided the data supporting hormonal intervention as an effective therapy and determined the optimal dose of diethylstilbestrol. In addition, orchiectomy was found to be equivalent to diethylstilbestrol but without the cardiovascular complications associated with estrogen administration. These studies focused on surgical or medical castration. With the understanding that prostate cancer is under hormonal regulation, blockade of the adrenal source of testosterone with agents such as ketoconazole or cyproterone acetate was used as second-line therapy with only limited success. The concept of complete androgen blockade was introduced by Labrie [37] and with the advent of both luteinizing hormone–releasing hormone (LHRH) agonists (or orchiectomy) and dihydrotestosterone receptor blockers, the question could be studied. A randomized, double-blind study evaluating the combination of flutamide and leuprolide with the combination of leuprolide and placebo demonstrated a statistically significant superior progression-free and overall survival in favor of total androgen blockade, although the advantage was small. Because leuprolide and goserelin are LHRH agonists, initial stimulation of the pituitary-testis axis may cause a disease flare resulting in worsening symptoms, or in extremely rare isolated cases it may cause sudden death. We suggest the addition of flutamide to begin concomitantly with LHRH agonists to prevent disease flare.

A recent meta-analysis performed by the Prostate Cancer Trialists' Collaborative Group analyzed 5710 patients from 22 randomized trials. They were unable to show any benefit of complete androgen blockade compared with surgical or medical castration [38]. A subsequent meta-analysis study by Caubet and coworkers [39] evaluated nine randomized studies demonstrating an improvement in overall survival and an increase in time-to-progression for maximum androgen blockade compared with monotherapy (orchiectomy vs LHRH). Furthermore, this study suggested an advantage for nonsteroidal antiandrogens over steroidal antiandrogens. These studies continue the ongoing controversy regarding the most appropriate hormonal therapy for metastatic prostate cancer.

There has been a suggestion of survival advantage with hormone therapy in the VACURG study, which compared placebo with three different doses of diethylstilbestrol in the treatment of advanced disease. A retrospective analysis of patients treated according to the Eastern Cooperative Oncology Group prostate protocols suggested that continued androgen blockade despite progression of disease was associated with better survival.

The discovery of receptors for other growth factors, such as epidermal growth factor receptor (EGFr), provides a foundation for alternative treatment strategies. Suramin sodium is a polysulfonated naphthylurea used to treat African trypanosomiasis and onchocerciasis and has been found to bind the EGFr and block growth. In addition, suramin has been shown to decrease circulating androstenedione, dihydroepiandrosterone, and dihydroepiandrosterone sulfate by 40% in patients with metastatic prostate cancer in whom previous hormone therapy had failed. In vitro, suramin can block the proliferation of prostate cancer cells as well as inhibit testosterone and fibroblast growth factor–induced proliferation. Pilot studies of this agent in hormonal-refractory patients have reported a response rate as high as 54% and suggest that suramin may be useful in the treatment of metastatic prostate cancer. Current trials used the observation of nonandrogen autocrine and paracrine growth factors as a rationale to test the combination of LHRH analogue, dihydrotestosterone receptor blockade, and EGFr blockade.

Finasteride, a 5-α-reductase, has been found to have moderate effects in patients with metastatic prostate carcinoma [40]. In a pilot study of 10 men with either stage C or D disease, the combination of finasteride and flutamide caused a significant decrease in prostate-specific antigen. Eighty percent of the men remained potent, however, suggesting that this combination of hormone therapy may provide clinical benefit while allowing the patient to maintain potency [41].

Single-agent chemotherapy has had little effect on the outcome of prostate cancer. Studies of doxorubicin, mitoxantrone, cisplatin, cyclophosphamide, methotrexate, estramustine, and 5-fluorouracil have demonstrated minimal single-agent activity, and combination chemotherapies have had no impact on this disease. The observation that estramustine inhibits mitosis through disrupting microtubules lead to a series of combination chemotherapies with excellent tolerance and activity in metastatic prostate cancer patients. Vinblastine (4 mg/m^2 IV weekly × 6 wk) and estramustine (600 mg/m^2 PO daily × 6 wk) gave a 30% response rate with improvement in symptoms [42]. Other combinations have included oral etoposide (50

mg/m^2/d) and estramustine (15 mg/kg/d) for 3 weeks. This combination produced a 53% response rate and was a well-tolerated regimen [43]. Most recently, paclitaxel (120 mg/m^2 over 96-h continuous infusion) with estramustine (600 mg/m^2 daily) caused a 53% response rate but with greater than grade 2 toxicity in approximately one third of patients [44]. Thus, it appears that estramustine-based combination therapies have a beneficial effect in patients with hormone-refractory prostate cancer.

One of the most devastating complications for prostate cancer is the pain and dysfunction from bone metastases. External beam irradiation is useful in palliating isolated bone metastases. Unfortunately, patients with metastatic prostate cancer usually have multiple bone metastases. Two new approaches to the treatment of bone disease using radiation include hemibody irradiation and the use of bone-seeking compounds such as ^{89}Sr or ^{186}Re-hydroxyethylidene diphosphonate. Phase I and II studies of hemibody irradiation explored doses from 6 to 10 Gy and found the most effective dose for pain control to be 6 Gy for the upper body and 8 Gy for the mid and lower body. Delay in progression of bone metastases and a delay in the appearance of new disease within the field of hemibody irradiation have been seen in patients with breast and prostate cancer. Toxicities included hematologic effects, nausea, vomiting, diarrhea, anorexia, xerostomia, and loss of taste.

^{89}Sr is a pure β-emitting radionuclide that follows the calcium metabolic pathways. The use of ^{89}Sr to treat malignant disease was first reported by Lawrence and colleagues, in 1950, for multiple myeloma. Robinson and colleagues [45] have reported palliative benefit in patients with osseous prostate cancer metastases. Porter and McEwan [46] confirmed the palliative nature of ^{89}Sr at 30 to 60 mCi/kg, a dose that does not result in toxicities.

Samarium-153 EDTMP (ethylenediaminetetramethylenephosphonic acid) is a new radiopharmaceutical bone-seeking agent that has been reported to cause significant improvement in bone pain from metastasis [47].

TRANSITIONAL CELL CARCINOMA OF THE UROTHELIUM

ETIOLOGY AND RISK FACTORS

There are three major histologic types of cancers that arise from the urothelium. Squamous cell and adenocarcinomas of the bladder present a different clinical and therapeutic problem and are not discussed here.

The major risk factor for transitional cell carcinoma remains tobacco use, particularly in association with a slow acetylator phenotype and exposure to β-naphthylamine (Table 14-9). Although dietary factors have been implicated in bladder cancer formation, there is no definitive evidence to date. Animal studies suggested that saccharin consumption is associated with the development of bladder tumors in the rat, but recent metaanalyses do not implicate this substance in bladder tumor formation in humans. Chlorine has been implicated in the carcinogenesis of bladder cancer. Metaanalysis has confirmed that the consumption of higher chlorinated water (chlorination by-products) is associated with a 1.21 relative risk for bladder cancer.

Screening tests for bladder cancer have not yet been developed fully. Preliminary results from the Drake Health Registry suggest that in high-risk people exposed to β-naphthylamine, screening with Papanicolaou cytology, fluorescence image analysis, measurement of urinary nuclear

Table 14-9. Risk Factors for Transitional Cell Carcinoma

ß-Napthylamine
Tobacco [47]
Slow acetylator phenotype [48]
Chlorination by-products [49]
Diet (questionable) [50–52]
   High caloric intake from fat in those < 65 y
   Decrease risk with consumption of carotenoid in those < 65 y
   High sodium intake

Table 14-10. Staging of Transitional Cell Carcinoma of Urinary Badder

Stage*	TNM Staging	Criteria
0	Tis	Carcinoma in situ
	Ta	Noninvasive papillary cancer
	N0	
	M0	
I (A)	T1	Invasion of subepithelial connective tissue
	N0	
	M0	
II (B1)	T2	Invasion of muscle not extending beyond the inner half
	N0	
	M0	
III (B2)	T3a	Invasion of deep muscle — outer half of the bladder wall
	T3b	Invasion of perivesical fat
	N0	
	M0	
IV (C)	T4	Invasion of neighboring anatomical structures: prostate, uterus, vagina, pelvic wall, abdominal wall
	N0	
	M0	
or		
(D)	Any T	
	N1	Metastasis to a single lymph node ≤ 2 cm
	N2	Metastasis to a single lymph node 2–5 cm in size or multiple lymph nodes < 5 cm in diameter
	N3	Metastasis in any lymph node > 5 cm in diameter
	M0	
or		
	Any T	
	Any N	
	M1	Distant metastasis

*American Urological Association staging in parentheses.

native proteins, and urinalysis may be capable of identifying early changes, although the specificity of these changes is uncertain.

STAGING AND PROGNOSIS

Transitional cell carcinoma of the bladder may be distinguished according to whether the tumor is superficial or invasive. Superficial tumors of the bladder represent local disease with little or no capability for metastasis and thus can be treated with local therapies. Histologic grading, tumor type (papillary or carcinoma in situ), muscle invasion, and differentiation are important clinicopathologic features that should be evaluated (Table 14-10).

Recurrence of superficial tumors (stage 0 or stage 1) and the need for intravesical therapy are determined by grade, tumor size, and whether there are multiple tumors [53–55]. True squamous differentiation in the tumor usually predicts for poor response to systemic chemotherapy.

Many genetic markers are being studied as indicators for progression of superficial tumors, EGFr, p53, pRB, c-*erb*-2, nuclear matrix, metalloproteinases, and E cadherin. Nuclear accumulation of p53 has been associated with tumor recurrences and tumor progression in transitional cell carcinoma of the bladder. A multivariable analysis of grade pathologic stage, lymph node status, and nuclear p53 status confirmed p53 overexpression as an independent predictor [56]. A recent study by Lacombe and coworkers [57] analyzed 196 tissue specimens from 98 patients (before and after treatment with intravesical Bacille Calmette–Guérin [BCG]) for mutant nuclear p53 overexpression using immunohistochemistry and the relative risk of disease progression in patients with > 20% expression of p53 in pretreatment samples. Although p53 expression could not predict response to BCG in patients who did not respond, it was strongly predictive of disease progression. Thus, patients with refractory tumors and mutant p53 overexpression should be considered candidates for cystectomy.

PRIMARY DISEASE THERAPY

Most uroepithelial tumors present with either gross or microscopic hematuria. Urinary cytology is an important part of the evaluation. Full assessment of the uroepithelium is indicated and is accomplished with cystoscopy and IV or retrograde pyelography. Transurethral resection of the bladder tumor (TURBT) is the initial treatment. Intravesical therapy is usually considered for high-grade tumors, carcinoma in situ, or recurrent low-grade tumors. Recent genetic evaluation of multiple simultaneous tumors arising in women suggests a clonal origin and the probability that tumors arose from a

single cell that seeded other areas of uroepithelium. This process is well established in experimental animal models.

Treatment for superficial bladder cancers is directed not only at tumor regression but also at reduction of the subsequent recurrence rate and prevention of tumor invasion. TURBT alone, for low-grade papillary transitional cell carcinoma, or in combination with intravesical chemotherapy and immunotherapy can control local superficial tumor and prevent recurrences and invasion. Many therapeutic agents have been used in the treatment of superficial disease. BCG is considered the best of these agents, though it is not without associated morbidity.

Herr and coworkers [58] performed a 10-year follow-up of a prospective randomized control trial comparing TURBT alone versus TURBT and intravesical BCG. The median time to progression had not been reached in the BCG-treated group, and 10-year progression-free survival was 61.9% versus 38% in the TURBT-alone group. It should be noted that all patients who receive BCG experienced cystitis. A recent 15-year update of this group, which was recently published, found no significant differences with regard to overall progression rates and disease-specific survival [59]. In addition, there was a 31% incidence of upper tract tumors after a median of 7.3 years of follow-up. Although small in size (86 patients), this study demonstrates the necessity of close follow-up for extended periods, in spite of the initial advantage shown in the BCG-treated group.

Thiotepa, mitomycin C, and doxorubicin are the most common intravesical chemotherapies employed today and have been shown to be effective and safe agents. Burnand and colleagues [60] reported a randomized trial demonstrating that a single dose of thiotepa (90 mg over 30 min) can reduce recurrences by 40% at 1 year of follow-up compared with TURBT alone. Weekly thiotepa given for established superficial tumor can cause complete regression in approximately 30% of cases. The low molecular weight of thiotepa allows absorption across the bladder epithelium and may cause toxicity, specifically mild leukoneutropenia.

Mitomycin C appears to give the same clinical results as thiotepa, with less risk of leukoneutropenia but with increased risk for bladder irritation. Among intravesical chemotherapy agents, doxorubicin appears to give the best response rates in patients with established tumors, with a CR rate as high as 66%.

A randomized study of 262 patients with stage Ta and T1 papillary tumors or carcinoma in situ treated with either doxorubicin or BCG was reported by Lamm and colleagues [61]. Estimated 5-year disease-free survival was 17% for the doxorubicin-treated patients and 37% for BCG-treated patients with Ta or T1 lesions without carcinoma in situ (P=0.015). The median time to treatment failure in patients with carcinoma in situ was 5.1 months for doxorubicin and 39 months for BCG. Estimated 5-year disease-free survival in patients with carcinoma in situ was 18% for doxorubicin and 45% for BCG.

In a randomized prospective trial of 337 patients with high-risk superficial bladder tumors, Krege and coworkers [62] compared TURBT alone versus resection with BCG or resection with mitomycin-C. All patients underwent complete resection before starting intravesical therapy. Both groups treated with intravesical therapy had a lower relative risk of recurrence. Although there was no significant difference in the rates of progression between the two treatment groups, mitomycin-C demonstrated an initial modest advantage in patients with recurrent tumors. Side effects were more common with BCG. Thus, it seems reasonable to consider mitomycin-C intravesical therapy, especially in the context of recurrence. Other forms of intravesical immunotherapy, specifically interferon α, appear to have benefits in superficial bladder cancer as well. We have conducted pilot studies of intravesical tumor necrosis factor. Although this agent can be given with a high degree of safety, clinical benefit has not yet been proven.

Phototherapy for superficial bladder tumors is an alternative treatment but has not been tested against standard agents. Phototherapy employs laser treatments with photosensitizing agents, such as photofrin polyporphyrin. This approach is under investigation in refractory superficial tumors.

ADJUVANT THERAPY FOR REGIONAL DISEASE

The current standard therapy for locally invasive transitional cell carcinoma of the bladder remains cystectomy. The patient's risk of relapse depends on the depth of invasion into the wall of the bladder. Overall, there is a 40% to 60% chance of failure from cystectomy alone, raising the question of the need and effectiveness of adjuvant therapies. New pathologic techniques are becoming available to help distinguish metastatic potential of invasive bladder cancers, which include measurements of p53, NM23 RNA levels, DNA ploidy, and expression of the antigen T138 on the cell surface. Much recent work has been published regarding the use of concomitant chemotherapy

with radiation and TURBT as a means of providing effective local and systemic therapy while preserving an intact bladder. Primary radiation therapy has a 5-year survival of 20% to 40% and results in dismal local control [63]. Based on in vitro data, the National Cancer Institute of Canada tested cisplatin plus radiation versus radiation alone in a randomized clinical trail [64]. Patients randomized to the chemotherapy group got three cycles of concomitant cisplatin at 100 mg/m² every 21 days with their radiation. There was no significant differences between the groups with regard to response, overall survival or progression-free survival, but there was significantly better local control with concomitant cisplatin and a trend toward better bladder preservation.

The role of radiotherapy combined with multiagent chemotherapy has been explored by Kaufman and coworkers [65]. A pilot study of 53 patients demonstrated a 77% survival rate at 54 months [66]. Pilot data from a protocol of complete transurethral resection, and outpatient multidrug chemotherapy followed by a short course of high-dose split-fraction radiotherapy, has shown similar excellent results with a 70% CR rate [67]. A phase I/II SWOG study demonstrated that combination TURBT systemic therapy (methotrexate, vinblastine, cisplatin) and pelvic radiation (with concurrent cisplatin) could result in a combined CR of 56% (19 of 34 patients in this series). Complete response and improved survival with this protocol was associated with minimally invasive disease (T2 > T3,4), lack of nodal involvement, complete resection at TURBT, and completion with as much planned chemotherapy as possible. However, local control was suboptimal in this trail with 11 of 19 complete responders experiencing local recurrence. Toxicity was acceptable.

The RTOG reported a phase II trial evaluation bladder preservation for invasive disease, using two cycles of MCV after incomplete resection followed by concomitant radiation and cisplatin in 91 patients [68]. Patients not entering a complete remission went to immediate cystectomy. If CR was achieved, the patient received a third cycle of cisplatin with consolidating radiation. The CR rate was 80% in this study, with an actuarial 4-year survival of 62% and an actuarial survival at 4 years of 44% with the bladder intact. Cystectomy ultimately was required in 40% (37 of 91). Toxicity was high, however, with 12% rate of leukopenia and 16 cases of severe delayed toxicity.

Finally, a group at MGH published a trial of 106 patients treated with as complete a TURBT as possible followed by the aforementioned RTOG regimen [69]. Only if the patients achieved T0 status, as in the RTOG trial, could they go on to cisplatin plus radiotherapy instead of cystectomy. The CR rate was 66%, and the 5-year actuarial survival was 52%, with 43% surviving with intact bladders. The 5-year freedom from invasive bladder recurrence was 79%. The survival figures were inversely proportional to stage with clinical T2 disease faring the best. In patients with T3 to T4 disease, the presence of hydronephrosis at study predicted poorer outcome. Toxicity, as in the RTOG trial, was substantial, with significant incidences of leukopenia and gastrointestinal toxicities.

Although large multicenter phase III trials remain to answer the questions regarding the ultimate utility of these combined-modality bladder-preserving approaches, it seems reasonable to offer this approach to patients unable or unwilling to undergo cystectomy. Common features of success from the above trials include resection of as much visible tumor as possible, completion of as much MCV as possible (given the toxicity), early stage (ie, T2), and lack of hydronephrosis. Should the patient not experience a CR, reconsideration of cystectomy is mandated. Although theoretical concerns regarding surgery after chemoradiation rationally exist, there are not current studies that demonstrate an increased complication rate [68], and none were reported in the above trials.

The role of adjuvant or neoadjuvant chemotherapy has not been definitively proven at this time, but preliminary reports of randomized trials suggest that cisplatin-based multiagent chemotherapy may have a significant impact on the treatment of high-risk invasive bladder cancer. Stockle and coworkers [70] reported a study of 49 patients with pathologically staged T3b and T4a bladder cancer with or without lymph node involvement randomized to receive methotrexate, vinblastine (or epirubicin), doxorubicin, and cisplatin following cystectomy or cystectomy alone. Although time of follow-up is limited, only three of 18 patients treated with adjuvant chemotherapy have relapsed compared to 18 of 23 patients in the control arm. Freiha and coworkers [71] conducted a randomized control trial comparing radical cystectomy alone to radical cystectomy followed by four cycles of MCV-like chemotherapy in patients with pT3b or pT4 disease with or without nodal involvement. Twenty-five patients from each group were evaluable at 5 years. Of note, patients in the observation group received MCV therapy at first sign of recurrence. The recurrence rate in the adjuvant group was 48% (12 of 25 patients) versus 76% in the observation group. Although there was significant freedom from progression in the chemotherapy group, there was no difference in overall survival. The authors contributed the latter finding to the crossover allowed in the design, indicating the benefit from chemotherapy could be seen with delayed treatment as well. Trials involving neoadjuvant multiagent cisplatin-based chemotherapy have not been complete as of this time. Preliminary data suggest that major pathologic responses of the primary tumor to chemotherapy is seen in approximately 40% of patients [74–76]. These patients have a much-improved survival compared to those patients who did not achieve a response to treatment prior to cystectomy.

CHEMOTHERAPY FOR ADVANCED DISEASE

Advances in chemotherapy have been sought in the setting of metastatic transitional cell carcinoma of the urinary bladder. Phase II studies of single agents demonstrated significant activity (> 15%) for methotrexate, vinblastine, doxorubicin, cisplatin, and 5-fluorouracil. Until quite recently, cisplatin had been the single best agent and is currently the cornerstone of combination chemotherapy regimens. The most commonly used combinations today are M-VAC and MCV. Although response rates to M-VAC were significantly lower than those reported in single-institution studies (33% vs 60%), M-VAC was found to be superior to cisplatin alone (objective response rates of 33% vs 15%, respectively; P=0.001) in a randomized trial evaluating the treatment of metastatic bladder cancer conducted by the Eastern Cooperative Oncology Group [75].

Concerns regarding the toxicity of cisplatin, especially in patients with baseline renal insufficiency, have led a number of investigators to explore the efficacy of carboplatin-based regimens. Based on phase II trials illustrating equivalent results with carboplatin and carboplatin-based therapies, Bellmunt and coworkers [70] published a randomized control trial comparing standard MVAC with the carboplatin-based regimen M-CAVI (methotrexate, carboplatin at dose AUC of 5, and vinblastine). This study was prematurely stopped when it was clear that MVAC had a clear survival advantage over M-CAVI. Response rates favored MVAC as well, but this was not significant (52% vs 39%, respectively, with 3 CRs in the MVAC

arm). Toxicity, however, was clearly more frequent with MVAC. Given the favorable toxicity of M-CAVI, it is possible that an AUC of 5 was inadequate. The absence of doxorubicin could have also played a role in the observed differences. More trials are anticipated.

In an attempt to improve the toxicity profile on M-VAC, colony-stimulating factors have been employed. Although granulocyte colony-stimulating factor and granulocyte-macrophage colony-stimulating factor can reduce the length of leukoneutropenia and improve mucositis, response and survival rates have not differed significantly.

Nevertheless, the search for more active agents has proceeded. A phase II trial published by ECOG studied the activity of paclitaxel (a novel agent that blocks depolymerization of microtubules) in patients with previously untreated advanced transitional cell carcinoma of the bladder [77]. Twenty-six patients were treated with paclitaxel 250 mg/m^2 by 24-hour continuous infusion and granulocyte–macrophage colony-stimulating hormone support every 21 days until disease progression or intolerance. Forty-two percent of these patients demonstrated a response (11 of 26) with seven of 26 patients obtaining CR (27%), making paclitaxel the most active single-agent against transitional cell carcinoma of the bladder studied thus far. Patients with visceral metastases had fewer responses than those with soft tissue or lymph node metastases. Toxicity was acceptable, with median number of four cycles completed (eight for those who respond). Twenty-three percent of patients developed grade 3 neutropenia, but only two had febrile neutropenia. Only two patients stopped treatment because of neuropathy, and the rest stopped because of malaise and fatigue. The estimated median survival of the group was 8.4 months with a projected 1-year survival of 37%. Furthermore, paclitaxel retains activity in patients with renal insufficiency without additional renal toxicity [78]. Given its high rate of activity, it seems reasonable to choose paclitaxel alone or in combination with carboplatin in patients with renal insufficiency or who have relapsed or proven refractory to MVAC. Further recommendations will depend on the results of future trials examining the use of paclitaxel and paclitaxel-based regimens.

RENAL CELL CARCINOMA

ETIOLOGY AND RISK FACTORS

In 1995, approximately 32,000 people in the United States were diagnosed with renal cell carcinoma (RCC) and nearly 50% of them had metastatic disease at presentation. Although there are reports of long-term survivors with metastatic disease, the 5-year survival curves predict that virtually all patients will die from their disease by that time. Radical nephrectomy for local disease remains the only curative approach. Investigation of systemic therapies for RCC has provided insights into new treatment methods that may affect survival of a subset of patients.

Molecular genetic evaluation has provided greater insight into the nature of RCC. The most common chromosomal abnormality has been the loss of heterozygosity of 3p14-26, which is found in 66% to 98% of clear cell RCC tumors. Papillary tumors do not appear to have this abnormality. Patients with Hippel-Lindau disease have similar loss of heterozygosity of 3p. Further molecular genetic studies may uncover markers for metastatic behavior [79].

There has been a causative relationship between tobacco use and the development of RCC. Beyond this major risk factor, obesity, analgesic abuse, and asbestos exposure have been linked with the development of RCC (Table 14-11). The use of Thorotrast as a contrast medium in the early part of this century to visualize the kidney and liver has also been linked to the development of RCC. Other risk factors include acquired cystic disease of the kidney and end-stage renal failure.

STAGING AND PROGNOSIS

Staging is presented in Table 14-12. Many prognostic schema have been used to attempt to predict survival and outcome (Table 15-13). The sarcomatoid variant of RCC tends to have a worse prognosis, with median survival of less than 1 year. Performance status, disease-free survival greater than 1 year (or in some schema > 2 y), number of sites of metastases (one vs more than one), and the presence of central nervous system metastases are common prognostic factors in most schema.

PRIMARY DISEASE THERAPY

A radical nephrectomy may be performed from a number of different approaches and includes complete resection of Gerota's fascia, kidney, and adrenal gland. The role of regional lymph node dissection remains unknown. Although no definitive proof exists that lymph node dissection will prolong survival, in the context of adjuvant therapy trials it is imperative that staging is accurately assessed. In the usual lymph node dissection, the ipsilateral nodes from the diaphragm to the origin of the common iliac arteries and the renal hilar lymph nodes are removed. Kidney-sparing operations are being performed that include partial nephrectomy and excisional resection of the tumor. Although reports of these less radical procedures appear good, a number of pathologic series suggest that renal cell tumors may be multicentric. Partial nephrectomies should be considered in patients in whom preservation of renal function is an important goal of therapy, including patients with Hippel-Lindau disease or unilateral kidney.

Radiation therapy for RCC has been directed at the palliation of metastatic sites, specifically, bone, spine, and brain. Stereotactic radiation or gamma knife therapy may be useful in conjunction with whole-brain radiation for palliation of single brain metastases of 2 cm or less. Initial reports on this modality suggest high sterilization rates. There is no clear evidence to date that adjuvant radiotherapy to the bed of the kidney improves survival, and we do not routinely give adjuvant radiation therapy to patients who have had a nephrectomy.

ADVANCED DISEASE THERAPY

Treatment of metastatic disease remains difficult. Biologic response modifiers have had the most impact on treatment of metastatic disease. High-dose interleukin-2 recently was approved by the United States Food and Drug Administration for the treatment of this condition.

Common toxic effects to interleukin-2 (> 50%) in patients treated with high doses include chills, pruritus, nausea, vomiting, diarrhea, hyperbilirubinemia, oliguria with increase in blood urea nitrogen and creatinine, weight gain, edema, hypotension, and lymphopenia with eosinophilia. Respiratory distress with pulmonary edema secondary to leaky capillary syndrome, bron-

Table 14-11. Risk Factors for Renal Cell Carcinoma

Genetic [75,80]
    von Hippel—Lindau disease
    Familial RCC
Acquired traits
    Cystic kidney disease
    End-stage renal failure requiring dialysis
Environmental factors [81–83]
    Tobacco use
    Asbestos exposure
    Analgesic abuse (phenactin)
    Obesity
    Thorotrast

Table 14-12. Staging of Renal Cell Carcinoma

Stage*	TNM Staging	Criteria
I (A)	T1	Limited to the kidney, ≤ 2.5 cm, surrounded by normal renal parenchyma
	N0	
	M0	
II (A)	T2	Tumor > 2.5 cm, limited to the kidney
	N0	
	M0	
III (C)	T1	Metastasis to a single lymph node ≤ 2 cm
	N1	
	M0	
or		
(C)	T2	Metastasis to a single lymph node 2–5 cm or multiple lymph nodes < 5 cm
	N2	
	M0	
or		
(B)	T3a	Tumor involving perinephric fat
	T3b	Tumor involving renal vein
	T3c	Involvement of infradiaphragmatic vena cava
	N0	
	M0	
or		
(C)	T3a	Tumor involving perinephric fat
	T3b	Tumor involving renal vein
	T3c	Involvement of infradiaphragmatic vena cava
	N1	
	M0	
or		
IV (D)	T4a	Tumor invasion beyond Gerota's fascia into surrounding organs
	T4b	Tumor involving supradiaphragmatic vena cava
	Any N	
	M0	
or		
	Any T	
	N2 or N3	Metastasis to a lymph node > 5 cm
	M0	
or		
	Any T	
	Any N	
	M1	Distant metastases

Robson staging in parentheses.

chospasm, pleural effusion, somnolence, disorientation, anemia, thrombocytopenia, hypothyroidism, and arrhythmias is seen in 10% to 50% of patients. Rare toxic effects include myocardial infarction, central line sepsis, severe hypotension, renal failure, and death. In centers that have experience with high-dose interleukin-2, much of the toxicity can be managed with noninvasive monitoring and fluid replacement, antibiotics, H-2 blockers, antiemetics, and antihistamines. Awareness of early warning signals, such as slight change in mental status and skipping one or two doses, has improved the overall toxicity profile of high-dose interleukin-2. Blood pressure support is maintained with fluid replacement and adrenergic agonists, such as dopamine and norepinephrine. Rarely, intubation and mechanical ventilatory support are required. The interleukin-2 dose is held until the patient has cardiopulmonary stabilization. Usually this requires skipping a dose or two over the course of 1 week.

Although response rates to high-dose interleukin-2, alone or with adoptively transferred lymphokine-activated killer cells, vary from 4% to 35%, the duration of the response in those achieving a complete remission is significantly long. There was no difference in overall survival in patients with metastatic RCC treated in a randomized study of high-dose interleukin-2 with and without lymphokine-activated killer cells [85]. Objective clinical responses using high-dose interleukin-2 in the treatment of metastatic RCC have been reported to occur in 4% to 35% of cases. The summary of 255 patients treated with high-dose interleukin-2 reported to the Food and Drug Administration that established interleukin-2 as a treatment for metastatic RCC demonstrated an overall response rate of 14%. Approximately one third of responses are complete and patients usually maintain their response for about 2 years.

Although preliminary studies using lower doses of interleukin-2 were discouraging, a more recent randomized study of high-dose interleukin-2 versus a log lower dose of IV interleukin-2 (72,000 IU/kg) given on the same schedule found similar overall response rates: 7% CR, and 8% PR for low-dose interleukin-2 versus 3% CR and 17% PR for high-dose interleukin-2 [86].

Trials employing interferon α suggest a response rate from 10% to 20%. Initial studies employing Cantell preparations of human leukocyte interferon reported by Quesada and colleagues [87] and Kirkwood and colleagues [88] suggested a clinical role for interferon α. These studies were limited by availability and specific activity of the material. Subsequent trials of recombinant

DNA–produced interferon α and lymphoblastoid interferon α have confirmed activity of this cytokine in metastatic RCC, with response rates of 18%.

Flu-like symptoms are the most common acute toxicity to the interferons and are seen in virtually 100% of patients. Flu-like symptoms begin about 1 to 2 hours following a dose of interferon α and include fever, chill or rigor, myalgias, low backache, arthralgias, headache, and malaise. Gastrointestinal symptoms such as nausea, vomiting, and diarrhea are rare. Acetaminophen pretreatment usually blunts the flu-like symptoms of interferon α. Tachyphylaxis of the flu-like symptoms occurs with repetitive doses. Chronically, patients may have low-grade fever and with the decrease in appetite associated with interferon α develop subclinical dehydration, which contributes to the malaise. We recommend vigorous fluid intake by mouth to improve the tolerance to the agent. Occasionally, IV hydration on an outpatient basis may be warranted.

Central nervous system toxicity includes slight confusion, minimal paranoia, stupor, and coma and is associated with diffuse slowing on the electroencephalogram. These effects are reversible, but stupor and coma may take as long as 3 to 4 weeks to resolve. Peripheral neuropathy is also uncommon and is associated with the typical hand-glove paresthesias with slowing of nerve conduction.

Cardiovascular toxicity is usually characterized by supraventricular tachyarrhythmias, which may be controlled with β blockers or calcium channel blockers. Cardiac toxicity is usually seen at dosages of over 10 mU/day, in older patients (> 70 y), and in patients with underlying heart disease.

Mild elevation in transaminases occurs in patients treated with interferon α and clinical hepatitis rarely is seen. Elevation in bilirubin is unusual and should make the clinician search for another cause. Elevations in transaminases rarely are associated with liver pain.

Common hematologic abnormalities seen in patients treated with interferon α are characterized by leukoneutropenia with a cellular marrow. Systemic infections are rare. Thrombocytopenia occasionally occurs.

Renal abnormalities include increase in protein excretion and the development of partially reversible nephrotic syndrome and renal failure. Metabolic abnormalities associated with high-dose interferon α treatment are unusual and include hypocalcemia, hyperkalemia, and hypoalbunemia. Prognostic features of responding patients have been identified, including tumor burden and performance status.

At present, interferon α is a reasonable alternative for treatment in patients with metastatic renal cell carcinoma. We recommend subcutaneous treatment with 3 mU/m² three times weekly, and dose escalation to 10 mU/m² three times weekly as tolerated. We continue treatment for a minimum 2 to 3 months when possible. Patients with non–life-threatening minimal progression of disease, stable disease, or evidence of response during the first 2 to 3 months continue on treatment for up to 1 year.

Although preliminary studies of combination interferon-α and interleukin-2 have been encouraging, a randomized study of the combination versus high-dose interleukin-2 alone failed to demonstrate any benefit from the addition of interferon α [89].

Table 14-13. Prognostic Factors in Renal Cell Carcinoma

Histology (sarcomatoid variant)
Performance status
Disease-free survival
Central nervous system disease
Number of metastatic sites

From Palmer and coworkers [84]; with permission.

REFERENCES

1. Sladden M, Dickinson J: Testicular cancer: how effective is screening? *Aust Fam Physician* 1993, 22:1350–1356.

2. Dieckmann KP, Klan R, Bunte S: HLA antigens, Lewis antigens, and blood groups in patients with testicular germ-cell tumors. *Oncol J Clin Exp Cancer Res* 1993, 50:252–258.

3. Pinczowski D, McLaughlin JK, Lackgren G, *et al.*: Occurrence of testicular cancer in patients operated on for cryptorchidism and inguinal hernia. *J Urol* 1991, 146:1291–1294.

4. Marselos M, Tomatis L: Diethylstilbestrol: I. Pharmacology, toxicology and carcinogenicity in humans. *Eur J Cancer* 1992, 28A:1182–1189.

5. Prener A, Hsieh CC, Engholm G, *et al.*: Birth order and risk of testicular cancer. *Cancer Causes Control* 1992, 3:265–272.

6. Zhang Z, Vena JER, Zielezny M, *et al.*: Occupational exposure to extreme temperature and risk of testicular cancer. *Arch Environ Health* 1995, 50:13–18.

7. Klepp O, Olsson AM, Henrikson H, *et al.*: Prognostic factors in clinical stage I nonseminomatous germ cell tumors of the testis: multivariate analysis of a prospective multicenter study. Swedish-Norwegian Testicular Cancer Group. *J Clin Oncol* 1990, 8:509–518.

8. Birch R, Williams S, Cone A, *et al.*: Southeastern Cancer Group: prognostic factors for favorable outcome in disseminated germ cell tumors. *J Clin Oncol* 1986, 4:400–407.

9. Aass N, Klepp O, Cavallin-Stahl E, *et al.*: Prognostic factors in unselected patients with nonseminomatous metastatic testicular cancer: a multicenter experience. *J Clin Oncol* 1991, 9:818–826.

10. Sesterhenn IA, Weiss RB, Mostofi FK, *et al.*: Prognosis and other clinical correlates of pathologic review in stage I and II testicular carcinoma: a report from the Testicular Cancer Intergroup Study. *J Clin Oncol* 1992, 10:69–78.

11. Lerner SE, Mann BS, Blute ML, *et al.*: Primary chemotherapy for clinical stage II nonseminomatous germ cell testicular tumors: selection criteria and long-term results. *Mayo Clin Proc* 1995, 70:821–828.

12. Horwich A, Norman A, Fisher C, *et al.*: Primary chemotherapy for clinical stage II nonseminomatous germ cell tumors of the testis. *J Urol* 1994, 151:72–77.

13. Baniel J, Roth BJ, Foster RS, *et al.*: Cost and risk benefit in the management of clinical stage II nonseminomatous testicular tumors. *Cancer* 1995, 75:2897–29903.

14. Culine S, Theodore C, Terrier-Lacombe MJ, *et al.*: Primary chemotherapy in patients with nonseminomatous germ cell tumors of the testis and biological disease only after orchiectomy. *J Urol* 1996, 155:1296–1298.

15. Bajorin DF, Sarosdy MF, Pfister DG, *et al.*: Randomized trial of etoposide and cisplatin versus etoposide and carboplatin in patients with good-risk germ cell tumors: multi-institutional study. *J Clin Oncol* 1993, 11:598–606.

16. Loehrer PJ Sr, Johnson D, Elson P, *et al.*: Importance of bleomycin in favorable-prognosis disseminated germ cell tumors: an ECOG trial. *J Clin Oncol* 1995, 13:470–476.

17. Levi JA, Raghavan D, Harvey V, *et al.*: The importance of bleomycin in combination chemotherapy for good-prognosis germ cell carcinoma. *J Clin Oncol* 1993, 11:1300–1305.

18. McAleer JJ, Nicholls J, Horwich A: Does extragonadal presentation impart a worse prognosis to abdominal germ-cell tumors? *Eur J Cancer* 1992, 28A:825–828.

19. Bosl GJ, Motzer RJ: Testicular germ cell cancer [review]. *N Engl J Med* 1997, 337:242–253.

20. Broun Erm Nichols CR, Gize G, *et al.*: Tandem high-dose chemotherapy with autologous bone marrow transplantation for initial relapse of testicular germ cell cancer. *Cancer* 1997, 79:1605–1610.

21. Pienta KJ, Esper PS: Risk factors for prostate cancer. *Ann Intern Med* 1993, 118:793–803.

22. DerSimonian R, Clemens J, Spirtas R, Perlman J: Vasectomy and prostate cancer risk: methodological review of the evidence. *J Clin Epidemiol* 1993, 46:163–172.

23. Hankin JH, Zhao LP, Wilkens LR, Kolonel LN: Attributable risk of breast, prostate and lung cancer in Hawaii due to standard fat. *Cancer Causes Control* 1992, 3:17–23.

24. Ross RK, Bernstein L, Lobo RA, *et al.*: 5-Alpha-reductase activity and risk of prostate cancer among Japanese and US white and black males. *Lancet* 1992, 339:887–889.

25. Bacquet CR, Horm JW, Gibbs T, *et al.*: Socioeconomic factors and cancer incidence among blacks and whites. *J Natl Cancer Inst* 1991, 83:551–557.

26. Elghany NA, Schumacher MC, Slattery ML, *et al.*: Occupation, cadmium exposure, and prostate cancer. *Epidemiology* 1990, 1:107–115.

27. Fleming C, Wasson JH, Albertsen PC, et al.: A decision analysis of alternative treatment strategies for clinically localized prostate cancer. Prostate Patient Outcome Research Team. *JAMA* 1993, 269:2650–2658.

28. Lu-Yao GL, McLerran D, Wasson J, Wennberg JE: An assessment of radical prostatectomy: time trends, geographic variation, and outcomes. The Prostate Patient Outcome Research Team. *JAMA* 1993, 269:2633–2636.

29. Littrup PJ, Lee F, Mettlin C: Prostate cancer screening: current trends and future implications. *CA* 1992, 42:198–211.

30. Gerber GS, Thompson IM, Thisted R, Chodak GW: Disease-specific survival following routine prostate cancer screening by digital rectal examination. *JAMA* 1993, 269:61–64.

31. McCormack RT, Rittenhouse HG, Finlay J, *et al.*: Molecular forms of prostate specific antigen and the human kallikrein gene family: a new era. *Urology* 1995, 45:729–744.

32. Thompson IM, Zeidman EJ: Current urological practice: routine urological examination and early detection of carcinoma of the prostate. *J Urol* 1992, 148:326–329.

33. Cama C, Olsson CA, Raffo AJ, *et al.*: Molecular staging of prostatic cancer: II. Comparison of application of enhanced reverse transcriptase polymerase chain reaction assay for PSA versus prostate specific membrane antigen. *J Urol* 1995, 153:1373–1378.

34. Sgrignoli AR, Walsh PC, Steinberg GD, *et al.*: Prognostic factors in men with stage D1 prostate cancer: identification of patients less likely to have prolonged survival after radical prostatectomy. *J Urol* 1994, 152:1077–1081.

35. Paulson DF, Lin GH, Hinshaw W: Radical surgery versus radiotherapy for adenocarcinoma of the prostate. *J Urol* 1982, 128:502–504.

36. Bolla M, Gonzalez D, Warde P, *et al.*: Improved survival in patients with locally advanced prostate cancer treated with radiotherapy and goserelin. *N Engl J Med* 1997, 337:295–300.

37. Labrie F, Luthy I, Veilleux R, *et al.*: New concepts on the androgen sensitivity of prostate cancer. *Prog Clin Biol Res* 1987, 243:145–172.

38. Prostate Cancer Trialists' Collaborative Group: Maximum androgen blockade in advanced prostate cancer: an overview of 22 randomized trials with 3283 deaths in 5710 patients. *Lancet* 1995, 346:265–269.

39. Caubet JF, Tosteson TD, Dong EW, *et al.*: Maximum androgen blockade in advanced prostate cancer: a meta-analysis of published randomized controlled trails using nonsteroidal antiandrogens. *Uroloy* 1997, 49:71–78.

40. Presti JC Jr, Fair WR, Andriole G, *et al.*: Multicenter, randomized, double-blind, placebo controlled study to investigate the effect of finasteride (MK-906) on stage D prostate cancer. *J Urol* 1992, 148:1201–1204.

41. Fleshner NE, Trachtenberg J: Treatment of advanced prostate cancer with the combination of finasteride plus flutamide: early results. *Eur Urol* 1993, 24(suppl):106–112.

42. Hudes GR, Greenberg R, Krigel RL, *et al.*: Phase II study of estramustine and vinblastine, two microtubule inhibitors, in hormone-refractory prostate cancer. *J Clin Oncol* 1992, 10:1754–1761.

43. Pienta LJ, Redman BG, Bandekar R, *et al.*: A phase II trial of oral estramustine and oral etoposide in hormone refractory prostate cancer. *Urology* 1997, 50:401–406.

44. Hudes GR, Nathan F, Khater C, *et al.*: Phase II trial of 96-hour paclitaxel plus oral estramustine phosphate in metastatic hormone-refractory prostate cancer. *J Clin Oncol* 1997, 15:3156–3163.

45. Robinson RG, Preston DF, Baxter KG, *et al.*: Clinical experience with strontium-89 in prostatic and breast cancer patients. *Semin Oncol* 1993, 20(suppl):44–48.

46. Porter AT, McEwan AJ: Strontium-89 as an adjuvant to external beam radiation improves pain relief and delays disease progression in advanced prostate cancer: results of a randomized controlled trial. *Semin Oncol* 1993, 20(suppl):38–43.

47. Marsh GM, Callahan C, Pavlock D, *et al.*: A protocol for bladder cancer screening and medical surveillance among high-risk groups: the Drake Health Registry experience. *J Occup Med* 1990, 32:881–886.

48. Kadlubar FF, Butler MA, Kaderlik KR, *et al.*: Polymorphisms for aromatic amine metabolism in humans: relevance for human carcinogenesis. *Environ Health Perspect* 1992, 98:69–74.

49. Vineis P, Ronco G: Interindividual variation in carcinogen metabolism and bladder cancer risk. *EHP Environmental Health Perspectives* 1992, 98:95–99.

50. Morris RD, Audet AM, Angelillo IF, *et al.*: Chlorination, chlorination by-products, and cancer: a meta-analysis. *Am J Public Health* 1992, 82:955–963.

51. Vena JE, Graham S, Freudenheim J, *et al.*: Diet in the epidemiology of bladder cancer in western New York. *Nutrition Cancer* 1992, 18:255–264.

52. Elcock M, Morgan RW: Update on artificial sweeteners and bladder cancer. *Regul Toxicol Pharmacol* 1993, 17:35–43.

53. Mills PK, Beeson WL, Phillips RL, Fraser GE: Bladder cancer in a low risk population: results from the Adventist Health Study. *Am J Epidemiol* 1991, 133:230–239.

54. Kiemeney LA, Witjes JA, Verbeek AL, *et al.*: The clinical epidemiology of superficial bladder cancer. Dutch South-East Cooperative Urological Group. *Br J Cancer* 1993, 67:806–812.

55. Tachibana M, Deguchi N, Baba S, *et al.*: Prognostic significance of bromodeoxyuridine high labeled bladder cancer measured by flow cytometry: does flow cytometric determination predict the prognosis of patients with transitional cell carcinoma of the bladder? *J Urol* 1993, 149:739–743.

56. Esrig D, Elmajian D, Groshen S, *et al.*: Accumulation of nuclear p53 and tumor progression in bladder cancer. *N Engl J Med* 1994, 331:1259–1264.

57. Lacombe L, Dalbagni G, Zhang Z, *et al.*: Overexpression of p53 in a high-risk population of patients with superficial bladder cancer before and after Bacillus Calmette-Guerin therapy: correlation to clinical outcome. *J Clin Oncol* 1996, 14:2646–2652.

58. Herr HW, Schwalb BM, Zhang Z, *et al.*: Intravesical Bacillus Calmette-Guerin therapy prevents tumor progression and death from superficial bladder cancer: ten-year follow-up of a prospective randomized trial. *J Clin Oncol* 1995, 13:1404–1408.

59. Cookson MS, Herr HW, Zhang Z, *et al.*: The treated natural history of high-risk superficial bladder cancer: 15-year outcome. *J Urol* 1997, 158:62–67.

60. Burnand KG, Boyd PJ, Mayo ME, *et al.*: Single dose intravesical thiotepa as an adjuvant to cystodiathermy in the treatment of transitional cell bladder carcinoma. *Br J Urol* 1976, 48:55–59.

61. Lamm DL, Crissmann J, Blumenstein B, *et al.*: Adriamycin versus BCG in superficial bladder cancer: a Southwest Oncology Group Study. *Prog Clin Biol Res* 1989, 310:263–270.

62. Krege S, Giani G, Meyer R, *et al.*: A randomized multicenter trial of adjuvant therapy in superficial bladder cancer: transurethral resection only versus transurethral resection plus mitomycin-C versus transurethral resection plus Bacillus Calmette-Guerin. *J Urol* 1996, 156:962–966.

63. Einstein AB Jr, Wolf M, Halliday KR, *et al.*: Combination transurethral resection, systemic chemotherapy, and pelvic radiotherapy for invasive (T2-T4) bladder cancer unsuitable for cystectomy: a phase I/II SWOG study. *Urology* 1996, 47:652–657.

64. Coppin CM Gospodarowica MK, James K, *et al.*: Improved local control of invasive bladder cancer by concurrent cisplatin and preoperative or definitive radiation: the NCI Canada Trials Group. *J Clin Oncol* 1996, 14:2901–2907.

65. Kaufman DS, Shipley WU, Griffin PP, *et al.*: Selective bladder preservation by combination treatment of invasive bladder cancer [see comments]. *New Engl J Med* 1993, 329:1377–1382.

66. Shipley WU, Kaufman DS, Heney NM, *et al.*: The integration of chemotherapy, radiotherapy and transurethral surgery in bladder-sparing approaches for patients with invasive tumors. *Prog Clin Biol Res* 1990, 353:85–94.

67. Zietman AL, Shipley WU, Kaufman DS: The combination of *cis*-platin based chemotherapy and radiation in the treatment of muscle-invading transitional cell cancer of the bladder. *Int J Rad Oncol Biol Phys* 1993, 27:161–170.

68. Tester W, Caplan R, Heany J, *et al.*: Neoadjuvant combined modality program with selective organ preservation for invasive bladder cancer: results of RTOG phase II trial 8802. *J Clin Oncol* 1996, 14:119–126.

69. Kachnic LA, Kaufman DS, Heney NM, *et al.*: Bladder preservation by combined modality therapy for invasive bladder cancer. *J Clin Oncol* 1997, 15:1022–1029.

70. Stockle M, Meyenburg W, Wellek S, *et al* Advanced bladder cancer (stages pT3b, pT4a, pN1, pN2): improved survival after radical cystectomy and 3 adjuvant cycles of chemotherapy. Results of a controlled prospective study. *J Urol* 1992, 148:302–306.

71. Freiha F, Reese J, Torti FM: A randomized trial of radical cystectomy versus radical cystectomy plus cisplatin, vinblastine, and methotrexate chemotherapy for muscle invasive bladder cancer. *J Urol* 1996, 155:495–499.

72. Splinter TA, Scher HI, Denis L, *et al.*: The prognostic value of the pathological response to combination chemotherapy before cystectomy in patients with invasive bladder cancer. European Organization for Research on Treatment of Cancer—Genitourinary Group. *J Urol* 1992, 147:606–608.

73. Wallace DM, Raghavan D, Kelly KA, *et al.*: Neo-adjuvant (pre-emptive) cisplatin therapy in invasive transitional cell carcinoma of the bladder. *Br J Urol* 1991, 67:608–615.

74. Skinner DG, Daniels JR, Russell CA, *et al.*: The role of adjuvant chemotherapy following cystectomy for invasive bladder cancer: a prospective comparative trial. *J Urol* 1991, 245:459–464; discussion 464–467.

75. Loehrer PJ Sr, Einhorn LH, Elson PJ, *et al.*: A randomized comparison of cisplatin alone or in combination with methotrexate, vinblastine, and doxorubicin in patients with metastatic urothelial carcinoma: a cooperative group study. *J Clin Oncol* 1992, 10:1066–1073.

76. Bellmunt J, Ribas A, Eres N, *et al.*: Carboplatin-based versus cisplatin-based chemotherapy in the treatment of surgically incurable advanced bladder carcinoma. *Cancer* 1997, 80:1966–1975.

77. Roth BJ, Dreicer R, Einhorn LH, *et al.*: Significant activity of paclitaxel in advanced transitional cell carcinoma of the urothelium: a phase II trial of the ECOG. *J Clin Oncol* 1994, 12:2264–2270.

78. Dreicer R, Gustin DM, See WA, *et al.*: Paclitaxel in advanced urothelial carcinoma: its role in patients with renal insufficiency and as salvage therapy. *J Urol* 1996, 156:1606–1608.

79. McCredie M, Stewart JH: Risk factors for kidney cancer in New South Wales: IV. Occupation. *J Indust Med* 1993, 50:349–354.

80. van der Hout AH, van den Berg E, van der Vlies P, *et al.*: Loss of heterozygosity at the short arm of chromosome 3 in renal-cell cancer correlates with the cytological tumor type. *Int J Cancer* 1993, 53:353–357.

81. McCredie M, Stewart JH, Day NE: Different roles for phenacetin and paracetamol in cancer of the kidney and renal pelvis. *Int J Cancer* 1993, 53:245–249.

82. McCredie M, Stewart JH: Risk factors for kidney cancer in New South Wales—I. Cigarette smoking. *Eur J Cancer* 1992, 28A:2050–2054.

83. La Vecchia C, Negri E, D'Avanzo B, Franceschi S: Smoking and renal cell carcinoma. *Cancer Res* 1990, 50:5231–5233.

84. Palmer PA, Vinke J, Philip T, *et al.*: Prognostic factors for survival in patients with advanced renal cell carcinoma treated with recombinant interleukin-2. *Ann Oncol* 1992, 3:475–480.

85. Rosenberg SA, Lotze MT, Yang JC, *et al.*: Prospective randomized trial of high-dose interleukin-2 alone or in conjunction with lymphokine-activated killer cells for the treatment of patients with advanced cancer. *J Nat Cancer Inst* 1993, 85:622–632.

86. Yang JC, Topalian SL, Parkinson D, *et al.*: Randomized comparison of high-dose and low-dose intravenous interleukin-2 for the therapy of metastatic renal cell carcinoma: an interim report. *J Clin Oncol* 1994, 12:1572–1576.

87. Quesada JR, Swanson DA, Gutterman JU: Phase II study of interferon alpha in metastatic renal cell carcinoma: a progress report. *J Clin Oncol* 1985, 3:1086–1092.

88. Kirkwood JM, Harris JE, Vera R, *et al.*: A randomized study of low and high doses of leukocyte alpha-interferon in metastatic renal cell carcinoma: the American Cancer Society Collaborative Trial. *Cancer Res* 1985, 45:863–871.

89. Atkins MB, Sparano J, Fisher RI, *et al.*: Randomized phase II trial of high-dose interleukin-2 either alone or in combination with interferon alfa-2b in advanced renal cell carcinoma. *J Clin Oncol* 1993, 11:661–670.

PEB
Cisplatin, Etoposide, and Bleomycin

The success of platinum-based multichemotherapy for the treatment of nonseminomatous testicular cancers has provided the foundation for the treatment of early-stage disease as well as metastatic testicular cancer. Randomized studies have demonstrated that three-drug combinations (PVB or PEB) are better than two-drug combinations (PV or PE).

Cisplatin's anticancer action is not exactly known but it is thought that its action is similar to that of a bifunctional alkylating agent. Cisplatin binds to plasma protein, and although serum half-life is calculated in hours, tissue levels have been detected as long as 4 mo after treatment. Cisplatin is excreted via the kidney.

Etoposide (VP16) is a podophyllotoxin from the mandrake plant. Although podophyllotoxins bind to tubulin, there is little discernible effect of etoposide on microtubular assembly. Etoposide blocks cell division at G_2. Stable ternary complexes are formed with DNA and topoisomerase II, causing single-strand DNA breaks. Elimination is principally renal although a significant amount of unchanged drug and metabolites can be found in the feces. Recent studies suggest that etoposide may be carcinogenic and lead to second malignancies.

Bleomycin is derived from the fungus *Streptomyces verticullus* and is classified as an antibiotic. The major isoform in the mixture is A_2. Bleomycin binds to DNA and ferrous ion. Ferrous ion oxidized, ultimately leading to oxygen radicals that cause DNA single- and double-strand breaks. The majority of the drug is excreted via the renal pathway.

CANDIDATES FOR TREATMENT
Patients with stage II nonseminomatous cancers (adjuvant) and those with metastatic seminoma and nonseminoma testicular malignancies

SPECIAL PRECAUTIONS
Dosage of PEB should be given on schedule regardless of CBC counts; for granulopenic fever, etoposide dosage is modified by a 25% reduction; for patients with granulocytopenia on d 1 of the second, third, or fourth cycle of therapy, daily blood cell counts are done and if leukocyte counts do not recover adequately, etoposide is held on d 5; bleomycin should be discontinued for signs of pulmonary fibrosis including respiratory lag, inspiratory rales, or radiographic changes; cisplatin can cause rash, magnesium wasting, Fanconi's syndrome, diabetes insipidus, peripheral neuropathy, hearing loss, and anaphylaxis

ALTERNATIVE THERAPIES
PVB (cisplatin, vinblastine, bleomycin); VAB-VI (vinblastine, dactinomycin, bleomycin, cyclophosphamide, cisplatin)

TOXICITIES
Cisplatin: leukopenia, thrombocytopenia, anemia, hemolytic anemia, nephrotoxicity, hyperuricemia, uric acid nephropathy, ototoxicity, anaphylaxis, neurotoxicity, optic neuritis, papilledema, stomatitis, syndrome of inappropriate diuretic hormone secretion, nausea, vomiting, diabetes insipidus, Fanconi's syndrome, magnesium wasting; **Bleomycin:** urticaria, Raynaud's phenomenon, pulmonary fibrosis, pneumonitis, burning at injection site, nail loss, fever, chills, anaphylaxis, stomatitis, confusion, wheezing, hepatotoxicity, pleuropericarditis, renal toxicity, cerebral arteritis, cerebral vascular accidents, myocardial infarction, thrombotic microangiopathy, rash, alopecia; **Etoposide:** anemia, leukopenia, thrombocytopenia, stomatitis, anaphylaxis, chemical phlebitis, neurotoxicity, anorexia, nausea, vomiting, lethargy, diarrhea, alopecia

DRUG INTERACTIONS
Cisplatin: allopurinol, colchicine, probenecid, sulfinpyrazone, antihistamines, buclizine, cyclizine, loxapine, meclizine, phenothiazines, thioxanthines, trimethobenzamid, bleomycin, radiation therapy, aminoglycosides, furosemide, vaccines, erythromycin, ethacrynic acid, salicylates, vancomycin; **Etoposide:** radiation therapy, vaccines; **Bleomycin:** general anesthetics, concurrent radiation, cisplatin, vincristine

DOSAGE AND SCHEDULING

	Day	1	2	3	4	5	6	7	8	9	10	11	12	13	14
Cisplatin 20 mg/m²/d x 5, q 3 wk		■	■	■	■	■									
Etoposide, 100 mg/m²/d x 5, q 3 wk		■	■	■	■	■									
Bleomycin 30 U/wk		■							■						
Chemistries, tumor markers with each cycle, d 1		□													
CBC weekly and daily on subsequent doses if CBC counts are low, d 1,8		□							□						
CXR prior to therapy every 2 mo															

DOSAGE MODIFICATIONS: *Maintain PEB schedule regardless of CBC counts; for granulopenic fever, reduce VP-16 dosage by 25%; for granulocytopenia on d 1 of 2nd, 3rd, or 4th cycle of therapy, do daily CBC counts and if WBC counts do not recover adequately, hold VP-16 on d 5; discontinue bleomycin if signs of pulmonary fibrosis develop*

PEB (Continued)

RECENT EXPERIENCES AND RESPONSE RATES

Study	Evaluable Patients, n	Dosage and Schedule	Complete Response Rates
Williams et al., N Engl J Med 1987, 316:1435–1440	121 nonseminoma	Cisplatin 20 mg/m^2/d x 5 q3 wk Vinblastine 0.15 mg/kg d1 & 2q3 wk Bleomycin 30 U/wk	61%
	123 nonseminoma	Cisplatin 20 mg/m^2/d x 5 q3 wk VP-16 100 mg/m^2/d x 5 q3 wk Bleomycin 30 U/wk	60%
Einhorn et al., J Clin Oncol 1989, 7:387–391	88 nonseminoma	Cisplatin 20 mg/m^2/d x 5 q3 wk VP-16 100 mg/m^2/d x 5 q3 wk Bleomycin 30 U/wk 3 cycles	66(75%)
	vs 96 nonseminoma	Cisplatin 20 mg/m^2/d x 5 q3 wk VP-16 100 mg/m^2/d x 5 q3 wk Bleomycin 30 U/wk 4 cycles	70(73%)

NURSING INTERVENTIONS

Give antiemetics, maintain adequate IV fluid intake, monitor input and output closely, monitor weight; assess patient performance, mental and pulmonary status; use antidiarrheals as needed; monitor blood counts, liver function, and renal function; patients should be aware of delayed nausea and treated appropriately; instruct patient regarding the development of fever and urinary symptoms; advise the patient to stop smoking

PATIENT INFORMATION

Patient may experience nausea, vomiting, allergic reactions; patient should inform the physician if allergic types of reaction have occurred in the past; risk for pulmonary toxicity increased in smokers; watch for fever, chills, change in urinary habits, tarry stool, blood in the stool, change in hearing, pins and needles, rash, diarrhea, and sore in the mouth

ADMINISTRATION NOTES

Cisplatin: supplied as a powder and reconstituted in sterile water for injection, which should be stored at room temperature and should be protected from freezing and light; if solutions more dilute than 1 mg/mL are used, cisplatin should be diluted in 5% dextrose and saline; platinum will precipitate if it comes into contact with aluminum; reconstituted cisplatin is stable for 20 h at room temperature; **Etoposide:** supplied as a solution in a benzyl alcohol, polysorbate, and alcohol and should be stored below 40°C; may be diluted into either 0.9% saline or 5% dextrose solutions to a final dilution of 0.2–0.4 mg/mL; may precipitate at high concentrations; **Bleomycin:** supplied as sterile bleomycin sulfate and stored at room temperature; diluents containing benzyl alcohol are not recommended for neonates; reconstituted solutions with saline or dextrose are stable for 24 h at room temperature and for 2 wk at 4°C.

VAB-6
Vinblastine, Cyclophosphamide, Dactinomycin, Bleomycin, Cisplatin

Vinblastine is an alkaloid from the plant *Vinca rosea*. Vinblastine will bind to tubulin and inhibit microtubule formation. It disrupts cells during the M phase of mitosis. The drug is metabolized in the liver and excreted in the bile. Dose modifications are required for hyperbilirubinemia. One mechanism of resistance to vinblastine is through the ATP-dependent efflux pump O-170 (MDR-1).

Cyclophosphamide is an alkylating agent that is activated in the hepatic microsomal system. 4-Hydroxycyclophosphamide enters the cell where it is converted to aldophosphamide and ultimately phosphoamide mustard and acrolein. Acrolein is excreted unchanged in the urine and is principally responsible for hemorrhagic cystitis. Phosphoamide mustard cross-links to strands of DNA and RNA, inhibiting cell division and protein synthesis. Up to 25% of the drug may be eliminated unchanged in the urine.

Dactinomycin is an antibiotic from *Streptomyces* species and is not cell cycle–specific in its antitumor mechanisms. Dactinomycin will intercalate into DNA and prevent RNA template formation as well as cause single-strand DNA breaks. Elimination is principally through the biliary tree with ~50% of the drug being excreted in the feces unchanged.

Bleomycin is derived from the fungus *Streptomyces verticullus* and is classified as an antibiotic. The major isoform in the mixture is A_2. Bleomycin binds to DNA and ferrous ion. Ferrous ion is oxidized, ultimately leading to oxygen radicals that cause DNA single- and double-strand breaks. The majority of the drug is excreted via the renal pathway.

Cisplatin's anticancer action is not exactly known but it is thought that its action is similar to that of a bifunctional alkylating agent. Cisplatin binds to plasma protein, and although serum half-life is calculated in hours, tissue levels have been detected as long as 4 months after treatment. Cisplatin is excreted via the kidney.

DOSAGE AND SCHEDULING

	Day 1	2	3	4	5	6	7
Vinblastine 4 mg/m² d 1	■						
Cyclophosphamide 600 mg/m² d 1	■						
Dactinomycin 1 mg/m² d 1	■						
Bleomycin 30 U IV push d 1	■						
Bleomycin 20 U/m² continuous infusion d 1,2,3	■■■						
Cisplatin 120 mg/m² d 4				■			
Chemistries, tumor markers with each cycle, d 1	□						
CBC, daily and on subsequent doses if CBC counts are low, d 1	□						
CXR prior to therapy q 2 mo							

Cycle repeated every 4 wk.

DOSAGE MODIFICATIONS: *Maintain VAB-6 schedule regardless of CBC counts; for granulocytic fever, reduce dactinomycin and vinblastine by 25%; discontinue bleomycin should signs of pulmonary fibrosis develop.*

SPECIAL PRECAUTIONS
Dosage of VAB-6 should be given on schedule regardless of CBC counts; for granulocytic fever, dactinomycin and vinblastine dosage is modified by a 25% reduction; bleomycin should be discontinued for signs of pulmonary fibrosis including respiratory lag, inspiratory rales, or radiographic changes; can cause rash, magnesium wasting, Fanconi's syndrome, diabetes insipidus, peripheral neuropathy, hearing loss, and anaphylaxis

TOXICITIES
Cisplatin: leukopenia, thrombocytopenia, anemia, hemolytic anemia, nephrotoxicity, hyperuricemia, uric acid nephropathy, ototoxicity, anaphylaxis, neurotoxicity, optic neuritis, papilledema stomatitis, syndrome of inappropriate diuretic hormone secretion, nausea, vomiting, diabetes insipidus, Fanconi's syndrome, magnesium wasting; **Bleomycin:** urticaria, Raynaud's phenomenon, pulmonary fibrosis, pneumonitis, burning at injection site, nail loss, fever, chills, anaphylaxis, stomatitis, confusion, wheezing, hepatotoxicity, pleuropericarditis, renal toxicity, cerebral arteritis, cerebral vascular accidents, myocardial infarction, thrombotic microangiopathy, rash, alopecia; **Dactinomycin:** aplastic anemia, leukopenia, esophagitis, pharyngitis, diarrhea, prostatitis, gastrointestinal ulceration, anaphylaxis, phlebitis, hepatitis, hyperpigmentation, nausea, vomiting, skin rash, and alopecia; **Cyclophosphamide:** gonadal depression, leukopenia, thrombocytopenia, myocarditis, hemorrhagic cystitis, pneumonitis, interstitial pulmonary fibrosis, syndrome of inappropriate diuretic hormone secretion, anaphylaxis, stomatitis, hyperglycemia, hyperpigmentation of skin and fingernails, nausea, vomiting, headache, skin rash, and alopecia; **Vinblastine:** leukoneutropenia, thrombocytopenia, cellulitis, stomatitis, jaw pain, loss of ankle jerk, peripheral neuropathy, nausea, vomiting, paralytic ileus, alopecia

DRUG INTERACTIONS
Cisplatin: allopurinol, colchicine, probenecid, sulfinpyrazone, antihistamines, buclizine, cyclizine, loxapine, meclizine, phenothiazines, thioxanthines, trimethobenzamid, bleomycin, radiation therapy, aminoglycosides, furosemide, vaccines, erythromycin, ethacrynic acid, salicylates, vancomycin; **Dactinomycin:** allopurinol, colchicine, probenecid, sulfinpyrazone, radiation therapy, vaccines, vitamin K; **Vinblastine:** radiation therapy, vaccines, allopurinol, colchicine, probenecid, sulfinpyrazone; **Bleomycin:** general anesthetics, concurrent radiation, cisplatin, vincristine; **Cyclophosphamides:** allopurinol, colchicine, probenecid, sulfinpyrazone, anticoagulants, radiation therapy, cocaine, hepatic enzyme inducers, lovastatin, succinylcholine, vaccines

RECENT EXPERIENCES AND RESPONSE RATES

Study	Evaluable Patients, n	Dose and Schedule	Complete Response Rates, %
Bosl et al., J Clin Oncol 1988, 6:1231–1238	82	VAB-6	83
	82 (good-risk pts) nonseminoma	vs Etoposide 100 mg/m^2/d x 5 Cisplatin 20 mg/m^2/d x 5 q 3–4 wk	88
Bosl et al., J Clin Oncol 1986, 4:1493–1499	125 met. nonsem. and 22 met. sem.	VAB-6	69
	19 extragonadal	VAB-6	53
Stanton et al., J Clin Oncol 1985, 3:336–339	28 sem.	VAB-6	86

NURSING INTERVENTIONS

Give antiemetics, maintain adequate IV fluid intake, monitor inputs and outputs closely, monitor weight; assess patient performance, mental and pulmonary status; use antidiarrheals as needed; monitor blood counts and liver, pulmonary, and renal function; patients should be aware of delayed nausea and treated appropriately; instruct patient regarding the development of fever and urinary symptoms; advise the patient to stop smoking; patient should be on adequate bowel regimen to prevent paralytic ileus, which may be caused by vinblastine

PATIENT INFORMATION

Patient may experience nausea, vomiting, allergic reactions; patient should inform the physician if allergic types of reactions have occurred in the past; risk for pulmonary toxicity increased in smokers; watch for fever, chills, change in urinary habits, tarry stool, blood in the stool, change in hearing, pins and needles, rash, diarrhea, and sore in the mouth; pins and needles may develop, as well as pain in the jaw; constipation may develop and should be treated aggressively but not from below because leukopenia may have developed

ADMINISTRATION NOTES

Cisplatin: supplied as a powder and reconstituted in sterile water for injection, which should be stored at room temperature and should be protected from freezing and light. If solutions more dilute than 1 mg/mL: are used, cisplatin should be diluted in 5% dextrose and saline; platinum will precipitate if it comes into contact with aluminum; reconstituted cisplatin is stable for 20 h at room temperature; **Vinblastine:** provided in a lyophilized powder and reconstituted in 0.9% sterile saline; final concentration of the drug is 1 mg/mL; once reconstituted, vinblastine folate has a shelf-life of 30 d at 2°C–8°C; **Cyclophosphamide:** for injection, comes either as a lyophilized or nonlyophilized powder; sterile water or bacteriostatic water may be used to prepare both formulations; reconstituted cyclophosphamide is stable for 24 h at room temperature or for 6 d refrigerated; **Bleomycin:** supplied as sterile bleomycin sulfate and stored at room temperature; diluents containing benzyl alcohol are not recommended for neonates; reconstituted solutions with saline or dextrose are stable for 24 h at room temperature and for 2 wk at 4°C; **Dactinomycin:** a powder that may be stored at room temperature and reconstituted with sterile water without preservative.

M-VAC
Methotrexate, Vinblastine, Doxorubicin, and Cisplatin

The M-VAC regimen was found to be superior to cisplatin alone (objective response rates of 33% vs 15%, respectively; P=0.001) in a randomized trial evaluating the treatment of metastatic bladder cancer conducted by the Eastern Cooperative Oncology Group. Patients eligible for treatment with M-VAC include those patients with metastatic transitional cell carcinoma (TCC) of the uroepithelium who have adequate renal function. The role of M-VAC in the treatment of metastatic TCC is well documented. The use of M-VAC or other combination chemotherapy for adjuvant treatment of high-risk local TCCs has not yet been proven, and patients should be encouraged to participate in randomized trials evaluating these therapies.

Methotrexate is an antimetabolite that inhibits dihydrofolic acid reductase, thus interfering with DNA synthesis. Methotrexate is polyglutamated within cells, which allows the compound to remain in cells for prolonged periods of time. Renal excretion by glomerular filtration and active tubular secretion is the principal route of elimination, with as much as 90% of the drug excreted in the first 24 h.

Vinblastine is an alkaloid from the plant *Vinca rosea*. Vinblastine will bind to tubulin and inhibit microtubule formation. It disrupts cells during the M phase of mitosis. The drug is metabolized in the liver and excreted in the bile. Dose modifications are required for hyperbilirubinemia. One mechanism of resistance to vinblastine is through the ATP-dependent efflux pump P-170 (MDR-1).

Doxorubicin is a anthracycline antibiotic from *Streptomyces peucetius* (variety *caesius*). All of doxorubicin's mechanisms of action have not been elucidated, but it will enter the cell quickly and intercalate with DNA, thus inhibiting cellular division. Forty percent to 50% of the drug is excreted in the bile over a 7-d period. Patients with liver dysfunction require dose reduction.

Cisplatin's anticancer action is not exactly known but it is thought that its action is similar to that of a bifunctional alkylating agent. Cisplatin binds to plasma protein, and although serum half-life is calculated in hours, tissue levels have been detected as long as 4 mo after treatment. Cisplatin is excreted via the kidney.

CANDIDATES FOR TREATMENT
Patients with metastatic transitional cell carcinoma with renal, liver, cardiac, and adequate bone marrow function under some circumstances; patients with high-risk for relapse from local resected disease may be candidates

SPECIAL PRECAUTIONS
Dosage of M-VAC should be adjusted for toxicity; full-dose methotrexate and vinblastine should be given on d 15 and 22 for leukocyte count > 1999 cells/mm^3 and platelet count > 74,999 mm^3; for worse hematologic toxicity, chemotherapy dose should be held and restarted at 67% when the counts return to normal; omit d 15 and 22 if recovery of blood counts takes > 2 wk to recover; on d 15 and 22 should be given on schedule regardless of CBC counts; for granulocytic fever, dactinomycin and vinblastine dosage is modified by a 25% reduction; bleomycin should be discontinued for signs of pulmonary fibrosis including respiratory lag, inspiratory rales, or radiographic changes; can cause rash, magnesium wasting, Fanconi's syndrome, diabetes insipidus, peripheral neuropathy, hearing loss, and anaphylaxis

TOXICITIES
Methotrexate: nausea, vomiting, gingivitis, pharyngitis, stomatitis, diarrhea, enteritis, leukopenia, thrombocytopenia, hypogammaglobulinemia, erythematous rash, pruritus, urticaria, photosensitivity, depigmentation, alopecia, acne, hepatic atrophy and necrosis, cirrhosis, renal failure, cystitis, defective oogenesis or spermatogenesis, menstrual dysfunction, infertility, fetal defects, abortion, nephropathy, blurred vision, seizures, arachnoiditis, leukoencephalopathy, conjunctivitis; **Vinblastine:** leukoneutropenia, thrombocytopenia, cellulitis, stomatitis, jaw pain, loss of ankle jerk, peripheral neuropathy, nausea, vomiting, paralytic ileus, alopecia; **Doxorubicin:** leukoneutropenia, cardiotoxicity, arrhythmias, phlebosclerosis, facial flushing, alopecia, hyperpigmentation of the nail beds and dermal creases, recall reaction to radiation, erythematous streaking at IV site, tissue necrosis from extravasation, mucositis, conjunctivitis, nausea, vomiting, allergy including anaphylaxis; **Cisplatin:** leukopenia, thrombocytopenia, anemia, hemolytic anemia, nephrotoxicity, hyperuricemia, uric acid nephropathy, ototoxicity, anaphylaxis, neurotoxicity, optic neuritis, papilledema, stomatitis, syndrome of inappropriate diuretic hormone secretion, nausea, vomiting, diabetes insipidus, Fanconi's syndrome, magnesium wasting

DRUG INTERACTIONS
Methotrexate: alcohol, acetaminophen, amiodarone, estrogens, erythromycin, isoniazid, methyldopa, phenothiazines, phenytoin, piperacillin, rifampin, allopurinol, colchicine, sulfinpyrazones, nonsteroidal antiinflammatory agents, folic acid, oral neomycin, salicylates, sulfonamides, vaccines; **Vinblastine:** radiation therapy, vaccines, allopurinol, colchicine,

(Continued on next page)

DOSAGE AND SCHEDULING

	Day											
	1	2	3	4	5	6	7	10	15	20	22
Methotrexate 30 mg/m^2 d 1, 15, 22	■								■		■
Vinblastine 3 mg/m^2 d 2, 15, 22		■							■		■
Doxorubicin 30 mg/m^2 d 2		■									
Cisplatin 70 mg/m^2 d 2		■									
Chemistries d 1	□										
BUN/creatinine d 1, 15, 22	□								□		□
24-h CrCl d 1	□										
CBC d 1	□										

Cycle repeated every 3 wk.

DOSAGE MODIFICATIONS: *Give full-dose methotrexate and vinblastine on d 15 and 22 if WBC count is 1999/mm^3 and platelet count is > 74,999/mm^3. If counts fall below, dose is held and restarted at 67% when counts return to normal. Omit d 15 and 22 if blood counts take more than 2 wk to recover. On d 15 and 22 methotrexate should be given on schedule regardless of CBC counts.*

M-VAC (Continued)

RECENT EXPERIENCES AND RESPONSE RATES

Study	Evaluable Patients, n	Dose and Schedule	Response Rates, % Complete/Partial
Sternberg et al., J Urol 1988, 139:461–69	92	Methotrexate 30 mg/m² d 1, 15, 22 Vinblastine 3 mg/m² d 2, 15, 22 Doxorubicin 30 mg/m² d 2 Cisplatin 70 mg/m² d 2	34/28
Sternberg et al., J Urol 1990, 144:396–397	121	Methotrexate 30 mg/m² d 1, 15, 22 Vinblastine 3 mg/m² d 2, 15, 22 Doxorubicin 30 mg/m² d 2 Cisplatin 70 mg/m²	36/36
Connor et al., J Urol 1990, 144:397	14	Methotrexate 30 mg/m² d 1, 15, 22 Vinblastine 3 mg/m² d 2, 15, 22 Doxorubicin 30 mg/m² d 2 Cisplatin 70 mg/m²	31/37
Scher et al., J Urol 1988, 139:470–477	41 neoadjuvant	Methotrexate 30 mg/m² d 1, 15, 22 Vinblastine 3 mg/m² d 2, 15, 22 Doxorubicin 30 mg/m² d 2 Cisplatin 70 mg/m²	24/39
Scher et al., J Urol 1988, 139:478–487	5 extragonadal	Methotrexate 30 mg/m² d 1, 15, 22 Vinblastine 3 mg/m² d 2, 15, 22 Doxorubicin 30 mg/m² d 2 Cisplatin 70 mg/m²	60/—

DRUG INTERACTIONS (Continued)

probenecid, sulfinpyrazone; **Doxorubicin:** allopurinol, colchicine, alcohol, amiodarone, estrogens, isoniazid, methyldopa, phenothiazines, phenytoin, piperacillin, rifampin, vaccines; **Cisplatin:** allopurinol, colchicine, probenecid, sulfinpyrazone, antihistamines, buclizine, cyclizine, loxapine, meclizine, phenothiazines, thioxanthines, trimethobenzamid, bleomycin, radiation therapy, aminoglycosides, furosemide, vaccines, erythromycin, ethacrynic acid, salicylates, vancomycin

NURSING INTERVENTIONS

Give antiemetics, maintain adequate IV fluid intact, monitor input and output closely, monitor weight. Assess patient performance, mental and pulmonary status. Use antidiarrheals as needed. Monitor blood counts and liver and renal function. Patients should be aware of delayed nausea and treated appropriately. Instruct patient regarding the development of fever and urinary symptoms. Patient should be on adequate bowel regimen to prevent paralytic ileus, which may be caused by vinblastine.

PATIENT INFORMATION

Patient may experience nausea, vomiting allergic reactions. Patient should inform the physician if allergic types of reaction have occurred in the past. Watch for fever, chills, change in urinary habits, tarry stool, blood in the stool, change in hearing, pins and needles, rash, diarrhea, and sore in the mouth. Pins and needles may develop, as well as pain in the jaw. Constipation may develop and should be treated aggressively but not from below because leukopenia may have developed.

ADMINISTRATION NOTES

Methotrexate: for IV use, provided as a preservative-free lyophilized powder, which is reconstituted in sterile 5% dextrose or 0.9% saline; concentration should not exceed 25 mg/mL; **Vinblastine:** provided in a lyophilized powder and is reconstituted in 0.9% sterile saline; final concentration of the drug is 1 mg/mL; once reconstituted, vinblastine sulfate has a shelf-life of 30 d at 2°C–8°C; **Doxorubicin:** provided as a sterile red-orange powder containing a 1:5 (w:w) ratio of lactose and a 1:0.1 ratio of methylparaben; powder may be stored at room temperature protected from light; doxorubicin is reconstituted with 0.9% sodium chloride injection to give a final concentration of 2 mg/mL; bacteriostatic diluents should be avoided; the reconstituted drug is stable for 15 d in the refrigerator and the dark; 5-fluorouracil and sodium heparin may cause doxorubicin to precipitate and should not be mixed with drug; the drug also may be obtained as a liquid with no preservatives; **Cisplatin:** supplied as a powder and reconstituted in sterile water for injection, which should be stored at room temperature and should be protected from freezing and light; if solutions more dilute than 1 mg/mL are used, cisplatin should be diluted in 5% dextrose and saline; platinum will precipitate if it comes into contact with aluminum; reconstituted cisplatin is stable for 20 h at room temperature.

Tumors of the female reproductive organs are heterogeneous with regard to histology, natural history, clinical behavior, and methods of treatment. Appropriate treatment requires careful diagnostic evaluation to distinguish them from other malignancies of the pelvis (eg, sigmoid, rectal, and bladder cancers) as well as from metastatic lesions (eg, Krukenburg's tumors). Accurate staging is critical because therapy is virtually always guided by extent of spread. Treatment of these malignancies requires a thorough understanding of their natural history and should not be attempted by those with little experience in this field. Optimal conditions for diagnosis, staging, and therapy require excellent communication between the medical and radiation oncologists, the radiologist, and the surgeon. This is particularly true when multimodality therapy is contemplated.

Tumors included in this section include the common tumors of the ovary, uterine cervix, uterus, vulva, and gestational trophoblastic neoplasms (Table 15-1).

OVARIAN CANCER

APPROACH TO THE THERAPY OF EPITHELIAL TUMORS OF THE OVARY

Etiology, Risk Factors, and Screening

These tumors comprise approximately 95% of all ovarian malignancies. The prevalence is 30 to 50 in 100,000 women, with a lifetime incidence of 1 in 70 women. They occur most commonly in women in their sixth and seventh decades. Etiology and risk factors for ovarian cancer include advanced age; nulliparity; prior history of endometrial, breast, or colon cancer; European or North American descent; and any history of the familial syndromes. Screening the general population is neither cost effective nor practical; however, certain subpopulations of patients (defined by the risk factors described above) may be candidates.

Three screening tests are currently employed: bimanual pelvic examination, CA-125, and transvaginal ultrasound. The pelvic examination is cost effective and reliable in experienced hands but lacks adequate sensitivity and specificity as a screening test. It is estimated that physical examination will detect only 1 in 10,000 ovarian carcinomas in asymptomatic women.

The radioimmunoassay for CA-125, a tumor-specific antigen, is elevated in 80% of ovarian carcinomas but in only 50% of women with cancer limited to the ovary. In addition, it may be elevated in women with benign ovarian disease and in otherwise healthy women, limiting its specificity. In postmenopausal women with a pelvic mass, however, a serum CA125 > 65 U/mL is predictive of cancer in up to 75% of cases.

Ultrasound techniques are expensive and also limited in their specificity and sensitivity. In a recent study of 8500 asymptomatic women who underwent transvaginal ultrasound, 121 underwent surgery. Fifty-seven patients had serous cystadenomas, and eight had primary ovarian cancers (6 stage IA, 1 stage IIC, 1 stage IIIB). Only one patient had palpable ovarian enlargement and one had an elevated CA-125 [1]. Combinations of CA-125 measurements and transvaginal ultrasound are promising in high-risk patients but should be considered experimental.

Recommendations for screening are controversial. The 1994 National Institutes of Health Consensus Conference concluded there is no effective method for screening and detecting early ovarian cancer [2]. Nevertheless, some authorities feel that a reasonable strategy would be to screen those patients with a strong familial history or a familial cancer syndrome (Table 15-2). Although the average woman has a lifetime risk of 1 in 70 of developing ovarian cancer, it increases to 1 in 20 in women with a first-degree relative with ovarian cancer, 1 in 14 to in women with two first-degree relatives, and 40% for the hereditary ovarian cancer syndrome. Although there is no data demonstrating that screening reduces the mortality of the disease even in the higher risk groups, women who are at the highest risk may at least have an annual bimanual pelvic examination, assay for CA-125, and transvaginal ultrasound. Prophylactic oophorectomy is a consideration for women with a history of familial ovarian cancer syndrome.

The role of screening for genetic mutations (see Role of Genetic Mutations section) remains undefined. It would not be advisable to offer genetic screening, which is now commercially available, without adequate guidance from a clinical geneticist to interpret the results and offer recommendations to patients.

Protective factors for women at risk for ovarian carcinoma include oral contraceptive use, full-term pregnancy, breast-feeding, and possibly tubal ligation. In women at high-risk who are undergoing abdominal surgery for other indications, prophylactic oophorectomy may be indicated. In this group, estrogen replacement should be discussed.

Table 15-1. Common Tumors of the Female Genital Tract

Ovary
  Epithelial
  Stromal
  Germ cell
  Metastatic
Uterus
  Adenocarcinoma
  Sarcoma
    Leiomyosarcoma
    Mixed mesodermal tumors
    Endometrial stromal sarcoma
Cervix
  Squamous cell carcinoma
  Adenocarcinoma
  Adenosquamous carcinoma
Vulva
Gestational trophoblastic neoplasm
  Hydatidiform mole
  Invasive mole
  Choriocarcinoma

Table 15-2. Strategies for Early Diagnosis and Prevention of Ovarian Cancer

Identification of risk factors, including family history
Annual bimanual rectovaginal examination
Annual CA-125, transvaginal ultrasound in selected patients
Prophylactic oophorectomy in selected patients
Risk reduction strategies in selected patients
Higher risk in Japanese who emigrate to the United States

Role of Genetic Mutations

Approximately 10% of all epithelial ovarian cancers are associated with inheritance of an autosomal-dominant genetic aberration, which confers cancer predisposition with a high penetrance. Perhaps the most important new dimension in understanding the etiology of some cancers of the ovary was the discovery of the role of mutations in the *BRCA1* gene. Located on chromosome 17q12-21, the *BRCA1* gene is a tumor-suppressor gene. Mutations of *BRCA1* are associated with a higher incidence of breast cancer (especially but not exclusively in women of Ashkenazi Jewish descent) and ovarian cancer. Germ-line mutations of the gene are associated with a lifetime risk of breast cancer (up to 85%) and ovarian cancer (up to 45%) for women with multiple family members who have ovarian and breast cancer over more than two generations. The incidence of germ-line mutations among women with ovarian cancer, however, is controversial ranging from less than 1 in 47 to 5 in 115 [3,4] but is higher than that found in the general population (0.0006) [5]. A recent study has detected probable germ-line mutations in *BRCA1* in 13 out of 374 women with epithelial ovarian cancer who are younger than 70 years of age [6]. Women with mutations in *BRCA1* may have a greater likelihood of having breast cancer, and mutations are linked to the breast–ovary syndrome, which is linked to a lesser extent with mutations in the *BRCA2* gene on chromosome 13q.

In additions to mutations in the *BRCA* genes, a higher incidence of ovarian cancer is observed in women who are members of families characterized by the Lynch II syndrome (hereditary nonpolyposis coli [HNPCC]). These families are characterized by a higher incidence of carcinomas of the ovary, breast, colon, and uterus, which occur more frequently than expected among a single generation, in multiple sequential generations, and in a younger age population. The HNPCC syndrome is characterized by mutations in any of four known genes (*hMSH2*, *hMLH1*, *hPMS1*, and *hPMS2*), which are the human homologues of genes associated with mismatch repair, or more simplistically, genes that "proofread" errors in DNA replication and correct errors in homopolymeric or dimeric repeats, which occur frequently in human genes. In patients with mutations in these genes, mutations build up in the human genome and can be characterized by instability in microsatellites (*ie*, portions of the genome with dimeric repeating sequences [*eg*, CACACACA...] or homopolymeric sequences [*eg*, AAAAAAA...]). These patients are characterized by familial clustering of colon, breast, and endometrial carcinomas as well as a variety of other carcinomas that are less common. Thus, women with a well-defined familial history for these malignancies should be followed more carefully for the development of these cancers.

For sporadic ovarian cancers, aberrations in various other protooncogenes, tumor suppressor genes, and signal transduction pathways have been characterized. These include *ras*, *erb*-B2, and p53. Mutations in Ki-*ras*-2 most frequently occur at codon 12 (but can also occur at codon 13) and are found in approximately 30% to 50% of mucinous tumors (both borderline and invasive) and with a lower frequency in serous tumors. Mutations in p53 occur rather late in the development of ovarian cancer, occurring in approximately 10% of early-stage cancers and 40% of late-stage tumors but not borderline tumors. These mutations may correlate with worse overall outcome.

DIAGNOSIS AND MANAGEMENT OF EARLY-STAGE DISEASE
Management of the Adnexal Mass

Detection of an adnexal mass either by physical or radiographic examination requires a management strategy. Although the vast majority of adnexal masses are benign, 13% to 21% of women undergoing surgery for a suspicious mass will have an ovarian malignancy. Recommendation for surgery depends on the degree of suspicion that this mass is malignant. Factors that should be considered include age, menopausal status, family history, size and type of mass, duration, characteristics of associated symptoms, CA-125, unilaterality versus bilaterality, and characteristics on ultrasound. Management may include observation with repeat examination, further radiographic tests, and laparoscopy or laparotomy (depending on the clinical circumstances).

Staging and Management of Early-Stage Epithelial Cancer of the Ovary
Overall Goals

The natural history of ovarian cancer is dominated by locoregional spread, with peritoneal involvement being most common. Precise histologic diagnosis and accurate staging are required prior to treatment. The International Federation of Gynecology and Obstetrics (FIGO) staging system (1989) is described in Table 15-3. Goals of therapy for early-stage disease (FIGO I–III) include cure; goals for later-stage disease (suboptimal III–IV) include prolongation of survival, palliation, particularly reduction of ascites, preservation of bowel function, adequate nutrition, and prevention of pain.

The cornerstone of treatment for epithelial ovarian tumors is surgery performed by an experienced gynecologic oncologist. Patients require a staging laparotomy with thorough inspection of the entire peritoneal cavity including the gutters, the pelvis and the domes of

---

Table 15-3. Staging and Prognosis of Ovarian Carcinoma

Stage	Characteristics
I	Disease confined to the ovaries
IA	One ovary, capsule intact, no ascites
IB	Both ovaries, capsule intact, no ascites
IC	IA or IB +: ascites, + washings, capsule ruptures, tumor on ovarian surface
II	Disease confined to the pelvis
III	Disease confined to the abdominal cavity, including surface of the liver, pelvic, inguinal or para-aortic lymph node, omentum, or bowel
IIIA	Negative nodes, + microscopic seeding of peritoneal surfaces
IIIB	Negative nodes, peritoneal implants ≤ 2 cm.
IIIC	Positive nodes and/or abdominal implants > 2 cm.
IV	Spread to liver parenchyma, lung (if effusion only, with positive cytology), or other extra-abdominal site

Prognosis

Stage	3-y Survival, %
IA, IB	90.4
IC, II	66.5
III	28.1
IV	10.4

Adapted from International Federation of Gynecology and Obstetrics [32].

---

the diaphragm, total abdominal hysterectomy and bilateral salpingo-oophorectomy, liver palpation and biopsy, lymph node sampling, omentectomy, and peritoneal washings. All gross disease should be removed if possible. If surgical debulking is incomplete, the surgeon must estimate the size and extent of residual tumor. Patients who have had a biopsy only or incomplete debulking may be referred to an experienced gynecologic oncologist for consideration for re-operation, as clinical outcome may be affected. Staging is performed per FIGO criteria.

RECOMMENDATIONS FOR TREATMENT OF EARLY-STAGE DISEASE

Approximately 25% of women with ovarian cancer will have disease confined to one or both ovaries. These women have a much more favorable prognosis. The primary therapy of patients with early stage ovarian cancer, either confined to the ovary (FIGO stage I) or confined to the pelvis (FIGO stage II), is surgery. Nevertheless, among selected subgroups, the failure rate is high enough to warrant adjuvant therapy with either radioisotopes, external beam irradiation or chemotherapy. The Gynecologic Oncology Group has attempted to precisely define the subgroups that would benefit from adjuvant therapy and determine the optimal form of therapy for these patients. Two clinical trials were initiated in 1976 in order to accomplish these goals.

Stage IA and IB

Gynecologic Oncoloy Group (GOG) study 7601 included patients with stage Ia or Ib disease (growth limited to one or both ovaries with no ascites and negative peritoneal washings) with well- or moderately-differentiated histologies. Patients were randomized to observation or to receive melphalan 0.2 mg/kg of body weight orally for 5 days every 4 to 6 weeks for 12 cycles. With a follow-up of 6 years, there was no difference between the two groups. Furthermore, the 5-year disease-free survival in the observation arm was 91%, and the overall survival was 94%, suggesting that this subset of patients does well and should not receive adjuvant therapy [7].

Stages IAii, IBii, IC–IIC, and IA or IB with poorly differentiated histology

GOG 7602 included patients with either a ruptured capsule or excrescences on the ovarian surface; high grade histology; positive ascites or peritoneal washings; or spread to the uterus, fallopian tubes, or other pelvic tissues [7]. Patients were randomized to receive melphalan as with stage IA and IB or 15 mCi of intraperitoneal ^{32}P as chromic phosphate. The failure rate with 6 years of follow-up was 20%, with failures distributed evenly between both groups. Toxicities were modest in both groups; however, the authors concluded that treatment with ^{32}P was preferred because of the limited toxicity and no risk of developing leukemia, which has been observed with alkylating agents. In the replacement trial for the GOG, treatment with ^{32}P is compared with three cycles of cyclophosphamide/cisplatin. Optimal therapy for these patients remains unknown. When feasible, they should be entered into clinical trials.

Currently, the Society of Gynecologic Oncologists recommends that most epithelial tumors, including early-grade ovarian carcinomas, receive adjuvant chemotherapy with the exception of grade 1, stage IA epithelial ovarian cancers [8].

RECOMMENDATIONS FOR TREATMENT OF OPTIMAL DISEASE

The largest single subgroup of women with ovarian carcinoma are those presenting with stage III disease [9]. Prognosis correlates well with extent of residual disease following primary debulking surgery. Patients with optimally debulked disease have a favorable prognosis versus those in whom the tumor was too extensive to be adequately debulked. The cut-off for optimal disease is usually determined as being either less than 1 cm or less than 2 cm, depending on the investigators. It is likely that this is a continuum with those with the least tumor burden following surgery having the best prognosis. Prognosis worsens as the diameter of the smallest residual lesion increases, with approximately 40% of those with residual microscopic disease alive at 8 years versus 25% with residual disease < 0.5 cm and 10% with residual disease 0.5 to 2.0 cm.

The overall survival for women with optimally debulked disease is around 25%; thus, there is an appreciable cure rate for women treated with aggressive initial surgery followed by platinum-based chemotherapy. Following surgery, all women should receive at least six cycles of platinum-based therapy, with either cisplatin or carboplatin in combination with paclitaxel. If cisplatin is employed, patients require careful monitoring of renal function and neurologic status. Doses will need to be modified for either azotemia or for new onset of sensory neuropathy because continued treatment at the same doses will likely lead to a worsening of both conditions. Systemic treatment with carboplatin is likely equivalent in this setting, although this remains to be proven definitively. Treatment with carboplatin does not result in permanent renal damage, ototoxicity, or neurologic deficits. Nevertheless, patients must be closely monitored for onset of neutropenic fevers and thrombocytopenia with attendant risk of hemorrhage.

For women receiving treatment with cisplatin, which is still considered the "gold standard," the major controversy concerns the optimal route—intravenous or intraperitoneal—by which the drug is administered. A recent intergroup trial, led by the Southwest Oncology Group (SWOG), compared treatment with intravenous cyclophosphamide in combination with either intraperitoneal or intravenous cisplatin. The results revealed a survival advantage for the group receiving intraperitoneal over intravenous cisplatin (49 mo vs 41 mo, respectively; P = 0.02), and there was a significant reduction in sensory neuropathy with intraperitoneal therapy [10]. The SWOG and the Eastern Cooperative Oncology Group (ECOG) are currently testing a more intensive intraperitoneal regimen incorporating paclitaxel and cisplatin in women with stage III ovarian cancer.

RECOMMENDATIONS FOR TREATMENT OF SUBOPTIMALLY DEBULKED AND STAGE IV DISEASE

Women who have residual disease of less than 2 cm after initial debulking surgery have a substantially worse prognosis than those with optimally debulked disease. Nevertheless, a small proportion of these women will enjoy long-term disease-free survival. In contrast, women with disease outside the abdominal cavity or in the liver parenchyma (stage IV) have a worse prognosis and rarely enjoy long-term disease-free survival. In addition to residual tumor volume, other factors are associated with a poor prognosis, including gross residual tumor after first-line chemotherapy, grade 3 histology, aneuploidy, and increased S-phase or elevated Her 2/neu.

Evidence strongly suggests that chemotherapy can prolong survival in women with stage III disease, whether optimally or suboptimally debulked, and possibly in stage IV disease. Thus, women in these disease categories should be encouraged to receive chemotherapy as a treatment option following surgery. There are many active agents (Table 15-4).

For patients with disease remaining after surgery, the most common treatment is combination therapy with paclitaxel and a platinum compound. The standard of care must be considered paclitaxel plus cisplatin as administered in GOG 111 [11], although combinations of carboplatin and paclitaxel are acceptable. The major toxicities of this regimen are emesis and myelosuppression. Emesis may be controlled with newer antiemetics, such as ondansetron or granisetron. A hematopoietic growth factor (eg, granulocyte or granulocyte–macrophage colony-stimulating factor) may decrease the duration of neutropenia and the number of days of administering antibiotics, but it has not been shown to improve survival or response duration and should not be considered standard therapy. Use of a single alkylating agent, such as melphalan, is suboptimal therapy and should only be considered in patients who cannot receive standard therapy.

A recent study, GOG 132, compared treatment with cisplatin (100 mg/m^2) as a single agent with paclitaxel (200 mg/m^2) as a single agent versus paclitaxel (135 mg/m^2) plus cisplatin (75 mg/m^2) administered concurrently (all regimens given every 3 wk for six cycles) in women with suboptimally debulked disease [11a]. The results of this trial failed to demonstrate the same median survival for women treated with the combination as in GOG 111. Furthermore, women who received cisplatin (either in combination with paclitaxel or as a single agent) did equally as well, demonstrating the superiority of platinum-based therapies. Women receiving paclitaxel alone had an inferior result.

Two issues are currently being studied with regard to combination paclitaxel plus platinum regimens. The first is the use of 3-hour paclitaxel versus the standard 24-hour infusion. The former is more cost effective and easier because drug can be administered in the outpatient setting; however, whether this is equivalent to 24-hour paclitaxel regarding toxicity and efficacy remains to be determined.

The second issue is whether carboplatin is an effective substitute for cisplatin. This is also of interest because the toxicity profile of carboplatin differs from that of cisplatin with fewer irreversible oto-, nephro- and neurotoxicities. In addition, it is easier to administer carboplatin in the outpatient setting because of the absence of a requirement for pretreatment hydration. A report from the SWOG demonstrated equal efficacy for the combination of cyclophosphamide plus carboplatin versus cyclophosphamide and cisplatin but a lower incidence of irreversible toxicities associated with cisplatin treatment, including nephrotoxicity and neurotoxicity.

Several early studies suggest that the combination of carboplatin and paclitaxel is equivalent in therapeutic outcome to cisplatin and paclitaxel. Two small studies from Nebraska [12] and the Netherlands [13] have employed 3-hour paclitaxel and carboplatin as a 30-minute infusion, with acceptable toxicities and reasonable therapeutic outcome. In addition, the ECOG has tested the combination of short-infusion paclitaxel and carboplatin, with essentially equivalent survival to that observed in women on GOG 132 who received standard therapy and with an overall improvement in quality of life (Schink, personal communication). Thus, combinations of short-infusion paclitaxel over 3 hours and carboplatin administered in the outpatient setting would currently be considered an acceptable alternative to regimens such as that employed in GOG 111 in women with suboptimally debulked and stage IV ovarian cancer.

Other considerations

Prior to treatment, levels of the ovarian tumor marker CA-125 should be measured and used as adjunctive evidence of response to therapy. Levels should be measured routinely during the course of treatment. A consistent rise in CA-125 can be used as a measure to failure of treatment in the absence of radiographic and clinical changes. Likewise, a linear fall in serum levels of CA-125 can be used as a measure of treatment success in the absence of radiographic and clinical changes. Recent data suggest that incorporation of CA-125 is a critical element in treatment. Levels of carcinoembryonic antigen and CA-19 may be elevated in women with mucinous carcinomas and may be potentially useful in following the course of the disease.

Treatment should consist of four to eight cycles of therapy administered every 3 weeks or monthly. Residual disease should be measured prior to initiation of therapy by visual inspection at the time of surgery, by computed tomography (CT) scan if bulk disease remains, or by physical examination or chest roentgenogram when appropriate. Levels of CA-125 are followed as described in the previous paragraph. If these levels rise or fail to decrease, resistance to treatment should be suspected.

EVALUATION OF THE PATIENT AFTER INITIAL THERAPY

Following four to eight cycles of initial chemotherapy, patients who are clinically responding should be reevaluated using CA-125 levels and CT scan. Patients who have clinically progressed through initial therapy have a poor prognosis [14]. Options for these patients include further treatment with a non–platinum-containing regimen or experimental therapy.

Table 15-4. Single-Agent Activity in Ovarian Cancer*

Drug	Patients, n	Response Rate, %
Cisplatin		
Low dose (30– mg/m^2)	71	45
Intermediate (60–90)	31	55
High dose (100–120)	21	52
Carboplatin	18	50
Cyclophosphamide		
Low dose	355	43
High dose	36	61
Melphalan	541	47
Thiotepa	337	48
Chlorambucil	40	23
Doxorubicin	58	34
Fluorouracil	92	20
Methotrexate	25	20
Hexamethylmelamine	59	34
Vinblastine	20	10
Taxol	124	24[†]
Ifosfamide	40	20[†]
Gemcitabine	38	13

*Previously untreated patients except as noted.
†Most patients heavily pretreated.

The information here is provided as guidance only. Prescribers should always consult the manufacturer's current prescribing information.

247

Patients with residual tumor on CT scan or markedly elevated CA-125 levels have a similar prognosis and may be offered additional platinum-based therapy, non-platinum therapy or experimental treatment. Patients who have a clinical complete response on CT scan with either a normal CA-125 or low level may be candidates for second-look surgery. The role of second-look surgery is controversial even though it clearly offers the most accurate assessment of response to chemotherapy and has important prognostic implications. The role of interval debulking, (ie, a second debulking at the time of second-look surgery) has been advocated by some as having therapeutic utility, although improvement in survival has not been demonstrated [15]. One trial by the EORTC, however, did demonstrate a survival advantage [16], but in the absence of effective second-line therapies, the entire therapeutic utility of second-look surgery remains unproven [17]. For patients who are enrolled in clinical trials and who require second-look, such an approach is reasonable. If aggressive second-line treatment is contemplated, this may also be a reasonable approach.

Treatment of Residual Disease

Patients who at second-look surgery have small-volume residual disease may be candidates for a variety of consolidation therapies. One reasonable approach would be six additional cycles of platinum-based chemotherapy. A second approach, currently experimental, would be treatment with high-dose chemotherapy and peripheral stem cell rescue. This is currently being tested in the intergroup study GOG 164. Studies of conventional chemotherapy have failed to demonstrate a survival benefit for dose intensification of standard therapy. The use of higher doses with stem cell support requires further testing. Several recent editorials have recommended caution with such an approach [18].

Another option for patients with minimal residual disease after second debulking is intraperitoneal chemotherapy. This remains an experimental approach, although there is much preclinical and clinical data to suggest that it is of interest. The ECOG is currently conducting a clinical trial of intraperitoneal floxuridine administered in combination with intraperitoneal cisplatin or carboplatin for women with minimal residual disease.

Salvage Chemotherapy

For patients who have failed initial therapy with either frank progressive disease, positive disease on CT scan after six to eight courses of treatment, or gross disease of more than 2 cm at time of second-look, second line chemotherapy may be an option. Currently, the topoisomerase I inhibitor topotecan is approved by the FDA for this use. In a European trial with 92 evaluable patients in which topotecan was administered in a 5-day schedule, the overall response rate was 16% with acceptable toxicities [19]. A second trial by the New York Gynecologic Oncology Group employed topotecan as a 21-day infusion as second-line therapy with a 43% response rate and acceptable toxicities (Hochster, unpublished). Furthermore, in another European trial, topotecan was slightly more effective than paclitaxel in the second-line setting with response rates of 20% versus 13% [20].

Other commercially available agents may also have modest activity in the second-line setting. These include gemcitabine, etoposide, hexamethylmelamine, 5-fluorouracil plus leucovorin, and doxorubicin. Experimental agents are being tested by the GOG, New York GOG, ECOG, and SWOG.

THERAPEUTIC TRIALS IN OVARIAN CANCER

E9622, ECOG phase II pilot study of prolonged topotecan infusion with cisplatin as first-line treatment of ovarian cancer—first-line therapy for women with suboptimally debulked disease and those with optimal disease who are not candidates for S9619 (see below); this study will test recent observations of substantial activity for infusional topotecan in ovarian cancer.

S9619, phase II trial of intraperitoneal cisplatin and intravenous and intraperitoneal paclitaxel in women with optimally debulked stage III epithelial ovarian carcinoma; this is an intergroup study of the SWOG and ECOG that tests the role of more intensive initial intraperitoneal therapy in women with optimally debulked disease.

E1E97, ECOG phase II study of consolidation therapy with intraperitoneal floxuridine and cisplatin in women with microscopic residual disease following second-look therapy; this tests intraperitoneal consolidation therapy in women in "complete clinical response" with laparotomy or laparoscopy-documented small volume (< 1 cm) disease after induction therapy and/or cytoreduction.

GO164, salvage therapy with paclitaxel plus carboplatin versus salvage therapy with stem cell supported high-dose carboplatin, mitoxantrone, and cyclophosphamide in patients with low-volume ovarian cancer; this is an NCI high-priority intergroup trial led by the GOG, with ECOG and SWOG participating; this study seeks to determine the efficacy of high-dose therapy in women with ovarian cancer who have had a good but not complete clinical response to first-line therapy; patients must have stage III disease, adequate initial staging and debulking, four to six cycles of platinum-based induction therapy, reassessment surgery with debulking, a documented partial response to initial therapy, disease of less than 1 cm at time of reassessment surgery, and agreement by third party to pay for transplant; no patients have been enrolled yet.

S9501, ECOG phase II study of 9-20-S-amino-camptothecin (9-AC) as second-line therapy in advanced ovarian carcinoma; this is a collaborative study of the ECOG and the New York GOG to test a novel topoisomerase-I inhibitor.

E2E96, ECOG phase II clinical trial of perillyl alcohol in the treatment of advanced ovarian cancer; this study tests the utility of the "cytostatic" compound perillyl alcohol, one of a family of monoterpenes in ovarian cancer.

UTERINE CERVICAL CARCINOMA

APPROACH TO TREATMENT
General Principles

Cervix cancer has a biphasic age distribution with peaks in the fourth to fifth decades and in the eighth to ninth decades. It affects nearly 14,000 women annually. Cervix cancer is more common in lower socioeconomic groups and in women who have been sexually active. It is more common in women who have had early first intercourse, multiple sexual partners, and multiple pregnancies. It is less common in women who are nulliparous and in those who are sexually inactive, such as nuns. There is a very close association between infection with specific subtypes of human papillomavirus (specifically types 16 and 18) and the development of cervical cancer and carcinoma in situ. The association with HIV infection is appreciable but not fully defined. Risk factors are listed in Table 15-5.

Screening, Early Detection, and Diagnosis

The Pap smear, or cytologic evaluation of cells obtained from the cervix, is one of the most sensitive, specific, and cost-effective screening test for human cancer. International studies have demonstrated a significant reduction in the death rate from cervix cancer since the introduction of this test. False-negative results are usually related to poor preparation of the smears or inadequate sampling. Combined with the relatively slow rate of development of invasive cervix cancer from the dysplastic lesions of the cervix, an annual Pap smear has a good probability of preventing the development of invasive cancer. The technique for obtaining an adequate smear has been well described [21].

The management of patients with dysplastic lesions of the cervix is complex and beyond the scope of this chapter. Low-grade lesions require careful follow-up, although the majority will regress spontaneously. The management of high-grade lesions is more controversial. Carcinoma in situ has an unacceptable rate of progression to invasive disease and requires either very close follow-up or immediate surgical management. Entry of these patients into chemoprevention studies with novel agents may also be appropriate.

The diagnosis of invasive cervical cancer requires examination of tissue obtained from a cervical biopsy specimen. In the case of an abnormal Pap smear, either a colposcopic biopsy or cone biopsy are adequate. For lesions that can be appreciated visually on speculum examination, a punch biopsy is adequate for diagnosis.

APPROACH TO THE PATIENT WITH EARLY-STAGE DISEASE

Goals of treatment in early-stage disease are cure; goals in late stage disease are to prevent pain, preserve renal function, and prevent disease progression that can result in fistula formation, malodorous discharge, and thromboembolic events. As opposed to carcinoma of the ovary, diagnosis is usually straightforward because the cervix can be visually inspected and easily biopsied. Thus, 75% of cervix cancers are diagnosed at early stages, whereas only 25% of ovarian carcinomas are diagnosed prior to abdominal spread.

Unlike ovarian cancer, the staging for cervix cancer is based on clinical findings (Table 15-6). Optimal examination is conducted under anesthesia. Other tests may be employed, including cervical biopsy, cystoscopy, proctosigmoidoscopy, chest radiography, and CT scan of the abdomen. Thus, unlike ovarian cancer, surgical staging for cervical cancer is not warranted; however, surgical staging is acknowledged to be more accurate.

As with ovarian cancers, precise staging is required because this correlates well with prognosis. Long-term survival rates are 76% for stage I (confined to the cervix), 55% for stage II (local spread to adnexa or upper vagina), 31% for stage III (spread to pelvic sidewalls or lower vagina), and 7% for stage IV (spread beyond the pelvis). Furthermore, accurate staging is the foundation for further approaches to therapy. In addition to clinical staging, a chest roentgenogram is required to rule out pulmonary spread, and a CT scan of the abdomen and pelvis is required to rule out lymph node and liver involvement. The role of nuclear magnetic resonance imaging remains unresolved.

For patients with disease confined to the pelvis, radiation therapy is recommended. Radiation consists of external beam therapy at doses of 5000 to 6000 cGy, followed by brachytherapy with a cesium source to deliver 6500 to 7200 cGy to Point A (the bulkiest portion of the tumor). The addition of chemotherapy to radiation therapy, either concurrently or in the neoadjuvant setting (prior to radiation therapy), is currently being studied and will likely become one new standard of care. Neoadjuvant therapy has consistently failed to demonstrate a clinical benefit. One randomized clinical trial demonstrated that the addition of neoadjuvant chemotherapy to radiation shortened survival.

One early randomized trial conducted by the GOG demonstrated a progression-free survival benefit for patients with stage III cervical carcinoma who were treated with the combination of oral hydroxyurea plus external-beam radiation therapy compared with radiation therapy and the radiation sensitizer misonidazole. A recent trial by the GOG compared standard radiation therapy in combination with either oral hydroxyurea or with concurrent administration of fluorouracil and cisplatin. Preliminary reports suggest a survival benefit for the latter. Thus, concurrent therapy with external beam radiation and chemotherapy appears to be an option for patients with advanced disease.

Early-stage cervical cancer (stage I or IIA) can be treated with radical hysterectomy yielding equivalent results to radiation therapy. Radical hysterectomy includes, in addition to total hysterectomy, en bloc resection of the parametrial connective tissues and the upper vagina, ureteral dissection, and total pelvic lymphadenectomy. The

Table 15-5. Risk Factors for Cervix Cancer

Lower socioeconomic status, underdeveloped countries
First coitus at early age
Multiple sexual partners
Human papillomavirus types 16, 18, 31, 33, 35
Acquired immunodeficiency syndrome—related malignancy
Carcinoma in situ

Table 15-6. Staging and Prognosis of Cervical Cancer

Stage	Characteristics
I	Microscopic or macroscopic disease confined to the cervix
II	Disease confined to the pelvis but not to the pelvic sidewall or to the lower one third of the vagina
III	Disease that has spread to the pelvic sidewall or the lower one third of the vagina or presents with hydronephrosis
IV	Disease that has involved the mucosa of the bladder or rectum or has spread outside the pelvis

Prognosis

Stage	Survival, %
I	76%
II	55%
III	31%
IV	7%

Adapted from Creasman [33].

risks of surgical complications is markedly increased as compared with total hysterectomy.

APPROACH TO THE PATIENT WITH METASTATIC OR RECURRENT DISEASE

For patients with positive para-aortic lymph nodes, therapy is controversial. Treatment of microscopic disease in para-aortic nodes with extended field radiation therapy prolonged survival in one study; however, this does not necessarily imply a clinical benefit for patients with macroscopic involvement. These patients may be considered candidates for treatment of advanced disease; control of the primary lesion is indicated in order to prevent local complications.

Patients who fail local radiation therapy and have no evidence of distant disease may be candidates for pelvic exenteration. This is a morbid procedure that should only be attempted by those with expertise in this area. Partial exenterative procedures (anterior or posterior) may be associated with less morbidity. Reconstructive procedures include construction of continent conduits, creation of a neovagina, and low rectal anastomosis.

Patients who have failed local therapy or present de novo with disease at distant sites (eg, the liver, bone, or lung) are candidates for systemic therapy. The utility of single agents is limited. The activity for selected single agents is shown in Table 15-7.

The GOG conducted a randomized trial of three different doses and schedules of cisplatin [22]. The higher dose (100 mg/m^2) produced higher response rates, but no improvement in duration of response or survival was seen.

The role of combination chemotherapy in cervical cancer is controversial. Although many prefer a cisplatin-based regimen, there is no standard therapy. Most combinations use cisplatin plus bleomycin with one or more additional agents, such as ifosfamide, often employed on an infusional schedule. However, combination chemotherapy has not been shown to be more effective than single-agent therapy and may accrue substantial toxicities. The introduction of ifosfamide and the use of infusional schedules has resulted in an increase in complete responses and high overall response rates [23]. This question is currently being tested by the GOG.

Recent results with the combination of the vitamin A derivative 13-cis-retinoic acid and the biologic response modifier interferon have been reported, and the combination has activity. This remains to be confirmed, but the activity of this combination may be equivalent to more toxic cisplatin-based treatments. Patients may be considered for experimental therapy once the risks and benefits have been fully explained.

Palliation of symptoms may be achieved with local radiotherapy. Surgical resection of late and isolated lung metastases may result in long-term survival in up to 25% of cases. Renal function may be preserved with a percutaneous renal stent; however, prolonged survival or palliation have not been demonstrated with this approach. Adequate pain control may be achieved with opiates, such as protracted-release morphine preparations or fentanyl patches. Patients with fistula formation often present with intractable problems (eg, malodorous discharge, which may be partially controlled with charcoal-impregnated pads) or with infection requiring antibiotic therapy. Cachexia requires dietary counseling and nutritional supplementation.

CLINICAL TRIALS IN ADVANCED CERVICAL CANCER

E1E96, ECOG trial of interleukin-12 with advanced carcinoma of the uterine cervix; based on studies that demonstrate that patients who can mount an immune response to human papillomaviral antigens can clear high-grade cervical dysplasias, this study tests the role of an immunopotentiating agent with concurrent measurements of cell-mediated immunity.

ENDOMETRIAL CARCINOMA

APPROACH TO TREATMENT

General Principles

Cancer of the endometrium is the most common tumor of the female genital tract, accounting for approximately 33,000 cases of cancer annually. Because endometrial carcinoma is usually detected in early stages, this disease accounts for fewer deaths than carcinoma of the ovary. At time of diagnosis 80% of cases fall into Stage I disease, confined to the uterine corpus. This disease is usually easily diagnosed; however, well-differentiated tumors may be difficult to distinguish from endometrial hyperplasia.

Screening, Early Detection, and Diagnosis

Risk factors are described in Table 15-8. Routine screening of asymptomatic, postmenopausal women is probably not warranted. However, women over 40 years of age with abnormal bleeding, massive obesity, or history of endometrial hyperplasia may require

ITable 15-7. Single-Agent Activity in Carcinoma of the Uterine Cervix		
Drug	Patients, n	Response Rate, %
Cisplatin	52	40
Vincristine	44	23
Doxorubicin	78	10
Bleomycin	172	10
Cyclophosphamide	228	14
5-Fluorouracil	348	20
Methotrexate	77	16
Paclitaxel	52	17

Table 15-8. Risk Factors for Endometrial Carcinoma	
Increased risk	Decreased risk
Obesity	Combination oral contraceptives
Nulliparity	
Late menopause	
Estrogen use	
Hypertension	
Diabetes	
Long-term tamoxifen use	
Familial cancer syndrome (Lynch II)	

routine screening because they are at higher risk. The most provocative data on risk for endometrial carcinoma comes from the recent National Surgical Adjuvant Breast and Bowel Project trials in women with breast cancer who received long-term tamoxifen therapy. There was an increased incidence of endometrial cancer among those women receiving tamoxifen, which was likely due to tamoxifen's estrogenic action on uterine tissue. The clinical, pathologic, and molecular characteristics of these tumors are now being analyzed and may offer some clues to the etiology of this disease. Women receiving long-term tamoxifen therapy require closer follow-up, which may indicate the development of a uterine carcinoma.

Among postmenopausal patients, the use of hormone replacement therapy (HRT) is increasing because of salutary effects on bone density and cardiovascular disease. There is some controversy about whether HRT increases the risk of endometrial carcinoma, with most recent studies suggesting that it does not among the general population. However, there does appear to be an increased risk of breast cancer among women with a previous history of or family history of breast cancer. Whether there is an increased risk of cancer among women with a prior history of endometrial cancer is currently being studied in an intergroup trial by the GOG and the ECOG. There is also a familial risk factor for endometrial carcinoma. Endometrial carcinoma is part of the HNPCC or Lynch II familial cancer syndrome (*see* Ovarian Cancer section)

The peak age group for the development of endometrial carcinoma is 60 to 70 years. The disease is associated with obesity and diabetes, making these patients somewhat older and less healthy than other patients with gynecologic malignancies. This accounts for the lesser role played by chemotherapy in the treatment of this disease.

The typical presentation of endometrial carcinoma is postmenopausal bleeding, which occurs in 80% of patients. Other symptoms include vaginal discharge and leukorrhea. Evaluation of postmenopausal bleeding includes fractional dilatation and curettage, with separation of cervical and endometrial specimens. Endometrial carcinoma must be distinguished from atypical hyperplasia. In addition to standard pathology, grading of the tumor is important in the subsequent management.

Staging and Prognosis

Staging of endometrial carcinoma is described in Table 15-9. Factors that adversely affect survival include clear cell, papillary, or adenosquamous histologies; increased grade; increased uterine size; myometrial invasion; positive peritoneal cytology; positive pelvic or paraaortic lymph nodes; or adnexal spread. There is a high percentage of patients with favorable factors; therefore, survival rates in endometrial carcinoma are higher than those of ovarian carcinoma.

Recommendations for Treatment of Endometrial Carcinoma

Treatment recommendations are summarized in Table 15-10. Specific recommendations are as follows.

Treatment of Stage I Disease

For patients with disease confined to the uterine corpus, the treatment is total abdominal hysterectomy and bilateral salpino-oophorectomy (TAH-BSO). The ovaries are removed because of occasional implants on ovaries or fallopian tubes. Suspicious pelvic nodes are also excised; if the frozen section is positive, para-aortic lymph node dissection is indicated. For patients at high risk of recurrence, adjuvant radiation therapy may be given. For patients who are not candidates for surgery, radiation therapy may provide equivalent results.

Treatment of Stage II–III Disease

For patients with gross involvement of the uterine cervix, either a radical hysterectomy or preoperative radiation therapy is indicated, followed by TAH-BSO. For patients with microscopic cervical spread, treatment includes TAH-BSO, followed by postoperative radiation therapy. For patients with spread to other pelvic tissues, treatment includes TAH-BSO, followed by pelvic irradiation.

Table 15-9. Staging and Prognosis of Endometrial Carcinoma

Stage	Characteristics
I	Disease confined to the corpus
IA	Confined to endometrium
IB	Invasion to < half of the myometrium
IC	Invasion to > half of the myometrium
II	Disease involves the corpus and cervix
IIA	Involves the endocervical gland
IIB	Invasion of the cervical stroma
III	Disease confined within the pelvis
IIIA	Invasion of serosa/adnexa or + peritoneal cytology
IIIB	Vaginal metastases
IIIC	+ Pelvic or paraaortic lymph nodes
IV	Advanced disease
IVA	+ Bladder or bowel mucosa
IVB	Distant metastases including abdominal or inguinal nodes

Prognosis

Stage	5-y Survival, %
I	72.3
II	56.4
III	31.5
IV	10.5

Adapted from International Federation of Gynecology and Obstetrics [32].

Table 15-10. Treatment Recommendation by Stage for Endometrial Carcinoma

Stage	Treatment
I, II	TAH-BSO (en bloc)
	Paraaortic lymph node sampling (myometrial invasion only) with or without pelvic node sampling
	Peritoneal washings
	Postoperative radiation therapy for:
	High-risk: positive lymph nodes or adnexal spread
	?Intermediate risk: myometrial invasion >1/2, spread to cervix or vascular space, positive peritoneal washings, grade 3, incomplete surgical staging
	Adjuvant chemotherapy for papillary serous histology
III	Radiation alone or surgery plus radiation therapy
IV	Radiation therapy with or without hormonal therapy with or without chemotherapy

Treatment of Stage IV Disease

For patients with disease that has spread beyond the pelvis, TAH-BSO plus pelvic irradiation may be required to prevent complications from hemorrhage. Systemic therapy would include either hormonal therapy or chemotherapy.

Hormonal Therapy

Hormonal therapy is most successful in patients with a long disease-free interval (≥ 2 y), well-differentiated tumors, and tumors rich in progesterone receptors. There is a high degree of progesterone-receptor positivity in endometrial carcinomas, ranging from 33% to 64% in undifferentiated tumors to 81% to 95% in well-differentiated tumors, with 70% to 72% overall [24]. The definition of "receptor rich" is unclear. Overall, response to hormonal therapy with progestational agents is observed in 71% of patients with positive cytosolic progesterone receptors and in 8% of patients without progesterone-receptor protein [24]. One caveat is that the assay for progesterone receptors must be performed properly and on fresh tissue that has been rapidly frozen at -70°C with appropriate controls.

The most commonly employed agent is the progestational agent megestrol acetate, which is administered at higher doses than are employed for breast cancer (320 mg daily). Progestational agents (eg, 17-hydroxyprogesterone caproate or 6-α-methyl-hydroxy progesterone acetate) are administered by injection. Toxicities with progestational agents are modest, with the most common side effects being fluid retention and weight gain. Response rates initially reported at 35% [25] have not been confirmed in later studies in which response rates in the range of 11% to 16% are more common [26]. The antiestrogenic agent tamoxifen also has activity in endometrial carcinoma that is comparable to that of progestational agents.

Chemotherapy

For patients who have failed treatment with progestational agents or who have life-threatening visceral involvement and are candidates for systemic chemotherapy, treatment with cytotoxic drugs is indicated. Single-agent activity is shown in Table 15-11.

Treatment with combination chemotherapy likely increases response rates over single-agent therapy with doxorubicin; however, the magnitude of the benefits are small, and toxicities are increased. Two-drug therapy with doxorubicin and cisplatin has resulted in

response rates of 33% [27]. A number of studies have employed CAP (cyclophosphamide, doxorubicin, and cisplatin) or cyclophosphamide, doxorubicin, and vinblastine with response rates of 31% to 47%. In a randomized phase II study of cisplatin versus CAP conducted by the North Central Cancer Treatment Group, 3 out of 14 responded to cisplatin and 5 out of 16 to CAP. Only 7% and 12% of patients survived two years, respectively, and the authors concluded that treatment with experimental phase II agents was warranted [28]. These recommendations are still reasonable. Combinations of cytotoxic agents plus progestational agents have been tested and do not appear more active than single agent chemotherapy.

New cytotoxic drugs appear to have activity in patients with advanced endometrial carcinoma. The ECOG trial E3E93 has demonstrated activity for topotecan, administered on a 5-day schedule but with significant toxicities mainly related to myelosuppression. Paclitaxel is also an active agent in the treatment of endometrial carcinoma. Trials studying combinations of these agents with doxorubicin and other conventional agents are in progress. Patients with advanced disease who are otherwise in good health may be candidates for clinical trials using experimental agents once the risk and benefits of such an approach are described to the patient.

CLINICAL TRIALS IN ENDOMETRIAL CARCINOMA

GO137, randomized double-blinded trial of estrogen replacement therapy versus placebo in women with stage I or II endometrial adenocarcinoma; this study, led by the GOG, seeks to determine whether women with endometrial cancer who receive hormone-replacement therapy have a higher risk of secondary cancers.

GESTATIONAL TROPHOBLASTIC NEOPLASM

APPROACH TO TREATMENT

General Principles

Gestational trophoblastic neoplasm (GTN) is a family of related neoplasms encompassing molar pregnancy, placental site trophoblastic tumor, and choriocarcinoma. Molar pregnancy may be classified as complete or partial based on histopathology and karyotype. The incidence of GTN varies widely among different parts of the world, being five times more common in Africa and Asia than Europe or North America. Although uncommon in North America, GTN is an important neoplasm to the medical oncologist because it is highly curable with chemotherapy. Even patients with high-risk disease will enter remission in approximately 70% of cases with modern, aggressive combination chemotherapy regimens.

The etiology of GTN is not well established. Patients with a prior molar pregnancy have a higher risk for developing trophoblastic disease. Risk factors (Table 15-12) for the development of a molar pregnancy include a uterus large for dates, although a molar pregnancy can occur in a normal sized uterus. Time of evacuation may also increase the incidence of malignant sequelae, with evacuations occurring earlier than 10 weeks being less likely to result in a malignancy.

Table 15-11. Single-Agent Activity in Carcinoma of the Endometrium

Agent	Response Rate, %
Cisplatin	42
Doxorubicin	37
Cyclophosphamide	21
5-Fluorouracil	23
Idarubicin	10
Mitoxantrone	5
Carboplatin	28
Megestrol acetate (high dose)	24
Hexamethylmelamine	9
Etoposide (oral)	0
Paclitaxel	36
Ifosfamide	24

Table 15-12. Risk Factors for Gestational Trophoblastic Neoplasms

Mole
  Asia greater risk than North America, Europe
  Age older than 50 y or younger than 16 y
  Prior hydatidiform mole
Postmolar gestational trophoblastic neoplasm
  Increased βhCG
  Increased maternal age
  Uterine enlargement
  Theca lutein cysts

Table 15-13. Prognostic Factors for Gestational Trophoblastic Neoplasm

Nonmetastatic GTN
Low risk
  Serum βhCG < 40,000 mIU/mL
  Duration < 4 mo
  No antecedent term pregnancy, prior chemotherapy, or brain or liver metastases
High risk
  Serum βhCG > 40,000 mIU/mL
  Duration > 4 mo
  Antecedent term pregnancy, failed prior chemotherapy, or brain or liver metastases

Screening and Early Diagnosis

Screening for GTN is not clinically indicated; however, it is important for the obstetrician and the internist who are caring for the patient to be aware of this entity. In women who have had an evacuated molar pregnancy, indications for treatment include failure of the hCG to normalize following evacuation of a molar pregnancy, evidence of locally invasive disease, or evidence of metastatic disease. The most common site of metastatic disease is the lung; in later stages the liver, abdominal cavity and brain can all be involved.

TREATMENT

The clinical features have been reviewed previously [29]. Prognosis and approach to treatment are directly related to the clinical and histopathologic features of this disease (Table 15-13). Clinical features include degree of invasiveness (localized to uterine cavity, invasion into uterine myometrium, or metastatic to lungs or vagina [low risk], or to brain or liver [high risk]), disease-free interval and bulk of tumor (best assessed by levels of the tumor marker human chorionic gonadotropin). The important histopathologic features include the presence of complete or partial mole and the presence of choriocarcinoma.

Methotrexate was first reported to be curative in patients with metastatic choriocarcinoma in 1956 and has remained the mainstay of therapy for low-risk disease. The most commonly employed regimen is the New England Trophoblastic Disease Center regimen (methotrexate 1 mg/kg IM every other day for 8 d, alternating with leucovorin rescue 0.1 mg/kg IM every other day for 8 d). Methotrexate has also been administered as a 12-hour intravenous infusion, orally, and as weekly intramuscular therapy. Cure rates are high with all regimens; however, the accepted regimen is the alternating 8-day treatment. Actinomycin is also an active drug in the treatment of GTN, but it is more toxic than the combination of methotrexate and leucovorin.

Patients with high-risk disease include those with brain or liver metastases, large tumor burdens or high human chorionic gonadotropin levels, prior failed chemotherapy, or long disease intervals. These patients require treatment with combination chemotherapy. Early regimens combined methotrexate and actinomycin with other agents. More recently, etoposide has been incorporated into GTN regimens, with equivalent results but less toxicity [30]. The two most important regimens are EMA/CO (etoposide with methotrexate/leucovorin and actinomycin plus cyclophosphamide with vincristine, each administered on alternate weeks) and EMA/EP, which substitutes etoposide and cisplatin for cyclophosphamide and vincristine. With EMA/CO, poor-risk patients had a survival rate of 84%, and those who had failed prior therapy had a response rate of 74%. In a subsequent series, responses were observed in 76% of chemotherapy-naive, high-risk patients and in 57% of patients who had failed prior treatment [31].

REFERENCES

1. Van Nagell JR, Gallion HH, DePriest PD: Ovarian cancer screening. *Cancer* 1995, 75:2642–2646.

2. 1994 National Institutes of Health Consensus Conference. *Gynecol Oncol* 1994, 55:S173.

3. Takahashi H, Behbakht K, McGovern PE, *et al.*: Mutation analysis of the BRCA1 gene in ovarian cancers. *Cancer Res* 1995, 55:2998–3002.

4. Merajver SD, Pham TM, Caduff RF, *et al.*: Somatic mutations in the BRCA1 gene in sporadic ovarian tumours. *Nat Genet* 1995, 9:439–443.

5. Ford D, Easton DF, Peto J: Estimates of the gene frequency of BRCA1 and its contribution to breast and ovarian cancer incidence. *Am J Hum Genet* 1995, 57:1457–1462.

6. Stratton JF, Gaythier SA, Russell P, *et al.*: Contribution of BRCA1 mutations to ovarian cancer. *N Engl J Med* 1997, 336:1125–1130.

7. Young RC, Walton LA, Ellenberg SS, *et al*: Adjuvant therapy in stage I and stage II epithelial ovarian cancer: results of two prospective randomized trials. *N Engl J Med* 1990, 322:1021–1027.

8. Society of Gynecologic Oncologists: Practice guidelines for gynecologic malignancies. *Oncology* 1997, 12:129–133.

9. American College of Surgeons' Commission on Cancer and the American Cancer Society: The National Cancer Database report on ovarian cancer treatment in United States hospitals. *Cancer* 1996, 78:2236–2246.

10. Alberts DS, Liu PY, Hannigan EV, *et al.*: Intraperitoneal cisplatin plus intravenous cyclophosphamide versus intravenous cisplatin plus intravenous cyclophosphamide for stage III ovarian cancer. *N Engl J Med* 1996, 335:1950–1955.

11. McGuire WP, Hoskins WJ, Brady MF, *et al.*: Cyclosphosphamide and cisplatin compared with paclitaxel and cisplatin in patients with stage III and stage IV ovarian cancer. *N Engl J Med* 1996, 334:1–6.

11a. Muggia FM, Braly PS, Brady MF, *et al.*: Phase III of cisplatin (P) or paclitaxel (T) versus their combination in suboptimal stage III and IV epithelial ovarian cancer (EOC): Gynecologic Oncology Group (GOG) study number 132 [abstract]. *Proc Annu Meet Am Soc Clin Oncol* 1997, 16:A1257.

12. Coleman RL, Bagnell KG, Townley PM: Carboplatin and short-infusion paclitaxel in high-risk and advanced-stage ovarian carcinoma. *Cancer J Sci Am* 1997, 3:246–253.

13. ten Bokkel Huinink WW, van Warmerdam LJC, *et al.*: Phase II study of the combination of carboplatin and paclitaxel in patients with ovarian cancer. *Ann Oncol* 1977, 8:351–354.

14. Eisenhauer EA, Vermorken JB, van Glabbeke M: Predictors of response to subsequent chemotherapy in platinum pretreated ovarian cancer: a multivariate analysis of 704 patients. *Ann Oncol* 1997, 8:963–968.

15. Tuxen MK, Straus G, Lund B, Hansen M: The role of second-look laparotomy in the long-term survival in ovarian cancer. *Ann Oncol* 1997, 8:643–648.

16. van der Burg MEL, van Lent, Kobierska A, *et al.*: Intervention debulking surgery (IDS) does improve survival in advanced epithelial ovarian cancer (EOC): an EORTC Gynecologic Cancer Cooperative Group (GCCG) study. *Proc Am Soc Clin Oncol* 1993, 12:258.

17. van der Burg MEL: More than 20 years second-look surgery in advanced epithelial ovarian cancer: what did we learn [review]. *Ann Oncol* 1997, 8:627–629.

18. Thigpen JT: Dose-intensity in ovarian carcinoma: hold, enough? *J Clin Oncol* 1997, 15:1291–1292.

19. Creemers GJ, Bolis G, Gore M, *et al.*: Topotecan, an active drug in the second-line treatment of epithelial ovarian cancer: results of a large European phase II study. *J Clin Oncol* 1996, 14:3056–3061.

20. ten Bokkel Huinink WW, Gore M, Carmichael J, *et al.*: Topotecan versus paclitaxel for the treatment of recurrent epithelial ovarian cancer. *J Clin Oncol* 1997, 15:2183–2193.

21. Wilkinson EJ: Pap smears and screening for cervical cancer. *Clin Obstet Gynecol* 1990, 33:817–821.

22. Bonomi P, Blessing JA, Stehman FB, *et al.*: Randomized trial of three cisplatin dose schedules in squamous cell carcinoma of the cervix: a Gynecologic Oncology Group study. *J Clin Oncol* 1985, 3:1079–1085.

23. Buxton EJ, Meanwell CA, Hilton C, *et al.*: Combination bleomycin, ifosfamide and cisplatin chemotherapy in cervical cancer. *J Natl Cancer Inst* 1989, 81:359–361.

24. Richardson GS, MacLaughlin DT.: The status of receptors in the management of endometrial cancer. *Clin Obstet Gynecol* 1986, 29:628–637.

25. Reifenstein EC: The treatment of advanced endometrial cancer with hydroxyprogesteron caproate. *Gynecol Oncol* 1974, 2:377–414.

26. Podratz KC, O'Brien PC, Malkasian GD: Effects of progestational agents in the treatment of endometrial carcinoma. *Obstet Gynecol* 1985, 66:106–115.

27. Seltzer V, Vogl SE, Kaplan BH: Adriamycin and cis-diamminedichloroplatinum in the treatment of metastatic endometrial adenocarcinoma. *Gynecol Oncol* 1984, 19:308–313.

28. Edmonson JH, Krook JE, Hilton JF, *et al.*: Randomized phase II studies of cisplatin and a combination of cyclophosphamide-doxorubicin-cisplatin (CAP) in patients with progestin-refractory advanced endometrial carcinoma. *Gynecol Oncol* 1987, 28:20–24.

29. Berkowitz RS, Goldstein DP: Gestational trophoblastic diseases. *Semin Oncol* 1989, 16:410–416.

30. Newlands ES, Bagshawe KD, Begent RJH, *et al.*: Developments in chemotherapy for medium- and high-risk patients with gestational trophoblastic tumors (1979-1984). *Br J Obstet Gynecol* 1986, 93:63–69.

31. Bolis G, Bonazzi C, Landoni F, *et al.* EMA/CO regimen in high-risk gestatational trophoblastic tumor. *Gynecol Oncol* 1988, 31:439–444.

32. International Federation of Gynecology and Obstetrics: Annual report on the results of treatment in gynecologic cancer. *Int J Gynecol Obstet* 1989, 28:189–190.

33. Creasman WT: New gynecologic cancer staging. *Gynecol Oncol* 1995, 55:157–158.

PLATINUM COMPOUND FOR SUBOPTIMAL OVARIAN CARCINOMA

Chemotherapy for advanced suboptimally debulked (> 1 cm) or metastatic ovarian carcinoma is based on the combination of paclitaxel and a platinum compound. Cisplatin forms DNA adducts composed of intrastrand cross-links that act much in the same way as classic alkylating agents, preventing DNA transcription and synthesis and causing DNA strand breaks. Carboplatin is a cisplatin analogue with a different toxicity profile and different pharmacokinetic profile, but carboplatin also forms platinum adducts.

Paclitaxel is a natural product of the Western yew, which has a complex biochemical structure. Paclitaxel inhibits depolymerization of tubulin, a unique mechanism of action for a chemotherapeutic agent. Paclitaxel was introduced into front-line therapy based on excellent clinical activity in the second-line setting. In the Gynecologic Oncology Group study GOG 111, paclitaxel plus cisplatin was compared with cyclophosphamide plus cisplatin and demonstrated a survival advantage.

A recent preliminary report by the GOG, in which single-agent cisplatin, single-agent paclitaxel, and the combination of the two were compared, revealed that combination therapy and single-agent cisplatin (given at a higher dose than was administered in the combination) offered equivalent survival, and both were better than single-agent paclitaxel. Furthermore, recent small phase II trials have demonstrated comparable survivals for combinations of paclitaxel and carboplatin. Thus, either combination would be accepted as a reasonable first-line therapy for women with advanced ovarian carcinoma.

INDICATIONS

Advanced (Stage III-IV) ovarian carcinoma; some patients with stage IC or II disease may be treated with this regimen

SPECIAL PRECAUTIONS

Patients must have adequate white blood cell and platelet counts and must not be dehydrated prior to initiating treatment; myelosuppression was more profound when paclitaxel was administered with cisplatin; ketoconazole may inhibit paclitaxel metabolism; caution should be employed when administering paclitaxel with these agents; cisplatin should be discontinued with evidence of nephrotoxicity, ototoxicity or neurotoxicity.

DRUG INTERACTIONS

Cisplatin: may potentiate renal effects of nephrotoxic compounds such as aminoglycoside

TOXICITIES

Paclitaxel: acute hypersensitivity reaction (with wheezing, shortness of breath, urticaria, and hypotension) occurred in 2% of patients receiving paclitaxel; alopecia, nausea and vomiting, profound granulocytopenia, myelosuppression, cardiac conduction abnormalities requiring a pacemaker, hypotension, bradycardia, peripheral neuropathy, arthralgias/myalgias, diarrhea, mucositis; **Cisplatin:** nephrotoxicity, ototoxicity, neurotoxicity, emesis, Coombs positive hemolytic anemia, electrolyte abnormalities; **Carboplatin:** granulocytopenia, thrombocytopenia, nausea, vomiting

RECENT EXPERIENCE AND RESPONSE RATES

Study	Regimen	Evaluable Patients, n	Response Rate, %	Median PFS, mo	Median OS, mo
McGuire et al. N Engl J Med 1996, 334:1	Paclitaxel 135 mg/m^2 (24-h infusion); Cisplatin 75 mg/m^2	184	73	18.0	38.0
Muggia et al. Proc ASCO 1997, 18:57	Cisplatin 100 mg/m^2	200	74	16.4	30.2
Muggia et al. Proc ASCO 1997, 18:57	Paclitaxel 200 mg/m^2	213	46	11.4	26.0
Muggia et al. Proc ASCO 1997, 18:57	Paclitaxel 135 mg/m^2; Cisplatin 75 mg/m^2	202	72	14.1	26.6
Coleman et al. Cancer J Sci Am 1997, 3:246	Paclitaxel 175 mg/m^2 (3-h infusion); Carboplatin AUC 7-7.5	22	84	—	—
ten Bokkel Huinink et al. Ann Oncol 1997, 8:351	Paclitaxel 200 mg/m^2 (3-h infusion); Carboplatin 550 mg/m^2	21	100	—	—
Schink, 1998*	Paclitaxel 150 mg/m^2 (3-h infusion); Carboplatin AUC 5.0	44	*	*	*

* Study is not yet complete.
AUC—area under the curve; OS—overall survival; PFS—progression-free survival.

PACLITAXEL PLUS A PLATINUM COMPOUND FOR SUBOPTIMAL OVARIAN CARCINOMA (Continued)

DOSAGE AND SCHEDULING

Cisplatin: 75–100 mg/m^2 over 1–2 h; patients require at least 2 L prehydration with normal saline or D51/2NS intravenously with good urine output prior to drug administration; antiemetic precautions can include granisetron 2 mg PO, dexamethasone 20 mg IV, and/or prochlorprazine 10 mg IV; lorazepam 1 mg IV or PO can be administered for refractory patients

Paclitaxel: 135–200 mg/m^2 can be administered as a 3-h infusion in the outpatient setting or as a 24-h infusion in the inpatient setting; premedication to prevent an allergic reaction should be administered, including cimetidine 300 mg IV, Benadryl (diphenhydramine) 50 mg IV, and Decadron 20 mg PO at 6 h and 12 h prior to administration of paclitaxel; appropriate antiemesis should be instituted because 50% of patients will develop nausea or vomiting; patients should be monitored closely at the initiation of paclitaxel therapy, and the infusion should be discontinued for any sign of an allergic reaction (especially flushing or dyspnea)

Carboplatin: can be dosed at 500–550 mg/m^2 or at 5.0–7.5 area under the curve (AUC), using the Calvert or other convenient formula to calculate the desired area under the curve; unlike cisplatin, the drug does not require prehydration and can be given in the outpatient setting over 15 min; treatment usually continues for 4–8 cycles; CBC, differential, platelet count, CA-125, BUN, and creatinine should be monitored prior to each cycle; failure of CA-125 to decrease suggests emerging resistance to drug treatment

NURSING INTERVENTIONS

Combined blood count, including platelets, should be checked prior to administering drugs; patients should be pretreated with adequate antiemetic therapy; renal function should be monitored; patients should be monitored for signs of neurotoxicity

PATIENT ASSESSMENT

Patients should be questioned regarding their fertility status; paclitaxel may be mutagenic and/or teratogenic

PATIENT INFORMATION

Patients should be cautioned regarding the development of fevers 8–14 d after administration of paclitaxel; patients should be informed about alopecia and cautioned regarding the hypersensitivity reactions, thrombocytopenia, and neutropenia

ADMINISTRATION NOTES

Paclitaxel is supplied in 30-mg/5-mL vials; paclitaxel should be diluted in 0.9% sodium chloride for injection or 5% dextrose solution USP at 0.3–1.2 mg/mL; because the vehicle reacts with polyvinyl chloride (PVC), administration of paclitaxel requires non-PVC bottles and polyethylene-lined tubing

COSTS

The cost to the pharmacist for each infusion of paclitaxel will probably be > $1000; the cost to the pharmacist for an infusion of cisplatin is ~$450.

INTRAPERITONEAL THERAPY FOR OPTIMALLY DEBULKED OVARIAN CANCER

Therapy for optimally debulked (< 1 cm) ovarian cancer may differ from that of suboptimal disease. A recent intergroup study has demonstrated a survival benefit for women receiving intraperitoneal therapy compared with intravenous therapy. Whether the benefits of intensified therapy delivered in this manner will outweigh the inconvenience of placing an intraperitoneal port and the cumbersome administration with uncertain distribution of the drug remains to be demonstrated. Nevertheless, the impressive improvement in survival observed (49 mo vs 41 mo) is important.

DOSAGE AND SCHEDULING

Cyclophosphamide 600 mg/m^2 IV d 1
Cisplatin mg/m^2 in 2 L of normal saline administered rapidly intraperitoneally
Intraperitoneal therapy is warmed to body temperature prior to infusion and instilled rapidly through an intraperitoneal Tenckhoff or Drum catheter or Portacath; simultaneously, patients receive 1 L of normal saline with 3 g magnesium sulfate and 40 g mannitol IV.
Courses are repeated every 3 wk for 6 cycles; doses were held or modified for azotemia, neuropathy, or myelosuppression

INDICATIONS

Optimally debulked (< 1 cm) stage III ovarian carcinoma

SPECIAL PRECAUTIONS

Patients must have adequate white blood cell and platelet counts and must not be dehydrated prior to initiating treatment; patients must have adequate renal function; the catheter must be functioning properly with no evidence of bowel perforation; treatment should be stopped for refractory abdominal pain

DRUG INTERACTIONS

Cisplatin: may potentiate renal effects of nephrotoxic compounds such as aminoglycoside

TOXICITIES

Cisplatin: nephrotoxicity, ototoxicity, neurotoxicity, emesis, Coombs positive hemolytic anemia, electrolyte abnormalities; **Cyclophosphamide:** granulocytopenia, thrombocytopenia, nausea, vomiting, hemorrhagic cystitis, pneumonitis, alopecia

NURSING INTERVENTIONS

Combined blood count, including platelets, should be checked prior to administering drugs; patients should be pretreated with adequate antiemetic therapy; renal function should be monitored; patients should be monitored for signs of neurotoxicity

PATIENT ASSESSMENT

Patients should be questioned regarding their fertility status, although it is unlikely that patients with ovarian cancer will be pregnant; cyclophosphamide may be mutagenic and/or teratogenic

PATIENT INFORMATION

Patients should be cautioned regarding the development of fevers 8–14 d after administration of chemotherapy; patients should be informed about alopecia and cautioned regarding the potential for development of acute leukemia in patients treated with alkylating agents

ADMINISTRATION NOTES

The intraperitoneal solution should be prewarmed prior to administration; the bag should be checked to ensure that the solution is running into the peritoneal cavity freely; the fluid does not need to be drained

COST

The cost to the pharmacist for the cyclophosphamide is ~$50; the cost to the pharmacist for an infusion of cisplatin is ~$450.

MEGACE FOR ADVANCED ENDOMETRIAL CARCINOMA

The mainstay of therapy for endometrial carcinomas are progestational agents. Megace (megestrol acetate) is available orally.

The precise mechanism of action is unknown. Progestins promote the differentiation and maintenance of endometrial tissues. In endometrial cancer, they probably act as negative growth regulators acting either directly or in concert with other growth factors, such as transforming growth factor β, which inhibits cell growth.

RECENT EXPERIENCES AND RESPONSE RATES

Study	Overall Response Rate ,%
Reifenstein *et al. Gynecol Oncol* 1974, 2:377	35
Podratz *et al. Obstet Gynecol* 1985, 66:106	11

DOSAGE AND SCHEDULING

Megace 40–80 mg/d PO
Liver function tests should be checked prior to treatment

INDICATIONS

Advanced endometrial and breast cancer

ELIGIBILITY AND EXCLUSIONS

Eligibility: advanced or refractory endometrial cancer; **Exclusions:** none

SPECIAL PRECAUTIONS

Reduce dose in patients with pre-existing liver disease; patients with congestive heart failure should be monitored carefully

DRUG INTERACTIONS

None

TOXICITIES

Fluid retention, weight gain, liver function abnormalities (uncommon), thromboembolic phenomena (rare)

NURSING INTERVENTIONS

None

PATIENT INFORMATION

Patients should be warned about possible fluid retention; Megace may be teratogenic

ADMINISTRATION

Available as 20-mg or 40-mg tablets.

Tumors of the central nervous system (CNS) occupy a unique position within the spectrum of human cancer, and the management of patients with primary neoplasms of the CNS presents a formidable challenge to clinicians involved in the care of cancer patients. Primary brain tumors represent approximately 2% of all adult cancers in the United States, and the American Cancer Society predicted that 17,200 new primary brain tumors would be diagnosed in 1995 [1]. Brain tumors are a heterogeneous group of neoplasms that can arise from any of the constituent elements of the CNS, including neurons, glia, endothelia, meninges, and the biologic behavior of a given brain tumor is predicated on its cells of origin. The most common primary brain tumors in adults are glial neoplasms; these account for approximately 65% of all primary CNS tumors. Important advances during the past 15 years in the fields of neuroimaging, neurosurgery, and neuropathology have greatly increased the accuracy of detection of brain tumors. Similar advances in the neurosciences have increased understanding of brain tumor neurobiology. Over that same interval, the development of chemotherapeutic agents with improved CNS penetration and the development of improved drug delivery systems have focused interest on the role of chemotherapy in the treatment of brain tumors. Despite these advances, the prognosis for patients with primary brain tumors has not improved significantly. New and promising protocols continue to be developed, however, and a review of the latest treatment strategies for patients with brain tumors is especially pertinent.

Glial cells, such as astrocytes, oligodendrocytes, and ependymocytes, are the support cells of the CNS. They perform important nutritive, metabolic, and electrophysiologic functions that are prerequisite for normal neuronal activity. Normal glial cells have a low rate of division except in response to brain injury. When these cells become malignant, their rate of proliferation increases markedly, and they can spread rapidly throughout the brain. Gliomas can originate from any cell of glial origin and include astrocytic neoplasms, such as astrocytomas and anaplastic astrocytomas, arising from astrocytes, oligodendrogliomas arising from oligodendrocytes, and ependymomas and choroid plexus papillomas arising from ependymocytes. The cell of origin of the glioblastoma, the most primitive and malignant of the gliomas, is not always clear. Evidence points to an astrocytic origin in most cases. In the usual sense, however, gliomas include only astrocytomas, anaplastic astrocytomas, and glioblastomas because these tumors constitute approximately 90% to 96% of all glial neoplasms. Gliomas exhibit characteristic age-specific incidence patterns. Both astrocytomas and glioblastomas have small peaks in incidence during childhood followed by a steady rise in incidence until larger adult peaks are reached in the fifth and sixth decades [2]. There is a slight male predominance without racial predilections in patients with gliomas.

ETIOLOGY AND RISK FACTORS

The environmental and genetic factors that may lead to the development of gliomas are incompletely understood. There is substantial evidence that previous cranial irradiation increases the incidence of malignant gliomas after a latent period of from 3 to 30 years [3]. Children are most vulnerable to the effects of ionizing radiation on the CNS. Head trauma has been cited, but most studies have failed to demonstrate an increased incidence of gliomas following head injury. The concurrence of gliomas with progressive multifocal leukoencephalopathy and multiple sclerosis has led to unconfirmed speculation regarding the role of demyelination in the genesis of gliomas. Smoking, alcohol consumption, and dietary patterns have not been shown to be risk factors for gliomas. Thirty-three percent of patients with glioblastoma have a family history of cancer, but instances of familial gliomas are rare. Certain genetic disorders are clearly associated with the occurrence of glial neoplasms. Patients with tuberous sclerosis, Turcot's syndrome, and the peripheral form of neurofibromatosis (NF, type I) are predisposed to subependymal astrocytomas, glioblastomas or medulloblastomas, and anterior optic nerve gliomas. The genetic basis of Turcot's syndrome has been identified. The association between glioblastoma and multiple colorectal adenomas in Turcot's syndrome results from a germ line mutation in a mismatch-repair gene, whereas patients with Turcot's syndrome and a germ line mutation in the adenomatous polyposis coli (APC) gene develop a different primary brain tumor, medulloblastoma, in association with multiple colonic adenomas [4]. The gene for NF I has also been identified and maps to chromosome 17q11.2. Its protein product, neurofibromin, has a putative role in a p21 ras-GTP signal transduction pathway that may be important for cell cycle regulation [5].

Vogelstein and Kinzler's [6] pioneering work with colorectal neoplasia has yielded the current paradigm of cancer as a multistep genetic disease resulting from a sequence of "hits" or alterations in the DNA sequence of critical cell cycle regulatory genes. In colon cancer, increasingly anaplastic clones of tumor cells are generated by a series of well-defined genetic mutations. Although the cause of gliomas is not known with similar precision, the molecular biology of gliomas also suggests clues regarding their pathogenesis. Specific oncogenes, genes that promote neoplastic cell transformation by encoding growth factors, growth factor receptors, intracellular transducers, or nuclear transcription factors, have been identified in astrocytomas. These include a homologue of c-erbB, which encodes the epidermal growth factor receptor (EGFR), and c-sis, which encodes the B-subunit of platelet-derived growth factor. Tumor suppressor genes, genes that suppress cell growth, are also believed to be important in glioma ontogeny. The two best-characterized tumor suppressor genes in human cancers, Rb and p53, are located on chromosomes 13 and 17. Deletion loci on chromosomes 13 and 17 as well as on chromosomes 9, 10, and 22 have been identified in gliomas; inactivation of tumor suppressor genes at these loci, either by deletion or by unmasking of a mutant allele, may be important in the pathogenesis of glial neoplasms. Although a specific sequence of genetic alterations leading to the anaplastic progression of gliomas has not yet been determined, it is clear that mutations accumulate with greater frequency in the genome of high-grade gliomas than low-grade gliomas. Most evidence points to an important role for the p53 tumor suppressor gene early in the ontogeny of gliomas. Mutations of p53 can be found in all grades of astrocytomas, whereas certain genetic mutations, such as loss of chromosome 10 or EGFR gene amplification, are largely restricted to high-grade gliomas [7]. Further, clonal expansion of cells expressing the p53 mutation has been shown to be associated with tumor progression [8]. Rb deletion may be a second important step in astrocytoma progression because recent work has demonstrated that Rb is inactivated in high-grade, but not low-grade, gliomas [9]. Finally, amplification of the EGFR oncogene, which occurs with the greatest frequency in glioblastoma and is less frequent in anaplastic astrocytoma and astrocytoma, may be a critical third genetic hit and one that may have prognostic significance. Some studies have shown than EGFR gene amplification correlates with shorter survival for patients with malignant gliomas, although the certainty of this correlation is not firmly established [10].

Patients with gliomas may develop a variety of clinical symptoms, which range from insidiously evolving cognitive impairment to the apoplectic onset of status epilepticus. In general, patients present with a change in mental function, headaches, seizures, focal neurologic signs such as hemiparesis or aphasia, or evidence of increased intracranial pressure. In such patients, and increasingly in asymptomatic patients, computed tomography (CT) and magnetic resonance imaging (MRI) of the brain provide sensitive, accurate detection of the tumor mass. The diagnosis of a glioma, as with other tumors, is established by surgical resection or biopsy and histopathologic examination.

GRADING AND PROGNOSIS

Identifying those factors that have an impact on survival is critical for determining the appropriate treatment and for counseling a given patient. Over the past 15 years, multiinstitutional, randomized clinical trials, including those conducted by the Brain Tumor Study Group (BTSG) and the Radiation Therapy Oncology Group–Eastern Cooperative Oncology Group (RTOG-ECOG), and other large retrospective surveys have established several factors as predictive of survival in patients with gliomas [11,12]. These factors can be divided into clinical, pathologic, and treatment categories.

The clinical factors that are of prognostic significance in patients with gliomas include age at the time of diagnosis, performance status, and seizures. Survival is longer for patients who are less than 40 at the time of diagnosis, patients who initially have a high performance status, and possibly for patients who present with seizures [11,12]. Performance status is rated using the Karnofsky Scoring System, a clinical grading scale that is based on the patient's ability to perform activities of daily living. Scores range from 10 to 100, and patients with normal or near-normal scores (80–100) have an improved prognosis.

The most important prognostic factor in predicting outcome for patients with glial neoplasms is the histopathologic appearance of the tumor. Multiple grading systems have been employed by neuropathologists in evaluating gliomas, and this has led to some confusion in determining which histologic features are most predictive of survival in patients with gliomas. The two most frequently employed grading systems are the three-tier system, such as those proposed by the World Health Organization (WHO) and Burger and Rubenstein [13], which divides astrocytic neoplasms into astrocytomas, anaplastic astrocytomas, and glioblastoma multiforme, and the Kernohan system [14], which grades astrocytomas from grade I through IV, grade IV astrocytomas being the most malignant. Kernohan grades I and II astrocytoma roughly correspond with the WHO designation of astrocytoma, whereas grades III and IV correspond with the classifications anaplastic astrocytoma and glioblastoma (Table 16-1). Low-grade (I–II) astrocytomas are better differentiated and show less evidence of cytologic atypia than high-grade astrocytomas (III–IV), which are more poorly differentiated and which show increasing evidence of such anaplastic features as nuclear atypism, mitoses, endothelial proliferation, or coagulative necrosis. Regardless of which grading system is employed, the presence of coagulative necrosis is the single histologic feature most predictive of survival [13]. Patients with astrocytomas containing necrosis on biopsy or resection have a median survival of 8 to 10 months; patients with anaplastic astrocytomas survive on average 18 to 24 months. Patients with astrocytomas lacking anaplastic features have a median survival of 5 to 7 years. High-grade astrocytomas are often called malignant gliomas and low-grade astrocytomas benign based on the degree of cellular differentiation these tumors display histologically. As can be seen from the survival data given, however, even low-grade astrocytomas behave in a clinically malignant fashion, regardless of their histopathologic appearance.

An inherent limitation in the histopathologic examination of gliomas, beyond the lack of consensus regarding grading systems, is that the tissue sampled may not be representative of the tumor. The histology of the gliomas can vary significantly within the boundaries of the tumor, and because brain resections or biopsy specimens are often limited so as to preserve neurologic function, the subsequent pathologic diagnosis may underestimate the actual degree of malignancy. Mention should also be made of two histologic variants, pilocystic astrocytomas and subependymal giant cell astrocytomas, whose biologic behavior is distinct from other astrocytomas. Pilocystic astrocytomas occur primarily in children or young adults, most frequently are located in the cerebellum, and have 20-year survival rates in excess of 75% [15]. Subependymal giant cell astrocytomas occur typically in patients with tuberous sclerosis, are periventricular in location, and are also associated with long-term survival following surgery. These two histologic variants are distinguished clinically and pathologically from other astrocytomas, and they should be regarded as separate entities when determining the treatment strategies for patients with gliomas.

The location of the glioma within the neuraxis is also important in predicting survival. The topography of a tumor is often closely related to its clinical behavior. For example, as many as 70% of cerebellar gliomas are pilocystic astrocytomas and are associated, as noted previously, with excellent 25-year survival rates. Even for cerebellar astrocytomas with anaplastic features, long-term survival rates are improved over patients with gliomas at other sites. In contrast, patients with localized low-grade gliomas of the brain stem have only a 50% chance of survival at 3 years [16]. The distinction between low-grade and high-grade gliomas remains critical, however, because tumor histology is predictive of survival independent of tumor location. In the series of localized brain stem gliomas just described, 3-year survival for patients with high-grade tumors was less than 10%.

Table 16-1. Histologic Classification of Gliomas

Kernohan classification	Three-Tier Classification	Median Survival
Grade I, II	Astrocytoma	5–7 y
Grade III	Anaplastic astrocytoma	18–24 mo
Grade IV	Glioblastoma multiforme	8–10 mo

Table 16-2. Prognostic Factors

Prognostic Factor	Increased Survival
Age	Age less than 40 y at diagnosis
Performance status	High performance status
Histology	Low-grade glioma
Location	Cerebellar glioma
Treatment	Postoperative radiation

Postoperative ionizing radiation is the treatment factor most important in predicting survival for patients with high-grade gliomas (Table 16-2). A BTSG trial randomizing patients with grade III and IV astrocytomas to treatment with surgery alone and treatment with surgery plus radiation showed that median survival was more than doubled from 14 to 36 weeks by the addition of radiation to surgery [11]. Similar results were recorded by the Scandinavian Glioblastoma Study Group (SGSG) with median survival increased from 5.2 months to 10.8 months by the addition of postoperative radiation. The extent of surgical resection may have an impact on survival. Some investigators have reported that survival is increased in patients who undergo extensive tumor resection at the time of diagnosis [17]. The prognostic significance of adjuvant chemotherapy for high-grade gliomas and radiation therapy for low-grade gliomas has not yet been determined. The impact of these and other treatment strategies on survival is discussed in the following section.

PRIMARY DISEASE THERAPY

Gliomas, similar to other CNS malignancies, are unique among human cancers. Gliomas have important anatomic and biologic characteristics that distinguish them from cancers of other organ systems. These characteristics have a great impact on the clinical behavior and treatment response of gliomas, and their significance should be well understood by clinicians involved in treatment of patients with glial neoplasms. They include the presence of the blood–brain barrier; the absence of conventional draining lymphatics; confinement in a fixed volume by a nondistensible skull; a partially privileged immunologic state; and a propensity for local, nonmetastatic growth.

The blood–brain barrier is a selectively permeable barrier between the plasma and the brain interstitium formed by specialized cerebral endothelial cells. Although the endothelia of extracerebral vessels permit essentially free passage of macromolecules into parenchymal tissues, the tight junctions of cerebral endothelia markedly limit the entry into the brain of molecules that are water soluble, ionized, or greater than 200 daltons. Although the new cerebral vessels that proliferate within the tumor bed often have an incomplete or inefficient blood–brain barrier the blood–brain barrier continues to limit significantly the penetration of chemotherapeutic drugs into glial tumors. Conversely, because endothelia supplying the glioma are in many cases abnormally permeable, some passage of plasma proteins into the brain interstitium occurs, and this leads to the development of vasogenic edema. The absence of conventional draining lymphatics accelerates edema formation. Because the cranial cavity has a restricted volume, increases in peritumoral edema and the tumor mass itself can result in deleterious increases in intracranial pressure. Fortunately, vasogenic edema responds well to treatment with corticosteroids. Corticosteroids are a major adjunct in the management of patients with gliomas, and their dose should be carefully titrated to maximize the reduction in morbidity from increased intracranial pressure and minimize the complications of prolonged corticosteroid use.

The incidence of seizures in patients with gliomas reaches 60% in some series, and therefore the prophylactic use of anticonvulsants is recommended [18]. Treatment usually is initiated with phenytoin (Dilantin) at a dose of 5 to 7 mg/kg/d and drug levels should be maintained in the therapeutic range, which is 10 to 20 µg/mL in most laboratories. Carbamazepine (Tegretol), phenobarbital, or valproic acid can also be used for prophylaxis against secondary generalized seizures. The incidence of deep vein thrombosis ranges from 40% to 45% in patients with high-grade gliomas; therefore

treatment with anticoagulants is often required. The prevention of pulmonary embolus has traditionally been accomplished by the use of infrarenal inferior vena cava (IVC) filter because of the fear of iatrogenic intracerebral hemorrhage in patients with brain tumors. A retrospective report found, however, that the complications from IVC filters in patients who are not anticoagulated is unacceptably high, reaching 62%, whereas the incidence of anticoagulant-associated intracerebral hemorrhage in patients with high-grade gliomas is no higher, approximately 2%, than in patients not receiving the anticoagulants [19]. Anticoagulants can be safely used in conjunction with IVC filters for the treatment of deep vein thrombosis and the prevention of pulmonary embolism in patients with gliomas, provided that anticoagulants effects are assiduously monitored.

Although the anatomic and biologic characteristics of glial neoplasms pose special problems for clinicians treating patients with gliomas, they also afford potential advantages. Because gliomas remain localized and rarely metastasize, involvement of other vital organ systems almost never occurs. Patients seldom suffer the systemic complications seen frequently with other cancers. The blood–brain barrier, as stated earlier, is abnormally permeable at the site of the tumor. As a result, it limits the penetration of chemotherapeutic drugs into normal brain tissue far more efficiently than into the tumor itself, and significantly higher doses of chemotherapy can be achieved in the tumor than in the adjacent brain parenchyma. Finally, although gliomas are immunologically privileged tumors, this privileged status makes them potentially susceptible to innovative immunologic therapies.

The primary therapies used in the treatment of gliomas are surgery, radiation, and chemotherapy. Brachytherapy may be a potentially useful adjunct therapy. Immunotherapy and gene therapy offer promise for the future but thus far have not proven to be clinically beneficial. Because high-grade gliomas and low-grade gliomas have such distinct natural histories, it is most appropriate to consider their management separately.

HIGH-GRADE GLIOMAS

Surgery is the primary therapy for patients with high-grade gliomas. High-grade gliomas are infiltrative tumors with indistinct margins, and they inevitably involve adjacent normal parenchyma. Although complete resection is not possible, most neurosurgeons favor subtotal resection of the tumor at the time of diagnosis. Subtotal resection improves diagnostic accuracy by providing sufficient tissue for histologic examination, relieves mass effect, and often improves performance status. Furthermore, several clinical trials have shown survival is increased in patients who undergo extensive surgical resection at the time of presentation [17,20]. Nonetheless, criticism regarding selection bias in these trials has been raised, and the benefit of subtotal resection over stereotactic biopsy for patients with newly diagnosed gliomas has not been definitely established.

Radiation following surgery is standard primary therapy for patients with high-grade gliomas. The value of postoperative radiation therapy has been proven by multiple large clinical trials [11,12,17]. Radiation improves or stabilizes neurologic function in approximately 90% of patients. Median survival, as stated previously, is more than doubled for patients receiving postoperative radiation therapy when compared with patients treated with supportive therapy following surgery.

Whole-brain irradiation is no longer considered mandatory for high-grade gliomas [21]. Studies have demonstrated that tumor extent on CT scan correlates well with the pathologic extent of glioblastomas at autopsy with a margin of 2 cm. Conventional radiotherapy now, therefore, includes the tumor and a 2- to 3-cm margin around the limits of peritumoral edema, as demonstrated on CT or MRI, in the radiation field. This approach minimizes damage to the adjacent normal parenchyma.

Studies have determined that the optimal dosing schedule for patients with high-grade gliomas is a total dose of approximately 6000 rad delivered in 172 to 200 rad fractions [11,17]. Larger total doses or the same total dose delivered in fewer, larger fractions result in an unacceptably high incidence of radionecrosis, a progressive late effect of radiation that begins from months to several years following radiotherapy and that results from damage to slowly dividing oligodendroglia and endothelia. Fewer fractions with larger fractionated doses also potentiate the acute effects of radiation, such as cerebral edema, scalp and cranial soft tissue irritation, and hair loss. Hyperfractionation, the use of two to three daily fractions that are smaller than conventional fractions, has not been shown to improve survival over conventional daily fractionation.

In contrast to radiotherapy, no standard chemotherapy has been established for the treatment of high-grade gliomas. The nitrosureas, BCNU, CCNU, and methyl-CCNU, are highly lipophilic chemotherapeutic agents specifically synthesized with characteristics to maximize blood–brain barrier penetration and are the drugs most frequently employed. Virtually every chemotherapeutic drug used to treat systemic malignancies has been used to treat high-grade gliomas, either as a single agent or in combination [22]. Drugs have been delivered by bolus or continuous IV infusion, intraarterial bolus, and direct topical application to tumor.

Chemotherapy typically is administered as adjuvant treatment after surgery either during radiotherapy or following the completion of radiotherapy. A survival benefit from adjuvant chemotherapy for patients with high-grade gliomas has not been unequivocally demonstrated. Studies comparing single-agent or combination chemotherapy in addition to radiotherapy with radiotherapy alone have shown either a limited beneficial effect or no beneficial effect of chemotherapy [11,12,17]. A metaanalysis of 16 large, prospective, randomized chemotherapeutic trials for high-grade gliomas involving more than 3000 patients compared the survival rates of patients who received radiation alone with those who received radiation and adjuvant chemotherapy [23]. Median survival in patients treated with radiation alone was 9.4 months; median survival was 12.6 months in patients treated with radiation and adjuvant chemotherapy. The authors concluded that "chemotherapy is advantageous for patients with malignant gliomas" [23]. However, questions concerning which subgroup of patients benefit the most from chemotherapy, which chemotherapeutic agent or agents are most effective, and what route of drug delivery is best remain unanswered, and the value of adjuvant chemotherapy remains unclear.

Important arguments against the use of adjuvant chemotherapy can be made. Adjuvant chemotherapy, as noted previously, is administered either concurrent with radiation or following the completion of radiation. Radiotherapy, in the process of reducing tumor volume, actively destroys the vascular supply to much of the tumor bed. Drug delivery to the tumor, which is already impaired by the presence of the blood–brain barrier, is further limited. Because most chemotherapeutic agents are given as a bolus infusion and many have short half-lives, the possibility of delivering therapeutic concentrations of chemotherapy to the tumor is markedly decreased in the setting of the atretic vascular supply produced by radiotherapy. Laboratory studies have demonstrated that sublethal doses of chemotherapeutic agents accelerate the development of resistant cell lines in culture, and therefore the use of adjuvant chemotherapy during or after radiotherapy potentially promotes tumor resistance to chemotherapy. In addition, radiotherapy reduces the growth fraction—the percentage of cells either synthesizing DNA or actively cycling—of high-grade gliomas. Because almost all chemotherapeutic agents are effective at killing only dividing, or soon to be dividing, cells and because the growth fraction of high-grade gliomas is low before treatment begins, radiotherapy potentially decreases the already limited effectiveness of chemotherapeutic agents when it is delivered before or during chemotherapy.

A promising and innovative chemotherapeutic strategy designed to minimize the inherent limitations of drug delivery to glial tumors and to circumvent the potential problems of chemotherapy when used as adjuvant treatment has been developed by investigators at the University of Pittsburgh Cancer Institute and the John Hopkins Oncology Center. This protocol administers BCNU and cisplatin chemotherapy as primary therapy for high-grade gliomas following surgery and before radiation. Patients receive three monthly cycles of chemotherapy and then are treated with a standard course of radiotherapy consisting of 6020 rad divided in 35 fractions. Each cycle of chemotherapy is delivered by continuous infusion over 72 hours. Continuous infusion of chemotherapeutic agents provides sustained plasma drug levels, permits drug to equilibrate more completely between plasma and interstitium, and results in a more homogeneous distribution and higher concentrations of drug within the tumor. Because chemotherapy is administered as neoadjuvant therapy, after surgery and before radiotherapy, the growth fraction of the tumor is relatively high, and the vascular supply of the tumor that persists postoperatively is intact. This strategy maximizes the potential tumor response to chemotherapy and minimizes the possibility of delivering sublethal concentrations of drug to the tumor. Results of two studies employing this protocol demonstrated substantial short-term and long-term survival benefits in patients with high-grade gliomas when compared with historical controls treated with standard radiotherapy and adjuvant chemotherapy [24,25]. These studies have formed the basis of a current ECOG–Southwest Oncology Group (SWOG) phase III trial comparing the efficacy of continuous infusion, neoadjuvant BCNU-cisplatinum followed by radiotherapy with radiotherapy and concurrent, adjuvant BCNU delivered by IV bolus in patients with newly diagnosed glioblastoma.

Other strategies designed to maximize drug delivery to glial neoplasms include intraarterial chemotherapy, blood–brain barrier disruption, and topical chemotherapy. Intraarterial administration of chemotherapy potentially permits increased delivery of drug to the tumor without increasing systemic toxicity. Local toxicities have limited the clinical usefulness of intraarterially administered BCNU. Retinal damage and blindness have followed the administration of BCNU in the carotid artery below the ophthalmic artery, and the supraophthalmic delivery of BCNU, while reducing eye toxicity, has produced coagulative necrosis of white matter and irreversible encephalopathy. A BTSG phase III trial comparing intraarterial BCNU with IV bolus BCNU showed a lack of efficacy in patients treated with intraarterial BCNU [26]. The major limitations of intraarterial chemotherapy may be related to a fluid dynamic phenomenon called streaming, which is essentially unequal arterial mixing of drug with plasma that results in a markedly heterogeneous distribution and delivery of drug. The development of new superselective arterial catheters may overcome this limitation by generating a more homogeneous arterial distribution of drug. The clinical effectiveness of intraarterial chemotherapy is yet to be demonstrated, however. Similarly, blood–brain barrier disruption and topical chemotherapy delivery by means of negatively charged liposomes or bioerodable polymers, although promising, have shown only small clinical benefit.

Brachytherapy is the stereotactic implantation of radiation sources, usually ^{125}iodine or ^{192}iridium, in a tumor for 4 to 6 days. This technique provides a local boost in the dose of radiation that can be delivered to the tumor beyond conventional radiotherapy while sparing surrounding parenchyma. Brachytherapy can be delivered following the completion of conventional radiotherapy or at the time of tumor recurrence. Although some studies have shown a clinical benefit in patients with high-grade gliomas treated with brachytherapy, demonstration that brachytherapy is a clinically useful adjunct therapy awaits confirmation in larger randomized trials [27].

Immunotherapy and gene therapy are potential biologic therapies for patients with high-grade gliomas. Laboratory success, however, has yet to be translated into clinical efficacy. Lymphokine-activated killer cells, produced by incubating lymphocytes with recombinant interleukin-2, although capable of lysing autologous glioblastoma cells in vitro, generally were ineffective and toxic when used in combination with interleukin-2 as intratumoral therapy for malignant gliomas [28,29]. A small proportion of patients did, nonetheless, manifest sustained clinical responses, and, in one study, long-term survival was reported in 4 of 29 patients [30]. Two of five patients treated with lymphokine-activated killer cells and interleukin-2 as primary therapy for newly diagnosed glioblastoma multiforme were alive and free of tumor 21 months after treatment [30]. These results indicate that, in some circumstances, exogenously delivered immune cells are, in fact, capable of exerting significant, durable antitumor activity against malignant gliomas. Other approaches to immunotherapy, including the use of tumor vaccines composed of autologous glioma cells as active, specific immunotherapy, have also met with limited clinical success [31,32]. Although no significant survival benefit was seen in early studies of autologous tumor vaccines with conventional adjuvant, most patients were capable of generating delayed-type hypersensitivity responses when challenged with glioma extracts. Further, in one trial randomizing 65 patients to treatment with supportive care, radiotherapy, immunotherapy with autologous tumor vaccines, and immunotherapy plus radiotherapy, equal survival for patients in the immunotherapy and radiotherapy groups (7.4- and 7.5-month median survivals) and improved survival in the combination therapy group (10.1-month median survival) were demonstrated [33].

These observations again support the hypothesis that effective immune responses can be generated against glial malignancies. They also provide a rationale for further exploring the role of active immunotherapy of brain tumors, especially in view of the rapidly developing molecular technologies that permit the use of cytokine gene transfer systems to potentiate the effectiveness of biologic therapies. One such preclinical model, in which rats treated with glioma cells transfected to express antisense insulin-like growth factor 1 were cured of their brain tumors, has formed the basis of a molecular brain tumor vaccine trial currently being conducted at Case Western Reserve University [34]. In this trial, patients with recurrent gliomas, after surgical resection of their tumors and ex vivo introduction of the insulin-like growth factor 1 antisense gene into the tumor cells, are vaccinated with their genetically modified tumor

cells in an attempt to stimulate immune-mediated rejection of their brain tumors. In an alternative approach to gene therapy for malignant gliomas, the in vivo retroviral-mediated gene transfer of the herpes simplex thymidine kinase gene into rat gliomas and subsequent treatment with gancyclovir produced a 77% cure rate in an animal model [35]. Based on the success of this preclinical model, and on the results of a pilot study at the National Institutes of Health demonstrating the feasibility of such an approach, a clinical trial of gene therapy in patients with high-grade gliomas using retroviral-mediated gene transfer is presently being conducted at multiple centers in the United States. Although not yet of demonstrated clinical benefit, immunotherapy and gene therapy offer great promise in the future for the treatment of gliomas.

LOW-GRADE GLIOMAS

Considerable controversy exists concerning the management of low-grade gliomas [36]. Most patients with low-grade gliomas present with a transient neurologic event, usually a seizure, and have a normal neurologic examination. The tumor is detected on brain CT or MRI as a nonenhancing mass lesion with little or no mass effect. The issue of when to biopsy or resect the mass has not been settled. Some studies have shown that deferring diagnosis and delaying therapy until the tumor progresses does not shorten survival, but other investigators recommend immediate diagnosis [36,37]. A diagnosis may be pursued by biopsy or resection. Several studies have shown that survival is increased in patients undergoing complete resection when compared with patients undergoing subtotal resection. No studies to date have randomized patients to biopsy or resection, however, and therefore the impact of the timing and extent of surgery on the natural history of low-grade gliomas remains unanswered.

There is no agreement either on the timing of radiotherapy. Some investigators favor immediate radiotherapy, especially for patients undergoing partial resection, whereas others recommend deferring radiotherapy in patients with low-grade gliomas, especially in view of the risk of delayed radionecrosis. The timing of radiotherapy in the treatment of low-grade gliomas is currently the subject of a national protocol being conducted by the BTCG and the SWOG.

Given the lack of consensus regarding the management of patients with low-grade gliomas, the timing of diagnosis and therapy must be made by the patient's physician based on the clinical impression. If a diagnosis is deferred, regular neurologic examinations and neuroimaging studies are required. If a diagnosis is pursued, the patient may be a candidate for entry into the national protocol, described previously, which is designed to determine the appropriate timing of radiotherapy for patients with low-grade gliomas.

REGIONAL AND ADVANCED DISEASE

High-grade gliomas, as noted earlier, rarely metastasize, and the concepts of regional and advanced disease cannot be applied to gliomas as they can to other systemic malignancies. Essentially all high-grade gliomas recur, however, and most low-grade gliomas progress. Unfortunately the management of recurrent or progressive disease is hampered by the lack of uniformity in the initial treatment of gliomas. Patients with recurrent disease may or may not have undergone tumor debulking, may or may not have received chemotherapy, and may or may not have been treated with brachytherapy. Developing well-controlled, randomized treatment trials of patients with recurrent glial neoplasms is made difficult by such variability, and the management of these patients often, of necessity, becomes individualized.

Despite these limitations, soundly conceived trials for patients with recurrent gliomas whose tumors have progressed after treatment with BCNU are being devised. BCNU is an alkylating agent that exerts its cytotoxic effect by forming DNA adducts, preferentially at the O^6 position of guanine, and cross-linking DNA. Normal and neoplastic cells are protected from BCNU cytotoxicity by the activity of O^6-alkylguanine-alkyltransferase (O^6-AGAT), an enzyme that removes BCNU adducts before cross-link formation. Pharmacologic agents that reduced O^6-AGAT activity have been shown to increase the efficacy of BCNU in in vitro cytotoxicity studies [38]. Based on these preclinical studies, phase I–II trials designed to restore BCNU sensitivity in patients with refractory gliomas by employing O^6-AGAT modulating drugs have been developed. In one clinical trial,

in which the O^6-AGAT modulating agents streptozocin and 6-mercaptopurine were administered before BCNU delivery, a 32% response rate was reported for patients with recurrent gliomas who had previously failed radiotherapy, surgery, and chemotherapy [39].

CONCLUSION

Gliomas are aggressive, lethal tumors. Survival is measured in months for patients with high-grade gliomas and in years for patients with low-grade gliomas. Advances in clinical neurooncology and in the neurosciences promise to improve this outlook, however. Ongoing multiinstitutional, randomized clinical trials will eventually result in a more uniform, effective approach to the treatment of glial neoplasms, and ongoing laboratory studies will continue to provide the new and innovative therapies that ultimately will result in long-term survival for patients with gliomas.

REFERENCES

1. Wingo PA, Tong T, Bolden S: Cancer statistics, 1995. *CA* 1995, 45:8–30.

2. Schoenberg BS: Epidemiology of primary intracranial neoplasms: disease distribution and risk factors. *Neurobiol Brain Tumors* 1991, 4:3–18.

3. Ron E, Modan B, Boice JD, *et al.*: Tumors of the brain and nervous system after radiotherapy in childhood. *N Engl J Med* 1988, 319:1033–1040.

4. Hamilton SR, Liu B, Parsons R, *et al.*: The molecular basis of Turcot's syndrome. *N Engl J Med* 1995, 332:839–847.

5. Gutmann DH, Collins FS: The neurofibromatosis gene and its protein product, neurofibromin. *Neuron* 1993, 10:335–343.

6. Vogelstein B, Kinzler KW: The multistep nature of cancer. *Trends Genet* 1993, 9:138–141.

7. von Deimling A, von Ammon K, Schoenfeld D, *et al.*: Subsets of glioblastoma multiforme defined by molecular genetic analysis. *Brain Pathol* 1993, 3:19–26.

8. Sidransky D, Mikkelsen T, Schwechheimer K, *et al.*: Clonal expansion of p53 mutant cells is associated with brain tumor progression. *Nature* 1992, 355:846–847.

9. Henson JW, Schnitker BL, Correa KM, *et al.*: The retinoblastoma gene is involved in malignant progression of astrocytomas. *Ann Neurol* 1994, 36:714–721.

10. Hurtt MR, Moossy J, Donovan-Peluso M, *et al.*: Amplification of epidermal growth factor receptor gene in gliomas: histology and prognosis. *J Neuropathol Exp Neurol* 1992, 51:84–90.

11. Walker MD, Alexander E, Munt WE, *et al.*: Evaluation of BCNU and/or radiotherapy in treatment of anaplastic gliomas. *J Neurosurg* 1978, 49:333–343.

12. Chang CH, Horton J, Schoenfield D, *et al.*: Comparison of post-operative radiotherapy and combined postoperative radiotherapy and chemotherapy in the multidisciplinary management of malignant gliomas. *Cancer* 1983, 52:997–1007.

13. Burger PC, Vogel FS, Green SB, *et al.*: Glioblastoma multiforme and anaplastic astrocytoma: pathologic criteria and prognostic implications. *Cancer* 1985, 56:1106–1111.

14. Kernohan JW, Moborn RF, Svien HJ, *et al.*: A simplified classification of gliomas. *Mayo Clin Proc* 1949, 24:71–75.

15. Hayostek CJ, Shaw EG, Scheithauer B, *et al.*: Astrocytomas of the cerebellum: a comparative clinicopathologic study of pilocytic and diffuse astrocytomas. *Cancer* 1993, 72:856–869.

16. Albright AL, Guthkelch AN, Packer RJ, *et al.*: Prognostic factors in pediatric brain stem gliomas. *J Neurosurg* 1986, 65:751–755.

17. Walker MD, Green SB, Byar DP, *et al.*: Randomized comparison of radiotherapy and nitrosoureas for the treatment of malignant glioma after surgery. *N Engl J Med* 1980, 303:1323–1329.

18. Shady JA, Black PM, Kupsky WJ, *et al.*: Seizures in children with supratentorial astroglial neoplasms. *Pediatr Neurosurg* 1994, 21:23–30.

19. Levin JM, Schiff D, Loeffler JS, *et al.*: Complications of therapy for venous thromboembolic disease in patients with brain tumors. *Neurology* 1993, 43:1111–1114.

20. Ammirati M, Vick N, Liao YL, *et al.*: Effect of the extent of surgical resection on survival and quality of life in patients with supratentorial glioblastomas and anaplastic astrocytomas. *Neurosurgery* 1987, 21:201–206.

21. Marks JE: Ionizing radiation. *Neurobiol Brain Tumors* 1991, 4:299–319.

22. Kornblith PL, Walker M: Chemotherapy for malignant gliomas. *J Neurosurg* 1988, 68:1–17.

23. Fine HA, Dear KB, Loeffler JS, *et al.*: Meta-analysis of radiation therapy with and without adjuvant chemotherapy for malignant gliomas in adults. *Cancer* 1993, 71:2585–2597.

24. Gilbert MR, Lunsford LK, Kondziolka L, *et al.*: A phase II trial of continuous infusion chemotherapy, external beam radiotherapy and local boost radiotherapy. *Proc Am Soc Clin Oncol* 1993, 12:176.

25. Gross SA, Sheidler VR, Ahn H, *et al.*: Complete and partial response of newly diagnosed malignant astrocytomas following continuous infusion of BCNU and cisplatin. *Proc Am Soc Clin Oncol* 1989, 8:344.

26. Shapiro WR, Green SB, Burger PC, *et al.*: A randomized comparison of intra-arterial (IA) versus intravenous BCNU for patients with malignant gliomas: interim analysis demonstrating lack of efficacy for IA BCNU. *Proc Am Soc Clin Oncol* 1987, 6:69.

27. Larsen DA, Gutin PH, Leibel SA, *et al.*: Stereotaxic irradiation of brain tumors. *Cancer* 1990, 65:792–799.

28. Jacobs SK, Wilson DJ, Kornblith PL: In vitro killing of human glioblastoma by interleukin-2–activated autologous lymphocytes. *J Neurosurg* 1986, 64:114–117.

29. Barbara D, Saris SC: Intratumoral LAK cell and interleukin-2 therapy of human gliomas. *J Neurosurg* 1989, 70:175–182.

30. Merchant RE, Ellison MD, Young HF: Immunotherapy for malignant glioma using human recombinant interleukin-2 and activated autologous lymphocytes. *J Neuro-Oncol* 1990, 8:173–188.

31. Grace JT, Perese DM, Metzhar RS, *et al.*: Tumor autograft responses in patients with glioblastoma multiforme. *J Neurosurg* 1961, 18:159.

32. Bloom HJG, Peckham MJ, Richardson AE, Alexander PA, Payne PM: Glioblastoma multiforme: a controlled trial to assess the value of specific active immunotherapy in patients treated by radical surgery and radiotherapy. *Br J Cancer* 1973, 27:253–567.

33. Trouillas P: Immunologie et immunotherapie des tumeurs cerebrales: etat actuel. *Rev Neurol [Paris]* 1973, 128:23–38.

34. Trojan J, Johnson TR, Rudin SD, *et al.*: Treatment and prevention of rat glioblastoma by immunogenic C6 cells expressing antisense insulin-like growth factor 1 RNA. *Science* 1993, 25:94–96.

35. Ram Z, Culver KW, Walbridge S, *et al.*: In situ retroviral-mediated gene transfer for the treatment of brain tumors in rats. *Cancer Res* 1993, 53:83–88.

36. Recht LD, Lew R, Smith TW: Suspected low-grade glioma: is deferring treatment safe? *Ann Neurol* 1992, 31:431–436.

37. Shapiro WR: Low-grade gliomas: when to treat? *Ann Neurol* 1992, 31:437–438.

38. Peiper RO, Futscher B, Dong Q, *et al.*: Effects of streptozotocin/bischloroethylnitrosourea combination therapy on O^6-methylguanine-DNA methyltransferase activity and mRNA levels in HT-29 cells in vitro. *Cancer Res* 1991, 51:1581–1585.

39. Gilbert MR, Matey L, Minhas T, *et al.*: Dual modulation of BCNU resistance in patients with refractory or recurrent glial neoplasms. *Proceedings of the Annual Meeting of the American Association for Cancer Research*, 1994, 35:A2153.

BCNU AND CISPLATIN

The ECOG-SWOG phase III study compared three cycles of infusional BCNU and cisplatin followed by radiation therapy with radiation therapy and concurrent BCNU for patients with newly diagnosed supratentorial glioblastoma multiforme. The primary objective was to compare survival and time to progression in adults with glioblastoma multiforme receiving standard therapy (BCNU and radiation therapy) with those receiving three cycles of BCNU and cisplatin followed by radiation therapy. Secondary objectives were to compare the proportion of patients who survive 1 year following institution of treatment with these therapies and to compare the frequency and severity of toxicities of these therapeutic approaches.

The role of adjuvant chemotherapy, which is chemotherapy delivered during or following the completion of radiotherapy, is of uncertain benefit in prolonging survival in patients with glioblastoma multiforme. The use of up-front continuous infusion chemotherapy maximizes the potential tumor response to chemotherapy by improving drug delivery to the tumor and has been shown in phase II trials to prolong survival when compared with historical controls receiving adjuvant chemotherapy.

RESPONSE RATES

Study	Evaluable patients, *n*	Complete response	Partial response	Progressive disease
ECOG-SWOG phase III	52	8 (16%)	33 (67%)	2 (4%)

Complete response = complete resolution of enhancing tumor by volumetric CT or MRI.
Partial response = > 50% reduction in tumor volumes.
Progressive disease = > 25% increase in tumor volume.

CANDIDATES FOR TREATMENT

Histologically confirmed supratentorial glioblastoma multiforme. Patients must be ≥ 14 d and ≤ 42 d from date of surgery at the time of study registration; patients having only a biopsy can be entered at 10 d poststereotactic biopsy; patients age ≥ 18 y; ECOG performance status of 0, 1, or 2; no concurrent malignancy except curatively treated basal cell or squamous cell carcinoma of the skin or carcinoma in situ of the cervix; patients with prior malignancies who have been disease-free for > 5 y are eligible

SPECIAL PRECAUTIONS

No prior antineoplastic therapy for the brain tumor or any other malignancy; must not be on increasing doses of steroid within 3 d of randomization; have adequate hematologic, renal, and liver function (WBC > 4000, platelet > 150,000, creatinine > 1.6, bilirubin > 2.0); laboratory values must be done within 2 wk before registration; no evidence of significant pulmonary disease; patients with symptomatic pulmonary disease or known chronic obstructive pulmonary disease must have a $D_{L_{CO}} \geq 50\%$ of predicted and an FVC $\geq 60\%$ of predicted; not pregnant or lactating; women of childbearing potential and sexually active men are strongly advised to use an accepted, effective method of contraception; pathology materials must be available for submission to the ECOG Coordinating Center for review; patients must give written informed consent

TOXICITIES

Hematologic: leukopenia and thrombocytopenia occur within 25–35 d, may last 60 d, and may be cumulative, anemia; **Gastrointestinal:** nausea and vomiting; **Hepatic:** reversible elevations of SGOT, SGPT, and bilirubin; **Pulmonary (BCNU):** infiltrates or fibrosis, especially with prolonged therapy and higher doses, cumulative doses of 1200 mg/m^2 should not be exceeded; **Renal:** elevated serum creatinine and BUN, cisplatin nephrotoxicity is dose-related and relatively uncommon with adequate hydration and diuresis; BCNU nephrotoxicity can produce a decrease in kidney size and renal failure with large doses; **Neurologic (cisplatin):** peripheral neuropathy common and dose-limiting when the cumulative cisplatin dose exceeds 400 mg/m^2; seizures are rare, ototoxicity, manifested initially by high-frequency hearing loss, common, vestibular toxicity uncommon, tetany (secondary to hypomagnesemia) and Lhermitte's sign rare; **Dermatologic (cisplatin):** alopecia uncommon; **Cardiovascular:** hypotension from rapid or concentrated infusion of BCNU, rare cisplatin-provoked coronary vasospasm; **Other:** Burning at injection site and facial flushing with BCNU, hypomagnesemia, hypocalcemia, hyponatremia, vein irritation, fatigue, and rare anaphylaxis with cisplatin

NURSING IMPLICATIONS

Assess laboratory test values before administration; patients may require potassium and magnesium supplementation in addition to fluids; assess urine output before each dose; maintain hydration; monitor intake and output; urine output should be 100 to 150 mL/h; diuretics may be ordered; premedicate with antiemetics; avoid skin contact with BCNU; assess for burning at IV site, stomatitis, signs of anaphylaxis, and signs of neurotoxicity; monitor CBC and liver and renal function tests.

CARMUSTINE (BCNU), STREPTOZOCIN, AND INTRAVENOUS 6-MERCAPTOPURINE

PCI phase II trials of carmustine (BCNU), streptozocin (STZ), and IV 6-mercaptopurine (6-MP) are being conducted in patients with refractory brain neoplasms. Primary objectives were to determine the toxicity and maximum tolerated dose of the STZ and IV 6-MP and continuous-infusion BCNU regimen and assess the clinical response of patients with refractory or recurrent malignant gliomas to the combination of BCNU, STZ, and IV 6-MP. Secondary objectives were to correlate clinical tumor response with changes in treatment-induced peripheral blood lymphocyte O^6-AGAT activity and assess changes in O^6-AGAT levels following exposure to STZ and during continuous infusion of BCNU.

Nitrosoureas are the most common chemotherapeutic agents used for the treatment of malignant gliomas. Unfortunately, standard administration of these agents, usually as adjuvant therapy after radiation treatment, has little impact on survival. The development of resistance in the tumor cells to alkylation by nitrosoureas may be the cause of the poor clinical response. The mechanism of resistance of tumor cells to nitrosoureas is thought to be mediated by an upregulation of the intracellular levels of O^6-AGAT. Strategies have been developed to modulate O^6-AGAT activity and increase the efficacy of nitrosourea therapy. Modulators of O^6-AGAT, such as STZ and 6-MP, enhance BCNU cytotoxicity in in vitro studies. Based on these preclinical data, this trial will explore the efficacy of combining STZ and 6-MP with BCNU as a treatment regimen for patients with malignant gliomas who have failed prior nitrosourea therapy.

RESPONSE RATES

Study	Evaluable patients, n	Partial response	Stable disease	Progressive disease
PCI phase II	28	7 (25%)	8 (28%)	13 (47%)

Partial response—> 50% reduction in tumor volume.
Stable disease—< 50% reduction in tumor volume but not > 25% increase in tumor volume.
Progressive disease—> 25% increase in tumor volume.

DOSAGE AND SCHEDULING

Day	1	1*	3	X
6-MP 750 mg/m²	X	2	X	1
STZ 500 mg/m²	2	X	X	5
BCNU 40 mg/m² qd CI	X	X	1	X
O^6-AGAT levels	X	1	4	11†

*Drawn before the first dose of STZ.
†Drawn at the conclusion of BCNU infusion.

CANDIDATES FOR TREATMENT

Histologic diagnosis of glioblastoma multiforme, anaplastic astrocytoma, gliosarcoma anaplastic oligodendroglioma, and mixed anaplastic glioma, with the exception of patients with primary brain stem tumors; patients with brain stem lesions must have unequivocal evidence of progressive disease following primary therapy; refractory or recurrent primary brain neoplasm following primary surgery, radiation, and chemotherapy; measurable disease ECOG performance status of 0, 1, or 2

SPECIAL PRECAUTIONS

Informed consent as documented by a signed consent form indicating the investigational nature of the treatment and its potential risks; absolute granulocyte count ≥ 1500, platelets ≥ 100,000, creatinine ≥ 2.0, bilirubin ≥ 2.0, and SGOT ≥ four times normal; patients with symptomatic pulmonary disease must have an $FEV_1 > 1$ L; patients with concurrent malignancies are excluded; any prior chemotherapy must be completed at least 4 wk before study entry (6 wk for nitrosoureas or mitomycin C); women of childbearing potential must be practicing an effective method of contraception, have a negative pregnancy test, and refrain from nursing

TOXICITIES

Hematologic: leukopenia and thrombocytopenia occur within 15–35 d, may last 60 d, and may be cumulative, anemia; **Gastrointestinal:** nausea and vomiting, STZ can cause diarrhea and abdominal cramping; **Hepatic:** reversible elevations of SGOT, SGPT, and bilirubin; **Pulmonary (BCNU):** infiltrates or fibrosis, especially with prolonged therapy and higher doses, cumulative doses of 1200 mg/m² should not be exceeded; **Renal:** elevated serum creatinine and BUN; renal tubular acidosis and proteinuria can be associated with STZ treatment, BCNU can produce a decrease in kidney size and renal failure with large doses; **Endocrine (STZ):** rare reactive hyperglycemia can follow insulin release; **Cardiovascular:** hypotension from rapid or concentrated infusion of BCNU; **Other:** Burning at injection site, conjunctivitis, and facial flushing with BCNU, mucositis, stomatitis, rash, and fever with 6-MP

NURSING IMPLICATIONS

Assess laboratory test values before administration; patients may require potassium and magnesium supplementation in addition to fluids; premedicate with antiemetics; avoid skin contact with BCNU; assess for burning at IV site, stomatitis, signs of anaphylaxis, and signs of neurotoxicity; monitor CBC and liver and renal function tests.

HERPES SIMPLEX THYMIDINE KINASE AND GANCICLOVIR

Genetic Therapy, Inc. (Gaithersburg, MD) is conducting a multicenter trial of herpes simplex thymidine kinase and ganciclovir gene therapy for surgically accessible recurrent glioblastoma multiforme and surgically inaccessible recurrent high-grade gliomas. The objective is to investigate the efficacy of retroviral gene therapy in patients with recurrent malignant gliomas.

In a pilot study performed at the National Institutes of Health, 15 patients with recurrent malignant gliomas were treated by genetically altering tumor cells with stereotactically injected herpes simplex thymidine kinase (HSV-tk) retroviral vector-producer fibroblasts. Ganciclovir, a drug that is toxic to any tumor cells incorporating the HSV-tk gene but nontoxic to normal cells, was then administered IV. Decreased tumor volume or loss of enhancement at the treated site was seen in follow-up MRI in several patients, suggesting that treatment with HSV-tk gene therapy had resulted in antitumor activity. Toxicity was minimal.

In protocol GTI 0103, patients with surgically accessible recurrent glioblastoma multiforme will undergo craniotomy and maximal resection of the tumor. The tumor cavity and any residual tumor will then be directed injected with HSV-tk vector producer cells. An Ommaya reservoir will be implanted at the site of surgery for later injection of additional vector producer cells. Two weeks after surgery, patients will receive a 14-d course of IV ganciclovir. Tumor response will be measured by MRI, and patients will receive additional cycles of vector producer cells and ganciclovir based on their response to the initial treatment.

In protocol GTI 0107, patients with recurrent malignant gliomas that are not accessible to conventional neurologic surgery will receive intratumoral injections of HSV-tk vector producer cells using stereotactic techniques. Two weeks after surgery, patients will receive a 14-d course of IV ganciclovir. Tumor response will be measured by serial MRI.

CANDIDATES FOR TREATMENT

Protocol GTI 0103—gene therapy for surgically accessible glioblastoma multiforme: patients must be > 18 y with recurrent glioblastoma multiforme; patients must have surgically accessible tumors; patients with tumors involving the brain stem, basal ganglia, or both hemispheres; patients with multifocal disease; and patients with diffuse subependymal tumor or cerebrospinal fluid dissemination are excluded; patients must have received primary surgical treatment and radiation treatment at least 12 wk before study entry; patients with a prior history of other local therapies including, but not limited to, brachytherapy, gamma knife treatment, stereotactic radiosurgery, or wafer implants are excluded; patients must have demonstrated evidence on contrast MRI scan of progressive disease while on a stable or increasing dose of steroids; Karnofsky performance status at the time of study enrollment must be > 60%

Protocol GTI 0107—gene therapy for surgically inaccessible malignant glioma: patients must be > 18 y of age with recurrent anaplastic astrocytoma or glioblastoma multiforme; MRI scan must demonstrates a contrast-enhancing tumor that is < 30 cm^3 in total volume and is stereotactically accessible; patients with tumors involving the brain stem, both hemispheres, or corpus collasum; patients with diffusely infiltrative or multifocal disease; and patients with diffuse subependymal tumor or cerebrospinal fluid dissemination are excluded; patients must have received primary surgical treatment and radiation treatment at least 12 wk before study entry; patients with a prior history of other local therapies including, but not limited to, brachytherapy, gamma knife treatment, stereotactic radiosurgery, or wafer implants are excluded; patients must have demonstrated evidence on contrast MRI scan of progressive disease within 14 d of study entry while on a stable or increasing dose of steroids; Karnofsky performance status at the time of study enrollment must be > 60%.

ADRENAL CORTICAL CARCINOMA

ETIOLOGY AND RISK FACTORS

Adrenal cortical carcinomas (ACC) are exceedingly rare tumors with an incidence of two cases per million population. There is a bimodal age distribution, with peak incidences in children under 5 years of age and in people in their fourth to sixth decade. Although no etiologic factors have been identified, ACC has been associated with certain hereditary syndromes (multiple endocrine neoplasia type I and a sarcoma, breast, and lung cancer syndrome).

Patients with ACC present with symptoms related to steroid hormone excess or an enlarging abdominal mass (Table 17-1). Women present more commonly with functioning ACC, whereas men are more likely to have nonfunctioning ACC. The most common hormone excess is hypercortisolism and associated Cushing syndrome. Children most commonly present with virilization. Aldosterone-secreting ACC occurs but is exceedingly rare.

STAGING AND PROGNOSIS

The endocrinologic evaluation of functional ACC includes assessment of steroid hormone synthesis. The initial evaluation should include a single-dose overnight dexamethasone test (a positive test is a urinary free cortisol level > 100 μg/d). The etiology of the hypercortisolism can be further delineated by the clinical situation and the low- or high-dose dexamethasone suppression tests (or ovine corticotropin-releasing hormone test) as indicated. The presence of elevated, nonsuppressible steroid hormone levels can serve as a useful tumor marker for subsequent follow-up. Patients with clinically silent adrenal tumors should have a judicious clinical and biochemical evaluation [1].

Computed tomography (CT) of the adrenal glands is the technique most commonly used for radiologic evaluation of an adrenal mass. CT scan has 80% sensitivity for adrenal masses less than 1 cm and a sensitivity of 95% for tumors 3 to 4 cm in diameter. Abdominal CT scan can also identify local and distant metastases. However, adrenal CT scan is nonspecific in delineating a benign versus malignant mass. There have been several reports suggesting that magnetic resonance imaging (MRI) may be helpful in distinguishing benign adenomas from ACC, pheochromocytoma, or metastases to the adrenal gland based on relative brightness of the T2-weighted scan. MRI may aid in equivocal cases to improve the specificity of adrenal CT scan [2–6]. In some cases, iodocholesterol scanning can be useful to functionally localize the unilateral or bilateral nature of functional adrenal tumors [6]. The only definitive radiologic criteria for malignancy of a mass are evidence of local invasion or distant metastases.

Conversely, the frequent use of CT imaging of the abdomen has led to the discovery of adrenal "incidentalomas" in 0.6% of abdominal CT scans. The adrenal incidentaloma is usually benign but requires assessment by a clinician familiar with an efficient clinical and biochemical work-up of this issue. Although fewer than 1% of adrenal tumors that are less than 6 cm in size represent ACC, the risk of malignancy of lesions greater than 6 cm ranges from 35% to 98%. Therefore, it is recommended that all nonfunctioning tumors greater than 5 cm in diameter undergo surgical resection. Adrenalectomy is also warranted for all functional tumors, regardless of size. Biochemical screening for urinary catecholamines to exclude pheochromocytoma is obligatory before any needle biopsy or operation for an adrenal mass; such an intervention might precipitate a fatal hypertensive crisis if the patient has an unrecognized pheochromocytoma. Fine-needle biopsy of an adrenal mass does not aid in the differential between benign and malignant tumors. Therefore, fine-needle aspiration (FNA) is not routinely performed unless metastatic cancer or lymphoma are suspected.

The most important factors in the staging of ACC are tumor size and local invasion at presentation (Table 17-2). Prognosis in ACC depends on disease stage at presentation. Historically, approximately 70% of patients present with advanced (stage III or IV) disease; however, more recent series have nearly 50% lower-stage (I or II) patients [7]. Patients have an overall median survival of 2 years, with 5-year and 10-year survival rates of 22% to 30% and 10%, respectively. Patients with stage I or II disease have substantially better prognosis overall (~50% at 5 y); however, survival drops off quickly at stage III (median, 12 months; only 20% alive at 5 y) and is very poor for patients with stage IV disease (median, 6 months; 5% alive at 5 y) [7].

In addition to tumor size (>100 g), other factors associated with poor prognosis are vascular invasion, mitotic rate, necrosis, and nuclear ploidy. Factors of limited significance include capsular invasion, immunohistochemical staining, and functional status of the tumor.

Table 17-1. Presenting Clinical Features of Adrenal Cortical Carcinoma

Symptom	Rate, %
Cushing's syndrome	40–60
Virilization or feminization	10–20
Hypertension and hypokalemia	1
Abdominal symptoms only	30

Table 17-2. Staging Criteria for Adrenal Cortical Carcinoma

	Stage			
	I	II	III	IV
TNM Components	T1, N0, M0	T2, N0, M0	T1 or T2, N1, M0 or T3, N0, M0	Any T, any N, M1 or T3–T4, N1

Criteria
T1 — Tumor ≤ 5 cm, no invasion
T2 — Tumor > 5 cm, no invasion
T3 — Tumor outside adrenal in fat
T4 — Tumor invading adjacent viscera
N0 — No involved lymph nodes
N1 — Positive lymph nodes
M0 — No distant disease
M1 — Distant disease

Adapted from Sullivan et al. [35].

PRIMARY DISEASE THERAPY

Complete surgical resection is the basis of effective treatment for ACC and offers the only curative therapy. The goal of the initial operation is en bloc resection, which may involve adjacent viscera, vena cava, or diaphragm. The tumors tend to be quite locally invasive and require meticulous yet radical extirpation. Less than half of patients are resectable at time of presentation. Steroid hormone replacement is critical perioperatively and is continued postoperatively at replacement doses until complete recovery of the hypothalamic–pituitary axis. This may take up to 2 years after surgery [8]. Patients should be counseled regarding the dangers of Addisonian crisis during acute illnesses that require exogenous steroid replacement. Patients with stage I and II disease at surgical resection have a median survival of 5 years, whereas patients with invasion of contiguous structures have a mean survival of 2.3 years.

ADJUVANT THERAPY FOR REGIONAL DISEASE

Although surgical resection can be curative, a majority of patients have recurrence, with a median disease-free interval of 3 to 12 months for those who do recur. Approximately one third recur locally, one third recur as distant metastases only, and one third demonstrate both local and distant disease at recurrence. There have been several studies recommending adjuvant mitotane after resection of localized disease. However, other studies have shown no increase in survival, and therefore, adjuvant therapy is not generally implemented. The disease-free interval was a significant prognostic factor in a report from the National Cancer Institute for select patients with recurrent or metastatic disease [9]. In this nonrandomized study, 15 patients treated with chemotherapy alone had a median survival from first recurrence of 11 months, whereas 18 patients whose recurrent disease was curatively re-resected in addition to chemotherapy had a median survival of 27 months. One third of the operated patients survived more than 5 years from initial re-resection. A more recent multicenter review of reoperative results demonstrated similar findings, ie, patients who presented with resectable recurrences and who were resected survived longer than those patients who recurred with unresectable disease or who elected to forgo re-resection [7]. These retrospective data would seem to support resection of local recurrences, or metastasectomy, when possible. Patients who have undergone curative resection should be followed for recurrences by urine

Table 17-3. Chemotherapy for Advanced Adrenal Cortical Cancer

Study	Agents	Response Rate
Decker et al. [10]	Mitotane, doxorubicin	19% = 3/16 PR
van Slooten et al. [11]	Cisplatin, doxorubicin, cyclophosphamide	18% = 2/11 PR
Schlumberger et al. [12]	Cisplatin, doxorubicin, 5-FU	23% =1/13 CR, 2/13 PR
Bukowski et al. [13]	Mitotane, cisplatin	30% = 1/37 CR, 10/37 PR
Johnson et al. [14]	Cisplatin, etoposide	2/2 PR
Hesketh et al. [15]	Cisplatin, etoposide, bleomycin	1/4 CR, 2/4 PR
Berruti et al. [16]	Cisplatin, etoposide, doxorubicin	2/2 PR

CR—complete remission; 5-FU—5-flurouracil; PR—partial remission.

steroid profiles and serial chest and abdominal CT scans. Of those who are unresectable at time of reoperation, palliative debulking of ACC has not been shown to have a survival benefit but significantly improves quality of life, especially in decreasing tumor bulk and functionality of the tumors.

THERAPY FOR ADVANCED DISEASE

Adrenal cortical carcinomas metastasizes to lung (71%), liver (42%), and bone (26%). The pesticide analogue o,p-DDD (mitotane) has been used for treatment because of its adrenolytic properties. Chemotherapy for ACC has been largely ineffective, with most responses anecdotal and with no clear efficacy or documented benefit (Table 17-3) [10–16]. Mitotane is poorly tolerated and has not been studied in a randomized setting. Although there are isolated reports of long-term survivors, most of the 20% to 30% of patients who respond to mitotane have partial response of short duration. Pulmonary metastasectomy, isolated liver resection, and local-recurrence re-resection have been shown to induce remission in some patients [7,9]. External beam radiotherapy is ineffective except in the management of painful bony metastases.

Other agents under investigation include suramin (an inhibitor of reverse transcriptase and growth factor binding) and gossypol (a mitochondrial uncoupler that inhibits tumor growth in mice), but responses have been limited. There is no information about immunotherapeutic strategies for metastatic ACC.

THYROID CANCER

ETIOLOGY AND RISK FACTORS

Thyroid cancer is the most common endocrine malignancy. Currently, there are 12,400 new cases of thyroid cancer diagnosed per year, with an estimated death toll of 1230. Thyroid cancer commonly presents as a thyroid nodule. Although 4% to 7% of the general population have thyroid nodules, only 10% of solid nodules are malignant. Important clinical factors that increase the likelihood of malignancy include patient age (< 20 y or > 50 y); growth on thyroid stimulating hormone (TSH) suppressive therapy; residence in an iodine-deficient geographic areas; and a history of thyroiditis, goiter, or head and neck irradiation. Worrisome but nonspecific clinical features include neck pain, dysphagia, hoarseness, dyspnea, and cervical adenopathy. Although prior exposure to head and neck radiation is an etiologic factor in the development of papillary thyroid cancer, it is not a prognostic factor in its outcome. Patients with a history of childhood neck irradiation have a 33% to 37% chance of malignancy. Age of exposure and a radiation dose up to 2000 cGy has been shown to have a linear relation with the increased risk associated with ionizing radiation.

Papillary thyroid cancer has also been associated with several inherited tumor syndromes (Gardner's syndrome, Cowden's disease, and familial polyposis coli). A family history of thyroid cancer or other endocrine tumors should elicit the possibility of a multiple endocrine neoplasia syndrome (MEN). Recent advances in the genetics of MEN type II allow direct DNA testing for mutation in ret protooncogene of individuals at risk for MEN type II. Subsequent prophylactic surgical management can be recommended in these patients.

Fine-needle aspiration biopsy has revolutionized the accuracy of diagnosing thyroid cancer. Thyroid scans are now largely unnecessary and the annual number of thyroidectomies has been substantially reduced with the advent of the FNA-cytology assessment. Between 70% and 94% of FNA biopsies give the correct cytologic diagnosis. FNA cytology is divided into categories of benign, suspicious or indeterminate, malignant, and insufficient sample. Patients with benign-appearing FNA cytology are placed on exogenous L-thyroxine therapy at a dose sufficient to suppress TSH to less than 0.4 mIU/mL. Approximately 20% to 40% of those who do not respond to this treatment will be diagnosed with thyroid cancer at time of surgery. FNA cannot reliably distinguish between follicular adenoma and follicular thyroid cancer; patients with indeterminate follicular lesions require thyroidectomy to document the pathologic presence of vascular or capsular invasion by cancer. The rate of follicular cancer at surgery is 24% by this method of management. CT scan and MRI can be helpful in selected cases to evaluate the degree of tracheal deviation and compression, extension into the mediastinum, and carotid artery involvement by tumor.

STAGING AND PROGNOSIS

The most important factors in staging of thyroid cancer are patient age, tumor size, and cell type. The staging system is outlined in Table 17-4.

There are four primary cell types of thyroid cancer, with varying natural histories, treatments, and outcome. Well-differentiated thyroid cancer is the most common type, accounting for 90% of all thyroid cancers. This category is further subdivided into papillary (75%) and follicular (10%–15%) cancer. Mixed papillary follicular cancer has been reclassified as a follicular variant of papillary thyroid cancer due to the similar behavior and prognosis to usual papillary cancer. Follicular cancers are increasingly uncommon, except in iodine-deficient geographic areas. Follicular cancer with capsular invasion alone may have a better prognosis; follicular lesions without vascular or capsular invasion are benign follicular adenomas.

Compared with papillary thyroid cancers, follicular cancer is less likely to metastasize to lymph nodes and more likely to pursue an aggressive course in older patients. The most important feature of a follicular cancer is the presence or absence of distant metastases at presentation in the elderly; when present, they portend a very poor, treatment-resistant course.

Prognosis for well-differentiated thyroid cancer is related primarily to risk group, although those of papillary histology have a slightly better prognosis than do the follicular cell types. Several widely-used systems for determining risk have been developed based on multivariate analysis (AMES, AGES, MACIS). All systems have documented that a very important factor in predicting survival is patient age at presentation. Tumor invasion, size of primary tumor, and presence of distant metastases are also significant factors. Nuclear DNA content also has been cited as an important prognostic variable. Table 17-5 presents the most recent scoring system for papillary thyroid cancer [17]. The prognostic significance of cervical lymph node involvement is controversial; some studies have reported an univariant survival advantage with local nodal involvement. In general, the presence of cervical lymph node metastases is a predictor of local recurrence but does not influence survival (Table 17-6).

Hürthle cell cancers account for 2% to 4% of all well-differentiated cancers, and exhibit a poorer prognosis. Other less fortuitous histologies include tall cell, insular, and diffuse sclerosing papillary variants. Although the relatively uncommon Hürthle cell variant is staged with the other well-differentiated tumors, in some cases they metastasize early to lymph nodes, lung, and bone.

Medullary thyroid cancer (MTC) (5%–10% of patients) arises from the neuroendocrine parafollicular C cells, which secrete calcitonin as part of the amine precursor uptake and decarboxylation system. The serum levels of calcitonin can thus serve as a biochemical marker for this disease. MTC appears in four unique clinical settings: 1) sporadic (80% of cases), 2) inherited in association with MEN type IIa, 3) inherited in association with MEN type IIb, and 4) familial MTC. The three inherited forms arise from precursor C-cell hyperplasia and usually are multifocal. MTC can present either as a clinical thyroid nodule or as occult disease detected by provocative

Table 17-4. Staging of Thyroid Cancers

Primary Tumor (T)	Nodal Involvement (N)	Metastases (M)
T1 — T ≤ 1 cm within thyroid	N0 — node negative	M0 — No distant metastases
T2 — 1 cm < T ≤ 4 cm	N1a — ipsilateral node(s) involved	M1 — Distant metastases
T3 — T > 4 cm	N1b — contralateral, midline, or mediastinal node(s) involved	
T4 — Any size extending beyond capsule		

Cancer Stage	Papillary or follicular, age < 45 y	Papillary or follicular, age ≥ 45 y	Medullary	Undifferentiated
I	Any T, any N, M0	T1, N0, M0	T1, N0, M0	—
II	Any T, any N, M1	T2, N0, M0	T2, N0, M0	—
		T3, N0, M0	T3, N0, M0	—
			T4, N0, M0	
III	—	T4, N0, M0	Any T, N1, M0	
		Any T, N1, M0		
IV	—	Any T, any N, M1	Any T, any N, M1	All stage IV

From Beahrs et al. [36].

Table 17-5. MACIS Prognostic Index for Papillary Thyroid Cancer

Variable	Points Assigned
Age < 39	+ 3.1
Age > 40	+ 0.08 × age
Diameter of primary tumor	+ 0.3 × cm
Incomplete resection	+ 1
Extrathyroidal invasion	+ 1
Distant metastases	+ 3

MACIS Score	Metastasis at 10 y, %	Mortality at 20 y, %
< 6	3	1
6–6.9	18	13
7–7.9	40	45
8 +	60	76

Adapted from Hay et al. [17].

pentagastrin-stimulated screening in a patient at risk for an inherited form. With the recent identification of specific germline mutations in the *ret* protooncogene in patients with inherited forms of MTC, direct DNA testing has replaced provocative testing and has led to early thyroidectomy in those patients at risk (18,19).

Anaplastic thyroid cancer (2% of patients) is a highly malignant tumor arising from thyroid epithelium and, in some cases, from preexisting well-differentiated thyroid cancer or long-standing goiter. With earlier and more effective treatment of differentiated cancer, the incidence of anaplastic cancer has dropped dramatically over the past 50 years. Over half of the small cell variants of anaplastic thyroid cancer diagnosed in the past are now believed to be thyroid lymphomas. This important distinction is made today by immunohistochemistry and flow cytometry and is crucial to prognosis (Table 17-7) and management. One third to one half of cases of non-Hodgkin's lymphoma of the thyroid gland occur in the setting of preexisting Hashimoto's thyroiditis.

Primary Disease Therapy

Primary treatment of thyroid cancer is based on histologic type. Surgical resection of well-differentiated cancers is the mainstay of treatment. Isolated papillary lesions smaller than 1 cm occur in 10% of thyroid glands at autopsy. After thyroid lobectomy is performed, these minimal thyroid cancers require no treatment other than expectant follow-up.

The extent of resection of papillary carcinomas remains controversial. At present there is a consensus that for low-risk, well-differentiated thyroid cancer, the minimal operation is a thyroid lobectomy and isthmectomy. Total or near-total thyroidectomy should be performed for lesions larger than 1.5 cm in angioinvasive follicular cancer, Hürthle cell cancer, or papillary cancer in association with prior neck irradiation or local invasion. A survival advantage for total thyroidectomy versus subtotal thyroidectomy or lobectomy has never been shown in a prospective randomized study but has been observed in retrospective series. Total thyroidectomy offers the significant advantage of simplifying postoperative surveillance and treatment of thyroid cancer. Major risks associated with total thyroidectomy include a 1% risk of permanent recurrent laryngeal nerve injury and a 1% to 3% chance of permanent hypoparathyroidism. These risks are demonstrably lower in the hands of expert surgeons. Neck dissection has no proven role in primary treatment of well-differentiated thyroid cancer, although some controversy does exist with the surgical management of lymph node involvement. Some advocate a formal dissection for clinically obvious lymph node metastases. Prognosis is noted in Table 17-6.

Surgical resection is the primary therapy for MTC. The operation of choice is total thyroidectomy and central node dissection. Modified or radical node dissection should be performed for palpable cervical disease. Patients with MEN type II should undergo total thyroidectomy on diagnosis of the syndrome because most patients will otherwise develop lethal MTC by their second decade. Prognosis is noted in Table 17-7.

Anaplastic cancer of the thyroid usually presents as a locally advanced tumor for which surgical intervention is not an curative option. Core or incisional biopsy may be required to definitely exclude lymphoma. An aggressive surgical debulking and tracheostomy may be warranted to forestall death from asphyxiation. Primary therapy for thyroid lymphoma is external radiation or combination chemotherapy, depending on stage (*see* Chapter 20).

ADJUVANT THERAPY FOR REGIONAL DISEASE

Postoperative management of patients with well-differentiated thyroid cancer includes hormonal therapy and radioactive iodine treatment (Table 17-8). Regardless of risk status, all patients with thyroid cancer should receive exogenous L-thyroxine suppressive therapy; considerable indirect evidence demonstrates that long-term TSH suppressive therapy favorably influences tumor recurrence, disease progression, and survival in well-differentiated thyroid cancer. Thyroglobulin is secreted by normal and cancerous thyroid cells and serves as a useful tumor marker for thyroid cancer persis-

Table 17-6. Survival Rates for Papillary and Follicular Thyroid Cancer

	5 y, %	10 y, %	Distant Metastases at Presentation, %
Papillary	95	92	20
Follicular	82	70	18

Table 17-7. Prognosis for Medullary Thyroid Cancer, Anaplastic Thyroid Cancer, and Thyroid Cancer

Thyroid Cancer Subtype	Associated Endocrinopathies	15-y Survival, %
Medullary		
Sporadic	None	70–80
MEN-IIa	Pheochromocytoma, parathyroid hyperplasia	85–90
MEN-IIb	Pheochromocytoma, mucosal neuromas	< 40–50
FMCT	None	100%
Anaplastic	None	4–6 mo median survival
Thyroid lymphoma	None	51 at 10-y survival

FMCT—familial medullary thyroid cancer; MEN-IIa and MEN-IIb—multiple endocrine neoplasia, types IIa and IIb.

Table 17-8. Adjuvant Management of Well-differentiated Thyroid Cancer

1. Postoperative withdrawal of L-thyroxine for 6 wk; administration of tri-iodothyronine (25–50 µg BID-TID) for first 4 wk. (Pregnancy should be prevented during this period.)

2. When TSH is > 35 mIU/mL, obtain ^{131}I scan and serum thyroglobulin level.

3. If, after total thyroidectomy, thyroid remnants or metastases are detected, or thyroglobulin level is > 10 mg/dL, administer calculated ablative/therapeutic dose of ^{131}I, with post-therapy whole-body scan.

4. Begin/resume long-term L-thyroxine replacement to completely suppress TSH to < 0.1 mIU/mL.

5. Repeat hypothyroid ^{131}I scan, thyroglobulin monitoring and radiotherapy every 6–12 mo until normal, then every 3–5 y (or until total ^{131}I dose of 500–800 mCi).

tence, recurrence, and progression. The sensitivity of this method is greatest when the patient is hypothyroid with high TSH levels. A poorly differentiated cancer may still secrete thyroglobulin after its iodine-concentrating ability has been lost.

Normal thyroid tissue concentrates radioiodine much more efficiently than thyroid cancer. Thus, any remaining thyroid tissue after thyroidectomy will decrease the efficacy of [131]I. Patients should have an ablative dose of ^{131}I while they are intentionally hypothyroid. [131]I is the treatment of choice for recurrent or metastatic differentiated thyroid cancer (20,21).

Radioiodine is not taken up by Hürthle cell, tall cell, medullary, or most anaplastic thyroid cancers and, thus, is not a therapeutic option. However, differentiated thyroid cancer that has lost affinity for radioiodine can still be treated successfully with large doses; 30% to 90% of patients with detectable thyroglobulin levels and a negative low-dose radioiodine scan who are treated with ^{131}I have uptake on their posttherapy scan. A treatment dose of 150 cGy delivers approximately 1000 cGy to the lesion. The risks of ^{131}I include temporary local pain, swelling, nausea and temporary myelotoxicity in up to a third of patients. Cases of leukemia and bladder cancer have been reported at high doses.

The most effective treatment for pulmonary metastases is ^{131}I, although it only offers palliation for bony metastases. External radiation therapy is reserved for palliation of bony metastases or for radioiodine-insensitive cases. Thyroid cancers that do not respond to radioiodine therapy are treated as advanced disease. Resection of recurrent regional disease offers no proven or theoretical advantage over [131]I. For locally advanced thyroid cancer, some have observed successful local control in a majority of patients treated with low-dose doxorubicin and hyperfractionated radiotherapy but no improvement in distant disease or in survival.

Treatment selection for regional MTC is based on the indolent growth of most of these tumors. Basal and stimulated calcitonin levels and serum carcinoembryonic antigen are followed postoperatively as indicators of recurrence and progression. With close surveillance and early reoperation, survival rates as high as 86% have been reported. Most experts recommend resection of clinically or radiologically evident disease, but some advocate aggressive search for residual MTC, using invasive imaging techniques followed by comprehensive resection in an attempt to obtain a biochemical cure [22,23]. MTC is insensitive to ^{131}I and external radiation.

THERAPY FOR ADVANCED DISEASE

There has not been substantial recent progress in the treatment of relapsed and metastatic thyroid cancer. In 33% to 42% of patients, metastatic disease does not take up radioiodine, and these patients have significantly decreased survival rates (at 10 years, 83% for those who do take up ^{131}I vs < 1% for those who do not). The most active chemotherapeutic agent is doxorubicin; at a dose up to 75 mg/m^2, it produces a 17% to 33% response rate in metastatic non-MTC. Responses are partial and of a moderate duration (up to ~2 y); most patients die of pulmonary (80%) and cerebral (20%) metastases. The combination of doxorubicin with other agents, such as cisplatin or bleomycin, have not improved efficacy. Although there is much indirect evidence that autoimmune mechanisms may favorably influence the outcome of patients with metastatic thyroid cancer, no trials employing biologic response modifiers have been reported.

Chemotherapy in advanced MTC is generally not administered until the development of debilitating diarrhea (the main symptom of advanced disease), which occurs with calcitonin levels greater than 10,000 pg/mL. Doxorubicin alone or in combination has the highest response rate (15%–30%), with mean duration of response of 21 months. There was no documented survival benefit. Octreotide therapy has produced palliation of symptoms and objective biochemical responses in several recent small studies; however, dose escalation usually was required to maintain the effect. Interferon α (IFN α) may provide similar palliative benefit as octreotide for advanced MTC.

Anaplastic thyroid cancer is stage IV by definition. Systemic chemotherapy has made no impact on the dismal prognosis. A protocol employing low-dose doxorubicin as a radiosensitizer for hyperfractionated external radiotherapy has been advocated. The multimodality therapy of radiotherapy, aggressive surgery, and combination chemotherapy may improve local control but offers no survival advantage.

CARCINOID TUMORS

ETIOLOGY AND RISK FACTORS

Carcinoid tumors arise from neuroendocrine enterochromaffin cells of neural crest origin and secrete the biogenic amine serotonin (5-hydroxytryptamine [5-HT]). Enterochromaffin cells are part of the amine precursor uptake and decarboxylation system, which is characterized by the potential for secretion of multiple amine and peptide hormones. Carcinoid tumors can also secrete adrenocorticotropic hormone (ACTH), somatostatin, α− and β−human chorionic gonadotropin, gastrin, and pancreatic polypeptide, which can disguise or complicate the clinical presentation of a carcinoid tumor. Precursor enterochromaffin cells are found submucosally throughout the gastrointestinal tract, bronchial tree, and genitourinary tract; carcinoid tumors arise from any of these sites.

Carcinoid tumors are clinically evident at a reported rate of 3.2 cases per 1 million, although this number underestimates their actual incidence according to autopsy studies. There are known associations of carcinoids with multiple endocrine neoplasia type I, of ampullary carcinoids with von Recklinghausen's disease, and of gastric carcinoids with hypergastrinemic states (*eg*, pernicious anemia, atrophic gastritis, and gastrinoma).

Carcinoid tumors have a characteristically indolent course that is heterogenous, depending on the histology and endocrine features of this diverse group of tumors. The median duration of symptoms prior to diagnosis is 21 months. Although one half of the symptomatic patients have unresectable disease at the time of diagnosis, over 50% of these patients will live 5 years or more after diagnosis. Median survival after onset of symptoms is 3.5 to 8.5 years.

The carcinoid syndrome is a spectrum of symptoms caused by the release of serotonin, histamine, and tachykinins into the systemic venous circulation. Symptoms include flushing, diarrhea, bronchospasm, and valvular heart disease (*ie*, tricuspid regurgitation, pulmonary stenosis). The severity of carcinoid syndrome is related directly to the bulk of tumor draining into the systemic circulation, which bypasses the first-pass effect of the portal circulation. The syndrome almost never occurs from midgut tumors unless they have metastasized to the liver. Rarely, carcinoid syndrome arises in patients with nonmetastatic gastrointestinal primary tumors, ovarian or testicular carcinoids, MTC, or pancreatic islet tumors. Precipitated by stress, FNA, alcohol, chemotherapy, or anesthesia, severe symptoms can present as carcinoid crisis associated with abdominal pain, hypotension, tachyarrhythmias, coma, and death. Carcinoid crisis is treated with parental (IV) octreotide in an emergent setting or administered prophylactically prior to FNA or surgery (100 μg SQ every 8 h).

In patients suspected to have a carcinoid tumor, the diagnosis is confirmed by measuring levels of 24-hour urine serotonin and 5-HIAA (serotonin metabolite). Measurement of platelet serotonin, serum chromogranin A, serotonin and substance P, and urinary 5-hydroxytryptophan (5-HTP, a serotonin precursor) can be helpful in ambiguous cases. Bronchial lavage for ACTH and thymic vein sampling are of little value in the diagnosis of bronchial carcinoid. Tumor localization can be difficult, relying on endoscopy, colonoscopy, CT scan, and other studies, as appropriate. The use of radiolabeled somatostatin receptor scintigraphy (SRS) has greatly improved the sensitivity and specificity in the localization of carcinoid tumors and regional or distant metastases; SRS should be applied in any patient with foregut or midgut carcinoid, carcinoid syndrome, or evidence of metastasis [24,25].

STAGING AND PROGNOSIS

Carcinoid tumors are generally classified by their primary location, which helps explain their heterogeneity in biologic behavior and prognosis (Table 17-9). Foregut carcinoids usually appear in the bronchial tree as classic "coin lesions" on chest radiographs. Foregut tumors also include tumors of the thymus, stomach, duodenum, and pancreas. They typically have a low 5-HT content and often secrete other agents, such as 5-HTP, histamine, or ACTH. Gastric carcinoids are commonly multifocal in sporadic cases. Midgut carcinoids secrete 5-HT and can arise from the appendix, ileum, and rarely from the jejunum or right colon. Over half of appendiceal carcinoids are diagnosed at surgery for acute appendicitis (1:250 appendicitis cases), and 90% are less than 1 cm in size. Appendiceal carcinoids occur predominantly at the tip of the appendix. Jejunoileal carcinoids are usually multiple in 25% to 35% of patients (~15% are < 1 cm). Of jejunoileal tumors, 40% are found within 2 ft of the ileocecal valve. Hindgut carcinoid tumors rarely secrete 5-HT; they arise from the rectum and rarely from the bladder, ovary, testis, and left colon (80% are < 1 cm). During screening with endoscopy for adeno-

matous lesions, rectal carcinoids are recognized frequently, typically as a small yellow nodule protruding from the anterior or lateral rectal wall.

Important prognostic factors for carcinoid tumors are site of primary tumor (see Table 17-9), histologic subtype, size of primary tumor, and extent of tumor at presentation. Of the four histologic subtypes, the insular variant is considered to have the best prognosis, trabecular is intermediate, and glandular and undifferentiated have the worst prognosis. No histologic criteria can differentiate benign from malignant neoplasms. The size of the primary tumor is indicative of malignant potential, whereas race, age, gender, nuclear DNA content, and hormonal function have not proven to be significant prognostic factors. The most important predictor of survival is the presence of metastases (Table 17-10).

PRIMARY DISEASE THERAPY

The only curative therapy for carcinoid tumors is operative resection. The extent of surgery is determined by the size and extent of the primary tumor. Lesions less than 1 cm in size are generally amenable to simple full-thickness excision. The extent of surgery is still somewhat controversial for lesions 1 to 2 cm in size; other prognostic factors (eg, site and histology) are commonly taken into account. Results of this treatment strategy have been reportedly curative for appendiceal and rectal carcinoids [25]. For patients with appendiceal lesions greater than 2 cm in the appendix, a right hemicolectomy is recommended. Rectal tumors of 2 cm or greater in size require an abdominoperineal or low anterior resection. Perioperative octreotide blockade is recommended for patients with carcinoid syndrome.

THERAPY FOR REGIONAL DISEASE

This indolent group of tumors recurs in patients after a median disease-free interval of 16 years. Primary resection of involved regional lymph nodes is reportedly associated with improved survival (80% at 5 y). Resection of isolated hepatic metastases may also improve prognosis [25]. However, only 2% to 5% of patients with carcinoid syndrome are candidates for hepatic resection.

As ileal carcinoids spread to the mesentery and lymph nodes, a marked fibrotic reaction can distort or infarct the bowel. Palliative resection is appropriate for bowel obstruction or bowel ischemia but has never been shown to prolong survival.

THERAPY FOR ADVANCED DISEASE

Carcinoid tumors metastasize to liver, bone, lymph nodes, and other less common sites (eg, the breast or heart). Resection of metastatic disease can be either curative or palliative. The benefit of palliative

Table 17-9. Prognosis of Carcinoid Tumors

Site	Relative Frequency, %	Rate of Metastasis, %	5-y Survival, %	Incidence of Carcinoid Syndrome, %
Foregut				
Bronchi	12	20	87	13
Stomach	2	22	52	9.5
Midgut				
Appendix	40	2	99	< 1
Ileum	25	35	54	9
Hindgut				
Rectum	15	15	83	1

Adapted from Norton et al. [37]; with permission.

Table 17-10. Prognosis for Carcinoid Tumors by Stage

	5-y Survival, %	10-y Survival, %
Localized disease	94	88
Regional lymph node metastasis	64	—
Distant metastases	18–30	0

resection should not be overlooked. As these tumors are often indolent, resection can provide a long interval of relative stability in spite of known residual disease.

Management of patients with the carcinoid tumor syndrome and unresectable disease should be separated into two distinct but related components. The syndrome should be managed by pharmacologic means, whereas the malignancy should be addressed by extirpative, embolic, or chemotherapeutic means. Management of the carcinoid syndrome can be helped by avoiding precipitating factors, such as caffeine or alcohol. In addition, there are a variety of pharmacologic agents that can be useful. Octreotide, in particular, can frequently provide outstanding palliation (Table 17-11).

Systemic treatment directed at the malignant component of the carcinoid tumor has been conventionally reserved until the tumor shows some evidence of progression. For metastatic disease mainly or completely confined to the liver, hepatic artery embolization (with or without concomitant chemotherapeutic agents) can have a substantial effect on the hormone production, although usually not on survival. Combination chemotherapeutic regimens of streptozotocin/5-fluorouracil or streptozotocin/adriamycin have similar, substantial partial response rates–particularly if hormone production is used as an endpoint—however, a survival advantage has not been evident (Table 17-12) [25]. Similarly, IFN α has been used extensively in some institutions with good results in managing patients over long periods of time; however, it is difficult to separate the effect of the therapy on survival from the indolent nature of the disease [26,27].

Immunotherapy of carcinoid metastases using leukocyte or recombinant IFN α has produced a good but variable biochemical response rate (29%–60%), with occasional complete remissions reported [28]. The median duration of response varies from 6 to 34 months. In addition, IFN α can offer excellent palliation of the carcinoid syndrome (30%–80% response rate). In a randomized study, therapy with IFN α had a significantly higher response rate and fewer side effects than did systemic 5-fluorouracil chemotherapy. Prior cytotoxic chemotherapy did not preclude effective treatment with IFN α [28]. The combination of IFN α and octreotide recently produced biochemical objective responses in 77% of patients, with median duration of remission of 12 months [29]. Therapy with IFN α has been less successful in reducing tumor size (15% response rate) [29].

PANCREATIC ENDOCRINE TUMORS

EPIDEMIOLOGY AND RISK FACTORS

Pancreatic endocrine tumors are rare human malignancies that are similar to carcinoid tumors; they are derived from enterochromaffin cells that are histologically classified as Apudoma (amine precursor uptake and decarboxylation). Although the incidence of clinically detected pancreatic islet cell tumors is approximately five cases per million population, autopsy series have revealed a prevalence of incidental pancreatic endocrine tumors up to 1.5%. Neoplasms of the endocrine pancreas are defined as functional when they secrete hormones that cause a clinical syndrome. A nonfunctional tumor is one not associated with a clinical syndrome despite the production of hormones. This latter category includes tumors secreting pancreatic peptide (PPoma) and neurotensin (neurotensinomas). Except for insulinomas, which are most commonly benign, pancreatic endocrine tumors have a high (60%–90%) malignant potential. Gastrinomas are the most common malignant pancreatic islet cell tumors and are well studied due to their association with Zollinger–Ellison syndrome and MEN type 1. The localization, surgical management, and therapies are similar for several of these rare tumors of the endocrine pancreas and are detailed together.

ZOLLINGER-ELLISON SYNDROME

In 1955, Zollinger and Ellison theorized a relationship between two patients with severe peptic ulcer disease and pancreatic tumors. At present, Zollinger–Ellison syndrome (ZES) is estimated to occur in 0.1% of patients with duodenal ulcer disease. Gastrinomas present commonly as sporadic cases but are associated with MEN type I syndrome in 25% of patients. The familial patients tend to present at younger ages and have multiple tumors.

The clinical presentation of ZES is a result of gastric acid hypersecretion secondary to hypergastrinemia. Patients typically present with abdominal pain, diarrhea, and peptic ulcer disease. The diagnosis of ZES is confirmed by a fasting hypergastrinemia and an elevated basal gastric acid secretion of at least 15 mEq/h. Other diagnoses that can mimic ZES (eg, retained gastric antrum syndrome, chronic gastric outlet obstruction, and antral G-cell hyperplasia) are excluded by history and provocative tests (eg, secretin stimulation test or standard meal test).

Gastrinomas occur in the head of the pancreas or duodenum up to 90% of the time in an area bounded by the sweep of the duode-

Table 17-11. Pharmacotherapy for Carcinoid Syndrome

Agent	Flush	Diarrhea	Dose
Phenoxybenzamine	Better	No change	10–30 mg/d
Chlorpromazine	Better	No change	10–25 mg q 8 h
Methyldopa	Somewhat better	No change	4–6 g/d
Cyproheptadine	No change	Better	4–8 mg q 8 h
Ketanserin	Somewhat better	Better	40–160 mg/d
Methysergide	No change	Better	3–8 mg/d
Octreotide	Better (89%)	Better (74%)	50–150 μg SQ q 8 h
rIFN α-2b	Better	Better	9–30 X 10_6 U/m^2/wk

Adapted from Norton et al. [37]; with permission.

Table 17-12. Adjuvant Therapy for Carcinoid Tumors

Agent	Response Rate, %
Doxorubicin	21
Streptopzocin	30
5-Fluorouracil	26
Streptozocin and 5-Fluorouracil	33
Streptozocin + doxorubicin	40
Interferon α	42–47 (median duration 36 months)

num, the neck of the pancreas, and the junction of the cystic and common bile ducts (*ie*, the gastrinoma triangle) [30]. Histologically indistinguishable, the malignant potential of pancreatic endocrine tumors is determined by the presence of metastases. Approximately 50% of patients with gastrinomas have metastasized to lymph nodes or liver at time of presentation.

Multiple modalities are used for the localization of pancreatic endocrine tumors. Abdominal CT scan locates primary tumors in approximately 50% of ZES cases, although this modality is dependent on tumor size and location. CT scan is more sensitive for pancreatic gastrinomas than it is for other typically smaller extrahepatic tumors. Visceral angiography can also be used to selectively focus on the arterial supply of the pancreas and peripancreatic area, with a variable success rate of 45% to 85%. Reports are small and variable regarding whether MRI is more sensitive than visceral angiography or CT scan for detecting metastases.

Somatostatin receptor scintigraphy is also a sensitive modality to localize primary gastrinomas (60%) and their metastases (90%). This technique is also useful for other pancreatic endocrine tumors except for insulinomas, which lack sufficient numbers of the type II somatostatin receptors [24,25]. In a small fraction of patients, the initial localization studies of CT scan, visceral angiography, and SRS will not identify the primary tumor. Portal venous hormone sampling and selective arterial secretin stimulation test may help localize the region of the functional tumor.

Other imaging modalities under ongoing evaluation are endoscopic and intraoperative ultrasonography (IOUS). A localization rate of 82% of primary gastrinomas using endoscopic ultrasonography has been reported in one institution; this modality has also been used for insulinoma [31–33]. Most authorities agree that IOUS is an important adjunct to the operative exploration for both gastrinoma and insulinoma [31,32]. A prospective study of the use of IOUS revealed a change in operative procedure in 10% of cases. Both of these techniques are sensitive for the detection of primary pancreatic neuroendocrine tumors but are highly user dependent. Intraoperative endoscopic duodenal transillumination may help in identification of small, duodenal gastrinomas, but duodenotomy and palpation of the lumen is standard now for most surgeons for gastrinoma [31].

TREATMENT OF ZOLLINGER-ELLISON SYNDROME
Medical Management
Treatment of ZES requires medical management of gastric acid hypersecretion and localization of primary tumor and metastatic disease. The peptic ulcer disease associated with ZES is successfully treated long-term with antisecretory medications: histamine H2 antagonists (cimetidine, famotidine), omeprazole, lansoprazole, or proton-pump inhibitors. These drugs should be adjusted to obtain a gastric pH > 5 during the hour prior to the next dose. These medications have been found to be efficacious and safe with long-term usage and have minimal side effects.

Surgical Management
With the success of antisecretory medications, the number of gastrectomies and their associated morbidity and mortality has drastically declined. Therefore, the factor most responsible for the prognosis of gastrinomas is their malignant potential. Once gastric acid hypersecretion is controlled, the goal of surgical management is resection of gastrinoma in patients with ZES. The survival rate for ZES is 62% to 87% at 5 years and 47% to 77% at 10 years. In patients who had undergone complete resection at the time of surgery, the rates improve to 90% and from 62% to 100% at 5 and 10 years, respectively [34]. There is controversy as to the role of surgical management of gastrinomas in patients in MEN type I.

TREATMENT OF METASTATIC GASTRINOMA
Chemotherapy, hepatic artery embolization, cytoreductive surgery, hormonal therapy with somatostatin analog octreotide, immunotherapy with IFN, hepatic transplantation, or combinations of these have been studied in small numbers. These modalities have been examined for patients with pancreatic and neuroendocrine tumors, including carcinoids, with varying success. Although there has been a low response rate, the combination of streptozotocin and doxorubicin is commonly recommended as treatment for metastatic pancreatic endocrine tumors, including gastrinomas [26]. There have been small studies that show that hormonal treatment with octreotide and immunotherapy with IFN α can seem to stabilize progressive disease. Additional studies are needed to evaluate the efficacy of these therapies for gastrinomas and other malignant pancreatic endocrine tumors [26].

INSULINOMAS
The most common pancreatic endocrine tumor is insulinoma whose clinical syndrome was characterized by Whipple in 1935. Whipple's triad includes 1) symptoms of hypoglycemia during fasting, 2) a documented blood sugar below 50 mg/dL, and 3) relief of symptoms once glucose is administered. Insulinomas occur predominantly in women in their fourth decade with an overall incidence of 0.8 per million population. The symptoms of patients with insulinomas are classified into two categories: neuroglycopenic and adrenergic symptoms. These symptoms include confusion, seizure, personality change, coma or palpitations, trembling, diaphoresis and tachycardia. The diagnosis of an insulinoma is confirmed by a monitored 72-hour fast that documents symptoms associated with a blood sugar less than 50 mg/dL and a plasma insulin-to-glucose ratio above 0.4. To exclude other causes of hyperinsulinism (*eg*, reactive hypoglycemia and surreptitious administration of insulin or oral hypoglycemic agents) elevated plasma levels of C-peptide and proinsulin are documented [32].

Once the biochemical diagnosis of an insulinoma is confirmed, radiologic studies can be performed for preoperative tumor localization. Insulinomas are almost exclusively found in the pancreas; similar localization studies as outlined for gastrinomas can be undertaken. However, given the small nature of these pancreatic tumors, the rare incidence of malignancy, and the high likelihood of the presence of the tumor in the pancreas, IOUS is the most sensitive and most useful technique for localization of the primary tumor.

Unlike gastrinomas, only 10% of insulinomas are malignant. Management of these tumors focuses on surgical resection of primary lesion for control of symptoms. Medical therapy prior to surgery can include dietary control and the administration of octreotide and diazoxide, both of which have been shown to decrease hyperinsulinemia; however neither method provides adequate control of hypoglycemia for most patients. Tumor debulking can be performed for accessible metastases as well as combined chemotherapy and immunotherapy, as discussed previously for all pancreatic neuroendocrine tumors.

UNCOMMON PANCREATIC ENDOCRINE TUMORS

These rare tumors of the pancreatic endocrine cells are most frequently malignant; metastases are present in more than half of the patients at the time of diagnosis. The surgical management and treatment for metastatic disease is common to all pancreatic endocrine tumors as discussed previously.

VIPOMAS

The VIPoma syndrome (Verner–Morrison syndrome) is characterized by profuse watery diarrhea that leads to hypokalemia and dehydration. This syndrome is also referred to as the acronym WDHA (watery diarrhea, hypokalemia, and achlorhydria). Vipomas are diagnosed by elevated fasting levels of plasma VIP (vasoactive intestinal polypeptide) associated with severe secretory diarrhea. Management initially includes correction of electrolyte imbalances, acidosis, and dehydration. Octreotide has been found to decrease volume of diarrhea in a majority of patients. Surgical excision of these tumors, predominantly located in the pancreas, is the mainstay of palliative and potentially curative treatment.

GLUCAGONOMA

The syndrome associated with glucagonomas includes a dermatitis known as necrolytic migratory erythema, diarrhea, diabetes, anemia, and stomatitis. This rare tumor usually occurs as a large tumor that can be anywhere in the pancreas. The diagnosis is established by the documentation of elevated levels of plasma glucagon. Octreotide treatment eliminates the rash associated with glucagonomas, although it is not effective in treatment for the diabetes. Surgical excision is recommended, although the majority are metastatic on presentation.

SOMATOSTATINOMA

This is the most uncommon pancreatic endocrine tumor. Symptoms are attributed to the various hormonal functions of somatostatin and include diabetes, gallbladder disease, diarrhea, steatorrhea, and hypochlorhydria. Somatostatinomas are biochemically diagnosed by elevated plasma levels of somatostatin and are associated with von Recklinghausen's disease if located in the duodenum. Surgery, if technically feasible, is warranted.

REFERENCES

1. Ross NS, Aron DC: Hormonal evaluation of the patient with an incidentally discovered adrenal mass. *N Engl J Med* 1990, 323:1401–1405.

2. Reinig JW, Doppman JL: Magnetic resonance imaging of the adrenal. *Radiology* 1986, 26:186–190.

3. Doppman JL, Reinig JW Dwyer AJ, *et al.*: Differentiation of adrenal masses by magnetic resonance imaging *Surgery* 1987, 102:1018–1026.

4. Reinig JW, Doppman JL, Dwyer AJ, Frank J: MRI of indeterminate adrenal masses *Am J Radiol* 1986, 147:493–496.

5. Doppman JL, Nieman LK, Travis WD, *et al.*: CT or MR imaging of massive macronodular adrenocortical disease: a rare cause of autonomous primary adrenal hypercortisolism. *J Comput Assist Tomogr* 1991, 15:773–779.

6. Yu KC, Alexander HR, Ziessman HA, *et al.*: Role of preoperative iodocholesterol scintiscanning in patients undergoing adrenalectomy for Cushing's syndrome. *Surgery* 1995, 118:981–987.

7. Bellantone R, Ferrante A, Boscherini M, *et al.*: Role of reoperation in recurrence of adreanl cortical carcinoma: results from 188 cases collected in the Italian national registry for adrenal cortical carcinoma. *Surgery* 1997, 122:1212–1218.

8. Doherty GM, Nieman LK, Cutler GB Jr, *et al.*: Time to recovery of the hypothalamic-pituitary-adrenal axis after curative resection of adrenal tumors in patients with Cushing's syndrome. *Surgery* 1990, 108:1085–1090.

9. Jensen JC, Pass HI, Sindelar WF, Norton JA: Aggressive resection of recurrent or metastatic disease in select patients with adrenocortical carcinoma. *Arch Surg* 1991, 126:457–461.

10. Decker RA, Elson P, Hogan TF, *et al.*: Eastern cooperative oncology group study 1989: mitotane and adriamycin in patients with advanced adrenocortical carcinoma. *Surgery* 1991, 110:1006–1013.

11. Van Slooten H, Moolenaar AJ, Van Seters AP, Smeek D: The treatment of adrenocortical carcinoma with o,p-DDD: prognostic implications of serum levels monitoring. *Eur J Clin Oncol* 1984, 20:47–53.

12. Schlumberger M, Brugieres L, Gicquel C, *et al.*: 5-Fluorouracil, doxorubicin, and cisplatin as treatment for adrenal cortical carcinoma. *Cancer* 1991, 67:2997–3000.

13. Bukowski RM, Wolfe M, Levine HS, *et al.*: Phase II trial of mitotane and cisplatin in patients with adrenal carcinoma: a Southwest Oncology Group study. *J Clin Oncol* 1993, 11:161–165.

14. Johnson DH, Creco A: Treatment of metastatic adrenal cortical carcinoma with cisplatin and etoposide (VP-16). *Cancer* 1986, 58:2198–2202.

15. Hesketh PJ, McCaffrey RP, Finkel HE, *et al.*: Cisplatin-based treatment of adrenocortical carcinoma. *Cancer Treat Rep* 1987, 71:222–224.

16. Berruti A, Terzolo M, Paccotti P: Favorable response of metastatic ACC to etoposide, adriamycin and cisplatin. *Tumor* 1992, 78:345–348.

17. Hay ID, Bergstralh EL, Goellner JR, *et al.*: Predicting outcome in papillary thyroid carcinoma: development of a reliable prognostic scoring system in a cohort of 1779 patients surgically treated at one institution during 1940 through 1989. *Surgery* 1993, 114:1050–1057.

18. Chi DD, Toshima K, Donis-Keller H, Wells SA Jr: Predictive testing for multiple endocrine neoplasia type 2A based on the detection of mutations in the *ret* proto-oncogene. *Surgery* 1994, 116:124–132.

19. Wells SA Jr, Chi DD, Toshima K, *et al.*: Predictive DNA testing and prophylactive thyroidectomy in patients at risk for multiple endocrine neoplasia type 2A. *Ann Surg* 1994, 220:237–247.

20. Wells SA Jr, Ontjes DA, Cooper CW, *et al.*: The early diagnosis of medullary carcinoma of the thyroid gland in patients with multiple endocrine neoplasia type II. *Ann Surg* 1975, 182:362–370.

21. Mazzaferri EL, Young RL: Papillary thyroid carcinoma: a 10-year follow-up report of the impact of therapy in 576 patients. *Am J Med* 1981, 70:511–518.

22. Moley JF, Wells SA Jr, Dilley WG, Tisell LE: Reoperation for recurrent or persistent medullary thyroid cancer. *Surgery* 1993, 114:1090–1096.

24. Moley JF, Dilley WG, DeBenedetti MK: Improved results of cervical reoperation for medullary thyroid carcinoma. *Ann Surg* 1997, 225:734–740.

25. Meko JB, Doherty GM, Siegel BA, Norton JA: Evaluation of somatostatin-receptor scintigraphy for detecting neuroendocrine tumors. *Surgery* 1996, 120:975–984.

26. Wiedenmann B, Jensen RT, Mignon M, *et al.*: General recommendations for the preoperative diagnosis and surgical management of neuroendocrine gastroenteropancreatic tumors. *World J Surg* 1998, in press.

27. Arnold R, Frank M, Kajdan U: Management of gastroenteropancreatic endocrine tumors: the place of somatostatin analogues. *Digestion* 1994, 55:107–113.

28. Oberg K, Norheim I, Lundqvist G, Wide L: Cytotoxic treatment in patients with malignant carcinoid tumors: response to streptozocin alone or in combination with 5-FU. *Acta Oncol* 1987, 26:429–432.

29. Oberg K, Norheim I, Lind E, *et al.*: Treatment of malignant carcinoid tumors with human leukocyte interferon: long term results. *Cancer Treat Rev* 1986, 70:1297–1304.

30. Tiensuu-Janson EM, Ahlstrom H, Andersson T, Oberg KE: Octreotide and interferon alfa: a new combination for the treamtent of malignant carcinoid tumours. *Eur J Cancer* 1992, 28A:1647–1650.

31. Stabile BE, Morrow DJ, Passaro E: The gastrinoma triangle: operative implications. *Am J Surg* 1984, 147:25–31.

32. Doherty GM, Norton JA: Preoperative and intraoperative localization of gastrinomas. *Probl Gen Surg* 1990, 7:521–532.

33. Doherty GM, Doppman JL, Shawker TH, *et al.*: Results of a prospective strategy to diagnose, localize and resect insulinomas. *Surgery* 1991, 110:989–997.

34. Thompson NW, Czako PF, Fritts LL: Role of endoscopic ultrasonography in the localization of insulinomas and gastrinomas. *Surgery* 1994, 116:1131–1138.

35. Sullivan M, Boileau M, Hodges CV: Adrenal cortical carcinoma *J Urol* 1978, 120:660–605.

36. Beahrs OH, Henson DE, Hutter RVP, Myers MH (eds): Manual for Staging of Cancer Philadelphia: JB Lippincott; 1988.

37. Norton JA, Doppman JL, Jensen RT: Curative resection in Zollinger-Ellison syndrome: results of a 10-year prospective study. *Ann Surg* 1992, 215:8–18.

MITOTANE AND CISPLATIN

Mitotane (o,p-DDD) is an isomer of the pesticide DDT that inhibits corticosteroid biosynthesis and, at high doses, causes selective adrenocortical atrophy and infarction. It is not effective in bulky retroperitoneal adrenal cortical cancer. Cisplatin is an alkylating agent that acts to cross-link DNA. In vitro, mitotane reverses the multidrug resistance mediated by MDR-1 expression that occurs in adrenal cortical cancer cells.

DOSAGE AND SCHEDULING

1. Prehydrate with saline 2 L IV and mannitol 12.5 g IV
2. Cisplatin 100 mg/m^2 IV, mannitol 25 g IV, and saline 1 L IV over 2 h, d 1
3. o,p-DDD 1 g PO four times daily, d 1 and daily while on regimen
4. Cortisone acetate and fludrocortisone acetate daily as needed

RECENT EXPERIENCE AND RESPONSE RATES

In a phase II clinical trial, these two agents in combination produced responses in 11 of 37 (30%) patients, with a median duration of response of 8 months and median time to response of 76 d[6]. Median survival from treatment was 11.8 mo. Although patients with complete surgical resection of tumor were not eligible for the study, a significant survival advantage was found for patients who had previously undergone surgical removal of primary tumor or bulky disease and for patients with a performance status of 0 or 1 [6]. Patients older than 65 y, those with extensive prior radiation, and those with poor tolerance to previous chemotherapy were considered high-risk and were given a lower dose of cisplatin.

CANDIDATES FOR TREATMENT

Patients with inoperable adrenal cortical cancer, regardless of tumor functionality

ALTERNATIVE THERAPIES

Dose escalation of mitotane to 8–16 g/d; possibly cisplatin and etoposide combination therapy, but currently insufficient data for recommendation [8–10]

SPECIAL PRECAUTIONS

Patients with significantly impaired renal function, myelosuppression, or hearing loss are ineligible

TOXICITIES

Drug combination: severe nausea and vomiting (22% of patients), mild mucositis, mild myalgias, weakness

Mitotane: dose-dependent anorexia, nausea, vomiting, diarrhea, confusion, somnolence, depression, dizziness, skin rash, cholestasis, male gynecomastia, visual disturbances

Cisplatin: nausea and vomiting, nephrotoxicity, irreversible paresthesias and neuropathies, cumulative ototoxicity, myelosuppression, anaphylaxis

DRUG INTERACTIONS

Anticonvulsants, aminoglycoside antibiotics, warfarin, exogenously administered steroids

NURSING INTERVENTIONS

Monitor renal function and obtain CBC, BUN, and creatine frequently throughout treatment; be prepared for anaphylactic reactions; provide proper antiemetics; hydrate well to prevent renal toxicity

PATIENT INFORMATION

Patient should be informed that mitotane may cause adrenal insufficiency.

LOW-DOSE DOXORUBICIN AND RADIATION THERAPY

Most anaplastic thyroid cancers are metastatic at presentation and, uncontrolled, produce death from suffocation in 4–6 mo. Conventional radiotherapy often fails to induce significant regression of tumor around the airway. Doxorubicin is the single most active agent against thyroid carcinoma and, in addition, acts as a radiosensitizer of radioresistant hypoxic tumor cells, particularly at low doses. A hyperfractionated radiation therapy schedule may deliver more efficacious therapy to rapidly dividing tissues, while minimizing tissue morbidity.

DOSAGE AND SCHEDULING

Doxorubicin 10 mg/m^2 IV administered 1 × wk 1.5 h prior to radiation therapy and hyperfractionated radiation dose of 160 cGy per treatment, 2 × d for 3 d/wk; total tumor dose 5760 cGy delivered over 40 d

DOSAGE MODIFICATIONS: 70% of patients require a 1-wk respite during therapy due to toxicity

LAB MONITORING: clinical examination and subjective dyspnea, WBC

RECENT EXPERIENCE AND RESPONSE RATES

Kim and Leeper reported that this regimen, which is under further investigation at the National Cancer Institute, resulted in complete tumor regression in 8 of 9 patients with anaplastic giant and spindle cell carcinoma of the thyroid gland [22]. Patients went on to die of distant metastatic disease (median survival from treatment 10 mo) without increased survival by comparison to historical controls. Findings were confirmed in a follow-up study published in 1987 (84% response rate) [18]. Median survival was 1 y from therapy.

CANDIDATES FOR TREATMENT

Patients with confirmed anaplastic thyroid cancer, patients with locally advanced well-differentiated thyroid cancer unresponsive to ^{131}I therapy.

ALTERNATIVE THERAPIES

Systemic chemotherapy (with adriamycin-based regimens). A phase II trial of doxorubicin and interferon alpha for metastatic nonmedullary thyroid cancer is currently ongoing at the Pittsburgh Cancer Institute

SPECIAL PRECAUTIONS

Airway must be secured first

TOXICITIES

Therapy combination: increased toxicity to the myocardium, mucosae, skin, and liver with this combination;
Doxorubicin: minimal at this dose;
Radiation: mild-to-moderate pharyngoesophagitis and tracheitis; skin erythema, hyperpigmentation and late desquamation, laryngeal edema, cervical myelopathy

PATIENT INFORMATION

Patient should be informed that therapy may cause local pain and swelling.

OCTREOTIDE AND INTERFERON α-2B

Octreotide, a long-acting analogue of the natural hormone somatostatin, suppresses the secretion of serotonin and gut peptides. It has been used effectively by many clinicians for the symptoms of carcinoid syndrome, but produces tumor regression at a low rate. Interferon α-2b (IFN α-2b) is believed to exert direct antiproliferative action against tumor cells as well as to modulate the host immune response to tumor. This protocol was designed to augment the response to octreotide by the addition of IFN α-2b, which itself has a 30%–60% response rate in malignant carcinoid tumors.

DOSAGE AND SCHEDULING

IFN α-2b 3×10^6 U SQ $3 \times$ wk and octreotide 100 μg SQ twice daily

DOSAGE MODIFICATIONS: Weeks 8–16 — dose escalation of IFN α-2b to 5×10^6 U SQ $3 \times$ wk, as allowed by side effects and leukocyte count ($> 4 \times 10^9$/l); after week 16 — further escalation of IFN α-2b to 10×10^6 U SQ $3 \times$ wk, as allowed by side effects and leukocyte count

LAB MONITORING: Urine 5-HIAA, plasma serotonin, and other tumor markers q 4 wk; CBC, platelet count, glucose, renal function, response q 4 wk; thyroid function, gallbladder ultrasound q 8 wk

RECENT EXPERIENCE AND RESPONSE RATES

In a recent phase II clinical trial, these two agents were administered together to 24 patients who, during initial treatment with octreotide (50–150 μg twice daily), had demonstrated progressive disease [30]. Administration of IFN α-2b together with octreotide produced an objective biochemical 77% response rate with median duration of response of 12 mo. Median survival from treatment was 58 mo. Symptoms of carcinoid syndrome were ameliorated in 10 of 18 patients (56%). No patient in this trial had significant objective tumor regression. No information is available concerning the efficacy of this regimen in patients not previously nonresponding to octreotide alone.

CANDIDATES FOR TREATMENT

Patients with inoperable metastatic carcinoid neoplasms, regardless of tumor functionality

SPECIAL PRECAUTIONS

Patients with significant preexisting cardiac disease or renal failure

ALTERNATIVE THERAPIES

Regimens with higher doses of octreotide (50–150 μg SQ TID) and IFN α-2b (10 mIUμ SQ daily); hepatic artery occlusion combined with chemotherapy or IFN α-2b (recently reported with comparable success rate)

TOXICITIES

Octreotide: changes in blood glucose mild and reversible, hypothyroidism, fat malabsorption, migratory thrombophlebitis; gallstones or sludge (15%–20% of patients) and acute cholecystitis (up to one third of patients with gallstones), prophylactic cholecystectomy may be appropriate;
IFN α-2b: flu-like syndrome and nausea and vomiting with first administration; may exacerbate preexisting cardiac disease; anorexia, mild weight loss, bone marrow suppression, disturbed thyroid function including hypothyroidism and autoimmune thyroiditis, depression

DRUG INTERACTIONS

Octreotide: H_2-antagonists, antidiarrheal agents, insulin, sulfonureas, β-blockers, antihypertensives, thyroid replacement hormone; **Interferon α:** unknown

NURSING INTERVENTIONS

Monitor for development of gallstones and biliary colic; instruct patient in self-injection

PATIENT INFORMATION

Patients may self-administer injection after learning technique

ACUTE MYELOID LEUKEMIA

Acute myeloid leukemia (AML) is the most common type of acute leukemia that occurs in adults, accounting for over 80% of the leukemias diagnosed in patients over age 20. AML can effect all ages but is rare in childhood. The incidence increases with age, with a median age at the time of diagnosis of approximately 55 years. AML is rare compared with other malignancies, accounting for approximately 3 cases per 100,000. Whereas certain environmental exposures (chemicals such as petroleum solvents or radiation exposure) and occupations (*eg*, rubber workers) have been associated with an increased risk of AML, the etiology in the vast majority of cases remains unclear. The molecular events leading to AML are now only beginning to be elucidated.

Several inherited genetic disorders and immunodeficiency states are associated with an increased risk of AML. These include disorders with defects in DNA stability, leading to random chromosomal breakage, such as Bloom's syndrome and Fanconi's anemia. Li-Fraumeni kindreds have mutated p53 on chromosome 17, which may alter tumor suppressor gene functions. Down syndrome (trisomy 21) is associated with an 18-fold increase in the risk of AML [1]. Congenital immunodeficiency states, such as ataxia-telangiectasia and X-linked agammaglobulinemia, are also associated with increased rates of AML (Table 18-1).

AML that has arisen out of a prior myelodysplastic syndrome or other bone marrow failure syndrome is termed secondary AML. A prior exposure to particular chemotherapy agents or radiation therapy for other diseases is being increasingly recognized as a risk factor for secondary AML [2]. Exposure to alkylating agents in regimens such as MOPP (mechlorethamine, vincristine, procarbazine, and prednisone) chemotherapy for Hodgkin's disease is associated with a cumulative risk of AML at 10 years that can be as high as 10% [3]. Exposure to epipodophyllotoxins is associated with the development of leukemia, often occurring within a few years of treatment and commonly having the specific chromosomal abnormality 11q23 [4,5]. Radiation therapy is also a risk factor for AML. The presence of prior myelodysplastic syndrome or other bone marrow failure syndrome is also associated with AML. An increasing incidence of myelodysplastic syndrome and associated secondary AML is being recognized following autologous bone marrow transplantation [6]. There is a 10% to 20% actuarial incidence of secondary AML/myelodysplasia after autologous bone marrow transplant when total body irradiation is part of the conditioning regimen for non-Hodgkin's lymphoma.

CLASSIFICATION AND PROGNOSIS

The diagnosis of AML is based on both the histologic and immunophenotypic evaluation of peripheral blood and bone marrow samples. Since 1976, the French-American-British (FAB) classification has been used to classify acute leukemia. Several modifications have been made since its creation, but the classification remains based on histologic appearance of the blasts and the use of histochemical stains. Eight subtypes of AML, designated M0 through M7, have been described. Currently, with the exception of the M3 (progranulocytic leukemia) subtype, initial therapy for remaining subtypes is similar. Various subtypes, however, may be associated with different prognoses.

Several prognostic factors have been identified in patients with AML (Table 18-2). These factors may be used to identify patients who have a high rate of cure with conventional chemotherapy alone. Conversely, patients with poor prognostic features may be considered for high-dose chemotherapy approaches (*eg*, bone marrow transplantation) early in the course of their disease, or they may be candidates for novel approaches to treat AML.

Older age has been demonstrated to be associated with inferior outcomes in numerous studies [7]. Patients over 60 years of age have a lower rate of complete remission following induction chemotherapy compared with patients younger than 60 years of age. The higher death rate in this population is related to an increase in treatment-related toxicity (*eg*, death from infection) but also to an increased risk of death related to leukemia. The increased incidence of secondary AML, which is often more refractory to chemotherapy, may provide a partial explanation for the inferior outcome in this population. The benefits of high dose post remission therapy in this population are also questionable.

Other adverse features of AML at the time of presentation include an elevated white blood cell count (WBC) of greater than 100,000. The reason for the impact of the high WBC on outcome is unclear but may suggest an increased proliferative capacity of the abnormal clone. Patients with high WBC are also at increased risk of leukostasis, which is an oncologic emergency created by the obstruction of the microvasculature by leukemic blasts. Patients with leukostasis may present with altered mental status or respiratory distress and have an increased early mortality [8].

Immunophenotypic analysis of leukemia cell surface antigens helps in the determination of myeloid or lymphoid lineage in cases in which histologic examination is not definitive [9]. The prognostic significance of particular cell surface antigens has not yet been fully defined [10]. Approximately 20% of myeloid leukemias may demon-

Table 18-1. Etiologic and Risk Factors in AML and ALL

AML	ALL
Chromosomal fragility syndromes	Chromosome fragility
Bloom's Syndrome	
Fanconi's Anemia	
Mutations of suppressor oncogenes (p53)	Down syndrome
Li-Fraumeni Syndrome	
Age	Radiation exposure
Myelodysplasia	
Radiation or chemotherapy	

ALL—acute lymphoblastic leukemia; AML—acute myeloid leukemia.

Table 18-2. Prognostic Factors in Acute Myeloid Leukemia

Factor	Good prognosis	Poor
White blood count	< 100,000	> 100,000
Age	< 60	> 60
Cytogenic SP Findings	Translocations 8;21 and 15;17 and inversion 16	Deletions of 5 and 7; trisomy 8; multiple cytogenic abnormalities

strate mixed-lineage antigens (both myeloid and lymphoid), and these leukemias are associated with a worse prognosis. AML with blasts expressing antigens that are associated with early hematopoietic development (eg, CD34) also have a poor outcome and may indicate the presence of a primitive malignant clone [11,12]. In one study, patients whose cells were CD14- or CD13-positive had a worse prognosis than those whose cells did not express these markers. Expression of CD2 may be associated with a better prognosis. The presence of certain cell surface markers in AML may serve as a target for emerging strategies using monoclonal antibodies as a part of treatment.

Specific cytogenetic abnormalities have been associated with clinical outcome. Translocations of 8;21, 15;17, and inversion 16 are associated with a good prognosis and an improved disease-free survival compared with patients with either normal chromosomes or other cytogenetic abnormalities [13]. Deletions of chromosomes 5 or 7 are associated with inferior outcomes, and these patients may be considered for early intensive therapy, such as bone marrow transplantation.

THERAPY

Chemotherapy

Treatment of AML has been divided into three stages: induction, post remission therapy, and therapy at the time of relapse. The goal of induction therapy is to achieve a complete remission (CR) and then to proceed to the administration of postremission therapy in an attempt to achieve the maximal disease-free survival and cure. Induction therapy for all types of AML includes the combination of cytosine arabinoside (cytarabine or Ara-C) with an anthracycline. Induction for M3 AML should be considered distinct and is discussed below. Typically, patients receive cytarabine as a continuous infusion of 100 to 200 mg/m^2/d for 7 days. This infusion is combined with an anthracycline (eg, daunorubicin [7], idarubicin [14,15], or mitoxantrone [16]) for 3 days (Table 18-3). Two trials have compared daunorubicin/Ara-C and idarubicin/Ara-C in AML induction [14,15]. Idarubicin was associated with superior remission rates in patients under 60 years of age compared with daunorubicin. Of note, the daunorubicin arm of one study demonstrated a worse CR rate than that noted in larger

comparative trials; therefore, the superiority of idarubicin has not been clearly demonstrated. Daunorubicin and idarubicin are both associated with cardiotoxicity at doses greater than 450 mg/m^2, whereas mitoxantrone is felt to be less cardiotoxic. A current Eastern Cooperative Oncology Group (ECOG) trial is comparing daunorubicin, idarubicin, and mitoxantrone in combination with cytarabine as induction therapy for AML. Combination chemotherapy is associated with an induction CR rate of approximately 60% to 70% in patients younger than 60 years of age and 40% in patients older than 60 years of age.

Alternative induction regimens include high-dose cytarabine [17], high-dose cyclophosphamide and etoposide [18], or standard-dose cytarabine and etoposide [19]. In a single-institution trial, the addition of high-dose cytarabine following standard "7+3" improved the remission rate in patients with AML to 86% in patients under age 63 years of age [20]. This regimen has not been directly compared with the standard "7+3" regimen in a randomized study.

There is debate about whether older patients (> 70 y of age) and patients with secondary AML benefit from intensive induction approaches because in this population the CR rates remain low, and the treatment-related toxicity is significant. Low-dose Ara-C (10–20 mg/m^2/d) has been advocated by some in the treatment of older patients in an attempt to avoid the acute side effects associated with standard induction [21,22]. Although responses can be seen with low-dose Ara-C, many weeks of therapy may be required, and complications related to prolonged pancytopenia can be noted just as when following standard induction chemotherapy. In a recent large Southwestern Oncology Group trial, elderly patients (median age, 68 y) with favorable or normal cytogenetics had CR rates comparable with younger patients, suggesting that these patients may benefit from more aggressive induction regimens [23].

It is estimated that 1×10^9 leukemia cells may remain when patients are in complete remission. Postremission therapy is designed to further reduce and eliminate these cells. Postremission therapy may include reiterations of standard-dose cytarabine and anthracycline for two more courses or the use of other doses of cytarabine. In a prospective trial, Cancer and Leukemia Group B (CALGB) compared three different doses of cytarabine as postremission therapy [24]. Patients younger than 60 years of age received either 100 mg/m^2 for 5 days, 400 mg/m^2 for 5 days, or 3 g/m^2 every 12 hours for a total of six doses, each given four times over 4 to 6 months. This is followed by four more cycles of subcutaneous cytarabine at 100 mg/m^2 twice daily for 10 doses and daunorubicin 45 mg/m^2. Patients under 60 years of age receiving the high-dose cytarabine arm had a superior disease-free survival compared with the other groups, whereas there was no difference between arms in patients over 60 years of age.

Despite induction CR rates of greater than 60%, the long-term disease-free survival in patients with AML remains approximately 30% to 40%. Choice of chemotherapy at the time of relapse may be based on the duration of the first remission interval. Patients with a remission interval of greater than 1 year may respond to a similar regimen at the time of relapse, whereas patients with a shorter duration of remission should be considered for alternative regimens. Options for treatment of relapse include high-dose cytarabine [25], mitoxantrone and etoposide [26], carboplatin [27], or high-dose cyclophosphamide and etoposide [18] (Table 18-4). A second remission rate of approximately 40% to 50% is noted in these patients; however, these remissions are rarely durable, and long-term disease-free survival is unusual.

Table 18-3. Initial Therapy of Acute Myeloid Leukemia

1. Cytarabine via continuous infusion (100–200 mg/m^2 × 7 d)
   +
   Daunorubicin (45 mg/m^2 × 3 d)
   or
   idarubicin (12 mg/m^2)
   or
   mitoxantrone (12 mg/m^2)
2. High-dose cytarabine and anthracycline
3. Cytarabine via continuous infusion
   +
   Daunorubicin
   +
   High-dose cytarabine
4. Cyclophosphamide and etoposide

Table 18-4. Salvage Therapy for Leukemia

Acute Myeloid Leukemia	Acute Lymphocytic Leukemia
Etoposide and mitoxantrone	High-dose cytarabine and anthracycline
High-dose cytarabine and anthracycline	Teniposide and cytarabine
Carboplatin	High-dose methotrexate
High-dose cyclophosphamide and etoposide	

Table 18-5. Treatment of Promyelocytic Leukemia

Induction
ATRA (45 mg/m^2/d) until CR
followed by
Daunorubicin (60 mg/m^2 × 3 d)
+
Ara-C via continuous infusion (200 mg/m^2 ×7 d)

Consolidation
Ara-C
+
Daunorubicin

ARTA — all trans-retonic acid; CR — complete response.

Promyelocytic leukemia (APML) represents a distinct subgroup of AML. This subtype is characterized by promyelocytic blasts containing the 15;17 chromosomal translocation. This translocation leads to the generation of the fusion transcript comprised of the retinoic acid receptor (α-RAR) and a sequence called PML. Prior to the recognition of this molecular abnormality, the clinical observation had been made that retinoic acid induced differentiation of blasts in patients with APML, and investigators in France and China used retinoic acid to treat patients with APML [28]. All *trans*-retinoic acid (ATRA) was found to be superior to *cis*-retinoic acid both in vitro and in vivo in APML and was capable of inducing complete remissions in patients with APML [29]. ATRA alone dose not produce long-term CRs and should be used in combination with chemotherapy (Table 18-5). The combination of ATRA and chemotherapy at the time of induction leads to CR rates in greater than 85% of patients [30–32]. The exact timing of administration of ATRA and chemotherapy has yet to be fully determined [33]. Use of ATRA reduces the complications associated with induction chemotherapy in patients with APML, such as disseminated intravascular coagulation. Approximately 20% of patients treated with ATRA may develop the "retinoic acid syndrome" characterized by fever, pulmonary infiltrates, and hypoxemia with and without leukocytosis [34]. Therefore, it is important to distinguish APML from other subtypes of AML because ATRA should be used as part of the treatment regimen. In addition, studies suggest that high-dose cytarabine as consolidation therapy may not be associated with the same benefit in patients with APML as compared with other types of AML. For this reason, many groups have adopted a strategy of using subsequent courses of daunorubicin-based chemotherapy during the postremission period.

In an attempt to ameliorate the toxicity of induction chemotherapy related to prolonged pancytopenia, the use of human hematopoietic growth factors has been investigated. Granulocyte–macrophage colony-stimulating factor (GM-CSF) following induction chemotherapy for AML accelerates recovery of granulocytes and is not associated with an increased incidence of recurrent leukemia. Two large cooperative group trials have examined the effect of GM-CSF after induction chemotherapy [35,36]. An ECOG study demonstrated a higher remission rate and more rapid recovery of neutrophils associated with GM-CSF use, whereas a CALGB study did not demonstrate a benefit of GM-CSF compared with placebo. Both trials initiated GM-CSF on day 8; however, the ECOG trial employed the use of GM-CSF only if aplasia on day 8 was achieved. This may account for the benefit seen in the ECOG trial. A randomized trial that compared granulocyte colony-stimulating factor with placebo in patients with AML demonstrated a shortened duration of neutropenia and a need for antifungal therapy during induction and remission therapy [37]. Other recent studies, however, have demonstrated no benefit from the addition of growth factors during induction [38].

Bone Marrow Transplantation

Bone marrow transplantation (BMT) offers the best option for long-term disease-free survival in patients with AML in second and third remission. Both allogeneic and autologous transplantation lead to overall disease-free survival in 30% to 50% of patients. Conditioning regimens used for transplantation include high-dose cyclophosphamide and total-body irradiation [39], cyclophosphamide and busulfan [40,41], as well as regimens containing high-dose cytarabine or etoposide [42]. To date, the superiority of one regimen over another has not been demonstrated. Survival is less than 20% after allogeneic bone marrow transplant in patients with refractory disease.

Bone marrow transplantation at the time of first remission is associated with a higher disease-free survival than chemotherapy alone. A large French study randomized patients to standard chemotherapy, autologous bone marrow transplantation, or to allogeneic bone marrow transplantation (if an HLA-identical sibling was available) [43]. There was no significant difference in survival between these three approaches. An improvement in disease-free survival was noted in the allogeneic BMT arm of the study compared with autologous BMT, and both transplantation approaches were better than standard chemotherapy. However, due to the increased treatment-related mortality associated with allogeneic BMT, as well as the ability to salvage patients who were treated with chemotherapy alone with autologous BMT, there was no significant difference in overall survival between the groups.

Allogeneic Bone Marrow Transplant

The best results of allogeneic BMT are reported in patients receiving transplants from HLA-identical siblings. Single-institution series suggest disease-free survival rates in patients with AML in first remission to be as high as 60% to 70%. Transplantation in second and third remissions is associated with a much lower disease-free survival rate [44]. Graft-versus-host disease (GVHD) remains the principle toxicity associated with BMT and reduces the overall effectiveness of this approach. The influence of the graft-versus-leukemia effect on disease-free survival does not appear to be as significant in AML as in chronic myelogenous leukemia (CML) [45]. Several groups have used T-cell depletion as a means to reduce the incidence of GVHD, an approach that does not appear to compromise disease-free survival [46,47]. Donor lymphocyte infusions may be used to treat patients who relapse after allogeneic BMT, but the complete response rate is only 20% [48].

For patients without a suitable sibling donor, the unrelated BMT registry may be used to identify a donor for up to 40% of patients [49]. The treatment-related mortality associated with an unrelated BMT remains significant, approaching 40% in registry series [50]. This approach may be considered for patients in second or subsequent remissions; however, its use in the first-remission setting remains controversial.

Autologous Bone Marrow Transplant

Autologous BMT is an option for patients without an HLA-matched sibling and for older patients. The treatment-related mortality associated with autologous transplantation is lower than allogeneic BMT, approaching 2% to 5%. Relapse after BMT remains the most significant complication of this approach. Both regimens containing chemotherapy only and those including total-body irradiation appear to be equally effective. Purging of the bone marrow to remove minimal residual disease can be performed by the use of either monoclonal antibodies, which are directed to antigens expressed on the surface of leukemia cells or by incubation of the marrow in cytotoxic drugs such as 4-hydroperoxycyclophosphamide [51–53]. To date, no clear benefit has been demonstrated by the purging of bone marrow by either technique. Long-term disease-free remission can be obtained in 30% to 50% of patients who receive autologous BMT in second or subsequent relapse.

ACUTE LYMPHOBLASTIC LEUKEMIA

ETIOLOGY AND RISK FACTORS

Acute lymphoblastic leukemia (ALL) is common in children but is rare in the adult population. Several factors, such as Down syndrome and radiation exposure, are associated with ALL, but the etiology is unknown in the majority of cases (*see* Table 13-1). Recent advances in the molecular genetics of ALL may allow for elucidation of the molecular events leading to ALL.

CLASSIFICATION AND PROGNOSIS

Acute lymphoblastic leukemia is a heterogeneous disease with distinct clinical features displayed by various subtypes. As with AML, the FAB classification is used to classify ALL. Three subtypes, L1 through L3, have been identified. Immunophenotyping identifies that the majority of cells are of B lineage and that most have characteristics consistent with a pre–B-cell phenotype. Approximately 25% of adult ALL are of T-cell lineage. Whereas earlier studies have suggested a worse prognosis associated with the T-cell phenotype, recent studies have not confirmed this finding [54–56].

Recurring cytogenetic abnormalities also have been demonstrated in ALL. The most common cytogenetic abnormality is the 9;22 translocation, which occurs in approximately 30% of adult ALL. Approximately one half of patients produce a fusion protein p190, whereas the remaining patients demonstrate a p210 similar to patients with CML. The Philadelphia chromosome is a very poor prognostic finding, and these patients should be treated with allogeneic BMT if a donor is available [57–59]. Other translocations include translocation of 11q23 and translocation of chromosomes 1;9. Both of these abnormalities also appear to be associated with an inferior outcome. The recently identified 12;21 translocation, which is not detected on routine cytogenetic analysis, appears to associated

with an improved prognosis in children with ALL [60–62]. The frequency of this translocation appears to be less in the adult ALL population compared with children. The prognostic importance of this translocation in adults has not been fully defined.

In addition to cytogenetic abnormalities, several clinical variables have also been associated with prognosis. These factors include age, sex, time to remission, and WBC at presentation [54] (Table 18-6). Extramedullary disease is common in these patients and treatment includes central nervous system (CNS) prophylaxis.

TREATMENT

Approximately one third to 40% of adults with ALL will be cured with modern chemotherapy. All induction regimens now include multiagent chemotherapy. The addition of anthracyclines to vincristine and prednisone alone or in combination with L-asparaginase has improved the induction CR rate in patients with adult ALL to over 70%. A CALGB study added cyclophosphamide to these four agents during induction, resulting in an 85% remission rate [54]. With intensive consolidation and CNS prophylaxis, the median survival in this study was 36 months. Prolonged maintenance therapy, which prevents relapse in children but has yet to be proven effective in adults, is standard in most ALL protocols and often includes methotrexate and 6-mercaptopurine in combination with "pulses" of vincristine and prednisone. A German multicenter study that used an induction phase containing eight drugs and an additional eight drugs during consolidation has been reported [55]. When combined with CNS prophylaxis, which includes both intrathecal methotrexate and cranial radiation, the remission rate was 74%. Treatment of the adult ALL L3 subtype using an intensive variation of this therapy over a short duration (six cycles) appears effective with a leukemia-free survival of 71% at 4 years [63].

Despite aggressive induction, the majority of adults with ALL relapse. A second remission may be obtained with chemotherapy in 10% to 70% of patients, depending on the regimen used. If relapse occurs after a prolonged remission, reinduction with similar agents used at the time of presentation may be used. The durability of second and subsequent remissions is poor, and these patients should be considered candidates for BMT.

BONE MARROW TRANSPLANTATION

Allogenic Bone Marrow Transplantation

Allogeneic BMT for adults with ALL is associated with a 5-year disease-free survival of approximately 40% in patients undergoing BMT in first remission and 20% to 30% for patients undergoing BMT in second remission [64,65]. The role of allogeneic BMT in

Table 18-6. Prognostic Factors in ALL

Factor	Good Prognosis	Poor Prognosis
Age	< 35 y	> 35 y
Sex	Female	Male
Time to complete remission	< 4 wk	> 4 wk
Cytogenetic finding	T-cell phenotype Hyperdiploid cytogenetics	Philadelphia chromosome, t(9;22), t(4;11)
White Blood Count	< 30,000/μL	> 30,000/μL

patients in first remission remains unclear. When results of allogeneic BMT in patients with ALL in first remission was compared with the results of chemotherapy alone, no clear benefit of early BMT was demonstrated [66]. The overall 5-year leukemia-free survival was 44% for patients who underwent BMT in first remission compared with 38% for patients receiving chemotherapy only. In this study, the treatment-related mortality in the patients undergoing BMT was high (39%); therefore, the benefits of transplantation may have been underestimated. In other series, allogeneic BMT in first remission in "high-risk" patients has been associated with a disease-free survival of over 60% [67]. Subgroups of patients with poor risk features may be considered for early consolidation with BMT.

Autologous Bone Marrow Transplantation

Autologous bone marrow transplantation provides an alternative source of stem cells for patients for whom no donor can be identified. Recent studies have shown that the residual leukemia cells infused at the time of marrow infusion can contribute to relapse [68]. A variety of approaches have been attempted to reduce the risk of marrow contamination by tumor cells, including immunologic purging using monoclonal antibodies, long-term culture strategies, and chemical purging in vitro. To date, no purging strategy has proved superior to the others, and some have been associated with prolonged time to engraftment [69,70].

Uncontrolled trials of autologous BMT in first and second remission have produced results superior to the disease-free survival often seen with chemotherapy alone. Prospective multicenter trials have not demonstrated a clear benefit in favor of autologous BMT in the treatment of adult patients in first remission. In one study, 96 patients were randomly assigned to autologous BMT, and 96 patients received chemotherapy alone. There was no significant difference in the incidence of treatment-related mortality, relapse, CR duration, or survival with a disease-free survival at 3 years of approximately 35% [71]. When autologous BMT is compared with allogeneic BMT, the treatment-related mortality associated with autologous BMT is much lower; however, the risk of relapse is significantly higher. Nonetheless, autologous BMT plays a significant role in the treatment of adult patients with ALL in second or subsequent remission in whom a donor is not available.

CHRONIC MYELOGENOUS LEUKEMIA

ETIOLOGY AND RISK FACTORS

Chronic myelogenous leukemia is a clonal myeloproliferative disorder of a pluripotent stem cell and is characterized by a specific chromosomal abnormality involving the translocation of chromosomes 9 and 22, creating the Philadelphia chromosome. The median age of patients at the time of diagnosis is 55, but CML can be seen in both children and young adults. The causative factor in the majority of cases of CML is not known. Ionizing radiation is associated with the development of CML.

CLASSIFICATION AND PROGNOSIS

Patients with CML have an elevated WBC and are often asymptomatic at the time of presentation. The peripheral smear demonstrates mature leukocytes as well as other myeloid precursors (particularly basophils). The bone marrow is hypercellular and demonstrates a myeloid predominance. Chronic-phase CML is characterized by a WBC that is stable or easily controlled with chemotherapy and bone marrow without a significant number of blasts. The median survival for patients in stable phase is approximately 4 years. Patients eventually progress to an accelerated phase characterized by an increasingly difficult-to-control WBC. Finally, patients develop blast crisis, which is similar to acute leukemia. The majority of patients in blast crises have myeloid leukemia; however, approximately 20% to 30% of cases are lymphoid in derivation. The median survival after developing blast crises is only 3 months. Chemotherapy agents appropriate to the derivation of the leukemia (myeloid or lymphoid) are used to treat blast crisis. If remission is obtained, it is often of short duration.

THERAPY

Treatment options for patients in stable phase CML are initially directed at controlling the elevated WBC. Hydroxyurea is very effective in controlling the majority of patients. Busulfan is now rarely used because of the unpredictable effect on stem cells and occasional episodes of prolonged pancytopenia. After the WBC is stabilized on hydroxyurea, interferon alpha (IFN α) may be initiated. A recent French study suggests both a survival benefit and an increased rate of major cytogenetic response (< 35% Ph+ cells in the bone marrow) from the combination of IFN α and subcutaneous Ara-C compared with interferon alone [72]. It is important to appreciate that the time to maximal cytogenetic response after the initiation of IFN α may be prolonged at least 6 to 9 months in some patients. The dose of IFN α used is titrated according to the WBC, with a goal of approximately 2000 to 4000 cells/mm^3. The side effects of IFN α can be significant and include fever, chills, malaise, headaches, anorexia, joint pains, and depression. Twenty percent to 30% of patients are not able to tolerate IFN α secondary to these side effects.

Allogeneic BMT offers the only option for long-term disease-free survival in patients with CML. Transplants using HLA-identical siblings may be associated with an overall disease-free survival of 60% to 70% at 5 years. Transplants from unrelated donors have a high treatment-related mortality but are still associated with overall survival rates of 40% to 50% at 5 years [50]. The development of GVHD remains the principal obstacle to higher success rates. The graft-versus-leukemia effect is significant in CML, and T-cell–depleted transplants are associated with a higher incidence of relapse after transplant [45]. Donor lymphocyte infusions (DLI) have emerged as a powerful treatment for patients who have relapsed after allogeneic BMT. When administered at the time of cytogenetic relapse, DLI leads to complete cytogenetic response in over 70% of patients [48]. Strategies of combining T-cell–depleted BMT with delayed DLI are now being explored. Autologous transplantation in CML is associated with a high relapse rate and remains investigational.

The timing of transplant in patients with CML is important. Patients treated in early chronic phase (< 1 y after diagnosis) appear to have an improved disease-free survival compared with patients treated in late chronic phase [73]. Disease-free survival rates are much lower when patients undergo transplantation in the second chronic phase (accelerated or blastic phase) compared with the early chronic phase. Transplantation in blast crisis is successful in approximately 10% of cases.

18-7. Therapy for Chronic Lymphocytic Leukemia

Agent	Overall Response Rate (CR), %
Chlorambucil	40–70 (rare)
Fludarabine (untreated)	80 (25–74)
Fludarabine (previously treated)	17–74 (0–20)

CR—complete response rate.

Table 18-8. Therapy for Hairy Cell Leukemia

Agent	Duration of Treatment	Overall Response Rate (CR), %
2-chlorodeoxyadenosine	1 wk	95 (80)
Pentostatin	3–6 mo	83 (57)
Interferon	12 mo	80 (9)

CR—complete response rate.

CHRONIC LYMPHOCYTIC LEUKEMIA

ETIOLOGY AND RISK FACTORS

Chronic lymphocytic leukemia (CLL) is the most common leukemia in the United States and occurs most often in patients older than 60 years of age. There are no known predisposing factors, although familial clustering has been reported.

CLASSIFICATION AND PROGNOSIS

A classification system developed by Rai (stages 0, I, II, III, and IV) has been used in the United States for many years. An alternative staging system (A, B, and C) has been proposed by Binet. Prognosis in CLL is linked to the stage of disease at presentation. Patients with lymphocytosis only (Rai stage 0 or Binet stage A) have a median survival of greater than 10 years from diagnosis. Patients presenting in more advanced stages have shorter survival expectancies (median survival: Rai stage I or II, 7 years; Rai stage III or IV, 4 years).

THERAPY

Treatment of chronic lymphocytic leukemia should be based on symptoms related to adenopathy or cytopenias. There is no benefit derived from treating patients solely to control the WBC. Patients may tolerate WBC > 300,000 without complications. Initial therapy can include the use of single alkylating agents. Chlorambucil may be administered chronically (often a daily dose of 6 to 8 mg) or by pulse dosing (0.4 to 0.8 mg/kg of body weight orally every 2 wk) usually for no less than 8 to 12 months. There appears to be no benefit from the addition of prednisone to chlorambucil. Patients treated with combination chemotherapy regimens have a higher response rate, but survival is not improved. Other agents to treat CLL include the fluorinated analogue of adenine, fludarabine, or with the deoxyadenosine analogue, 2-chlorodeoxyadenosine [74,75] (Table 18-7). Recent data suggest that fludarabine is associated with a higher response rate, longer duration of response, and improved progression-free survival in a randomized trial of previously untreated patients compared with chlorambucil [76]. There is no benefit to the addition of prednisone to fludarabine, and it is actually associated with an increased risk of opportunistic infections [77]. Fludarabine leads to profound depression of T-cell subsets, particularly CD4+ cells. Patients receiving fludarabine should be considered candidates to receive prophylaxis for *Pneumocystis carinii* pneumonia. For young patients with advanced stage disease, both autologous and allogeneic BMT may be considered.

HAIRY CELL LEUKEMIA

Hairy cell leukemia is a chronic lymphoproliferative disease with a good prognosis. It is most commonly diagnosed in middle-aged men who present with pancytopenia and an enlarged spleen. A dry marrow aspiration in a patient with these symptoms is typical. Hairy cells have cytoplasmic projections that are fine or hair-like. Tartrate-resistant acid phosphatase (Trap stain) is present in the leukemic cells of most patients. Flow cytometry may be used to make the diagnosis because hairy cells express CD103.

Treatment options for patients with hairy cell leukemia have included splenectomy, chlorambucil, androgens, and interferons (Table 18-8). Formerly, treatment was often initiated when patients were symptomatic or had hematologic indications, such as anemia, thrombocytopenia, or neutropenia. With the recent availability of multiple systemic agents that are capable of inducing durable and complete hematologic remissions in a high percentage of patients, consideration should be given to treating patients early in the course of their disease. A single course of 2-chlorodeoxyadenosine appears to results in excellent long-term survival in more than 90% of patients with newly diagnosed hairy cell leukemia [78]. A second course of 2-chlorodeoxyadenosine, pentostatin, or interferon can be considered for patients who have evidence of recurrent disease [79].

REFERENCES

1. Watson MS, Carroll AJ, Shuster JJ, *et al.*: Trisomy 21 in childhood acute lymphoblastic leukemia: a Pediatric Oncology Group study (8602). *Blood* 1993, 82:3098–3102.

2. Curtis RE, Boice JD Jr, Stovall M, *et al.*: Risk of leukemia after chemotherapy and radiation treatment for breast cancer [see comments]. *N Engl J Med* 1992, 326:1745–1751.

3. Pedersen-Bjergaard J, Larsen SO: Incidence of acute nonlymphocytic leukemia, preleukemia, and acute myeloproliferative syndrome up to 10 years after treatment of Hodgkin's disease. *N Engl J Med* 1982, 307:965–971.

4. Pui CH, Ribeiro RC, Hancock ML, *et al.*: Acute myeloid leukemia in children treated with epipodophyllotoxins for acute lymphoblastic leukemia. *N Engl J Med* 1991, 325:1682–1687.

5. Hudson MM, Raimondi SC, Behm FG, Pui CH: Childhood acute leukemia with t(11;19)(q23;pl3). *Leukemia* 1991, 5:1064–1068.

6. Stone RM: Myelodysplastic syndrome after autologous transplantation for lymphoma: the price of progress [editorial]. *Blood* 1994, 83:3437–3440.

7. Champlin R, Gale RP: Acute myelogenous leukemia: recent advances in therapy. *Blood* 1987, 69:1551–1562.

8. Ventura GJ, Hester JP, Smith TL, Keating MJ: Acute myeloblastic leukemia with hyperleukocytosis: risk factors for early mortality in induction. *Am J Hematol* 1988, 27:34–37.

9. Chan LC, Pegram SM, Greaves MF: Contribution of immunophenotype to the classification and differential diagnosis of acute leukemia. *Lancet* 1985, 1:475–479.

10. Griffin JD, Davis R, Nelson DA, *et al.*: Use of surface marker analysis to predict outcome of adult acute myeloblastic leukemia. *Blood* 1986, 68:1232–1241.

11. Borowitz MJ, Gockerman JP, Moore JO, *et al.*: Clinicopathologic and cytogenic features of CD34 (My 10)-positive acute nonlymphocytic leukemia. *Am J Clin Pathol* 1989, 91:265–270.

12. Campos L, Guyotat D, Archimbaud E, *et al.*: Surface marker expression in adult acute myeloid leukaemia: correlations with initial characteristics, morphology and response to therapy. *Br J Haematol* 1989, 72:161–166.

13. Bloomfield C, Lawrence D, Arthur D, *et al.*: Curative impact of intensification with high-dose cytarabine (HIDAC) in acute myeloid leukemia (AML) varies by cytogenetic group [abstract]. *Blood* 1994, 1(suppl):A431.

14. Wiemik PH, Banks PL, Case DC Jr, *et al.*: Cytarabine plus idarubicin or daunorubicin as induction and consolidation therapy for previously untreated adult patients with acute myeloid leukemia. *Blood* 1992, 79:313–319.

15. Berman E, Heller G, Santorsa L, *et al.*: Results of a randomized trial comparing idarubicin and cytosine arabinoside with daunorubicin and cytosine arabinoside in adult patients with newly diagnosed acute myelogenous leukemia. *Blood* 1991, 77:1666–1674.

16. Hiddemann W, Kreutzmann H, Straif K, *et al.*: High-dose cytosine arabinoside and mitoxantrone: a highly effective regimen in refractory acute myeloid leukemia. *Blood* 1987, 69:744–749.

17. Phillips GL, Reece DE, Shepherd JD, *et al.*: High-dose cytarabine and daunorubicin induction and postremission chemotherapy for the treatment of acute myelogenous leukemia in adults. *Blood* 1991, 77:1429–1435.

18. Brown RA, Herzig RH, Wolff SN, *et al.*: High-dose etoposide and cyclophosphamide without bone marrow transplantation for resistant hematologic malignancy. *Blood* 1990, 76:473–479.

19. Bishop JF, Lowenthal RM, Joshua D, *et al.*: Etoposide in acutenonlymphocytic leukemia: Australian Leukemia Study Group. *Blood* 1990, 75:27–32.

20. Mitus Aj, Nfiller KB, Schenkein DP, *et al.*: Improved survival for patients with acute myelogenous leukemia [see comments]. *J Clin Oncol* 1995, 13:560–569.

21. Tilly H, Castaigne S, Bordessoule D, *et al.*: Low-dose cytarabine versus intensive chemotherapy in the treatment of acute nonlymphocytic leukemia in the elderly. *J Clin Oncol* 1990, 8:272–279.

22. Bolwell BJ, Cassileth PA, Gale RP: Low-dose cytosine arabinoside in myelodysplasia and acute myelogenous leukemia [review]. *Leukemia* 1987, 1:575–579.

23. Estey E, Thall P, Beran M, *et al.*: Effect of diagnosis (refractory anemia with excess blasts, refractory anemia with excess blasts in transformation, or acute myeloid leukemia [AML]) on outcome of AML-type chemotherapy. *Blood* 1997, 90:2969–2977.

24. Mayer Rj, Davis RB, Schiffer CA, *et al.*: Intensive postremission chemotherapy in adults with acute myeloid leukemia: Cancer and Leukemia Group B [see comments]. *N Engl J Med* 1994, 331:896–903.

25. Rudnick SA, Cadman EC, Capizzi RL, *et al.*: High-dose cytosine arabinoside (HDARAC) in refractory acute leukemia. *Cancer* 1979, 44:1189–1193.

26. Lazzarino M, Morra E, Alessandrino EP, *et al.*: Mitoxantrone and etoposide: an effective regimen for refractory or relapsed acute myelogenous leukemia. *Eur J Haematol* 1989, 43:411–416.

27. Martinez JA, Martin G, Sanz GF, *et al.*: A phase 11 clinical trial of carboplatin infusion in high-risk acute nonlymphoblastic leukemia. *J Clin Oncol* 1991, 9:39–43.

28. Degos L: [All-*trans*-retinoic acid in the treatment of acute promyelocytic leukemia]. *Presse Med* 1990, 19:1483–1484.

29. Warrell RP Jr, Frankel SR, Nhller WH Jr, *et al.*: Differentiafion therapy of acute promyelocytic leukemia with tretinoin (all-*trans*-retinoic acid). *N Engl J Med* 1991, 324:1385–1393.

30. Fenaux P, Castaigne S, Dombret H, *et al.*: All-*trans*-retinoic acid followed by intensive chemotherapy gives a high complete remission rate and may prolong remissions in newly diagnosed acute promyelocytic leukemia: a pilot study on 26 cases. *Blood* 1992, 80:2176–2181.

31. Fenaux P, Le Deley MC, Castaigne S, *et al.*: Effect of all *trans*retinoic acid in newly diagnosed acute promyelocytic leukemia: results of a multicenter randomized trial: European APL 91 Group. *Blood* 1993, 82:3241–3249.

32. Tallman MS, Andersen JW, Schiffer CA, *et al.*: All-*trans*-retinoic acid in acute promyelocytic leukemia [see comments]. *N Engl J Med* 1997, 337:1021–1028.

33. Fenaux P, Chastang C, Sanz M, *et al.*: ATRA followed by chemotherapy (CT) vs ATRA plus CT and the role of maintenance therapy in newly diagnosed acute promyelocytic leukemia(APL): first interim results of APL 93 trial [abstract]. *Blood* 1997, 90:A533.

34. Frankel SR, Eardley A, Lauwers G, *et al.*: The "retinoic acid syndrome" in acute promyelocytic leukemia [see comments]. *Ann Intern Med* 1992, 117:292–296.

35. Rowe JM, Andersen JW, Mazza JJ, *et al.*: A randomized placebo-controlled phase III study of granulocyte-macrophage colony-sfimulating facotr in adult patients (>55 to 70 years of age) with acute myelogenous leukemia: a study of the Eastern Cooperative Oncology Group (El490). *Blood* 1995, 86:457–462.

36. Stone RM, Berg DT, George SL, *et al.*: Granulocyte-macrophage colony-stimulating factor after initial chemotherapy for elderly patients with primary acute myelogenous leukemia: Cancer and Leukemia Group B [see comments]. *N Engl J Med* 1995, 332:1671–1677.

37. Heil G, Hoelzer D, Sanz MA, *et al.*: A randomized, double-blind, placebocontrolled, phase III study of filgrastim in remission inducfion and consolidation therapy for adults with de novo acute myeloid leukemia: the Intemational Acute Myeloid Leukemia Study Group. *Blood* 1997, 90:4710–4718.

38. Lowenberg B, Boogaerts MA, Daenen SM, *et al.*: Value of different modalities of granulocyte-macrophage colony-stimulating factor applied during or after induction therapy of acute myeloid leukemia. *J Clin Oncol* 1997, 15:3496–506.

39. Clift RA, Buckner CD, Appelbaum FR, *et al.*: Allogeneic marrow transplantation in patients with acute myeloid leukemia in first remission: a randomized trial of two irradiation regimens [see comments]. *Blood* 1990, 76:1867–1871.

40. Copelan EA, Biggs JC, Thompson JM, *et al.*: Treatment for acute myelocytic leukemia with allogeneic bone marrow transplantation following preparation with BuCy2. *Blood* 1991, 78:838–843.

41. Copelan EA, Biggs JC, Szer J, *et al.*: Allogeneic bone marrow transplantation for acute myelogenous leukemia, acute lymphocytic leukemia, and multiple myeloma following preparation with busulfan and cyclophosphamide (BuCy2) [review]. *Semin Oncol* 1993, 20:33–38.

42. Blume KG, Long GD, Negrin RS, *et al.*: Role of etoposide (VP-16) in preparatory regimens for patients with leukemia or lymphoma undergoing allogeneic bone marrow transplantation. *Bone Marrow Transplant* 1994, 14(suppl 4):S9–S10.

43. Zittoun RA, Mandelli F, Willemze R, *et al.*: Autologous or allogeneic bone marrow transplantation compared with intensive chemotherapy in acute myelogenous leukemia: European Organization for Research and Treatment of Cancer (EORTC) and the Gruppo Italiano Malattie Ematologiche Mahgne dell'Adulto (GIMEMA) Leukemia Cooperative Groups [see comments]. *N Engl J Med* 1995, 332:217–223.

44. Clift RA, Buckner CD, Thomas ED, *et al.*: The treatment of acute nonlymphoblastic leukemia by allogeneic marrow transplantation. *Bone Marrow Transplant* 1987, 2:243–258.

45. Horowitz MM, Gale RP, Sondel PM, *et al.*: Graft-versus-leukemia reactions after bone marrow transplantation. *Blood* 1990, 75:555–562.

46. Papadopoulos EB, Carabasi MH, Castro-Malaspina H, *et al.*: T-cell-depleted allogeneic bone marrow transplantation as postremission therapy for acute myelogenous leukemia:freedom from relapse in the absence of graft-versus-host disease. *Blood* 1998, 91:1083–90.

47. Soiffer RJ, Fairclough D, Robertson M, *et al.*: CD6-depleted allogeneic bone marrow transplantation for acute leukemia in first complete remission. *Blood* 1997, 89:3039–3047.

48. Kolb HJ, Schattenberg A, Goldman JM, *et al.*: Graft-versus-leukemia effect of donor lymphocyte transfusions in marrow grafted patients: European Group for Blood and Marrow Transplantation Working Party Chronic Leukemia [see comments]. *Blood* 1995, 86:2041–2050.

49. Beatty PG. Hansen JA, Longton GM, *et al.*: Marrow transplantation from HLA matched unrelated donors for treatment of hematologic malignancies. *Transplantation* 1991, 51:443–447.

50. Szydlo R, Goldman JM, Klein JP, *et al.*: Results of allogeneic bone marrow transplants for leukemia using donors other than HLA-identical siblings. *J Clin Oncol* 1997, 15:1767–1777.

51. Yeager AM, Kaizer H, Santos GW, *et al.*: Autologous bone marrow transplantation in patients with acute nonlymphocytic leukemia, using ex vivo marrow treatment with 4-hydroperoxycyclophosphamide. *N Engl J Med* 1986, 315:141–147.

52. Selvaggi Kj, Wilson JW, Mills LE, *et al.*: Improved outcome for high-risk acute myeloid leukemia patients using autologous bone marrow transplantation and monoclonal antibody-purged bone marrow. *Blood* 1994, 83:1698–705.

53. Robertson MJ, Soiffer RJ, Freedman AS, *et al.*: Human bone marrow depleted of CD33-positive cells mediates delayed but durable reconstitution of hematopoiesis: clinical trial of MY9 monoclonal antibody-purged autografts for the treatment of acute myeloid leukemia. *Blood* 1992, 79:2229–2236.

54. Larson RA, Dodge RK, Burns CP, *et al.*: A five-drug remission induction regimen with intensive consolidation for adults with acute lymphoblastic leukemia: Cancer and Leukemia Group B study 8811. *Blood* 1995, 85:2025–2037.

55. Hoelzer D, Thiel E, Loffler H, *et al.*: Prognostic factors in a multicenter study for treatment of acute lymphoblastic leukemia in adults. *Blood* 1988, 71:123–131.

56. Linker CA, Levitt LJ, O'Donnell M, *et al.*: Treatment ofadult acute-lymphoblastic leukemia with intensive cyclical chemotherapy: a follow-up report. *Blood* 1991, 78:2814–2822.

57. Barrett AJ, Horowitz MM, Ash RC, *et al.*: Bone marrow transplantation for Philadelphia chromosome-positive acute lymphoblastic leukemia. *Blood* 1992, 79:3067–3070.

58. Forman SJ, O'Donnell MR, Nademanee AP, *et al.*: Bone marrow transplantation for patients with Philadelphia chromosome-positive acute lymphoblastic leukemia. *Blood* 1987, 70:587–588.

59. Sierra J, Radich J, Hansen JA, *et al.*: Marrow transplants from unrelated donors for treatment of Philadelphia chromosome-positive acute lymphoblastic leukemia. *Blood* 1997, 90:1410–1414.

60. Golub TR, Barker GF, Bohlander SK, *et al.*: Fusion of the TEL gene on 12pl3 to the AML1 gene on 2lq22 in acute lymphoblastic leukemia. *Proc Natl Acad Sci U S A* 1995, 92:4917–4921.

61. Rubnitz JE, Shuster JJ, Land VJ, *et al.*: Case-control study suggests a favorable impact of TELrearrangementin patients with B-lineage acute lymphoblastic leukemia treated with antimetabolite-based therapy: a Pediatric C)ncology Group study. *Blood* 1997, 89:1143–1146.

62. McLean TW, Ringold S, Neuberg D, *et al.*: TEL/AML-1 dimerizes and is associated with a favorable outcome in childhood acute lymphoblastic leukemia. *Blood* 1996, 88:4252–4258.

63. Hoelzer D, Ludwig WD, Thiel E, *et al.*: Improved outcome in adult B-cell acute lymphoblastic leukemia. *Blood* 1996, 87:495–508.

64. Barrett AJ: Bone marrow transplantation for acute lymphoblasti-cleukaemia. *Baillieres Clin Haematol* 1994, 7:377–401.

65. Barrett AJ, Horowitz MM, Gale RP, *et al.*: Marrow transplantation for acute lymphoblastic leukemia: factors affecting relapse and survival. *Blood* 1989, 74:862–871.

66. Horowitz MM, Messerer D, Hoelzer D, *et al.*: Chemotherapy compared with bone marrow transplantation for adults with acute lymphoblastic leukemia in first remission. *Ann Intern Med* 1991, 115:13–18.

67. Snyder DS, Chao NJ, Amylon MD, *et al.*: Fractionated total body irradiation and high-dose etoposide as a preparatory regimen for bone marrow transplantation for 99 patients with acute leukemia in first complete remission. *Blood* 1993, 82:2920–2928.

68. Brenner MK, Rill DR, Moen RC, *et al.*: Gene-marking to trace origin of relapse after autologous bone-marrow transplantation. *Lancet* 1993, 341:85–86.

69. Gilmore MJ, Hamon MD, Prentice HG, *et al.*: Failure of purgedautologous bone marrow transplantation in high risk acute lymphoblastic leukaemia in first complete remission. *Bone Marrow Transplant* 1991, 8:19–26.

70. Uckun FM, Kersey JH, Vallera DA, *et al.*: Autologous bone marrow transplantation in high-risk remission T-lineage acute lymphoblastic leukemia using immunotoxins plus 4-hydroperoxycyclophosphamide for marrow purging. *Blood* 1990, 76:1723–1733.

71. Fiere D, Lepage E, Sebban C, *et al.*: Adult acute lymphoblastic leukemia: a multicentric randomized trial testing bone marrow transplantation as postremission therapy: the French Group on Therapy for Adult Acute Lymphoblastic Leukemia. *J Clin Oncol* 1993, 11:1990–2001.

72. Guilhot F, Chastang C, Michallet M, *et al.*: Interferon alfa-2b combined with cytarabine versus interferon alone in chronic myelogenous leukemia: French Chronic Myeloid Leukemia Study Group [see comments]. *N Engl J Med* 1997, 337:223–229.

73. Goldman JM, Szydlo R, Horowitz NM, *et al.*: Choice of pretransplant treatment and timing of transplants for chronic myelogenous leukemia in chronic phase [see comments]. *Blood* 1993, 82:2235–2238.

74. Keating MJ, Kantarjian H, O'Brien S, *et al.*: A new agent with marked cytoreducfive activity in untreated chronic lymphocyfic leukemia. *J Clin Oncol* 1991, 9:44–49.

75. Piro LD, Carrera CJ, Beutler E, Carson DA: 2-Chlorodeoxyadenosine: an effecfive new agent for the treatment of chronic lymphocytic leukemia. *Blood* 1988, 72:1069–1073.

76. Rai K, Peterson B, Elias L, *et al.*: A randomized comparison of fludarabine and chlorambucil for patients with previously untreated chronic lymphocytic leukemia: a CALGB, SWOG, CTG /NCI-C and ECOG intergroup study [abstract]. *Blood* 1996, 88:A552.

77. Anaissie E, Kontoyiannis DP, Kantarjian H, *et al.*: Listeriosis in patients with chronic lymphocytic leukemia who were treated with fludarabine and prednisone. *Ann Intern Med* 1992, 117:466–469.

78. Piro LD, Carrera Cj, Carson DA, Beutler E: Lasting remissions in hairy-cell leukemiainduced by a single infusion of 2-chlorodeoxyadenosine. *N Engl J Med* 1990, 322:1117–1121.

79. Saven A, Piro LD: Treatment of hairy cell leukemia. *Blood* 1992, 79:1111–1120.

CYTOSINE ARABINOSIDE AND ANTHRACYCLINE

The combination of cytosine arabinoside and one of the anthracycline antibiotics has become the standard induction regimen for acute myeloid leukemia around the world.

Cytosine arabinoside is an antimetabolite that interferes with DNA synthesis after conversion to ara-CTP, which is a potent inhibitor of DNA polymerase. In addition, metabolites of ara-CTP accumulate in DNA, causing a defect in ligation of newly synthesized fragments of DNA. Cytarabine may be inactivated by two intracellular enzymes, cytidine deaminase and deoxycytidine deaminase.

The anthracycline antibiotics are a class of drug that mediate their effects by binding to DNA and intercalation. The anthracyclines enter cells through a passive transport process and can be pumped out of cells through the multidrug resistance protein MDR1 or P glycoprotein. The natural substance daunorubicin has been used in the treatment of leukemia for over 20 years. More recently, a synthetic anthracycline, idarubicin, appears to have greater activity than daunorubicin, largely because of the persistence of an active metabolite. Another synthetic compound, mitoxantrone, has been used in the treatment of acute leukemia and has the advantage of possibly being less cardiotoxic.

CANDIDATES FOR TREATMENT

Newly diagnosed patients with AML or relapsed AML (especially if first remission lasted 1 y)

SPECIAL PRECAUTIONS

Rapid cell turnover and hyperuricemia with possible renal damage (start patients on allopurinol 300 mg/d if necessary)

ALTERNATIVE THERAPIES

None is standard

TOXICITIES

Drug combination: extremely myelotoxic, resulting in marrow aplasia with attendant pancytopenia; neutropenia 2–4 wk following induction; overwhelming sepsis possible (institute antibiotics); platelet transfusions if platelet count < 20,000/mL; mucositis, alopecia; **ara-C:** hepatotoxicity, with transaminasemia and/or jaundice in some patients; **Anthracyclines:** cardiotoxicity (monitored with MUGA scans)

DRUG INTERACTIONS

None

NURSING INTERVENTIONS

Observe patients for any signs of infection; provide antimetics, particularly during the daunorubicin phase of the protocol; monitor blood counts and liver function tests daily; wash hands carefully

PATIENT INFORMATION

Patients undergoing induction therapy for AML are often quite ill prior to therapy. Considerable counseling and reassurance are necessary at this phase of the patient's disease. The patient needs to be informed rapidly about the various treatment options available once remission is achieved (consolidation with chemotherapy, BMT).

DOSAGE AND SCHEDULING

STANDARD REGIMEN

Ara-c 100–200 mg/m² /d continuous infusion, d1–7	▬▬▬	
Daunorubicin 45–50 mg/m²/d, IV bolus, d1–3	▬▬	
Bone marrow		☐

SECOND COURSE

Ara-c 100–200 mg/m²/d continuous infusion, d1–5	▬▬▬
Daunorubicin 45–50 mg/m²/d, IV bolus, d1–2	▬

Following achievement of complete remission: one or more courses of ara-C at high-dose (1.5–3 g/m² x 12 doses, lower for patients ≥ age 60 y) with daunorubicin daily for 3 d at completion of ara-C are recommended.

3 7 3 INDUCTION REGIMEN (ALTERNATIVE)

Cytarabine 100 mg/m²	▬▬▬▬
Daunorubicin 45 mg/m²	▬▬
Cytarabine 2 g/m²	▬▬

CYCLE 1 AND 3

Cytarabine 200 mg/m²	▬▬▬
Daunorubicin 60 mg/m²	▬

CYCLE 2

Cytarabine 2 g/m²	▬▬
Etoposide 100 mg/m²	▬
Day	1 2 3 4 5 6 7 8 9 10 11 12 13 14

RECENT EXPERIENCE AND RESPONSE RATES

Most studies report complete remission rates of 60%–70% (lower in patients older than 60 y)

INDUCTION AND CONSOLIDATION FOR PROMYELOCYTIC LEUKEMIA

All *trans*-retonic acid (ATRA) has emerged as an important component in the treatment of patients with promyelocytic leukemia (APML). ATRA reduces the acute complications associated with the administration of chemotherapy, such as disseminated intravascular coagulation. ATRA is combined with daunorubicin-based chemotherapy, and studies are currently being performed to optimize the time of administration of this agent. Administration of ATRA may be associated with the development of the retinoic acid syndrome. Fenaux and coworkers [31] has reported a regimen that combines ATRA and chemotherapy and results in a complete response rate of 91% in patients with APML.

DOSAGE AND SCHEDULING

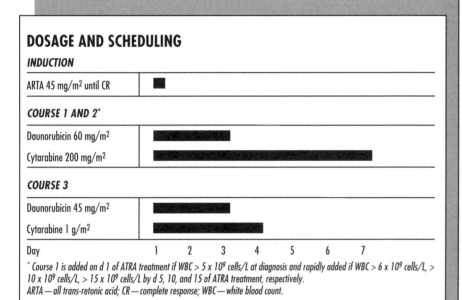

INDUCTION

ARTA 45 mg/m² until CR	■

*COURSE 1 AND 2**

Daunorubicin 60 mg/m²	
Cytarabine 200 mg/m²	

COURSE 3

Daunorubicin 45 mg/m²	
Cytarabine 1 g/m²	

Day	1	2	3	4	5	6	7

* Course 1 is added on d 1 of ATRA treatment if WBC > 5 x 10⁹ cells/L at diagnosis and rapidly added if WBC > 6 x 10⁹ cells/L, > 10 x 10⁹ cells/L, > 15 x 10⁹ cells/L by d 5, 10, and 15 of ATRA treatment, respectively.
ARTA — all trans-retonic acid; CR — complete response; WBC — white blood count.

CANDIDATES FOR TREATMENT
Newly diagnosed patients with APML

SPECIAL PRECAUTIONS
Retinoic acid syndrome with rapidly increasing white blood count, hypoxia, and diffuse pulmonary infiltrates; coagulopathy may develop; treatment includes platelet transfusion; other considerations include heparin, tranexamic acid, and fresh frozen plasma; fibrinogen transfusions may be considered

ALTERNATIVE THERAPIES
Standard induction chemotherapy for acute myeloid leukemia

TOXICITIES
Drug combinations: extremely myelotoxic, resulting in marrow aplasia with attendant pancytopenia; neutropenia 2–4 wk following induction; sepsis possible; platelet transfusions in platelet count < 30,000/mL; mucositis; alopecia; **Ara-C:** hepatotoxicity with elevated transaminasemia and/or jaundice in some patients; **Antracycline:** cardiotoxicity. **ATRA:** retinoic acid syndrome

DRUG INTERACTIONS
None

NURSING INTERVENTIONS
Same as for acute myeloid leukemia (*see* Cytosine Arabinoside and Anthracycline section)

PATIENT INFORMATION
Same as for acute myeloid leukemia (*see* Cytosine Arabinoside and Anthracycline section).

HIGH-DOSE CYTOSINE ARABINOSIDE

In an effort to increase the efficacy and durability of remissions, regimens containing cytosine arabinoside in high doses have been studied. High doses of ara-C give rise to higher levels of intracellular ara-C and increase the efficacy of the agent. As an induction regimen, high-dose ara-C is accompanied by an anthracycline antibiotic or L-asparaginase.

DOSAGE AND SCHEDULING

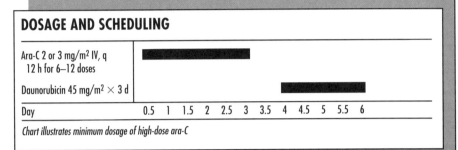

	0.5	1	1.5	2	2.5	3	3.5	4	4.5	5	5.5	6
Ara-C 2 or 3 mg/m² IV, q 12 h for 6–12 doses												
Daunorubicin 45 mg/m² × 3 d												
Day												

Chart illustrates minimum dosage of high-dose ara-C

RECENT EXPERIENCE AND RESPONSE RATES

Complete responses are seen in about 50% of patients tested in relapse

CANDIDATES FOR TREAMENT
AML in relapse

SPECIAL PRECAUTIONS
Tumor lysis syndrome with release of uric acid and phosphorus alkalinization of the urine should be induced and allopurinol, 300 mg/d, started immediately

ALTERNATIVE THERAPIES
Standard-dose ara-C; Carboplatin

TOXICITIES
Drug combination: neutropenia and thrombocytopenia; nausea, vomiting, diarrhea; elevated liver function tests; **High-dose ara-C:** cerebellar toxicity (slurred speech, ataxia), ototoxicity, conjunctivitis; extreme myelotoxicity resulting in narrow aplasia and pancytopenia

DRUG INTERACTIONS
None

NURSING INTERVENTIONS
Observe patients for signs of infection; give antiemetic; monitor blood counts and liver function tests daily; wash hands carefully; watch for ataxia daily; manage conjunctivitis with glucocorticoid eyedrops every 6–8 h

PATIENT INFORMATION
Patients should be informed that this regimen is myelotoxic and that prolonged myelosuppresion is expected.

MITOXANTRONE AND ETOPOSIDE

Both mitoxantrone and etoposide have shown activity as single agents in acute myeloid leukemia (AML). A combination of the two agents is a relatively effective therapy for patients with relapsed disease. The regimen is relatively well tolerated.

DOSAGE AND SCHEDULING

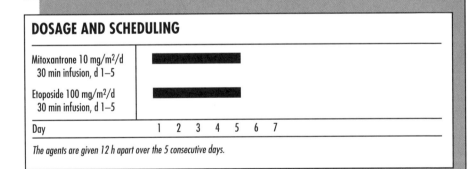

	1	2	3	4	5	6	7
Mitoxantrone 10 mg/m²/d 30 min infusion, d 1–5							
Etoposide 100 mg/m²/d 30 min infusion, d 1–5							
Day							

The agents are given 12 h apart over the 5 consecutive days.

RECENT EXPERIENCE AND RESPONSE RATES

Complete response rate of 45%–50%; as with most regimens used in relapse for AML, the duration of remission achieved is relatively brief. In a study by Lazzarino and colleagues [17]; 61% of patients achieved complete remission including several patients with disease refractory to other therapy; the median CR duration was 5 mo with a range of 2 to 12 + mo.

CANDIDATES FOR TREATMENT
AML in relapse

SPECIAL PRECAUTIONS
Possibility of cardiotoxicity: obtain baseline MUGA scan

ALTERNATIVE THERAPIES
Ara-C and anthracycline, carboplatin, high-dose ara-C

TOXICITIES
Drug combination: myelosuppression; severe oral mucositis; reactivation of herpes virus (administer acyclovir); mild nausea and vomiting, diarrhea, transaminasemia, alopecia

DRUG INTERACTIONS
None

NURSING INTERVENTIONS
Parental hyperalimentation for grade 3 oral mucositis; monitor for myelosuppression

PATIENT INFORMATION
Patients undergoing induction therapy for AML are often quite ill prior to therapy. Considerable counseling and reassurance are necessary at this phase of the patient's disease. The patient needs to be informed rapidly about the various treatment options available once remission is achieved (consolidation with chemotherapy, BMT).

The information here is provided as guidance only. Prescribers should always consult the manufacturer's current prescribing information.

BFM INTENSIFIED INDUCTION AND CONSOLIDATION THERAPY

A significant advance in the treatment of acute lymphocytic leukemia (ALL) in adults has come from a series of German multicenter studies, the BFM regimens (Berlin, Frankfurt, Munich). This intensive multiagent regimen has an induction phase with prednisone, vincristine, daunorubicin, and L-asparaginase followed by cyclophophamide, cytarabine, 6-mercaptopurine, and methotrexate given over a period of 52 days. Following this, a reinduction phase is begun using dexamethasone, vincristine, doxorubicin, cyclophosphamide, ara-C, and thioguanine over the next 42 days. Then a maintenance phase with 6-mercaptopurine and methotrexate is started for up to 130 weeks. Central nervous system (CNS) prophylaxis consists of cranial irradiation with 24 Gy and intrathecal methotrexate (10 mg/m², maximum single dose 15 mg), once weekly for 4 wk during phase 2 when complete remission is achieved after phase 1. If complete remission is delayed until after completion of phase 2, CNS prophylaxis is given immediately thereafter.

Several important prognostic factors were uncovered during this study. Favorable outcome was seen in patients who achieved complete remission in less than 4 wk, who were younger than 35 years, whose initial leukocyte count was less than 30,000, and whose immunophenotype was T-ALL. The absence of these good prognostic factors resulted in an adverse outcome; that is, the presence of two or three adverse factors was associated with a median remission duration of 9.6 mo, whereas the absence of these factors resulted in a better outcome.

CANDIDATES FOR TREATMENT
Patients with ALL at diagnosis

SPECIAL PRECAUTIONS
Patients should have urine alkalinized (place on allpurinol 300 mg/dL)

ALTERNATIVE THERAPIES
Bone marrow transplantation after induction

TOXICITY
Myelosuppression with attendant problems

DRUG INTERACTIONS
None

NURSING INTERVENTIONS
Neutropenia is expected, therefore observe for any signs of infection; give antiemetics, particularly during daunorubicin phase of protocol; monitor blood counts and liver function tests daily; wash hands carefully

PATIENT INFORMATION
Patients undergoing induction therapy for ALL are often quite ill prior to therapy. Considerable counseling and reassurance are necessary at this phase of the patient's disease. The patient needs to be informed rapidly of the various treatment options available once remission is achieved (consolidation, BMT).

DOSAGE AND SCHEDULING

DRUG	DOSE AND DAYS
Induction	
Phase 1	
Prednisone	60 mg/m² d 1–28
Vincristine	1.5 mg/m² IV* d 1,8,15,22
Daunorubicin	25 mg/m² IV d 1,8,15,22
L-Asparaginase	5000 U/m² IV d 1–14
Phase 2	
Cyclophosphamide	650 mg/m² IV d 29,43,57
ara-C	75 mg/m² IV d 31–34,38–41,45–48,52–55
6-Mercaptopurine	60 mg/m² PO d 29–57
Methotrexate	10 mg/m² IT d 31,38,45,52
Consolidation	
Phase 1	
Dexamethasone	10 mg/m² PO d 1–28
Vincristine	1.5 mg/m² IV* d 1,8,15,22
Doxorubicin	25 mg/m² IV d 1,8,15,22
Phase 2	
Cyclophosphamide	650 mg/m² IV d 29
ara-C	75 mg/m² IV d 31–34,38–41
Thioguanine	60 mg/m² PO d 29–42
Maintenance	
6-Mercaptopurine	60 mg/m² PO/d, wk 10–18
Methotrexate	20 mg/m² PO/IV/wk and d 29–130

Maximum dose of 2 mg/m².
CNS prophylaxis consisted of cranial irradiation with 24 Gy and intrathecal methotrexate, 10/mg² (maximum single dose, 15 mg/m²), once weekly for 4 wk during phase II when complete remission was achieved.

RECENT EXPERIENCE AND RESPONSE RATES
Complete remission of 74%, with 34% of patients in continuous complete remission at 5 y; median survival is 28 mo.

ECOG INTENSIFIED INDUCTION AND CONSOLIDATION THERAPY

Modifications of the BFM protocol have been used by cooperative groups such as the Cancer and Leukemia Group. The Eastern Cooperative Oncology Group (ECOG) is joining with MRC of the UK to examine the role of bone marrow transplantation in the first remission of ALL. Patients receive the following induction regimen and are then randomized to autologous BMT (or assigned to allogenic BMT if a donor is available). Both groups receive intensification before either transplantation or conventional consolidation and maintenance.

DOSAGE AND SCHEDULING

DRUG	DOSE AND DAYS
Induction	
Phase 1	
Daunorubicin	60 mg/m² IV push d 1,8,15,21
Vincristine	1.4 mg/m² IV push* d 1,8,15,21
Prednisolone	60 mg/m² PO qd d 1–28
L-Asparaginase	10,000 U IM or IV in 100 ml D5W over 30 min qd d 17–28
Methotrexate	12.5 mg IT d 15 *only*

If CNS leukemia is present at diagnosis, methotrexate IT or via an Ommaya reservoir is given weekly until blasts are absent. 24 Gy cranial irradiation and 12 Gy to the spinal cord are administered concurrent with phase 2.

Phase 2 (weeks 5–8)	
Cyclophosphamide	650 mg/m² IV in 250 cc normal saline for 30 min, d 1,14,28
ara-C	75 mg/m² IV in 100 cc D5W for 30 min, d 1–4, 8–11, 15–18, 22–25
6-Mercaptopurine	60 mg/m² PO qd d 1–28
Methotrexate	12.5 mg IT d 1, 8, 15, 22

Postponed if total WBC count < 3 x 10⁹/L

Intensification (weeks 13–16)	
HD Methotrexate	3 g/m² IV in NS 500 mL over 2 h, d 1,8,22
L-Asparaginase	10,000 Lu/m² IV in 100 mL D5W over 30 min, d 2,9,23
Leucovorin rescue	10 mg/m² IV D5W 50 mL q 6 h x 4 doses beginning 22–24 h after completion of methotrexate; then 10 mg/m² PO q 6 h x 72 h

Begin 4 wk from d 28 of induction, phase 2; postpone if WBC < 3 x 10⁹/L.
If randomized to autologous BMT or assigned to allogenic BMT, perform harvest (1–3 x 10⁸/kg nucleated cells) within 3–7 wk from start of intensification. Postpone harvest until marrow cellularity on biopsy ≥ 30%.

Day -6 to day -4: fractioned TBI total dose 1320 cGy; **For males only:** 400 cGy testicular boost; **Day -3:** etoposide 60 mg/kg IV; **Day 0:** allogeneic or autologous marrow infusion; **Day 0—+27:** GM-CSF 250 µg/m²/day over 4–6 h IV

If randomized to chemotherapy, start conventional consolidation maintenance (beginning 1–2 mo after intensification).

Cycle I Consolidation	
ara-C	75 mg/m² IV in 500 mL D5W
Etoposide	100 mg/m² IV in 500 mL NS over 1 h, d 1–5
Vincristine	1.4 mg/m²,* d 1, 8, 15, 22
Dexamethasone	10 mg/m² PO, d 1–28

Cycles II, IV Consolidation	
ara-C	75 mg/m² IV in 500 mL D5W over 30 min, d 1–5
Etoposide	100 mg/m² IV in 500 mL normal saline x 60 min, d 1–5

Begin 4 wk from day 1 of each cycle or when WBC count > 3.0 x 10⁹/L, except cycle IV which begins 2 mo from day 1 following cycle III or when WBC count > 3.0 x 10⁹/L.

Cycle III Consolidation	
Daunorubicin	25 mg/m² IV push, d 1, 8, 15, 22
Cyclophosphamide	650 mg/m² IV in 250 mL normal saline over 30 min, d 29
ara-C	75 mg/m² IV 100 mL D5W over 30 min, d 31–34, 38–41
6-Thioguanine	60 mg/m² PO, d 29–42

Begin 4 weeks from day 1 of cycle II or when WBC count > 3.0 x 10⁹/L.

Maintenance Therapy	
Vincristine	1.4 mg/m² IV* every 3 mo
Prednisolone	60 mg/m² PO x 5 d every 3 mo
6-Mercaptopurine	75 mg/m² PO/d
Methotrexate	20 mg/m² PO or IV/wk for 2.5 y
Interferon alpha	3 MU SC 3 times/wk — Ph+ patients only

All drug doses are based on the lesser of the actual/corrected ideal body weight.
*Maximum dose of 2 mg/m².

CANDIDATES FOR TREATMENT
ALL at diagnosis

SPECIAL PRECAUTIONS
Patients should have their urine alkalinized (place on allopurinol 300 mg/d)

ALTERNATIVE THERAPIES
Bone marrow transplant after induction

RECENT EXPERIENCE AND RESPONSE RATES
60% complete response rate

TOXICITY
Myelosuppression with attendant problems

DRUG INTERACTIONS
None

NURSING INTERVENTIONS
Neutropenia is expected, therefore, observe for any signs of infection; give antiemetics, particularly during daunorubicin phase of the protocol; monitor blood counts and liver function tests daily; wash hands carefully

PATIENT INFORMATION
Patients undergoing induction therapy for ALL are often quite ill prior to therapy. Considerable counseling and reassurance are necessary at this phase of the patient's disease. The patient needs to be informed rapidly about the various treatment options available once remission is achieved (consolidation with chemotherapy, BMT).

CHAPTER 19: HODGKIN'S DISEASE
Alan R. Yuen, Sandra J. Horning

Hodgkin's disease is uncommon. The annual incidence is two per 100,000 people in the United States, accounting for about 14% of all newly diagnosed lymphomas. In developed countries, there is a bimodal age distribution with one peak in the late 20s and a second peak after age 45 years [1,2].

The etiology of Hodgkin's disease has not been definitively established. Immunologic and molecular evidence shows that the Epstein–Barr virus is highly associated with histologic subtypes. However, a direct causal relationship has not yet been shown.

Pathologically, Hodgkin's disease is characterized by the presence of large abnormal cells with prominent nucleoli (Reed–Sternberg cells or mononuclear variants). However, most of the tumor is composed of a mixture of normal-appearing inflammatory cells. Hodgkin's disease can be divided into several histologic subtypes. The widely endorsed Rye classification specifies four categories: lymphocyte predominant, nodular sclerosis, mixed cellularity, and lymphocyte depleted. Nodular sclerosis accounts for approximately 75% of Hodgkin's disease cases; lymphocyte depletion is extremely rare.

The diagnosis of Hodgkin's disease requires examination of a histologic sample by an experienced hematopathologist. Material from an excisional biopsy specimen usually is necessary to establish the initial diagnosis because fine needle aspiration often provides insufficient material or architectural information to render a definite diagnosis. Hodgkin's disease should be differentiated from non-Hodgkin's lymphomas, some of which may have a similar histologic appearance. Special immunohistochemical stains to test for cell surface markers may assist in establishing the diagnosis.

Most patients present with painless enlargement of the lymph nodes. The most common sites of involvement include the neck and the mediastinum. Other common sites are the axillae, spleen, and para-aortic lymph nodes. In most cases, the disease spreads in a nonrandom fashion to involve contiguous nodal sites. In advanced stages, the disease may spread to involve the liver, bone marrow, bone, or other extranodal sites. Constitutional symptoms, such as fevers, sweats, and weight loss, are also more common with advanced disease.

Accurate staging is crucial in planning the treatment of patients with Hodgkin's disease so that specific treatment can be tailored to the extent and location of disease. For example, radiotherapy alone can treat patients effectively with a limited extent of disease determined through careful and systemic staging. The widely accepted Ann Arbor Staging Classification System has been modestly revised. The Cotswold revision of the Ann Arbor Staging Classification System [3] is shown in Table 19-1. Staging evaluation requires a careful history to determine the duration and presence of fever, night sweats, and weight loss; a careful physical examination with special attention to sites of lymph nodes, liver, and spleen; laboratory evaluation including a complete blood count, erythrocyte sedimentation rate, alkaline phosphatase and lactate dehydrogenase levels, and tests for renal and hepatic function; and radiographic studies, including a chest radiograph and computed tomography (CT) scans of the chest, the abdomen, and the pelvis. A lower-extremity lymphangiogram may yield additional information about the architecture and size of retroperitoneal adenopathy beyond that provided by the CT scan. It also provides an inexpensive and simple way to monitor response to treatment. Bone marrow biopsies are indicated in patients with systemic symptoms and those with extensive or bulky clinical disease. Staging laparotomy (with splenectomy, liver biopsy, and retroperitoneal lymph node sampling) has been incorporated in staging when radiation therapy alone was being considered for primary therapy.

Laparotomy currently is used more selectively. Patients with supradiaphragmatic presentations who are young, asymptomatic, and have both nonbulky involvement of two lymph node regions and a normal erythrocyte sedimentation rate often are treated with extended-field radiotherapy without laparotomy. A laparotomy is not necessary if chemotherapy is planned as part of the treatment.

TREATMENT MODALITIES
Radiation
Radiotherapy was the first modality demonstrated to be curative for Hodgkin's disease. There is a dose-response curve to therapy (greater rate of control with higher doses of radiation for a given tumor burden). Doses of 4000 to 4400 cGy are required for identifiable tumor masses, whereas subclinical disease in apparently uninvolved areas can be controlled with doses of 3000 to 3500 cGy [4]. Radiotherapy alone is curative in carefully staged patients with limited, asymptomatic disease and is a useful component of treatment in patients with bulky disease. The success of radiotherapy in favorable, limited disease is based on an understanding of the patterns of spread of disease and the inclusion of identifiable sites of disease as well as contiguous nodal sites in the radiation fields.

Chemotherapy
The development of MOPP (mechlorethamine, vincristine, procarbazine, prednisone) chemotherapy in the 1960s represented a major advance in the treatment of patients with advanced-stage Hodgkin's disease, which to that time had been largely fatal. About 85% of patients achieved a complete response and over 50% were continuously free of disease at a median of 14 years' follow-up [5]. In the early 1970s, a second major advance came with the introduction of ABVD (doxorubicin, bleomycin, vinblastine, dacarbazine), a

---

Table 19-1. Cotswold Revision of the Ann Arbor Stage in Classification of Hodgkin's Disease

Stage I: Involvement of a single lymph node region (*eg*, cervical, axillary, inguinal, mediastinal) or lymphoid structure, such as spleen, thymus, and Waldeyer's ring, or involvement of a single extralymphatic site (IE)

Stage II: Involvement of ≥ 2 lymph node regions or lymph node structures on the same side of the diaphragm; extralymphatic involvement on one side of the diaphragm by limited direct extension from an adjacent nodal site (IIE)

Stage III: Involvement of lymph node regions or lymphoid structures on both sides of the diaphragm, which may be accompanied by limited contiguous involvement of one extralymphatic site (IIIE)

Stage III$_1$: Spleen or splenic, hilar, celiac, or portal node involvement

Stage III$_2$: Paraaortic, iliac, or mesenteric node involvement

Stage IV: Extensive extranodal disease
  A: Asymptomatic
  B: Unexplained weight loss >10% of body weight in the previous 6 mo, or unexplained fever > 38°C during the previous month, or recurrent drenching night sweats during the previous month
  X: Bulky disease

From Lister and coworkers [3].

chemotherapy regimen containing drugs non–cross-resistant to those in MOPP. The activity of the ABVD regimen was demonstrated first in patients in whom MOPP failed and later as effective initial therapy [6].

A number of randomized, controlled trials have tested the efficacy of MOPP, ABVD, and various combinations of MOPP with ABVD (Table 19-2). The results from the Cancer and Leukemia Group B (CALGB) [7], Milan [8], and the European Organization for the Research and Treatment of Cancer [9] show that ABVD or an ABVD combination with MOPP yields superior response rates and freedom from progression compared with MOPP alone. However, the results with MOPP in these randomized studies are less favorable than those from the National Cancer Institute (NCI), possibly because of deviation from the dosing guidelines as specified by the original investigators. MOPP/ABV hybrid and MOPP-ABV alternating were equivalent in efficacy in studies from NCI Canada [10] and from Milan [11]. A superior response rate, relapse-free survival, and overall survival were seen with MOPP/ABV hybrid compared with a sequence of MOPP followed by ABVD in the Intergroup trial [11a].

The results of the various randomized studies suggest that ABVD or a combination of ABVD and MOPP is superior to MOPP alone. An Intergroup trial has compared MOPP/ABV hybrid to ABVD alone. Preliminary results showed no difference in complete response rate, freedom from progression, or overall survival between treatments thus far. However, there was a significantly greater incidence of pulmonary, hematologic, and infectious toxicities with the hybrid treatment [12]. Longer follow-up is needed, however, before final conclusions can be made.

Investigators at the German Hodgkin's Lymphoma Study Group reported preliminary results of a time-condensed regimen, BEACOPP, in patients with advanced-stage disease. In this large, randomized, three-arm study, BEACOPP and intensified BEACOPP were compared to COPP/ABVD. Early analysis resulted in early closure of the COPP/ABVD arm because of superior complete remission rates, freedom from failure, and overall survival among the BEACOPP arms. Longer follow-up is needed to assess the long-term effects of these various treatments and to ascertain whether the intensified BEACOPP arm is superior to the standard dosing regimen [13].

TREATMENT STRATEGIES

Early-Stage, Favorable Disease

The current standard of treatment for patients with stage I or IIA nonbulky disease is radiotherapy alone. Clinically, stage I or IIA patients with *favorable* features (*ie*, nonbulky disease, absence of systemic symptoms, normal erythrocyte sedimentation rate, young age, fewer than four nodal sites) may be treated with mantle irradiation with extension to the para-aortic fields. *Less favorable* stage I or IIA patients or those with constitutional symptoms may be approached with treatment directed by staging laparotomy or with combined chemotherapy and radiotherapy. Recent results of radiotherapy in early-stage disease are shown in Table 19-3. Most patients enter a sustained remission, and overall survival is very high, in part because of effective second-line treatments at relapse.

Extended courses of treatment with chemotherapy alone, such as ABVD, have been tested in patients with early-stage disease. As expected, response rates and overall survival are excellent, although patients are exposed to higher doses of potentially toxic agents [14].

A number of centers are studying the use of less toxic or abbreviated chemotherapy and limited-volume radiotherapy in early-stage favorable-disease patients to avoid the complications associated with staging laparotomy (including splenectomy) and those associated with extended-field radiotherapy. Although these early results are encouraging, longer follow-up and comparison with established ther-

Table 19-2. Treatment of Advanced-Stage Hodgkin's Disease

Study	Evaluable Patients, *n*	Regimen	% (at 1y) CR	% (at 1y) FFS	% (at 1y) OS
Santoro *et al.* [8]	43	MOPP x 12	74	37 FPP	58 (10)
	45	MOPP/ABVD x 6/6	89	61* FFP	69
Somers *et al.* [9]	96	MOPP x 8	57	43	57 (6)
	96	MOPP/ABVD x 4/4	59	60*	65
Canellos *et al.* [7]	123	MOPP x 6–8	67	50	66 (5)
	115	ABVD x 6–8	82*	61*	73
	123	MOPP/ABVD x 6/6	83*	65*	75
Vivani [11]	204	MOPP/ABV x 6	89	69 FFP	72 (10)
	211	MOPP/ABVD x 3/3	91	67 FFP	74
Glick *et al.* [11a]	737	MOPP/ABV x 8	82*	77*	89* (2.5)
	total	MOPP x 6–8/ABVD x 3 (sequential)	73	65	82
Connors *et al.* [10]	146	MOPP/ABV x 8	85	75 FFP	84 (4)
	141	MOPP/ABVD x 4/4	83	70 FFP	84

*P<0.05
CR—complete response; FFP—freedom from progression; FFS—failure-free survival; OS—overall survival.

apies are necessary before these strategies can be considered standard. Recent results of some of these new approaches to treatment of early-stage disease also are listed in Table 19-3.

Bulky Mediastinal Disease

Patients with stage I or II disease with bulky mediastinal involvement (defined as the ratio of the maximum mediastinal diameter to the greatest internal transthoracic diameter greater than one third) should be treated with combination chemotherapy and radiation. Treatment of bulky disease with either radiation or combination chemotherapy alone is associated with a substantial relapse rate. In addition, using chemotherapy prior to radiotherapy will in most patients reduce the volume of required radiation and decrease the toxicity to adjacent organs.

Advanced-Stage Disease

Patients with stage III or IV disease should be treated with doxorubicin-containing combination chemotherapy. Highly selected stage IIIA patients with upper abdominal disease and no or only minimal splenic involvement may be treated with total lymphoid irradiation. As noted earlier, either ABVD or an ABVD combination is appropriate. The selection of the particular regimen should be based on the potential toxicities expected and the tolerance of the individual patient. Consolidative radiotherapy should be considered in patients with bulky mediastinal involvement to decrease the chance of recurrence in that site.

SECOND-LINE TREATMENT

The majority of patients with Hodgkin's disease are cured with initial therapy. However, a small portion of patients treated with radiotherapy alone for limited favorable disease, and a larger subset of patients treated with combination chemotherapy alone or with radiotherapy for advanced-stage or unfavorable disease, relapse after attaining an initial remission.

Patients relapsing after radiotherapy alone do as well with salvage combination chemotherapy as patients with advanced-stage disease who have never received radiation. Salvage treatment after relapse from combination chemotherapy is less successful. Retreatment with the initial chemotherapy regimen or employment of a non–cross-resistant regimen offers high response rates among patients with favorable characteristics at relapse, particularly those with a long duration of remission. Among this group, however, long-term disease-free survival is achieved in a minority of patients, and it is achieved in even fewer among those with early relapses or other unfavorable characteristics. Wide-field radiotherapy as a salvage treatment can result in long remissions, but the number of optimal candidates for this treatment is limited.

High-dose therapy with autografting shows the greatest promise in the treatment of patients at relapse, with as many as half of patients event-free at several years follow-up. In addition, with greater experience, the morbidity and mortality associated with the procedure continue to decline. Predictors of improved outcome include less disease at time of transplant [15,16], fewer relapses [16–18], sensitive disease at time of transplant [16,18], better performance status [16], nodal disease, and absence of B symptoms at relapse [19]. The series by Reece and coworkers [19] consists only of patients in first relapse. With a median follow-up of 2.3 years, it is notable that 64% of the entire group is free from progression (FFP), with over 80% FFP among those patients with an initial remission greater than a year. Results such as these suggest that high-dose therapy and autografting should be used early after first relapse when more favorable characteristics are

Table 19-3. Treatment of Early-Stage Hodgkin's Disease

Study	Evaluable patients, n	Regimen	Stage	% (at 1 y) CR	% (at 1 y) FFP	% (at 1 y) OS
Bates et al. [33]	30	VBM x 6-XRT	I-IIA	90	87	93 (2.5)
Hagemeister et al. [34]	79	NOVP x 3-XRT	I-II	95	87	98 (2.5)
Brusamolino et al. [35]	88	STNI	PS I-II (F)	94	69	96 (5)
	76	CT-XRT	I-II (U)	99	91	93
Noordijk et al. [36]	130	STNI	I-II (F)	94	81	99 (3)
	124	vs EBVP-IF XRT	I-II (F)	90	79	100
	156	MOPP/ABV x 6-IF XRT	I-II (U)	85	88*	92 (3)
	160	vs EBVP x 6-IF XRT	I-II (U)	82	72*	92
Horning et al. [37]	35	VBM x 6-IF XRT	I-II		87 (5)	
	43	STNI			92	
Colonna et al. [38]	262	ABVD x 1–4-XRT	MMR < 1/3		94	93 (10)
			MMR > 1/3, < 0.45		87	87
			MMR > 0/45		63	78
Bonfante et al. [39]	37	ABVD x 4-STNI	I-II	100	100	100 (2)
	36	ABVD x 4-IF XRT		100	100	100

*P<0.01 CT:MOPP x 6 or ABVD x 3.

CR—complete response; EBVP—epirubicin, bleomycin, vinblastine, prednisone; F—favorable; FFP—freedom from progression; NOVP—novantrone, vincristine, vinblastine, prednisone; OS—overall survival; STNI—subtotal nodal irradiation; U—unfavorable; VBM—vinblastine, bleomycin, methotrxate, VF— very favorable.

likely to be present. In spite of the favorable results with high-dose therapy and autografting, very few randomized studies have confirmed the apparent superiority of this approach. Yuen and coworkers [20] compared a group of patients treated with high-dose therapy who developed refractory disease or who were at first relapse with a matched group of patients who received conventional treatment. The group that received high-dose therapy had a better outcome overall and among patients who had refractory disease or an early relapse. However, there was no significant difference in outcome among patients who relapsed more than a year after initial therapy. Longer follow-up is needed to see if the apparent improvements will be sustained over time and also to better characterize long-term side effects associated with high-dose therapy and autografting.

SIDE EFFECTS OF TREATMENT

The satisfaction with success in the treatment of Hodgkin's disease over the last several decades must be tempered by increasing recognition of long-term side effects that limit the quality of life and survival of patients cured of their disease. Leukemias and second malignancies are among the most problematic of treatment-related side effects. Cardiac, pulmonary, and other organ toxicities also limit the quality of life of long-term survivors.

The risk of secondary leukemia is related to the extent of prior alkylator therapy. Recent estimates from Van Leeuwen and coworkers [21] show an eightfold risk of leukemia among patients treated with six or fewer cycles of nitrogen mustard plus procarbazine, with an increase to 40-fold among patients treated with more than six cycles. Whether or not the addition of radiotherapy to chemotherapy increases the leukemia risk is controversial [22,23], as is that of additional increased risk among patients who have had a splenectomy or splenic radiation [21,23,24]. Most patients in the series that reported an increased incidence of leukemia were treated with six or more cycles of MOPP chemotherapy, which is not currently favored. The incidence of leukemia among patients treated in the 1980s [21] or

with ABVD [22] appears to be significantly less, though longer follow-up is needed to characterize the risk more completely.

The relative risks for non-Hodgkin's lymphoma, lung cancers, gastrointestinal cancers, urogenital cancers, melanoma, soft tissue sarcomas, and thyroid cancer [25] also are increased among Hodgkin's disease patients compared with the general population. Van Leeuwen and coworkers [26] found that the risk of lung cancer was related to the use of radiotherapy without additional risk from chemotherapy. Hancock and coworkers [27] found a sevenfold relative risk for breast cancer among patients younger than 30 years of age who had received radiation. The addition of MOPP increased the relative risk even further. Mauch and coworkers [28] confirmed the dramatically increased risk for breast cancer among younger women and showed that the risk of all second solid tumors continued to rise even after 15 years follow-up.

Hancock and coworkers [29] found about a threefold risk of cardiac death and acute myocardial infarction among patients who received more than 3000 cGy of mediastinal irradiation. The relative risk also increased for patients less than 20 years of age and for those with minimal cardiac blocking.

The risk of infertility is related to the chemotherapy regimen employed. MOPP chemotherapy is associated with a very high rate of azoospermia in males and amenorrhea in females. ABVD is associated with a much lower rate of infertility. MOPP/ABVD combinations have been associated with about 50% azoospermia even after prolonged follow-up [30].

Pulmonary toxicity associated with mantle radiation and chemotherapy has been found in up to 70% of patients by CT scanning shortly after starting radiotherapy [31]. Horning and coworkers [32] found a 20% decrease in pulmonary function tests at less than 15 months' follow-up among patients treated with mediastinal radiation.

In summary, the improvements in the treatment of Hodgkin's disease have come with a number of side effects that limit the quality and quantity of life after successful treatment of the disease. Increasing recognition of these effects should help to guide the development of safer and equally effective treatments.

REFERENCES

1. Medeiros L, Greiner T: Hodgkin's disease. *Cancer* 1995, 75:357–369.

2. MacMahon B: Epidemiological evidence of the nature of Hodgkin's disease. *Cancer* 1957, 10:1045–1054.

3. Lister TA, Crowther D, Sutcliffe SB, *et al.*: Report of a committee convened to discuss the evaluation and staging of patients with Hodgkin's disease: Cotswolds meeting. *J Clin Oncol* 1989, 7:1630–1636.

4. Vijayakumar S, Myrianthopoulos L: An updated dose-response analysis in Hodgkin's disease. *Radiother Oncol* 1992, 24:1–13.

5. Longo DL, Young RC, Wesley M, *et al.*: Twenty years of MOPP therapy for Hodgkin's disease. *J Clin Oncol* 1986, 4:1295–1306.

6. Bonadonna G, Santoro A, Gianni AM, *et al.*: Primary and salvage chemotherapy in advanced Hodgkin's disease: the Milan Cancer Institute experience. *Ann Oncol* 1991, 1:9–16.

7. Canellos GP, Anderson JR, Propert KJ, *et al.*: Chemotherapy of advanced Hodgkin's disease with MOPP, ABVD, or MOPP alternating with ABVD. *N Engl J Med* 1992, 327:1478–1484.

8. Santoro A, Bonfante V, Viviani S, *et al.*: Decrease in mortality rate by Hodgkin's disease after ABVD vs MOPP: 10-year results. *Proc ASCO* 1991, 10:281.

9. Somers R, Carde P, Henry-Amar M, *et al.*: A randomized study in stage IIIB and IV Hodgkin's disease comparing eight courses of MOPP versus an alteration of MOPP with ABVD: a European Organization for Research and Treatment of Cancer Lymphoma Cooperative Group and Groupe Pierre-et-Marie-Curie controlled clinical trial. *J Clin Oncol* 1994, 12:279–287.

10. Connors JM, Klimo P, Adams G, *et al.*: Treatment of advanced Hodgkin's disease with chemotherapy—comparison of MOPP/ABV hybrid regimen with alternating courses of MOPP and ABVD: a report from the National Cancer Institute of Canada Clinical Trials Group. *J Clin Oncol* 1997, 15:1638–1645.

11. Viviani S, Bonadonna G, Santoro A, *et al.*: Alternating versus hybrid MOPP and ABVD combinations in advanced Hodgkin's disease: ten-year results. *J Clin Oncol* 1996, 14:1421–1430.

11a. Glick J, Tsiatis A, Schilsky R, *et al.*: A randomized phase III trial of MOPP/ABV hybrid vs sequential MOPP/ABVD in advanced Hodgkin's disease: preliminary results of the Intergroup trial. *Proc ASCO* 1991, 10:271.

12. Duggan D, Petroni G, Johnson J, *et al.*: MOPP/ABV versus ABVD for advanced Hodgkin's disease: a preliminary report of CALGB 8952 (with SWOG, ECOG, NCIC). *Proc Am So Clin Oncol* 1997 16:5a.

13. Diehl V, Tesch H, Lathan B, *et al.* on behalf of the German Hodgkin's Lymphoma Study Group (GHSG): BEACOPP, a new intensified hybrid regimen, is at least equally effective compared with copp/abvd in patients with advanced. *Proc Am So Clin Oncol* 1997, 16:43a.

14. Rueda A, Alba E, Ribelles N, *et al.*: Six cycles of ABVD in the treatment of stage I and II Hodgkin's lymphoma: a pilot study. *J Clin Oncol* 1997, 15:1118–1122.

15. Rapoport AP, Rowe JM, Kouides PA, *et al.*: One hundred autotransplants for relapsed or refractory Hodgkin's disease and lymphoma: value of pretransplant disease status for predicting outcome. *J Clin Oncol* 1993, 11:2351–2361.

16. Anderson JE, Litzow MR, Appelbaum FR, *et al.*: Allogeneic, syngeneic, and autologous marrow transplantation for Hodgkin's disease: the 21-year Seattle experience. *J Clin Oncol* 1993, 11:2342–2350.

17. Armitage J: Early bone marrow transplantation in Hodgkin's disease. *Ann Oncol* 1994, 5:161–163.

18. Weaver CH, Petersen FB, Appelbaum FR, *et al.*: High-dose fractionated total-body irradiation, etoposide, and cylcophosphamide followed by autologous stem-cell support in patients with malignant lymphoma. *J Clin Oncol* 1994, 12:2559–2566.

19. Reece DE, Connors JM, Spinelli JJ, *et al.*: Intensive therapy with cyclophosphamide, carmustine, etoposide ± cisplatin, and autologous bone marrow transplantation for Hodgkin's disease in first relapse after combination chemotherapy. *Blood* 1994, 83:1193–1199.

20. Yuen AR, Rosenberg SA, Hoppe RT, *et al.*: Comparison between conventional salvage therapy and high-dose therapy with autografting for recurrent or refractory Hodgkin's disease. *Blood* 1997, 89:814–822.

21. van Leeuwen FE, Chorus AM, van den Belt-Dusebout AW, *et al.*: Leukemia risk following Hodgkin's disease: relation to cumulative dose of alkylating agents, treatment with teniposide combinations, number of episodes of chemotherapy, and bone marrow damage. *J Clin Oncol* 1994, 12:1063–1073.

22. Biti G, Cellai E, Magrini S, *et al.*: Second solid tumors and leukemia after treatment for Hodgkin's disease: an analysis of 1121 patients from a single institution. *Int J Radiation Oncol Biol Biophysics* 1994, 29:25–31.

23. Dietrich PY, Henry-Amar M, Cosset JM, *et al.*: Second primary cancers in patients continuously disease-free from Hodgkin's disease: a protective role for the spleen? *Blood* 1994, 84:1209–1215.

24. Hudson B, Hudson V, Linch D, Anderson L: Late mortality in young BNLI patients cured of Hodgkin's disease. *Ann Oncol* 1994, 5:65–66.

25. Sankila R, Garwicz S, Olsen JH, *et al.*: Risk of subsequent malignant neoplasms among 1641 Hodgkin's disease patients diagnosed in childhood and adolescence: a population-based cohort study in the five Nordic countries. *J Clin Oncol* 1996, 14:1442–1446.

26. van Leeuwen FE, Klokman WJ, Hagenbeek A, *et al.*: Second cancer risk following Hodgkin's disease: a 20-year follow-up study. *J Clin Oncol* 1994, 112:312–325.

27. Hancock SL, Tucker MA, Hoppe RT: Breast cancer after treatment of Hodgkin's disease. *J Natl Cancer Inst* 1993, 85:25–31.

28. Mauch PM, Kalish LA, Marcus KC, *et al.*: Second malignancies after treatment for laparotomy staged IA-IIIB Hodgkin's disease: long-term analysis of risk factors and outcome. *Blood* 1996, 87:3625–3632.

29. Hancock SL, Donaldson SS, Hoppe RT: Cardiac disease following treatment of Hodgkin's disease in children and adolescents. *J Clin Oncol* 1993, 11:1208–1215.

30. Viviani S, Ragni G, Santoro A, *et al.*: Testicular dysfunction in Hodgkin's disease before and after treatment. *Eur J Cancer* 1991, 27:1389–1392.

31. Mah K, Keane T, Van Dyk J, *et al.*: Quantitative effect of combined chemotherapy and fractionated radiotherapy on the incidence of radiation-induced lung damage: a prospective clinical study. *Int J Radiation Oncol Biol Biophysics* 1994, 28:563–574.

32. Horning SJ, Adhikari A, Rizk N, *et al.*: Effect of treatment for Hodgkin's disease on pulmonary function: results of a prospective study. *J Clin Oncol* 1994, 12:297–305.

33. Bates NP, Williams MV, Bessell EM, *et al.*: Efficacy and toxicity of vinblastine, bleomycin, and methotrexate with involved-field radiotherapy in clinical stage IA and IIA Hodgkin's disease: a British National Lymphoma Investigation pilot study. *J Clin Oncol* 1994, 12:288–296.

34. Hagemeister F, Purugganan R, Fuller L, *et al.*: Treatment of early stages of Hodgkin's disease with novantrone, vincristine, vinblastine, prednisone and radiotherapy. *Semin Hematol* 1994, 31:36–43.

35. Brusamolino E, Lazzarino M, Orlandi E, *et al.*: Early-stage Hodgkin's disease: long-term results with radiotherapy alone or combined radiotherapy and chemotherapy. *Ann Oncol* 1994, 5:101–106.

36. Noordijk E, Carde P, Mandard A-M, *et al.*: Preliminary results of the EORTC-GPMC controlled clinical trial H7 in early-stage Hodgkin's disease. *Ann Oncol* 1994, 5:107–112.

37. Horning SJ, Hoppe RT, Mason J, *et al.*: Stanford-Kaiser Permanente G1 study for clinical stage I to IIA Hodgkin's disease: subtotal lymphoid irradiation versus vinblastine, methotrexate, and bleomycin chemotherapy and regional irradiation. *J Clin Oncol* 1997, 15:1736–1744.

38. Colonna P, Jais JP, Desablens B, *et al.*: Mediastinal tumor size and response to chemotherapy are the only prognostic factors in supradiaphragmatic Hodgkin's disease treated by ABVD plus radiotherapy: ten-year results of the Paris-Ouest-France 81/12 trial, including 262 patients. *J Clin Oncol* 1996, 14:1928–1935.

39. Bonfante V, Santoro A, Viviani S, *et al.*: ABVD plus radiotherapy (subtotal nodal vs involved field) in early-stage Hodgkin's disease (HD). *Proc Am So Clin Oncol* 1994, 13:373.

ABVD
Doxorubicin, Bleomycin, Vinblastine, Dacarbazine

The ABVD regimen was developed to treat patients in whom MOPP chemotherapy had failed, and thus includes agents non–cross-resistant to the components of MOPP. The efficacy of ABVD was proven first as a second-line therapy in MOPP failures and later as superior to MOPP in randomized trials. The additional advantage of ABVD is in a lower incidence of sterility and very rare incidence of secondary leukemia. However, cardiac and pulmonary toxicities are associated with the use of doxorubicin and bleomycin components of the regimen.

CANDIDATES FOR TREATMENT
Patients with bulky disease or stage III or IV Hodgkin's disease

SPECIAL PRECAUTIONS
Patients with abnormal left ventricular function or history of coronary artery disease, significantly impaired respiratory function, or elevated bilirubin

ALTERNATIVE THERAPIES
MOPP/ABVD, MOPP/ABV, ABVD, Stanford V.

DOSAGE AND SCHEDULING

	1	2	3	4	5	6	7	8	9	10	11	12	13	14	15
Doxorubicin 25 mg/m² IVP d 1, 15	■														■
Bleomycin 10 U/m² IVP d 1, 15	■														■
Vinblastine 6 mg/m² IVP d 1, 15	■														■
Dacarbazine 375 mg/m² IVP d 1, 15	■														■
CBC with diff. d 1,15	☐														☐
SMAC d 1	☐														
Day	1	2	3	4	5	6	7	8	9	10	11	12	13	14	15

28-d cycle. Pulmonary function tests with DLCO approximately q 2–3 cycles or sooner if new, noninfectious pulmonary signs or symptoms develop; PA and lateral CXR q 2 cycles.

DOSAGE MODIFICATIONS

WBC	Platelets	Dose Adjustment [25]
>4000	>130,000	100% of all drugs
3000–3999	100,000–129,000	50% doxorubicin, vinblastine, & dacarbazine
2000–2999	80,000–99,000	50% dacarbazine & 25% doxorubicin & vinblastine
1500–1999	50,000–79,000	25% dacarbazine & NO doxorubicin or vinblastine
<1500	<50,000	NO doxorubicin, vinblastine or dacarbazine

RECENT EXPERIENCE AND RESPONSE RATES

Study	Evaluable Patients	CR, %	FFS, %	OS, %
Bonadonna et al. [6]	118	92*	81 (FFP)	77 (7 y)
Canellos et al. [7]	115	82	61	73 (5 y)

Includes use of radiotherapy.
CR—complete response; FFS—failure-free survival; FFP—freedom from progression; OS—overall survival.

MOPP AND ABVD

The proven activity of MOPP and ABVD as non–cross-resistant regimens led researchers to combine the two regimens in alternating fashion. The strategy was based on the Goldie-Coldman hypothesis that concludes that as many active drugs as possible should be administered as early in treatment as possible to prevent cells resistant to one drug from developing resistance to others. A superior response rate and failure-free survival of alternating MOPP and ABVD over MOPP alone has been observed in a number of studies, but a superior outcome of MOPP with ABVD over ABVD alone has not been observed.

CANDIDATES FOR TREATMENT

Patients with bulky disease or stage III or IV Hodgkin's disease

SPECIAL PRECAUTIONS

Patients with abnormal ventricular function or history of coronary artery disease, significantly impaired respiratory function, or elevated bilirubin

ALTERNATIVE THERAPIES

MOPP/ABVD, MOPP/ABV, ABVD, Stanford V.

DOSAGE AND SCHEDULING

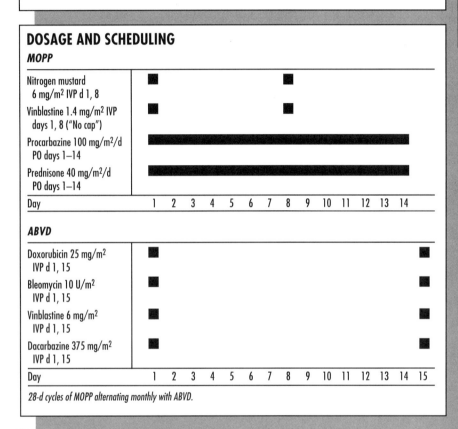

MOPP

	1	2	3	4	5	6	7	8	9	10	11	12	13	14
Nitrogen mustard 6 mg/m² IVP d 1, 8	■							■						
Vinblastine 1.4 mg/m² IVP days 1, 8 ("No cap")	■							■						
Procarbazine 100 mg/m²/d PO days 1–14	██
Prednisone 40 mg/m²/d PO days 1–14	██
Day														

ABVD

	1	2	3	4	5	6	7	8	9	10	11	12	13	14	15
Doxorubicin 25 mg/m² IVP d 1, 15	■														■
Bleomycin 10 U/m² IVP d 1, 15	■														■
Vinblastine 6 mg/m² IVP d 1, 15	■														■
Dacarbazine 375 mg/m² IVP d 1, 15	■														■
Day															

28-d cycles of MOPP alternating monthly with ABVD.

RECENT EXPERIENCES AND RESPONSE RATES

Study	Evaluable Patients	CR, %	FFS, %	OS, %
Santoro et al. [8]	45	89	61 (FFP)	69 (10 y)
Connors et al. [10]	141	83	70 (FFP)	84 (4 y)
Canellos et al. [7]	123	83	65	75 (5 y)
Somers et al. [9]	96	59	60	65 (6 y)

CR—complete response; FFS—failure-free survival; FFP—freedom from progression; OS—overall survival.

MOPP/ABV HYBRID

The MOPP/ABV regimen was also developed according to the Goldie-Coldman theory. In this regimen, all agents are given by day 8 of the 28-d cycle, in contrast to MOPP alternating with ABVD, in which all agents are not introduced until the second month. The hybrid regimen was shown to be as effective as alternating MOPP-ABVD by Connors and coworkers [10] and superior to sequential MOPP-ABVD in regard to response and survival.

CANDIDATES FOR TREATMENT
Patients with bulky disease or stage III or IV
  Hodgkin's disease

ALTERNATIVE THERAPIES
MOPP/ABVD, MOPP/ABV, ABVD, Stanford V.

DOSAGE AND SCHEDULING

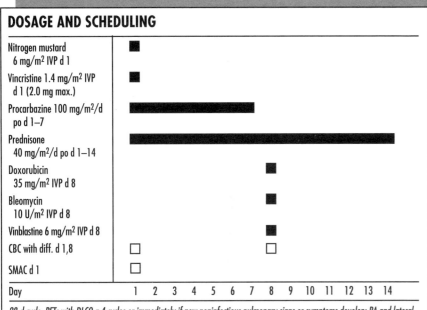

Nitrogen mustard
  6 mg/m² IVP d 1

Vincristine 1.4 mg/m² IVP
  d 1 (2.0 mg max.)

Procarbazine 100 mg/m²/d
  po d 1–7

Prednisone
  40 mg/m²/d po d 1–14

Doxorubicin
  35 mg/m² IVP d 8

Bleomycin
  10 U/m² IVP d 8

Vinblastine 6 mg/m² IVP d 8

CBC with diff. d 1,8

SMAC d 1

| Day | 1 | 2 | 3 | 4 | 5 | 6 | 7 | 8 | 9 | 10 | 11 | 12 | 13 | 14 |

28-d cycle. PFTs with DLCO q 4 cycles or immediately if new noninfectious pulmonary signs or symptoms develop; PA and lateral CXR q 2 cycles

RECENT EXPERIENCES AND RESPONSE RATES

Study	Evaluable Patients	CR, %	FFS, %	OS, %
Glick *et al.* [11]	370	82	77	89 (2.5 y)
Conners *et al.* [10]	146	85	77 (FFP)	84 (4 y)

CR — complete response; FFP — freedom from progression; FFS — failure-free survival; OS — overall survival.

STANFORD V

This novel chemotherapy regimen was designed to shorten the period of treatment, decrease the total doses of agents with the most significant long-term toxicities (alkylating agents, doxorubicin, and bleomycin), and maintain dose intensity. Adjuvant radiotherapy was administered to sites of bulky disease. The investigators at Stanford have reported excellent results in patients with bulky mediastinal involvement or with stage III or IV disease [12]. However, longer follow-up is needed, and the regimen should be tested in other centers and in a randomized comparison to confirm the very favorable results thus far.

CANDIDATES FOR TREATMENT

Patients with bulky disease or stage III or IV Hodgkin's disease

SPECIAL PRECAUTIONS

Patients with abnormal left ventricular function or history of coronary artery disease, significantly impaired respiratory function, or elevated bilirubin; elderly patients (constipation, obstipation)

ALTERNATIVE THERAPIES

MOPP/ABVD, MOPP/ABV, ABVD

TOXICITIES

Etoposide: moderately severe nausea and vomiting, hair loss

DRUG INTERACTIONS

As with ABVD regimen

NURSING INTERVENTIONS

As with ABVD regimen

PATIENT INFORMATION

As with ABVD regimen.

DOSAGE AND SCHEDULING

Drug	Day 1	Day 8	Day 15	Day 22	Day 28
Doxorubicin 25 mg/m² IV d 1,15	■		■		
Vinblastine† 6 mg/m² IV d 1,15	■		■		
Mechlorethamine 6 mg/m² IV d 1	■				
Vincristine†‡ 1.4 mg/m² IV d 8,22		■		■	
Bleomycin 5 U/m² IV d 8,22		■		■	
Etoposide 60 mg/m² IV d 15,16			■		
Prednisone§ 40 mg/m² PO qod	████████████████████████				

*Treatment repeated every 28 d for a total of 3 cycles.
†Vinblastine dose decreased to 4 mg/m², and vincristine dose decreased to 1 mg/m² during cycle 3 for patients ≥ 50 y of age.
§Tapered by 10 mg qod starting at week 10.
‡Maximum dose, 2.0 mg

RECENT EXPERIENCES AND RESPONSE RATES

Study	Evaluable Patients	FFS, %	OS, %
Bartlett et al. [12]	65	87	96 (3 y)

CR—complete response; FFS—failure-free survival; OS—overall survival.

CHAPTER 20: NON-HODGKIN'S LYMPHOMA
Craig H. Moskowitz, Carol S. Portlock

The non-Hodgkin's lymphomas are a group of monoclonal lymphoid malignancies defined by their characteristic lymph node pattern and cytology. Each pathologic entity has a distinctive clinical presentation, natural history, response to treatment, and survival pattern. Many histologic classifications have been proposed to encompass the diversity of non-Hodgkin's lymphomas. The Working Formulation proposed by the National Cancer Institute for classification of non-Hodgkin's lymphoma has been widely adopted in the United States [1]. This classification recognizes three prognostic groups of non-Hodgkin's lymphomas (low-, intermediate-, and high-grade categories), which are identified by the shape of survival curves generated from 1971 to 1975 clinical data.

The non-Hodgkin's lymphomas represent the seventh most common cause of death from cancer in the United States. The aggressive lymphomas, diffuse large cell lymphoma and, in particular, small, noncleaved cell lymphomas, are increasing in frequency with the AIDS epidemic.

ETIOLOGY AND RISK FACTORS

The cause of most non-Hodgkin's lymphomas is unknown. The rare entity HTLV-1–associated lymphoma is clearly linked to retroviral infection, but the specific molecular events leading to lymphomagenesis are not completely known. The risk of lymphoma is low among infected individuals and other host factors may play a role [2].

AIDS-associated lymphomas are also linked to retroviral infection, but in these cases the emergence of lymphoma is more likely secondary to virus-associated immunodeficiency rather than to a direct tumor-promoting effect of the HIV infection. Excessive B-cell proliferation, often stimulated by the Epstein–Barr virus, is thought to be the milieu necessary for lymphomagenesis [3]. The specific molecular events await definition. Whether similar mechanisms are pertinent to the etiology of other non-Hodgkin's lymphomas is speculative. Other established causes include genetic factors (such as X-linked lymphoproliferative syndrome, in which genetically linked immunodeficiency results in B-cell lymphomas) and environmental exposures (Epstein–Barr virus and malaria in Burkitt's lymphoma; irradiation).

DIAGNOSIS

The diagnosis of a non-Hodgkin's lymphoma requires expert hematopathologic evaluation, often in conjunction with immunophenotypic, genotypic, and karyotypic studies (Table 20-1). The architectural pattern of diffuse or follicular involvement is evaluated on lymph node, not extranodal, material. Specialized studies often require fresh or frozen tissue and should be planned in advance of lymph node biopsy.

Demonstration of B-cell monoclonality can usually be performed on fixed tissue using immunoperoxidase methods. T-cell monoclonality requires molecular studies of fresh tissue (T-cell receptor gene rearrangement).

Some immunophenotypic patterns may identify specific disease entities, such as Ki-1 antigen in T-cell DLCL, or IgM immunophenotype with small lymphocytic lymphoma (Waldenström's macroglobulinemia). Chromosomal translocations may be associated with certain histologic patterns: t(2;5) in Ki-1 lymphomas; t(8;14) in Burkitt's lymphoma; t(11;14) in mantle zone lymphoma; and t(14;18) in follicular lymphomas. These chromosomal changes cannot be used in isolation to diagnose lymphoma. Rather, they add weight to a histologic diagnosis, and their specificity remains an area of current investigation. A new pathologic classification, the Revised European American Lymphoma (REAL) classification, has been proposed that takes into account immunotyping and genotyping to help classify lymphomas [4].

Serum antibody studies of associated retroviral infection may be appropriate. HIV-associated lymphomas are those of intermediate and high-grade histologies, as are HTLV-1–associated lymphomas. Evidence of positive antibody titers with lymphadenopathy does not confer the diagnosis of lymphoma without histologic documentation.

STAGING

Once a diagnosis of non-Hodgkin's lymphoma is established, a full staging evaluation must be undertaken to plan treatment. Although the Ann Arbor staging classification for Hodgkin's disease is used in non-Hodgkin's lymphomas, it is not completely applicable. Recently, proposals for other staging systems have been made for low-grade, lymphoblastic, and small, noncleaved cell lymphomas to account for the high frequency of extranodal involvement and indicators of tumor bulk and cell proliferation. The standard staging studies for the lymphomas are provided in Table 20-2. In general,

---

Table 20-1. Diagnostic Studies in Non-Hodgkin's Lymphoma

1. Lymph node biopsy; extranodal site biopsies as indicated
2. Expert hematopathology using Working Formulation classification
3. Frozen tissue stored for special studies
4. Immunophenotyping by flow cytometry and and or immunoperoxidase of fixed or frozen tissue
5. Karotype performed on fresh tissue culture
6. Genotype performed on fresh tissue

Table 20-2. Studies Used for Staging Non-Hodgkin's Lymphomas

1. History
2. Blood work
   a. Complete blood count, platelets, review of smear
   b. Liver function tests
   c. Renal function tests
   d. Lactic dehydrogenase
3. Imaging
   a. Chest radiography
   b. CT scan of chest (if chest radiograph is positive), abdomen, and pelvis
   c. Lymphogram, if CT of abdomen or pelvis is negative
   d. Selected CNS, GI, bone studies depending on symptoms
   e. Gallium scan in intermediate-grade immunoblastic lymphoma and SNCL
4. Histology
   a. Lymph node biopsy
   b. Bone marrow biopsy (bilateral in low-grade histologies)
   c. CSF cytology in intermediate-grade and immunoblastic lymphoma with bone marrow; testicular disease and in lymphoblastic lymphoma and SNCL

CT—computed tomography; CNS—central nervous system; CSF—cerebrospinal fluid; GI—gastrointestinal; LL—lymphoblastic lymphomas; SNCL—small noncleaved cell lymphomas.

---

decisions regarding therapy may be based on full clinical staging with appropriate percutaneous biopsies.

LOW-GRADE LYMPHOMAS

According to the Working Formulation for classification of the non-Hodgkin's lymphomas, there are three histologic subtypes of low-grade lymphoma: small lymphocytic, follicular small cleaved, and follicular mixed small and large cell. A fourth subtype is often included within this category by many investigators, although it was not originally described in the Working Formulation. It is alternatively termed diffuse intermediate differentiation lymphoma, mantle zone lymphoma, or diffuse small cleaved cell lymphoma—centrocytic type.

The low-grade lymphomas are monoclonal B-cell diseases, presenting most often with generalized adenopathy with or without bone marrow involvement. Hepatosplenomegaly, other extranodal involvement (gastrointestinal tract, lung, skin, bone), and epidural or nerve compression may occur. Despite frequent bone marrow disease, meningeal involvement does not occur and central nervous system (CNS) prophylaxis is not required during therapy.

Approximately 10% of patients with low-grade lymphoma will be found to have clinical stage I or II disease after complete clinical staging. These patients are often candidates for regional radiation therapy [5] (Table 20-3). Treatment outcome may be excellent with low morbidity. Prognostic factors include age, disease site, tumor bulk, and histology.

The majority of patients with low-grade lymphoma have advanced disease at presentation (intraabdominal stage II or stage III or IV). There are many management options for such patients, and the criteria for selection among them remain controversial, because curative treatment is not established [6]. Despite high rates of complete response, relapse is usually noticed within 2 to 4 years of completing therapy [7]. Consolidative radiation therapy or maintenance with interferon may prolong disease-free intervals in some series.

The single-agent regimen pulse chlorambucil (16 mg/m^2 PO qd × 5 days) is well tolerated and effective in the palliative therapy of low-grade lymphoma. Objective responses are achieved in approximately 65% of patients, with median disease-free survival of 2 years [8]. Prompt tumor responses (in less than 3 mo) make this regimen more useful clinically than continuous daily chlorambucil. Hematologic toxicity is mild, although cumulative platelet depression may be encountered.

More recently, autologous stem cell transplantation (ASCT) has been used in patients with low-grade lymphoma. This intensive approach has been studied primarily in second or later remission and is limited to use in younger patients. Promising preliminary results have led to investigation of this modality in first remission [9,10]. Critical to ASCT is the collection of uninvolved normal hematopoietic stem cells. Technologies to purge tumor cells from involved marrow or to positively select normal stem cells are under investigation [11]. Bone marrow harvest and storage are often recommended in first remission; the value of ASCT in first remission remains to be determined.

INTERMEDIATE-GRADE LYMPHOMAS

The intermediate-grade lymphomas are a group of four diseases, the most prevalent being diffuse large cell lymphoma. Immunoblastic lymphoma, classified as a high-grade tumor, is usually managed as an intermediate-grade lesion and is often combined with diffuse large cell lymphoma in outcome data. These five malignancies share common clinical characteristics: slight male predominance, presentation in middle age, rapidly enlarging adenopathy with approximately one half of patients presenting with stage I and II.

Masses may be bulky, particularly in the mediastinum (sometimes with associated superior vena cava obstruction or tracheobronchial compression) or abdomen. Involved extranodal sites are often symptomatic, such as ulcerated and hemorrhagic gastrointestinal tract disease or lytic bone lesions. Lymphomatous meningitis may be detected at diagnosis or may develop during treatment, particularly when there is involvement of the bone marrow. CNS prophylaxis lessens this risk and should be incorporated into most treatment protocols if bone marrow disease is identified. A curative treatment outcome is possible in approximately one half of patients with intermediate-grade lymphoma. The International NHL Prognostic Factor Project, a model to determine complete remission rates and overall survival in patients with intermediate grade NHL determined five prognostic variables that had independent statistical significance in multivariate analysis [12]. These were age, serum LDH, performance status, stage, and number of extranodal sites. . Patients with regional disease presentations (stage I or II) require combination chemotherapy with or without regional radiation therapy because relapses are frequent with radiation alone [13]. An ECOG randomized phase III study of CHOP versus CHOP and involved field radiotherapy in early stage disease determined that

Table 20-3. Treatment Strategy for Low-Grade Lymphoma

1. Stages I and peripheral II: regional radiation therapy
2. Stages II (intraabdominal), III and IV
   a. Patient's age ≤ 55 y
      i. Consider intensive therapy protocols
      ii. Bone marrow harvest in patients with complete responses
      iii. Autologous stem cell transplantation in first or second remission (on protocol study)
   b. Patient's age ≥ 55 y
      i. Consider observation
      ii. Palliative chemotherapy (chlorambucil or CVP) or regional irradiation

Table 20-4. Independent Prognostic Factors in Intermediate Grade NHL

Factor	Relative Risk	P Value
Age ≤ 60 versus > 60	1.96	< .001
Serum LDH normal versus ABN	1.85	< .001
Performance Status 0,1 or 2–4	1.80	< .001
Stage I, II, versus III or IV	1.47	< .001
Extranodal sites ≤ 1 versus > 1	1.48	< .001

Each factor that a patient has is equal to 1; maximum number is 5.

Table 20-5. Outcome According to the International Prognostic Index

Risk Group	Number of Factors	Complete Remission, %	Two-Year RFS, %	Five-Year RFS, %	Two-Year Survival, %	Five-Year Survival, %
Low	0 or 1	87	79	70	84	73
Low int.	2	67	66	50	66	51
High int.	3	55	59	49	54	43
High	4	44	58	40	34	26

the 6-year disease-free survival rate was significantly better in the radiotherapy arm [14]. When radiation therapy is employed, it is often possible to shorten the period of chemotherapy. In patients who are found to be in the poorest IPI prognostic categories, intensification of initial treatment with high-dose chemotherapy plus hematopoietic growth factors with or without autologous stem cell support is currently under investigation. Slow responders to CHOP (cyclophosphamide, doxorubicin, vincristine, and prednisone) defined by an incomplete response to four cycles of CHOP were randomized to receive four more cycles of CHOP versus high dose therapy and autologous stem cell transplantation. In this setting there was no difference in the two treatment programs; however, patients were not stratified according to the international index (Tables 20-4 and 20-5).

There is no single standard chemotherapy regimen for intermediate-grade lymphomas [15–18] (Table 20-6). Many multiagent regimens are in use. A recent prospective clinical trial comparing four such regimens in patients with advanced disease revealed that complete response rates, and disease-free rates, and overall survival rates were similar for each chemotherapeutic protocol. These preliminary data establish a contemporary standard by which new regimens must be compared [19,20].

Results of the United States High Priority Lymphoma Study indicated that over 50% of patients either fail to achieve a complete remission or relapse after receiving standard front-line therapy. These patients are destined to die of intermediate grade non-Hodgkin's lymphoma, usually within 3 to 6 months, unless they respond to second-line therapy. The most successful therapeutic modality for these patients has been autologous stem cell transplantation (ASCT) [21–23]. The most significant predictor of a favorable outcome following ASCT is tumor chemosensitivity at the time of transplant. Results are poor in patients with primary refractory disease who do not attain a complete remission with salvage chemotherapy and in patients with recurrent disease that is not chemosensitive with second-line therapy. Cytoreductive therapy prior to the conditioning regimen and ASCT serves several purposes: it makes it possible to determine which patients have chemosensitive disease and benefit from ASCT; effective reinduction therapy allows ASCT to be done in a setting of minimal disease burden; it may decrease the likelihood that the stem cell product is contaminated with lymphoma cells by acting as an in vivo purge; and when chemotherapy is combined with hematopoietic growth factors, peripheral blood progenitor cells may be collected more efficiently.

There is no standard approach to second-line therapy for patients with relapsed and refractory intermediate grade NHL. Factors to consider before treatment is instituted include the patient's age, performance status, histopathology, sites of disease, bone marrow status, types of previous therapy, and success rates of available second-line therapies. The chemotherapeutic agents that have substantial salvage activity include ifosfamide, etoposide, cytosine arabinoside, cisplatin, carboplatin, methotrexate, and dexamethasone [24].

HIGH-GRADE LYMPHOMAS

The Working Formulation recognizes three high-grade lymphomas, although one, immunoblastic lymphoma, is treated as an intermediate-grade lesion. Lymphoblastic lymphoma and the small, noncleaved cell lymphomas (Burkitt's and non-Burkitt's) are characterized by young age, male gender predominance, rapidly enlarging adenopathy that is often bulky, frequent bone marrow disease, and a high incidence of meningeal involvement if prophylaxis is not successfully carried out [25,26]. Almost all cases of lymphoblastic lymphoma are T-cell type, whereas small noncleaved cell lymphoma is B-cell phenotype.

Small, noncleaved cell lymphoma has been increasing in incidence during the past decade with the AIDS epidemic. This lymphoma is often seen in association with immunodeficiency states, and in this setting, sites of disease often may be unusual (gastrointestinal tract, parenchymal brain, soft tissue) [27].

Treatment of high-grade lymphomas is rapidly initiated, typically with high-dose, short-course combination chemotherapy, with CNS prophylaxis. Bulky disease may be associated with tumor lysis syndrome when rapid response occurs. Attention to hydration, alkalinization, prophylactic allopurinol, and monitoring of renal function, calcium, electrolytes, and phosphate balance is necessary.

In the setting of HIV infection, the use of intensive chemotherapy is controversial because treatment may be significantly compli-

Table 20-6. Treatment Strategy for Intermediate-Grade Lymphoma

1. Stages I and peripheral II: combination chemotherapy with or without adjuvant radiation therapy
2. Stages II, III, and IV: combination chemotherapy
   a. CNS prophylaxis for patients with multiple sites of extranodal disease, bone, bone marrow, testicular, or paranasal sinus tumor
   b. Tumor lysis precautions with treatment initiation of bulky disease
   c. GI tract disease may require surgical resection
   d. Consider autologous stem cell transplantation for patients with histologically documented partial responses or in second remission

CNS—central nervous system; GI—gastrointestinal.

cated by opportunistic infections [28]. Nevertheless when the T-cell count is adequate, therapy may be well tolerated and excellent outcomes achieved.

HTLV-1–associated lymphomas are not identified separately in the Working Formulation. Most patients present clinically with a high-grade disease characterized by rapid onset, lytic bone lesions, subcutaneous nodules, hypercalcemia, and leukemic phase. Pathology is usually that of diffuse large cell lymphoma or immunoblastic lymphoma. In southern Japan, where HTLV-1 is endemic, a broader clinical spectrum is seen with indolent and aggressive clinical and histologic subtypes. Prognosis for patients with aggressive presentations is poor, with only transient responses to intensive regimens. Moreover, HTLV-1–infected patients are also at greater risk for opportunistic infection [2].

REFERENCES

1. National Cancer Institute: Summary and description of a working formulation for clinical usage. The non-Hodgkin lymphoma pathologic classification project. *Cancer* 1982, 49:2112–2135.

2. Shimoyama M: Diagnostic criteria and classification of clinical subtypes of adult T-cell leukemia-lymphoma. The Lymphoma Study Group. *Br J Haematol* 1991, 79:428–437.

3. Straus SE: Epstein–Barr virus infections: biology, pathogenesis, and management. *Ann Intern Med* 1993, 118:45–58.

4. Harris NL, Jaffe ES, Stein H, et al.: A revised European-American Classification of lymphoid neoplasms: a proposal from the International Lymphoma Study Group. *Blood* 1994, 84:1361–1392.

5. Paryani SB, Hoppe RT, Cox RS, *et al.*: Analysis of non-Hodgkin's lymphomas with nodular and favorable histologies, stage I and II. *Cancer* 1983, 52:2300.

6. Portlock CS: Management of the low-grade non-Hodgkin's lymphomas. *Sem Oncol* 1990, 17:51–59.

7. Gribben JG, Freedman AS, Woo SD, *et al.*: All advanced stage non-Hodgkin's lymphomas with a polymerase chain reaction amplifiable breakpoint of bcl-2 have residual cells containing the bcl-2 rearrangement at evaluation and after treatment. *Blood* 1991, 78:3275–3280.

8. Portlock CS, Fischer DS, Cadman E, *et al.*: High dose pulse chlorambucil in advanced low-grade non-Hodgkin's lymphoma. *Cancer Treat Rep* 1987, 71:1029–1031.

9. Weisdorf DJ, Andersen JW, Glick JH, Oken MM: Survival after relapse of low grade non-Hodgkin's lymphoma: Implications for marrow transplantation. *J Clin Oncol* 1992, 10:942–947.

10. Freedman AS Ritz J, Nouberg D, *et al.*: Autologous bone marrow transplantation in 69 patients with a history of low-grade B cell non-Hodgkin's lymphoma. *Blood* 1991, 77:2524.

11. Gribben JG, Saporito L, Barber M, *et al.*: Bone marrows of non-Hodgkin's lymphoma patients with a bcl-2 translocation can be purged of polymerase chain reaction-detectable lymphoma cells using monoclonal antibodies and immunomagnetic bead depletion. *Blood* 1992, 80:1083–1089.

12. Shipp M, Harrington D, Anderson J, *et al.*: Predictive model for aggressive non-Hodgkin's lymphomas. The International NHL Prognostic Factor Project. *N Engl J Med* 1993, 329:987–992.

13. Yahalom J, Varsos G, Fuks Z, *et al.*: Adjuvant cyclophosphamide, doxorubicin, vincristine, and prednisone chemotherapy after radiation therapy in stage I low-grade and intermediate-grade non-Hodgkin lymphoma: results of a prospective randomized study. *Cancer* 1992, 71:2342–2350.

14. Glick JH, Kim K, *et al.*: An ECOG randomized phase III trial of CHOP versus CHOP plus radiotherapy for intermediate grade early stage NHL. *Proc ASCO* 1995:14;391.

15. Mckelvey EM, Gottlieb JA, Wilson HE, *et al.*: Adriamycin combination chemotherapy in malignant lymphoma. *Cancer* 1976, 38:1494–1493.

16. Skarin AT, Canellos GP, Rosenthal DS, *et al.*: Improved prognosis of diffuse histiocytic and undifferentiated lymphoma by use of high dose methotrexate alternating with standard agent (M-BACOD). *J Clin Oncol* 1983, 1:91–98.

17. Klimo P, Conners JM: MACOP-B chemotherapy for the treatment of diffuse large-cell lymphoma. *Ann Int Med* 1985, 102:596–602.

18. Longo DL, Devita VT, Duffey PL, *et al.*: Superiority of ProMACE-CytaBOM over ProMACE-MOPP in the treatment of advanced diffuse aggressive lymphoma: Results of a prospective randomized trial. *J Clin Oncol* 1991, 9:25–38.

19. Miller TP, Dana BW, Weick JK, *et al.*: SWOG clinical trials for intermediate and high grade non-Hodgkin's lymphomas. *Sem Hematol* 1988, 25(Suppl 2):17–22.

20. Fisher RI, Gaynor E, Dahlberg S, *et al.*: Comparison of a standard regimen CHOP with three intensive chemotherapy regimens for advanced NHL. *N Engl J Med* 1993, 328:1002–1006.

21. Meyer RM, Hryniuk WM, Goodyear MD: The role of dose intensity in determining outcome in intermediate-grade non-Hodgkin's lymphoma. *J Clin Oncol* 1991, 9:339.

22. Haioun C, Lepage E, Gisselbrecht C, *et al.*: Autologous bone marrow transplantation (ABMT) versus sequential chemotherapy in first complete remission aggressive non-Hodgkin's lymphoma (NHL): First interim analysis on 370 patients (LNH87 protocol). *Proc ASCO* 1992, 11:316.

23. Gulati S, Yahalom J, Acaba L, *et al.*: Treatment of patients with relapsed and resistant non-Hodgkin's lymphoma using total body irradiation, etoposide, and cyclophosphamide and autologous bone marrow transplantation. *J Clin Oncol* 1992, 10:936–941.

24. Velasquez WS, Cabanillas F, et al.: Effective salvage therapy for lymphoma with cisplatin in combination with high dose ara-C and dexamethasone (DHAP). *Blood* 1988, 71:117–122.

25. Picozzi VJ, Coleman CN: Lymphoblastic lymphoma. *Sem Oncol* 1990, 17:96–103.

26. McMaster ML, Greer JP, Greco FA, *et al.*: Effective treatment of small-noncleaved-cell lymphoma with high intensity, brief duration chemotherapy. *J Clin Oncol* 1991, 9:941.

27. Knowles DM, Chamulak GA, Subar M, *et al.*: Lymphoid neoplasias associated with the acquired immunodeficiency syndrome (AIDS): The New York University Medical Center Experience with 105 patients (1981–1986). *Ann Intern Med* 1988, 108:744.

28. Kaplan LD, Kahn JO, Crowe S, *et al.*: Clinical and virologic effects of recombinant human granulocyte-macrophage colony stimulating factor in patients receiving chemotherapy for human immunodeficiency virus-associated non-Hodgkin's lymphoma: results of a randomized trial. *J Clin Oncol* 1991, 9:929.

29. Luce JK, Gamble JF, Wilson HE, *et al.*: Combined cyclophosphamide, vincristine and prednisone therapy of malignant lymphoma. *Cancer* 1971, 28:306–317.

30. Armitage JO, Dick FR, Corder MP, *et al.*: Predicting therapeutic outcome in patients with diffuse histiocytic lymphoma treated with CHOP. *Cancer* 1982, 50:1695–1702.

CVP
Cyclophosphamide, Vincristine, Prednisone

CVP is a well-tolerated palliative regimen [28]. Monthly cycles are repeated to maximum response plus 2 cycles. Randomized studies have demonstrated no response or survival advantage with the use CVP over continuous daily alkylating agent therapy. Responses are more rapid with CVP (within 3 mo), but not more durable.

Toxicity is primarily hematologic with drug-induced neutropenia. Hemorrhagic cystitis may occur and hydration reduces its frequency. Vinca-associated neurologic toxicity is mild with a capped 2-mg dose. Corticosteroid toxicities are infrequent with monthly cycles.

DOSAGE AND SCHEDULING

	Day 1	2	3	4	5	6	7
Cyclophosphamide 400 mg/m² PO qd x 5 d	███████████						
Vincristine 1.4 mg/m² IV, d 1 (max 2 mg IV)	█						
Prednisone 100 mg/m² PO qd x 5 d	███████████						

Cycles are repeated every 28 d.

RECENT EXPERIENCES AND RESPONSE RATES

Study	Evaluable Patients, n	Complete Responses, %	Median Survival, y
Hoppe RT, *Blood* 1981, 58:592	40	85	7.5
Anderson T, *Cancer Treat Rep* 1977, 61:1057	49	67	7

CANDIDATES FOR TREATMENT
Patients with low-grade non-Hodgkin's lymphoma

ALTERNATIVE THERAPIES
Single-agent chlorambucil or cyclophosphamide; CHOP

TOXICITIES
Prednisone: acne, thrush, thinning of the skin and striae; suppression of the adrenal–pituitary axis, hypokalemia, loss of muscle mass, increased appetite, myopathy, osteoporosis, cushingoid appearance, gastitis, peptic ulcer disease; euphoria, depression, psychosis, increased risk of infections and cataracts; **Cyclophosphamide:** myelosuppression with platelet sparing; nausea and vomiting, alopecia, darkening of skin and nails, mucositis (rare), hemorrhagic or sterile cystitis (5%–10% of patients, usually reversible, but can lead to fibrosis and bladder cancer), immunosuppression, SIADH; infertility, **Vincristine:** severe local inflammation possible if extravasated, alopecia, peripheral neuropathies, ileus

DRUG INTERACTIONS
Cyclophosphamide: allopurinol, drugs that induce or block hepatic microsomal enzymes, sulfhydryl agents (*eg*, mesna); **Vincristine:** cisplatin, paclitaxel, and other drugs that affect peripheral nervous system

NURSING INTERVENTIONS
Give cyclophosphamide in the morning; administer vincristine as slow IV push to avoid extravasation; evaluate for neurologic deficit before each vincristine dose; maintain high fluid intake and encourage frequent voiding, stool softeners, and bulk diet

PATIENT INFORMATION
The most common side effects reported are leukopenia, hyperglycemia, weight gain, insomnia, alopecia, sensory neuropathy.

CHOP
Cyclophosphamide, Hydroxydaunorubicin, Vincristine, Prednisone

CHOP is a potentially curative regimen in intermediate-grade lymphoma [13]. It is also used in low-grade lymphoma, particularly with evidence of histologic transformation. Responses are prompt (usually complete in less than 4 mo), and chemotherapy is continued for 2 cycles beyond maximal response or for a minimum of 6 cycles. Complete remission is achieved in 60%–75% of patients [29].

Recent prospective comparison with more intensive, "second- and third-generation" regimens has shown no significant differences to date in response rates or survival outcome of patients with advanced intermediate-grade lymphomas. CHOP therefore, has, become the standard drug program in this setting [18].

Toxicity is moderate and reasonably well tolerated, even in the elderly. Total alopecia is the most distressing side effect to patients. Other adverse effects are similar to those outlined for CVP. Potential cardiac toxicity secondary to hydroxy-daunorubicin (doxorubicin) should be monitored closely, and doses ≥ 450 mg/m^2 should be avoided whenever possible.

DOSAGE AND SCHEDULING

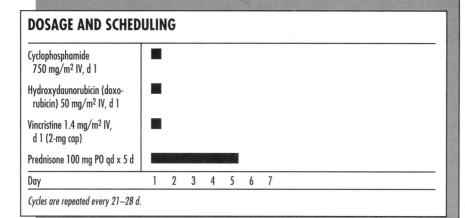

Cyclophosphamide 750 mg/m^2 IV, d 1	■							
Hydroxydaunorubicin (doxo-rubicin) 50 mg/m^2 IV, d 1	■							
Vincristine 1.4 mg/m^2 IV, d 1 (2-mg cap)	■							
Prednisone 100 mg PO qd x 5 d	▬▬▬▬▬							
Day	1	2	3	4	5	6	7	

Cycles are repeated every 21–28 d.

RECENT EXPERIENCES AND RESPONSE RATES

Study	Evaluable Patients, n	Complete Responses, %	Median Survival
Armitage JD, J Clin Oncol 1984, 2:898	75	51	31% at 4–9 y
Gams RA, J Clin Oncol 1985, 3:1188	90	54	35% at 6 y
Dixon DO, J Clin Oncol 1986, 5:197	412	53	30% at 12 y

CANDIDATES FOR TREATMENT
Patients with low-grade or intermediate-grade non-Hodgkin's lymphoma

SPECIAL PRECAUTIONS
Patients with hepatic dysfunction; patients with impaired cardiac function (contraindicated)

ALTERNATIVE THERAPIES
m-BACOD, MACOP-B, ProMACE-CytaBOM, COP-BLAM

TOXICITIES
Prednisone: acne, thrush, thinning of the skin and striae, suppression of the adrenal–pituitary axis, hypokalemia, loss of muscle mass, increased appetite, myopathy, osteoporosis, cushingoid appearance, gastritis, peptic ulcer disease, euphoria, depression, psychosis, increased risk of infections and cataracts; **Cyclophosphamide:** myelosuppression with platelet sparing, nausea and vomiting, alopecia, darkening of skin and nails, mucositis (rare), hemorrhagic or sterile cystitis, immunosuppression, SIADH, infertility; **Vincristine:** severe local inflammation possible if extravasated, alopecia, peripheral neuropathies, ileus; **Hydroxydoxorubicin:** myelosuppression (leukocytes and platelets, cumulative dose should not exceed 550 mg/m^2), nausea and vomiting; mucositis, alopecia, radiation recall, local tissue damage progressing to necrosis if extravasated, hyperpigmentation, phlebitis, irreversible congestive heart failure (dose-dependent), acute arrhythmias

DRUG INTERACTIONS
Cyclophosphamide: allopurinol, drugs that induce or block hepatic microsomal enzymes, sulfhydryl agents (*eg*, mesna); **Vincristine:** cisplatin, taxol, and other drugs that affect peripheral nervous system; **Hydroxydaunorubicin:** heparin, mediastinal radiation, interferon

NURSING INTERVENTIONS
Give cyclophosphamide in the morning; administer vincristine and hydroxydoxorubicin as slow IV push to avoid extravasation; evaluate for neurologic deficit before each vincristine dose; maintain high fluid intake and encourage frequent voiding, stool softeners, and bulk diet

PATIENT INFORMATION
The most common side effects reported are leukopenia, alopecia, nausea, vomiting, hyperglycemia, sensory neuropathy, insomnia.

PROMACE-CYTABOM

Prednisone, Doxorubicin, Cyclophosphamide, Etoposide, Cytosine Arabinoside, Bleomycin, Vincristine, Methotrexate, Leucovorin

This third-generation drug regimen developed at the National Cancer Institute is well-suited to growth factor support and dose intensification [16]. Although the prospective Intergroup study revealed no statistically significant progression-free survival (45% vs 36%) or survival advantage for this regimen over CHOP, follow-up remains short and in younger patients this is often a highly effective regimen with low morbidity. Because mortality was greater with ProMACE-CytaBOM (4% vs 1%) than with CHOP, reflecting poor tolerance in the elderly, this program should only be used in young, otherwise well patients.

DOSAGE AND SCHEDULING

Prednisone 60 mg/m^2 PO, d 1–14

Doxorubicin 25 mg/m^2 IV, d 1

Cyclophosphamide 650 mg/m^2 IV, d 1

Etoposide 120 mg/m^2 IV, d 1

Cytosine arabinoside (ara-C) 300 mg/m^2 IV, d 8

Bleomycin 5 mg/m^2 IV, d 8

Vincristine 1.4 mg/m^2 IV, d 8

Methotrexate 120 mg/m^2 IV, d 8

Leucovorin 25 mg/m^2 PO, d 9–10 q 6 hr x 4

Day: 1 2 3 4 5 6 7 8 9 10 11 12 13 14

One double-strength co-trimoxazole is given BID throughout treatment. Cycles are repeated every 21 d until complete remission followed by 2 consolidation cycles (min 6 cycles).

DOSAGE MODIFICATIONS: *Reduce bleomycin if renal failure develops, withhold methotrexate if creatinine clearance ≤ 60 mL/min.*

RECENT EXPERIENCES AND RESPONSE RATES

Study	Evaluable Patients, *n*	Complete Responses, %	Median Survival
Fisher RI, In *Advances in Cancer Chemotherapy.* Skarin AT, NY, 1986	37	80	Not reached
Miller TP, *Sem Hematol* 1988, 25 (suppl2):41	48	69	70% at 15 mo

CANDIDATES FOR TREATMENT

Patients with intermediate-grade non-Hodgkin's lymphoma

SPECIAL PRECAUTIONS

Patients with renal dysfunction
Patients with impaired cardiac function (contraindicated)

ALTERNATIVE THERAPIES

CHOP, MACOP-B, m-BACOD

TOXICITIES

Cyclophosphamide, prednisone, vincristine, doxorubicin: see CHOP protocol for list of toxicities; **ara-C:** myelosuppression (leukopenia and thrombocytopenia), nausea and vomiting, stomatitis, flulike syndrome, transient transaminitis, infertility; **Bleomycin:** alopecia, stomatitis, nail bed thickening, hyperpigmentation and skin desquamation (common); acute anaphylaxis with ARDS, dose-related pneumonitis progressing to pulmonary fibrosis (max cumulative dose of 200 U/m^2); frequent severe fevers; **Methotrexate:** myelosuppression nausea and vomiting, severe mucositis with ulceration and bloody diarrhea, irreversible cirrhosis (rare), pneumonitis, alopecia, renal tubular necrosis; **Etoposide:** myelosuppression (leukopenia and thrombocytopenia), nausea and vomiting, alopecia, mucositis

DRUG INTERACTIONS

Cyclophosphamide, prednisone, vincristine, doxorubicin: see CHOP protocol list of interactions; **ara-C:** cisplatin, thiopurines, methotrexate, hydroxyurea; **Bleomycin:** radiation therapy, nephrotoxic drugs; **Etoposide:** ara-C, methotrexate, cisplatin, calcium antagonists, coumadin; **Methotrexate:** aspirin, NSAIDs, alcohol, 5-FU, L-asparaginase

NURSING INTERVENTIONS

See CHOP protocol for list of interventions; in addition, test dose of bleomycin (1 U IM) prior to first dose; use glass containers for infusion of bleomycin; administer etoposide over 1 h to avoid hypotension and extravasation; monitor methotrexate levels if renal dysfunction develops; maintain leucovorin every 6 hr until methotrexate levels are nontherapeutic

PATIENT INFORMATION

The most common side effects reported are alopecia, nausea, vomiting, weight gain, leukopenia, hyperglycemia, insomnia.

DHAP

DHAP is a second-line, salvage regimen for patients with intermediate grade or immunoblastic non-Hodgkin's lymphoma who have not attained a complete remission from up-front therapy or who have relapsed. Because only 45%–50% of patients are cured with their initial chemotherapy treatment program, many patients need to receive salvage chemotherapy. Depending on the patient's age, comorbidity, and performance status, the goals of second-line therapy vary. Transplant-eligible patients require only cytoreduction, whereas in transplant-ineligible patients a complete remission is desired.

DHAP is a treatment program that has the best reported efficacy in this setting. In the original report, 90 patients with progressive recurrent lymphoma were treated: 28 patients achieved a complete remission and 22 a partial remission for an overall response rate 56%.

Vigorous hydration with mannitol-induced diuresis was given in all patients. The acute tumor lysis syndrome was observed in 5 patients, emphasizing the need for frequent monitoring of electrolytes. Toxicity was severe with neutropenia, thrombocytopenia, renal, cerebellar, and gastroinstestinal dysfunction common.

DOSAGE AND SCHEDULING

Cisplatin: 100 mg/m^2 IV continuous infusion (CI) x 24 h, day 1 *or* 50 mg/m^2 as 1 h-infusion daily x 2
Ara-C: 2 g/m^2 x 2 IV: each infusion over 3 h q12 x 2 day 2
Dexamethazone: 40 mg IV or PO daily days 1–4

Patients are hospitalized to undergo treatment. Hydration with normal saline at 150–250 mL/h is administered for a 36-h period and after the first 6 hours of hydration cisplatin can be administered. Therapy is repeated every 3–4 weeks for a maximum of 4 cycles after maximal tumor response. Patients aged older than 70 years received ara-C are treated with a dose of 1 g/m^2.

TOXICITIES

Profound myelosuppression with marked neutropenia and thrombocytopenia, especially in patients with lymphomatous involvement of the bone marrow or previous pelvic irradiation. Documented infections were seen in 30% of patients with a mortality of 33% in these patients. Tumor lysis syndrome occurred in 5% of patients. Renal insufficiency is seen in 20% and can be irreversible. Acute cerebellar dysfunction and tinnitus has been reported.

Neutropenia can be shortened by growth factor support (G-CSF or GM-CSF).

CANDIDATES FOR TREATMENT

Patients with refractory or relapsed intermediate grade or immunoblastic non-Hodgkin's lymphoma

SPECIAL PRECAUTIONS

Patients who are elderly; patients with renal or neurological dysfunction; patients with compromised bone marrow reserve

ALTERNATIVE THERAPIES

Ifosamide and etoposide alone or with cisplatin or carboplatin C-MOPP

DRUG INTERACTIONS

Aminoglycoside antibiotics should be avoided; any drugs that have renal or ototoxicity must be used with caution

NURSING INTERVENTIONS

Monitor renal function and obtain BUN, creatinine and 12-h urine collection for creatinine clearance; provide proper antiemetics, hydrate well; observe for signs of infection; neutropenia is expected; severe thrombocytopenia occurs, and signs for bleeding should be monitored

PATIENT INFORMATION

The most common side effect include fever when the blood counts are low, nausea, vomiting, and alopecia.

VANDERBILT REGIMEN
Cyclophosphamide, Etoposide, Vincristine, Bleomycin, Methotrexate, Leucovorin, Prednisone

Small noncleaved cell lymphomas—Burkitt's and non-Burkitt's types—are rare high-grade lymphomas. When associated with HIV infection, this phenotype is one of the most common histologies. HIV-negative small, noncleaved cell lymphoma is a highly curable disease with high-dose, short-course therapy [24]. CNS prophylaxis is essential. As with lymphoblastic lymphoma, tumor lysis is a serious complication of effective initial therapy and must be anticipated with initiation of hydration, alkalinization, and allopurinol, and frequent monitoring of electrolytes, renal function, and calcium and phosphate balance.

Severe myelosuppression is to be expected with this drug protocol. Even with growth factor support, nadir fever should be anticipated as well as the need for platelet support. Mucositis may occur in up to half of all patients. Nevertheless, maintaining treatment schedule is important whenever possible to combat this rapidly growing neoplasm.

DOSAGE AND SCHEDULING

Agent	Cycle 1						Cycle 2					
	Day 1	Day 2	Day 3	Day 8	Day 15	Day 22	Day 29	Day 30	Day 31	Day 36	Day 43	Day 50
CTX	X	X					X					
ETOP	X	X	X				X	X	X			
ADR							X	X				
VCR				X		X				X		X
BLEO				X		X				X		X
MTX					X						X	
LV			X		X						X	
PRED	X	X		X			X	X	X	X		

REGIMEN

In cycle 1, CTX—cyclophosamide 1500 mg/m²; ETOP—etoposide 400 mg/m²; VCR—vincristine 1.4 mg/m² (2 mg max), BLEO—bleomycin 10 U/m²; MTX—methotrexate 200 mg/m²; LV—leucovorin 15 mg/m² (q 6 h x 6); PRED—prednisone 60 mg/m². In cycle 2, etoposide dose is reduced to 100 mg/m² and ADR (doxorubicin) is added at 45 mg/m². Allopurinol is routinely given. Patients with meningeal involvement at diagnosis receive methotrexate 12 mg/m² IT weekly x 5 and whole-brain radiation 2000 cGy in 10 fractions. Prophylactic intrathecal therapy is recommended.

DOSAGE MODIFICATIONS: Cycle 2 can be delayed if ANC < 1000. Reduce bleomycin, if renal failure develops; withhold methotrexate if creatinine clearance ≤ 60 mL/min.

RECENT EXPERIENCE AND RESPONSE RATES

Study	Evaluable Patients, n	Complete Responses, %	Disease-Free Survival
McMaster et al., J Clin Oncol 1991; 9:941–946	20	85	65% at 29 mo

CANDIDATES FOR TREATMENT
Patients with high-grade non-Hodgkin's lymphoma

SPECIAL PRECAUTIONS
Patients with renal dysfunction

ALTERNATIVE THERAPIES
Stanford regimen using combined modality

TOXICITIES
Cyclophosphamide, prednisone, vincristine: see CVP protocol for list of toxicities; **Bleomycin:** alopecia, stomatitis, nail bed thickening, hyperpigmentation and skin desquamation (common), acute anaphylaxis with ARDS, dose-related pneumonitis progressing to pulmonary fibrosis (max cumulative dose of 200 U/m²); frequently severe fever; **Methotrexate:** myelosuppression, nausea and vomiting, severe mucositis with ulceration and bloody diarrhea, irreversible cirrhosis (rare), pneumonitis, alopecia, renal tubular necrosis, **Etoposide:** myelosuppression (leukopenia and thrombocytopenia), nausea and vomiting, alopecia, mucositis

DRUG INTERACTIONS
Cyclophosphamide, prednisone, vincristine: see CVP protocol for list of interactions; **Bleomycin:** radiation therapy, nephrotoxic drugs; **Etoposide:** ara-C, methotrexate, cisplatin, calcium antagonists, coumadin; **Methotrexate:** aspirin, NSAIDs, alcohol, 5-FU, l-asparaginase

NURSING INTERVENTIONS
See CVP protocol for list of interventions; test dose of bleomycin (1 U IM) prior to first dose; use glass containers for infusion of bleomycin; administer etoposide over 1 h to avoid hypotension and extravasation; mix intrathecal methotrexate with buffered nonbacteriostatic solution; monitor methotrexate levels if renal dysfunction develops and maintain leucovorin every 6 h until methotrexate levels are nontherapeutic

PATIENT INFORMATION
These most common side effects reported are pancytopenia, infections, alopecia, bleeding, mucositis, peripheral neuropathy

CHAPTER 21: MYELOMA
James R. Berenson

INCIDENCE AND ETIOLOGY

The incidence for multiple myeloma in the United States exceeds 3 people per 100,000 and appears to be increasing. Myeloma accounts for 1% of malignant disease and over 10% of hematologic malignancies. The occurrence of myeloma is more common in men than in women and more common in African Americans than in whites (Table 21-1). It most commonly presents in the seventh decade, with fewer than 2% of patients younger than age 40 years.

The cause of multiple myeloma remains unknown. Monoclonal gammopathy of undetermined significance (MGUS) may offer a clue to its pathogenesis [1]. More than 33% of patients with apparent benign monoclonal gammopathy will develop myeloma, another lymphoplasmacellular malignancy, or progression of their monoclonal gammopathy. The incidence of myeloma in patients with MGUS is 25% after 20 to 35 years of follow-up. These observations implicate MGUS as a premalig-

nant clonal disorder that, on further transforming damage to the clone, can give rise to multiple myeloma.

Genetic predisposition, radiation exposure, chronic antigenic stimulation, and various environmental or occupational conditions have been observed as factors but account for only a small percentage of all myeloma. Recent reports demonstrate the importance of autocrine stimulation of the malignant clone by IL-6 and the apparent role of oncogene activation at various stages of the disease. The recent identification of the human herpesvirus 8 in the bone marrow of myeloma patients provides a possible new etiologic factor in this disease [2,3]. Interestingly, these studies showed this virus to be present in nonmalignant dendritic cells, suggesting a novel mechanism by which viruses in general may stimulate malignant transformation and growth. If this virus proves etiologic, it may also become a new target for therapeutic approaches in the future. These and other recently appreciated factors provide insight into the pathogenesis of myeloma, but their relationship to the original malignant event is not yet spelled out.

DIAGNOSIS AND STAGING

Diagnosis of myeloma is made by the presence of malignant plasma cells in the bone marrow (usually > 10%) or by biopsy proof of a plasmacytoma plus either protein evidence of myeloma with a monoclonal serum or urine protein or characteristic osteolytic lesions. For the past 20 years, the most commonly used staging system has been that proposed by Durie and Salmon (Table 21-2). It correlates tumor burden with the presence or absence of severe anemia, hypercalcemia, advanced skeletal disease, and the amount of monoclonal protein detected in serum or urine [4].

Clinical stage has proved to be predictive of survival in many series. Stage I patients generally survive over 5 years, whereas the median survival for Stage II patients is 3 to 4 years and for Stage III rarely more than 2 years. The presence of renal failure has an important negative prognostic significance in myeloma. More recent studies have demonstrated that elevated plasma ß-2 microglobulin and elevated plasma cell labeling index are also important adverse prognostic signs that may at times override the significance of clinical stage [5]. Although renal dysfunction will result in elevated serum β-2 microglobulin levels, this protein is an independent prognostic factor in myeloma [6]. The presence of both low plasma ß-2 microglobulin and elevated plasma cell labeling index appears to be a strong predictor of long survival in patients with myeloma.

Table 21-1. Risk Factors for the Development of Multiple Myeloma

African-American race
Male gender
Advanced age
Monoclonal gammopathy of undetermined significance (MGUS)
Chronic immune stimulation
Exposure to ionizing radiation
Occupational exposure to pesticides, paints, and solvents
Genetic predisposition

Table 21-2. Clinical Staging System for Myeloma

Stage	Criteria	Myeloma Cell Mass, cells/m²

I	All of the following:
	1. Hemoglobin > 10 g/dL
	2. Serum calcium value normal (≤ 12 mg/100 mL)
	3. On x-ray, normal bone structure or solitary bone plasmacytoma only
	4. Low M-component production rates
	  a. IgG value < 5 g/100 mL
	  b. IgA value < 3 g/100 mL
	  c. Urine light chain M-component on electrophoresis < 4 g/24 h
		< 0.6 x 10¹² (low)

II	Fitting neither stage I nor III	0.6–1.2 x 10¹² (intermediate)

III	One or more of the following:
	1. Hemoglobin < 8.5 g/100 mL
	2. Serum calcium value > 12 mg/100 mL
	3. Advanced lytic bone lesions
	4. High M-component production rates
	  a. IgG value > 7 g/100 mL
	  b. IgA value > 5 g/100 mL
	  c. Urine light chain M-component on electrophoresis > 12 g/24 h
		1.2 x 10¹² (high)

Subclass		
A	Serum creatine < 2 mg/100 mL	
B	Serum creatine ≥ 2 mg/100 mL	

Modified from Durie, Salmon [4]; with permission.

Table 21-3. Prognostic Factors

Patient factors	Tumor biology
Age	Plasma cell labeling index (PCLI)
Performance status	C reactive protein (CRP)
Concomitant illness	Circulating soluble IL-6 receptor (sIL-6R)
Renal function	Lactic dehydrogenase
Serum albumin	ras Gene mutations
	p53 and p16 abnormailities
Factors reflecting tumor burden	Plasmablastic subtype
Clinical stage (Table 22-2), including component factors Hb, M-component concentration, serum calcium, Osteolytic lesions	Chromosomal abnormalities
	Circulating tumor cells
β 2-microglobulin	
Bone marrow plasma cell percent	

Several other factors have been found to have prognostic importance in myeloma (Table 21-3). They relate to patient factors, tumor burden and tumor biology. Recently, specific chromosomal abnormalities (especially those involving chromosomes 11 and 13) have portended poor outcome in these patients [7]. In one study [3], multivariate analysis identified serum creatinine, B2M, plasma cell percent (by immunofluorescent technique) along with 3 biologic factors, PCLI, CRP and sIL-6R as the independent prognostic variables. The presence of abnormalities on magnetic resonance imaging in early-stage disease may also suggest an adverse outcome [9].

PRIMARY DISEASE THERAPY

Although high-dose therapy followed by hematopoietic support may result in long-term survival in a few cases, the goals of treatment in most cases are to extend survival several years, to produce objective disease regression with its attendant relief from pain and other disease symptoms, and to protect the patient's ability to lead an active life for as long as possible. For the past three decades the standard treatment for multiple myeloma has been widely considered to be use of the single alkylating agent, melphalan, or a combination of melphalan and prednisone (MP), which is usually given in a high-dose, intermittent, outpatient regimen (Fig. 21-1) [10]. When this treatment is used, objective responses, documented by a 50% or greater decrease in serum M-protein levels and control of other major manifestations of disease, are seen in 50% of patients. Unfortunately, response duration is generally less than 2 years and the median duration of survival is 30 months. Survival durations exceeding 5 years are achieved in fewer than 20% of patients.

Numerous combination chemotherapy regimens have been developed in an attempt to improve on the results obtained from use of the MP regimen (Table 22-4). Most resemble either the vincristine, carmustine (BCNU), melphalan, cyclophosphamide, and prednisone (VBMCP) regimen or the VMCP/VBAP regimen, consisting of alternating cycles of vincristine plus prednisone combined with either melphalan plus cyclophosphamide or with BCNU plus doxorubicin. Because of promising preliminary results, several randomized clinical trials have been conducted to compare MP with more aggressive multidrug regimens. However, most randomized trials and metaanalyses have suggested that these more aggressive combination chemotherapy regimens with their added toxicity may slightly improve response rates, but these therapies have made no significant impact on overall survival. Results of the recent Eastern Cooperative Oncology Group (ECOG) trial comparing VBMCP (vincristine, carmustine [BCNU], melphalan, cyclophosphamide, and prednisone) with MP (melphalan and prednisone) showed response rates of 72% and 51%, respectively; but more importantly, no difference was found in overall survival between patients receiving these two regimens [10].

Other commonly used combination chemotherapy regimens include VMCP (vincristine, melphalan, cyclophosphamide, and prednisone) alternating with VBAP (vincristine, BCNU, doxorubicin, and prednisone) [11], ABCM (doxorubicin, BCNU, cyclophosphamide, and melphalan) [12], and VMCPP alternating with VBAPP [13]. Recent studies show the efficacy of high-dose oral glucocorticosteroids alone in these patients without the bone marrow toxicity produced by use of alkylating agents. A recent promising, newer steroid-containing combination without alkylator therapy from MD Anderson Cancer Center that consists of VAD (infusional vincristine and adriamycin with oral dexamethasone)

results in both rapid and high response rates [14]. Although an historical comparison of this combination to oral dexamethasone alone showed an improvement in response rate, it did not produce an improvement in overall survival [15].

In determining what type of therapy to initiate in the newly diagnosed patient, it is important to consider the extent of disease, other clinical conditions, and whether the patient is a candidate for highdose therapy regimens. For example, several small randomized trials have demonstrated no benefit to treating asymptomatic early-stage patients with chemotherapy. A "wait and watch" approach is warranted in this group of patients until more effective therapies become available. In patients who are candidates for high-dose therapy followed by autologous hematopoietic support, regimens without alkylating agents are preferable because of the difficulty in collecting adequate stem cells in patients exposed to these agents prior to stem cell mobilization. Thus, VAD is ideally suited for initial therapy in these patients. In elderly patients or in those persons unable to tolerate more aggressive chemotherapy, oral dexamethasone alone or MP is the preferred form of treatment.

Initial chemotherapy is generally given for 6 to 12 months and rarely results in complete responses. Responding patients demonstrate a reduction in tumor mass as reflected in decreases in paraprotein levels, and enter a plateau phase, at which point the monoclonal protein level remains constant despite continued chemotherapy.

MAINTENANCE THERAPY

The use of continued chemotherapy during plateau phase does not improve overall survival as demonstrated in several large randomized trials. In fact, continuation of therapy leads to a permanent reduction in bone marrow reserve and increases the risk of secondary leukemia. Recent attempts to prolong survival with maintenance therapy have largely involved the use of interferon α-2 (IFN α-2). Used alone as initial therapy, this agent has little demonstrated antimyeloma activity, which may in fact reflect its ability to reduce immunoglobulin production by plasma cells without actually reducing tumor cell growth [16]. Although some single-arm trials have suggested a benefit with the addition of this agent to other chemotherapy, several large randomized trials have not shown an improvement in overall survival with the addition of IFN α-2 to other initial chemotherapeutic regimens. However, an early large randomized Italian study suggested that this drug may have a role in maintenance therapy as demonstrated by its ability to prolong plateau and possibly prolong overall survival in certain subgroups [17]. Patients with stable disease during induction chemotherapy did not appear to benefit from treatment. Unfortunately, most subsequent trials with the exception of the Canadian study have shown little impact on overall survival with maintenance IFN α-2 therapy [13,18–21]. A recent unpublished meta-analysis of randomized trials suggests a slight but significant benefit in both progression-free and overall survival with use of maintenance IFN α-2 therapy; but included in the analysis, were several positive studies that have not been published in peer-reviewed publications. As a result, one must weigh the considerable toxicity and expense against the minimal possible benefit of this agent before using it in patients responding to initial chemotherapy. A recently published Southwest Oncology Group (SWOG) trial comparing maintenance therapy of IFN plus prednisone versus IFN alone showed a survival advantage for patients receiving the combination treatment [22].

Whether this simply reflects the activity of glucocorticosteroids in maintenance therapy will be answered in the current SWOG 9210 trial.

HIGH-DOSE THERAPY

Based on the higher response rates achieved with more aggressive combinations of alkylating agents, high-dose chemotherapy with or without hematopoietic support has been studied. Initial trials involved patients with resistant multiple myeloma who were treated with melphalan in doses of 70 to 140 mg/m². Although dramatic responses were noted, these responses were short-lived and associated with significant morbidity related to protracted myelosuppression. Hematopoietic support using autologous bone marrow was added to shorten the duration of granulocytopenia, allowing for more intensive preparative conditioning with higher doses of melphalan (200 mg/m²) alone or lower doses (140 mg/m²) combined with total body irradiation (TBI) or busulfan and cyclophosphamide. In these early studies, despite treatment eligibility based on resistance to conventional chemotherapy, impressive cytoreduction was achieved, but progression-free survival was brief. Several favorable prognostic factors for sustained response were identified and included chemotherapy-sensitive myeloma and a shorter duration of primary treatment.

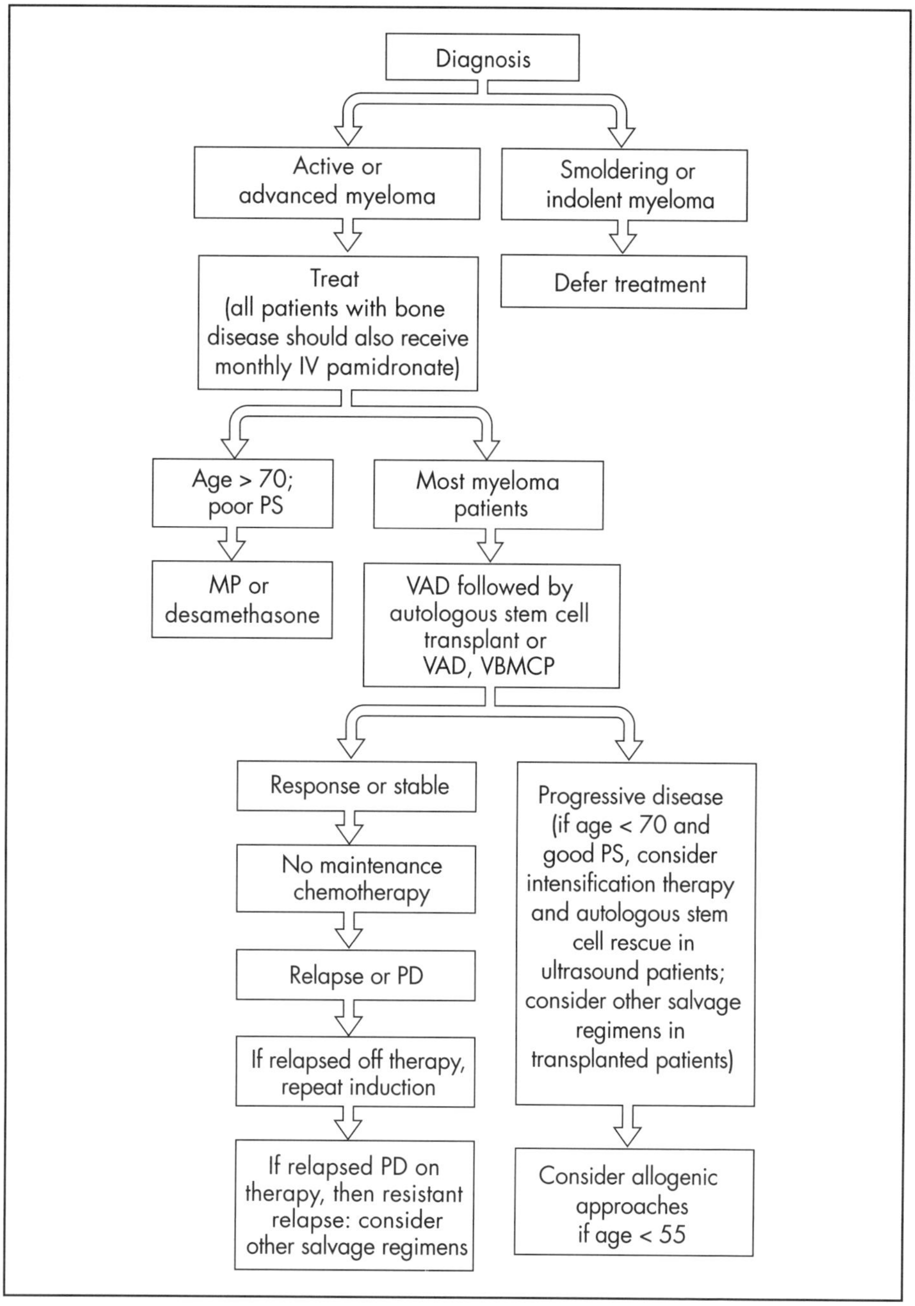

FIGURE 21-1.

Treatment strategy for myeloma. MP—melphelan and prednisone; PD—progressive disease; PS—performance status; VAD—vincristine, doxorubicin, and dexamethasone; VBMCP—vincristine, carmustine (BCNU), melphalan, cyclophosphamide, and prednisone.

Based on these results, autologous bone marrow transplantation was used on recently diagnosed patients with chemotherapy-responsive disease. These studies showed very high response rates with a high frequency of complete remissions, and suggested improved long-term myeloma-free survival compared with patients treated with conventional chemotherapy alone.

In a recent randomized French study of 200 untreated patients with intermediate- to high-stage multiple myeloma, patients assigned to high-dose chemotherapy and autologous bone marrow transplantation achieved higher overall response rates and better progression-free and overall survival than that achieved by patients continued on conventional chemotherapy [23]. A recent update of this study continues to show similar benefits in patients on the high-dose arm [24]. Several other similar, large randomized trials comparing patients receiving high-dose therapy with those patients obtaining conventional treatment are also currently in progress. A potential problem unresolved by the use of autologous bone marrow support is the presence of clonogenic plasma cells in the autologous bone marrow product. One approach to overcome this problem has been to change the source of hematopoietic support from bone marrow to autologous peripheral blood progenitor cells obtained by leukaphereses. This latter product contains much less tumor contamination than what is found in bone marrow harvests. A further possible way to reduce the risk of tumor cell contamination in the autograft is through purification of the leukapheresis material by negatively purging with a battery of anti–B-cell antibodies or by positive selection for hematopoietic progenitor cells.

The lack of uniform expression of B-cell antigens on malignant plasma cells reduces the efficacy of the former technique. On the other hand, in a recent single-arm study of positive hematopoietic progenitor cells selected by their expression of the early hematopoietic CD34 antigen, residual tumor cell contamination of the autograft was markedly reduced by this procedure, and yet these CD34-selected progenitor cells produced rapid hematologic recovery of neutrophils and platelets [25]. A recently completed randomized trial using this selection technique in 134 patients confirmed these results, and showed most patients receiving CD34-enriched autografts contained tumor-free products to the sensitivity of the assay [26]. Whether the achievement of a tumor-free autograft will result in improvement in overall survival is unknown and may require more effective high-dose therapy regimens.

Given the high response rate and likelihood of prolonged progression-free survival with relatively low treatment-related mortality (< 2%) in patients undergoing high-dose chemotherapy with autologous progenitor cell support, this treatment modality should be considered for patients aged 70 years or less with intermediate- to advanced-stage multiple myeloma responsive or stable following conventional chemotherapy.

Because of the encouraging results from the French Intergroup trial, several groups have conducted trials involving multiple courses of high-dose therapy. Although a nonrandomized trial from the University of Arkansas suggested a survival benefit in patients undergoing two courses of high-dose therapy [27], early results from the randomized French Intergroup trial show no survival difference between patients undergoing two courses versus one course of high-dose therapy [28].

Allogeneic bone marrow transplantation has also been used in myeloma. Its potential advantage includes the complete absence of malignant cells in the infused product as well as a possible therapeutic form of adoptive immunotherapy or graft-versus-tumor effect mediated by the allogeneic bone marrow. Occasionally, patients relapsing after autologous transplantation have been treated with this procedure, but the outcome has been generally poor. Due to age restrictions and lack of available donors, very few studies have been published, and most contain small numbers of patients. The results have been disappointing, with a high risk of treatment-related mortality attributable to early transplant-related organ toxicity and graft-versus-host disease. Although early results from the largest study of allogeneic transplants from the European Bone Marrow Transplant Registry were encouraging [29], a recently published update showed that many patients have relapsed, with very few patients alive and free of disease. Thus, there has been no demonstrated clinical advantage of allogeneic transplantation as hematopoietic support following myeloablative chemotherapy in multiple myeloma.

A new possible approach has been the use of donor leukocyte infusions (DLIs) with a possible graft-versus-myeloma effect observed in several patients undergoing this procedure [30]. However, many of these patients died from opportunistic infections soon after DLI. In addition, many of these patients also were receiving glucocorticosteroids as immunosuppressive therapy, so some of the responses may have resulted from these agents rather than the DLIs. Recently, the MD Anderson group developed an allogeneic transplantation procedure involving lower doses of conditioning chemotherapy, which may allow the graft-versus-myeloma effect to occur without the high treatment-related mortality [31].

THERAPY FOR REFRACTORY OR RELAPSED DISEASE

Thirty percent to 50% of multiple-myeloma patients will have progressive disease despite conventional therapy and have a particularly poor prognosis. Even in patients who do achieve an initial response, nearly all will ultimately relapse and develop disease unresponsive to initial therapy. When these patients relapse, repeat use of the original induction regimen may achieve remissions (usually lasting < 1 y) especially in patients with a long duration of their initial remission. Numerous studies of standard-dose alkylating agents, anthracyclines, spindle toxins, and other drugs have failed to produce results in refractory patients. Likewise, nucleoside antagonists, taxanes, and nitrosoureas have been tried without therapeutic effect. A recent SWOG study suggests topotecan may have some activity in previously treated patients [32]. High-dose glucocorticosteroids (eg, prednisone 200 mg every other day [or pulse 60 mg/m^2 daily for 5 d every 8 d] or dexamethasone 40 mg daily for 4 d repeated every 8–14 d) may produce excellent responses even in refractory patients. However, the duration of response is usually less than 1 year. Toxicities include insomnia, hyperglycemia, mental status changes, and increased risk of infections. VAD may be used in patients who initially failed MP, but its efficacy in patients who previously failed high-dose dexamethasone therapy alone is less impressive. This salvage regimen remains one of the most active treatments even in patients relapsing after high-dose therapy and is very well tolerated by most patients.

Recently, use of another anthracycline (idarubicin) with dexamethasone (both given orally) has produced encouraging results in preliminary studies. Etoposide with cyclophosphamide or in other regimens, such as EDAP (etoposide, dexamethasone, cytarabine, and cisplatin) or ICE (etoposide, cyclophosphamide and idarubicin), have also demonstrated some activity in refractory myeloma.

Intravenous cyclophosphamide alone may also produce responses in patients with resistant myeloma [33].

Because patients relapsing frequently develop expression of a protein involved in multidrug resistance, P-glycoprotein approaches to block the expression of this protein have been developed [34]. Early approaches involved the addition of cardiotoxic drugs (eg, quinine and verapamil or the nephrotoxic agent cyclosporine) to patients receiving VAD-type regimens after failing a similar type of chemotherapy initially. With the newer multidrug resistance inhibitor PSC 833, encouraging results have been observed in small single-arm trials, but significant neurotoxicity was also found in some patients [35]. This agent is now being investigated in several large randomized trials.

Intensive treatment with high-dose alkylating agents and radiation may produce dramatic response in patients with refractory disease. However, these responses are short-lived and cannot be considered a standard form of salvage treatment. A recent French study suggests that high-dose therapy may be more effective when done at the time of first relapse than as part of the patient's initial treatment plan. Thus, this certainly is an option in patients who have relapsed following conventional therapy. However, induction of disease stabilization or response with conventional chemotherapy should be achieved prior to attempting a high-dose program, otherwise the outcome is extremely poor. In patients relapsing following high-dose therapy, another high-dose treatment regimen may be used if the initial therapy resulted in a relatively long remission following the first transplant. Alternatively, in patients who previously underwent autologous transplantation, allogeneic support may be tried, but the high risk of treatment-related mortality must be considered in any decision regarding this form of treatment.

BONE DISEASE

Bone disease is the major cause of morbidity in multiple myeloma, resulting from stimulation of osteoclasts by bone-resorbing cytokines (tumor necrosis factor, interleukin-1-β and interleukin-6), which are overabundant in the myeloma bone marrow. Osteolytic lesions and generalized osteoporosis may lead to severe pain, pathologic fractures, and spinal cord compression and collapse. These complications often require radiation therapy to relieve pain or to treat actual or impending pathologic fractures or spinal cord compression. Plasma cell tumors are relatively responsive to radiation treatment. Responses typically occur rapidly, with most lesions treated with approximately 3000 cGy. However, it is important to avoid unnecessary radiotherapy because its myelosuppressive effect may limit the ability to deliver cytotoxic doses of systemic chemotherapy. Often the latter treatment alone will be effective for relieving skeletal pain. High doses of analgesics may be necessary until pain control is achieved with radiation treatment or chemotherapy. Surgery may be necessary to treat actual fractures or prevent large lytic lesions from developing fractures. The placement of intramedullary rods is usually the surgical procedure of choice. Spinal disease may require surgical decompression or stabilization of the spine. Previous attempts to reduce the development of these skeletal complications with calcium, sodium fluoride, androgenic steroids, or combinations of the three have been unsuccessful.

Bisphosphonates inhibit osteoclastic activity and are effective in the treatment of hypercalcemia associated with myeloma. Previous attempts to use relatively weak first-generation bisphosphonates (etidronate or clodronate) orally as an adjunct to chemotherapy had no significant effect on the development of skeletal complications in myeloma patients. A recent large randomized trial compared the effect of the more potent second-generation agent pamidronate (given as a 90-mg 4-h infusion every 4 wk for 21 cycles) with placebo on the development of bony complications in patients on chemotherapy [36,37]. At study entry, patients were stratified according to whether they were receiving first-line chemotherapy or had already failed initial chemotherapy. In both strata, pamidronate was successful in both reducing the percentage of patients developing at least one skeletal event as well as reducing the number of events experienced by the patient. In addition, patients experienced less pain after beginning pamidronate therapy, their requirement for analgesic usage was less than that of placebo-treated patients, and individuals treated with the bisphosphonate showed a better ECOG performance status. Interestingly, pamidronate also led to a significant improvement (50%) in overall survival in the stratum of patients who entered the trial having failed initial chemotherapy. Several recent in vitro studies suggest that these agents may have both a direct and indirect antitumor effect on myeloma. Although the clinical trial involved patients with Durie-Salmon stage III myeloma, it is likely that this drug will also be efficacious in reducing these complications in patients at earlier stages of the disease.

NEW THERAPY APPROACHES

A number of new therapeutic strategies for myeloma are now in clinical development. Specifically, use of antagonists to interleukin-6 have been evaluated in early phase I trials. In one myeloma patient, vaccination of an allogeneic donor with purified paraprotein induced an immune response to the monoclonal protein by the donor, and these donor cells were used clinically in the patient [38]. Whether this approach will prove generally useful awaits larger clinical trials, which have been initiated. Use of ex vivo–generated dendritic cells specifically armed with part of the monoclonal protein is another new immunologic approach that is being explored. However, the presence of a possible etiologic agent (human herpesvirus-8) for myeloma in these types of immune cells must be considered in these therapeutic strategies. Because of the encouraging results on overall survival from the recent pamidronate trial, higher doses of bisphosphonates alone are being used to treat previously treated patients in clinical trials.

In summary, many regimens will produce responses in patients with myeloma, but long-term disease control is uncommon. High-dose therapy with peripheral blood stem cell support seems to offer both longer progression-free and overall survival than conventional treatment but is not curative in the vast majority of patients. Use of intravenous pamidronate reduces the bony complications while improving the quality of life of these patients; it may even improve overall survival in some patients. Newer immunologic or other novel approaches will be required to improve these patients' outcomes.

MYELOMA

REFERENCES

1. Kyle RA: "Benign" monoclonal gammopathy after 23 years of follow-up. *Mayo Clinic Proc* 1993, 68:26–36.
2. Rettig MB, Ma HJ, Vescio RA, *et al.*: Kaposi's sarcoma-associated herpesvirus infection of bone marrow dendritic cells from multiple myeloma patients. *Science* 1997, 276:1851–1854.
3. Said JW, Rettig MR, Heppner K, *et al.*: Localization of kaposi's sarcoma-associated herpesvirus in bone marrow biopsy samples from patients with multiple myeloma. *Blood* 1997, 90:4278–4282.
4. Durie BGM, Salmon SE: A clinical staging system for multiple myeloma. *Cancer* 1975, 36:842–854.
5. Greipp PR, Lust JA, O'Fallon M, *et al.*: Plasma cell labeling index and beta2-microglobulin predict survival independent of thymidine kinase and c-reactive protein in multiple myeloma. *Blood* 1993, 91:3382–3387.
6. Durie B, Stock-Novack D, Salmon S, *et al.*: Prognostic value of pretreatment serum beta2 microglobulin in myeloma: a Southwest Oncology Group Study. *Blood* 1990, 75:823–830.
7. Tricot G, Barlogie B, Jagannath S, *et al.*: Poor prognosis in multiple myeloma is associated only with partial or complete deletions of chromosome 13 or abnormalities involving 11q and not with other karyotype abnormalities. *Blood* 1995, 86:4250–4256.
8. Greipp PR, Gaillard JP, Klein B, *et al.*: Independent prognostic value for plasma cell labeling index, immunofluorescence microscopy plasma cell percent, beta 2-microglobulin, soluble interleukin-6 receptor and C-reactive protein in myeloma trial E9487. *Blood* 1994, 84:385.
9. Kusumoto S, Jinnai I, Itoh K, *et al.*: Magnetic resonance imaging patterns in patients with multiple myeloma. *Br J Haematol* 1997, 99:649–655.
10. Oken MM, Harrington DP, Abramson N, *et al.*: Comparison of melphalan and prednisone with vincristine, carmustine, melphalan, cyclophosphamide, and prednisone in the treatment of multiple myeloma. *Cancer* 1997, 79:1561–1567.
11. Salmon SE, Tesh D, Crowley J, *et al.*: Chemotherapy is superior to sequential hemibody irradiation for remission consolidation in multiple myeloma: a Southwest Oncology Group Study. *J Clin Oncol* 1990, 8:1575–1584.
12. MacLennan ICM, Chapman C, Dunn J, *et al.*: Combined chemotherapy with ABCM vs melphalan for treatment of myelomatosis. *Lancet* 1993, 339:200–205.
13. Salmon SE, Crowley JJ, Grogan TM, *et al.*: Combination chemotherapy, glucocorticoids, and interferon alpha in the treatment of multiple myeloma: a Southwest Oncology Group study. *J Clin Oncol* 1994, 12:2405–2414.
14. Barlogie B, Smith L, Alexanian R: Effective treatment of advanced multiple myeloma refractory to alkylating agents. *N Engl J Med* 1984, 3:1353–1356.
15. Alexanian R, Dimopoulos MA, Delasalle K, *et al.*: Primary dexamethasone treatment in multiple myeloma. *Blood* 1992, 80:887–890.
16. Palumbo A, Battaglio S, Napoli P, *et al.*: Recombinant interferon-gamma inhibits the in vitro proliferation of human myeloma cells. *Br J Haematol* 1994, 86:726–732.
17. Mandelli F, Avvisati G, Amadori S, *et al.*: Maintenance treatment with recombinant interferon alfa-2b in patients with multiple myeloma responding to conventional induction chemotherapy. *N Engl J Med* 1990, 322:1430–1434.
18. Powles R, Raje N, Cunningham D, *et al.*: Maintenance therapy for remission in myeloma with intron A following high-dose melphalan and either an autologous bone marrow transplantation or peripheral stem cell rescue. *Stem Cells Daytona* 1995, 13:114–117.
19. Browman GP, Rubin S, Walker I, *et al.*: Interferon alpha-2b maintenance therapy prolongs progression-free and overall survival in plasma cell myeloma: results of a randomized trial. *Proc Am Soc Clin Oncol* 1994, 13:408.
20. Peest D, Deicher H, Coldewey R, *et al.*: A comparison of polychemotherapy and melphalan/prednisone for primary remission induction, and interferon-alpha for maintenance treatment, in multiple myeloma: a prospective trial of the German Myeloma Treatment Group. *Eur J Cancer* 1995, 31A:146–151.
21. The Nordic Myeloma Study Group: Interferon alpha-2b added to melphalan-prednisone for initial and maintenance therapy in multiple myeloma: a randomized, controlled trial. *Ann Intern Med* 1996, 124:212–222.
22. Salmon S, Crowley J: Alpha interferon plus alternate day prednisone (IFN/P) improves remission maintenance duration in multiple myeloma (MM) compared to IFN alone. *Proc Am Soc Clin Oncol* 1997, 16:46.
23. Attal M, Harousseau J-L, Stoppa A-M, *et al.*: A prospective, randomized trial of autologous bone marrow transplantation and chemotherapy in multiple myeloma. *N Engl J Med* 1996, 335:91–97.
24. Attal M, Harousseau JL, Stoppa AM, *et al.*: Autologous transplantation-clinical results in multiple myeloma. *Blood* 1997, 90:1858.
25. Schiller G, Vescio R, Freytes C, *et al.*: Transplantation of CD34+ peripheral blood progenitor cells after high-dose chemotherapy for patients with advanced multiple myeloma. *Blood* 1995, 86:390–397.
26. Vescio R, Stewart A, Ballester O, *et al.*: Myeloma cell tumor reduction in PBPC autografts following CD34 selection: the results of a phase III trial using the CEPRATE device. *Blood* 1997, 90:1872.
27. Barlogie B, Jagannath S, Vesole DH, *et al.*: Superiority of tandem autologous transplantation over standard therapy for previously untreated multiple myeloma. *Blood* 1997, 89:789–793.
28. Attal M, Payen C, Facon T, *et al.*: Single versus double transplant in myeloma: a randomized trial of the Inter Groupe Francais du Myelome (IFM). *Blood* 1997, 90:1859.
29. Gahrton G, Tura S, Ljungman P, *et al.*: European Group for bone marrow transplantation: allogeneic bone marrow transplantation in multiple myeloma. *N Eng J Med* 1991, 325:1267.
30. Tricot G, Vesole DH, Jagannath S, *et al.*: Graft-versus-myeloma effect: proof of principle. *Blood* 1996, 87:1196–1198.
31. Giralt S, Estey E, van Besien K, *et al.*: Induction of graft-versus-leukemia without myeloablative therapy using allogeneic PBSC after purine analog containing regimens. *Blood* 1996, 88:2444.
32. Kraut EH, Crowley JJ, Wade JL, *et al.*: Evaluation of topotecan in resistant and relapsing multiple myeloma: a Southwest Oncology Group Study. *J Clin Oncol* 1998, 16:589–592.
33. Lenhard RE Jr, Oken MM, Barnes JM, *et al.*: High-dose cyclophosphamide: an effective treatment for advanced refractory multiple myeloma. *Cancer* 1984, 53:1456–1460.
34. Grogan TM, Spier CM, Salmon SE, *et al.*: P-glycoprotein expression in human plasma cell myeloma: correlation with prior chemotherapy. *Blood* 1993, 81:490–495.
35. Sonneveld P, Marie J-P, Huisman C, *et al.*: Reversal of multidrug resistance by SDZ PSC 833, combined with VAD (vincristine, doxorubicin, dexamethasone) in refractory multiple myeloma: a phase I study. *Leukemia* 1996, 10:1741–1750.
36. Berenson J, Lichtenstein A, Porter L, *et al.*: Long-term pamidronate treatment of advanced multiple myeloma patients reduces skeletal events. *J Clin Oncol* 1998, 16: 593–602.
37. Berenson J, Lichtenstein A, Porter L, *et al.*: Efficacy of pamidronate in reducing skeletal events in patients with advanced multiple myeloma. *N Eng J Med* 1996, 334:488–493.
38. Kwak LW, Taub DD, Duffey PL, *et al.*: Transfer of myeloma idiotype-specific immunity from an actively immunised marrow donor. *Lancet* 1995, 345:1016–1020.

MP
Melphalan and Prednisone

Melphalan and prednisone is the prototype regimen in the single-alkylating-agent therapy for multiple myeloma. The high-dose intermittent schedule has proved a simple, relatively safe way to administer melphalan. A 1972 study reported that prednisone doubled the response rate to melphalan and that it produced modest improvement in survival. MP became, and for some, remains, the standard chemotherapy for multiple myeloma. Treatment is generally administered in cycles of 3–6 wk duration and is continued for 1–2 y, although it sometimes has been continued it until disease progression.

An important problem with this protocol is the erratic absorption of oral melphalan, which sometimes leads to inadequate bioavailability in some patients who take apparently adequate oral doses.

DOSAGE AND SCHEDULING

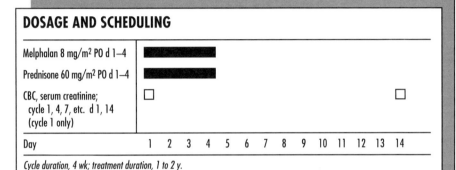

	Day	1	2	3	4	5	6	7	8	9	10	11	12	13	14
Melphalan 8 mg/m² PO d 1–4															
Prednisone 60 mg/m² PO d 1–4															
CBC, serum creatinine; cycle 1, 4, 7, etc. d 1, 14 (cycle 1 only)															

Cycle duration, 4 wk; treatment duration, 1 to 2 y.

DOSAGE MODIFICATIONS: After first cycle, modify melphalan dose for depressed blood counts as follows: ANC 1000–2000/μL — give 75%; ANC 750–1000 or platelets 50,000–100,000/μL — give 50%; delay treatment for ANC < 750/μL or platelets < 50,000/μL.

RECENT EXPERIENCES AND RESPONSE RATES

Study	Evaluable Patients, n	Dosage and Scheduling	Objective Response (%)	Median Survival (mo)
Alexanian, et al., Cancer 1972, 30:382–389.	77	Melphalan 0.25 mg/kg PO d 1–4 Prednisone 2 mg/kg PO d 1–4 Cycle duration, 6 wk	47*	24
Abramson, et al., Cancer Treat Rep 1982, 66:1273–1277.	72	Melphalan 8 mg/m² PO d 1–4 Prednisone 75 mg PO d 1–7 Cycle duration, 4 wk	43‡	25
Oken, et al., Proc ASCO 1987, 6:203	217	Melphalan 8 mg/m² PO d 1–4 Prednisone 60 mg/m² PO d 1–4	51†	30
Bergsagel, et al., N Engl J Med 1979, 301:743–748.	125	Melphalan 9 mg/m² PO d 1–4 Prednisone 100 mg PO d 1–4 Cycle duration, 4 wk	40*	28

*Response requires ≥ 75% decrease in M-protein production.
†Response requires ≥ 50% decrease in M-protein value.
‡Response evaluated at 6 mo only.

CANDIDATES FOR TREATMENT
Patients with active or advanced myeloma, particularly those who are elderly and frail

SPECIAL PRECAUTIONS
Risk for infection greater during early cycles (use allopurinol to prevent hyperuricemia during early months); treatment-associated myelodysplastic syndrome and acute leukemia occur in some

ALTERNATIVE THERAPIES
Melphalan alone, VMCP/VBAP, ABCM

TOXICITIES
Melphalan: bone marrow suppression leading to neutropenia with increased risk for infection, thrombocytopenia with risk for bleeding, erythroid hypoplasia with risk for symptomatic anemia; long-term toxicity: testicular atrophy, amenorrhea, risk for treatment-induced acute leukemia; **Prednisone:** immunosuppression, infection, edema, exacerbation of diabetes, weight gain, menstrual abnormalities, mental status dysfunction (especially in elderly)

DRUG INTERACTIONS
None

NURSING INTERVENTIONS
Instruct patient to seek medical attention if fever or other specific or subjective symptoms develop that could represent infection; monitor blood glucose if diabetic; antacid therapy may be used

PATIENT INFORMATION
Patient should take melphalan on empty stomach, prednisone after meals; anticipate possibility of mood and appetite changes or fluid retention; be alert to early signs of bleeding or infection.

VBMCP
Vincristine, BCNU, Melphalan, Cyclophosphamide, Prednisone

VBMCP is a prototype combination chemotherapy regimen that is more intensive than standard MP. Initial reports of a markedly increased response rate in comparison with MP were confirmed in a large randomized trial. The regimen is one of multiple alkylating agents plus the vinca alkyloid, vincristine, and prednisone. Full-dose melphalan plus prednisone is part of the regimen but is administered at 5-wk rather than 4-wk intervals. Part of the increase in response rate may be attributed to the addition of three intravenous drugs to the sometimes erratically absorbed, orally administered melphalan.

BCNU, or carmustine, is a nitrosourea that is primarily an alkylating agent, as are both cyclophosphamide and melphalan. Vincristine is a vinca alkyloid and is cell cycle–specific for the M phase, interfering with the mitotic spindle formation.

DOSAGE AND SCHEDULING

Vincristine 1.2 mg/m² IV d 1

BCNU 20 mg/m² IV d 1

Melphalan 8 mg/m² PO d 1–4

Cyclophosphamide 400 mg/m² IV d 1

Prednisone 40 mg/m² PO

CBC, LFTs d 1 and every 6 mo
Creatinine cycle 1, 4, 7, etc. d 1

Prednisone 20 mg/m² PO
cycle 1–3 20 d 8–14

Day: 1 2 3 4 5 6 7 8 9 10 11 12 13 14

Cycle duration, 5 wk; treatment duration, 1 to 2 y.

DOSAGE MODIFICATIONS: After first cycle, modify melphalan, BCNU, cyclophosphamide for depressed blood counts as follows: ANC 1000–2000/µL—give 75%; ANC 750–1000 or platelets 50,000–100,000/µL—give 50%; delay treatment for ANC < 750/µL or platelets < 50,000/µL vincristine dose reduction required for hepatic insufficiency.

RECENT EXPERIENCES AND RESPONSE RATES

Study	Evaluable Patients, n	Dosage and Scheduling	Response, %	Median Survival, mo	5-Y Survival, %
Case, et al., Am J Med 1977, 63:897–903. Lee, et al., In Wiernik (ed.) Controversies in Oncology 1982, pp 61–79.	81	Vincristine 0.03 mg/kg IV d 1 BCNU 0.5 mg/kg IV d 1 Melphalan 0.25 mg/kg PO d 1–4 Cyclophosphamide 10 mg/kg IV d 1 Prednisone 1 mg/kg PO d 1–7, then 0.5 mg/kg d 8–14, then taper	78*	38	—
Oken, et al., Proc ASCO 1987, 6:203	214	Vincristine 1.2 mg/m² IV d 1 BCNU 20 mg/m² IV d 1 Melphalan 8 mg/m² PO d 1–4 Cyclophosphamide 400 mg/m² IV d 1 Prednisone 60 mg/m² PO d 1–7; (20 mg/m² PO d 8–14 cycle 1–3)	72*	31	26

*Response requires ≥ 50% decrease in M-protein value.

CANDIDATES FOR TREATMENT
Patients with active myeloma unless they are elderly (> 70 years) and frail

SPECIAL PRECAUTIONS
Risk for infection greater during early cycles (use allopurinol to prevent hyperuricemia during early months); treatment-associated myelodysplastic syndrome and acute leukemia occur in some; VBMCP poorly tolerated by patients > 70 years of age and frail—MP is better choice

ALTERNATIVE THERAPIES
MP, VMCP/VBAP, ABCM, melphalan alone, VBMCP and interferon

TOXICITIES
Drug combination: long-term toxicity: testicular atrophy, amenorrhea, risk for treatment-induced acute leukemia; **Melphalan:** bone marrow suppression leading to neutropenia with increased risk for infection, thrombocytopenia with increased risk for bleeding, erythroid hypoplasia with risk for symptomatic anemia; **Prednisone:** immunosuppression, infection, exacerbation of diabetes, weight gain, edema, mental status dysfunction—especially in elderly; **BCNU:** bone marrow suppression possibly longer than that with melphalan or cyclophosphamide, pain in injected extremity or at IV site, nausea, vomiting, liver or renal dysfunction; pulmonary fibrosis (rare); **Cyclophosphamide:** bone marrow suppression but relatively platelet sparing, nausea, vomiting, hemorrhagic cystitis, alopecia; rarely, pulmonary fibrosis, liver dysfunction; **Vincristine:** peripheral neuropathy, cranial nerve neuropathy, constipation, alopecia, vesicant if extravasated; SIADH (rare)

DRUG INTERACTIONS
Cyclophosphamide: barbiturates, phenytoin, chloral hydrate

NURSING INTERVENTIONS
Push fluids for 24 hours after cyclophosphamide to reduce risk for hemorrhagic cystitis; give antiemetic before administration; monitor blood glucose if diabetic; antacid therapy may be used

PATIENT INFORMATION
Maintain good fluid intake; take melphalan on empty stomach, prednisone after meals; anticipate possibility of mood and appetite changes or fluid retention; be alert to early signs of bleeding or infection; call physician for blood in urine; vincristine may cause severe constipation: monitor bowel pattern carefully, use mild laxatives, seek medical attention if persistent or severe.

VMCP/VBAP AND ABCM

Vincristine, Melphalan, Cyclophosphamide, Prednisone/Vincristine, BCNU, Doxorubicin, Prednisone; and Doxorubicin, BCNU, Cyclophosphamide, Melphalan

This regimen consists of alternating cycles of vincristine plus prednisone combined with either melphalan plus cyclophosphamide or with BCNU plus doxorubicin. The strategy of rapid alternating cycles provides maximum early exposure to active combinations and theoretically could prevent or delay the emergence of resistant clones. An alternative strategy of giving three cycles of VMCP followed by three cycles of VBAP yielded essentially identical results in a SWOG study. Therefore, these results are pooled. A third variation on VMCP/VBAP, the ABCM regimen, eliminates vincristine and prednisone and yields similar results.

DOSAGE AND SCHEDULING

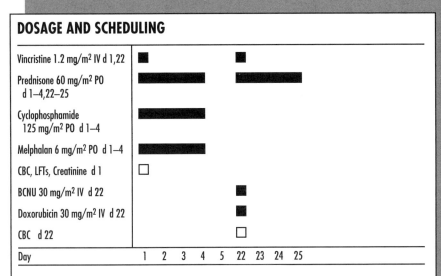

| | Day | 1 | 2 | 3 | 4 | 5 | 22 | 23 | 24 | 25 |

Vincristine 1.2 mg/m² IV d 1,22
Prednisone 60 mg/m² PO d 1–4,22–25
Cyclophosphamide 125 mg/m² PO d 1–4
Melphalan 6 mg/m² PO d 1–4
CBC, LFTs, Creatinine d 1
BCNU 30 mg/m² IV d 22
Doxorubicin 30 mg/m² IV d 22
CBC d 22

DOSAGE MODIFICATIONS: *reduce dose of vincristine and doxorubicin for impaired liver function or significant treatment-induced cytopenias*

RECENT EXPERIENCES AND RESPONSE RATES

Study	Evaluable Patients, n	Dosage and Scheduling	Response, %	Median Survival, mo	5-Y Survival, %
VMCP/VBAP Durie, *et al.*, J Clin Oncol 1986, 4:1227–1237; Salmon, *et al.*, J Clin Oncol 1990, 8:1575–1584.	614	Vincristine 1.0 mg IV d 1, 22 Prednisone 60 mg/m² PO d 1–4, 22–25 Melphalan 6 mg/m² d 1–4 Cyclophosphamide 125 mg/m² PO d 1–4 BCNU 30 mg/m² IV d 22 Doxorubicin 30 mg/m² IV d 22	38*	30	27
ABCM Maclennan, *et al.*, Lancet 1992, 339:200–205.	314	Doxorubicin 30 mg/m² IV d 1 BCNU 30 mg/m² IV d 1 Cyclophosphamide 100 mg/m² PO d 22–25 Melphalan 6 mg/m² PO d 22–25	61†	32	25

Response requires ≥ 75% decrease in M-protein production.
†Response — achievement of plateau phase.*

CANDIDATES FOR TREATMENT

Patients with active myeloma who are elderly and frail (partially or totally bedridden)

SPECIAL PRECAUTIONS

Risk for infection greater during early cycles (use allopurinol to prevent hyperuricemia during early months); treatment-associated myelodysplastic syndrome and acute leukemia occur in some; do not use doxorubicin in patients with significant cardiac decompensation (ejection fraction < 45%, signs of congestive heart failure [CHF], recent myocardial infarction [MI], or unstable angina); do not exceed cumulative doxorubicin dose of 450 mg/m²

ALTERNATIVE THERAPIES

MP, melphalan alone, VMCP/VBAP, ABCM

TOXICITIES

Melphalan: bone marrow suppression leading to neutropenia with increased risk for infection, thrombocytopenia with increased risk for bleeding, erythroid hypoplasia with risk for symptomatic anemia; **Prednisone:** immunosuppression, infection, Cushing's syndrome, exacerbation of diabetes, weight gain, edema, mental status dysfunction—especially in elderly; **BCNU:** bone marrow suppression possibly longer than that with melphalan or cyclophosphamide, pain in injected extremity or at IV site, nausea, vomiting, liver or renal dysfunction; pulmonary fibrosis rare at this dose range; **Cyclophosphamide:** bone marrow suppression but relatively platelet sparing, nausea, vomiting, alopecia, hemorrhagic cystitis, pulmonary fibrosis (rare), liver dysfunction (rare); **Vincristine:** peripheral neuropathy, cranial nerve neuropathy, constipation, alopecia, vesicant if extravasated; SIADH (rare); **Doxorubicin:** myelotoxicity, nausea, vomiting, alopecia, cardiotoxicity—generally at higher doses, vesicant if extravasated; **long-term toxicity:** testicular atrophy, amenorrhea, risk for treatment-induced acute leukemia

DRUG INTERACTIONS

Cyclophosphamide: barbiturates, phenytoin, chloral hydrate

NURSING INTERVENTIONS

Push fluids for 24 h after cyclophosphamide to reduce risk for hemorrhagic cystitis; give antiemetic before administration; monitor blood glucose if diabetic; antacid therapy may be used

PATIENT INFORMATION

Patient should maintain good fluid intake; take melphalan on empty stomach, prednisone after meals; anticipate possibility of mood and appetite changes or fluid retention; be alert to early signs of bleeding or infection; seek medical attention for blood in urine; vincristine may cause severe constipation: monitor bowel pattern carefully, use mild laxatives, seek medical attention if persistent or severe.

The information here is provided as guidance only. Prescribers should always consult the manufacturer's current prescribing information.

VAD
Vincristine, Doxorubicin, Dexamethasone

The VAD regimen combines vincristine and adriamycin by 4-d infusion with high-dose oral dexamethasone. It is primarily a salvage regimen in patients who have relapses but has gained an additional application as a treatment to be used prior to autologous bone marrow transplant harvest when alkylating agents are to be avoided. Responses to this regimen usually occur within 2 mo, making VAD more rapid than MP or VMCP/VBAP and, possibly, VBMCP. The repeated cycles of high-dose corticosteroids are an important component in this regimen's effectiveness and may generate most of the activity in patients with refractory disease.

DOSAGE AND SCHEDULING

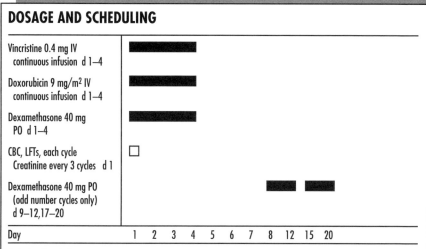

	Day	1	2	3	4	5	6	7	8	12	15	20

Vincristine 0.4 mg IV
  continuous infusion d 1–4

Doxorubicin 9 mg/m^2 IV
  continuous infusion d 1–4

Dexamethasone 40 mg
  PO d 1–4

CBC, LFTs, each cycle
  Creatinine every 3 cycles d 1

Dexamethasone 40 mg PO
  (odd number cycles only)
  d 9–12,17–20

Cycle duration, 4 wk.
Trimethoprim/sulfamethoxazole 1 DS PO daily and clortrimazole troches, 10 mg 3×d as prophylaxis while receiving therapy.
During dexamethasone, patients should receive an H$_2$-receptor antagonists; such as ranitidine, at full dose.

DOSAGE MODIFICATIONS: *Reduce dose of vincristine and doxorubicin for impaired liver function; reduce dexamethasone for severe dyspepsia, edema refractory to diuretics, myopathy, severe hypertension, severe corticosteroid withdrawal symptoms or cushingoid changes, steroid psychosis or hallucinations; after first cycle, reduce doxorubicin for myelotoxicity: 75% if ANC is 1500–1000/mm^3, 50% if ANC is 750–1000 or platelets are 50,000–100,000/μL.*

RECENT EXPERIENCES AND RESPONSE RATES

Study	Evaluable Patients, n	Dosage and Scheduling	Cycle Duration, wk	Objective Response, %
Alexanian, et al., Ann Intern Med 1986, 105:8–11.	39	Vincristine 0.4 mg IV d 1–4 Doxorubicin 9 mg/m^2 IV d 1–4; both by continuous infusion Dexamethasone 40 mg PO d 1–4, 9–12, 17–20, 25–28	6	46[†]
Lokhorst, et al., Br J Haemotol 1989, 71:25–30.	31	Vincristine 0.4 mg IV d 1–4 Doxorubicin 9 mg/m^2 IV d 1–4; both by continuous infusion Dexamethasone 40 mg PO d 1–4, 9–12, 17–20 (odd # cycles) Dexamethasone 40 mg PO d 1–4, (even # cycles)	4	60[‡]

*In previously treated patients
[†]Response requires ≥ 75% decrease in M-protein production.
[‡]Response requires ≥ 50% decrease in serum M-protein level.

CANDIDATES FOR TREATMENT
Alternative primary regimen for patients under consideration for stem cell harvest. Most often used in patients with relapsed myeloma.

SPECIAL PRECAUTIONS
Regimen is contraindicated in patients with poor liver function; prophylactic trimethoprim/sulfamethoxazole and clortrimazole troches advised during therapy; use allopurinol to prevent hyperuricemia during early months; doxorubicin is contraindicated in patients with significant cardiac decompensation (ejection fraction < 45%, signs of CHF, recent MI, or unstable angina); do not exceed cumulative doxorubicin dose of 450 mg/m^2; to prevent dyspepsia or ulcer, administer an H$_2$-receptor agonist at full dosage during dexamethasone

TOXICITIES
Vincristine: peripheral neuropathy, cranial nerve neuropathy, constipation, alopecia, vesicant if extravasated; SIADH (rare); **Doxorubicin:** myelotoxicity, nausea, vomiting, alopecia, flare, cardiotoxicity (generally at higher doses), vesicant if extravasated; **Dexamethasone:** immunosuppression, infection, Cushing's syndrome, osteoporosis, exacerbation of diabetes, weight gain, hypertension, edema, mental status dysfunction—especially in elderly

DRUG INTERACTIONS
Doxorubicin and vincristine are compatible

NURSING INTERVENTIONS
Carefully place venous access catheter before initiating VAD; do not use a peripheral IV site—would expose patient to excessive risk for doxorubicin or vincristine extravasation injury; if right atrial catheter or central venous port is in place, administer doxorubicin and vincristine in an ambulatory outpatient setting with portable infusion pump; doxorubicin and vincristine may be mixed together; monitor regularly for hypertension, CHF, severe fluid retention, behavioral changes, symptoms of ulcer or dyspepsia, infections—including local Candida infections

PATIENT INFORMATION
Patient should anticipate possibility of mood and appetite changes or fluid retention; be alert to early signs of infection; vincristine may cause severe constipation: monitor bowel pattern carefully, use mild laxatives, seek medical attention if persistent or severe.

The accumulation of fluid in the pleural or pericardial space, as a result of either cancer or its treatment, leads to a progressive reduction in the ability of the patient to oxygenate. This inability to oxygenate, first manifested as dyspnea on exertion, is a result of reduced cardiac output or compromised pulmonary reserve. Although the end result of progressive respiratory failure is the same, the presenting signs and symptoms of malignant pleural or pericardial effusions differ (Table 22-1) [1,2].

PATHOPHYSIOLOGY

The causes of both effusions are essentially identical, reflecting a profound imbalance in the production and clearance of normal fluid through the respective space. In both instances, the presence of active malignancy in either space leads to the production of an exudative effusion that exceeds the capacity of normal lymphatic channels to clear it. The presence of significant amounts of tumor in the mediastinal lymph nodes, or the obstruction of mediastinal lymphatics by radiation-induced fibrosis, greatly exacerbates the clinical problem. Although reduced oncotic pressure due to hypoproteinemia or concurrent infection can exacerbate a malignant effusion, the direct presence of malignancy and the obstruction of mediastinal lymphatic flow are the primary contributing factors to the development of clinically significant, malignant pleural, and pericardial effusions.

In the case of the pericardium, the development of symptoms is a function of the rapidity with which the fluid accumulates, the amount of fluid produced, and the premorbid condition of the underlying myocardium [1]. Slowly accumulating fluid can produce no symptoms until a relatively massive amount of fluid has developed because the pericardium has time to stretch. Eventually, the combination of volume of fluid and speed of onset results in resistance to ventricular filling during diastole and a progressive compromise of cardiac output [6].

In the pleural space, the pathway is similar, but the speed of onset is of less importance in determining the onset of symptoms. However, the development of dyspnea is a function of the amount of fluid produced and the condition of the lungs prior to the onset of the effusion. At a point that varies among patients, the increase in accumulated fluid and the degree of prior pulmonary compromise intercept to produce a sense of dyspnea.

CLINICAL PRESENTATION

The interplay between volume and underlying organ function leads to a wide spectrum of presenting symptoms and signs. Radiographically obvious but clinically silent pleural and pericardial effusions are common. In both instances, the initial presentation is usually shortness of breath on exertion. It is important to remember that patients with malignant pericardial effusions present with dyspnea on exertion, but the critical diagnostic test—the echocardiogram—usually is done at rest. This can result in a delay in therapy when the echo shows no evidence of tamponade. As outlined in Table 22-1, the two syndromes go on to manifest different signs and symptoms, reflecting the primarily cardiac or pulmonary organ systems being stressed. In malignant pleural effusions the progression of symptoms usually is linear and relatively predictable. On the other hand, pericardial effusions can lead to a rapid change in clinical status as critical pressures are exceeded [3]. Consequently, the presence of the classical findings of a positive Kussmaul's sign and pulsus paradoxus are actually very late findings indicative of the potential for rapid clinical deterioration in patients with malignant pericardial effusions. The use of potent diuretics, therefore, can impact rapidly on ventricular filling pressures and exacerbate the symptoms of pericardial tamponade.

DIAGNOSTIC ALGORITHMS

Figures 22-1 and 22-2 outline recommended diagnostic and treatment algorithms for malignant pleural and pericardial effusions. These are predicated on the assumption that the patient in question either has or is highly suspected to have a malignancy known to cause malignant effusions. These algorithms do *not* apply to the general medical patient who presents with a wider spectrum of possible diagnoses.

The approach to the patient with a suspected malignant pleural effusion is outlined in Figure 22-1 [4]. Most cases are detected during a routine chest radiograph or during computed tomography (CT) done to assess disease response or stability. The presence of new or worsening dyspnea often leads to the radiograph study. Obvious infection, heart failure, or an immunologic disorder usually can be excluded by the history and physical examination. The diagnostic thoracentesis can then complete the initial evaluation. Although literally hundreds of pleural fluid markers have been described, the diagnosis can be made by the simple use of cytologic examination and a comparison of serum and pleural fluid levels of lactate dehydrogenase and protein (Table 22-2). In my practice, the

Table 22-1. Signs and Symptoms of Malignant Effusions in the Chest

	Pleural	Pericardial
Common	Dyspnea (exertion)	Dyspnea (exertion)
	Dyspnea (rest)	Dyspnea (rest)
	Cough	Jugular venous distension
	Dullness to percussion	Distant heart sounds
	Egophony	
Uncommon	Cyanosis	Cyanosis
	Anorexia	Peripheral vasoconstriction
	Chest pain	Pulsus paradoxus
		Narrow pulse pressure (Kussmaul's sign)
		Electrical alterans

Table 22-2. Diagnostic Test for Confirming Presence of Malignant Pleural Effusion

Test	Positive Predictive Value, %
Cytology	100
Fluid LDH > 200 U	100
Fluid/blood LDH ratio > 0.6	99
Fluid/protein ratio > 3 g	95
Fluid/blood protein ratio > 0.5	99

Adapted from Health and Public Policy Committee, American College of Physicians [5].

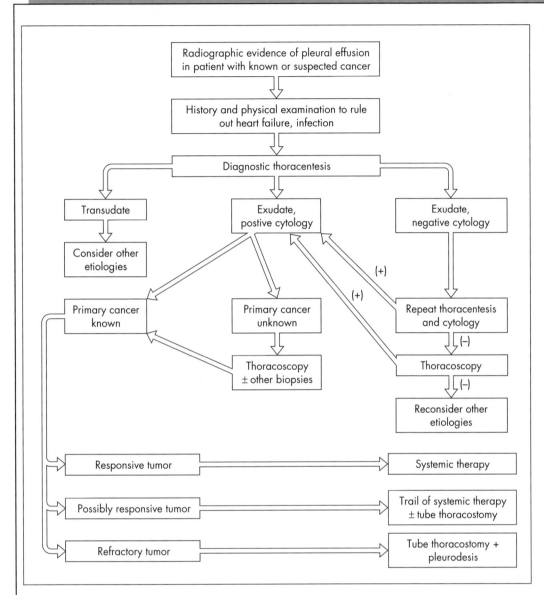

FIGURE 22-1.

Approach to the diagnosis and therapy of malignant pleural effusion. (*From* Ruckdeschel [4]; with permission.)

use of blind, transcutaneous needle biopsies as a next step has been virtually abandoned. If a transudate is present, there is no evidence of a malignant effusion. A cytologically negative exudate can present diagnostic dilemmas for the physician, but if a second diagnostic thoracentesis is negative I usually move directly to thoracoscopy, which allows direct visualization of the pleural space and biopsy of any suspicious area directly.

The approach to the patient with a suspected malignant pericardial effusion is outlined in Figure 22-2. Many cases are detected by changes on the chest radiograph. The "water bottle" cardiac silhouette is the most common change, although any significant change in cardiac width is important. At least 1- to 1.5-cm differences in cardiac width between films must be allowed for cardiac-cycle–related variation, but beyond 2 cm there is rarely any question about the diagnosis. Patients often have chest CT scans done for purposes of measuring tumor response, and this, too, can be an effective means of diagnosing a malignant pericardial effusion, especially one with an associated thick layer of tumor "cake." The history

and physical examination rule out most instances of heart failure, infection, and recent myocardial infarction. The optimal diagnostic test is the echocardiogram, which can both establish the presence of fluid and determine if diastolic filling is impaired. Pericardiocentesis to ascertain the cytologic nature of the fluid is usually less important because the diagnosis can be made rapidly during therapy. In unusual settings, the pericardiocentesis is the preferred procedure (*eg*, when the patient has such a poor prognosis from their systemic cancer that an operative procedure is believed to be relatively or absolutely contraindicated).

THERAPY OF MALIGNANT EFFUSIONS IN THE THORAX

Figures 22-1 and 22-2 also outline the recommended therapeutic approach to patients with malignant intrathoracic effusions. The decision to treat or not to treat must be individualized for each patient. Only in the moribund or rapidly progressive end-stage patient do I proceed with either no treatment or needle aspiration

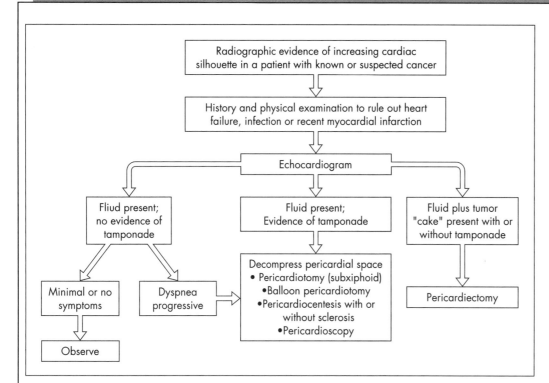

FIGURE 22-2.

Approach to the diagnosis and therapy of malignant pericardial effusion.

only. In both the pleural and pericardial spaces, it is associated with a relatively rapid recurrence of fluid and little prolonged palliative benefit. On the other hand, I take a relatively aggressive approach to the patient who is asymptomatic but who has a significant effusion. For the patient with a pericardial effusion, the prolonged presence of an exudative effusion can increase the risk of a more constrictive presentation, requiring a more extensive surgical procedure later. The patient who will live more than 3 to 4 months following their systemic disease is a good candidate for early intervention to prolong the palliative effect.

The therapy of malignant pleural effusions depends on the responsiveness of the underlying cancer to systemic chemotherapy. Newly diagnosed responsive tumors such as lymphomas or small cell lung cancer can be treated directly with systemic therapy unless the volume of the effusion is life-threatening. During relapse, these cancers often migrate to the occasionally or rarely responsive subgroups. Patients with breast cancer typify a group of patients that are often responsive to systemic therapy. They can be treated by simple drainage followed by a trial of systemic therapy. During failure, they too often migrate to the refractory group. For patients whose effusion is caused by a tumor that is generally refractory to therapy, the treatment of choice is tube thoracostomy followed by pleurodesis. Several of the more commonly employed agents for pleurodesis are listed in Table 22-3 [1,7,8].

There are, however, some general points to be made about intrapleural therapy. The effusion should not be tapped to total dryness during the diagnostic thoracentesis because this may lead to an increased risk of lung puncture and the possibility of adhesions that prevent full reexpansion of the lung. The lung must fully reexpand for therapy to be effective. A conventional chest tube or smaller bore tubes can be used, although good trials have not been done comparing them. Drainage by suction is required. There is some controversy about how much control of the drainage is needed. Most

reports suggest getting the daily drainage down to 100 to 250 mL per 24 hours before introducing the sclerosing agent, but hard data have been elusive. There are studies of shorter drainage periods with little attention paid to the volume of drainage.

Historically, a wide array of agents have been employed for intrapleural therapy. Tetracycline in its parenteral form was the most common agent employed until it was taken off the market by its manufacturer [9–11]. Several tetracycline derivatives (doxycycline, minocycline) have been proposed as alternatives, but it is not clear that they work as well as tetracycline did; several reports describe the need for multiple injections before control is achieved [12–14]. Bleomycin, an anticancer drug, was shown to be superior to tetracycline in one of the few randomized trials in this area, but concerns have been raised about its cost [15,16]. Many surgeons prefer the use of talc as an intrapleural agent, but it requires an operative procedure for insufflation or the use of a slurry of sterile talc that can be difficult to obtain [17–19]. Several large clinical trials are addressing this issue.

The predominant therapy for malignant pericardial effusions should be subxiphoid pericardiotomy [20,21], although many centers

Table 22-3. Agents Commonly Employed as Intrapleural Therapy for Malignant Effusions

Bleomycin	60 U*
Doxycycline	1–1.5 g
Talc	4–5 g

Also used for malignant pericardial effusions.

persist in using needle pericardiocentesis with insertion of a drainage catheter and sclerosing agent [22,23]. I reserve needle pericardiocentesis for the urgent clinical situation when a surgeon or operating room is not available and for the patient with an extremely limited prognosis. The increasing availability of video-assisted thoracoscopic equipment has led to an increased use of pericardioscopy to drain the pericardial space and make a more certain diagnosis when the etiology is in question [24]. As in the pleural space, the thoracoscopic approach allows better visibility of lesions for direct biopsy. A new procedure has been described, percutaneous balloon pericardiotomy, that allows for the nonsurgical creation of a pericardial window [25]. Although its potential is exciting, the role of this procedure in managing pericardial effusions has yet to be fully assessed. Severe right ventricular failure after relief of tamponade has been described and is one more reason to treat as early as possible [26].

Talc controls the effusion in about 90% of cases, but the issues of patient selection have not been addressed, and clinical trials that address this are just getting underway. Pericardiotomy by the traditional surgical approach controls nearly all effusions except those with a significant tumor cake, for which a pericardiectomy is required. (Whether to escalate to a full thoracic operation in this setting is unclear, and the risks must be balanced against the potential benefits for each patient.) The usage of balloon pericardiotomy is too new to have a sense of its comparative efficacy.

Whatever the therapy for malignant effusions involving either the pleural or pericardial spaces, it must be stressed that the purpose of the therapy is strictly palliative. Survival is short for both groups, particularly for those with pericardial effusions. Consequently, the therapy of this disorder must be sensitive to the balance of risk and benefit.

OUTCOME

Therapy for malignant pleural effusions controls the effusion in nearly 70% of cases treated with bleomycin or tetracycline derivatives.

ACKNOWLEDGMENT

The author gratefully acknowledges the expert secretarial assistance of Mrs. Janet Whalen.

REFERENCES

1. Mills SA, Graeber GM, Nelson MG: Therapy of malignant tumors involving the pericardium. In *Thoracic Oncology*, edn 2. Edited by Roth J, Ruckdeschel JC, Weisenburger T. Philadelphia: WB Saunders, 1995:492–513.

2. Moores DWO, Ruckdeschel JC: Pleural effusions in patients with malignancy. In *Thoracic Oncology*, edn 2. Edited by Roth J, Ruckdeschel JC, Weisenburger T. Philadelphia: WB Saunders, 1995:556–566.

3. Hankins JR, Satterfield JR, Aisner J, *et al.*: Pericardial window for malignant pericardial effusion. *Ann Thorac Surg* 1980, 30:465.

4. Ruckdeschel JC: Management of malignant pleural effusion: an overview. *Semin Oncol* 1988, 15(suppl 3):24–28.

5. Health and Public Policy Committee, American College of Physicians: Diagnostic thoracentesis and pleural biopsy in pleural effusions. *Ann Intern Med* 1985, 103:799–802.

6. Hancock EW: Neoplastic pericardial disease. *Card Clin* 1990, 8:673.

7. Anderson CB, Philpott GW, Ferguson TB: The treatment of malignant pleural effusions. *Cancer* 1974, 33:916–922.

8. Tattersall MHN, Boyer MJ: Management of malignant pleural effusions. *Thorax* 1980, 45:81–82.

9. Wallach HW: Intrapleural therapy with tetracycline and lidocaine for malignant pleural effusions (letter). *Chest* 1975, 73:246.

10. Gupta M, Opfell RW, Padova J, *et al.*: Intrapleural bleomycin versus tetracycline for control of malignant pleural effusion: a randomized study. *Proc Am Assoc Cancer Res Am Soc Clin Oncol* 1980, 21 (abstract):189.

11. Johnson CE, Curzon PGD: Comparison of intrapleural bleomycin and tetracycline in the treatment of malignant pleural effusion. *Proc Br Thorac Soc Thorax* 1985, 40:210.

12. Robinson LA, Fleming WH, Gailbraith TA: Intrapleural doxycycline control of malignant pleural effusions. *Ann Thorac Surg* 1993, 55:1115–1121.

13. Vaughn LM, Walker PB, Sahn SA: Alternatives to tetracycline pleurodesis. *Ann Pharmacol* 1992, 26:562.

14. Manson T: Treatment of malignant pleural effusion with doxycycline. *Scand J Infect Dis* 1988, 53(suppl):29–34.

15. Ruckdeschel JC, Moores D, Lee JY, *et al.*: Intrapleural therapy for malignant pleural effusions: a randomized comparison of bleomycin and tetracycline. *Chest* 1991, 100:1528–1535.

16. Ostrowski MJ: An assessment of the long-term results of controlling the reaccumulation of malignant effusions using intracavitary bleomycin. *Cancer* 1986, 57:721–727.

17. Jones GR: Treatment of recurrent malignant pleural effusion by iodized talc pleurodesis. *Thorac* 1969, 24:69–73.

18. Adler RH, Sayek I: Treatment of malignant pleural effusion: a method using tube thoracostomy and talc. *Ann Thorac Surg* 1976, 22:8–15.

19. Fentiman IS, Rubens RD, Hayward JL: A comparison of intracavity talc and tetracycline for the control of pleural effusions secondary to breast cancer. *Eur J Cancer Clin Oncol* 1986, 22:1079–1081.

20. Little AG, Kremser PC, Wade JI, *et al.*: Operation for diagnosis and treatment of pericardial effusions. *Surgery* 1984, 96:738.

21. Appelqvist P, Maamies T, Grohn P: Emergency pericardiotomy as primary diagnostic and therapeutic procedure in malignant pericardial tamponade: report of three cases and review of the literature. *J Surg Oncol* 1982, 21:18.

22. Wong B, Murphy J, Chang CJ, *et al.*: The risk of pericardiocentesis. *Am J Cardiol* 1979, 44:1110.

23. Gatenby RA, Hertz WH, Kessler HB: Percutaneous catheter drainage for malignant pericardial effusion. *J Vasc Interv Radiol* 1991, 2:151.

24. Millaire A, Wurtz A, deGroote P, *et al.*: Malignant pericardial effusions: usefulness of pericardioscopy. *Am Heart J* 1992, 124:1030.

25. Ziskind AA, Pearce AC, Lemon CC, *et al.*: Percutaneous balloon pericardiotomy for the treatment of cardiac tamponade and large pericardial effusions: description of the technique and report of the first 50 cases. *J Am Coll Cardiol* 1993, 21:1–5.

26. Anguera I, Pare C, Perez-Villa F: Severe right ventricular dysfunction following pericardiocentesis for cardiac tamponade. *Int J Cardiol* 1997, 59:212–214.

MALIGNANT PLEURAL EFFUSIONS

Malignant pleural effusions are a common consequence of advanced solid tumors that lead to significant morbidity and mortality. They can be diagnosed and treated readily. Treatment depends on the condition of the patient and the potential responsiveness of the underlying cancer to systemic chemotherapy.

MANAGEMENT OR INTERVENTION

1. If responsive tumor, treat systemically.
2. If an unresponsive tumor, drain through tube thoracostomy, then ensure complete lung expansion, instill bleomycin 60 U, or talc 4–5 g, or tetracycline substitute 1–1.5 g. Consider drainage with a small-bore catheter in patients with good performance status.

CAUSATIVE AGENTS
Tumor in the pleural space or tumor extensively involving mediastinal lymph drainage

PATHOLOGIC PROCESS
Excessive production of exudative fluid with reduced clearance due to blocked mediastinal lymphatics; radiation fibrosis may exacerbate

DIFFERENTIAL DIAGNOSIS
Infection, including tuberculosis, mesothelioma, congestive heart failure, parapneumonic effusion, lymphatic obstruction, and rheumatologic disorders

PATIENT ASSESSMENT
History and physical examination thoracentesis: cytology; LDH and protein.

MALIGNANT PERICARDIAL EFFUSIONS

Malignant pericardial effusions are less common and cause symptoms by reducing cardiac output. They are much more sensitive to speed of onset. Treatment depends on adequate drainage of pericardial space.

MANAGEMENT OR INTERVENTION

Drain pericardial space
Pericardiocentesis with sclerosis (bleomycin) if poorer prognosis
Subxiphoid pericardiotomy
Video-assisted pericardioscopy
Balloon pericardiotomy
Pericardiectomy if large tumor cake and otherwise better prognosis

CAUSATIVE FACTORS
Tumor in the pericardial space or tumor obstructing mediastinal lymph nodes

PATHOLOGIC PROCESS
Excessive fluid production in pericardial space with reduced clearance due to blocked mediastinal lymphatics; radiation fibrosis may exacerbate

DIFFERENTIAL DIAGNOSIS
Infection (especially viral), cardiomyopathy, recent myocardial infarction, rheumatologic disorders, and congestive heart failure

PATIENT ASSESSMENT
History and physical examination: pulsus paradoxus, Kussmaul's sign, echocardiogram.

Despite the sophisticated diagnostic tools available to establish the diagnosis of human neoplasia, oncologists frequently are asked to evaluate and treat a subset of patients with metastatic cancer in whom detailed investigations fail to identify a primary anatomic site. The reported prevalence of unknown primary carcinoma (UPC) varies with the practice setting and the definition used from 0.5% to 9% of all patients who are diagnosed with cancer [1,2]. Because identification of the primary has formed the basis for predicting the expected behavior and assigning appropriate therapy of malignant diseases, the absence of a primary poses a major challenge. The inability to identify a primary generates anxiety for the patient, who may believe that the physician's evaluation has been inadequate or that the prognosis would be improved if a primary could be established.

As suggested by the aforementioned prevalence statistics, the definition of UPC has not been standardized, varying in published reports primarily with regard to the extent of evaluation required to accept this diagnosis. A recent definition includes patients with UPC as those who have a biopsy-proven malignancy for which the anatomic origin remains unidentified after history and physical examination, including breast palpation and pelvic examination in women and testicular and prostate examination in men; laboratory studies, including liver and renal function tests; hemogram; chest radiograph; computed tomography of abdomen and pelvis; and mammography in women. Only positive findings on this initial evaluation are then investigated in detail [3,4]. Depending on the clinical situation, additional studies might include sputum cytology, computed tomography of the chest, breast ultrasonography, or gastrointestinal endoscopy.

In practice, however, considerable controversy surrounds the evaluation of patients with UPC. It is clear that despite understanding their limitations, unnecessary studies are often carried out because treatment planning is based on both the anatomic origin and the histologic type of the malignancy. The arguments for an exhaustive versus directed evaluation of patients with UPC have been outlined by many authors [5–15]. The most effective strategy takes into account the projected natural history and duration of survival and provides a reasonable probability of locating the primary anatomic site without compromising quality of life with difficult and time-consuming diagnostic studies. The overall goal is to identify the treatable patient subsets or occult primaries through a rapid, rational, calculated approach.

BIOLOGIC ASPECTS

Patients with UPC are heterogeneous and composed of numerous underlying primary cancers that remain occult during observation of patient. Many different primary cancers can remain occult during observation of the patient. This concept is supported by studies showing that a detailed postmortem anatomic investigation frequently establishes a primary in patients [5,16]. Detailed clinical and biochemical study of UPC cells, although heterogeneous in their origins, may represent a valuable resource for understanding fundamental aspects of the metastatic phenotype [17–20]. As is the case for the specific well-defined primary neoplasms discussed elsewhere in this book, it is the phenomenon of metastasis, as purely exemplified by the patient with UPC, that causes the majority of cancer deaths.

The fact that numerous occult anatomic sites can give rise to carcinomas that present with only metastatic disease supports the possibility that specific interactions of genetic and environmental insults

could give rise to genomic and biochemical changes that lead to the early development of the metastatic phenotype without the associated changes supporting local growth in the organ of origin [21]. Although this concept must be considered highly speculative, it is an hypothesis that can be tested through analysis of available biomarkers, such as oncogenes and tumor suppressor genes, which have been characterized for cancers with known anatomic origins, such as lung, pancreatic breast, and colorectal carcinomas. Either the absence of genetic changes typical for malignancies with established primaries or the presence of unusual variants of known genetic alterations support this hypothesis.

Whether the biology of UPC is fundamentally different from known primary carcinoma with systemic metastases remains controversial. Nystrom and coworkers [22] have argued that the distribution of metastatic sites in patients with UPC in which the primary subsequently is found is sufficiently different from known primary carcinoma to support the hypothesis that UPC is biologically unique. A preliminary analysis of a consecutive series of UPC patients shows that there are no significant differences in the patterns of metastases [23], although overall survival for UPC patients was inferior to patients in whom the primary was found [4]. Continued study of UPC patients is necessary to resolve this controversy.

The reason the primary organ site cannot be diagnosed remains unknown. Previous investigators have speculated that the tumor may remain below the limits of clinical or radiographic detection or that it spontaneously regressed [21]. Another possibility is that a clinically detectable primary never develops because of the development of specific genetic changes that support metastatic over local growth.

PATHOLOGY

An early, accurate pathologic assessment of biopsy material is essential in the initial evaluation of the patient with suspected UPC. In this context, the pathologist usually is able to confirm that the lesion is neoplastic and may be able to judge if the lesion is primary or metastatic. In some situations, however, it may be impossible to determine if the tumor has arisen from the biopsied organ site. This problem often complicates the cytologic evaluation of fine-needle aspirate specimens and emphasizes the need for close communication between the clinician and the pathologist.

The initial pathologic assessment of the biopsied material usually is initiated by light microscopic examination of paraffin sections stained with hematoxylin and eosin. Based on established cytologic criteria [24], the pathologist usually can place the tumor into broad groups, such as carcinoma, sarcoma, or lymphoma. Additionally, many carcinomas are immediately recognized as manifesting at least some glandular differentiation (adenocarcinoma). When glandular differentiation is absent, patients with UPC frequently are diagnosed with poorly differentiated carcinoma or undifferentiated carcinoma. Other specimens lack any cytologically distinguishing features, in which case a diagnosis of an undifferentiated malignancy is reported. In these groups with poorly differentiated carcinoma, undifferentiated carcinoma, or undifferentiated malignancy, additional pathologic studies, including histochemistry, immunohistochemistry, and electron microscopy, are employed most frequently and productively. A vast array of tissue markers is available; however, in practice, regular use is limited to a few [25]. Emphasis should be placed on the identification of patients with lymphoma because these neoplasms are curable with therapy.

Because special studies usually are not performed routinely unless there is a reasonable suspicion that they will be contributory, direct discussions between the pathologist and clinician are critical to ensure the most focused pathologic characterization possible. Random use of large numbers of tissue markers are rarely helpful for establishing a diagnosis or planning therapy.

CLINICAL CHARACTERISTICS AND NATURAL HISTORY

The clinical presentations of UPC are extremely varied. Historically, patients have been characterized as to whether they have disease above or below the diaphragm [26]. Given the heterogeneity and widespread metastases that characterize this disease, however, this arbitrary division is of doubtful value. Other investigators have begun to subclassify patients based largely on clinicopathologic criteria of histology, involved organ sites, and responsiveness to therapy. This approach has led to the definition of well-characterized patient subsets, which are discussed subsequently. Despite these efforts at subclassification, the majority of patients present with solitary or multiple areas of involvement in a variety of visceral sites. In most cases, the presenting symptoms and physical signs simply reflect the neoplastic involvement of these organ sites.

The demographics of the UPC patient population mirror those of the general population of patients referred to a large cancer center, except for an excess of men among the UPC patients [2]. The median age is approximately 60 years. The family history frequently identifies additional cancers with established origins in other family members; however, no clearly familial instances of UPC have been reported. Table 23-1 shows the distribution of metastatic sites and histologic classification of 1196 UPC patients from one series. These data have remained unchanged as compared with the original series reported in 1994 [2].

The clinical features outlined have been analyzed to determine their effect on survival. There are considerable differences in survival for the four most frequently encountered pathologic

subtypes of UPC. The median survival for patients with squamous carcinoma (exclusive of patients with mid-high cervical adenopathy) was 13 months; adenocarcinoma, 6 months; carcinoma 11 months; and neuroendocrine carcinoma, 27 months. The state of differentiation or mucin production does not significantly influence the poor survival of patients with adenocarcinoma. The influence of other clinicopathologic features of UPC on survival has been assessed using univariate and multivariate analyses. These data are summarized in Table 23-2. Other studies have documented similar results [27].

Table 23-1. Major Sites of Tumor Involvement and Histologic Diagnoses Identified in 1196 Patients With Unknown Primary Carcinoma

	Patients, n	%
Histologic diagnosis		
Adenocarcinoma	706	59.0
Carcinoma	335	28.0
Squamous carcinoma	75	6.3
Neuroendrocine carcinoma	54	4.5
Unknown/other*	26	2.2
Major metastatic sites		
Lymph nodes	519	43.4
Liver	404	33.8
Bone	334	27.9
Lung	315	26.3
Pleura and pleural space	129	10.8
Peritoneum	118	9.9
Brain	84	7.0
Adrenal	71	5.9
Skin	41	3.4

*Includes malignant neoplasm, 5; and unknown, 21.
Adapted from Abbruzzese and coworkers [2].

Table 23-2. Univariate and Multivariate Survival Analyses

Univariate Survival Analysis

Variable	Grouping	P*	Effect on Survival
Age, years	20–39, 40–49, 50–59, 60–69, 70+	.43	None
Sex	Male, female	.0018	Decreased survival for men
Race	White, other	.86	None
No. of organ sites	1, 2, 3+	.0018	Decreased survival with more organ sites
Involved organ sites			
Lung	—	.0014	Deleterious
Bone	—	.0005	Deleterious
Liver	—	.0050	Deleterious
Pleura	—	.0019	Deleterious
Brain	—	.014	Deleterious
Lymph nodes	—	<.0001	Advantageous
Axillary	—	.0003	Advantageous
Supraclavicular	—	.44	None
Peritoneum	—	.59	None
Skin	—	.69	None
Histology			
Adenocarcinoma	—	<.0001	Deleterious
Carcinoma	—	.0058	Advantageous
Squamous carcinoma	—	.058	Advantageous
Neuroendocrine	—	.0009	Advantageous

Multivariate Survival Analysis

Variable	Relative Risk†	P*	Effect on Survival
Male sex	1.39	.0007	Deleterious
Increasing no. of organ sites	1.23	<.0001	Deleterious
Involved organ sites			
Liver	1.33	.0064	Deleterious
Lymph nodes	0.46	<.0001	Advantageous
Suprclavicular	1.56	.013	Deleterious
Peritoneum	0.59	.0099	Advantageous
Histology			
Adenocarcinoma	1.46	.0001	Deleterious
Neuroendocrine carcinoma	0.30	.0005	Advantageous

*Log-rank test.
†Calculated from the Cox proportional hazards regression.
Adapted from Abbruzzese and coworkers [2]; with permission.

THERAPEUTIC APPROACH AND RESPONSE TO THERAPY

Unknown primary carcinomas are a heterogeneous group of tumors with widely varying natural histories; therefore, in discussing treatment and survival, it is imperative to understand the patient population studied. When all patients are considered, UPC is a highly aggressive neoplasm with an overall median survival of 3 to 4 months in older series [6,22]. Most recent studies have documented median survivals of 9 to 12 months [28–30]. In a series of 657 consecutive patients, the median survival was 11 months [2], and this number has remained consistent in the expanded series of 1196 patients.

The treatment of UPC continues to evolve. Although the majority of patients are treated with systemic chemotherapy, the careful integration of surgery, radiation therapy, and even periods of observation is important in the overall management of these patients [12]. Observation is particularly important for patients with single sites of disease that have received adequate local therapy.

The most common problem is treatment of the patient with progressive metastatic carcinoma or adenocarcinoma involving two or more organ sites [31–55]. Table 25-3 outlines the results from five trials. Recently, Hainsworth and coworkers [56] reported that a combination of carboplatin, paclitaxel, and etoposide was effective for some patients with UPC. Use of a chemosensitivity assay may help guide the selection of the optimal combination [57]. Treatment of these patients remains suboptimal and awaits discovery of novel strategies applicable to other highly resistant adenocarcinomas, such as those originating in the lung or gastrointestinal tract. This situation is contrasted with the management of the favorable subsets described. These patients have been grouped together primarily on the basis of their responsiveness to therapy or favorable natural histories. The number of patients who fall into these groups is small; however, they are important to recognize because specific treatment may significantly extend survival.

Table 23-3. Selected Chemotherapeutic Trials in Unknown Primary Carcinoma

Author	Histology	Regimen	Patients, n	Response, %	Median Survival, mo
Pasterz et al. [27]	Adenocarcinoma and undifferentiated carcinoma	5-FU/adria/cytoxan/cisplatin	44	28	NS
Greco et al. [28]	Poorly differentiated carcinoma and adenocarcinoma	CDDP/vinblastine bleo ± doxorubicin	68	56 (22% CR)	18*
Moertel et al. [31]	Adenocarcinoma	5-FU	88	16	NS
Woods et al. [34]	Adenocarcinoma and undifferentiated carcinoma	Adria/mito-C	25	36	4.5
Raber et al. [41]	Adenocarcinoma and undifferentiated carcimoma	CDDP/VP-16/5-FU	36	22	NS
Lenzi et al. [43]	Adenocarcinoma and poorly differentiated carcinoma	CDDP/5-FU/folinic Acid	31	30	18
Hainsworth et al. [44]	Poorly differentiated carcinoma	CDDP/etoposide	32	60 (32% CR)	NS
Hainsworth et al. [56]	Adenocarcinoma and poorly differentiated carcinoma and adenocarcinoma	Paclitaxel/carboplatin/etoposide	55	47	13.4

*Calculated from data presented.
NS—Not stated.

REFERENCES

1. Greco FA, Hainsworth JD: Cancer of unknown primary site. In *Cancer: Principles and Practice of Oncology*, edn 4. Edited by De Vita VT Jr, Hellman S, Rosenberg SA. Philadelphia: JB Lippincott, 1993:2072–2092.

2. Abbruzzese JL, Abbruzzese MC, Hess KR, *et al.*: Unknown primary carcinoma: natural history and prognostic factors in 657 consecutive patients. *J Clin Oncol* 1994, 12:1272–1280.

3. Abbruzzese JL: An effective strategy for the evaluation of unknown primary tumors. *Cancer Bull* 1989, 41:157.

4. Abbruzzese JL, Abbruzzese MC, Lenzi R, *et al.*: Analysis of a diagnostic strategy for patients with suspected tumors of unknown origin. *J Clin Oncol* 1995, 13:2094–2103.

5. Nystrom JB, Weiner JM, Wolf RM, *et al.*: Identifying the primary site in metastatic cancer of unknown origin: inadequacy of roentgenographic procedures. *JAMA* 1979, 241:381.

6. Newman KH, Nystrom JS: Metastaic cancer of unknown origin: nonsquamous cell type. *Semin Oncol* 1982, 9:427.

7. Stewart JF, Tattersall MHN, Woods RL, *et al.*: Unknown primary adenocarcinoma: incidence of over investigation and natural history. *Br Med J* 1979, 1:1530.

8. Karsell PR, Sheedy PF II, O'Connell MJ: Computed tomography in search of cancer of unknown origin. *JAMA* 1982, 248:340–343.

9. Didolkar MS, Fanous N, Elias EG, *et al.*: Metastatic carcinoma from occult primary tumors: a study of 254 patients. *Ann Surg* 1977, 186:625.

10. McMillan JH, Levine E, Stephens RH: Computed tomography in the evaluation of metastatic adenocarcinoma from an unknown primary site. *Radiology* 1982, 143:143–146.

11. Walsh JW, Rosenfield AT, Jaffe CC, *et al.*: Prospective comparison of ultrasound and computed tomography in the evaluation of gynecologic pelvic masses. *AJR Am J Roentgenol* 1978, 131:955–960.

12. Raber MN, Abbruzzese JL, Frost P: Unknown primary tumors. *Curr Opin Oncol* 1992, 4:3.

13. Shahangian S, Fritsche HA: Serum tumor markers as diagnostic aids in patients with unknown primary tumors. *Cancer Bull* 1989, 41:152.

14. Koch M, McPherson TA: Carcinoembryonic antigen levels as an indicator of the primary site in metastatic disease of unknown origin. *Cancer* 1981, 48:1242.

15. Abbruzzese J, Raber M, Frost P: The role of CA-125 in patients with unknown primary tumors. *Proc Am Soc Clin Oncol* 1990, 9:118.

16. Le Cesne A, Le Chevalier T, Caille P, *et al.*: Metastases from cancers of unknown primary site: data from 302 autopsies. *Pesse Med* 1991, 20:1369–1373.

17. Motzer RJ, Rodriguez E, Reuter VE, *et al.*: Genetic analysis of an aid in diagnostic for patients with midline carcinomas of uncertain histologies. *J Natl Cancer Inst* 1991, 83:341.

18. Ilson DH, Motzer RJ, Rodriguez F, *et al.*: Genetic analysis in the diagnosis of neoplasms of unknown primary site. *Semin Oncol* 1992, 20:229–237.

19. Motzer RJ, Rodriguez E, Reuter VE, *et al.*: Molecular and cytogenetic studies in the diagnosis of patients with poorly differentiated carcinomas of unknown primary site. *J Clin Oncol* 1995, 13:274–182.

20. Bar-Eli M, Abbruzzese JL, Lee-Jackson D, *et al.*: p53 Mutation spectrum in human unknown primary tumors. *Anticancer Res* 1993, 13:1619–1624.

21. Frost P, Raber M, Abbruzzese J: Unknown primary tumors—are they a unique subgroup of neoplastic disease? *Cancer Bull* 1987, 39:216.

22. Nystrom JS, Weiner JM, Heffelfinger-Juttner J, Irwin LE: Metastatic and histologic presentations in unknown primary cancer. *Semin Oncol* 1977, 4:53.

23. Abbruzzese JL, Raber MN: Unknown primary carcinoma. In *Clinical Oncology*. Edited by Abeloff MD, Armitage JO, Lichter AS, Niederhuber JE. New York: Churchill Livingstone; 1995, 1822–1845.

24. Mackay B, Ordoñez NG: The role of the pathologist in the evaluation of poorly differentiated tumors and metastatic tumors of unknown origin. In *Poorly Differentiated Neoplasms and Tumors of Unknown Origin*. Edited by Fer MF, Greco AF, Oldham RK. Orlando; Grune & Stratton, 1986:3.

25. Hainsworth JD, Wright EP, Johnson DH, Davis BW, Greco FA: Poorly differentiated carcinoma of unknown primary site: clinical usefulness of immunoperoxidase staining. *J Clin Oncol* 1991, 9:1931–1938.

26. Ultmann JE, Phillips TL: Cancer of unknown primary site. In *Cancer: Principles and Practice of Oncology*. Edited by DeVita VT Jr, Hellman S, Rosenberg SA. Philadelphia: JB Lippincott, 1989: 1941–1950.

27. Pasterz R, Savaraj N, Burgess M: Prognostic factors in metastatic carcinoma of unknown primary. *J Clin Oncol* 1986, 4:1652.

28. Greco FA, Vaughn WK, Hainsworth JD: Advanced poorly differentiated carcinoma of unknown primary site: recognition of a treatable syndrome. *Ann Intern Med* 1986, 104:547.

29. Sporn JR, Greenberg BR: Empiric chemotherapy in patients with carcinoma of unknown primary site. *Am J Med* 1990, 88:49.

30. Kambhu SA, Kelsen D, Fiore J, Niedzwiecki D, *et al.*: Metastatic adenocarcinomas of unknown primary site. *Am J Clin Oncol* 1990, 13:55.

31. Moertel CG, Reitmeier RJ, Schutt AJ, *et al.*: Treatment of patient with adenocarcinomas of unknown origin. *Cancer* 1972, 30:1469.

32. McKeen E, Smith F, *et al.*: Fluorouracil (F), Adriamycin (A), and mitomycin (M), FAM for adenocarcinoma of unknown origin. *Proc AACR ASCO* 1980, 21:358.

33. Rodnick S, Tremont S, *et al.*: Evaluation and therapy for adenocarcinoma of unknown primary (ACUP), *Proc AACR ASCO* 1981, 22:379.

34. Woods RL, Fox RM, *et al.*: Metastatic adenocarcinomas of unknown primary site. *N Engl J Med* 1980, 303:87–89.

35. Valentine J, Rosenthal S, *et al.*: Combination chemotherapy for adenocarcinoma of unknown primary origin. *Cancer Clin Trials* 1979, 2:265–268.

36. Bedikian AY, Bodley GP, *et al.*: Sequential chemotherapy for adenocarcinoma of unknown primary. *Am J Clin Oncol* 1983, 6:219–224.

37. Goldberg R, Smith F, Veno W, Ahlgren J, Schein P: Treatment of adenocarcinoma of unknown primary with fluorouracil, adriamycin, and mitomycin-C (FAM). *Am Soc Clin Oncol* 1986, 5:129.

38. Walach N: Treatment of adenocarcinoma of unknown origin with cyclophoshamide (C), Oncogin (O), Methotrexte (M), and 5-fluorouracil (F), (COMF). *Proc Am Soc Clin Oncol* 1986, 5:125.

39. Shildt RA, Kennedy PS, Chen TT, *et al.*: Management of patients with metastatic adenocarcinoma of unknown origin: a Southwest Oncology Group study. *Cancer Treat Rep* 1983, 67:77–79.

40. Anderson H, Thatcher N, Rankin E, *et al.*: VAC (Vincristine, Adriamycin, Cyclophosphamide) chemotherapy for metastatic carcinoma from an unknown site. *Eur J Cancer Clin Oncol* 1983, 19:49–52.

41. Raber MN, Faintuch J, Abbruzzese JL, *et al.*: Continuous infusion 5-fluorouracil, etoposide and cis-diamminedichloroplatinum in patients with metastatic carcinoma of unknown primary origin. *Ann Oncol* 1991, 2:519.

42. LeChevalier T, Tremblay J, Rouesse J; *et al.*: Phase II trial of methotrexate-FAM in adenocarcinoma of unknown primary. *Proc ASCO* 1987, 6:130.

43. Lenzi R, Raber MN, Frost P, Schmidt S, Abbruzzese JL: Phase II study of cisplatin, 5FU, and folinic acid in patients with tumors of unknown primary origin. *Eur J Cancer* 1993, 29A:1634.

44. Hainsworth JD, Johnson DH, Greco FA: The role of etoposide in the treatment of poorly differentiated carcinoma of unknown primary site. *Cancer* 1991, 67:310.

45. Lenzi R, Raber MN, Gravel D, Frost P, Abbruzzese JL: Phase I and II trials of a laboratory derived synergistic combination of cisplatin and 2'-deoxy-5-azacytidine. *Int J Oncol* 1995, 6:447–450.

46. Kelsen D, Martin DS, Coloriore J, *et al.*: A Phase II trial of biochemical modulation using *N*-phosphonacetyl-L-aspartate, high-dose methotrexate, high-dose 5-flourouracil, and leucovorin in patients with adenocarcinoma of unknown primary site. *Cancer* 1992, 70:1988.

47. Gill I, Guaglianone P, Gruneberg SM, *et al.*: High dose intensity of cisplatin and etoposide in adenocarcinoma of unknown primary. *Anticancer Res* 1991, 11:1231–1235.

48. Porta C, Moroni M, Nastasi G, *et al.*: COMF combination chemotherapy for the treatment of adenocarcinoma of unknown primary origin. *Ann Oncol* 1992, 3(suppl):48.

49. Trudeau M, Thirlwell MP, Boos G, *et al.*: Cancer of unknown primary syndrome (CUPS): Predictive value of CA-125 in patients treated with 5-fluorouracil, doxorubicin and cisplatin (FAP) [abstract]. *Proc Am Soc Clin Oncol* 1993, 12:399.

50. Ahlgren JD, Bern M, Booth B, *et al.*: Protracted infusional 5FU (PIF): An active, well-tolerated regimen in metastatic adenocarcinoma of undetermined primary (AUP): a mid-Atlantic oncology program (MOAP) study [abstract]. *Proc Am Soc Clin Oncol* 1993, 12:401.

51. Colleoni M, Buzzoni R, Bajetta E: Fluorouracil plus folinic acid in metastatic adenocarcinoma of unknown primary site suggestive or a gastrointestinal primary. *Tumori* 1993, 79:116–118.

52. van der Gaast A, Henzen-Logmans SC, Planting AS, *et al.*: Phase II study of oral administration of etoposide for patients with well- and moderately-differentiated adenocarcinomas of unknown primary site. *Ann Oncol* 1993, 4:789–790.

53. de Campos ES, Menasce LP, Radford J, *et al.*: Metastatic carcinoma of uncertain primary site: a retrospective review of 57 patients treated with vincristine, doxorubicin, cyclophosphamide (VAC) or VAC alternating with cisplatin and etoposide (VAC/PE). *Cancer* 1994, 73:470–475.

54. Akerley W, Thomas A, Miller M, *et al.*: Phase II trial of oral etoposide for carcinoma of unknown primary (CUP) [abstract]. *Proc Am Soc Clin Oncol* 1994, 13:406.

55. Merrouche Y, Lasset C, Trillet-Lenoir V, *et al.*: Phase II study of cisplatin and etoposide in a subgroup of patients with carcinoma of unknown primary [abstract]. *Proc Am Soc Clin Oncol* 1994, 13:401.

56. Hainsworth JD, Erland JB, Kalman LA, *et al.*: Carcinoma of unknown primary site: treatment with 1-hour paclitaxel, carboplatin, and extended-schedule etoposide. *J Clin Oncol* 1997, 15:2385–2393.

57. Hanauske AR, Clark GM, Von Hoff DD: Adenocarcinoma of unknown primary: retrospective analysis of chemosensitivity of 313 freshly explanted tumors in a tumor cloning system. *Invest New Drugs* 1995, 13:43–49.

58. Jesse RH, Perez CA, Fletcher GH: Cervical lymph node metastases: unknown primary cancer. *Cancer* 1973, 31:854.

59. Wang RC, Geopfert H, Barber AE, Wolf P: Unknown primary squamous cell carcinoma metastatic to the neck. *Arch Otolaryngol Head Neck Surg* 1990, 116:1388.

60. Weir L, Keane T, Cummings B, *et al.*: Radiation treatment of cervical lymph node metastases from an unknown primary: an analysis of outcome by treatment volume and other prognostic factors. *Radiother Oncol* 1995, 35:206–211.

61. Marcial-Vega VA, Cardenes H, Perez CA, *et al.*: Cervical metastases from unknown primaries: radiotherapeutic management and appearance of subsequent primaires. *Int J Radiat Oncol Biol Phys* 1990, 19:919.

62. Carlson LS, Fletcher GH, Oswald MJ: Guidelines for the radiotherapeutic techniques for cervical metastases from an unknown primary. *Int J Radiat Oncol Biol Phys* 1986, 12:2101.

63. Talmi YP, Wolf GT, Hazuka M, *et al.*: Unknown primary of the head and neck. *J Laryngol Otol* 1996, 110:353–356.

64. De Braud F, Heilbrun LK, Ahmed K, *et al.*: Metastatic squamous cell carcinoma of an unknown primary localized to the neck: advantages of an aggressive treatment. *Cancer* 1989, 64:510.

65. Lee NK, Byers RM, Abbruzzese JL, Wolf P: Metastatic adenocarcinoma to the neck from an unknown primary. *Am J Surg* 1991, 162:306.

66. Patel J, Nemoto T, Rosner D, *et al.*: Axillary lymph node metastasis from an occult breast cancer. *Cancer* 1981, 47:2923.

67. Ashikari R, Rosen PP, Urban JA, Senoo T: Breast cancer presenting as an axillary mass. *Ann Surg* 1976, 183:415.

68. Ellerbrook N, Holmes F, Singletary E, Evans H, *et al.*: Treatment of patients with isolated axillary nodal metastases from an occult primary carcinoma consistent with breast origin. *Cancer* 1990, 66:1461.

69. Jackson B, Scott-Conner C, Moulder J: Axillary metastasis from occult breast carcinoma: diagnosis and management. *Am Surg* 1995, 61:431–434.

70. Rosen PP: Axillary lymph node metastases in patients with occult noninvasive breast carcinoma. *Cancer* 1980, 46:1298.

71. August CA, Murad TM, Newton M: Multiple focal extraovarian serous carcinoma. *Int J Gynaecol Pathol* 1985, 4:11.

72. Dalrymple JC, Bannatyne P, Russell P, *et al.*: Extraovarian peritoneal serous papillary carcinoma: a clinicopathologic study of 31 cases. *Cancer* 1989, 64:110.

73. Strnad CM, Grosh WN, Baxter J, *et al.*: Peritoneal carcinomatosis of unknown primary site in women. *Ann Intern Med* 1989, 111:213.

74. Ransom DT, Patel SR, Keeney GL, *et al.*: Papillary serous carcinoma of the peritoneum: a review of 33 cases treated with platin-based chemotherapy. *Cancer* 1990, 66:1091.

75. Lenzi R, Hess KR, Abbruzzese MC, *et al.*: Poorly differentiated carcinoma and poorly differentiated adenocarcinoma of unknown origin: favorable subsets of patients with unknown primary carcinoma? *J Clin Oncol* 1997, 15:2056–2066.

76. Farrugia DC, Norman AR, Nicolson MC, *et al.*: Unknown primary carcinoma: randomised studies are needed to identify optimal treatments and their benefits. *Eur J Cancer* 1996, 32A:2256–2261.

77. van der Gaast A, Verweij J, Henzen-Logmans SC, Rodenburg CJ, *et al.*: Carcinoma of unknown primary: identification of a treatable subset? *Ann Oncol* 1990, 1:119.

78. Jones A, Farrow G, Richardson FL: The extragonadal germ cell cancer syndrome: the Mayo Clinic experience. *Poorly Differentiated Neoplasms and Tumors of Unknown Origin*. Edited by Fer MF, Greco FA, Oldham RK. Orlando: Grune & Stratton, 1986:203.

79. Richardson RL, Shoumacher RA, Fer MF, *et al.*: The unrecognized extragonadal germ cell cancer syndrome. *Ann Intern Med* 1981, 94:181.

80. Fox RM, Woods RL, Tattersall MHN: Undifferentiated carcinoma in young men: the atypical teratoma syndrome. *Lancet* 1979, 1:1316.

81. Currow DC, Findlay M, Cox K, *et al.*: Elevated germ cell markers in carcinoma of uncertain primary site do not predict response to platinum based chemotherapy. *Eur J Cancer* 1996, 32A:2357–2359.

82. Hainsworth JD, Johnson DH, Greco FA: Cisplatin-based combination chemotherapy in the treatment of poorly differentiated carcinoma and poorly differentiated adenocarcinoma of unknown primary site: results of a 12-year experience. *J Clin Oncol* 1992, 10:912–922.

83. Hainsworth JD, Johnson DH, Greco FA: Poorly differentiated neuroendocrine carcinoma of unknown primary site. A newly recognized clinicopathologic entity. *Ann Intern Med* 1988, 109:364–371.

84. Moertel CG, Kvols LK, O'Connell MJ, Rubin J: Treatment of neuroendocrine carcinomas with combined etoposide and cisplatin: evidence of major therapeutic acitivty in the anaplastic variants of these neoplasms. *Cancer* 1991, 68:227.

85. Hess K, Abbruzzese MC, Lenzi R, *et al.*: Classification and regression tree analysis of 1000 consecutive patients with unknown primary carcinoma [abstract]. *Proc Am Soc Clin Oncol* 1996, 15:452.

SQUAMOUS CARCINOMA INVOLVING MID-HIGH CERVICAL LYMPH NODES

High cervical adenopathy with squamous carcinoma is an important clinical subset because of its well-defined natural history and responsiveness to therapy [58–61]. With appropriate evaluation, including direct visualization of the hypopharynx, nasopharynx, larynx, and upper esophagus, an occult primary lesion will be frequently identified. When no primary is found, aggressive local therapy is applied to the involved neck [60–62]. Thirty percent to 50% of 5-year survivals have been reported with radical neck surgery, high-dose radiotherapy, or a combination of both modalities. A potential advantage of radiation therapy is that the suspected primary anatomic sites (nasopharynx, oropharynx, and hypopharynx) can be included in the radiation port [60,62]. Recent studies suggest that the eventual emergence of the primary site adversely affects the prognosis [63]. The role of chemotherapy in these patients is unclear. One randomized study, however, suggested that chemotherapy with cisplatin and 5-fluorouracil improved the response rate and median survival relative to radiation alone [64].

Patients with adenocarcinoma involving mid-high cervical nodes and patients with lower cervical or supraclavicular adenopathy of all histologies have a much poorer prognosis [65]. These patients are managed with local measures (usually radiation therapy) or may be candidates for systemic chemotherapy protocols.

RECOMMENDED THERAPY

Low N-stage (NX, N1, or N2A): surgery followed by radiation therapy (> 50 Gy) or radiation therapy alone (minimum 50 Gy) to ipsilateral neck with or without nasooropharynx.
High N-stage (N2B, N3A, N3B) or poorly differentiated tumors: cisplatin 100 mg/m^2 d 1, 22, and 43 with concurrent radiation therapy **or** cisplatin 100 mg/m^2 d 1 plus 5-FU 1000 mg/m^2/d by continuous infusion d 1–5. Repeat courses of cisplatin and 5-FU every 3–4 wk for three courses followed by radiation therapy.

WOMEN WITH ISOLATED AXILLARY ADENOPATHY

Isolated axillary adenopathy secondary to metastatic adenocarcinoma usually occurs in women and has unique clinical features. Many of these women have occult breast primaries, which can be identified in 40% to 70% of these patients who undergo mastectomy [66,67]. In this setting, rebiopsy of involved axillary nodes for estrogen and progesterone levels should be considered in view of the influence of this information on diagnosis and management. Management is based on the treatment of stage II breast cancer, and this should include both local and systemic therapies. Prognosis following treatment is comparable to women with stage II breast cancer [68,69]. Older series have advocated modified radical mastectomy and axillary dissection for primary treatment [66,67,70]. A series of 42 patients suggested that survival was superior in patients receiving systemic chemotherapy, and local control was improved by irradiating the breast and the axilla [68]. The actuarial disease-free survival in this study was 71% at 5 years and 65% at 10 years.

Patients with axillary adenopathy and involvement of additional sites (usually liver or bone) or with nonadenocarcinoma histology constitute a much more heterogeneous group composed of equal numbers of men and women as well as a broader histologic spectrum with poorly differentiated carcinoma and neuroendocrine carcinomas represented in addition to adenocarcinoma. The survival of patients with axillary adenopathy and other involved organ sites is intermediate between that of the overall UPC population and women with isolated axillary adenopathy [23].

The management of patients with involvement of the axilla as well as other sites or nonadenocarcinoma histology is less certain. These patients generally are approached using a combination of local and systemic modalities and again may be good candidates for novel systemic chemotherapy protocols.

RECOMMENDED THERAPY

General principles are based on the management of women with stage II breast cancer. Tamoxifen is added to the systemic therapy of patients with estrogen receptor–positive neoplasms.

Modified radical mastectomy with axillary nodal dissection followed by systemic chemotherapy with 5-FU, doxorubicin, FAC or similar regimen for six courses **or** chemotherapy with FAC, or similar regimen for six to eight courses followed by radiation therapy to the ipsilateral breast and axillary nodes. (Axillary dissection can be considered before chemotherapy to assess receptor status and complete nodal staging but increases the risk of arm edema following radiation therapy.)

PERITONEAL CARCINOMATOSIS

Women with diffuse peritoneal carcinomatosis with adenocarcinoma constitute another recently recognized subset. These patients form a distinctive subset because of their clinical similarities to typical ovarian carcinoma. Often, papillary histology and evaluations in CA-125 are found, but exploratory laparotomy fails to document a primary [71,72]. Other workers have also recognized this patient subset, terming this syndrome peritoneal papillary serous carcinoma or multifocal extraovarian serous carcinoma. These patients frequently respond to platinum-based chemotherapy [72–74]. Many patients in these series also underwent exploratory laparotomy with surgical debulking followed by chemotherapy. Median survivals are reported to be 16 months to 2 years.

The natural histories of men with isolated peritoneal carcinomatosis or patients with histologies inconsistent with ovarian carcinoma (*eg*, mucin-positive adenocarcinoma) or additional metastatic sites are much more poorly characterized, but overall survival, even with therapy, is poor.

RECOMMENDED THERAPY

Papillary serous carcinoma of the peritoneum: surgical debulking followed by systemic chemotherapy with carboplatin AUC=6 d 1 plus paclitaxel 175 mg/m^2 both IV d 1, repeat every 3–4 wk.
Adenocarcinoma of the peritoneum: systemic chemotherapy using cisplatin 75 mg/m^2 IV d 1; folinic acid 500 mg/m^2 in 200 mL normal saline IV over 2 h d 1–5; 5-FU 375 mg/m^2 IV after 1 h of folinic acid d 1–5; carboplatin AUC=6 d 1 plus paclitaxel 175 mg/m^2 both IV d 1, repeat every 3–4 wk; or a similar regimen.

POORLY DIFFERENTIATED AND UNDIFFERENTIATED CARCINOMA

Approximately one third of patients with UPC are defined as having this histologic picture. In this subset, detailed histochemical or immunohistochemical studies are most likely to identify highly treatment-responsive patients with lymphoma (leukocyte common antigen), germ cell (β-HCG, AFP), or neuroendocrine (neuron-specific enolase, chromogranin) neoplasms [25]. Additionally, Greco and coworkers [28] have identified a group of patients with poorly differentiated carcinoma or poorly differentiated adenocarcinoma that are responsive to platinum-based chemotherapy. Other investigators, however, conclude that these highly responsive patients are infrequently encountered in a consecutive series of UPC patients [75,76]. Most of these patients had clinical features (young age, mediastinal and retroperitoneal involvement, and rapid growth) of the extragonadal germ cell syndrome [77–80]. Many of these patients are male and have elevated β-HCG or AFP, although the usefulness of these serum tumor markers in predicting response is in question [75,81]. Motzer and coworkers [17] identified abnormalities in chromosome 12 specific for germ cell neoplasms in a group of male patients with poorly differentiated carcinoma involving midline structures confirming the germ cell origin of these tumors.

Combination chemotherapy regimens specific for germ cell carcinoma of testicular origin have usually been employed in the treatment of these patients [28,82]. These regimens have produced documented complete responses and an actual 10-year disease-free survival of 16% [82].

RECOMMENDED TREATMENT

Cisplatin 20 mg/m^2 d for 5 d plus etoposide 100 mg/m^2 d for 3–5 d with or without bleomycin 30 U/wk. Assess response after two courses of therapy; total of four to six courses for responding patients. Alternative approaches include carboplatin AUC=6 plus paclitaxel 200 mg/m^2 by 1-h infusion plus oral etoposide 50 mg/m^2 in 200 mL normal saline IV over 2 h d 1–5, 5-FU 375 mg/m^2 IV after 1 h of folinic acid d 1–5.

POORLY DIFFERENTIATED NEUROENDOCRINE CARCINOMA

Poorly differentiated (anaplastic) neuroendocrine carcinoma is an emerging clinicopathologic entity recognized primarily for its responsiveness to therapy. There is probably considerable overlap with extrapulmonary small cell carcinomas, anaplastic carcinoid, anaplastic islet cell tumors, Merkel's cell tumors, and paragangliomas. Histologically, these tumors are poorly differentiated, but histo-chemical stains are positive for chromogranin or neuron-specific enolase. These patients often present with diffuse hepatic or bone metastases but do not have the indolent histologic or clinical features of typical carcinoid tumors, islet cell tumors, or paragangliomas, and thus observation may not be appropriate. These tumors are also highly responsive to cisplatin-based chemotherapy [83,84].

RECOMMENDED THERAPY

Etoposide 130 mg/m^2 daily for 3 d plus cisplatin 45 mg/m^2 on d 2 and 3; courses repeated every 4 wk.

PATIENTS WITH ADENOCARCINOMA OR CARCINOMA OF UNKNOWN ORIGIN

The optimistic results for the favorable patients described previously do not apply to the vast majority of patients with UPC. Two thirds of UPC patients have metastatic adenocarcinoma with involvement of two or more visceral sites, usually some combination of liver, lung, lymph nodes, or bone. In addition, many men and women with poorly differentiated carcinoma or poorly differentiated adenocarcinoma have none of the clinical features outlined and respond poorly to chemotherapy [75]. Even in series showing optimistic results for selected patients with poorly differentiated carcinoma or poorly differentiated adenocarcinoma, the overall median survival remains poor at 12 months [82].

For unselected patients, numerous empiric chemotherapy combinations have been reported. Many have been based on doxorubicin (Adriamycin), 5-fluorouracil, or cisplatin. A recent report using carboplatin, paclitaxel, and etoposide reported that 47% (25 of 53 patients) had objective responses [56]. In this series, seven patients (13%) experiences complete responses. The actuarial median survival for the entire group, however, was 13.4 months. The disappointing aspect of this survival statistic is that it is not substantially different from the 11-month median survival reported in large consecutive series of UCP patients [2,85]. There is little information on the use of biologic agents alone or with chemotherapy. Response rates generally range from 20% to 30%; however, most responses are partial and brief, resulting in little or no impact on median survival. Newer regimens continue to be tested; however, there has been no substantial progress in the treatment of these patients to date (*see* Table 23–3).

RECOMMENDED THERAPY

Cisplatin 20 mg/m^2 for 5 d plus etoposide 100 mg/m^2 for 3–5 days **or** cisplatin 100 mg/m^2 plus etoposide 100 mg/m^2 for 3 d (repeat courses administered every 3–4 wk); **or** paclitaxel 200 mg/m^2 by 1 h IV infusion d 1, carboplatin calculated AUC=6 IV d 1, etoposide 50 mg alternated with 100 mg/m^2 PO d 1–10 (repeat courses administered every 21 d); **or** cisplatin 75 mg/m^2 IV d 1, folinic acid 500 mg/m^2 in 200 mL normal saline IV over 2 h d 1–5, 5-FU 375 mg/m^2 IV after 1 h of folinic acid 1–5, or similar regimen (repeat courses administered every 28 d).

In 1981, the appearance of Kaposi's sarcoma (KS) and *Pneumocystis carinii* pneumonia in homosexual men on the East and West coasts of United States, respectively, heralded the onset of the AIDS epidemic. A year later the first cases of non-Hodgkin's lymphoma (NHL) were reported. The first cases of primary central nervous system (CNS) lymphoma were reported in New York City in 1983. By 1985, the Centers for Disease Control and Prevention (CDC) revised the case definition for AIDS-surveillance reporting to include NHL. In 1993, invasive cervical carcinoma was also added to this list by the CDC as an index AIDS-defining neoplasm. These AIDS-defining neoplasms are characterized by aggressive clinical behavior with higher-grade lesions, more advanced stage, and shortened survival when compared with similar neoplasms in HIV-seronegative or HIV-indeterminate individuals [1].

More recently, reports from follow-up of the Multicenter AIDS Cohort Study and other epidemiological studies in the United States, Europe, Africa, and Australia have identified several neoplasms that are increased in incidence in patients with underlying HIV infection [2–4]. These neoplasms include intraepithelial anogenital neoplasia; Hodgkin's disease; seminoma; pediatric leiomyosarcoma and other soft tissue sarcomas; squamous cell carcinoma of the conjunctiva in Africa; and plasma cell neoplasms inclusive of multiple myeloma and perhaps plasmacytoma. In addition, other well-characterized neoplasms are encountered in this particular patient population and include squamous cell carcinoma of the skin, nonseminoma germ cell tumors, oral mucosa carcinoma, head and neck carcinoma, lung cancer, and malignant melanoma [5–7].

There is a paucity of a particular neoplasm that one might surmise would be seen in increased incidence in HIV-infected populations. Hepatitis B infection has long been linked to the development of hepatocellular carcinoma. Patients at risk for HIV and hepatitis B infection share common risk behaviors. The emergence of hepatocellular carcinoma as a significant malignant complication of HIV infection has not been seen. This may be attributable to the long latency period of hepatitis B infection prior to the development of hepatocellular carcinoma in patients without HIV infection. As we near the end of the second decade of the epidemic, the spectrum of malignancy in HIV-infected patients is clearly expanding (Table 24-1). This chapter will briefly comment on putative pathogenetic mechanisms of neoplasia in HIV infection. The major focus will be on the evolving therapeutic approach to patients with AIDS-related KS and NHL and also the diagnostic approach in patients with AIDS-related primary CNS lymphoma. A limited discussion about salient clinical aspects and treatment of other HIV-associated neoplasms is also included.

PATHOGENESIS

The clinical paradigm for analyzing these observations on HIV-associated malignancy includes the development of neoplastic complications in patients who have undergone solid organ transplantation [8]. It is known that KS and NHL are seen in increased incidence in patients with other immunodeficient states, whether congenital or acquired. What is less well recognized is that other tumors—especially squamous cell carcinoma of the skin and lips, cervical carcinoma, and other anogenital tract neoplasms—are also seen in increased incidence in patients who have undergone organ transplantation. Gastric carcinoma has been described in increased incidence in other immunodeficient states as well. It may not be surprising, therefore, to see increased numbers of HIV-infected patients develop solid tumors other than those that have been so characteristic since the inception of the epidemic.

Progressive immunologic deterioration is the hallmark of HIV infection, and malignancy evolves in this context in the majority of HIV-infected patients. The pathogenesis of AIDS-defining and HIV-associated neoplasia is no doubt complex and multifactorial, and much remains to be elucidated. The HIV virus is generally not thought to be an oncogenic virus [9]. However, a recent report suggests a more direct pathogenetic role for HIV infection because HIV viral genome has been found incorporated into the *fur*-gene complex on chromosome 15 in non–B-cell malignant lymphoma cells [10]. This suggestion warrants further study. What is known is that the HIV *tat*-gene protein product is a growth factor for KS [11]. These observations lend further support to a more direct link between HIV infection and malignancy.

Other concurrent viral infections in HIV-infected patients (eg, Epstein–Barr virus [EBV], human papillomavirus, and hepatitis B) are likely implicated in the development of malignancy as well. There are well-recognized epidemiologic links to malignancy, capacity for oncogenic transformation, or both for each of these viruses. A recent study has identified EBV viral genome in smooth muscle cells in leiomyosarcomas in pediatric patients and another young man, all of whom were HIV-infected [12]. In another study of HIV infection and Hodgkin's disease, 78% of cases were associated with EBV [13]. Sequences of an apparently new herpes-like virus have also been identified in patients with AIDS-related KS, body cavity–based NHL, and multicentric Castleman's disease [14–17]. In addition, this virus has also been demonstrated to infect bone marrow cells in HIV-seronegative patients with multiple myeloma [18]. Other reports have suggested that patients receiving prolonged antiretroviral (zidovudine) therapy with progressive and severe underlying immunosuppression (CD4 lymphocyte count < 50/μL) may have an increased probability of developing malignant lymphoma [19,20]. It is paradoxical that as HIV-infected patients live longer because of improvements in antiretroviral therapy and the recognition, management, and prophylaxis of opportunistic infections, they will be at

Table 24-1. Spectrum of Neoplastic Disease in HIV Infection

AIDS-defining neoplasms
  Kaposi's sarcoma
  Primary central nervous system lymphoma
  Non-Hodgkin's lymphoma
  Cervical carcinoma
Neoplasms with an increased incidence
  Anogenital neoplasia and squamous cell carcinoma of the anus
  Squamous cell carcinoma conjunctiva (newly reported in Africa)
  Hodgkin's disease (newly reported)
  Seminoma (newly reported)
  Pediatric leiomyosarcoma (newly reported)
  Plasmacytoma and multiple myeloma (likely)
Neoplasms that are well characterized
  Squamous cell carcinoma of the skin
  Nonseminomatous germ cell tumors
  Oral mucosa and head and neck carcinoma
  Lung cancer
  Malignant melanoma

increased risk for the development of neoplastic disease. The spectrum of malignancy in HIV infection is complex and heterogeneous. Improved understanding of the pathogenesis of HIV infection will likely lead to better insight of malignant transformation.

KAPOSI'S SARCOMA

EPIDEMIOLOGY

At the outset of the HIV epidemic, up to 40% to 50% of patients presented with KS as their index AIDS-defining illness. Nearly half of patients presented with disseminated disease; survival was very short, and their therapy was complicated by the underlying immunosuppression of HIV infection [21]. Many of these clinical features of AIDS (epidemic) KS were akin to those initially described in the African endemic form in children in the 1960s. It is well recognized that HIV-infected homosexual men have a 75,000-fold increased risk of developing KS versus the U.S. general population and that this risk is approximately 7 times greater than that for other HIV-risk-behavior groups. Presently, the incidence of AIDS-related KS is declining, which may be a manifestation of the changing risk-behavior profile of HIV-infected patients, new surveillance case definition (with CD4 lymphocyte count < 200/μL meeting clinical criteria for AIDS), and the development of wasting or other illnesses that may precede a diagnosis of KS.

The impact of current highly active antiretroviral therapies (HAART) employed in the clinic on the incidence of KS is under investigation. Presently, the annual risk of developing KS remains fairly constant over the duration of HIV infection, and as patients live longer, it is more likely they will develop the disease. It is projected that 15% to 20% of patients with HIV infection are destined to develop KS. Given the global implications of the AIDS epidemic, KS is now recognized as the leading cancer in males (48% of registered cases) and the second most common cancer in females (18%) in Kampala, Uganda; these percentages parallel the evolution of the epidemic [22]. There appears to be an early peak of KS in African children as well. The incidence of childhood disease has risen more than 40-fold in the era of AIDS, and 78% of cases tested were HIV-seropositive [22].

VIROLOGY OF KAPOSI'S SARCOMA–ASSOCIATED HERPESVIRUS/HUMAN HERPESVIRUS-8

By the end of 1994, Chang and coworkers [14] were the first to report a unique DNA sequence associated with KS in patients with AIDS, using representational difference analysis. These sequences were of nonhuman origin and were closely homologous to minor capsid and tegument protein genes of the Gammaherpesvirinae (rhadinovirus subgroup), herpesvirus saimiri, and EBV virus. It was soon recognized that this new virus was also present in KS patients without HIV infection. With the discovery of KS-associated herpesvirus/human herpesvirus-8 (KSHV/HHV-8), it is now known that 1) KSHV is found in essentially all forms of KS (95% of patients) regardless of HIV serostatus; 2) the virus is localized to KS lesions/spindle cell and not normal skin; 3) the virus also infects peripheral blood and is found in semen; 4) KSHV-antibody seroprevalence matches KS risk groups and geographic distribution with higher rates in the Mediterranean, Eastern Europe, and Africa; 5) background seroprevalence in areas with a lower incidence of KS (eg, the United Kingdom and the United States) are 2% to 3%; and 6) approximately 50% of AIDS-associated KS patients seroconvert within 3 to 4 years prior to developing the disease [15,23–27]. All of these epidemio-

logic and biologic features of KSHV not only link this virus to the disease but are suggestive of a more direct pathogenetic role. This virus has also been implicated in the pathogenesis of the emerging and distinct clinicopathologic entity of body-cavity-based or primary effusion lymphoma and multicentric Castleman's disease in HIV-infected patients [16,17].

PATHOGENESIS

It has been well established that the HIV *tat*-gene protein product is a potent growth factor for KS [11,28–30]. This protein increases bFGF and promotes migration and adhesion of vascular endothelial cells, which are deemed to be important in the development of the spindle tumors characteristic of KS [31,32]. Additional pathogenetic mechanisms involved include HIV-associated immune activation, dysregulation of cytokine modulatory pathways—with both inflammatory cytokines (interleukin-1 [IL-1], IL-6, tumor necrosis factor α [TNF α], and interferon) and angiogenic cytokines (basic fibroblast growth factor and vascular endothelial growth factor) having pivotal roles—and coexisting viral infection [33–35].

The KSHV/HHV-8 virus is no doubt implicated in the development of KS, but presently there is no direct proof that the virus in oncogenic or capable of immortalizing infected B cell or endothelial cell lines (*ie*, a transforming virus). This is substantiated by the lack of any animal or in vitro models, and it is noteworthy that the KS Y-1 cell line—an immortal neoplastic KS cell line—is without evidence of HHV-8 infection [36]. Nonetheless, the virus does contain numerous homologous genes that 1) stimulate cellular proliferation (v-cyclin, v–G-protein–coupled receptor/v–IL-8–receptor, and v–interferon regulatory factor); 2) inhibit apoptosis (vbcl-2, v–FLICE inhibitory protein, and vIL-6); and 3) play a role in recruitment of inflammatory cells and angiogenesis (vIL-6 and v–macophage inflammatory protein) [37,38]. The virus is potentially equipped to maintain a latent state in B cells or KS-associated endothelial cells but does not contain the necessary genes as seen in other rhadinoviruses (Stp, Tip), which can result in malignant transformation. In addition, there are no corresponding EBV nuclear antigens or latent membrane proteins, which are crucial for the maintenance of viral latency and for growth transformation of the host cell.

In summary, likely infection of normal mesenchymal progenitor cells by KSHV/HHV-8 results in activation/transformation to a "pre-KS" cell. Unlike normal mesenchymal progenitors, these cells acquire responsiveness to HIV *tat* and various cellular cytokines (eg, bFGF, IL-1, IL-6, oncostatin-M, and TNF alpha) [33]. The resultant cytokine dysregulation, secondary to the underlying HIV infection, promotes the proliferation and differentiation of the KS tumor by various endogenous and exogenous (autocrine and paracrine) growth factors. Proliferation is further stimulated by progressive immunosuppression, cytokine perturbations associated with HIV infection, and modulation by HIV *tat*. Ultimately, these cells grow in an uncontrolled manner that may be clonal in nature and recognized clinically as KS. Androgen-receptor-fragment analysis suggests that in some instances the transformation process may proceed to clonal proliferation [39]. An improved understanding of the pathogenesis of KS will no doubt lead to pathogenesis or mechanistically based therapeutic interventions, some of which are currently being investigated in the clinic.

THERAPEUTIC APPROACH

It is important to briefly mention that prospective follow-up and validation of the AIDS Clinical Trials Group (ACTG) clinical staging system of T (tumor, ulceration, edema, nodular oral disease, or visceral involvement), I (immune status and CD4 lymphocyte count ≥ 200/μL), and S (systemic illness, KPS > 70%, and B symptoms [inclusive of fever, weight loss, night sweats or diarrhea, and prior AIDS-defining opportunistic infection]) have recently confirmed its prognostic value [40,41]. This TIS system gives a score of 0 (good risk) or 1 (poor risk) for each of these factors. Tumor stage and CD4 lymphocyte count (especially < 150/μL) provide the most predictive information. AIDS-related KS is much more aggressive, associated with shortened duration of response, and generally pursues a relentless progressive course (the tempo of which may be variable at the outset when compared with de novo disease). For this reason it is often not desirable to "watch and wait" or delay treatment. In addition, there are clearly acceptable cosmetic indications to pursue some form of therapy, inclusive of liquid nitrogen cryotherapy, intralesional chemotherapy, or interferon. In patients with AIDS-related KS, radiation is usually reserved as a last resort for palliative intervention because it often precludes the administration of effective doses of systemic therapy into the tumor bed. Nonetheless, radiation can provide effective palliation [42].

Numerous chemotherapeutic agents have documented efficacy in KS and primarily include bleomycin, doxorubicin, etoposide, and the vinca alkaloids (eg, vinblastine and vincristine) [43,44]. Single-agent chemotherapy is clearly better tolerated with a broad range of response rates ranging between 10% to 75% [43]. Newer agents, such as the liposomal anthracyclines (doxorubicin and daunorubicin as first-line therapy) and paclitaxel (as salvage therapy), are efficacious [45–49]. Vinorelbine is a new vinca alkaloid that is currently undergoing evaluation in KS as well. Combination chemotherapy regimens—historically BV (bleomycin and vincristine) and ABV (doxorubicin, bleomycin, and vincristine)—are known to yield higher response rates (40%–85%) with more toxicity [43,50]. Results from recent randomized clinical trials suggest that single-agent liposomal anthracyclines have an improved therapeutic index over ABV [45,47]. For many patients, liposomal anthracyclines constitute appropriate first-line therapy. In patients with severe pulmonary disease, it may be prudent to administer ABV because this regimen has been demonstrated to be helpful in this setting [51]. Perhaps more importantly, with the improved understanding of the pathogenesis of KS, therapeutic interventions are evolving that are mechanistically based [52]. It will be helpful 1) to define the impact of current protease inhibitors and HAART regimens on the natural history of the disease [53], 2) to explore the impact of antiviral therapy on the underlying viral disease (and if this may result in prophylaxis of KS in high-risk patient populations) [54], and 3) to begin to tailor treatment strategies that modulate the various cytokine perturbations that have been demonstrated to promote tumor growth (eg, angiogenesis inhibitors [55], thalidomide → ↓ TNF α, IL-4 → ↓ IL-6, metalloprotease inhibitors → ↓ bFGF, neutralizing Ab → ↓ IL-1, topical retinoids, β human chronic gonadotropin [56], and antiviral therapy → HHV-8 [53,54]).

NON-HODGKIN'S LYMPHOMA

EPIDEMIOLOGY

Shortly after the onset of the AIDS epidemic, systemic B-cell NHL was seen in increased incidence in HIV-infected patients and was added to the case definition list. Approximately 5% to 10% of HIV-infected patients are destined to develop lymphoma [57]. NHL is the AIDS-defining illness in approximately 3% of HIV-infected

patients. As experience with nucleoside analog antiretroviral monotherapy (zidovudine) was gained, there was some initial concern about long-term administration and risk of developing NHL [19,20,58,59]. Clearly, the risk of developing lymphoma steadily increases with duration of HIV infection and advancing immunosuppression. It is now possible with the discovery of the protease inhibitors and emergence of HAART to achieve near-complete suppression of HIV viral load and obtain more sustained elevations in CD4 lymphocyte counts, both of which appear important in achieving at least partial immune restoration. The significance of this remains to be sorted out, but it is conceivable that long-term survivors of HIV infection will likely remain at increased risk for NHL. This would be reminiscent of the experience with patients undergoing solid organ transplantation and the life-long increased risk of lymphoma (among other tumors) because of attendant iatrogenic immunosuppression.

PATHOGENESIS

The pathogenesis of lymphoma in the setting of HIV infection is no doubt complex, and much remains to be elucidated. What is known is the following factors are all implicated:progressive immune suppression; chronic antigen stimulation and B-cell proliferation; associated immune activation and dysregulation of cytokine modulatory pathways (IL-6 and IL-10 in particular); altered bcl-6, p53 and c-myc protooncogene expression; and coexisting viral infections [1,60–63]. Several recent developments have further unveiled the potential role of viral oncogenesis in the pathogenesis of AIDS-related lymphoma and perhaps other B-cell neoplasms:1) EBVs long-standing association with systemic and CNS NHL; 2) HIV viral genome has been found incorporated into the fur-gene complex on chromosome 15 in non–B-cell lymphoma cells upstream to c-fes (a proto-oncogene) [10,64]; 3) KSHV/HHV-8 has recently been identified in HIV-infected patients with body-cavity-based NHL or primary effusion lymphoma and multicentric Castleman's disease and also in bone marrow dendritic cells of HIV-seronegative multiple myeloma patients [16–18,65].

THERAPEUTIC APPROACH

In general, AIDS-related NHL is characterized by higher grade (40%–60%), greater predilection for extranodal disease (80%), more advanced clinical stage (60%–70% stage III/IV) and shortened survival (median, 7–8 mo) when compared with lymphomas in HIV-seronegative patients [57,66,67]. At the time of presentation, the median CD4 lymphocyte count is 100/μL [68]. It was recognized early on that the clinical course was much more aggressive [69]. This in fact lead to the evaluation of more aggressive and dose-intensive combination chemotherapy regimens in this disease at the outset. Early results were dismal, regimens were poorly tolerated, and there was a trend for shortened survival [70]. More traditional NHL combination chemotherapy regimens were then evaluated in conjunction with 1) antiretroviral therapy [71], 2) the incorporation of colony-stimulating factors (CSFs) (of which granulocyte–macrophage CSF [GM-CSF] is known to upregulate HIV viral replication) [72], and 3) use of various CNS prophylaxis strategies because of the proclivity of AIDS-related lymphoma to disseminate or relapse in the CNS [71]. Complete responses ranged between 20% and 60%, with median survival durations of between 4 and 7 months [67,73].

Most recently, the ACTG completed the largest randomized clinical trial in AIDS-related NHL. The ACTG 142 study compared standard dose (SD) m-BACOD (methotrexate, bleomycin, doxorubicin, cyclophosphamide, vincristine, dexamethasone) plus GM-CSF with a dose-modified (low-dose [LD]) m-BACOD [68]. All patients received intrathecal cytosine arabinoside for meningeal prophylaxis during the first cycle of chemotherapy. The results of this study confirm that hematologic toxicity was significantly less, and overall, the dose-modified regimen was better tolerated with equivalent efficacy (complete response [CR] was 39% LD and 52% SD [$P = 0.56$], with median survival durations of 35 wk LD and 31 wk SD [$P = 0.25$]). Poor prognostic factors were identified inclusive of age over 35 years, history of injection drug use, stage III/IV disease, and (most important) a CD4 lymphocyte count of less than 100/µL [68,74]. A 3% CNS relapse rate was observed.

The longest median survival reported for AIDS-related NHL is 18 months in a single-institution study [75–77]. These patients were treated with a 96-hour continuous infusion of CDE (cyclophosphamide, doxorubicin, and etoposide), which is in the midst of confirmatory evaluation in both HIV-seronegative/positive patients with NHL in the Eastern Cooperative Oncology Group setting. An oral combination chemotherapy regimen has been developed inclusive of lomustine (CCNU), etoposide, cyclophosphamide, and procarbazine (also in a single-institution study) [78,79]. The rationale for this regimen was straightforward and took advantage of oral administration, in vitro synergy, and known first-line efficacy of the drugs in NHL; also two of the agents (CCNU and procarbazine) cross the blood-brain barrier. This regimen precluded the potential cardiotoxicity of doxorubicin-based regimens and avoided the additional immunosuppressive effects of corticosteroids. The addition of G-CSF to the regimen decreased the frequency of hospitalization for febrile neutropenia and decreased the incidence of leukopenia-related discontinuation of chemotherapy [79]. Thrombocytopenia, however, was more severe. The overall objective response rate with this regimen is 66% (CR 34%), with a 5% CNS relapse rate and median survival duration of 7 months [78,79]. In addition, 33% of patients survived one year, 11% survived two years, and 50% survived free from progression of their lymphoma.

The National Cancer Institute has recently reported a pilot study of EPOCH (etoposide, prednisone, vincristine, cyclophosphamide, doxorubicin) combination chemotherapy, the bulk of which is administered as a continuous infusion, with an objective CR of 60% and median survival of 5.6 months [80]. In this study, HIV viral burden was monitored closely in eight patients on days 1 and 6 of each cycle and at 3 and 6 weeks after chemotherapy. Antiretroviral therapy was withheld during chemotherapy because of overlapping toxicity. There was no apparent worsening of viral burden during chemotherapy administration, and in fact, there was a trend for lower viral burden between days 1 and 6 (median d 1 [17,000 RNA copies/muL plasma] vs median d 6 [8150 RNA copies/µL plasma]; $P < 0.01$) [80]. These observations suggest that cytotoxic chemotherapy may not adversely effect underlying HIV viral burden and clearly needs to be extended to larger numbers of patients with AIDS-related NHL. In a report of CEOP (cyclophosphamide, epirubicin, vincristine, prednisone) combination chemotherapy in Australia, similar results were obtained with an 82% objective response rate (47% CR) and median survival of 10 months [81].

It is important to note that from observation of recent clinical trials, approximately 10% to 20% of patients may be cured or, more appropriately, survive free from progression of their lymphoma. In patients with good prognostic factors at presentation, up to 30% may survive 3 years, and select patients may be appropriate candidates for more traditional or aggressive cytotoxic therapy [74]. As a result, salvage therapy (which has been very discouraging to date) may be increasingly important. Nonetheless, preliminary results with mitoguazone have been promising [82].

Treatment recommendations can be summarized as follows. The results of ACTG 142 imply that a dose-modified chemotherapy approach is appropriate for the majority of patients with AIDS-related NHL. However, it remains to be established which therapeutic regimen is the optimal. All patients should receive *P. carinii* pneumonia prophylaxis. It is probably preferable to continue effective antiretroviral regimens with chemotherapy, although this is under investigation. CSF support is likely warranted in the majority of patients. The role of routine CNS prophylaxis has yet to be defined and should be discouraged; exceptions may include patients with high-grade histologies, bone marrow involvement, and bulky lesions (particularly of the head and neck/paranasal sinus and epidural areas) that may invade the CNS. Patients with no adverse prognostic factors may be candidates for standard treatment approaches to improve the overall survival.

PRIMARY CENTRAL NERVOUS SYSTEM LYMPHOMA

EPIDEMIOLOGY AND PATHOGENESIS

Since the inception of the AIDS epidemic, primary CNS lymphoma (PCL) was regarded as an AIDS-defining neoplasm. Approximately 1% to 2% of HIV-infected patients develop PCL [57]. The overall incidence of this neoplasm in the general population is increasing, which is independent of the AIDS epidemic. Invariably, this tumor is encountered in patients with profound immunodeficiency (CD4 lymphocyte counts < 50/µL) and there is the ubiquitous association of this tumor with EBV infection. This latter observation may in fact be of considerable diagnostic importance.

DIAGNOSTIC EVALUATION

The diagnosis of AIDS-related PCL is challenging because of its protean manifestations. The lack of focal findings and the broad differential diagnosis in HIV-infected patients who present with soft neurologic findings often contribute to a delayed or missed diagnosis [83,84]. In one series of AIDS patients with PCL, an antemortem diagnosis was established in only half of patients [85]. The initial evaluation of an HIV-infected patient with suspected CNS lymphoma should establish whether the disease is systemic or primary. This can often be established by a complete physical examination, routine blood work, and a chest radiograph. If these limited clinical staging procedures reveal no obvious pathology, then further systemic evaluations (*eg*, body computed tomography [CT] and magnetic resonance imaging [MRI] scans, gallium scan, and bone marrow aspiration and biopsy) are of low yield and often can be avoided.

In the majority of cases, single and multiple contrast-enhancing lesions may be seen on head CT and MRI scans [83]. In AIDS-related PCL, lesions are usually hypodense in the absence of contrast; involve the basal ganglia, cerebellum, brain stem, and cerebral hemispheres; may demonstrate classic ring enhancement in up to 40% of cases; and may show no contrast enhancement at all in up to 10% of cases [83]. MRI is thought to be more sensitive than CT in identifying PCL. These radiographic findings are too inconsistent to be the only method of diagnosis. The differential diagnosis of a space-occupying CNS mass lesion in an HIV-infected patient is broad and principally includes toxoplasmosis, which may be on the decline as a result of the HAART therapy era. Progressive multifocal leukoencephalopathy, fungal and bacterial abscess, tuberculosis, gummatous lesions, infarct, hemorrhage, and glioma can also present as focal lesions. Because serologic techniques for diagnosis of toxoplasmosis are unreliable in a significant number of AIDS patients and ring enhancement is often an accompanying radiographic sign, biopsy is necessary to establish a diagnosis. Tissue can be obtained by a variety of methods inclusive of brain parenchyma via stereotactic brain biopsy, lumbar puncture for CSF cytology (between 20%–25% of AIDS cases have positive cytol-

ogy [83]), or orbit via aqueous tumor cytology. A careful ophthalmologic and slit-lamp examination may prove helpful to establish vitreal involvement. The preferable approach is dependent on the available expertise at any treatment center.

It is often appropriate to embark on a course of empiric treatment for toxoplasmosis for many patients in whom clinical status is stable and in whom CNS lymphoma is not the AIDS-defining illness. In this instance antitoxoplasma therapy is administered for 7 to 14 days, and head CT/MRI is repeated to document resolution of CNS mass lesions, thus establishing a diagnosis of toxoplasmosis. If the lesions are persistent, it is appropriate to proceed to biopsy. For patients in whom CNS mass lesion *is* the AIDS-defining event (and/or those with clinically significant intracranial disease [eg, mass effect]), it is generally advisable to attempt biopsy to offer diagnosis-specific therapy [83]. Current investigational modalities, which may greatly

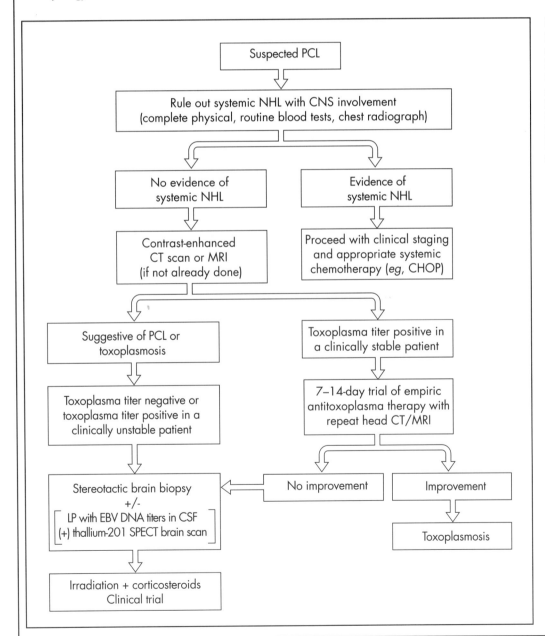

FIGURE 24-1.

Diagnostic algorithm in HIV-infected patients with central nervous system (CNS) mass lesion(s) and suspected primary CNS lymphoma (PCL). CHOP—cyclophosphamide, doxorubicin, vincristine, prednisone; CSF—colony-stimulating factor; CT—computed tomography; EBV—Epstein–Barr virus; MRI—magnetic resonance imaging; LP—lumbar puncture; NHL—non-Hodgkin's lymphoma; SPECT—single-photon emission computed tomography.

facilitate diagnostic evaluation in this setting, include detection of EBV DNA in CSF and thallium single-photon emission CT (SPECT) scanning [86]. Initial studies suggest that the presence of EBV DNA in CSF as detected by polymerase chain reaction has a specificity of 100% and a sensitivity of 98.5% [87]. In a large series of 61 patients, investigators at the University of Miami have reported that 95.2% of AIDS-related PCL cases have positive SPECT scans [88]. In another smaller study, thallium-brain SPECT scanning had a sensitivity of 100% and a specificity of 90% [89]. These modalities may prove to be very valuable in establishing a diagnosis of PCL and in complementing or replacing current diagnostic methods. The diagnostic approach for HIV-infected patients with a CNS mass lesion is summarized in Figure 24-1.

THERAPEUTIC APPROACH

Overall median survival for AIDS-related PCL ranges between 2 and 3 months [83,84]. Survival is likely to be improved in patients without prior AIDS-defining opportunistic infections and good performance status (KPS > 70%) [83,84,90]. This aspect of the natural history of the disease is important to consider in clinical decision-making because up to 20% of patients may survive a year following a course of radiotherapy [90]. For patients suspected of PCL with profound immunosuppression, advanced AIDS, and poor clinical status, it may be moot to establish a diagnosis or offer therapy because survival is so poor (ranging between 1–2 mo) [57,83].

Radiotherapy historically has been the primary treatment modality for PCL. It appears that combined-modality chemotherapy and radiation in HIV-seronegative/indeterminate PCL improves median survival by approximately 3 years and is the preferred approach [84]. This clearly must be regarded an investigational approach in the HIV setting, and trials are currently underway to define feasibility, toxicity, and efficacy. In the absence of a clinical trial, the authors generally offer definitive radiation therapy or sequential combined modality therapy (ie, 1 cycle of chemotherapy followed by radiation in "good-risk" patients) and attempt to wean any corticosteroids as rapidly as possible.

OTHER TUMORS

Hodgkin's disease, testicular cancer, lung cancer, anogenital neoplasms, and cervical carcinoma are increasingly recognized in HIV-infected patients. A more detailed discussion about the therapeutic approach to these neoplasms is beyond the scope of this discussion. Key points regarding the natural history and therapeutic approach are briefly summarized below.

HODGKIN'S DISEASE

It has recently been established that Hodgkin's disease is clearly seen in increased incidence in HIV-infected patients [2–4]. This tumor has been well characterized, especially in injecting drug users in Europe [13]. Several features of the natural history of this disease in this setting are worthy of comment. The majority of patients present with stage III and IV disease (often with extranodal disease), and as a result, systemic chemotherapy is the mainstay of treatment [13,91]. There is a paucity of mediastinal involvement that can be explained by the predominance of mixed cellularity and lymphocyte depletion histologies and lack of nodular sclerosis subtype. The frequency of

EBV-genome expression appears to be higher in HIV-related Hodgkin's disease versus de novo disease. Current treatment approaches generally have focused on traditional chemotherapy for Hodgkin's disease with the greatest experience reported for the ABVD (doxorubicin, bleomycin, vincristine, and dacarbazine) regimen. The complete remission rate is approximately 50%, and median survival is approximately 18 months [91]. The optimal chemotherapy regimen remains to be established, and a variety of regimens are currently under investigation. It also remains to be established whether a dose-modified approach akin to that for non-Hodgkin's disease is appropriate, and prospects for progression-free and long-term survival need to be identified.

TESTICULAR NEOPLASMS

Seminoma has recently been described in increased incidence in HIV infection [2,3]. Nonseminomatous germ cell tumors (NSGCT) are less commonly encountered. It appears on review of reported cases of testicular neoplasms in the HIV-infected patient population that the histopathologic subtype and clinical stage are no different than in the general population (50% seminoma vs 50% NSGCT; 40% stage I, 40% stage II, and 20% stage III) [5,6]. It is very important to recognize that HIV-infected patients with testicular cancer may be inappropriately down-staged (ie, moved from stage I to II) because of benign retroperitoneal lymphadenopathy, which is secondary to their underlying HIV infection and not metastasis [56]. This has obvious prognostic and therapeutic implications that are difficult to sort out in otherwise healthy asymptomatic HIV-infected patients with relatively high CD4 lymphocyte counts. There is no correlation of CD4 count and clinical stage of testis cancer in these patients. Sound clinical judgment regarding the staging of these patients is imperative. What is interesting is that the majority of HIV-infected testicular cancer patients reported in the literature tolerate standard systemic combination chemotherapy, radiotherapy, or both very well [56]. This contrasts with the toxicity encountered in the majority of HIV-infected patients with other neoplasms who generally present with advanced underlying immunodeficiency. A 95% complete remission rate was observed in 20 patients (approximately half received chemotherapy and the other half radiation) [92]. Less than 50% of these patients experienced severe grade 3 and 4 hematologic toxicity. Median survival approaches 40 months for patients with CD4 counts greater than 200/μL and 26 months for patients with CD4 counts less than 200/μL [5,6].

LUNG CANCER

As the HIV epidemic advances, it is apparent that lung cancer is more commonly recognized. Review of AIDS surveillance and cancer registry databases has not yet identified a true increased incidence of this neoplasm in HIV infection. Nonetheless, there are several features of lung cancer that develop in this setting that are suggestive of an altered natural history of the disease, eg, a clear correlation of cigarette smoking and risk of lung cancer in HIV-infected patients, a significantly younger age at time of diagnosis (median, 45 y), a predominance of adenocarcinoma histology (> 50%) and paucity of small cell carcinoma (< 10%), a significant number of patients (~85%; the majority of whom are male) presenting with stage III and IV disease versus 20% stage I disease in HIV-seronegative or indeterminate patients, and a clinical course that is more aggressive with shortened survival [5–7]. The median CD4 lymphocyte count is 233/μL, which suggests that profound immuno-

The information here is provided as guidance only. Prescribers should always consult the manufacturer's current prescribing information.

342

suppression and symptomatic HIV infection may not be significant cofactors in the pathogenesis of lung cancer in these patients [7]. The most important clinical implication of these observations is that lung cancer must be included in the differential diagnosis of an abnormal chest radiograph in HIV-infected patients, especially a solitary mass lesion. Patients with good medical/operative risk and stage I disease are best managed with surgical resection. HIV-seropositivity alone is not a contraindication to resection. There is, however, limited published data on the follow-up of HIV-infected lung cancer patients with stage I disease. For patients with regionally advanced disease and good clinical status, it would be prudent to offer sequential rather than concurrent chemotherapy and irradiation because of the enhanced toxicity. Patients with metastatic disease are managed similarly to HIV-seronegative or indeterminate patients, and clinical performance status may be of particular prognostic value as well. It would be interesting to identify the activity of the novel topoisomerase I inhibitors (eg, topotecan, 9-aminocamptothecin), which are known to have antiretroviral activity and are currently being evaluated in AIDS-related KS [93]. Overall median survival for HIV-infected lung cancer patients is 3 months; no 5-year survival rates have been published and, unfortunately, treatment and survival results are inconsistently reported [5–7].

ANOGENITAL TUMORS AND INVASIVE CERVICAL CARCINOMA

These neoplasms are clearly encountered in increased incidence in HIV-infected individuals. As immunodeficiency advances in HIV infection and patients live longer, there appears to be increased risk for the development of high-grade intraepithelial lesions both of the anus (especially in homosexual men who practice anoreceptive intercourse) and cervix. Consequently, appropriate anogenital tract surveillance (including gynecologic examination with PAP smear and colposcopy in women, anal examination and colposcopy in high-risk HIV-seropositive men, and provision of local modalities for treatment of high-risk lesions) is warranted and must be incorporated into primary care. The precise strategy of surveillance for anal intraepithelial neoplasia is currently being identified. The therapeutic approach to HIV-infected patients with invasive cervical carcinoma is identical to that for HIV-seronegative women; surgery and radiation remain the cornerstones of therapy. There is very little published chemotherapy data for patients with systemic disease, and overall, the clinical course is much more aggressive [94]. HIV-infected patients with anal squamous cell carcinoma are managed similarly to HIV-seronegative patients, with combined modality therapy. Chemotherapy with mitomycin (15 mg/m² IV, d 1) and 5-fluorouracil (1000 mg/m² as a 24-h continuous infusion, d 1–4) plus radiotherapy (3000 cGy over 3 wk) has been administered concomitantly to patients who are not HIV-infected. Up to 80% of patients have a complete remission, and abdominoperineal resection can be avoided. In the HIV setting, toxicity is much more pronounced, and it may be advisable to do sequential therapy [95]. There are as yet no AIDS-specific or dose-modified therapeutic approaches for HIV-infected patients with invasive cervical or anal cancer.

CONCLUSION

As the HIV epidemic advances and patients live longer (because of improvement in antiretroviral therapy and recognition, management, and prophylaxis of opportunistic infections), it becomes apparent that various neoplasms—both AIDS and non–AIDS-defining—will likely be of increasing clinical concern. It is important to continue to define the spectrum and biology of malignant disease in this setting with attention to the underlying HIV infection, quality of life, and prospects for improved survival. General supportive-care recommendations for the majority of patients with AIDS-related neoplasms include 1) optimizing protease inhibitor–based combination antiretroviral therapy to achieve complete or near complete HIV viral load suppression, 2) providing adequate prophylaxis for opportunistic infection (usually all patients receiving cytotoxic chemotherapy should receive preventative treatment for P. carinii pneumonia), and 3) close monitoring for myelosuppression with a low threshold to add cytokine/growth factor support. At present, a dose-modified chemotherapy approach has been confirmed to be efficacious only in AIDS-related NHL. In many instances, patients with AIDS-related malignancies are more susceptible to the toxicity of antineoplastic therapy or become too ill to withstand the therapy for which a dose-modified approach may be warranted. More importantly, patients with AIDS-related malignancies should always be considered appropriate candidates for participation on clinical trials to help resolve and improve the therapeutic approach for these diseases. Current chemotherapeutic regimens for the treatment of AIDS-related KS and NHL are summarized on the following pages.

REFERENCES

1. Levine AM:AIDS-related malignancies:the emerging epidemic. *J Natl Cancer Inst* 1993, 85:1382–1397.

2. Lyter DW, Bryant J, Thackeray R, *et al*.:Incidence of human immunodeficiency virus-related and nonrelated malignancies in a large cohort of homosexual men. *J Clin Oncol* 1995, 13:2540–2546.

3. Rabkin CS:Epidemiology of malignancies other than Kaposi's sarcoma and non-Hodgkin's lymphoma in HIV infection [abstract]. *J Acquir Immune Defic Syndr Hum Retrovirol* 1997, 14:A12.

4. Grulich A, Wan X, Law M, *et al*.:Rates of non-AIDS defining cancers in people with AIDS [abstract]. *J Acquir Immune Defic Syndr Hum Retrovirol* 1997, 14:A18.

5. Remick SC:The spectrum of non-AIDS-defining neoplastic disease in HIV infection. *J Investig Med* 1996, 44:205–215.

6. Remick SC:Non-AIDS-defining cancers. *Hematol Oncol Clin North Am* 1996, 10:1203–1213.

7. Vyzula R, Remick SC.:Lung cancer in patients with HIV infection. *Lung Cancer* 1996, 15:325–339.

8. Penn I:Cancer in the immunosuppressed organ recipient. *Transplant Proc* 1991, 23:1771.

9. Cremer KJ, Spring SB, Gruber J:Role of human immunodeficiency virus type 1 and other viruses in malignancies associated with acquired immunodeficiency disease syndrome. *J Natl Cancer Inst* 1990, 82:1016–1024.

10. Shiramizu B, Herndier BG, McGrath MS.:Identification of a common clonal human immunodeficiency virus integration site in human immunodeficiency virus associated lymphoma. *Cancer Res* 1994, 54:2069–2072.

11. Vogel J, Hinrichs SH, Reynolds RK, *et al.*:The HIV *tat* gene induces dermal lesions resembling Kaposi's sarcoma in transgenic mice. *Nature* 1988, 335:606–611.

12. McClain KL, Leach CT, Jenson HB, *et al.*:Association of Epstein–Barr virus with leiomyosarcomas in young people with AIDS. *N Engl J Med* 1995, 332:12–18.

13. Tirelli U, Errante D, Dolcetti R, *et al.*:Hodgkin's disease and human immunodeficiency virus infection:clinicopathologic and virologic features of 114 patients from the Italian Cooperative Group on AIDS and Tumors. *J Clin Oncol* 1995, 13:1758–1767.

14. Chang Y, Cesarman E, Pessin MS, *et al.*:Identification of herpesvirus-like DNA sequences in AIDS-associated Kaposi's sarcoma. *Science* 1994, 266:1865–1869.

15. Moore PS, Chang Y:Detection of herpesvirus-like DNA sequences in Kaposi's sarcoma in patients with and those without HIV infection. *N Engl J Med* 1995, 332:1181–1185.

16. Cesarman E, Chang Y, Moore PS, *et al.*:Kaposi's sarcoma-associated herpesvirus-like DNA sequences in AIDS-related body-cavity-based lymphomas. *N Engl J Med* 1995, 332:1186–1191.

17. Cesarman E, Knowles D:Herpes-like DNA sequences, AIDS-related tumors, and Castleman's disease. *N Engl J Med* 1995, 333:798–799.

18. Rettig MB, Ma HJ, Vescio RA, *et al.*:Kaposi's sarcoma-associated herpesvirus infection of bone marrow dendritic cells from multiple myeloma patients. *Science* 1997, 276:1851–1854.

19. Moore RD, Kessler HD, Richman DD, *et al.*:Non-Hodgkin's lymphoma in patients with advanced HIV infection treated with zidovudine. *JAMA* 1991, 265:2208–2211.

20. Pluda JM, Yarchoan R, Jaffe ES, *et al.*:Development of non-Hodgkin's lymphoma in a cohort of patients with severe human immunodeficiency virus (HIV) infection on a long-term antiretroviral therapy. *Ann Intern Med* 1990, 113:276–282.

21. Dezube BJ. Clinical presentation and natural history of AIDS-related Kaposi's sarcoma. *Hematol Oncol Clin North Am* 1996, 10:1023–1029.

22. Wabinga HR, Parkin DM, Wabwire-Mangen F, *et al.*:Cancer incidence in Kampala, Uganda, in 1989–91:changes in incidence in the era of AIDS. *Int J Cancer* 1993, 54:26–36.

23. Gao S-J, Kingsley L, Hoover DR, *et al.*:Seroconversion to antibodies against Kaposi's sarcoma-associated herpesvirus-related latent nuclear antigens before development of Kaposi's sarcoma. *N Engl J Med* 1996, 335:233–241.

24. Huang YO, Li JJ, Kaplan MH, *et al.*:Human herpesvirus-like nucleic acid in various forms of Kaposi's sarcoma. *Lancet* 1995, 345:759–761.

25. Miller G, Rigsby MO, Heston L, *et al.*:Antibodies to butyrate-inducible antigens of Kaposi's sarcoma-associated herpesvirus in patients with HIV-1 infection. *N Engl J Med* 1996, 334:1292–1297.

26. Purvis SF, Katongole-Mbidde E, Johnson J, *et al.*:High incidence of Kaposi's sarcoma-associated herpesvirus and Epstein–Barr virus in tumor lesions and peripheral blood mononuclear cells from patients with Kaposi's sarcoma in Uganda. *J Infect Dis* 1997, 175:947–950.

27. Whitby D, Howard MR, Tenant-Flowers M, *et al.*:Detection of Kaposi's sarcoma associated herpes virus in peripheral blood of HIV-infected individuals and progression to Kaposi's sarcoma. *Lancet* 1995, 346:799–802.

28. Nakamura S, Salahuddin SZ, Biberfeld P, *et al.*:Kaposi's sarcoma cells:long-term culture with growth factor from retrovirus-infected CD4+ T cells. *Science* 1988, 242:426–430.

29. Salahuddin SZ, Nakamura S, Biberfeld P, *et al.*:Angiogenic properties of Kaposi's sarcoma-derived cells after long-term culture in vitro. *Science* 1988, 242:430–433.

30. Ensoli B, Barillari G, Salahuddin SZ, *et al.*:Tat protein of HIV-1 stimulates growth to cells derived from Kaposi's sarcoma lesions of AIDS patients. *Nature* 1990, 345:84–86.

31. Ensoli B, Gendelman R, Markham P, *et al.*:Synergy between basic fibroblast growth factor and HIV-1 tat protein in induction of Kaposi's sarcoma. *Nature* 1994, 371:674–680.

32. Ensoli B, Markham P, Kao V, *et al.*:Block of AIDS-Kaposi's sarcoma (KS) cell growth, angiogenesis, and lesion formation in nude mice by antisense oligonucleotide targeting basic fibroblast growth factor:a novel strategy for the therapy of KS. *J Clin Investig* 1994, 94:1736–1746.33.   Miles SA:Pathogenesis of AIDS-related Kaposi's sarcoma:evidence of a viral etiology. *Hematol Oncol Clin North Am* 1996, 10:1011–1021.

34. Miles SA, Martinez-Maza O, Rezai A, *et al.*:Oncostatin-M as a potent mitogen for AIDS-Kaposi's sarcoma-derived cells. *Science* 1992, 255:1432–1434.

35. Miles SA, Rezai A, Salazar-Gonzalez JF, *et al.*:AIDS Kaposi's sarcoma-derived cells produce and respond to IL-6. *Proc Natl Acad Sci USA* 1990, 87:4068–4072.

36. Lunardi-Iskandar Y, Gill PS, Lam VH, *et al.*:Isolation and characterization of an immortal neoplastic cell line (KS Y-1) from AIDS-associated Kaposi's sarcoma. *J Natl Cancer Inst* 1995, 87:974–981.

37. Neipel F, Albrecht J-C, Fleckenstein B:Cell-homologous genes in the Kaposi's sarcoma-associated rhadinovirus human herpesvirus-8:determinants of its pathogenicity. *J Virol* 1997, 71:4187–4192.

38. Russo JJ, Bohenzky RA, Chen MC, *et al.*:Nucleotide sequence of the Kaposi's sarcoma-associated herpesvirus (HHV-8). *Proc Natl Acad Sci USA* 1996, 93:14862–14867.

39. Rabkin CS, Janz S, Lash A, *et al.*:Monoclonal origin of multicentric Kaposi's sarcoma lesions. *N Engl J Med* 1997, 336:988–993.

40. Krown SE, Metroka C, Wernz JC:Kaposi's sarcoma in the acquired immune deficiency syndrome:a proposal for uniform evaluation, response, and staging criteria. *J Clin Oncol* 1989, 7:1201–1207.

41. Krown SE, Testa MA, Huang J, *et al.*:AIDS-related Kaposi's sarcoma: prospective validation of the AIDS Clinical Trials Group staging classification. *J Clin Oncol* 1997, 15:3085–3092.

42. Swift PS. The role of radiation therapy in the management of HIV-related Kaposi's sarcoma. *Hematol Oncol Clin North Am* 1996, 10:1069–1080.

43. Lee F-C, Mitsuyasu RT. Chemotherapy of AIDS-related Kaposi's sarcoma. *Hematol Oncol Clin North Am* 1996, 10:1051–1068.

44. Remick SC, Reddy M, Herman D, *et al.*:Continuous infusion bleomycin in AIDS-related Kaposi's sarcoma. *J Clin Oncol* 1994, 12:1130–1136.

45. Northfelt DW, Dezube B, Miller B, *et al.*:Randomized comparative trial of Doxil vs Adriamycin, bleomycin, and vincristine (ABV) in the treatment of severe AIDS-related Kaposi's sarcoma (AIDS-KS) [abstract]. *Blood* 1995, 86:382A.

46. Northfelt DW, Dezube BJ, Thommes JA, *et al.*:Efficacy of pegylated-liposomal doxorubicin in the treatment of AIDS-related Kaposi's sarcoma after failure of standard chemotherapy. *J Clin Oncol* 1996, 15:653–659.

47. Gill PS, Wernz J, Scadden D, *et al.*:Randomized phase III trial of liposomal daunorubicin versus doxorubicin, bleomycin, and vincristine in AIDS-related Kaposi's sarcoma. *J Clin Oncol* 1996, 14:2353–2364.

48. Saville MW, Lietzau J, Pluda JM, *et al.*:Treatment of HIV-associated Kaposi's sarcoma with paclitaxel. *Lancet* 1995, 346:26–28.

49. Gill PS, Tulpule A, Reynolds T, *et al.*:Paclitaxel (Taxol) in the treatment of relapsed or refractory advanced AIDS-related Kaposi's sarcoma. *Proc ASCO* 1996, 15:306.

50. Gill PS, Rarick M, McCuthan JA, *et al.*:Systemic treatment of AIDS-related Kaposi's sarcoma:results of a randomized trial. *Am J Med* 1991, 90:427–433.

51. Gill PS, Akil B, Colletti P, *et al.*:Pulmonary Kaposi's sarcoma:clinical findings and results of therapy. *Am J Med* 1989, 87:57–61.

52. Karp JE, Pluda JM, Yarchoan R:AIDS-related Kaposi's sarcoma:a template for the tranlation of molecular pathogenesis into targeted therapeutic approaches. *Hematol Oncol Clin North Am* 1996, 10:1031–1049.

53. Routy J-P, Urbanek A, MacLeod J, *et al.*:Significant regression of Kaposi's sarcoma following initiation of an effective antiretroviral combination treatment [abstract]. *J Acquir Immune Defic Syndr Hum Retrovirol* 1997, 14:22A.

54. Mocroft A, Youle M, Gazzard B, *et al.*:Anti-herpesvirus treatment and risk of Kaposi's sarcoma in HIV infection. *AIDS* 1996, 10:1101–1105.

55. Dezube B, von Roenn JH, Holden-White J, *et al.*:Fumagillin analog (TNP-470) in the treatment of Kaposi's sarcoma:a phase I ACTG study. *J Clin Oncol* 1998, in press.

56. Gill PS, Lunardi-Iskandar Y, Louie S, *et al.*:The effects of preparations of human chorionic gonadotropin on AIDS-related Kaposi's sarcoma. *N Engl J Med* 1996, 335:1261–1269.

57. Remick SC. Acquired immunodeficiency syndrome-related non-Hodgkin's lymphoma. *Cancer Control* 1995, 2:97–103.

58. Levine AM, Bernstein L, Sullivan-Halley J, *et al.*:Role of zidovudine antiretroviral therapy in the pathogenesis of acquired immunodeficiency syndrome-related lymphoma. *Blood* 1995, 86:4612–4616.

59. Pluda JM, Venzon DJ, Tosaro G, *et al.*:Parameters affecting the development of non-Hodgkin's lymphoma in patients with severe human immunodeficiency virus infection receiving antiretroviral therapy. *J Clin Oncol* 1995, 11:1099–1107.

60. Ballerini P, Gaidano G, Gong J, *et al.*:Molecular pathogenesis of HIV-associated lymphomas. *AIDS Res Hum Retrovirus* 1992, 8:731–735.

61. Herndier BG, Kaplan LD, McGrath MS:Pathogenesis of AIDS lymphoma. *AIDS* 1994, 8:1025–1049.

62. Folks TM, Justement J, Kinter A, *et al.*:Cytokine-induced expression of HIV-1 in a chronically infected promonocyte cell line. *Science* 1987, 238:800–802.

63. Gaidano G, LoCoco F, Ye BH, *et al.*:Rearrangements of the *bcl*-6 gene in AIDS-associated non-Hodgkin's lymphoma:association with diffuse large-cell subtype. *Blood* 1944, 84:397–402.

64. Mack KD, Wei R, Herndier B, *et al.*:HIV insertional *cis*-activation of the proto-oncogene *c-fes* in AIDS asociated lymphomagenesis [abstract]. *J Acquir Immune Defic Syndr Hum Retrovirol* 1997, 14:A44.

65. Nador RG, Cesarman E, Chadburn A, *et al.*:Primary effusion lymphoma:a distinct clinicopatholgical entity associated with the Kaposi's sarcoma associated virus. *Blood* 1996, 88:646–656.

66. Knowles DM, Chamulak GA, Subar M, *et al.*:Lymphoid neoplasia associated with the acquired immunodeficiency syndrome (AIDS):the New York University Medical Center experience with 105 patients (1981–1986). *Ann Intern Med* 1988, 108:744–753.

67. Levine AM. Acquired immunodeficiency syndrome-related lymphoma. *Blood* 1992, 80:8–20.

68. Kaplan LD, Straus DJ, Testa M, *et al.*:Low-dose compared with standard-dose m-BACOD chemotherapy for non-Hodgkin's lymphoma associated with human immunodeficiency virus infection. *N Engl J Med* 1997, 336:1641–1648.

69. Ziegler JL, Beckstead JA, Volberding PA, *et al.*:Non-Hodgkin's lymphoma in 90 homosexual men:relation to generalized lymphadenopathy and acquired immunodeficiency syndrome. *N Engl J Med* 1984, 311:565–570.

70. Gill PS, Levine AM, Krailo M, *et al.*:AIDS-related malignant lymphoma:results of prospective treatment trials. *J Clin Oncol* 1987, 5:1322–1328.

71. Levine AM, Wernz JC, Kaplan L, *et al.*:Low-dose chemotherapy with central nervous system prophylaxis and zidovudine maintenance in AIDS-related lymphoma:a prospective multi-institutional trial. *JAMA* 1991, 266:84–88.

72. Kaplan LD, Kahn JO, Crowe S, *et al.*:Clinical and virologic effects of recombinant human granulocyte-macrophage colony-stimulating factor in patients receiving chemotherapy for human immunodeficiency virus-associated non-Hodgkin's lymphoma:results of a randomized trial. *J Clin Oncol* 1991, 9:929–940.

73. Freter CE:Acquired immunodeficiency syndrome-associated lymphoma. *Monogr Natl Cancer Inst* 1990, 10:45–54.

74. Straus DJ, Huang J, Testa MA, *et al.*:Prognostic factors in the treatment of HIV-associated non-Hodgkin's lymphoma (HANHL):analysis of ACTG 142 (low-dose vs. standard-dose m-BACOD + GM-CSF) [abstract]. *J Acquir Immune Defic Syndr Hum Retrovirol* 1997, 14:A38.

75. Sparano JA:Treatment of AIDS-related lymphomas. *Curr Opinion Oncol* 1995, 7:442–449.

76. Sparano JA, Wiernik PH, Hu X, *et al.*:Pilot trial of infusional cyclophosphamide, doxorubicin, and etoposide plus didanosine andfilgrastim in patients with human immunodeficiency virus-associated non-Hodgkin's lymphoma. *J Clin Oncol* 1996, 14:3026–3035.

77. Sparano JA, Wiernik PH, Strack M, *et al.*:Infusional cyclophosphamide, doxorubicin, and etoposide in human immunodeficiency virus type 1-related non-Hodgkin's lymphoma:a highly active regimen. *Blood* 1993, 81:2810–2815.

78. Remick SC, McSharry JS, Wolf BC, *et al.*:Novel oral combination chemotherapy in the treatment of intermediate-grade and high-grade AIDS-related non-Hodgkin's lymphoma. *J Clin Oncol* 1993, 11:1691–1702.

79. Remick SC, Bibighaus MR, Reddy M, *et al.*:Oral combination chemotherapy (CT) in conjunction with filgrastim (G-CSF) in the treatment of AIDS-related non-Hodgkin's lymphoma (NHL) [abstract]. *J Acquir Immune Defic Syndr Hum Retrovirol* 1997, 14:A37.

80. Little R, Franchini G, Pearson D, *et al.*:HIV viral burden (VB) during EPOCH chemotherapy (CT) for HIV-related lymphomas [abstract]. *J Acquir Immune Defic Syndr Hum Retrovirol* 1997, 14:A42.

81. Davis AJ, Goldstein D, Milliken S:Long-term follow-up of CEOP in the treatment of HIV-related NHL [abstract]. *J Acquir Immune Defic Syndr Hum Retrovirol* 1997, 14:A40.

82. Levine AM, Tulpule A, Tessman D, *et al.*:Mitoguazone therapy in patients with refractory or relapsed AIDS-related lymphoma:results from a multicenter phase II trial. *J Clin Oncol* 1997, 15:1094–1103.

83. Remick SC, Diamond C, Migliozzi JA, *et al.*:Primary central nervous system lymphoma in patients with and without the acquired immune deficiency syndrome:a retrospective analysis and review of the literature. *Medicine* 1990, 69:345–360.

84. Fine HA, Mayer RV. Primary central nervous system lymphoma. *Ann Intern Med* 1993, 119:1093–1104.

85. So YT, Beckstead JH, Davis RL. Primary central nervous system lymphoma in acquired immune deficiency syndrome:a clinical and pathological study. *Ann Neurol* 1986, 20:566–572.

86. Ruiz A, Post MJ, Bundschu C, *et al.*:Primary central nervous system lymphoma in patients with AIDS. *Neuroimaging Clin North Am* 1997, 7:281–296.

87. Cinque P, Brytting M, Vago L, *et al.*:Epstein–Barr virus DNA in cerebrospinal fluid from patients with AIDS-related primary CNS lymphoma of the central nervous system. *Lancet* 1993, 342:398–401.

88. Patel P, Raez LE:Primary central nervous system lymphomas in patients with acquired immunodeficiency syndrome (AIDS) [abstract]. *J Acquir Immune Defic Syndr Hum Retrovirol* 1997, 14:A40.

89. Lorberboym M, Estok L, Machac J, *et al.*:Rapid differential diagnosis of cerebral toxoplasmosis and primary central nervous system lymphoma by thallium-201 SPECT:*J Nucl Med* 1996, 37:1150–1154.

90. Baumgartner JE, Rachlin JR, Beckstead JH, *et al.*:Primary central nervous system lymphoma:natural history and response to radiation therapy in 55 patients with acquired immunodefciency syndrome. *J Neurosurg* 1990, 73:206–211.

91. Levine AM. HIV-associated Hodgkin's disease. Biologic and clinical aspects. *Hematol Oncol Clin North Am* 1996, 10:1135–1148.

92. Bernardi D, Salvioni R, Vaccher E, *et al*.:Testicular germ cell tumors and human immunodeficiency virus infection:a report of 26 cases. *J Clin Oncol* 1995, 13:2705–2711.

93. Li CJ, Zhang LJ, Dezube BJ, *et al*.:Three inhibitors of type 1 human immunodeficiency virus long terminal repeat-directed gene expression and virus replication. *Proc Natl Acad Sci USA* 1993, 90:1839–1842.

94. Klevins PM, Fleming PL, Mays MA, *et al*.:Characteristics of women with AIDS and invasive cervical cancer. *Obstet Gynecol* 1996, 88:269–273.

95. Chadha M, Rosenblatt EA, Malamud S, *et al*.:Squamous-cell carcinoma of the anus in HIV-positive patients. *Dis Colon Rectum* 1994, 37:861–865.

ABV THERAPY FOR KAPOSI'S SARCOMA
Single-Agent and Combination Doxorubicin, Bleomycin, and Vincristine

Single-agent chemotherapy in the management of AIDS-related Kaposi's sarcoma (AIDS-KS) is clearly easier to administer and less toxic than combination chemotherapy. In the absence of a requirement for immediate cytoreduction, single-agent chemotherapy is an attractive initial therapeutic intervention for many patients. Early studies of vinca alkaloids, bleomycin, podophyllotoxins, and anthracyclines established the activity of these agents in classical KS disease. It is important to mention that early studies of AIDS-KS used traditional solid-tumor and often disease-specific response criteria to varying degrees, which makes it difficult to analyze and compare clinical trial data. Clinical trial reporting will be streamlined with the adoption of the AIDS Clinical Trials Group (ACTG) clinical staging and response criteria across current generation and future studies.

Vinblastine, which has very high response rates in classical KS (90%), has a response rate of 30%–50% in AIDS-KS when administered at a dose of 4–8 mg/wk. Vincristine at a dose of 2 mg/wk as a single agent has been reported to have a response rate of 20%–60%. Doxorubicin (Adriamycin) alone in low weekly to biweekly doses (10–20 mg/m^2) has been associated with response rates of 10%–50%. Single-agent bleomycin administered on various dose schedules, including 72-h continuous infusion (20 mg/m^2/d), yielded response rates ranging between 40%–70%. Paclitaxel has substantial activity in AIDS-KS. At doses up to 100–175 mg/m^2 IV 3-h infusion every 2–3 wk, paclitaxel induces partial and complete responses in more than 50% of previously treated patients. Its effect appears to be qualitatively different from those of other agents, with a rapid, substantial reduction in tumor-associated edema. Moderate neutropenia requiring granulocyte–macrophage colony-stimulating factor (GM-CSF) is common. The various single and combination chemotherapy regimens that have been reported have response rates ranging between 30%–84%. Randomized controlled studies stratified by tumor stage have not been conducted with any of these regimens to date, and impact on survival has not been clearly demonstrated. There is, however, clear documentation of effective palliation with systemic cytotoxic chemotherapy and likely improved survival in many settings.

It is important to briefly touch on the supportive care issues in managing patients with AIDS-KS. These therapeutic principles are apropos for all HIV-infected patients with neoplastic complications of their disease. For a variety of AIDS-related neoplasms, clinical trials are addressing the issue of concurrent antiretroviral therapy with cytotoxic chemotherapy regimens. Published reports from the ACTG trial 075 defined 10 mg/m^2 of doxorubicin as the maximum tolerated dose (MTD) when used in combination with zidovudine (600 mg/d), vincristine (2 mg), and bleomycin (10 U/m^2) every other week. Hematologic and immunologic toxicity were the primary side effects. A later study adding GM-CSF to this regimen (ACTG 094) showed an overall better response rate, but it was the same MTD for doxorubicin. The ACTG 163 study administered ABV as follows: 20 mg/m^2 doxorubicin, 10 mm^2 bleomycin, 1 mg vincristine IV every 2 wk with dideoxyinosine (200 mg twice daily if ≥ 60 kg or 125 mg twice daily if < 60 kg) or with dideoxycytidine (0.75 mg three times daily if ≥ 50 kg or 0.375 mg three times daily if < 50 kg) with comparable and acceptable toxicity and response rates of 58% and 60%, respectively.

In the protease-inhibitor era, it is clearly preferable to maximize antiretroviral therapy prior to embarking on systemic cytotoxic chemotherapy because significant objective tumor regression may be encountered. It may be important to continue effective antiretroviral therapy with maximal viral suppression in conjunction with chemotherapy until further clinical studies address this issue. Because many patients are likely to have very complicated medical regimens, it is imperative to closely monitor for potential drug interactions and be alert for myelosuppression, immunologic side effects with emergence of opportunistic infectious complications, and other side effects commonly seen with cytotoxic chemotherapy. As a result, all patients should receive *Pneumocystic carinii* pneumonia prophylaxis when receiving cytotoxic chemotherapy irrespective of CD4 lymphocyte count. Other prophylactic strategies and interventions need to be made on an individual patient basis. In many instances of myelosuppression, it may be prudent to administer cytokine CSFs (*eg*, G-CSF, GM-CSF [generally given in conjunction with antiretroviral therapy to offset HIV upregulation], and erythropoietin). Thrombopoietin and other platelet factors are currently under investigation.

RECENT EXPERIENCES AND RESPONSE RATES

Study	Regimen	Evaluable Patients, n	Response Rate	Median Duration of Response, mo
Gill *et al.* (ACTG 075). *AIDS* 1994, 8:1695.	ABV + ZDV	24	71%	Not specified
Mitsuyasu *et al.* (ACTG 163). *Proc ASCO* 1995, 14:289.	ABV (ddl/ddC)	81	58% (ddl) 60% (ddC)	20 wk (ddl) 19 wk (ddC)
Saville *et al. Lancet* 1995, 346:26.	Paclitaxel	20	65%	34 wk
Gill *et al. Proc ASCO* 1996, 15:306.	Paclitaxel	30	53%	Not specified

ABV—doxorubicin, bleomycin, and vincristine; ddC—dideoxycytodine; ddl—dideoxyinosine; ZDV—zidovudine.

ABV THERAPY FOR KAPOSI'S SARCOMA (Continued)

DOSAGE AND SCHEDULING

Chemotherapy	Dose	Interval
Single agents		
Doxorubicin	10–15 mg/m2 IV	Every wk
	20.0 mg/m² IV	Every 2 wk
Bleomycin	20.0 mg/m²/d as 72-h continuous infusion	Every 3 wk
Vincristine	1.4 mg/m² IV (maximum 2.0 mg)	Every 2 wk
	1.0 mg IV	Every wk
Paclitaxel	100.0 mg/m² IV (3 h)	Every 2 wk
	135.0 mg/m² IV (3 h)	Every 3 wk
ABV regimen		
Doxorubicin	10.0–20.0 mg/m² IV, d 1	Every 2 wk
Bleomycin	10.0 mg/m² IV, d 1	
Vincristine	1.0–2.0 mg IV, d 1	
BV regimen		
Bleomycin	10.0 mg/m² IV, d 1	Every 2 wk
Vincristine	2.0 mg (total) IV, d 1	

CANDIDATES FOR TREATMENT

Management of patients with AIDS-KS should take into consideration not only prospects for symptomatic palliation and tumor regression but also the potential for myelotoxicity and immunosuppressive side effects of the therapeutic regimen; for patients with symptomatic disease or life-threatening organ involvement, prompt and effective cytoreductive treatment is required; patients with moderate disease (> 25 cutaneous lesions and no tumor edema or pulmonary involvement) can be treated with single agents; patients may also have fewer lesions but in cosmetically strategic locations, for which systemic therapy may also be appropriate; vinblastine, vincristine, doxorubicin, or bleomycin are appropriate in these situations; recent published data on liposomal anthracycline formulations (*see* Liposomal Anthracyclines section) for AIDS-KS suggest these agents may be suitable first-line alternatives; patients with rapidly progressing disease and/or significant visceral disease, especially symptomatic pulmonary involvement, should be treated with higher doses of liposomal anthracyclines or preferably the ABV combination regimen; paclitaxel is currently approved as second-line therapy

SPECIAL PRECAUTIONS AND NURSING INTERVENTIONS

Anthracyclines (including the liposomal formulations): patients with underlying cardiac disease (eg, HIV-related cardiomyopathy); **Bleomycin** chronic lung disease; **Vinca alkaloids and paclitaxel:** HIV-related peripheral neuropathy and constipation; in many of these circumstances it may be appropriate to avoid the offending cytotoxic agent altogether or closely monitor the functional status of the patient (eg, left ventricular ejection fraction by radionuclide scanning, diffusion capacity for carbon monoxide, and careful neurologic examination)

TOXICITIES

HIV-infected patients may be more susceptible and/or have more pronounced mucosal toxicity; for the majority of patients, the ABV regimen is not particularly troublesome in terms of nausea and vomiting; an occasional patient may require aggressive antiemetic support; myelosuppression remains the most important side effect for any cytotoxic agent and is generally more severe with combination regimens; bone marrow function and reserve is certainly compromised for the majority of HIV-infected patients with late-stage disease secondary to underlying disease, opportunistic infection, and myelotoxic antiretroviral therapy; complete blood counts (including platelets) need to be monitored and neutropenia, in particular, closely followed; it is advisable to have a low threshold to add G-CSF (usually 5 µg/kg administered subcutaneously) to the cytotoxic regimen between periods of chemotherapy administration and to maintain appropriate neutrophil counts, ideally > 1500/µL). Alternatively, GM-CSF (usually in conjunction with concurrent antiretroviral therapy) and erythropoietin can also be administered (*see* Chapter 4 for guidelines). Myelosuppression, neuropathy, and alopecia are all problematic with paclitaxel; myalgias are also commonly encountered; the optimal dose and schedule of this agent are to be determined; lower doses of this agent may lessen the toxicity and improve therapeutic index

PATIENT INFORMATION

General instructions for all HIV-infected patients receiving chemotherapy for AIDS-KS and other related neoplasms include the following: patients should at all times maintain adequate fluid intake and maximize good nutrition as feasible; patients should maintain excellent oral hygiene throughout therapy; it is appropriate to aggressively screen patients prior to embarking on systemic cytotoxic therapy for poor oral hygiene, dentition, and periodontal disease; patients need to be alerted for the prospects of mucosal and gastrointestinal side effects from the various regimens; blood counts need to be monitored closely and patients instructed to report and monitor signs and symptoms suggestive of infection (eg, fever, chills, cough, dyspnea, and sore throat); patients also need to be alerted for potential exacerbation of symptoms secondary to peripheral neuropathy while receiving vinca alkaloids and constipation, especially if receiving concurrent analgesic drugs; most regimens will likely lead to alopecia, and it is important to educate patients about this; myalgias may also be troublesome for patients receiving paclitaxel; finally, because many patients are bound to be taking multiple medications, there are no clear contraindications or specific drug-interactions that preclude the coadminstration of the various antineoplastic agents and the currently available antiretroviral agents inclusive of the protease inhibitors; pharmacokinetic studies are underway to help identify some of these issues.

LIPOSOMAL ANTHRACYCLINES

Liposomal formulations (microscopic phospholipid spheres) of some anthracyclines [doxorubicin (Doxil; Sequus Pharmaceuticals, Menlo Park, CA) and daunorubicin (DaunoXome; Nexstar, San Dimas, CA)] have been shown in animal models and early clinical trials in human patients to improve the therapeutic index when compared with the native anthracycline preparation, with less toxicity and comparable and/or improved efficacy in patients with AIDS-KS. Pharmacokinetic advantages of these formulations include a several-fold increase in plasma half-life with resultant prolonged circulation time, reduced clearance, a small volume of distribution, and markedly increased area under the curve. A putative advantage of the pegylated liposomal formulation (*eg*, liposomal doxorubicin) over the simple liposomal formulations is that the pegylated liposome reduces liposome opsonization and inhibits uptake by the reticuloendothelial system. The clinical significance of this remains to be sorted out, and to date, there are no comparative data of the two newly approved liposomal formulations of doxorubicin and daunorubicin. It is advisable for the clinician to become familiar and knowledgeable with one of the two agents. It is noteworthy in the trial data outlined below that both liposomal formulations were compared with an ABV (doxorubicin, bleomycin, and vincristine) combination regimen; however, for liposomal daunorubicin, the ABV regimen was dose-modified when compared with the traditional regimen.

Liposomal doxorubicin was investigated in an early phase II setting in patients with advanced KS. All 34 patients had poor prognostic disease as judged by AIDS Clinical Trials Group criteria. Patients were treated with 20 mg/m^2 of liposomal doxorubicin IV every 3 wk on an outpatient basis. Nineteen of 34 patients had received prior chemotherapy for KS, although no patient had received prior anthracyclines. An overall response rate of 73.5 % was observed with a complete response rate of 5.8%. In patients who had received previous chemotherapy, the response rate was 68.4%. Median duration of response was 9 wk. The major toxicity was neutropenia. Liposomal doxorubicin has also been investigated in patients with advanced KS who have failed standard chemotherapy. While receiving standard ABV or BV (bleomycin and vincristine) chemotherapy, fifty-three patients who experienced disease progression or intolerable toxicity received liposomal doxorubicin at a dose of 20 mg/m^2 IV every 3 wk. Nineteen patients (36%) had a partial response and one patient had a clinical complete response. The most common adverse effect was leukopenia, which occurred in 40% of patients.

Preliminary results of the largest randomized phase III clinical trial of liposomal doxorubicin versus ABV in 258 AIDS-KS patients have been reported [45]. In this study, the liposomal doxorubicin yielded a superior response rate of 43.0% versus 24.5% (*a much lower response rate than previously reported for the ABV regimen*). The toxicity profile also favored the liposomal formulation with 1) less alopecia, nausea/vomiting, and peripheral neuropathy; 2) comparable leukopenia; and 3) more stomatitis/mucositis. Liposomal daunorubicin has also been investigated in a prospective randomized phase III trial. In this study, 232 patients were randomized to receive liposomal daunorubicin (40 mg/m^2) or an ABV regimen (10 mg/m^2, 15 mg, and 1 mg, respectively, which is reduced vs standard ABV) both given IV every 2 wk. The overall response rate for liposomal daunorubicin was 25%, similar to the 28% in the ABV group. There was significantly less alopecia and peripheral neuropathy but significantly more grade 4 neutropenia in patients treated on the liposomal daunorubicin arm.

RECENT EXPERIENCES AND RESPONSE RATES

Study	Drug	Evaluable Patients, *n*	Dosage Schedule	Complete and Partial Response Rate, %
Harrison *et al. J Clin Oncol* 1995, 13:914.	Liposomal doxorubicin	34	20 mg/m^2 every 3 wk	73.5
Gill *et al. J Clin Oncol* 1996, 14:2353.	Liposomal daunorubicin	116	40 mg/m^2 every 2 wk	25.0
Northfelt *et al. J Clin Oncol* 1996, 15:653.	Liposomal doxorubicin	53	20 mg/m^2 every 3 wk	38.0

DOSAGE AND SCHEDULING

Chemotherapy	Dose	Interval
Liposomal doxorubicin	20 mg/m^2 IV (30 min)	Every 2–3 wk
Liposomal daunorubicin	40 mg/m^2 IV (1 h)	Every 2 wk

LIPOSOMAL ANTHRACYCLINES (Continued)

CANDIDATES FOR TREATMENT

Patients with rapidly progressive disease, extensive disease with edema, or pulmonary involvement, should be treated aggressively; liposomal anthracyclines may be used in this setting; clinicians should be alert to opportunistic infections; all patients should receive prophylaxis for *Pneumocystis carinii* pneumonia

ALTERNATIVE THERAPIES

ABV combination chemotherapy regimen

SPECIAL PRECAUTIONS AND NURSING INTERVENTIONS

Experience with liposomal anthracyclines is limited in patients with cardiac disease or risk factors; until further experience is recorded with these agents, the recommended total cumulative dose of liposomal doxorubicin is identical to that reported for doxorubicin; liposomal daunorubicin is perhaps less cardiotoxic; the drug with appropriate monitoring of left ventricular function (at 320 mg/m^2, 480 mg/m^2, and then 240 mg/m^2 increments thereafter) can be escalated. The pharmacokinetics of the liposomal anthracyclines have not been studied in patients with hepatic impairment and renal insufficiency, and dose modifications are recommended in these settings; both agents are not as likely as either native drug to cause severe extravasation; caution is advised, however, in both the administration and monitoring of infusion to avoid extravasation

TOXICITIES

In summary, liposomal formulations, when compared with ABV regimens, appear to be characterized by 1) significantly less alopecia, neurotoxicity, and gastrointestinal toxicity; 2) more stomatitis/mucositis; and 3) comparable myelosuppression, especially neutropenia; principal clinical toxicities include myelosuppression (60% risk of leukopenia) and an approximate 10% chance of thrombocytopenia and cardiotoxicity; infusion reactions occurring with the first cycle of therapy are not uncommon with liposomal doxorubicin (6.8% incidence); these are characterized by flushing, shortness of breath, facial swelling, headache, chest tightness, and back pain; the reactions generally do not recur with later cycles; palmar-plantar erythrodysesthesia occurs in 3.4% of patients receiving liposomal doxorubicin and is characterized by swelling, pain, erythema, and (in some circumstances) desquamation of the skin of the hands and feet; the incidence may be increased with higher dosage or more frequent administration; similarly, a triad of back pain, flushing, and chest tightness has been reported in 13.8% of patients receiving liposomal daunorubicin; this usually occurs during the first 5 minutes of the infusion and subsides with interruption of the infusion; in both situations, reduction of the infusion rate may be helpful, and these reactions do not preclude further therapy

DRUG INTERACTIONS

No formal drug-interaction studies have been conducted with liposomal anthracyclines; until specific compatibility data are available, it is not recommended that liposomal anthracyclines be mixed with other drugs; liposomal anthracyclines may interact with drugs known to interact with the conventional formulation of doxorubicin or daunorubicin

PATIENT INFORMATION

The liposomal anthracycline formulations compared with ABV regimens in controlled clinical trials cause significantly less alopecia; this is likely an important consideration for many patients.

DOSE-MODIFIED M-BACOD THERAPY FOR NHL
Methotrexate, Bleomycin, Doxorubicin, Cyclophosphamide, Vincristine, and Dexamethazone

In an attempt to ascertain if "less is better," the AIDS Clinical Trials Group (ACTG) recently completed the largest randomized trial in AIDS-related non-Hodgkin's lymphoma, comparing a standard dose of m-BACOD and a low dose (less cyclophosphamide, doxorubicin, and dexamethasone) of the same regimen. Patients treated with low-dose m-BACOD had significantly fewer hematologic toxic effects and spent fewer days in the hospital than patients treated with conventional doses of m-BACOD. These results justify the treatment of most patients who have AIDS-related lymphoma with reduced doses of cytotoxic chemotherapy. This study also demonstrated that CD4 lymphocyte count is a more important predictor of survival than dose intensity of chemotherapy. Febrile neutropenia was an infrequent complication in this trial, perhaps because granulocyte–macrophage colony-stimulating factor (GM-CSF), which was administered concurrently, shortened the duration of severe neutropenia. Opportunistic infections occurred in 20% of patients. Intrathecal cytosine arabinoside (ara-C) was used to prevent CNS relapse and resulted in a CNS relapse rate of 3.4%. The ACTG also explored the use of GM-CSF with escalating doses of m-BACOD, noting that full dose m-BACOD could be given safely without clinical progression of HIV disease.

RECENT EXPERIENCES AND RESPONSE RATES

Study	Regimen	Evaluable Patients, n	CR, %	Median Survival, mo
Levine et al. JAMA 1991, 266:84	Low-dose m-BACOD	35	46	6.50
Kaplan et al. N Engl J Med 1997, 336:1641.	Low-dose m-BACOD + GM-CSF	94	41	8.75
	Standard-dose m-BACOD + GM-CSF	81	52	7.75

CR—complete response rate; GM-CSF—granulocyte–macrophage colony-stimulating factor.

DOSAGE AND SCHEDULING

Chemotherapy*	Dose
Methotrexate	200 mg/m² IV d 15
Bleomycin	4 U/m² IV d 1
Doxorubicin	25 mg/m² IV d 1 (45 mg/m² standard dose)
Cyclophosphamide	300 mg/m² IV d 1 (600 mg/m² standard dose)
Vincristine	1.4 mg/m² IV d 1 (maximum 2 mg)
Dexamethasone	3 mg/m² PO d 1–5 (6 mg/m² standard dose)
GM-CSF	5 mug/kg SC d 4–13 as needed
CNS prophylaxis (ara-C)	50 mg IT d 1,8,15,22

* Cycle length every 21 d (minimum of 4 cycles; 2 after complete response).
Ara-C—cytarabine; CNS—central nervous system; GM-CSF—granulocyte–macrophage colony-stimulating factor; IT—intrathecally.

CANDIDATES FOR TREATMENT
The optimal therapy for AIDS-lymphoma remains to be defined; therapy must be tailored to the individual patient; for the majority of patients, a dose-modified approach may be appropriate, and the greatest experience has been reported for low-dose m-BACOD; individuals with favorable prognostic factors (none or one of the following: age > 35 y, history of injecting drug use, stage III/IV disease, and CD4 lymphocyte count < 100/μL) may be candidates for full-dose/standard chemotherapy in the hope of improving the complete response rate and prospect for long-term survival; a stratified therapeutic approach based on risk factors has yet to be applied in the management of AIDS-related lymphoma; furthermore, there are no data on the substitution of liposomal formulations in anthracycline-based combination chemotherapy regimens; finally, the role of routine central nervous system prophylaxis has not been definitively addressed in well-controlled clinical trials and may not be warranted in all patients (see chapter text for details); in any event, most patients with AIDS-lymphoma should be offered a trial of chemotherapy; although not curative of the lymphoma in most individuals, chemotherapy may result in significant palliation of symptoms and improve quality of life; if there is no response after 2 cycles of therapy or if there is a decline in performance status, discontinuation of chemotherapy is appropriate

ALTERNATIVE THERAPIES
Infusional CDE (cyclophosphamide, doxorubicin, and etoposide), oral combination chemotherapy, CEOP, EPOCH, or CHOP (cyclophosphamide, doxorubicin, vincristine, and prednisone); a suggested dose-modified CHOP regimen is as follows—Cyclophosphamide: 375 mg/m² IV d 1; Doxorubicin: 25 mg/m² IV d 1; Vincristine: 1.4 mg/m² (maximum 2.0 mg) IV d 1; Prednisone: 100 mg PO d 1–5 (cycle length every 21 d)

SPECIAL PRECAUTIONS AND NURSING INTERVENTIONS
Special precautions are needed for patients with underlying cardiac disease (eg, HIV-related cardiomyopathy) for the anthracyclines, chronic lung disease for bleomycin, and HIV-related peripheral neuropathy and constipation for the vinca alkaloids; in many of these circumstances, it may be appropriate to avoid the offending cytotoxic agent altogether or to closely monitor the functional status of the patient (eg, left ventricular ejection fraction by radionuclide scanning, diffusion capacity for carbon monoxide, and careful neurologic examination); given the immunosuppressive effects of chemotherapy regimens for lymphoma, the majority of which include corticosteroids, all patients should receive Pneumocystis carinii pneumonia prophylaxis regardless of CD4 lymphocyte count

TOXICITIES
Fifty-one percent of the patients receiving dose-modified m-BACOD will experience grade 3 or higher toxic effects; 50% will develop grade 4 neutropenia; episodes of febrile neutropenia will complicate approximately 6% of the cycles administered; 11% will develop grade 3 or higher thrombocytopenia; grade 3 or higher anemia will occur in 32% of patients; opportunistic infection will complicate the course of treatment in ~20% of patients

PATIENT INFORMATION
Traditional cytotoxic chemotherapy regimen dose-modified for AIDS patients with lymphoma.

INFUSIONAL CDE
Cyclophosphamide, Doxorubicin, Etoposide

Investigators at Albert Einstein initially reported this regimen in a pilot study with 12 patients. The regimen consists of a continuous 96-h infusion of cyclophosphamide, doxorubicin, and etoposide. Patients with small noncleaved-cell lymphoma and those with bone marrow involvement received central nervous system (CNS) prophylaxis consisting of intrathecal chemotherapy and whole-brain radiotherapy. This study and their subsequent reports demonstrated a response rate of 58%–93%. Their initial study had a long median survival of 17.4 mo. Therapy was generally well tolerated and was given on an outpatient basis using a portable infusion pump. The Eastern Cooperative Oncology Group is currently conducting a phase II pilot study of infusional CDE, coupled with dideoxyinosine (ddI) and granulocyte–macrophage colony-stimulating factor (protocol E1494-NHL). Regardless of CD4 count, all patients should receive prophylaxis for *Pneumocystic carinii* pneumonia during treatment.

ALTERNATIVE THERAPIES

Low dose m-BACOD, oral combination chemotherapy, CEOP, EPOCH or CHOP (cyclophosphamide, doxorubicin, vincristine, and prednisone)

TOXICITIES

Opportunistic infection is of primary concern, especially if CD4 lymphocyte counts are < 25/μL; concomitant use of steroids increases this risk; the combination of this regimen and ddI is associated with significantly less neutropenia and thrombocytopenia and fewer erythrocyte and platelet transfusions; CDE results in a significant decrease in CD4 and CD8 lymphocytes, an effect not abrogated by coadministration with ddI; nonhematologic toxicity consists of nausea and vomiting (72%) and stomatitis (56%); one patient has developed heart failure due to this regimen

PATIENT INFORMATION

This regimen requires placement of a central venous access device and patients will likely have to be hospitalized for 4 d in the absence of appropriate home-care support or if clinician is not familiar with the regimen; nonetheless, this regimen has resulted in the longest survival reported for patients with AIDS-related lymphoma; confirmatory multi-institutional trials are underway.

RECENT EXPERIENCES AND RESPONSE RATES

Study	Evaluable Patients, n	Response Rate, %	Median CD4 Count	Median Survival, mo
Sparano et al. Blood 1993, 81:2810	14	93	Not specified	17.4
Sparano et al. Leuk Lymphoma 1994, 14:263	21	86	84	18.0
Sparano et al. J Clin Oncol 1996, 14:3026	25	58	85	18.0

DOSAGE AND SCHEDULING

Chemotherapy*	Dose	Interval
Cyclophosphamide	800 mg/m² as 96-h CIV	Every 4 wk
Doxorubicin	50 mg/m² as 96-h CIV	Every 4 wk
Etoposide	240 mg/m² as 96-h CIV	Every 4 wk
G-CSF	5 μg/kg SC d 6 until ANC > 10,000/μL	
CNS prophylaxis (in select patients; *see* above)		
Cytarabine	45 mg/m² IT d 1, cycle 1	
Methotrexate	12 mg IT d 3 & 5, cycles 1 & 2	

* Maximum of 6 cycles (2 cycles after complete response).
ANC—absolute neutrophil count; CIV—continuous infusion; CNS—central nervous system; G-CSF—granulocyte colony-stimulating factor; IT—intrathecal.

ORAL-COMBINATION CHEMOTHERAPY

Recent studies have been investigating novel methods of drug scheduling and delivery, including protracted infusion and oral administration of chemotherapy in the treatment of AIDS-related lymphoma. An oral-combination chemotherapy regimen has been reported in 38 patients; it achieved complete remission in 13 of 38 patients (34%), an overall objective response rate of 66%, and an overall median survival of 7 mo. The 1-y, 18-mo, and 2-y survival rates are 34%, 21%, and 11%, respectively. Two of 38 patients (5%) developed CNS relapse or progression without prescribed CNS prophylaxis, which raises the possibility of CNS activity of lomustine and procarbazine. Although significant myelotoxicity was observed, the protocol was convenient and less costly to administer than standard intravenous chemotherapy. Interestingly, the incidence of clinically significant ($\geq$ grade 2) nausea, vomiting, diarrhea, and stomatitis seen with other intravenous chemotherapy is low with this regimen. Treatment is self-administered, and consequently, patient compliance is a very important consideration. A dose-modified oral regimen is being developed.

ALTERNATIVE THERAPIES

Low dose m-BACOD, infusional CDE (cyclophosphamide, doxorubicin, and etoposide), CEOP, EPOCH, and CHOP(cyclophosphamide, doxorubicin, vincristine, and prednisone)

TOXICITIES

The overall toxicity of this regimen compares favorably with that of others; myelosuppression is the most frequent and severe toxicity encountered, with leukopenia being more pronounced than thrombocytopenia; there is a 57% incidence of $\geq$ grade 3 neutropenia and 49% incidence of $\geq$ grade 3 thrombocytopenia with the oral chemotherapy regimen; a total of 21 episodes of febrile neutropenia (21% of treatment cycles) have occurred; The coadministration of granulocyte colony-stimulating factor significantly reduced both the number of hospitalizations for febrile neutropenia and the incidence of discontinuation of chemotherapy because of neutropenia; thrombocytopenia was, however, more severe with the administration of granulocyte colony-stimulating factor; interestingly, the incidence of clinically significant ($\geq$ grade 2) nausea, vomiting, diarrhea, and stomatitis seen with other regimens is low with this regimen

PATIENT INFORMATION

Administration of oral chemotherapy may be attractive to patients for a variety of reasons; some patients are often receiving complicated antiretroviral regimens and many other medications, a situation that may be cumbersome; if a patient's compliance cannot be assured, perhaps it is best to offer IV chemotherapy for their lymphoma; this regimen does not require CNS prophylaxis; the CNS relapse rate observed with this regimen is clinically acceptable.

RECENT EXPERIENCES AND RESPONSE RATES

Study	Regimen	Evaluable Patients, n	CR, n	Median Survival, mo
Remick et al. J Clin Oncol 1993, 11:191	Oral chemotherapy	18	39	7
Remick et al. J Acquir Immune Defic Syndr Hum Retrovirol 1997, 14:A37	Oral chemotherapy + G-CSF	20	30	7

CR—complete response rate; G-CSF—granulocyte colony-stimulating factor.

DOSAGE AND SCHEDULING

Chemotherapy*	Dosage
Lomustine	100 mg/m^2 (cycles 1 & 3) d 1
Etoposide	200 mg/m^2 d 1–3
Cyclophosphamide	100 mg/m^2 d 22–31
Procarbazine	100 mg/m^2 d 22–31
G-CSF	5 µg/kg SC d 5–21, 33–42
CNS prophylaxis	Not given

* Cycles administered every 6 wk for a total of 3 cycles; all chemotherapy drugs given orally.
CNS—central nervous system; G-CSF—granulocyte colony-stimulating factor.

CHAPTER 25: MYELOSUPPRESSION
Michael Gordon

Myelosuppression as a toxicity of cancer therapy is among the most common complications seen [1]. All forms of cancer treatment (including radiation therapy, immunotherapy, and especially chemotherapy) affect peripheral blood counts either by reducing bone marrow production or increasing peripheral blood destruction. Myelosuppression can affect all lineages of peripheral blood, although the myeloid series tends to be most commonly and significantly affected (Table 25-1). This results in neutropenia with the associated risks of bacterial or fungal infections. In most cases, neutropenia is short-lived, and the risk of infectious complications is low. Infection risk appears to be related to both the depth and duration of neutropenia. Other lineages can also be affected by the myelosuppressive effects of therapy. Anemia, most often cumulative in nature, can be seen in patients receiving treatment. This complication most often results in a reduction in quality of life due to fatigue and poorer energy. Finally, a small number of patients will develop thrombocytopenia from cancer therapy. The risk of clinically severe bleeding in patients with thrombocytopenia is low, and it is generally only the most myelosuppressed patients who develop severe thrombocytopenia. Overall, the development of myelosuppression as a complication of cancer therapy can be related to a range of variables that are addressed in Table 25-2.

PATHOPHYSIOLOGY

The production of blood cells by the bone marrow is an orderly process controlled by both positive and negative regulators called hematopoietic growth factors (HGFs) and cytokines, respectively (Table 26-3) [2]. These include both early-acting factors (primarily the interleukins) and late-acting factors (the colony-stimulating factors [CSFs]). These agents control the proliferation, differentiation, and maturation of multipotential precursor cells, which can be directed to various lineages based upon the relative expression of specific factors and clinical need. Overall, blood cell production is centered around the earliest of stem cells (the multipotential stem cell), which has the ability to self-replicate and ensure that adequate precursor cells are always present. The exhaustion of this stem cell supply, although hypothetical, could lead to severe bone marrow depletion and the total underproduction of blood cells. This is one concern with regard to the effects of cancer therapy on the bone marrow.

The ability of the bone marrow to produce blood cells is related not only to the availability of blood stem and precursor cell, but also to the health of the marrow microenvironment, which is primarily responsible for the production of the HGFs and cytokines. Damage to the marrow microenvironment, such as with radiation therapy, can produce a second mechanism for the development of myelosuppression.

Kinetically, the myelosuppressive effects of cancer therapy tend to be related to the stage of development that is damaged by the agent in question. Neutrophils, which usually survive 7 hours in the circulation, are most sensitive to treatment effects. Similarly, platelets, which last 7 to 10 days, are more commonly affected than red blood cells, which last 120 days in the circulation. The timing of new blood cell production is similar for all lineages, with approximately 7 days from stem cell to committed precursor and another week from committed elements to mature cells that are ready to be released into the circulation. These time lines can be significantly accelerated by the application of HGFs and CSFs to blood cell production.

CAUSES

The principle forms of anticancer therapy that result in myelosuppression are chemotherapy and radiation therapy. Radiation therapy damages not only the cellular component but also the marrow microenvironment. Biologic therapy such as immunotherapy may induce myelosuppression either by direct bone marrow suppression or by the induction of peripheral destruction. The latter of these two most commonly resolves quickly following discontinuation of these agents.

Chemotherapy

The effect of chemotherapy on bone marrow cells is similar to that which is desired on cancer cells. Different chemotherapy drugs can be classified into categories based upon their mechanism of action. Alkylating agents typically bind to nucleotide bases of DNA and thereby inhibit protein synthesis and replication. This effect is similar to that of the antitumor antibiotics, eg, doxorubicin, which intercalates into DNA strands preventing DNA synthesis. Vinca alkaloids and the taxanes inhibit microtubular synthesis and functions, which inhibits spindle formation, preventing cells from actively undergoing mitosis. Finally antimetabolites frequently substitute themselves for purine or pyrimidine nucleotides and block DNA or RNA synthesis. These latter agents may also block specific enzymes required for nucleotide synthesis. Much in the same manner that chemotherapy drugs are taken up by cancer cells, so are they used by bone marrow cells. Hence, the bone marrow, because of its rapidly proliferating state, tends to be affected in a manner similar to that of the cancer cells. An outline of cancer chemotherapeutic agents and their relative effects on different lineages is shown in Table 26-4. Several agents (eg, vincristine, low-dose methotrexate, L-asparaginase, and oral cyclophosphamide) generally do not cause myelosuppression; however some agents (eg, the nitrosureas and mitomycin C) frequently induce a delayed and prolonged myelosuppression.

Table 25-1. Categories of Cytopenias

Leukopenia: a reduction in circulating levels of white blood cells
Neutropenia: decrease in the number of circulating myeloid infection-fighting cells
Anemia: decrease in the number of red blood cells or hemoglobin concentration
Thrombocytopenia: decrease in the number of circulating platelets

---

Table 25-2. Factors Associated With Myelosuppression

Therapy
    Choice of chemotherapy agents and dose-intensity planned
    Radiation therapy including dose planned and volume irradiated
Bone marrow reserve
    Patient's age and nutritional status
    Prior therapy
    Bone marrow involvement with malignancy or other process

Table 25-3. Hematopoietic Growth Factors and Cytokines

	Name	Lineage	Approval Status
Colony-stimulating factors	C-CSF	m	Approved
	GM-CSF	m, mo	Approved
	EPO	e	Approved
	TPO	p	Investigational
	M-CSF	mo	No longer under study
Interleukins	Interleukin-11	p	Approved
	Interleukin-3	m, e, p	No longer under study
	Interleukin-6	p	No longer under study
	Interleukin-1	m, e, p	No longer under study

e—erythroid; G-CSF—granulocyte colony-stimulating factor; GM-CSF—granulocyte–macrophage colony-stimulating factor; EPO—erythropoietin; m—myeloid; mo—monocytic; M-CSF—macrophage colony-stimulating factor; p—platelet; TPO—thrombopoietin.

Immunotherapy

Biologic agents can be divided into two specific groups. The first, which includes the immunotherapeutic agents (eg, the interferons [α, β, and γ] and interleukin-2), can induce myelosuppression by reducing bone marrow cellular production. This occurs at modest doses of interferon and is one of the desired effects in its use in chronic myeloid leukemia. In contrast, the lymphopenia and neutropenia associated with interleukin-2 appears to be predominantly related to peripheral consumption by immunostimulated cells or by margination of related pools of cells. Both of these side effects are rapidly reversible, appear to be dose related, and generally are not associated with infectious complications. In addition to the interleukin-2–mediated neutropenia, this agent has the ability to induce a neutrophil dysfunction that lasts longer than the quantitative neutropenia.

The second form of immunotherapy is associated with monoclonal antibodies. These agents are generally not associated with myelosuppression. In specific cases in which the antibody is "tagged" with a radioactive particle, this combination may induce some degree of myelosuppression.

Radiation Therapy

Radiation therapy induces cell death by causing lethal double-stranded DNA breaks. These DNA breaks result in cell death/apoptosis when the cell enters the cell cycle. For this reason, it is cells in G_0 that tend to be most sensitive to DNA damage as opposed to those in G- or S-phase, which tend to be more resistant due to their ability to enzymatically correct damage. Hence, the myelosuppression associated with radiation therapy is often related to the volume of bone marrow irradiated, the total radiation dose, and the patients overall bone marrow reserve. This latter point is important because irradiated bone marrow space tends to not repopulate with hematopoietic cells for prolonged periods of time. This is distinctly different from the myelosuppression induced by chemotherapy, in which 1) bone marrow microenvironmental damage is generally not severe or long lasting, and 2) hematologic recovery is more rapid. The depth and duration of myelosuppression is somewhat dependent upon the volume of bone marrow irradiated, and hence, therapy to the long bones, sternum, vertebral bodies, or pelvis is associated with more myelosuppression than that to other regions.

DIAGNOSIS

Bone Marrow

Evaluation of the bone marrow's function is generally performed via a bone marrow aspiration and biopsy. This simple bedside procedure enables the physician to assess not only the overall cellularity of the bone marrow space but also the cellular components of the bone marrow compartment. It is particularly useful when determination of etiology for cytopenias is required. For example, patients with isolated thrombocytopenia may have a superimposed immune-mediated consumptive process that can be inferred based upon the presence of adequate or increased numbers of megakaryocytes in the bone marrow because patients with myelosuppression frequently have megakaryocytic hypoplasia. In addition, bone marrow assessments enable physicians to determine overall bone marrow reserve and assess for complicating issues such as bone marrow involvement by malignancy (both hematologic and nonhematologic).

Bone marrow aspirates can be performed in a variety of locations including the sternum (~2–3 cm below the sternomanubrial joint) and the anterior and posterior iliac crest. The posterior iliac crest is the ideal location for a bone marrow biopsy because the other two locations do not lend themselves to biopsy due to the thinness of the bone in these locations. Occasionally, bone marrow aspirates may be unsuccessful, resulting in either a lack of bone spicules for assessment or a "dry tap" with no aspirate specimen obtained. This may be due to any of the following causes: bone marrow hypoplasia or aplasia, involvement with malignancy, bone marrow fibrosis, or prior irradiation to the procedural site (which is important because it represents an error with regard to chosen location). Frequently, bone marrow regions will remain hypoplastic for years following irradiation to the location. Under the circumstances of an unsuccessful aspirate, it is critical that an adequate biopsy be obtained to assess the bone marrow pathophysiology. Newer methods to investigate bone marrow disorders, such as the use of magnetic resonance, are under investigation; however, even though these methods are unable to determine morphology, they can provide some information regarding cellularity and signal normalcy.

Table 25-4. Drug-Induced Myelosuppression

	Route of administration	Degree of suppression*	Time to nadir (wk)*	Time to recovery (wk)*	Affected cell type
Alkylating agents					
Busulfan	PO	Moderate–marked	2–4	6–8	L,P
Chlorambucil	PO	Moderate	2–3	4–8	L
Cyclophosphamide	IV,PO	Mild–moderate	1–2	2–4	L
Ifosfamide	IV	Moderate	1–2	2–4	L,P
Melphalan	PO	Moderate	2–3	4–7	L,P
Thiotepa	IV	Moderate–marked	2–3	4–6	P,L
Antibiotics					
Bleomycin	IV	0–mild	1–2	2–3	P,L
Daunorubicin	IV	Marked	2	3–4	L,P
Doxorubicin	IV	Marked	2	3–4	L,P
Idarubicin	IV	Marked	2	3–4	L,P
Mitoxantrone	IV	Marked	1–2	3	L,P
Mitomycin	IV	Moderate	Up to 8	Up to 10	L,P
Antimetabolites					
2-Chlorodeoxyadenosine	IV	Moderate	1–2	3–4	L,P
Cytosine arabinoside	IV	Moderate–marked	2	3	L,P
Fludarabine	IV	Mild–moderate	2–3	3–5	L,P
Fluorouracil	IV	Mild–moderate	1–2	2–3	L,P
Mercaptopurine	IV	Moderate	1–2	3–4	L,P
Methotrexate	PO	Moderate–marked	1–2	2–3	L,P
Vinca alkaloids/ Epipodophyllotoxins					
Etoposide	IV,PO	Mild–moderate	1–2	3	P
Teniposide	IV	Moderate–marked	1	2–3	L,P
Vinblastine	IV	Moderate	1–2	2–3	L
Vincristine	IV	Mild	1–2	2	L
Vinorelbine	IV	Moderate–marked	1–2	3–4	L
Miscellaneous					
L-asparaginase	IV	0–mild	1–2	—	L
Cisplatin	IV	Moderate	2–3	4–6	G,P,E
Carboplatin	IV	Moderate	2–3	4–6	G,P,E
Dacarbazine	IV	Mild	2–3	4–5	G,P
Hydroxurea	PO	Moderate — marked	1	2–3	G,P
Plalitaxel	IV	Moderate–marked	1–2	2–3	L,P
Procarbazine	PO	Moderate	3–4	4–6	P,G

*Dependent on dose, administration, and scheduling.
E—erythrocytes; L—leukocytes; P—platelets.

Peripheral Blood

Evaluation of the peripheral blood (PB) is the simplest tissue biopsy available under any circumstances. A PB smear can be made from a simple finger-stick, and its review allows assessment of leukocytes, erythrocytes, and thrombocytes, with regard to morphology and number. A manual differential count of the PB leukocytes can allow determination of the number of circulating neutrophilic granulocytes (segmented neutrophils [segs] and band forms). This number is critical because the determination of severe neutropenia is associated with an inherent risk of infection. The calculation of the absolute neutrophil count (ANC) is based upon the following equation, in which total WBC is the total number of white blood cells:

$$ANC = total\ WBC \times (\%segs + \%bands)$$

In addition to a quantitative evaluation of PB cells, a qualitative assessment can be performed, which can lend support to clinical diagnoses. These assessments include erythrocyte morphology (size, shape), leukocyte activation (presence of Dohle bodies or toxic granulation), and platelet size. Finally, PB evaluation can give insight into early signs of recovery from myelosuppression because an early wave of PB monocytes is characteristic of early myeloid recovery.

HEMATOLOGIC TOXICITIES

Neutropenia

Neutropenia is a deficiency of circulating polymorphonuclear leukocytes—the classic infection-fighting cell of the body. It tends to be readily suppressed by chemotherapy and is often the only lineage affected during chemotherapy-induced myelosuppression. Some ethnic groups have characteristically lower normal neutrophil counts due to a increase in the number of marginated cells present in their circulation. Most patients typically have a small marginated pool that can be demarginated by stress or drugs (corticosteroids or epinephrine). In the former cases, the percentage of cells existing in the marginated state is greater than usual. These patients are not at an increased risk of infectious complications regardless of the depth of their neutropenia. In some instances, neutropenia can fall to levels characteristically associated with an increased risk of infection (eg, < 1000 cells/µL. In other cases, a bone marrow hypoproduction of neutrophils (either idiopathic or cyclical in nature) can be associated with dangerously low neutrophil counts to levels < 100 cells/µL. These patients often have associated severe infectious complication, which may even be life threatening. Finally, the group of patients with underlying bone marrow disorders (eg, the myelodysplastic syndromes or leukemic processes) may have adequate or low numbers of neutrophils, which function poorly and therefore place these patients, even with adequate numbers of cells, at a relatively higher risk of infection.

Neutropenia associated with chemotherapy classically occurs approximately 1 to 2 weeks following most cytotoxic agents. The depth and duration of neutropenia is highly associated with the risk of infectious complications [3]. Fevers in the setting of severe neutropenia (ANC < 1000 cells/µL) is considered an oncologic emergency requiring rapid intervention with broad-spectrum antibiotics and aggressive medical management because immunocompromised neutropenic patients are at high risk for rapidly progressive and life-threatening infectious complications.

Appropriate antibiotic coverage includes either an antipseudomonal penicillin or a third-generation cephalosporin (ceftazidime) as initial monotherapy with expansion of coverage based upon microbiological cultures or response with regard to defervescence of fever. Antibiotics should be continued until the ANC has exceeded 500 cells/µL during recovery and patients are afebrile. Patients with a central venous access device and positive blood cultures are generally treated for a prolonged course (minimum 14 d) of antibiotics to sterilize their device regardless of ANC recovery. The use of white blood cell transfusions from HLA-identical donors has been used in patients and is reserved for those cases in which prolonged neutropenia is associated with gram-negative bacteremia or fungemia.

In the early 1990s, two hematopoietic CSFs were approved for the treatment of neutropenia associated with anticancer therapy. The first, granulocyte CSF (G-CSF or filgrastim [Neupogen; Amgen Inc., Thousand Oaks, CA]) is lineage-specific for neutrophils and induces bone marrow and PB increases in this lineage. The second factor, granulocyte-macrophage CSF (GM-CSF or sargramostim [Leukine; Immunex, Seattle, WA]) affects myeloid and monocytic lineages. Both agents have demonstrated the ability to accelerate myeloid recovery following chemotherapy, shortening the period of neutropenia and incidence of infection in both the standard and high-dose (bone marrow transplantation) setting [4,5]. The use of these agents in the management of radiation-induced neutropenia is investigational. At least one study showed that chemoradiotherapy patients with non–small cell lung cancer who were treated with GM-CSF demonstrated worse myelosuppression compared with patients treated without the support of growth factors. This outcome raises concerns over the use of CSFs with radiation therapy.

Anemia

Anemia or low hemoglobin concentration occurs when the hemoglobin falls below the lower limit of normal. In most centers, this is the area of 12 g/dL. Most patients are only mildly symptomatic from these minimal degrees of anemia, so no therapy is required. With continued chemotherapy, a progressive cumulative anemia frequently develops, which may become more severe and may event require red blood cell transfusions. Symptoms indicative of anemia include fatigue, tachycardia, dyspnea on exertion, and exacerbation of underlying cardiopulmonary disease (in extreme cases). Similar to the issues regarding thrombocytopenia and the possible peripheral destructive mechanisms involved, anemia can be induced by either hypoproduction or increased destruction. Increased destruction may be related to an immune-mediated process (eg, a Coombs' positive hemolytic anemia in lymphoma) or a microangiopathic process (eg, as in disseminated intravascular coagulation in solid cancers). The determination of the etiology may be important with regard to options for management. Correcting underlying causes is important for etiologies other than hypoproduction. In addition, because cancer patients may have poor nutrition, confirmation of adequate amounts of iron and vitamin stores (especially folate and B_{12}) are important components of the anemia work-up.

Transfusion of red blood cells, generally to keep the hemoglobin level above 8 g/dL is the standard for management of these patients. The use of subcutaneously administered erythropoietin has become more widespread based upon the data demonstrating reduced red blood cell transfusions requirements and improved quality of life for treated patients. It is important to note that for optimal effect, erythropoietin therapy should be initiated when anemia is developing and prior to the need for initial transfusions [6].

Thrombocytopenia

Thrombocytopenia is a deficiency in the number of circulating platelets. Like neutrophils, platelets exist in both marginated and demarginated pools. In addition, approximately one third of the circulating platelet pool is stored in the spleen at any given time. Normal platelet counts are generally in the range of 150,000 to 400,000/µL. Levels below 150,000/µL are considered low, though studies have demonstrated that modest reductions in the number of platelets are not associated with an increased risk of bleeding. In fact, it is generally accepted that platelet counts > 50,000/µL are acceptable for major or minor procedures and that adequate hemostasis can be obtained with these levels. Minor bleeding often does not occur until platelet counts fall below 20,000/µL , and in the average patient, the risk of major bleeding does not increase significantly until the platelet count falls below 10,000/µL.

Patients at higher risk of bleeding include those with increased peripheral destruction of platelets (eg, those with infection or DIC) or those on medications that may affect platelet function (eg, aspirin or nonsteroidal anti-inflammatory agents). These latter drugs should be avoided in patients with thrombocytopenia.

A recent debate has raged over the appropriate threshold for platelet transfusions. Traditionally, 20,000/µL has been used as the indicator for the transfusion of platelets to prevent bleeding. Recent studies, however, indicate that the use of a lower threshold of 10,000/µL is safe and apparently equally effective in preventing bleeding. This lower threshold has the benefit of avoiding transfusions in a percentage of patients and reducing the inherent risks associated with transfusions (eg, infectious [viral and bacterial], cost, and immunoreactive [transfusion reactions]). Recently, a new thrombopoietic growth factor, interleukin-11 (IL-11 or oprelvekin [Neumega; Genetics Institute, Cambridge, MA]) was approved for use in patients at high risk for the development of chemotherapy-induced thrombocytopenia [7]. Like the myeloid CSFs, this agent must be administered following chemotherapy until adequate platelet recovery has occurred. Other agents (*eg*, thrombopoietin) are also being studied for this indication.

OTHER INTERVENTIONS
Progenitor Cell Infusions

The use of either bone marrow cells or peripheral blood stem or progenitor cells (PBPCs) has become more and more widespread over the past several years. The availability of CSFs to improve the mobilization of the cells in to the PB where they can be isolated by leukopheresis has contributed significantly to this increase. In general, it is dose-intensive chemo- or chemoradiotherapy that require the use of this technology and for which it is most commonly applied. The use of PBPCs can accelerate not only myeloid recovery but platelet recovery as well, reducing the number of transfusions and the length of stay in the hospital. In addition, it is the incorporation of PBPC infusions into high-dose chemotherapy that has allowed transplantation procedures to move into the outpatient arena, which has cut costs and improved patient acceptance.

Although the use of PBPC has been routine for the past number of years in the autologous transplantation setting, it is relatively recent that it has been explored in the allogeneic setting. There appears to be an acceleration of hematologic recovery and possibly immune reconstitution with the use of PB compared to bone marrow progenitors, but it is unclear if unwanted side effects (*eg*, increased incidence of graft-versus-host disease) will be seen.

Obtaining PBPCs can be accomplished either with the static use of CSFs in the stead-state patient (CSFs alone) or following the administration of dose-intensive chemotherapy (*eg*, high-dose cyclophosphamide). The latter method has the advantage of using the chemotherapy to cytoreduce the patient's volume of disease prior to the transplant itself. It is also associated with an inherent risk of complications from the myelosuppression that follows the chemotherapy, which can occasionally be life threatening or jeopardize the planned transplant itself. Therefore, decisions regarding these approaches should be made on a case-by-case basis.

REFERENCES

1. DeVita V Jr: Principles of cancer management: chemotherapy. In *Cancer: Principles and Practice of Oncology*. Edited by DeVita V, Hellman S, Rosenberg S. Philadelphia: Lippincott-Raven; 1997:333–348.

2. Bagby G Jr, Segal G: Growth factors and the control of hematopoiesis. In *Hematology: Basic Principles and Practice*. Edited by Hoffman B Jr, Shattil S, *et al*. New York: Churchill Livingstone; 1995:207–241.

3. Bodey G, Buckley M, Sathe Y, *et al.*: Quantitative relationships between circulating leukocytes and infection in patients with acute leukemia. *Ann Intern Med* 1966, 64:328–340.

4. 4. Crawford J, Ozer H, Stoller R, et al: Reduction by granulocyte colony-stimulating factor of fever and neutropenia by chemotherapy in patients with small cell lung cancer. *N Engl J Med* 1991, 325:164–170.

5. Nemunaitis J, Rabinowe S, Singer J, *et al.*: Recombinant granulocyte-macrophage colony- stimulating factor after autologous bone marrow transplantation for lymphoid cancer. *N Engl J Med* 1991, 324:1773–1778.

6. Oster W, Herrmann F, Gamm H, *et al.*: Erythropoietin for the treatment of anemia of malignancy associated with neoplastic bone marrow infiltration. *J Clin Oncol* 1990, 8:956–962.

7. Tepler I, Elias L, Smith J II, *et al.*: A randomized, placebo-controlled, trial of recombinant human interleukin-11 in cancer patients with severe thrombocytopenia due to chemotherapy. *Blood* 1996, 87:3607–3614.

NEUTROPENIA

Neutropenia is defined as a deficiency in the number of functional neutrophil granulocytes. The criterion for neutropenia is an absolute neutrophil count less than 1000/μL. Patients with neutropenia are at greater risk of developing infections, particularly if they are undergoing dose-intensified or prolonged chemotherapy.

INTERVENTIONS

1. Prevention
   a. Avoid concurrent myelosuppressive agents and radiation therapy
   b. Chemotherapy dose reduction, if appropriate, maintaining schedule
   c. Delay interval between treatment cycles until neutrophil recovery
   d. Interrupt radiation therapy until neutrophil recovery
   e. Hematopoietic growth factor support (G-CSF, GM-CSF)
   f. Nutritional support
2. Prevention and treatment of sequelae
   a. Avoid exposure to infection and reverse isolation
   b. Meticulous personal hygiene
   c. Early antimicrobial treatment for associated fevers (broad-spectrum antibiotics, with staphylococcal and gram-negative coverage; biliary tree–enteric anaerobe; bowel-enteric anaerobe)
   d. Transfusion of neutrophils

GRANULOCYTE–COLONY-STIMULATING FACTOR (G-CSF) OR FILGRASTIM

1. **Indications:** Patients with malignancies receiving myelosuppressive chemotherapy associated with a significant (minimal 40%) incidence of severe neutropenia and fever (contraindicated in patients with known hypersensitivity to *E. coli*–derived proteins)
2. **Dosage and administration:** 5 μg/kg/d SC or IV to begin ≥ 24 h after chemotherapy; continue administration for up to 2 wk until ANC ≥ 10,000/mm^3 following neutrophil nadir
3. **Lab monitoring:** Baseline CBC and platelet counts, biweekly thereafter
4. **Adverse reactions:** medullary bone pain, increased uric acid, alkaline phosphatase, LDH, transient decreased blood pressure (rare)

GRANULOCYTE-MACROPHAGE–COLONY-STIMULATING FACTOR (GM-CSF) OR SARGRAMOSTIM

1. **Indications:** Patients with non-Hodgkin's lymphoma, acute lymphocyte leukemia, and Hodgkin's disease undergoing high-dose chemotherapy with progenitor cell support and elderly patients with acute myeloid leukemia receiving chemotherapy (contraindicated in patients with known hypersensitivity to GM-CSF, yeast-derived products or any component of the product)
2. **Dosage and administration:** 250 μg/m^2/d for 21 d by 2-h IV infusion beginning 2–4 h after ABMT; discontinue therapy when neutrophil count is > 20,000/mm^3
3. **Lab monitoring:** If blast cells appear, discontinue therapy; biweekly monitoring of renal and hepatic function and CBC with differential
4. **Adverse reactions:** > 5% incidence over placebo; diarrhea, exacerbation of preexisting asthma, renal or hepatic dysfunction, rash, exacerbation of arrhythmia, malaise, fever, headache, bone pain, hives, myalgia, dyspnea, peripheral edema

CAUSATIVE FACTORS

Primary: benign; chronic—severe, congenital, cyclic, idiopathic; **secondary:** neoplastic—hematologic malignancy, metastatic tumor; nonneoplastic—autoimmune, drug-related (chemotherapy, antibiotics, anticonvulsants, antidepressants); infection (bacterial, viral, mycobacterial); radiation; hematologic disease (aplastic anemia, myelofibrosis, paroxysmal nocturnal hemoglobinuria, T-gamma syndrome), organomegaly, nutritional deficiency

PATHOLOGIC PROCESS

Many unknown, possibly overproduction of cytokine suppressors or loss of growth factor receptors on progenitors, inhibition of nucleic acid and protein syntheses, maturation arrest, overproduction of hematopoietic inhibitors, antibody-induced destruction, drug-induced destruction, replacement of bone marrow by tumor or fibrosis, defective folate metabolism

DIFFERENTIAL DIAGNOSES

See Causative Factors

PATIENT ASSESSMENT

Leukocyte count and differential, review of smear for morphology, bone marrow aspiration and biopsy, karyotype, culture bone marrow, special bone marrow stains, including reticulin and acid-fast bacilli; serum B$_{12}$ and folate levels, analysis for T-cell receptor gene rearrangement.

TOXICITY GRADING

	0	1	2	3	4
WBC x 10^3	> 4.5	3.0– < 4.5	2.0– < 3.0	1.0– < 2.0	< 1.0
Neutrophil x 10^3	> 1.9	1.5– < 1.9	1.0– < 1.5	0.5– < 1.0	< 0.5

THROMBOCYTOPENIA

Thrombocytopenia is a shortage of functional platelets due to decreased production, increased consumption, defective function, or splenic pooling. The condition is often exacerbated by cancer therapy and can place the patient at risk of hemorrhage.

INTERVENTIONS

1. Prevention
   a. Avoid antiplatelet agents (*eg*, ASA)
   b. Chemotherapy dose adjustment, maintaining schedule
2. Prevention and treatment of sequelae
   a. Avoid invasive procedures
   b. Use progesterones to prevent menses
   c. GI tract prophylaxis (*ie*, antacids, stool softeners)
   d. Platelet transfusion (see below)

PLATELET TRANSFUSION

1. **Indications:** Prophylaxis for patients with platelet counts < 10,000–20,000/mm^3, prophylaxis for surgery if counts < 50,000/mm^3, treatment of hemorrhage if < 50,000–100,000/mm^3; signs and symptoms indicating need for transfusion: easy bruisability, petechiae, mucous membrane bleeding
2. **Preparations:** All are ABO compatible and may be leukocyte-depleted at the bedside; from whole blood (random donor), ≥ 5.5 × 10^{10}/bag; apheresis (single donor), > 3 × 10^{11}/bag; leukocyte-poor and single donor delay development of alloimmunization; HLA matched—for patients already alloimmunized
3. **Dose and administration:** 6 U (random donor) or 1 bag (single donor) IV infusion. Count should increase 5,000–10,000/μl/random donor bag. A poor response in platelet increment may be due to splenomegaly, fever, sepsis, disseminated intravascular coagulation (DIC), alloimmunization (1-h increment < 50% of expected suggests alloimmunization)
4. **Risks and adverse reactions:** *immune*—fever, allergic reaction, graft-versus-host reaction; *nonimmune*—volume overload, transmission of infection

INTERLEUKIN-11 (IL-11)

1. **Indications:** Patients with nonmyeloid malignancies receiving dose-intensive chemotherapy and at a high risk for the development of severe chemotherapy-induced thrombocytopenia (contraindicated in patients with known hypersensitivity to *E. coli*–derived products)
2. **Dosage and administration:** 50 μg/kg/d SC to begin following chemotherapy (no sooner than 6 h after chemotherapy) and continued until a postnadir platelet count of 50,000/μL is achieved or for a maximum of 21 d
3. **Lab monitoring:** Twice weekly complete blood and platelet counts
4. **Adverse reactions:** Asthenia, edema, dyspnea, rare incidence of atrial arrhythmias

CAUSATIVE FACTORS

Quantitative: *decreased production*—congenital, acquired: alcoholism, drug-related (chemotherapy and radiation, diuretics, H2 blockers), infections (viral), nutritional deficiency, tumor involvement of bone marrow, myelofibrosis, primary hematologic disorder; *increased consumption*—autoimmune (ITP, TTP, hematologic malignancy), DIC, drug-related (heparin, antibiotics, infection); **qualitative:** *drug-related*—nonsteroidal antiinflammatory agents, antimicrobials, psychiatric drugs, alcohol; *concomitant illness*—uremia, chronic liver disease, myeloproliferative disorders

PATHOLOGIC PROCESS

Clot formation, antibody-induced destruction, inhibition of nucleic acid synthesis, bone marrow replacement with tumor or fibrosis, sequestration in enlarged spleen, defective maturation, drug-induced acetylation of platelet cyclooxygenase

DIFFERENTIAL DIAGNOSES

See Causative factors

PATIENT ASSESSMENT

CBC, peripheral blood smear, mean platelet volume, bone marrow aspiration or biopsy, karyotype, platelet aggregation studies, bleeding time (if platelet count adequate).

TOXICITY GRADING

	0	1	2	3	4
Platelet					
x 10^3	> 130	90– < 130	50– < 90	25– < 50	< 25

ANEMIA

The patient with anemia has an abnormally low concentration of erythrocytes and hemoglobin. The potential risks of anemia are less serious than those of neutropenia and thrombocytopenia; however, with the trend toward intensified therapy doses and BMT, the incidence and severity of anemia are increasing. Transfusion continues to be the conventional method of support.

INTERVENTIONS

1. Prevention—erythropoietin support
2. Prevention and treatment of sequelae; transfusion of erythrocytes; management of fatigue

TRANSFUSION OF ERYTHROCYTES

1. **Indications:** Patients with symptomatic anemia requiring increased red cell mass and improved oxygen-carrying capacity. Symptoms may include tachycardia, dyspnea, angina, decreased mentation, transient ischemic attacks, syncope, postural hypotension, inability to maintain reasonable level of daily activity (contraindicated in asymptomatic patients with vitamin-responsive anemia, Fe-responsive anemia, erythropoietin-responsive anemias)
2. **Preparations:** *All ABO-compatible and cross-matched* —PRBC is blood component of choice, majority of plasma removed, 50–75 mL remain in each unit; preservative solution added; Hct = 70%–80%; 1 U increases Hb in 70 kg adult by 1–1.5 g/dL; *leukocyte-poor erythrocytes*—used to prevent febrile transfusion reactions and alloimmunization to leukocyte, antigen and platelet transfusion; *washed erythrocytes*—for patients with history of transfusion-related allergic reactions (usually due to plasma proteins), Hct = 50%–70%
3. **Dosage and administration:** Dose based on severity. In otherwise healthy patients, transfuse to Hb ≥ 8 g/dL. In patients with cardiac disease, frequently transfuse to Hb ≥ 10 g/dL. Infuse over 4 h via IV catheter with normal saline for flushing
4. **Risks and adverse reactions:** *Nonimmune*—volume overload, Fe overload, transmission of infections: hepatitis (1–2:100 transfusions), cytomegalovirus, HIV, HTLV-1, Epstein–Barr virus, bacterial infections (rare), Lyme disease, babesiosis, Chagas' disease, brucella, malaria, possibly TB; *immune*—acute or delayed hemolysis, fever (most common reaction with transfusion), allergic (urticaria, wheezing, angioedema), graft-versus-host (prevented by radiation therapy of blood product with 1500–3000 cGy)

ERYTHROPOIETIN (EPO)

1. **Indications:** Patients with chronic renal failure (CRF), patients with anemia due to chemotherapy (contraindicated in patients with uncontrolled hypertension or with hypersensitivity to mammalian cell–derived products of human albumin)
2. **Dose and administration:** *CRF*—50–100 U/kg IV three times pre week, reduce dose if target Hct is reached or if Hct increases > 4% in 2 wk; increase dose if target not reached or no increase of 5%–6% in 8 wk; maintenance dose is individualized; *chemotherapy*— 150 U/kg SC three times per week; can be increased to 300 U/kg three times per week after 8 wk; decrease if hematocrit > 40%
3. **Lab monitoring:** blood pressure, Hct 1–2 × wk during dose adjustment, Fe and Fe-binding capacity
4. **Adverse reactions:** *CRF patients*—hypertension, thrombotic events, headache, shortness of breath, tachycardia, hypercalcemia, nausea and vomiting, diarrhea (most frequent); flu-like symptoms, rash, urticaria, and seizures (rare); *patients receiving chemotherapy*: diarrhea, edema; fever, shortness of breath, paresthesia, URI (less frequent)

CAUSATIVE FACTORS

Blood loss, chemotherapy and radiation, chronic disease: tumor, infection, drug-related (zidovidine), hemolysis: autoimmune—tumor (CLL, lymphoma), drug-related; mechanical—chemotherapy (mitomycin C), DIC (tumor- or infection-related); nutritional deficiency: poor nutrition, postsurgery of gastrointestinal tract; bone marrow involvement: hematologic malignancy, metastatic tumor, myelofibrosis; concomitant illness: renal insufficiency, endocrine deficiencies

PATHOLOGIC PROCESS

Defective hemoglobin production, defective glucolysis, defective DNA synthesis, defective iron and B_{12} absorption, defective purine and pyrimidine synthesis, blockade in folate metabolism, erythrocyte parasites, bacterial toxins, antibody-induced destruction, erythropoietin deficiency, production of cytokines that inhibit hematopoiesis, replacement of bone marrow by tumor or fibrosis

DIFFERENTIAL DIAGNOSES

See Causative Factors

PATIENT ASSESSMENT

Erythrocyte count, hemoglobin concentration, hematocrit, mean corpuscular hemoglobin, mean corpuscular volume, mean corpuscular hemoglobin concentration, reticulocyte count, erythrocyte morphology, additional tests based on clinical evaluation: total and fractionated bilirubin, serum iron, total iron binding capacity, stool hematocrit, serum vitamin B_{12}, red cell folate, hemoglobin electrophoresis, direct and indirect Coombs' test, bone marrow aspiration and biopsy, thyroid function tests.

TOXICITY GRADING

	0	1	2	3
Hbg g%,	> 11,	9.5–10.9,	< 9.5,	Transfusion required
Hct%	> 32	28–31.9	< 28	Transfusion required

The information here is provided as guidance only. Prescribers should always consult the manufacturer's current prescribing information.

The gastrointestinal tract is a common site of treatment-related toxicity, which may contribute to profound patient morbidity and limit the dose or intensity of cancer therapy. Gastrointestinal dysfunction may cause pain, the inability to eat or properly digest food with progressive malnutrition, nausea and vomiting, perforation, and bleeding, and it may lead to serious infection. This chapter describes the side effects of systemic cancer therapy on the gastrointestinal tract and outlines current methods of prevention and management.

MUCOSITIS

It is estimated that approximately 1 million Americans are diagnosed with cancer each year, and 400,000 of these patients develop oral complications associated with cancer treatment [1]. Oral complications of chemotherapy occur through two interrelated pathophysiologic mechanisms. Because cells of the upper digestive tract undergo turnover on a 7- to 14-day cycle, they are susceptible to chemotherapy-induced direct stomatotoxicity. The resultant mucosal atrophy may lead to stomatitis, cheilosis, glossitis, and esophagitis. Indirect stomatotoxicity results from chemotherapy-induced myelosuppression and infections from the many potential pathogens that colonize the oral cavity. The greater the degree and duration of neutropenia, the greater the risk of infection. In addition, the direct cytotoxic effect of chemotherapy may disrupt the protective barrier of the oral epithelium and further enhance the predisposition to secondary infection. The mouth has been identified as the source of sepsis in 25% to 54% of neutropenic patients [2].

Assessment and Diagnosis

The frequency and severity of mucositis depend on the particular antineoplastic drug and its dose, schedule, and regimen (*ie*, given alone or in combination with other cytotoxic agents or radiation therapy). However, patients differ markedly in their ability to tolerate a given chemotherapeutic regimen. Patients who develop oral toxicity with the first course of therapy invariably show similar side effects during subsequent courses unless the doses are decreased or the drugs are changed. The state of oral health, performance status, and age are critical factors for the risk of complications. Young patients are reported to experience more toxicity than older patients. This may be related to a high incidence of hematologic malignancies and intent to deliver the most intensive therapies to young patients [3].

Preexisting oral disease unrelated to the cancer increases the risk of oral complications. At a National Institute of Health Consensus Development Conference [1] it was strongly recommended that all patients receiving chemotherapy undergo pretreatment dental evaluation with the following objectives: establish baseline data with which all subsequent examinations can be compared; identify risk factors for the development of oral complications; develop strategies to avoid treatment-related complications; and perform necessary dental treatment to reduce the likelihood of oral complications induced by cancer therapy. Invasive prophylactic dental procedures should be performed well before the onset of chemotherapy-induced neutropenia and thrombocytopenia. Bacterial and fungal surveillance cultures are not necessary, but suspicious lesions should be cultured.

Patients suffering from mucositis often describe a burning sensation in the mouth within 3 to 10 days of the initiation of chemotherapy. This frequently precedes objective signs and should alert the clinician to the problem. Any of the mucosal surfaces may then develop erythema and progress to erosion and ulceration over the next 3 to 5 days. Intense pain, inability to handle secretions, and

severe reduction in oral intake may ensue. The damage is usually reversible, with self-healing occurring over the 1 to 2 weeks following cessation of therapy.

Infection often follows mucositis but also may occur in the absence of direct stomatotoxicity. Oral infections with bacteria, especially gram-negative organisms, are the most frequent, although fungal and viral infections are common. With oral bacterial infections, the mucosa often has a necrotic appearance along with painful red ulcerations. Patients with chronic periodontal disease may develop acute periodontal or gingival bacterial infections that are edematous and painful, although in myelosuppressed patients the signs of inflammation often are absent. Fever is common in patients suffering from oral bacterial infections, and cultures from affected intraoral locales and blood may be positive. The sites of oral candidiasis are the sides and top of the tongue; the buccal, gingival, and palatal mucosa; and the commissures of the lips. The infection is manifest as painless, white, raised, curd-like strands or patches that tend to coalesce and adhere to the underlying mucosa. Forceful removal of the plaque reveals an erythematous or ulcerated mucosal surface. Diagnosis should be made by microscopic evaluation using a potassium hydroxide preparation and tissue cultures. Herpes simplex virus and varicella zoster are the two most common viral pathogens causing oral infection in immunocompromised patients. The characteristic vesicular lesions usually rupture within a day, resulting in diffuse ulceration that eventually crusts over. Diagnosis rests with viral cultures or the demonstration of characteristic intranuclear inclusions in the epithelial cells of stained smears.

Management

Patients likely to experience chemotherapy-induced mucositis should begin a program of routine oral hygiene and prophylaxis at the outset of chemotherapy. Patient and family education and continued guidance and motivational support are important to the success of preventative treatment. Components of a comprehensive oral care regimen include daily brushing and flossing; mouthwashing with saline, hydrogen peroxide, or sodium bicarbonate solution; and lip lubrication with petroleum jelly. Flossing is contraindicated during periods of severe thrombocytopenia, but brushing should continue unless significant bleeding occurs. Ongoing oral care depends on the severity of symptoms and patient tolerance.

A variety of topical agents and oral rinses are used to prevent or minimize mucositis in patients receiving chemotherapy (Table 26-1). Chlorhexidine, a broad-spectrum topical antimicrobial agent, has been studied in several randomized, placebo-controlled, double-blind, prophylactic trials producing varying results. Interpretation of these studies is difficult due to differences in the concentration and dosage schedules of chlorhexidine and the patient populations. However, a number of trials in patients undergoing induction chemotherapy for acute leukemia or bone marrow transplantations for hematologic malignancies have shown that chlorhexidine (0.12%) mouth rinses significantly reduce the incidence and severity of mucositis and candidiasis [4]. They should be considered for prophylactic use in patients undergoing intensive chemotherapy. Although both nystatin oral suspension and clotrimazole troches are commonly used for antifungal prophylaxis in patients with leukemia and bone marrow transplantations, the clinical results have been disappointing. In contrast, retrospective studies have shown a 50% to 80% incidence of severe herpes simplex (HSV) oral infection in severely myelosuppressed patients who are seropositive for the HSV antibody. Thus, patients undergoing induction treatment for acute leukemia or bone

Table 26-1. Topical Agents for Prevention and Treatment of Mucositis

Class	Agents	Dosage/Schedule	Guidelines and Comments
General cleaning	Hydrogen peroxide and saline 1:2	15 mL, qid, swish	Following toothbrushing
	Sodium bicarbonate and water—1 tsp in 500 mL	15 mL, qid, swish	Following toothbrushing
Antimicrobials	Chlorhexidine gluconate 0.12%	Mouth rinse bid (do not swallow)	Clinical trials do not show benefit
Antifungals	Nystatin oral suspension or lozenge	200,000 U qid	Preventive use unproven; for treatment of candidiasis
	Clotrimazole troche	10 mg qid	
Topical agents for generalized mucositis	Viscous Xylocaine 2%	15 mL q 4 h, swish	Limited duration of effect
	Dyclonine hydrochloride 0.5%	15 mL q 4 h, swish	
	Maalox, Benadryl, viscous Xylocaine in equal parts (MBX)	15 mL q 4 h, swish	
	Diphenhydramine and kaolin	15 mL q 4 h, swish	
	Sucralfate (1 g/10 mL)	10 mL qid swish and swallow	Clinical trials do not show benefit
Clinical			
Topical agents for localized mucositis	Benzocaine 15% gel or ointment	Apply to affected area qid	Avoid if coexisting oral infection
	Vitamin E (400 mg/mL)	Apply to affected area bid	Under investigation for this use

marrow transplantation should be tested for the presence of HSV antibody. Such patients are likely to benefit from prophylactic treatment with acyclovir [5]. Other agents that have been investigated for prophylaxis include allopurinol mouth wash, benzydamine hydrochloride, beta carotene, and sucralfate. Evidence of efficacy is lacking, therefore none of these agents can be recommended for routine use.

Prophylactic oral cryotherapy is being used increasingly in clinical practice. Patients are instructed to suck on ice chips for 30 minutes, 5 minutes prior to each dose of 5-fluorouracil (5-FU). A randomized study of 95 patients receiving 5-FU plus leucovorin demonstrated that oral cryotherapy resulted in a significant reduction in mucositis, as judged by physician and patient [6]. The low cost and ease of administration make oral cryotherapy an attractive preventative measure and should be considered for all patients receiving bolus 5-FU therapy. Pilot studies of hematologic growth factors had shown promise in decreasing the incidence of mucositis and accelerating the healing process [7]. However, randomized studies with granulocyte colony-stimulating factor (G-CSF) and granulocyte-macrophage colony-stimulating factor (GM-CSF) in patients receiving chemotherapy have not shown a benefit in reducing the incidence or severity of mucositis [8,9]. A pilot study of GM-CSF mouthwash showed efficacy in reducing the severity and duration of chemotherapy induced mucositis; this approach appears promising and deserves further study [10].

The management of overt mucositis is palliative and supportive. The frequency of general oral care procedures should be increased if possible. Pain relief is essential to allow for adequate oral intake, and systemic analgesics (oral or IV) are indicated when local therapy alone is insufficient. Early diagnostic and therapeutic intervention for infection may improve outcome. Bacterial and significant viral infections usually require systemic antibiotics. Although oral candidiasis may be treated with topical antifungal agents, fluconazole or amphotericin B may be necessary for refractory or disseminated infection. When mucositis is generalized throughout the oral surfaces, frequent swishing with a variety of topical anesthetics results in amelioration of pain, albeit for a limited period of time (see Table 26-1). A solution of equal parts diphenhydramine, Maalox, and viscous Xylocaine is easily prepared, inexpensive, and well tolerated. Based on its mechanism of action of adhering to duodenal ulcers, sucralfate suspension has been used empirically in a small number of patients with chemotherapy-induced mucositis with encouraging results in terms of pain relief and enhanced healing [11,12]. However, most randomized studies have not shown sucralfate to be effective in treating 5-FU–induced stomatitis and cannot be recommended for routine use [13]. For localized mucosal ulcerations, the application of bioadhesive topical gels [14], vitamin E [15], or capsaicin preparations [16] to desensitize pain receptors appears promising. Laser treatments have been used to treat mucositis, and preliminary studies show encouraging results in reducing the severity and duration of mucositis due to chemotherapy [17]. The treatment of chemotherapy-induced mucositis is still far from satisfactory, and new agents and novel therapies need to be explored.

NAUSEA AND VOMITING

Cancer patients identify nausea and vomiting as one of the most distressing and feared side effects of their illness and therapy. Complications of nausea and vomiting include weight loss, dehydration, electrolyte abnormalities, esophageal tears and gastrointestinal bleeding, aspiration pneumonia, psychological distress, diminished quality of life, and reduced patient compliance with anticancer therapy.

Almost 75% of cancer patients undergoing chemotherapy may experience nausea and vomiting during the course of chemotherapy. However, acute vomiting can be controlled in the majority of patients with the newer generation of drugs, such as the serotonin type 3 (5-HT3) receptor antagonists. Patient perception of vomiting due to chemotherapy may be changing as shown by a recent study in which 155 patients undergoing chemotherapy during 1993 completed a survey of their experiences. Nausea was the most severe side effect, but vomiting took fifth place unlike a similar survey done in 1983 in which vomiting was the most severe symptom reported [18].

The pathophysiology of chemotherapy-induced nausea and vomiting is the result of a complex neuronal reflex arch (Fig. 26-1). Two anatomically distinct regions of the brain are involved: the chemoreceptor trigger zone, a richly vascularized area located in the area postrema on the caudal margin of the fourth ventricle, and the vomiting center in the medulla oblongata. Because it is located outside the blood–brain barrier, the chemoreceptor trigger zone may be directly activated by a variety of noxious stimuli, such as chemotherapeutic agents and their metabolites, other drugs, or humoral factors. The vomiting center receives afferent input from the chemoreceptor trigger

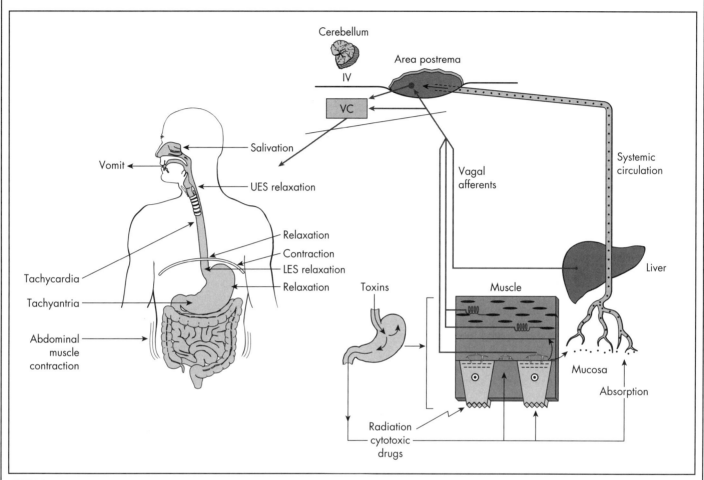

FIGURE 26-1.

Pathways involved in chemotherapy-induced nausea and vomiting. LES—lower esophageal sphincter; UES—upper esophageal sphincter. *From* Andrews and colleagues [54]; with permission.

zone, the limbic system, the higher cortical centers, the vestibular system, and the visceral afferent fibers from the gastrointestinal tract. The connections to the limbic system and cerebral cortex have been postulated as one explanation for the conditioned response of anticipatory vomiting. Through efferent neuronal pathways in the vagus nerve, the vomiting center mediates the autonomic and somatic reflexes culminating in nausea and vomiting, such as vasoconstriction, tachycardia, diaphoresis, diaphragmatic and abdominal muscle contraction, and intestinal retroperistalsis.

A variety of neurotransmitters are involved in the vomiting reflex. The chemoreceptor trigger zone is rich in dopamine, cholinergic, and serotonin receptors. Antagonism of these receptors forms the basis of action of many of the antiemetics currently in use [19]. Serotonin appears to be the principal neurotransmitter in the emetic reflex in humans [20]. A current hypothesis, supported by clinical data, suggests that highly emetogenic chemotherapy and radiation treatment induces cellular changes in the gastrointestinal tract. Damaged enterochromaffin cells of the upper gastrointestinal tract release serotonin locally, resulting in activation of the serotonin receptors on vagal and splanchnic afferent fibers originating within the intestinal wall. These visceral afferents activate receptors within the chemoreceptor trigger zone and the vomiting center, thus initiating the emetic reflex arch (Fig. 26-1).

Classification

Chemotherapy-induced nausea and vomiting can be classified as anticipatory, acute, and delayed based on the time of occurrence relative to chemotherapy administration.

Anticipatory Nausea and Vomiting

This is a conditioned response seen in 10% to 44% of patients receiving chemotherapy. It occurs before or during administration of chemotherapy but earlier than expected with the particular regimen being administered. The onset of anticipatory vomiting varies, but the pattern often becomes apparent after the first few courses of chemotherapy. Young adults (especially women) are more prone to develop anticipatory nausea and vomiting. Anxiety appears to be a component in the development of this syndrome; behavioral modification techniques and antianxiolytic agents, such as lorazepam, are useful in treating this condition.

Acute Nausea and Vomiting

Acute nausea and vomiting is seen generally within the first 24 hours of drug administration. The onset of nausea and vomiting after drug administration varies from a few minutes to several hours for each particular drug. Serotonin and 5-HT3 receptors appear to be the most important in the pathogenesis of acute nausea and vomiting though other neurotransmitters are also implicated. The clinician needs to familiar with the pharmacology of the antiemetic agents and the emetogenic potential of chemotherapeutic agents to effectively design a regimen to combat nausea and vomiting.

Delayed Nausea and Vomiting

Delayed nausea and vomiting is seen 24 hours or later after the administration of chemotherapeutic agents and may last for several days. The mechanism of delayed nausea and vomiting is unclear and still remains a difficult clinical problem with few effective therapeutic options.

Assessment and Diagnosis

Although chemotherapy is the most frequent cause of nausea and vomiting in patients with cancer, other causes are sufficiently common to warrant consideration in the differential diagnosis. Careful evaluation, including physical examination, measurement of serum electrolytes, and liver and renal function tests, is mandatory. Radiographic studies to evaluate the gastrointestinal or biliary tract or a computed tomography scan of the brain may be necessary.

The emetogenic properties of chemotherapeutic agents vary greatly and are influenced by dose, schedule, concomitant drugs, and radiation therapy (Table 26-2). Acute chemotherapy-induced nausea or vomiting typically begins 6 to 8 hours after the IV administration of an alkylating agent and may persist for up to 36 hours. Cisplatin and dacarbazine elicit nausea and vomiting in virtually every patient, with symptoms usually commencing very shortly after drug administration. Symptoms usually resolve within 24 hours but may persist for many days. This delayed nausea and vomiting is most commonly seen with cisplatin administration and is notoriously difficult to treat. Moreover, there is wide variation in patient tolerance to the emetic potential of chemotherapeutic agents. Certain characteristics influence the frequency and severity of symptoms, and recognition of these factors may help to individualize antiemetic therapy. A history of heavy alcohol intake, for instance, decreases the risk of nausea and vomiting. Young patients are more likely to develop the extrapyramidal side effects seen with many of the commonly used antiemetic agents. Patients with poor previous emetic control are at especially high risk of subsequent anticipatory nausea and vomiting, which underscores the importance of adequate prevention during the initial chemotherapy treatment.

Management

The clinical management of chemotherapy-induced nausea and vomiting requires a comprehensive strategy of pharmacologic intervention, patient and family support, and psychological and behavioral adjustment. A major principle is the prophylactic administration of antiemetic drugs (Table 26-3). Knowledge of the mechanisms of action, routes of administration, and adverse reactions of the various classes of currently available antiemetics is mandatory for effective therapy.

Phenothiazines

Prochlorperazine and thiethylperazine are the most commonly prescribed antiemetic agents and are adequate when given with chemotherapy of mild emetic potential. Both appear to be marginally more effective than chlorpromazine and may be administered orally or rectally. When either is given IV, hypotension is a dose-limiting side effect. The mechanism of action is blockade of dopamine receptors in the chemoreceptor trigger zone; hence extrapyramidal side effects, especially in young patients, are common.

Table 26-2. Emetic Potential of Common Cytotoxic Agents

High (> 90%)	Moderate (30%–60%)	Moderately High (60%–90%)	Low (10%–30%)
Cisplatin	Carboplatin	Cyclophosphamide	Bleomycin
Dacarbazine	Doxorubicin	Cytosine arabinoside	Fluorouracil
Nitrogen mustard	Daunorubicin	Ifosfamide	Vincristine
Streptozotocin	Mitomycin-C	Hexamethylmelamine	Vinblastine
	Procarbazine	Nitrosoureas	Melphalan
			Chlorambucil
			Methotrexate
			Etoposide
			Paclitaxel

Butyrophenones

Haloperidol and droperidol are structurally related to the phenothiazines. They are useful agents for the prevention and treatment of mild-to-moderate emetogenic chemotherapy. Although some studies have demonstrated the efficacy of butyrophenones in cisplatin-induced chemotherapy, they have been replaced by more effective antiemetics for this application. One disadvantage of droperidol is that it is only available as an IV formulation. Side effects include sedation, occasional dystonic reactions, and other extrapyramidal events.

Metoclopramide

Although metoclopramide, a substituted benzamide, is ineffective in low doses, at high doses it prevents and reduces cisplatin-induced nausea and vomiting in approximately 50% of patients. It is also beneficial when used with other highly emetogenic agents. Although metoclopramide originally was thought to be a dopamine antagonist, evidence suggests that at its effective high-dose range it acts principally through blockade of serotonin receptors. Prior to the introduction of specific serotonin antagonists, high-dose metoclopramide formed the basis of the most frequently prescribed combination therapy used with highly emetogenic chemotherapy. Adverse reactions to metoclopramide include sedation, diarrhea, and akathisia (restlessness). Parkinsonian-like symptoms, such as tremor and rigidity, are more likely to occur in the elderly, whereas major dystonic reactions occur most frequently in patients younger than 30 years of age. These neurologic side effects can be distressing and are to a great extent preventable with concomitant administration of diphenhydramine or a benzodiazepine.

Cannabinoids

The active constituent of dronabinol is delta-9-tetrahydrocannabinol, the principal psychoactive substance in marijuana. Dronabinol has mild to moderate antiemetic properties, although the mechanism of action is unknown. It is indicated for the treatment of chemotherapy-associated nausea and vomiting in patients who do not respond adequately to other antiemetic regimens. Toxicities include euphoria and dysphoria, mild sedation, dry mouth, and dizziness. The elderly are at greater risk for these unpleasant side effects, and the drug should be reserved for younger patients.

Table 26-3. Frequently Used Antiemetic Agents

Class/Action	Agent	Dosage/Schedule	Side Effects
Phenothiazines-dopamine antagonist	Prochlorperazine	10–20 mg PO q 4–5 h 25 mg PR q 4–6 h 10 mg IV q 4–6 h	Dystonic reaction
	Thiethylperazine	10 mg PO or PR, q 6–8 h	
	Chlorpromazine	10–25 mg PO q 4–6 h 10–25 mg IV q 3–4 h	
	Promethazine	25 mg PO, PR, IM q 4–6 h	Dystonic reaction
Butyrophenones-dopamine antagonist	Haloperidol	1–3 mg IV q 2–4 h	Sedation
	Droperidol	1–2.5 mg IV q 4 h	Dystonic reaction
Substituted benzamides-serotonin antagonist	Metoclopramide	1–3 mg/kg IV q 2 h × 2–3	Sedation
			Diarrhea
Cannabinoids-unknown	Dronabinol	10 mg PO before meals	Dysphoria
			Sedation
			Dry Mouth
5-HT$_3$ receptor antagonists	Ondansetron	8–15 mg IV × 1 8 mg PO q 8 h	Headache
	Granisetron	10 µg/kg IV × 1, 1–3 mg IV × 1 1 mg PO q 12 h, 2 mg PO × 1	Diarrhea
	Dolasteron	100 mg PO × 1, 1.8–2.4 mg/kg IV × 1	
Adjunctive agents	Dexamethasone	10–20 mg IV × 1	
	Lorazepam	1–2 mg IV × 1	
	Diphenhydramine	25–50 mg IV or PO q 4 h	

Serotonin Receptor Antagonists

Elucidation of the role of serotonin in the pathophysiology of chemotherapy-induced emesis has led to the development of a new and highly effective class of agents that probably exert their principal antiemetic activity by competitive antagonism of serotonin type 3 receptors in the afferent nerve fibers of the proximal gastrointestinal tract. These agents have greatly enhanced the quality of life of patients receiving highly emetogenic chemotherapy. Ondansetron, granisetron, and dolasteron are commercially available, but many other agents in this class are under active clinical investigation.

Randomized studies using a variety of doses and schedules have consistently shown both ondansetron, granisetron, and dolasteron to be significantly more effective than metoclopramide-containing regimens for the prevention of cisplatin-induced nausea and vomiting [21,22]. Approximately 65% to 75% of patients obtain major emetic control with either of these serotonin antagonists. When compared with regimens consisting of metoclopramide plus dexamethasone, the serotonin antagonists generally result in a longer time to first emetic episode, fewer side effects, decreased need for salvage antiemetics, and substantial patient preference. There is no definite evidence that one agent is active when another agent has failed to prevent emesis. The half-life of these agents range from 3 to 11 hours, and oral formulations are effective due to high bioavailability.

The relatively high cost of ondansetron and granisetron has necessitated evaluation of appropriate dosing schedules. The optimum doses of these serotonin agents and the best route of administration are not yet known. Oral formulations appear to be equally efficacious as intravenous administration. Ondansetron in doses of 8 to 15 mg, granisetron in doses of 10 µg/kg, and dolasteron in doses of 100 mg appear to be as active as higher doses in preventing emesis [23–26].

In cisplatin induced emesis the combination of a 5-HT3 antagonist and steroids appears to offer the best protection against emesis. Two hundred and thirty seven patients undergoing cisplatin chemotherapy were randomized to either ondansetron (8 mg) and dexamethasone (20 mg) or to metoclopramide (3 mg/kg twice daily), dexamethasone (20 mg), and lorazepam (1.5 mg/m^2). In patients who received ondansetron, complete protection from emesis was seen in 73% of patients and was significantly higher compared with 56% of those who received high-dose metoclopramide. The incidence of adverse events was also less in patients who received ondansetron [27]. In patients who have acute emesis with the regimen of ondansetron and dexamethasone, the addition of metopimazine (a dopamine antagonist not available in the United States) appears effective in reducing the incidence of emesis in subsequent cycles of chemotherapy [28].

The relative efficacy of ondansetron compared with granisetron has been studied in several randomized clinical trials and has recently been reviewed [29,30]. However, only one study utilized doses of these agents currently approved in the United States. Navari and colleagues [31] compared ondansetron, 0.15 mg/kg IV for three doses, with a single IV dose of granisetron at 10 or 40 µg/kg in 987 patients receiving moderate- to high-dose cisplatin. There were no differences in efficacy or toxicity. Complete emetic control was 51% for ondansetron and 47% and 48% for granisetron, 10 and 40 µg/kg, respectively. The most frequently reported side effects with either drug were a mild to moderate headache and diarrhea, seen in 15 and 8% of patients, respectively. Dolasteron is another 5-HT3 agent that can be used in patients receiving cisplatin chemotherapy. A randomized study showed that a single intravenous dose of dolasteron (either 1.8 or 2.4 mg/kg) had comparable safety and efficacy to a single 32-

mg dose of ondansetron given intravenously in patients receiving cisplatin chemotherapy [32]. Oral granisetron appears to be a viable alternative for patients receiving highly or moderately emetogenic therapy. Two randomized studies have compared oral granisetron (given in a single dose of 2 mg or 1 mg twice daily) with intravenous ondansetron (32 mg) in patients receiving moderately emetogenic or cisplatin chemotherapy [33,34]. Patients also received corticosteroids in addition to either granisetron or ondansetron. In both these studies, the oral granisetron and intravenous ondansetron provided comparable efficacy in preventing acute emesis with low toxicity.

The serotonin antagonists are also effective when used with moderately emetogenic therapy. The combination of a 5-HT3 antagonist and dexamethasone is better at preventing acute emesis than the combination of metoclopramide and dexamethasone [35,36]. In spite of these newer drugs, the treatment of delayed nausea and vomiting is still unsatisfactory; and despite the best regimen of metoclopramide and dexamethasone, 50% of patients who receive cisplatin-based chemotherapy will have delayed vomiting.

A double-blind study randomized 322 patients on the completion of cisplatin chemotherapy to oral ondansetron (8 mg twice daily) or oral metoclopramide (20 mg every 6 h) [37]. All patients received intramuscular dexamethasone for 3 days. All patients received acute emesis prophylaxis with ondansetron (8 mg) and dexamethasone (20 mg). Complete protection of delayed vomiting was seen in 62% of patients treated with ondansetron and was similar to that seen in patients who received metoclopramide (60%). However, in patients who vomited in the first 24 hours, ondansetron was better in preventing delayed vomiting (28.6%) than metoclopramide (8.8%). The combination of metoclopramide and dexamethasone has the advantage of lower cost and should be the treatment of choice for prevention of delayed nausea and vomiting. In patients who have adverse effects due to metoclopramide or have acute nausea and vomiting, ondansetron and dexamethasone should be prescribed.

In patients who receive moderately emetogenic therapy, routine prophylaxis for delayed nausea and vomiting appears unnecessary. Patients who have acute vomiting or moderate to severe acute nausea due to moderately emetogenic therapy should be treated for delayed nausea and vomiting [38].

Adjunctive Agents

Lorazepam, the most studied benzodiazepine, has only minimal activity as a single agent. However, its anxiolytic and amnestic properties serve both to diminish anticipatory nausea and reduce the memory of unpleasant emetic episodes. Steroids have mild antiemetic activity as single agents, although the mechanism is not well defined. Side effects of single-dose or short-course steroid treatment are negligible. Both benzodiazepines and steroids are commonly used in multidrug antiemetic regimens.

Combination Antiemetic Therapy

The pathophysiologic complexity of acute chemotherapy-induced nausea and vomiting suggests that combining antiemetics with differing mechanisms of actions and differing side effects may enhance efficacy and tolerance. Several randomized studies have shown that dexamethasone added to high-dose metoclopramide or the serotonin antagonists improves the emetic control compared with the single agents [39–42]. In practice the emetogenic potential of the chemotherapy and the patient's individual characteristics must be considered. Recommendations for commonly used combination antiemetic regimens are given in Table 26-4.

DIARRHEA

Chemotherapy-induced diarrhea results from a direct toxic effect on the rapidly proliferating mucosal cells of the small and large intestine. The antimetabolites are the most common class of drugs causing diarrhea, although it may be the clinical manifestation of any of the drugs implicated in direct stomatotoxicity. Between 25% and 65% of patients with metastatic colon cancer experience some degree of diarrhea associated with 5-FU therapy. There appears to be no significant difference in the incidence or severity of 5-FU–induced diarrhea between bolus or infusional administration of comparable doses. However, the addition of leucovorin or other biomodulators to 5-FU resulted in increased frequency and severity of diarrhea in a number of randomized trials. It is important to note that chemotherapy-induced diarrhea may be extremely severe and the cause of fatal toxicity, especially in elderly patients.

Assessment and Diagnosis

Diarrhea occurring in patients receiving chemotherapy is usually the result of the direct effect of treatment but also may be related to gastrointestinal infection, malabsorption, mechanical obstruction, or ancillary drug therapy, particularly antibiotics. It is extremely important that patients be evaluated promptly and the severity of symptoms and volume status assessed. With weekly boluses of 5-FU, the onset of diarrhea is usually after the fourth week of therapy; when it is administered as a 5-day bolus, symptoms may commence toward the conclusion of a treatment or any time thereafter.

Management

Mild to moderate diarrhea may be treated symptomatically with strict attention to adequate fluid intake to prevent dehydration. It is recommended that patients with severe watery or bloody diarrhea, crampy abdominal pain, fever, or overt dehydration be admitted to the hospital for IV fluids, antibiotics, and antidiarrheal medications. All chemotherapy should be stopped immediately, and further treatment at a reduced dose should be delayed until complete resolution of symptoms.

A number of drugs that slow peristalsis are available for the management of drug-induced diarrhea (Table 26-5). These drugs should be started at the onset of diarrhea and given only when other causes have been reasonably excluded. Octreotide acetate and

Table 26-4. Recommendations for Combinations Antiemetic Therapy

Highly Emetogenic Chemotherapy

Odansetron 8–15 mg IV *or* granisetron 10 µg/kg IV *or* 1–3 mg IV *or* dolasteron 1.8–2.4 mg/Kg IV, and dexamethasone 20 mg IV	Metoclopramide 3 mg/kg IV q 2 h × 3 and dexamethasone 20 mg IV × 1 and lorazepam 1–2 mg IV

Moderately Emetogenic Chemotherapy

Ondansetron 8–24 mg IV *or* 8 mg PO tid *or* Granisetron 10 µg/kg IV *or* 1 mg PO BID *or* 2 mg PO qd *or* dolasteron 100 mg PO qd and dexamethasone 20 mg IV	Prochlorperazine 10 mg PO q 4 h × 4 and dexamethasone 20 mg IV

Table 26-5. Medical Therapy for Chemotherapy-Induced Diarrhea

Agent	Dosage/Schedule	Guidelines and Comments
Kaolin and pectin	30–40 mL after each loose bowel movement	Acts as an intestinal absorbent, useful for mild diarrhea
Diphenoxylate with useful atropine	2.5 mg, 1–2 tablets after each loose bowel movement	Not to exceed 12 tablets in 24 h; for mild to moderate diarrhea
Loperamide useful	2 mg, 1–2 tablets after each loose bowel movement	Not to exceed 12 tablets in 24 h; for mild to moderate diarrhea
Camphorated opium tincture	5–10 mL qid	Acute toxicity may be CNS depression
Tincture of opium	0.6 mL qid	Contains 25 times more morphines than paregoric; do not confuse preparations
Somatostatin analogue	150 µg/h by continuous venous infusion	Effective for 5-FU–induced diarrhea

somatostatin analogue have been shown to be effective for the treatment of severe diarrhea caused by 5-FU that is refractory to more conservative therapy [43].

The optimum dose of octreotide for treatment of 5-FU induced diarrhea is not yet known. An ongoing three- arm Eastern Cooperative Oncology Group study randomized patients with 5-FU–induced diarrhea to either octreotide 150 µg or 1500 µg given subcutaneously three times a day for 5 days to standard therapy with loperamide. Irinotecan (CPT-11) is notorious for causing diarrhea. Patients who receive this drug should be educated about possible side effects and antidiarrheal measures. Loperamide 4 mg orally should be taken at the first sign of diarrhea, followed by 2 mg every 2 hours (4 mg orally every 4 h at night) until diarrhea has completely resolved for 12 hours [44].

CONSTIPATION

The differential diagnosis of constipation in patients with cancer is diverse. Subacute constipation may be multifactorial, resulting from alteration in diet, decreased fluid intake, physical inactivity, and use of narcotics or drugs with anticholinergic action (antidepressants). The onset of new constipation may be the harbinger of serious complications of the underlying cancer, such as hypercalcemia, uremia, intestinal obstruction, or spinal cord compression. Among the chemotherapeutic agents, only vincristine and vinblastine cause drug-induced autonomic nerve dysfunction with resultant reduction in gastrointestinal peristalsis. The clinical manifestations include constipation, obstipation, colicky abdominal pain, and adynamic ileus. This presentation may be particularly difficult to differentiate from acute intestinal obstruction or other causes of a surgical abdomen. Symptoms generally appear a few days after drug administration. Geriatric patients or those taking significant doses of narcotic analgesics are most susceptible. Treated conservatively this condition usually resolves over 1 to 2 weeks. However, great care should be taken to avoid constipation with the judicious use of mild laxatives and stool softeners in all patients receiving narcotics and vinca alkaloids.

HEPATOTOXICITY

Surprisingly, hepatotoxicity is an unusual complication for most chemotherapeutic agents used singly or in standard-dose combinations. The hepatotoxic reaction most commonly seen is an incidental elevation of transaminases, although cholestasis, frank hepatic necrosis, and fibrosis may occur. In addition, hepatic venoocclusive disease has been reported rarely with some chemotherapeutic agents at conventional doses and occurs much more frequently at the higher doses used in allogeneic or autologous bone marrow transplantation.

Assessment and Diagnosis

Among chemotherapeutic agents available, plicamycin (mithramycin) is the most hepatotoxic. In past decades, plicamycin was used for the treatment of a variety of malignancies, and elevations of transaminases, often to very high levels, occurred in virtually 100% of patients. With the advent of less toxic and more efficacious chemotherapeutic agents, plicamycin is used only for the treatment of hypercalcemia of malignancy, in which lower doses are partially effective. In this clinical setting, the drug produces an approximately 15% incidence of mild reversible hepatic dysfunction.

Other chemotherapeutic agents that cause elevations of hepatic enzymes include the nitrosoureas (carmustine, lomustine, streptozocin), cytosine arabinoside, and methotrexate. The hepatic dysfunction is usually mild, reversible, and clinically insignificant. Long-term oral methotrexate, as used for nonmalignant conditions such as psoriasis and rheumatoid arthritis, may result in hepatic fibrosis, which tends to remain stable or regress when therapy is discontinued. Frank cirrhosis, a much more serious complication, also may occur. A high cumulative dose, rather than the duration of therapy, is most clearly associated with this toxicity. 5-FU, although largely catabolized by the liver, does not result in hepatotoxicity. In contrast, however, when fluorodeoxyuridine is given as an intraarterial hepatic infusion, chemical hepatitis and sclerosis of the intra- and extrahepatic ducts may be seen. The hepatitis is almost always reversible with temporary cessation of the intraarterial therapy, whereas sclerosis of intrahepatic and extrahepatic bile ducts accompanied by cholestatic jaundice is often irreversible and mandates discontinuation of treatment.

Management

As a rule, liver function tests should be evaluated prior to each cycle of chemotherapy. Drugs that are extensively metabolized by the liver or are excreted into the bile should be used with great caution in the presence of hepatic dysfunction due to the likelihood of altered drug pharmacokinetics and resultant increased toxicity. Although based in large part on empirical data, guidelines for dose modifications of chemotherapeutic agents have been summarized (Table 26-6) [45]. Paclitaxel, the newest chemotherapeutic agent approved in the United States, requires dose modification in patients with preexisting hepatic dysfunction. Preliminary guidelines are available from a recent phase 1 study in this patient population (*see* Table 26-6) [46]. At serum bilirubin levels above 5 mg/dL, excessive clinical toxicity is likely to be encountered with all of these drugs and they should not be used. However, prudent clinical judgment is required in this clinical setting. Use of the drug may be warranted if the hepatic dysfunction is due primarily to direct effects of the underlying malignancy, and a rapid antitumor effect may be expected by the

Table 26-6. Suggested Dose Modifications for Preexisting Hepatic Dysfunction

	Bilirubin Level		
	1.5–3.0	3.0–5.0	> 5.0
Doxorubicin	50%	25%	Omit
Vincristine	50%	Omit	Omit
Vinblastine	50%	Omit	Omit
Etoposide	50%	Omit	Omit
Cyclophosphamide	100%	75%	Omit
Methotrexate	100%	75%	Omit
Paclitaxel	75 mg/m^2	50 mg/m^2	50 mg/m^2

Expressed as % of standard dose
Adapted from Perry [45].

administration of some or all of these drugs, as in certain hematologic and lymphoid malignancies.

GASTROINTESTINAL BLEEDING

Gastrointestinal bleeding is a frequent clinical problem in cancer patients. Upper gastrointestinal bleeding due to esophagitis or gastric or duodenal ulceration may be induced or exacerbated by cytotoxic agents, steroids, and nonsteroidal antiinflammatory drugs commonly prescribed for patients with cancer. Primary tumors of the esophagus, stomach, and colon may be the source of both massive and subacute gastrointestinal hemorrhage. Among nongastrointestinal cancers, melanoma that has metastasized to the bowel wall is the most common cause of bleeding. Bleeding may accompany gastrointestinal infections, such as candidal or herpetic esophagitis, and is common in severe graft-versus-host disease. Chemotherapy-induced severe thrombocytopenia and coagulation defects will complicate any gastrointestinal bleeding.

Assessment and Diagnosis

Initial evaluation requires rapid assessment of the magnitude of the bleeding and the status of the circulatory system. Impending or frank hypovolemic shock due to massive bleeding must be treated with immediate volume replacement. Transfusions of packed red blood cells are necessary to maintain the serum hematocrit at approximately 30%. Platelet transfusion is indicated for clinically significant bleeding when the platelet count is less than 50,000. Fresh frozen plasma should be given to correct abnormalities of the partial thromboplastin or prothrombin time.

The appropriate choice of invasive diagnostic procedures should be based on the history and physical examination. Hematemesis almost always indicates upper gastrointestinal blood and loss and can be easily confirmed by nasogastric tube aspiration. This procedure also enables therapeutic gastric lavage with saline solution for ongoing bleeding. Bright red blood per rectum indicates bleeding from the sigmoid colon or rectum and can be assessed by sigmoidoscopy. Maroon-colored stools are suggestive of bleeding from the lower small bowel or right colon. Fiberoptic endoscopy of the upper or lower gastrointestinal tract is the most useful and accurate diagnostic procedure in most cases of gastrointestinal bleeding. Technetium-

labeled red cell scans and angiography may be diagnostic when the source of the bleeding is out of the reach of endoscopic procedures and the rate of bleeding is approximately 1 mL/min.

Management

Acute diffuse upper gastrointestinal bleeding initially often is managed conservatively with IV administration of H$_2$ blockers. Fastidious patient monitoring of volume status and appropriate blood replacement are mandatory. If bleeding does not stop, an IV infusion of vasopressin may be added. However, caution and experience are needed with this approach because serious side effects, such as acidosis, hypertension, and visceral ischemia, may ensue.

A variety of specifically directed therapeutic interventions may be employed, depending on the nature of the lesion. Sclerotherapy is frequently effective in the treatment of bleeding esophageal varices. Single or multiple bleeding sites that are accessible are often controlled by therapeutic endoscopy, including electrocoagulation and laser photocoagulation. Such procedures are frequently useful for bleeding tumors of the esophagus and stomach and may obviate surgery. External beam radiation therapy may also be palliative in this setting. Arterial lesions demonstrated by angiography may be suitable candidates for selective radiologic embolization. This therapy is reserved for bleeding sites in the upper gastrointestinal tract because embolization of the colon is accompanied by an unacceptable incidence of bowel infarction and perforation. Surgery is indicated only when nonoperative treatment has failed to control the bleeding and when a discrete source has been identified that is amenable to a limited surgical procedure. In general, cancer patients with active gastrointestinal hemorrhage are poor operative candidates due to significant comorbidity; consideration of surgery must be individualized.

GASTROINTESTINAL TOXICITY FROM BIOLOGIC AGENTS

Interferon α

Interferon α, which is currently approved only for the treatment of hairy cell leukemia and AIDS-related Kaposi's sarcoma, also has activity in myeloproliferative syndromes, indolent lymphomas, myeloma, renal cell cancer, and melanoma. Toxicity is generally restricted to a transient flu-like syndrome seen in virtually all patients consisting of fever, myalgias, chills, and anorexia. Nausea is occasionally a significant problem. Some patients complain of a metallic taste, especially when therapy is initiated. Infrequently, high-dose regimens of interferon have been associated with profound watery diarrhea. Dose-related, reversible, mild to moderate elevations in hepatic transaminase levels occur in approximately 30% of patients and are more common in patients with preexisting abnormalities of liver function [47]. In patients with preexisting hyperbilirubinemia, cases of cholestatic jaundice and hepatic failure with death have been observed rarely.

Interleukins

Interleukin-2 (IL-2), a human recombinant glycoprotein cytokine, is approved for the treatment of metastatic renal cell cancer and has activity in the treatment of advanced melanoma. At its recommended high-dose bolus schedule significant nausea, vomiting, and diarrhea occur in approximately 75% of treated patients and stomatitis occurs in 30% [48,49]. The incidence appears to be dependent on dose and schedule, as lower dose and continuous-infusion regimens are associated with nausea, diarrhea, and stomatitis in only 25% of patients [50]. The standard antiemetics and antidiarrheals to treat these toxicities are of variable efficacy and often are required in combination [51]. Elevation of serum bilirubin levels above 5 mg/dL occurs in approximately 20% of patients and is usually associated with modest increases in hepatic transaminase levels. Studies suggest this increase is due to reversible cholestasis and usually is not dose limiting [51].

Bowel perforation is an unusual complication with high-dose IL-2, and in one large series was seen in 4 of 315 treated patients [52]. The exact pathophysiology remains unknown. Interruption of IL-2 treatment and surgical intervention are required for treatment.

Interleukin-4 (IL-4), a lymphokine that modulates the proliferation of activated T cells, has recently been studied in early clinical trials. In phase I testing, 12 of 84 treatment courses were complicated by significant gastroduodenal erosion or ulceration, associated with abdominal pain and occasional gastrointestinal bleeding. We suggest that the pathophysiology may result from IL-4–induced alterations in prostaglandin synthesis in the gastric mucosa. In contrast, upper gastrointestinal ulceration due to IL-2 is distinctly uncommon [53].

REFERENCES

1. National Cancer Institute: *Consensus Development Conference on Oral Complications of Cancer Therapies: Diagnosis, Prevention, and Treatment.* National Cancer Institute Monograph, vol 9. Bethesda, MD: National Cancer Institute, 1990:1–10.

2. Peterson DE: Toxicity of chemotherapy induced oral lesions. In Perry MC, Yarbro SW: *Toxicity of Chemotherapy.* New York: Grune and Stratton, 1984:155–180.

3. Sonis S, Clark J: Prevention and management of oral mucositis induced by antineoplastic therapy. *Oncology* 1991, 5:11–18.

4. Peterson DE: Oral toxicity of chemotherapeutic agents. *Semin Oncol* 1992, 19:478–491.

5. Redding SW:National Cancer Institute: *Role of Herpes Simplex Virus Reactivation in Chemotherapy-Induced Oral Mucositis.* National Cancer Institute Monograph, vol 9. Bethesda, MD: National Cancer Institute, 1990:103–105.

6. Mahood DJ, Dose AM, Loprinzi CL, *et al.*: Inhibition of fluorouracil-induced stomatitis by oral cryotherapy. *J Clin Oncol* 1991, 9:449–452.

7. Gabrilove JL, Jakubowski A, Scher H, *et al.*: Effect of G-CSF on neutropenia and associated morbidity due to chemotherapy for transitional cell carcinoma of the urethelium. *N Engl J Med* 1988, 318:1414–1422.

8. Pettengell R, Gurney H, Radford JA, *et al.*: Granulocyte colony -stimulating factor to prevent dose-limiting neutropenia in non-Hodgkin's lymphoma: a randomized controlled trial. *Blood* 1992, 80:1430–1436.

9. Atkinson K, Biggs JC, Downs K, *et al.*: GM-CSF after allogenic bone marrow transplantation: accelerated recovery of neutrophils, monocytes and lymphocytes. *Aust NZ J Med* 1991, 21:686–692.

10. Ibrahim EM, al-Mulhim FA: Effect of granulocyte-macrophage colony-stimulating factor on chemotherapy-induced oral mucositis in non-neutropenic cancer patients. *Med Oncol* 1997, 14:47–5 1.

11. Soloman MA: Oral sucralfate suspension for mucositis. *N Engl J Med* 1986, 315:459–460.

12. Pfeiffer P, Hansen O, Madsem EL, May O: Effect of prophylactic sucralfate suspension on stomatitis induced by cancer chemotherapy: a randomized, double-blind cross over study. *Acta Oncol* 1990, 29:171–173.

13. Loprinzi CL, Ghosh C, Camoriano J, *et al.*: Phase III controlled evaluation of sucralfate to alleviate stomatitis in patients receiving fluorouracil-based chemotherapy. *J Clin Oncol* 1997, 15:1235–1238.

14. LeVeque FG, Parzuchowski JB, Farinacci GC, *et al.*: Clinical evaluation of MGI 209, an anesthetic, film-forming agent for relief from painful oral ulcers associated with chemotherapy. *J Clin Oncol* 1992, 10:1963–1968.

15. Wadleigh RG, Redman RS, Graham ML, *et al.*: Vitamin E in the treatment of chemotherapy-induced mucositis. *Am J Med* 1992, 92:481–484.

16. Berger A, Henderson M, Nadoolman W, *et al.*: Oral capsaicin provides temporary relief for oral mucositis pain secondary to chemotherapy/radiation therapy. *J Pain Symptom Manage* 1995, 10:243–248.

17. Pourreau-Schnelder N, Soudry M, Franquin JC, *et al*: Soft-laser therapy for iatrogenic mucositis in cancer patients receiving high-dose fluorouracil: a preliminary report. *J Natl Cancer Inst* 1992, 84:358–359.

18. Griffin AM, Butow PN, Coastes AS, *et al.*: On the receiving end V: patient perceptions of the side effects of cancer chemotherapy in 1993. *Ann Oncol* 1995, 7:189–195.

19. Mitchell EP: Gastrointestinal toxicity of chemotherapeutic agents. *Semin Oncol* 1992, 19:566–579.

20. Cobbedu LX, Hoffman IS, Fuenmayor NT, *et al.*: Efficacy of ondansetron and the role of serotonin in cisplatin induced nausea and vomiting. *N Engl J Med* 1990, 322:810–816.

21. Marty M, Pouillart P, Scholl S, *et al.*: Comparison of the 5-hydroxy-tryptamine 3 (serotonin) antagonist ondansetron with high dose metoclopramide in the control of cisplatin-induced emesis. *N Engl J Med* 1990, 322:816–821.

22. Hainsworth J, Harvey W, Pendegress K, *et al.*: A single blind comparison of intravenous ondansetron, a selective serotonin antagonist, with intravenous metoclopramide in the prevention of nausea and vomiting associated with high dose cisplatin chemotherapy. *J Clin Oncol* 1991, 9:721–728.

23. Seynaeve C, Schullier J, Buser K, *et al.*: Comparison of the anti-emetic efficacy of different doses of ondansetron given as either a continuous infusion or a single intravenous dose in acute cisplatin-induced emesis: a multicentre, double-blind, randomized, parallel group study. *Br J Cancer* 1992, 66:192–197.

24. Ruff P, Paska W, Goedhals L, *et al.*: Ondansetron compared with granisetron in the prophylaxis of cisplatin-induced acute emesis: a multicentre, double-blind, randomized, parallel group study. *Oncology* 1994, 5:113–118.

25. Perez EA, Gandra DR. The clinical role of granisetron (Kytril) in the prevention of chemotherapy-induced emesis. *Semin Oncol* 1994, 21(3 suppl 5):15–21.

26. Rubenstein EB, Gralla RJ, Hainsworth JD, *et al.*: Randomized, double blind, dose response trial across four oral doses of dolasetron for the prevention of acute emesis after moderately emetogenic chemotherapy. *Cancer* 1997, 79:1216–1224.

27. Cunningham D, Dicato M, Verwey J, *et al.*: Optimal anti-emetic therapy for cisplatin induced emesis over repeat courses: ondansetron plus dexamethasone compared to with metoclopramide, dexamethasone plus lorazepam. *Ann Oncol* 1996, 7:277–282.

28. Depierre A, Lebeau B, Chevellier B, *et al.*: Efficacy of ondansetron, methylprednisolone plus metopimazine in patients previously uncontrolled with dual therapy in cisplatin containing chemotherapy [abstract]. *Ann Oncol* 1996 7(suppl 5):134.

29. Perez EA: Review of the preclinical pharmacology and comparative efficacy of 5-hydroxytryptamine-3 receptor antagonists for chemotherapy-induced emesis. *J Clin Oncol* 1995, 13:1036–1043.

30. Morrow Gr, Hickok JT, Rosenthal SN: Progress in reducing nausea and emesis: comparisons of ondansetron, granisetron, and tropisetron. *Cancer* 1995, 76:343–357.

31. Navari R, Gandara D, Heskth S, *et al*.: Comparative clinical trial of granisetron and ondansetron in the prophylaxis of cisplatin-induced emesis. *J Clin Oncol* 1995, 13:1242–1248.

32. Hesketh P Navari R, Grote T, *et al*.: Double-blind randomized comparison of the antiemetic efficacy of intravenous dolasteron mesylate and intravenous ondansetron in the prevention of acute cisplatin-induced emesis in patients with cancer. *J Clin Oncol* 1996, 14:2242–2249.

33. Gralla RJ, Popovic W, Strupp J, *et al*.: Can an oral antiemetic regimen be as effective as intravenous treatment against cisplatin: results of a 1054-patient randomized study of oral granisetron versus IV ondansetron [abstract]. *Proc Am Soc Clin Oncol* 1997, 16:178.

34. Perez EA, Chawla SP, Kayvin PK, *et al*.: Efficacy and safety of oral granisetron versus IV ondansetron in prevention of moderately emetogenic chemotherapy-induced nausea and vomiting [abstract]. *Proc Am Soc Clin Oncol* 1997, 16:A141.

35. The Italian Group for Antlemetic Research: Dexamethasone, granisetron, or both for the prevention of nausea and vomiting during chemotherapy for cancer. *N Engl J Med* 1995, 322:1–5.

36. The Italian Group for Antiemetic Research: Persistence of efficacy of three antiemetic regimens and prognostic factors in patients undergoing moderately emetogenic chemotherapy. *J Clin Oncol* 1995, 13:2417–2426.

37. Roila F, De Angelis V, Contu A, *et al*.: Ondansetron vs metoclopramide both combined with dexamethasone in the prevention of cisplatin-induced delayed emesis [abstract]. *Proc Am Soc Clin Oncol* 1996, 15:528.

38. The Italian Group for Antiemetic Research: Delayed emesis induced by moderately emetogenic chemotherapy: do we need to treat all patients? *Ann Oncol* 1997, 89:1252–1255.

39. Parikh PM, Charaak BS, Banavali SD, *et al*.: A prospective, randomized double-blind trial comparing metoclopramide alone with metoclopramide plus dexamethasone in preventing emesis induced by high-dose cisplatin. *Cancer* 1988, 62:2263–2266.

40. Roila F, Tonato M, Cognetti F, *et al*.: Prevention of cisplatin-induced emesis: a double blind multicenter randomized crossover study comparing ondansetron and ondansetron plus dexamethasone. *J Clin Oncol* 1991, 9:675–678.

41. Hesketh PJ, Harvey WH, Harker TM, *et al*.: A randomized, double-blind comparison of intravenous ondansetron alone and in combination with intravenous dexamethasone in prevention of high-dose cisplatin-induced emesis. *J Clin Oncol* 1994, 12:596–600.

42. Latreille J, Stewart D, Laberge F, *et al*.: Dexamethasone improves the efficacy of granisetron in the first 24 hours following high dose cisplatin chemotherapy [abstract]. *Proc Am Soc Clin Oncol* 1993, 12:133.

43. Petrelli N, Rodriquez-Bigos M, Creaven P, *et al*.: Efficacy of somatostatin analogue for treatment of chemotherapy induced diarrhea in colorectal cancer [abstract]. *Proc Am Soc Clin Oncol* 1992, 11:170.

44. Rothenbergh ML, Eckardt JR, Kuhn JG, *et al*.: Phase II trial of irinotecan in patients with progressive or rapidly recurrent colorectal cancer. *J Clin Oncol* 1996, 14:1128–1135.

45. Perry MC: Hepatotoxicity of chemotherapeutic agents. In *The Chemotherapy Source Book*. Edited by Perry MC. Baltimore: Williams & Wilkins; 1992:635–647.

46. Venook AP, Egorin M, Brown TD, *et al*.: Paclitaxel (Taxol) in patients with liver dysfunction (CALGB 9264) [abstract]. *Proc Am Soc Clin Oncol* 1994, 13:139.

47. Quesada JR, Talpaz M, Rios A: Clinical toxicity of interferons in cancer patients: a review. *J Clin Oncol* 1986, 4:234–243.

48. Lotze MT, Matory MD, Raynor AA, *et al*.: Clinical effects and toxicity of interleukin-2 in patients with cancer. *Cancer* 1986, 58:2764–2772.

49. Margolin KA, Rayner AA, Hawkins MJ, *et al*.: Interleukin-2 and lymphokine activated killer cell therapy of solid tumors: analysis of toxicity and management guidelines. *J Clin Oncol* 1989, 7:486–498.

50. West WH, Tauer KW, Yannelli JR, *et al*.: Constant-infusion recombinant interleukin-2 in adoptive immunotherapy of advanced cancer. *N Engl J Med* 1987, 316:898–905.

51. Lotze MT, Rosenberg SA: Interleukin-2: clinical applications. In *Biologic Therapy of Cancer*. Edited by DeVita VT, Hellman S, Rosenberg SA. Philadelphia: JB Lippincott; 1991.

52. Schwartzentruber D, Lotze MT, Rosenberg SA: Colonic perforation: an unusual complication of therapy with high-dose interleukin-2. *Cancer* 1988, 62:2350–2353.

53. Rubin JT, Lotze MT: Acute gastric mucosal injury associated with the systemic administration of interleukin-4. *Surgery* 1992, 111:274–280.

54. Andrews PL, Rapeport WG, Sanger GJ: Neuropharmacology of emesis induced by anti-cancer therapy. *Trends Pharmcol Sci* 1988, 9:334–341.

MUCOSITIS

Mucositis is a common side effect of chemotherapy and radiation therapy and may result in significant pain, dehydration, malnutrition, poor quality of life, limitation in cancer therapy, and secondary systemic infection. Radiation and certain chemotherapeutic agents cause direct damage to the oral mucosa, the severity of which depends on dose intensity, schedule, and concomitant treatment. In addition, chemotherapy-induced myelosuppression increases the risk for serious intraoral infections. Effective management requires thorough pretreatment assessment, correction of preexisting oral pathology, a comprehensive preventative oral hygiene program, treatment of infection, and attention to pain control.

PREVENTION AND MANAGEMENT

1. Pretreatment measures
   a. Complete oral and dental evaluation
   b. Correction of underlying pathology
2. Routine oral hygiene
   a. Daily brushing with soft brush and fluoride toothpaste
   b. Daily flossing unless severely thrombocytopenic
   c. Mouthwash four times daily
   d. Lip lubrication
3. Prophylactic measures
   a. Chlorhexidine gluconate 0.12% mouth rinse bid for intensive chemotherapy
   b. Severely myelosuppressed or HSV antibody positive patients should receive oral acyclovir, 200 mg five times per day
   c. Oral cryotherapy with ice chips for 30 min immediately before and after 5-FU
4. Mild to severe mucositis
   a. Complete examination and culture of oral cavity if indicated
   b. Patients should be on bland diet and instructed to pay strict attention to adequate fluid intake
   c. Administer topical anesthetics
   d. Administer topical or systemic antibiotics based on findings
   e. Administer systemic analgesics as needed

CAUSATIVE AGENTS

Antimetabolites: methotrexate, fluorouracil, cytosine arabinoside, mercaptopurine, hydroxyurea; **Alkylating agents:** nitrogen mustard, cyclophosphamide, ifosfamide, procarbazine; **Antibiotics:** bleomycin, doxorubicin, daunorubicin, plicamycin, mitomycin; **Vinca alkaloids:** vincristine, vinblastine; **Biologics:** IL-2, IFN-α

PATHOLOGIC PROCESS

Direct stomatotoxicity of chemotherapeutic agents due to high proliferative rate of mucosal cells of the upper digestive tract, resulting in mucosal atrophy that may lead to frank ulceration, and indirect stomatotoxicity due to chemotherapy or biologic-induced myelosuppression and oral infections from bacterial, fungal, and viral colonizing pathogens

DIFFERENTIAL DIAGNOSES

Bacterial: *Pseudomonas, Klebsiella, Escherichia coli, Serratia, Enterobacter, Proteus, Staphylococcus, Streptococcus;* **Fungal:** *Candida;* **Viral:** herpes simplex, varicella zoster

PATIENT ASSESSMENT

Baseline assessment: clinical evaluation of oral health, identify risk factors (performance status, age, agents given), education of family and other care providers; **Overt symptoms:** complete oral examination and grading of toxicity, CBC, culture of lesions if appropriate, attention to fluid status.

TOXICITY GRADING

1	2	3	4
Painless erythema	Painful erythema	Painful erythema	Requires parenteral or enteral support
Ulcers	Edema	Edema	
Mild soreness	Ulcers	Ulcers	
	Can eat	Cannot eat	

NAUSEA AND VOMITING

Nausea and vomiting are among the most distressing and feared side effects of cancer treatment. Elucidation of the pathophysiology of chemotherapy-induced nausea and vomiting and the role of a variety of neurotransmitters have greatly enhanced prevention and treatment. Chemotherapeutic agents differ markedly in their emetic potential, and symptoms depend on dose, schedule, and concomitant medications. There is also considerable interpatient variability. Effective management requires patient and family education and early prophylactic treatment. Combinations of antiemetics with differing mechanisms of actions and side effects are more effective than single agents alone.

PREVENTION AND MANAGEMENT

1. Prophylactic administration of antiemetic therapy based on emetogenic potential of the chemotherapy (*see* Table 26-4)
2. Provide patient support and guidelines for psychological and behavioral adjustments

TOXICITY GRADING

1	2	3	4
Vomiting	2–5 episodes in 24 h	6–10 episodes in 24 h	> 10 episodes in 24 h or requiring parenteral support
1 episode in 24 h			
Nausea			
Able to eat, reasonable intake	Intake significantly reduced	No significant intake	

CAUSATIVE AGENTS

Highly emetogenic: cisplatin, dacarbazine, nitrogen mustard, streptozocin; **Moderately emetogenic:** cyclophosphamide, ifosfamide, cytosine arabinoside, hexamethylmelamine, carboplatin, doxorubicin, mitomycin C, procarbazine, etoposide, paclitaxel; **Minimally emetogenic:** fluorouracil, bleomycin, methotrexate, vincristine, vinblastine

PATHOLOGIC PROCESS

Neuronal reflex arch mediated by the chemoreceptor trigger zone rich in serotoninergic and dopaminergic receptors. After further coordination in the vomiting center in the central nervous system, efferent neuronal pathways mediate autonomic and somatic responses that result in nausea and vomiting.

DIFFERENTIAL DIAGNOSES

Chemotherapy; narcotics; radiation to brain, abdomen, chest, spine; brain metastasis; gastrointestinal or biliary tract obstruction; hypercalcemia; hyponatremia; uremia

PATIENT ASSESSMENT

Increased risk of severe symptoms if history of "nervous stomach," motion sickness, poor emetic control with previous chemotherapy; patients with a history of heavy alcohol tolerate chemotherapy with less nausea and vomiting; young patients experience more anticipatory nausea and vomiting and are more susceptible to the extrapyramidal side effects of many antiemetics.

DIARRHEA

Diarrhea results from a direct toxic effect on the gastrointestinal mucosa. It is most frequently seen with antimetabolites and is related to dose and intensity of drug administration. There is considerable interpatient variability. Symptoms may range from mild to severe. All chemotherapy should be stopped at the first signs of significant diarrhea. Appropriate management requires strict attention to hydration and the institution of antidiarrheals and antibiotics if the diarrhea is severe or bloody or there is concomitant fever or neutropenia. For patients experiencing severe diarrhea, all subsequent chemotherapy should be given with great caution and at reduced dose intensity.

CAUSATIVE AGENTS

Antimetabolites, particularly 5-FU, methotrexate, cytosine arabinoside

PATHOLOGIC PROCESS

Direct toxic effect on rapidly proliferating mucosal cells of the small and large intestine

DIFFERENTIAL DIAGNOSES

Direct toxic effect of chemotherapeutic agent; gastrointestinal infection—*C. difficile*, gramnegative enteritis, viral enteritis, parasitic infection; other drugs, especially antibiotics; malabsorption; large bowel obstruction; dumping syndrome.

PATIENT ASSESSMENT

For moderate or severe diarrhea: evaluation of volume status; CBC, electrolytes, liver function tests; abdominal radiographic studies; blood cultures; stool leukocytes; stool cultures for enteric pathogens, ova, parasites; stool *Clostridium difficile* toxin titer

MANAGEMENT AND INTERVENTION

1. Mild to moderate diarrhea
   a. Maintain adequate fluid intake
   b. Provide antidiarrheal medication (*see* Table 26-5)
2. Severe diarrhea
   a. Stop chemotherapy until resolution
   b. Admit to hospital if bloody stools, severe crampy abdominal pain, fever, dehydration
   c. Provide IV fluids, antibiotics, antidiarrheal medication

TOXICITY GRADING

1	2	3	4
Increase of 2–3 stools/d over pretreatment	Increase of 4–6 stools/d, or nighttime stools, or moderate cramping	Increase of 7–9 stools/d, or incontinence, or severe cramping	Increase of > 10 stools/d, or grossly bloody diarrhea, or need for parenteral support

A classification of cancer-associated renal and metabolic abnormalities is shown in Table 27-1. Acute and chronic renal failure; proteinuria (the hallmark of glomerular involvement); hemorrhagic cystitis; fluid and electrolyte disorders, including hypercalcemia, hyponatremia, and syndrome of inappropriate antidiuresis (SIAD); and ectopic adrenocorticotropic hormone (ACTH) syndrome may all be associated with cancer or the treatment of malignant diseases (or both). This chapter highlights these renal and metabolic abnormalities, focusing on the clinical features, causes, and treatment of these disorders.

RENAL COMPLICATIONS

ACUTE RENAL FAILURE

Prerenal Azotemia

Cancer-associated acute renal failure affects the clinical management of patients and has an impact on patient morbidity and mortality. Acute renal failure can be classified into prerenal, postrenal, and intrinsic causes of renal dysfunction (see Table 27-1). This classification serves as a framework for diagnostic and therapeutic management.

Table 27-1. Cancer-Associated Renal Abnormalities

Acute renal failure
Prerenal
Obstruction
   Urethral
   Bladder neck — prostatic or bladder cancer
   Bilateral ureteral — cervical or testicular cancer
Intrinsic
   Vascular
   Interstitial nephritis
      Allergic interstitial nephritis
      Tumor infiltration
      Radiaiton nephritis
   Glomerulonephritis
   Acute tubular necrosis
      Nephrotoxic
         Endogenous — uric acid, myoglobin, immunoglobulins, hypercalcemia
         Exogenous — contrast, antibiotics, analgesics, antineoplastic agents
      Ischemic (sepsis, prolonged prerenal)
   Associated with bone marrow transplantation

Chrnoic renal failure
Prolonged obstruction — prostate, cervical, uterine, testicular, primary renal cancers or retroperitoneal lymphoma; stones
Nephrotoxic — antineoplastic agents and radiation

Glomerulonephropathies (proteinuria)
With Hodgkin's disease (minimal change GN)
With solid tumors (membranous GN)
With antineoplastic agents
Hemorrhagic cystitis

Metabolic disorders
Hyponatremia and SIAD
Hypercalcemia
Ectopic ACTH syndrome

ACTH — adrenocorticotropic hormone; GN — glomerulonephritis; SIAD — syndrome of inappropriate antidiuresis.

Anorexia, nausea and vomiting, and diarrhea associated with either tumor involvement or chemotherapy may cause volume depletion resulting in prerenal azotemia. Clues to the development of acute renal failure (manifested by a rising or elevated serum creatinine) because of volume depletion include a history suggesting volume loss, signs of volume depletion on physical examination, an elevated BUN-to-creatinine ratio (> 20:1), and a low urinary sodium value and fractional excretion of sodium (< 20 mEq/L and < 1%). Patients with cardiomyopathy causing decreased renal perfusion and patients with a reduced effective circulating volume (as in cirrhosis, nephrotic syndrome, or sepsis with vasodilation) also may develop prerenal acute renal failure characterized by an elevated BUN-to-creatinine ratio and low urinary sodium. Nonsteroidal antiinflammatory drugs may potentiate acute renal failure in patients with reduced effective circulating volume and should be avoided in such patients. The treatment of prerenal acute renal failure is volume repletion or correction of the reduced renal perfusion (eg, improving cardiac function).

Obstruction

Obstruction may occur at any site along the urinary tract and cause postrenal acute renal failure. Common causes of postrenal acute renal failure in patients with cancer are cervical and testicular (especially seminoma) carcinomas that cause ureteral obstruction, lymphoma with periaortic lymphadenopathy causing ureteral obstruction, and prostate and bladder carcinomas causing bladder outlet obstruction. Metastatic carcinoma also may infiltrate the retroperitoneal space and tissues and obstruct the ureters [1]. A history of urinary urgency, frequency, and reduced urine output with physical findings of a distended bladder and abdominal or pelvic mass suggests obstruction of the lower urinary tract, such as bladder outlet obstruction. The acute onset of flank pain may occur with rapid dilation of the renal pelvis and ureter proximal to an obstruction. Many cases of obstruction, however, are asymptomatic and diagnosed serendipitously by routine radiographic studies done for tumor monitoring (eg, bone scan, computed tomographic [CT] scan).

In acute renal failure caused by obstruction, the BUN-to-creatinine ratio is usually elevated. Obstruction is confirmed by finding hydronephrosis on ultrasound examination of the kidneys. On rare occasions postrenal acute renal failure may result from ureteral encasement. In such cases, obstruction may occur without hydronephrosis. Clinically suspected obstruction requires further urologic investigation, usually by contrast retrograde radiologic studies. Relief of obstruction can be accomplished by placement of either ureteral stents or nephrostomy tubes. The degree of resolution of the acute renal failure depends in part on the duration of the obstruction. In some cases, such as far advanced cervical carcinoma, uremia may develop. Aggressive intervention for the renal failure (relief of obstruction, dialysis) must be discussed candidly in view of the overall prognosis.

Once prerenal and postrenal causes for acute renal failure are excluded in the azotemic patient with cancer, intrinsic causes of acute renal failure must be considered (see Table 27-1). Intrinsic acute renal failure is characterized by a preserved BUN-to-creatinine ratio (10–20:1) and can be due to thrombosis or infarction of the renal vessels (a rare cause for acute renal failure), interstitial inflammation (acute allergic interstitial nephritis or lymphomatous infiltration), glomerulonephritis (characterized by proteinuria), or acute tubular necrosis (ATN) caused by ischemia or nephrotoxins [1]. ATN due to either ischemic (prolonged prerenal failure or sepsis) or nephrotoxic (aminoglycoside or contrast agent) causes is the most common form of acute renal failure. Certain types of intrinsic acute renal failure are more common to patients with cancer and are discussed briefly.

TUMOR INFILTRATION AND RADIATION NEPHRITIS

Tumor and lymphomatous infiltration of the kidneys rarely cause renal failure but should be considered in cases of unexplained acute renal failure in predisposed patients [2]. Renal biopsy may be required to make the diagnosis. Treatment of the underlying malignancy may improve renal function [2]. Radiation can cause a spectrum of renal problems, including malignant hypertension and acute and chronic renal failure. Radiation-induced chronic renal failure occurs with exposure to more than 2500 rads and is characterized by hypertension, anemia, fatigue, and proteinuria more than 1 g per 24 hours [3]. Histologically, interstitial nephritis accompanied by widespread glomerular sclerosis, tubular atrophy, and arteriolar fibrinoid necrosis is seen [3]. The recognition of radiation nephritis and limiting renal exposure to radiation have reduced the incidence of this form of renal failure.

ACUTE TUBULAR NECROSIS

ATN can be characterized etiologically as ischemic or nephrotoxic. The classic finding in either type of ATN is dirty brown casts on urinalysis. Because with ATN renal tubular function is impaired, little tubular reabsorption of sodium occurs. Thus, urinary sodium concentration and fractional excretion of sodium are high in ATN. The endogenous toxins associated with intrinsic acute renal failure include hypercalcemia, myoglobin (seen in cases of rhabdomyolysis), uric acid (as in the tumor lysis syndrome), and immunoglobulins, such as in multiple myeloma and amyloidosis, in which light chains, for unexplained reasons, are nephrotoxic. Acute renal failure associated with hypercalcemia is likely multifactorial in origin but includes a direct effect of hypercalcemia that reduces glomerular filtration and volume depletion as a result of the natriuretic effect of hypercalcemia [1]. Reduction of serum calcium and repair of volume deficits generally reverse the acute renal failure. The pathophysiologic contribution of myoglobin to the development of acute renal failure in rhabdomyolysis is poorly understood. Nontraumatic rhabdomyolysis may occur in the cancer patient in a variety of settings, including electrolyte disorders (hypokalemia and hypophosphatemia) and prolonged immobilization [1]. Appropriate treatment includes urinary alkalinization and maintenance of urinary output with mannitol or diuretics, or both.

Exposure to exogenous renal toxins is perhaps the most common cause of acute renal failure in patients with cancer. The widespread use of intravenous contrast agents, aminoglycoside antibiotics, amphotericin, and potentially nephrotoxic antineoplastic agents may contribute to the development of ATN in patients with cancer. The elderly (serum creatinine underestimates renal impairment caused by nephron loss with age) and those with baseline renal functional impairment from any cause are at particular risk for ATN with contrast agent or aminoglycoside exposure. Appropriate dosing of medications and hydration before contrast administration may reduce the potential for nephrotoxic ATN.

The nephrotoxicity of antineoplastic agents is shown in Table 28-2. Acute renal failure is the most commonly seen nephrotoxic complication of antineoplastic agents but cases of chronic renal failure occurring distant to chemotherapy exposure have been seen in a dose-related fashion with the nitrosureas and cisplatin. Cisplatin and high-dose methotrexate are the agents that most often cause acute renal failure. Biologic response modifiers, particularly interleukin, also may cause acute renal failure through a variety of mechanisms, including prerenal factors and glomerular and interstitial involvement [1] (see Table 28-2). Brief discussions of the specific antineoplastic agents causing nephrotoxicity follow.

ALKYLATING AGENTS
Cisplatin and Carboplatin

Cisplatin (cis-diamminedichloroplatinum II) is among the most widely used chemotherapeutic agents with efficacy against germ cell and solid tumors [1]. Nephrotoxicity is the limiting factor in the use of cisplatin and undoubtedly is related to the renal excretion of the drug [1,4]. Reduced glomerular filtration rate and polyuria and hypomagnesemia caused by renal magnesium wasting frequently are seen with cisplatin administration [1,4]. The risk of cisplatin-induced acute renal failure can be reduced by hypertonic saline hydration and forced diuresis with mannitol or furosemide, or both [1,4]. Careful attention to baseline renal function before treatment with cisplatin is required for appropriate dosing (Table 27-3). Carboplatin appears to be less nephrotoxic than cisplatin but also can cause acute renal failure and requires careful monitoring of renal function with appropriate predosage adjustment for renal insufficiency in addition to pretreatment hydration [5].

Cyclophosphamide

Cyclophosphamide has been used for many years to treat hematologic malignancies, lymphomas, and various solid tumors. The main nephrologic-related toxicities of cyclophosphamide are hemorrhagic cystitis and impaired water excretion after high-dose (50 mg/kg body weight) therapy [1]. A sustained diuresis after high-dose cyclophosphamide therapy is needed to avoid hemorrhagic cystitis. Because of the risk of hyponatremia secondary to cyclophosphamide-induced water retention, half-normal saline infusion before and throughout cyclophosphamide administration is recommended [1].

Nitrosureas

Streptozotocin is unique among the nitrosureas for its effects on the proximal tubule and the development of Fanconi's syndrome [1,6]. Monitoring of proteinuria is required when streptozocin is given (usually in the treatment of islet cell carcinoma of the pancreas and carcinoid tumor) [6]. Discontinuation of the drug is recommended when proteinuria develops to avoid permanent impairment of renal function [1,6]. Hypophosphatemia may be an initial manifestation of renal tubular dysfunction caused by streptozocin [1,6], and hypericosuria without hyperuricemia has been postulated as a causative event in streptozotocin-induced renal failure [7].

Chronic renal failure is the primary manifestation of nephrotoxicity of the other nitrosureas (BCNU, CCNU, methyl-CCNU), which vary in their potential for renal dysfunction, with semustine (methyl-CCNU) most commonly causing renal failure (see Table 27-2). Cumulative doses of nitrosureas more than 1200 to 1400 mg/m^2 are associated with irreversible renal failure that can progress to end-stage renal disease and the need for dialysis [8,9]. Such cases of renal failure may present months to years after the completion of treatment with nitrosureas, particularly with methyl-CCNU, and often in the absence of underlying or transient acute renal failure [8,9].

ANTIMETABOLITES

High-Dose Methotrexate

Although conventional dose methotrexate rarely causes nephrotoxicity, high-dose methotrexate (25–50 mg/kg to 1–7 g/m^2) has been associated with nonoliguric acute renal failure [1]. Because methotrexate primarily is excreted renally, any alteration in renal function affects plasma methotrexate levels and the rate of methotrexate elimination. With prolonged elevation of plasma methotrexate levels, bone marrow and gastrointestinal toxicity may occur [10]. Maintaining a high urinary volume and pH by alkalinization of the urine reduces the nephrotoxicity of high-dose methotrexate [11] and is integral to therapy with this agent. Methotrexate is poorly dialyzed [12], making management of patients with elevated methotrexate levels and renal insufficiency difficult and emphasizing the need for careful dosing of methotrexate in patients with renal dysfunction (*see* Table 27-3).

Other Antimetabolites

Table 27-2 shows the other antimetabolites capable of causing nephrotoxicity; renal dysfunction is much less common with these agents than with high-dose methotrexate. 5-Fluorouracil has been reported to cause acute renal failure as a result of hemolytic-uremic syndrome but only when given in combination with mitomycin [1].

Abnormalities of both proximal and distal tubular function may occur with 5-azacytidine. These are manifested by hypophosphatemia, low serum bicarbonate, polyuria or glucosuria, and renal salt wasting, which can result in volume depletion with hypotension and mild azotemia [13]. Supportive therapy with replacement of the lost electrolytes and minerals is required. Resolution of the acquired defects of tubular function occurs with discontinuation of 5-azacytidine [13].

ANTITUMOR ANTIBIOTICS

Mitomycin

Two patterns of mitomycin C–associated renal failure occur: a relatively uncommon dose-related acute renal failure seen with administration of mitomycin C alone [14] and a hemolytic-uremic type of renal failure seen when a combination of mitomycin C and 5-fluorouracil is given [1,15]. The latter is characterized by a microangiopathic hemolytic anemia and thrombocytopenia with acute renal failure, which on renal biopsy shows microthrombi [1,15]. Renal failure may persist and result in end-stage renal disease; fatal cases are not unusual [15]. Plasma exchange may be useful in some cases [16]. The renal failure seen with high-dose mitomycin C alone is characteristically less fulminant and related to cumulative drug dosage [1,15]. Microangiopathic hemolytic anemia is less frequent with this type of mitomycin C–induced renal dysfunction, but renal

Table 27-2. Possible Nephrotoxicity of Antineoplastic Agents

Drug	Risk High	Int	Low	Renal Effects
Alkylating agents				ARF
Carboplatin			X	ARF: decrease risk with hydration and forced diuresis, mannitol; CRF dose related
Cisplatin	X			Doses > 50 mg/kg: impaired water excretion; hemorrhagic cystitis
Cyclophosphamide			X	
Nitrosureas				
Streptozotocin	X			Fanconi's syndrome; may cause CRF
Carmustine (BCNU)			X	CRF: delayed effects, dose related
Lomustine (CCNU)			X	CRF: delayed effects, dose related
Semustine (MethylCCNU)		X		CRF: delayed effects with cumulative dose > 1200 mg/m^2
Antimetabolites				
High-dose methotrexate	X			ARF
Cytosine arabinoside			X	ARF
5-Fluorouracil*			X	ARF
5-Azacytidine			X	ARF: proximal and distal tubular dysfunction
6-Thioguanine			X	ARF
Vincristine, vinblastine				Impaired water excretion
Antitumor antibiotics				
Mitomycin			X	Hemolytic-uremic syndrome
Mithromycin	X			ARF: dose related; rare in doses used for hypercalcemia
Doxorubicin			X	ARF: case with proteinuria, glomerular proliferation
Biologic agents				
Interferon α			X	AFT: interstitial nephritis; proteinuria—minimal change; MPGN
Interferon γ		X		ARF: ATN; proteinuria
Interleukin-2		X		RF: prerenal azotemia with low fractional excretion of Na
Corynebacterium Parvum			X	ARF: proliferative GN

*Given with mitomycin C.
ARF—acute reanl failure; CRF—chronic renal failure; Int—intermediate; RF—renal failure.
Adapted from Massry and Glassock [113]; with permission.

biopsy shows similar changes [15]. Mortality with this type of renal failure is also high, usually occurring within 3 to 8 months [15].

Mithromycin

Nonrenal toxicity generally limits the use of high-dose (25–50 µg/kg daily for 5 days) mithramycin [1]. Nephrotoxicity, defined as a BUN more than 25 mg/dL or a reduction in creatinine clearance was noted in 22 of 54 patients (40%) given high-dose mithramycin for a variety of tumors [17]. Qualitative proteinuria (1+ on urine dipstick) also was noted in 78% of the patients. Underlying renal insufficiency and higher cumulative doses of mithramycin increased the risk of nephrotoxicity [17]. Histopathologic examination of renal tissue was consistent with ATN. Currently, low-dose mithramycin (25 µg/kg) is more commonly used (to treat hypercalcemia) [1]. Renal failure is much less likely with this dosage regimen. There are case reports of renal failure associated with single doses of mithramycin used to treat hypercalcemia [18]. Renal function should be monitored with mithramycin therapy, especially in patients with underlying renal dysfunction.

Despite the development of specific renal lesions (glomerular vacuolation) in animals given anthracycline antibiotics, such as doxorubicin (Adriamycin) and daunomycin [19], nephrotoxicity rarely occurs in humans. A single case report suggested that doxoru-

bicin causes renal toxicity [20], but there are no confirming data. Cardiac toxicity is the dose-limiting factor for doxorubicin administration and may occur at lower cumulative doses than the nephrotoxicity, thereby limiting the development of renal toxicity [1].

BIOLOGIC AGENTS
Interferons

The literature on interferon α–induced nephrotoxicity consists primarily of case reports documenting proteinuria and renal failure [21–23] or immune complex membranoproliferative glomerulonephritis [24]. Proteinuria and renal failure with focal segmental glomerulosclerosis and ATN on renal biopsy have been reported in a child treated with interferon-gamma [25]. In addition, one of the cases of interferon α nephrotoxicity described acute interstitial nephritis with minimal change nephropathy on biopsy [23]. Interferons are unique in that glomerular involvement is a common feature of their nephrotoxicity. Immune complex glomerulonephritis in a human immunodeficiency virus (HIV)–positive patient treated with interferon α was reported [26]. The authors suggested that a disruption in immunoregulation at the renal tissue level may underlie the observed pathologic responses seen with interferon therapy [26]. Additional study of the renal effects of interferons is needed.

Table 27-3. Dosing of Antineoplastic Agents in Patients with Renal Failure

Drug	Excreted Unchanged, %	Half-Life (Normal/ESRD Hours)	Dose for Normal Renal Function	Dose Adjustment for Renal Failure as % Reduction		
				GFR		
				> 50	10–50	< 10
Bleomycin	60	9/20	10–20 U/m^2	100	75	50
Carboplatin	50–70	6/increased	360 mg/m^2	100	75	50
Cisplatin	27–45	0.3–0.5/unknown	20–50 mg/m^2/d	100	50	25
Cyclophosphamide	10–15	4–7.5/10	1.5 mg/kg/d	100	75	50
Hyroxyurea	Substantial	Unknown	20–30 mg/kg/d	100	100	75
Melphalan	12	1.1–1.4/4–6	6 mg/d	100	50	20
Methotrexate	80–90	8–12/increased	15 mg/d to 12 g/m^2	100	75	50
Mitomycin C	Unknown	0.5–1/unknown	20 mg/m^2 q 6–8 wk	100	50	Avoid
Nitrosureas	Substantial	Short/unknown	Varies	100	100	75
Prototype — methylCCNU		Metabolites with variable T 1/2	Irreversible toxicity at dose more than 1500 mg/m^2	100	75	25–50
Streptozotocin	None	0.25/unknown	500 mg/m^2/d	100	75	50

Adapted from Bennett and coworkers [114]; with permission.
ESRD — end-stage renal disease.

Table 27-4. Treatment of Hypercalcemia

Treatment	Onset of Action	Duration of Action	Normalization, %	Advantages	Disadvanteges
Saline	Hours	During infusion	10	Rehydration	Cardiac compromise, intensive monitoring, hypokalemia, hypomagnesemia
Saline and loop diuretic	Hours	During treatment	10	Enhanced renal calcium excretion	Cardiac compromise, intensive monitoring, hypokalemia, hypomagnesemia
Calcitonin	Hours	2–3 d	10–20	Nontoxic, rapid onset of action in life-threatening hypercalcemia	Only lowers calcium by 2 mg/dL, tachyphylaxis
Mithramycin	24–48 h	5–7 d	40–60	Effective	Renal insufficiency, liver abnormalities, thrombocytopenia
Gallium nitrate	48–72 h	10–14 d	70–80	Potent	Length of intravenous administration, renal impairment
Pamidronate	24–48 h	10–14 d	70–100	Potent, relatively nontoxic	Fever, hypophosphatemia, hypomagnesemia, hypocalcemia

Interleukin-2, with or without lymphokine-activated killer cells, can cause prerenal azotemia characterized by oliguria, hypotension, and a low fractional excretion of sodium [27]. Fluid retention with edema formation also occurs, suggesting a leaky capillary syndrome associated with renal hypoperfusion [1]. The rapid development and resolution of the renal failure in most patients suggests a hemodynamic cause [28]. A case study showing reduced renal prostaglandin synthesis in the setting of increased plasma renin activity supports this theory [29]. Patients particularly at risk for interleukin-2 acute renal failure are those with underlying renal insufficiency; the degree of renal failure was greater and the duration of renal impairment was longer in such patients [27]. Recognition of the syndrome and appropriate fluid resuscitation are required. Nephrotoxicity is less likely with constant infusion of interleukin [30].

Treatment with *Corynebacterium parvum* immunotherapy caused an immune complex proliferative glomerulonephritis acute renal failure in a small number (3 of 87) of patients [31]. The renal failure resolved in all patients with discontinuation of the immunotherapy. Although *C. parvum*–induced acute renal failure is uncommon, attention to the renal function of patients treated with this antineoplastic agent is needed.

RENAL FAILURE ASSOCIATED WITH BONE MARROW TRANSPLANTATION

Renal failure that occurs in the setting of bone marrow transplantation may be caused by entities unique to this patient population. The timing of the development of acute renal failure following bone marrow transplantation may be important in defining the causative events and subsequent treatment related to the renal failure. In addition to prerenal azotemia and ATN, bone marrow transplant recipients may develop acute renal failure as a result of tumor lysis and stored marrow infusion, a hepatorenal-like acute renal failure associated with hepatic venoocclusive disease, or hemolytic-uremia syndrome as a result of cytoreductive therapy [32]. The hepatorenal-like form of acute renal failure typically occurs 10 to 21 days following transplant and often is associated with amphotericin therapy and sepsis [32]. This is the most common form of acute renal failure unique to the bone marrow transplant patient. Diagnosis of this syndrome can be difficult, and dialysis is often needed. Despite such measures, mortality remains high.

CHRONIC RENAL FAILURE

As noted previously, chronic renal failure in the cancer patient may result from nephrotoxic exposure, notably from radiation and certain antineoplastic agents, particularly the nitrosureas and cisplatin (*see* Table 27-2). Chronic renal failure in the cancer patient, however, is much more likely to be caused by obstruction. As with acute renal failure secondary to obstruction, cervical, testicular, bladder, and prostate cancers most commonly cause chronic renal failure by obstruction. The extent and duration of the obstruction are the primary factors affecting the degree of renal functional recovery with relief of the obstruction. As with obstruction-induced acute renal failure, diagnosis usually is made by ultrasound examination showing hydronephrosis. Treatment is relief of the obstruction through urologic intervention.

GLOMERULONEPHROPATHIES

The nephrotic syndrome can occur as a paraneoplastic manifestation in patients with solid tumors and lymphomas. Proteinuria is the cardinal finding, and the nephrotic syndrome (> 3.5 g protein in 24-h urine collection, hypoalbuminemia, edema) confirms glomerular involvement. The type of glomerulopathy tends to be related to the cancer: membranous glomerulopathy often is seen in patients with solid tumors (*eg*, colon and lung cancer), and minimal-change glomerulopathy occurs in patients with Hodgkin's lymphoma [33,34]. Nephrotic syndrome also has been reported in patients with non-Hodgkin's lymphomas but occurs less commonly [33,35] and often is associated with more extensive glomerular involvement and renal failure [36]. Leukemias are less frequently associated with nephrotic syndrome; chronic lymphocytic leukemia is the type of leukemia most often associated with the nephrotic syndrome [35]. The nephrotic syndrome may precede, occur concurrently, or follow the diagnosis of cancer or lymphoma and is unrelated to the stage of the disease [35]. There is some evidence for tumor-related antigens as pathogenetic triggers in the glomerulopathies of cancer, but the precise mechanisms for the development of these syndromes are not understood [33]. Frequently, remission of the tumor results in resolution of the proteinuria, and tumor recurrence is accompanied by relapse of the proteinuria [33,35].

As discussed previously, some antineoplastic agents have been associated with the development of proteinuria (*see* Table 27-2). The interferons and *C. parvum* are the agents most often associated with the development of proteinuria. The single case report of glomerulonephritis in a patient given doxorubicin has not been confirmed by additional reports.

UROLOGIC COMPLICATIONS

HEMORRHAGIC CYSTITIS

Uncontrolled urinary tract hemorrhage in the cancer patient is less common today because of improvements in radiation therapy dosing and the use of reducing agents such as mensa cyclophosphamide or ifosfamide therapy [37]. With both alkylating agents and radiation therapy, urothelial damage is the initiating event resulting in hemorrhagic cystitis. Underlying bleeding diathesis or the concomitant use of anticoagulants may potentiate urothelial damage and exacerbate medication-induced or radiation-induced genitourinary bleeding. Other antineoplastic agents implicated in the development of hemorrhagic cystitis include L-asparaginase, dactinomycin, mitomycin C, mithramycin, and 6-mercaptopurine [37]. The management of hemorrhagic cystitis from cancer therapy includes bladder catheterization for drainage and continuous irrigation. Intravesical cauterization and surgical intervention also may be required in refractory cases [37].

METABOLIC COMPLICATIONS

SYNDROME OF INAPPROPRIATE ANTIDIURESIS

Although there are multiple causes for this syndrome, including abnormalities of the central nervous system, various respiratory diseases, and certain pharmacologic agents, the most common cause remains malignancies, particularly small cell carcinoma of the lung.

In 1957, Schwartz and coworkers described 2 patients with bronchogenic cancer who manifested hyponatremia and continued urinary loss of sodium [38] and postulated that this syndrome may be caused by inappropriate secretion of an antidiuretic substance. In several instances, inappropriately high circulating levels of antidiuretic hormone (ADH) have been reported, hence the original term, inappropriate secretion of antidiuretic hormone (SIADH). Because in some cases ADH may not be the causative agent, the syndrome is best referred to as SIAD.

The diagnosis requires the presence of hyponatremia, hypoosmolality, inappropriately concentrated urine, and exclusion of other conditions that can cause hyponatremia, such as renal, adrenal, thyroid, cardiac, and hepatic abnormalities and volume depletion, edematous states, and diuretic use. Other features that are characteristic but not necessary for the diagnosis include a low blood concentration of urea and uric acid and continued renal excretion of sodium [39].

PHYSIOLOGY OF ANTIDIURETIC HORMONE SECRETION

Antidiuretic hormone, also called arginine vasopressin, is a peptide that is synthesized within the hypothalamus and stored in the posterior lobe of the pituitary gland. ADH release is regulated by hypothalamic osmoreceptors. An increase in plasma osmolality triggers release of ADH, which acts at the renal distal tubule and collecting duct to promote retention of free water and restore normal plasma osmolality. Conversely, a decrease in plasma osmolality suppresses ADH release. Increases in plasma osmolality of 2% to 3% above the normal (282 mOsm/kg) trigger ADH release. In humans this generally occurs at a plasma osmolality of 287 mOsm/kg, which is termed the osmotic threshold for ADH release [40].

Volume stimuli also regulate ADH release. A decrease in plasma volume as a result of hemorrhage, peripheral vasodilation, sustained quiet standing, and positive pressure ventilation all stimulate release of ADH by decreasing the left atrial inhibitory impulses directed at the hypothalamus. This compensatory mechanism restores plasma volume. In contrast, increases in plasma volume inhibit ADH release by increasing left atrial inhibitory input to ADH release. In the absence of ADH, diuresis occurs. Other conditions that inhibit ADH release include negative pressure ventilation, recumbency, lack of gravity, submersion in water, and exposure to cold. Volume stimulation overrides osmotic stimuli. Thus, the osmotic threshold for ADH release is increased by volume expansion and decreased by volume contraction.

In addition to volume and osmotic stimuli several pharmacologic agents can stimulate ADH release, such as chlorpropamide [41], clofibrate [42], carbamazepine, nicotine, certain tricyclic antidepressants [43], and the chemotherapeutic agents cyclophosphamide [44,45], vinblastine [46], and vincristine [47]. ADH release also can be triggered by nausea, pain, and surgery [40].

Pathophysiology

The hallmark of SIAD is the inability to dilute the urine maximally in the presence of hyponatremia. Urinary osmolality in SIAD is typically higher than plasma osmolality. Because the inability to dilute the urine maximally in the face of hyponatremia also can occur in the absence of abnormalities in ADH secretion, such as in elderly patients, patients with renal disease, or patients using diuretics, these conditions must be excluded before making the diagnosis of SIAD. Assessment of volume status is critical to differentiate volume contraction from SIAD. Patients with SIAD are euvolemic. In volume-contracted patients, the decrease in effective blood volume provides a nonosmotic, volume-responsive stimulus for ADH release. As a result of ADH release, hyponatremia can occur, and the urine can become inappropriately concentrated.

Ingestion of water in patients with SIAD leads to a prompt natriuresis [48]. Although it was originally thought that the natriuresis was the result of aldosterone suppression by expansion of the extracellular volume [38], it was shown subsequently that circulating levels of aldosterone are normal and respond normally to stimuli [49,50]. Atrial natriuretic factor levels, which increase with modest volume expansion following acute water ingestion and correlate with the prompt increase in sodium excretion [51], may cause natriuresis in this syndrome. It is worth pointing out that patients with SIAD who have low sodium intake or who develop extracellular volume contraction are able to conserve sodium. In these instances, patients with SIAD may have low urinary concentrations of sodium. Once the volume contract is corrected, urinary sodium excretion increases. By monitoring the response to isotonic saline infusion, patients with simple dehydration can be differentiated from patients with dehydration superimposed on SIAD. The former dilute their urine, whereas the latter do not dilute their urine once the volume deficit is corrected.

Patients with SIAD develop hyponatremia only if water intake is excessive. Although these patients rarely report excessive thirst, continued ingestion of water during hypoosmolality is considered to be inappropriate. Hypoosmolality should suppress thirst and thus prevent hyponatremia. The factors that lead to the continued ingestion of water in this syndrome have not yet been identified, but ADH itself is not dipsogenic.

In some cases of SIAD, especially in patients with cancer who develop this syndrome, frank hyponatremia may not develop. Rather patients may manifest excess ADH secretion with impairment of urinary dilution but without hyponatremia. In these instances, water intake appears to be more appropriate for the degree of hyponatremia. Why this should occur more often in cancer-related than other causes of SIAD remains unknown.

SYNTHESIS AND SECRETION OF ANTIDIURETIC HORMONE

Peptide and messenger RNA for ADH have been identified in the tumors of several patients with clinical SIAD, and circulating plasma levels of ADH are frequently increased. ADH is synthesized and processed in these tumors in a manner similar to its synthesis in the hypothalamus [52,53]. Only a small percentage of patients with SIAD have undetectable levels of plasma ADH, and in these instances their tumors may make other antidiuretic substances that have not yet been identified. Although small cell (oat cell) carcinoma of the lung is most frequently associated with SIAD [53], carcinomas of the head and neck [54,55], bladder [56], cervix [57,58], colon [59,60], ovary [61,62], pancreas [63], and prostate [64,65], as well as neuroblastomas [66–68], Ewing's sarcoma [69], reticulum cell carcinoma [70], mesothelioma [71], and histiocytosis [72] have been associated with this syndrome. The list is not inclusive, but it highlights the diversity of cancers reported with SIAD. In patients with malignancies and SIAD, the source of the ADH may not invariably be the tumor but may arise from the posterior pituitary gland via nonosmotic stimuli, such as nausea, pain, drugs, or chemotherapeutic agents.

Treatment

Because elevated levels of ADH lead to hyponatremia only if water intake exceeds its excretion, restriction of water intake is the cornerstone of therapy. To achieve a negative water balance, fluid intake should be restricted to approximately 800 mL/day. Correction of hyponatremia should be done slowly. Overzealous correction can lead to the rare but disabling condition known as central pontine myelinolysis [73,74]. Patients are at risk for this disorder if serum sodium is corrected more rapidly than 2 mEq/L/h, especially if the hyponatremia is chronic. More rapid correction can take place if the hyponatremia has been acute. The correction of hyponatremia with isotonic (0.9%) saline is usually ineffective because the sodium is excreted and the water is retained, which results in a paradoxic lowering of the serum sodium. Saline should be used only when given together with a loop diuretic, which impairs urine concentrating ability by facilitating free water excretion. The use of hypertonic (3%) saline should be reserved for emergencies in which neurologic symptoms such as seizures or coma occur or if the sodium level is below 110 mEq/L. The following are a list of guidelines for therapy. First, hyponatremia can be corrected at a rate of 0.5 mEq/L/h when not emergent. Second, in emergent situations the rate of correction should not exceed 2 mEq/L/h. Third, once the serum sodium is above 120 mEq/L the rate of correction can be slowed. During correction, the serum sodium must be monitored frequently.

Outpatient long-term treatment is directed at fluid restriction, but in instances of noncompliance or if impractical because of obligate fluid requirements, long-term daily furosemide with sodium chloride tablets to compensate for sodium loss can be used [75]. An alternate approach is to use an agent such as demeclocycline in doses of 600 to 1200 mg/d, which produces ADH-resistant nephrogenic diabetes insipidus, which is fully reversible on withdrawal of the medication [76]. Nonsteroidal antiinflammatory agents also should be discontinued because they potentiate the effect of ADH by blocking prostaglandin synthesis.

Other therapies are directed at decreasing tumor synthesis and secretion of ADH by reducing tumor burden with surgery, radiotherapy, or chemotherapy. Because several of the chemotherapeutic agents may themselves promote ADH release, careful attention to fluid management is necessary. For example, cyclophosphamide can cause SIAD and is used with large volumes of fluid to prevent bladder toxicity. Thus, it is necessary to monitor serum sodium and fluid status carefully during such regimens. If large volumes of fluid must be given with chemotherapy, the coadministration of demeclocycline or furosemide may be useful to lessen or prevent hyponatremia. In addition, because the nausea that may accompany chemotherapy is a potent stimulus to ADH release, antiemetic agents may be administered to diminish this side effect.

HYPERCALCEMIA ASSOCIATED WITH MALIGNANCY

Clinical Features

Hypercalcemia is the most common life-threatening metabolic disorder associated with malignancy and typically results in neuromuscular, renal, and gastrointestinal symptoms as well as impaired cognitive function. Marked dehydration and severe mental status changes accompany greater degrees of hypercalcemia. Hypercalcemic crisis with dehydration, renal insufficiency, and obtundation may be the first clinical manifestation of malignancy. More often, hypercalcemia of malignancy occurs late in the course of the disease. The symptoms of hypercalcemia may mimic those of the underlying malignancy, such as anorexia, weight loss, muscle weakness, and altered mental status. The severity of the hypercalcemic symptoms often correlates with the degree of hypercalcemia.

Causes

The cause of hypercalcemia of malignancy can be divided into two pathophysiologic mechanisms: local osteolytic hypercalcemia (LOH) and humoral hypercalcemia of malignancy (HHM), which account for 20% and 80% of cases, respectively. In certain patients, both of these mechanisms may be operative.

Humoral hypercalcemia of malignancy is associated with the production of a factor termed parathyroid hormone (PTH)–related peptide (PTHrP) by the tumor [77–80]. PTHrP is secreted into the circulation [77–82] and leads to osteoclastic bone resorption. The clinical HHM syndrome is characterized by hypercalcemia, hypercalciuria, hypophosphatemia, reduced levels of PTH, increased nephrogenous cyclic AMP, reduced plasma 1,25-vitamin D levels, and increased levels of PTHrP. Skeletal biopsy reveals a marked increase in osteoclastic bone resorption with a marked reduction in osteoblastic activity [83,84]. This dissociation of osteoclastic and osteoblastic activities contrasts with the bone morphology in primary hyperparathyroidism, in which osteoclastic and osteoblastic activities are increased in a coupled fashion. The tumors that usually are associated with HHM are squamous cell carcinomas of the lung, skin, ears, nose and throat, esophagus, and cervix [85]. HHM also is associated with renal, breast, bladder, ovarian, and endometrial carcinomas and HTLV-1 lymphomas. In contrast, prostate, colon, stomach, and pancreatic adenocarcinomas are rarely associated with HHM.

The absence of PTHrP in the sera of some patients with hypercalcemia of malignancy coupled with the observations that tumors are capable of making many factors that increase osteoclastic resorption of bone indicates that PTHrP is not the sole mediator of hypercalcemia of malignancy [86–88]. Several growth factors have been proposed as osteoclast-activating factors, including interleukins 1 and 2, tumor necrosis factor α, transforming growth factors, and prostaglandins [89–92]. A number of these factors may lead to local bone resorption in LOH.

Treatment

Treatment of hypercalcemia is summarized in Table 28-4. Severe hypercalcemia requires emergent treatment [93,94]. Patients with hypercalcemic crisis are severely dehydrated and require intravascular volume repletion with forced saline diuresis. Infusion of as much as 4 to 6 L of 0.9% NaCl in the first 24 hours is often necessary to restore intravascular volume. The addition of a loop diuretic should not be done until volume is first restored. Loop diuretics given before volume restoration may worsen dehydration and increase serum calcium because of enhanced proximal sodium and calcium reabsorption. Serum calcium is rarely normalized by saline diuresis alone, however, and is a short-term, not long-term, treatment. Because the mechanism of hypercalcemia of malignancy is due to increased bone resorption, patients require an antiresorptive agent, such as a biphosphonate, gallium nitrate, mithramycin, or calcitonin. The most effective treatment for hypercalcemia of malignancy is to treat the underlying disease.

Biphosphonates are analogues of pyrophosphate that bind to bone hydroxyapatite. The compounds are taken up by osteoclasts and inhibit osteoclast action by mechanisms that are not completely understood [95,96]. Pamidronate represents a new generation of aminobiphosphonates that are potent in their inhibition of osteoclast-mediated bone resorption yet do not cause mineralization defects. Current recommendations are for a single 45 to 60–mg IV dose over 24 hours [96,97]. Serum calcium levels gradually decline beginning 24 to 48 hours after the dose and remain normal for weeks. Serum calcium is monitored serially after treatment. The duration of effects appears to be shorter in patients with HHM than in patients with LOH [98,99]. Hypocalcemia and hypomagnesemia occur in 10% of patients and hypophosphatemia in 10% to 30% of patients. Transient fever is also a side effect.

Calcitonin therapy has its greatest utility within the first 24 to 36 hours of the treatment of severe hypercalcemia and should be used in conjunction with more potent, slower therapies while waiting for these effects. For example, the combined use of calcitonin with biphosphonates reduces serum calcium more quickly than if biphosphonates are used alone [93,94]. It is given as a dose of 4 U/kg body weight intramuscularly or subcutaneously every 12 hours. Tachyphylaxis often develops with calcitonin therapy. Calcitonin is considered only as an adjunctive therapy because calcium usually falls only by 2 mg/dL.

Gallium nitrate is another bone antiresorptive agent for the treatment of hypercalcemia. Normocalcemia ensues for 10 to 14 days after a 5-day infusion [93,94,100]. A disadvantage is the need for 5-day infusion and the concern for its adverse effects on renal function. It is less favored than biphosphonates.

Glucocorticoids have their greatest efficacy in patients with glucocorticoid responsive diseases, such as myeloma or lymphoma, or in patients whose hypercalcemia is associated with increased 1,25-vitamin D absorption of calcium and resorption of bone. A dose of 200 mg of hydrocortisone or its equivalent is given IV for 3 to 5 days [93,94].

Mithramycin previously was considered first-line treatment for hypercalcemia but has been replaced by biphosphonates. A dose of 12 to 25 μ/kg through 4 hours of intravenous infusion results in a fall in serum calcium in 6 to 12 hours [93,94]. The dose can be repeated daily several times if needed. Maximum calcium reduction occurs 48 to 72 hours later. The reduction is usually not sustained, and significant side effects of thrombocytopenia and nephrotoxicity limit its use. The drug is now used only in unusual or especially difficult situations.

ADRENOCORTICOTROPIC HORMONE

Cushing's syndrome resulting from the ectopic production and secretion of ACTH by a tumor accounts for about 10% to 15% of all patients diagnosed with Cushing's syndrome [101]. As a result of the excess secretion of ACTH by the nonpituitary source, the adrenal gland becomes hyperplastic, and overproduction of cortisol ensues. Cortisol inhibits the biosynthesis and secretion of hypothalamic corticotropin-releasing factor (CRF) and pituitary ACTH in a classic fashion that exemplifies the negative feedback of hormones. The secretion of ACTH by the nonpituitary tumor, however, is usually not suppressed by the excess cortisol. This feature of nonsuppressibility of ACTH by the tumor is useful to differentiate ACTH secretion from a pituitary source, which is suppressible. ACTH in the normal pituitary as well as in nonpituitary tumors is derived from processing of the proopiomelanocortin (POMC) gene. POMC mRNA from an ectopic tumor is usually longer than normal POMC mRNA from the pituitary, suggesting that ectopic secretion of ACTH likely results from abnormal gene expression [102].

Clinical Features

The first step in the diagnosis is to establish that the patient has signs and symptoms compatible with Cushing's syndrome. The clinical presentation of patients with this disorder is varied and appears to reflect the tumor type and the rapidity and severity of the hypercortisolism. The acute syndrome consists of rapid onset of hypertension, hypokalemia, edema, and glucose intolerance, and is most often associated with small cell lung carcinoma, which accounts for about three fourths of all cases of ectopic ACTH secretion [103,104]. In contrast, the chronic syndrome is indistinguishable from Cushing's syndrome and is associated with indolent tumors, most frequently bronchial carcinoids but also pancreatic or thymic carcinoids, medullary carcinoma of the thyroid, pheochromocytoma, or other neuroendocrine tumors [105].

Biochemical and Radiologic Diagnosis

The diagnosis involves demonstrating hypercortisolism by elevated 24-hour urinary free cortisol excretion and failure of cortisol suppression following a standard low-dose dexamethasone suppression test (Fig. 27-1). To distinguish ectopic ACTH from other forms of Cushing's syndrome requires additional tests (see Fig. 27-1). Distinguishing ACTH-dependent from non–ACTH dependent causes of Cushing's syndrome usually is done easily with determination of serum ACTH and cortisol levels. In ACTH-dependent causes, such as ectopic ACTH syndrome, serum levels of ACTH are measurable to elevated, whereas in the latter, ACTH levels are suppressed. The major differential diagnosis is distinguishing pituitary-dependent Cushing's syndrome from the ectopic ACTH syndrome. Patients with rapidly progressive ectopic ACTH syndrome usually can be diagnosed without difficulty. Patients who harbor more indolent nonpituitary tumors present a diagnostic challenge. Differentiation of these two entities requires the use of dynamic tests that are based on the assumption that pituitary-dependent disease retains some degree of responsiveness to cortisol feedback, whereas ACTH produced ectopically in nonpituitary tumors is not responsive to this feedback regulation.

The dynamic tests that are used include the cortisol response to high-dose dexamethasone suppression, the ACTH response to CRF during inferior petrosal sinus sampling, and the cortisol response to metyrapone. Typically, patients with pituitary-dependent Cushing's syndrome demonstrate suppression of ACTH and cortisol in response to high-dose dexamethasone suppression. In contrast, the expected response in patients with the ectopic ACTH syndrome is no suppression. Typically, malignant ectopic ACTH-secreting neoplasms, such as small cell lung carcinoma, almost always fail to suppress with high-dose dexamethasone. More indolent ectopic ACTH-secreting tumors, especially bronchial carcinoids, frequently demonstrate suppression [102,106].

Inferior petrosal sinus sampling has been proposed because of this latter problem. The test involves placing cannulae in the bilateral inferior petrosal sinuses that drain the pituitary gland. During the test, concurrent ACTH levels before and after CRH stimulation in both petrosal veins and at a distant peripheral site are obtained. The ratio of basal petrosal to peripheral ACTH of more than 2 is highly predictive (> 95%) of pituitary-dependent disease. Ratios of more than 3 obtained 5 minutes after CRH stimulation have an even greater sensitivity and specificity of nearly 100% [103].

Once a diagnosis of ectopic ACTH syndrome is considered, radiographic studies, including chest radiograph, CT scan, or magnetic resonance (MR) imaging of the chest, are indicated. Small cell carcinoma of the lung is usually apparent on plain film or CT scan. Bronchial carcinoids, because of their small size, may require MR imaging of the thorax, which is a more sensitive technique than CT scanning. Ectopic ACTH-secreting tumors may not become clinically apparent for as many as 5 to 10 years after the diagnosis of Cushing's syndrome has been established.

Treatment

Management of this syndrome must be done in light of the severity of the illness and the long-term prognosis because of the underlying tumor. Management is directed at both the ACTH-secreting tumor and the hypercortisolism. Malignant neoplasms responsible for the ectopic ACTH syndrome, such as small cell carcinoma, are usually

unresectable and have extensive metastases at the time of diagnosis. Surgical and medical interventions have been used to control the hypercortisolism associated with inoperable ectopic ACTH production. Bilateral adrenalectomy is a highly effective palliative measure in patients whose projected life span, based on the underlying tumor, would justify such a procedure. Bilateral adrenalectomy is of ques-

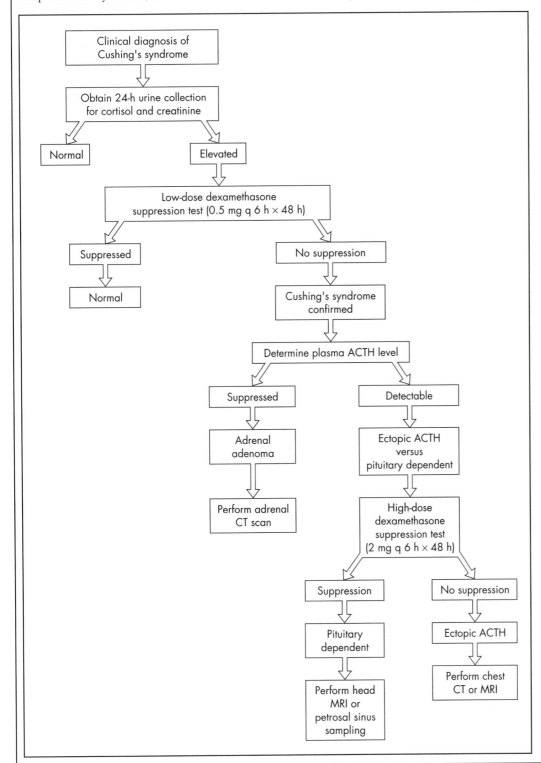

FIGURE 27-1.

Diagnosis of Cushing's syndrome and its causes. *Occassional patient with indolent ectopic ACTH—producing tumor (eg, bronchial carcinoid) will not suppress.

tionable benefit in patients with malignant ectopic ACTH syndrome whose life expectancy is measured in months from the time of diagnosis. The prognosis of small cell carcinoma of the lung also appears to be worse when the tumor is associated with the ectopic ACTH syndrome, perhaps because of increased aggressiveness of these tumors as well as many of the complications secondary to hypercortisolism (eg, weakness, hypokalemia, secondary infection).

Medical therapy of hypercortisolism is directed at the adrenal gland and involves use of both inhibitors of steroid biosynthesis (ketoconazole, metyrapone, aminoglutethamide) and adrenolytic (mitotane) agents. Ketoconazole, an antifungal agent that inhibits P-450 enzymes that are involved in the synthesis of cortisol, aldosterone, and sex steroids, has been used with variable results [107]. In general, patients with mild hypercortisolism are easier to control with this agent than those with severe disease. Metyrapone can also block steroidogenesis, but it is associated with gastrointestinal side effects and allergic reactions. Aminoglutethamide is also associated with skin rash, sedation, dizziness, ataxia, and gastrointestinal irritation. Adrenolytic agents, such as mitotane, have been reported to result in biochemical and clinical improvement in a few cases. This agent, however, has a slow onset of action and significant side effects. Another agent that has been tried in a small number of patients is octreotide, a long-acting somatostatin analogue. Few patients have been studied, and results are highly variable [108–111]. A glucocorticoid receptor antagonist, such as RU486, offers a method of alleviating excessive glucocorticoid action [112]. Little information is available regarding its effectiveness in this syndrome, and further studies are necessary to determine its efficacy.

REFERENCES

1. Rieselbach RE, Garnick MB: Renal diseases induced by antineoplastic agents. In *Diseases of the Kidney*, edn 3. Edited by Schrier RW, Gottschalk CW. Boston: Little Brown & Co, 1993:1165–1186.

2. Kanfer A, Vandewalle A, Morel-Maroger L, et al.: Acute renal insufficiency due to lymphomatous infiltration of the kidneys: report of six cases. *Cancer* 1976, 38:2588–2592.

3. Luxton RW: Radiation nephritis: a long-term study of 54 patients. *Lancet* 1961, 2:1221–1223.

4. Safirstein R, Winston J, Goldstein M, et al.: Cisplatin nephrotoxicity. *Am J Kidney Dis* 1986, 8:356–367.

5. Reed E, Jacob J: Carboplatin and renal dysfunction. *Ann Intern Med* 1989, 110:409.

6. Weiss RB: Streptozotocin: a review of its pharmacology, efficacy, and toxicity. *Cancer Treat Rep* 1982, 66:427–438.

7. Hricik DE, Goldsmith GH: Uric acid nephrolithiasis and acute renal failure secondary to streptozotocin nephrotoxicity. *Am J Med* 1988, 84:153–156.

8. Schacht RG, Feiner HD, Gallo GR, et al.: Nephrotoxicity of nitrosureas. *Cancer* 1981, 48:1328–1334.

9. Micetich KC, Jensen-Akula M, Mandard JC, Risher RI: Nephrotoxicity of semustine (methyl-CCNU) in patients with malignant melanoma receiving adjuvant chemotherapy. *Am J Med* 1981, 71:967–972.

10. Pitman SW, Parker LM, Tattersall MHN, et al.: Clinical trial of high-dose methotrexate (NSC-740) with citrovorum factor (NSC-3590)—toxicologic and therapeutic observations. *Cancer Chemother Rep* 1975, 6:43–49.

11. Pitman SW, Frei III E: Weekly methotrexate-calcium leucovorin rescue: Effect of alkalinization on nephrotoxicity; pharmacokinetics in the CNS; and use in CNS non-Hodgkin's lymphoma. *Cancer Treat Rep* 1977, 61:695–701.

12. Thierry FX, Vernier I, Dueymes JM, et al.: Acute renal failure after high-dose methotrexate therapy: role of hemodialysis and plasma exchange in methotrexate removal. *Nephrology* 1985, 51:416–417.

13. Peterson BA, Collins AJ, Vogelzang NJ, Bloomfield CD: 5-Azacytidine and renal tubular dysfunction. *Blood* 1981, 57:182–185.

14. Hamner RW, Verani R, Weinman EJ: Mitomycin-associated renal failure: case report and review. *Arch Intern Med* 1983, 143:803–807.

15. Hanna WT, Krauss S, Regester RF, Murphey WM: Renal disease after mitomycin C therapy. *Cancer* 1981, 48:2583–2588.

16. Price TM, Murgo AJ, Keveney JJ, et al.: Renal failure and hemolytic anemia associated with mitomycin C: a case report. *Cancer* 1985, 55:51–56.

17. Kennedy B: Metabolic and toxic effects of mithramycin during tumor therapy. *Am J Med* 1970, 49:494–503.

18. Benedetti RG, Heilman KJ, Gabow PA: Nephrotoxicity following single-dose mithramycin therapy. *Am J Nephrol* 1983, 3:277–278.

19. Fajardo LF, Eltringham JR, Stewart JR, Klauber MR: Adriamycin nephrotoxicity. *Lab Invest* 1980, 43:242–253.

20. Burke JF, Laucins JF, Brodovsky HS, Soriano RZ: Doxorubicin hydrochloride associated renal failure. *Arch Intern Med* 1977, 137:385–388.

21. Selby P, Kohn J, Raymond J, Judson I: Nephrotic syndrome during treatment with interferon. *Br Med J* 1985, 290:1180.

22. Lederer E, Truong L: Unusual glomerular lesion in a patient receiving long-term interferon alpha. *Am J Kidney Dis* 1992, 20:516–518.

23. Averbuch SD, Austin HA, Sherwin SA, et al.: Acute interstitial nephritis with the nephrotic syndrome following recombinant leukocyte A interferon therapy for mycosis fungoides. *N Engl J Med* 1984, 310:32–35.

24. Hermann J, Gabriel F: Membranoproliferative glomerulonephritis in a patient with hairy-cell leukemia treated with alpha II interferon. *N Engl J Med* 1987, 316:112–113.

25. Ault BH, Stapleton FB, Gaber L, et al.: Acute renal failure during therapy with recombinant human gamma interferon. *N Engl J Med* 1988, 319:1397–1400.

26. Kimmel PL, Abraham AA, Phillips TM: Membranoproliferative glomerulonephritis in a patient treated with interferon-alpha for human immunodeficiency virus infection. *Am J Kidney Dis* 1994, 24:858–863.

27. Bellegrun A, Webb DE, Austin HA, et al.: Effects of interleukin-2 on renal function in patients receiving immunotherapy for advanced cancer. *Ann Intern Med* 1987, 106:817–822.

28. Textor SC, Margolin K, Blayney D, et al.: Renal, volume, and hormonal changes during therapeutic administration of recombinant interleukin-2 in man. *Am J Med* 1987, 83:1055–1061.

29. Christiansen NP, Skubitz KM, Nath K, et al.: Nephrotoxicity of continuous intravenous infusion of recombinant interleukin-2. *Am J Med* 1988, 84:1072–1075.

30. West WH, Tauer KN, Yannelli JR, et al.: Constant infusion recombinant interleukin-2 in adoptive immunotherapy of advanced cancer. *N Engl J Med* 1987, 316:898–905.

31. Dosik GM, Gutterman JU, Hersh EM, et al.: Nephrotoxicity from cancer immunotherapy. *Ann Intern Med* 1978, 89:41–46.

32. Zager RA: Acute renal failure in the setting of bone marrow transplantation. *Kidney Int* 1994, 46:1443–1458.

33. Martinez-Maldonado M, Benabe JE: Nonrenal neoplasms and the kidney. In *Diseases of the Kidney*, edn 5. Edited by Schrier RW, Gottschalk CW. Boston: Little Brown & Co, 1993:2265–2285.

34. Dabbs DJ, Morel-Maroger L, Mignon F, Striker G: Glomerular lesions in lymphomas and leukemias. *Am J Med* 1986, 80:63–70.

35. Zimmerman SW, Vishnu-Moorthy A, Burkholder PM, *et al.*: Glomerulopathies associated with neoplastic disease. In *Cancer and the Kidney*. Edited by Rieselbach RE, Garnick MB. Philadelphia: Lea & Febiger, 1982:306–378.

36. Rault R, Holley JL, Banner BF, El-Shawy M: Glomerulonephritis and non-Hodgkin's lymphoma: a report of two cases and review of the literature. *Am J Kidney Dis* 1992, 20:84–89.

37. Garnick MB: Renal and metabolic complications. In *Current Cancer Therapeutics*. Edited by Kirkwood JM, Lotze MT, Yasko JM. Philadelphia: Current Medicine, 1994:264–269.

38. Schwartz WB, Bennett W, Curelop S, *et al.*: A syndrome of renal sodium loss and hyponatremia probably resulting from inappropriate secretion of antidiuretic hormone. *Am J Med* 1957, 23:529–542.

39. Beck LH: Hypouricemia in the syndrome of inappropriate secretion of antidiuretic hormone. *N Engl J Med* 1979, 301:528–530.

40. Reeves BW, Andreoli TE: The posterior pituitary and water metabolism. In *Williams Textbook of Endocrinology*. Edited by Wilson JD, Foster DW. Philadelphia: WB Sanders; 1992:311–356.

41. Garcia M, Miller M, Moses AM: Chlorpropamide-induced water retention in patients with diabetes mellitus. *Ann Intern Med* 1971, 75:549–554.

42. Moses AM, Howanitz J, van Gemert M, *et al.*: Clofibrate-induced antidiuresis. *J Clin Invest* 1973, 52:535–542.

43. Moses AM: Drug-induced states of impaired water excretion. In *The Posterior Pituitary: Hormone Secretion in Health and Disease*. Edited By Baylis PH, Padfield RL. New York: Marcel-Dekker, 1985:227–260.

44. DeFronzo RA, Braine H, Colvin OM, *et al.*: Water intoxication in man after cyclophosphamide therapy: time course and relation to drug activation. *Ann Intern Med* 1973, 78:861–869.

45. Stahel RA, Oelz O: Syndrome of inappropriate ADH secretion secondary to vinblastine. *Cancer Chemother Pharmacol* 1982, 8:253–254.

46. Berghmans T: Hyponatremia related to medical anticancer treatment. *Support Care Cancer* 1996, 4:341–350.

47. Stuart MJ, Cuaso C, Miller M, *et al.*: Syndrome of recurrent increased secretion of antidiuretic hormone following multiple doses of vincristine. *Blood* 1975, 45:315–320.

48. Goldberg M: Hyponatremia and the inappropriate secretion of antidiuretic hormone. *Am J Med* 1963, 35:293–298.

49. Bartter FC, Schwartz WB: The syndrome of inappropriate secretion of antidiuretic hormone. *Am J Med* 1967, 42:790–806.

50. Fichman MP, Michaelakis AM, Horton R: Regulation of aldosterone in the syndrome of inappropriate antidiuretic hormone secretion (SIADH). *J Clin Endocrinol Metab* 1974, 39:136–144.

51. Cogan E, DeBieve MF, Pepersack T, *et al.*: Natriuresis and atrial natriuretic factor secretion during inappropriate antidiuresis. *Am J Med* 1988, 84:409–418.

52. North WG, Ware J, Chahinian AP, *et al.*: Clinical evaluation of the neurophysins as tumor markers in small cell lung cancer. *Recent Res Cancer Res* 1985, 99:187–193.

53. Sorensen JB, Anderson MK, Hansen HH: Syndrome of inappropriate secretion of antidiuretic hormone (SIADH) in malignant disease. *J Intern Med* 1995, 238:97–110.

54. Ferlito A, Rinaldo A, Devaney KO: Syndrome of inappropriate antidiuretic hormone secretion associated with the head neck cancers: review of the literature. *Ann Otol Rhinol Laryngol* 1997, 106:878–883.

55. Talmi YP, Wolf GT, Hoffman HT, Krause CJ: Elevated arginine vasopressin levels in squamous cell cancer of the head and neck. *Laryngoscope* 1996, 106:317–321.

56. Kaye SB, Ross EJ: Inappropriate antidiuretic hormone (ADH) secretion in association with carcinoma of the bladder. *Postgrad Med J* 1977, 53:274.

57. Kothe MJC, Prins J, Dewit R, *et al.*: Small-cell carcinoma of the cervix with inappropriate antidiuretic-hormone secretion—case report. *Br J Obstet Gynecol* 1990, 97:647.

58. Ishibashi-Ueda H, Imakita M, Yutani C, *et al.*: Small cell carcinoma of the uterine cervix with syndrome of inappropriate antidiuretic hormone secretion. *Mod Pathol* 1996, 9:397–400.

59. Cabrijan T, Skreb F, Suskovic T: Syndrome of inappropriate secretion of antidiuretic hormone (SIADH) produced by an adenocarcinoma of the colon: Report of one case. *Rev Rheum Med Endocrinol* 1985, 23:213.

60. Elisaf MS, Konstantinides A, Siamopoulous KC: Chronic hyponatremia due to reset osmostat in a patient with colon cancer. *Am J Nephrol* 1996, 16:349–351.

61. Lam SK, Cheung LP: Inappropriate ADH secretion due to immature ovarian teratoma. *Aust N Z J Obstet Gynaecol* 1996, 36:104–105.

62. Taskin M, Barker B, Calanog A, Jormark S: Syndrome of inappropriate antidiuresis in ovarian serous carcinoma with neuroendocrine differentiation. *Gynecol Oncol* 1996, 62:400–404.

63. Nagashima Y, Iino K, Oki Y, *et al.*: A rare case of ectopic antidiuretic hormone-producing pancreatic adenocarcinoma: new diagnostic approach. *Intern Med* 1996, 35:280–284.

64. Ghandur-Mnaymneh L, Satterfield S, Block NL: Small cell carcinoma of the prostate gland with inappropriate antidiuretic hormone secretion: Morphological, immunohistochemical and clinical expressions. *J Urol* 1986, 135:1263–1266.

65. Gasparini ME, Broderick GA, Narayan P: The syndrome of inappropriate antidiuretic hormone secretion in a patient with adenocarcinoma of the prostate. *J Urol* 1993, 150:978–980.

66. Ahwal M, Jha N, Nabholtz JM, *et al.*: Olfactory neuroblastoma: report of a case associated with inappropriate antidiuretic hormone secretion. *J Otolaryngol* 1994, 23:437–439.

67. Asada Y, Marutsuka K, Mitsukawa T, *et al.*: Ganglioneuroblastoma of the thymus: an adult case with the syndrome of inappropriate secretion of antidiuretic hormone. *Hum Pathol* 1996, 27:506–509.

68. Argani P, Erlandson RA, Rosai J: Thymic neuroblastoma in adults: report of three cases with special emphasis on its association with the syndrome of inappropriate secretion of antidiuretic hormone. *Am J Clin Pathol* 1997, 108:537–543.

69. Zimbler H, Robertson GL, Bartter FC, *et al.*: Ewing's sarcoma as a cause of the syndrome of inappropriate secretion of antidiuretic hormone. *J Clin Endocrinol Metab* 1975, 41:390–391.

70. Miller R, Ashkar FS, Rudzinski DJ: Inappropriate secretion of antidiuretic hormone in reticulum cell sarcoma. *South Med J* 1971, 64:763–764.

71. Siafakas NM, Tsirogiannis K, Filadeitaki B, *et al.*: Pleural mesothelioma and the syndrome of inappropriate secretion of antidiuretic hormone. *Thorax* 1984, 39:872–873.

72. Simpson CD, Aitken SE: Malignant histiocytosis associated with SIADH and retinal hemorrhages. *Can Med Assoc J* 1982, 127:302–303.

73. Sterns RH, Riggs JE, Schochet SS: Osmotic demyelination syndrome following correction on hyponatremia. *N Engl J Med* 1986, 314:1535–1542.

74. Ayus JC, Krothapalli RK, Arieff AI: Treatment of symptomatic hyponatremia and its relation to brain damage: a prospective study. *N Engl J Med* 1987, 317:1190–1195.

75. Decaux G, Waterlot Y, Genette F, *et al.*: Treatment of the syndrome of inappropriate secretion of antidiuretic hormone with furosemide. *N Engl J Med* 1981, 304:329–330.

76. Cherril DA, Stote RM, Birge JR, *et al.*: Demeclocycline treatment in the syndrome of inappropriate antidiuretic hormone secretion. *Ann Intern Med* 1975, 83:654–656.

77. Heath DA, Senior PV, Varley VM, *et al.*: Parathyroid hormone–related protein in tumors associated with hypercalcemia. *Lancet* 1990, 335:66–69.

78. Ratcliff WA, Hutchesson ACJ, Bundred NJ, *et al.*: Role of assays for parathyroid-hormone-related protein in investigation of hypercalcemia. *Lancet* 1992, 339:164–167.

79. Burtis WJ, Brady TG, Orloff JJ, *et al.*: Immunochemical characterization of circulating parathyroid hormone–related protein in patients with humoral hypercalcemia of malignancy. *N Engl J Med* 1990, 32:1106–1112.

80. Goltzman D, Henderson JE: Parathyroid hormone-related peptide and hypercalcemia of malignancy. *Cancer Treat Res* 1997, 89:193–215.

81. Rankin W, Grill V, Mardin JJ: Parathyroid hormone-related protein and hypercalcemia. *Cancer* 1997, 80(suppl):1564–1571.

82. Guise TA: Parathyroid hormone-related protein and bone metastases. *Cancer* 1997, 80(suppl):1572–1580.

83. Stewart AF, Vignery A, Silverglate A, *et al.*: Quantitative bone histomorphometry in humoral hypercalcemia of malignancy: uncoupling of bone cell activity. *J Clin Endocrinol Metab* 1982, 55:219–227.

84. Nakayama K, Fukumoto S, Takeda S, *et al.*: Differences in bone and vitamin D metabolism between primary hyperparathyroidism and malignancy-associated hypercalcemia. *J Clin Endocrinol Metab* 1996, 81:607–611.

85. Stewart AF, Horst R, Deftos LJ, *et al.*: Biochemical evaluation of patients with cancer associated hypercalcemia: evidence for humoral and non-humoral groups. *N Engl J Med* 1980, 303:1377–1383.

86. Mundy GR: Malignancy and the skeleton. *Horm Metab Res* 1997, 29:120–127.

87. Roodman GD: Mechanisms of bone lesions in multiple myeloma and lymphoma. *Cancer* 1997, 80:1557–1563.

88. Mundy GR: Mechanisms of bone metastasis. *Cancer* 1997, 80:1546–1556.

89. Bertolini DR, Nedwin GE, Bringman TS, *et al.*: Stimulation of bone resorption and inhibition of bone formation in vitro by human tumor necrosis factor. *Nature* 1986, 319:516–518.

90. Black KS, Mundy GR, Garrett IR: Interleukin-6 causes hypercalcemia in vivo and enhances the bone resorbing potency of interleukin-1 and tumor necrosis factor by two orders of magnitude in vitro. *J Bone Min Res* 1990, 5(suppl):S271.

91. Mundy GR: Hypercalcemic factors other than parathyroid hormone–related protein. *Endocrinol Metab Clin North Am* 1989, 18:795–806.

92. Sato K, Fujii Y, Kasono K, *et al.*: Parathyroid hormone–related protein and interleukin 1β synergistically stimulate bone resorption in vitro and increase serum calcium concentration in mice in vivo. *Endocrinology* 1989, 24:2172–2178.

93. Bilezikian JP: Management of acute hypercalcemia. *N Engl J Med* 1992, 326:1196–1203.

94. Chisholm MA, Mulloy AL, Taylor AT: Acute management of cancer-related hypercalcemia. *Ann Pharmacother* 1996, 30:507–513.

95. Canfield RE: Rationale for diphosphonate therapy in hypercalcemia of malignancy. *Am J Med* 1987, 82(suppl):1–5.

96. Merlini G, Turesson I: Utility of bisphosphonates in treating bone metastases. *Med Oncol* 1996, 13:215–221.

97. Vinholes J, Guo CY, Purohit OP, *et al.*: Evaluation of new bone resorption markers in a randomized comparison of pamidronate or clodronate for hypercalcemia of malignancy. *J Clin Oncol* 1997, 15:131–138.

98. Dodwell DJ, Abbas SK, Morton AR, *et al.*: Parathyroid hormone–related protein and response to pamidronate therapy for tumor-induced hypercalcemia. *Eur J Cancer* 1991, 27:1629–1633.

99. Gurney H, Kefford R, Stuart-Haarris R: Renal phosphate threshold and response to pamidronate in humoral hypercalcemia of malignancy. *Lancet* 1989, 2:241–244.

100. Warrell RP Jr.: Gallium nitrate for the treatment of bone metastases [review]. *Cancer* 1997, 80(suppl):1680–1685.

101. Findling JW, Tyrrell JB: Occult ectopic secretion of corticotropin. *Arch Intern Med* 1986, 146:929–933.

102. DeKeyzer Y, Bertagna X, Lenne F, *et al.*: Altered proopiomelanocortin gene expression in adrenocorticotropin-producing nonpituitary tumors: comparative studies with corticotropic adenomas and normal pituitaries. *J Clin Invest* 1985, 76:1892–1898.

103. Tsigos C, Chrousos GP: Differential diagnosis and management of Cushing's syndrome. *Annu Rev Med* 1996, 47:443–461.

104. Gizza G, Chrousos GP: Adrenocorticotropic hormone-dependent Cushing's syndrome. *Cancer Treat Res* 1997, 89:25–40.

105. Orth DN: Ectopic hormone production. In *Endocrinology and Metabolism*, ed 2. Edited by Felig P, Baxter JD, Broadus AE, Frohman LA. New York: McGraw-Hill, 1987:1692–1735.

106. Malchoff CD, Orth DN, Abboud C, *et al.*: Ectopic ACTH syndrome caused by a bronchial carcinoid tumor responsive to dexamethasone, metyrapone, and corticotropin-releasing tumor. *Am J Med* 1988, 84:760–764.

107. Farwell AP, Devlin JT, Stewart JA: Total suppression of cortisol excretion by ketoconazole in the therapy of the ectopic adrenocorticotropic hormone syndrome. *Am J Med* 1988, 84:1063–1066.

108. Woodhouse NJW, Dagog-Jack S, Ahmed M, *et al.*: Acute and long-term effects of octreotide in patients with ACTH-dependent Cushing's syndrome. *Am J Med* 1993, 95:305–308.

109. de Herder WW, Lamberts SW: Is there a role for somatostatin and its analogues in Cushing's syndrome? *Metabolism* 1996, 45:830.

110. Vignati F, Loli P: Additive effect of ketoconazole and octreotide in the treatment of severe adrenocorticotropin-dependent hypercortisolism. *J Clin Endocrinol Metab* 1996, 81:2885.

111. Christin-Maitre S, Bouchard P: Use of somatostatin analog for localization and treatment of ACTH secreting bronchial carcinoid tumor. *Chest* 1996, 109:845–846.

112. Sartor O, Cutler GB Jr: Mifepristone: treatment of Cushing's syndrome. *Clin Obstet Gynecol* 1996, 39:506–510.

113. Weber B, Gasnick MB, Rieselbach R: Nephropathies due to antineoplastic agents. In *Textbook of Nephrology*, ed 2. Edited by Massry SC, Glassock RJ. Baltimore: Williams & Wilkins; 1989.

114. Bennett WM, Arnoff GR, Golpher TA: *Drug Prescribing in Renal Failure: Dosing Guidelines for Adults*, ed 3. Philadelphia: American College of Physicians, 1994.

URINARY TRACT OBSTRUCTION

Retroperitoneal tumors causing ureteral obstruction can occur with any solid neoplasm. Urologic and gynecologic cancers, together with lymphomas, are the most common causes of obstruction. The effects of obstruction on kidney function result in an early inability to concentrate the urine maximally. Renal blood flow is also markedly diminished, particularly in the setting of unilateral obstruction. Regardless of the precipitating neoplasm, the presenting clinical manifestation is usually excruciating pain.

MANAGEMENT OR INTERVENTION

1. Establish histologic diagnosis of the underlying neoplasm
2. Introduce appropriate therapeutic modalities based on primary disease and obstruction:
   a. For prostate cancer causing bilateral obstruction, consider urethral catheterization, suprapubic cystostomy, immediate bilateral orchiectomy, or other endocrine therapeutic approaches
   b. For lymphomas causing retroperitoneal obstruction, radiation therapy or combination chemotherapy can be employed
   c. For isolated metastases, localized radiation therapy can be effective
   d. For retroperitoneal metastases or lymphoma with loss of renal function, if the neoplasm has not been controlled, immediate percutaneous nephrotomy with placement of antegrade or retrograde stents in the immediate future, should be considered
   e. For sensitive neoplasms and testicular cancer, the presence of renal function abnormalities mandates consideration of temporary percutaneous nephrotomies
3. Inhibit xanthine oxidase with allopurinol to prevent a surge of uric acid, which could compromise renal function during systemic treatment
4. Minimize likelihood of infectious complications during manipulation of the obstructed urinary tract
5. Carefully manage postobstructive diuresis and natriuresis with intensive metabolic monitoring

CAUSATIVE FACTORS

Retroperitoneal tumors; urologic cancers, gynecologic cancers, and lymphomas causing lymphadenopathy in the paraaortic, paracaval, and periureteral locations; prostate and advanced cervical cancers commonly causing distal urinary tract obstruction; testicular cancers, especially seminoma, capable of obstructing both ureters simultaneously; metastatic neoplasms forming a plaque-like sheet of tumor

PATHOLOGIC PROCESS

Dilatation of proximal anatomic regions due to obstruction; kidney increases in weight and size and gradually atrophies; inability to concentrate urine maximally and marked dimunition of renal blood flow

DIFFERENTIAL DIAGNOSES

Retroperitoneal fibrosis, ureteral metastases, bladder neck obstruction, lymphadenopathy, kidney stones

PATIENT ASSESSMENT

Ultrasonography (method of choice); radionuclide studies; bone scans with technetium concentration to quantify renal blood flow; on occasion, retrograde and antegrade pyelography; cystoscopy and other interventional approaches for staging purposes; FEna to determine duration of obstruction.

TOXICITY GRADING

	0	1	2	3	4
BUN or serum creatinine	$\leq 1.25 \times N$	$1.26–2.5 \times N$	$2.6–5 \times N$	$5.1–10 \times N$	$> 10 \times N$
Proteinuria	No change	1+ < 0.3 mg/dL < 3 g/L	2–3+ 0.3–1.0 mg/dL 3–10 g/L	4+ > 1.0 mg/dL > 10 g/L	Nephrotic syndrome
Hematuria	No change	Microscopic	Gross	Gross + clots	Obstructive uropathy

N—upper limit of normal value of population under study.

GENITOURINARY HEMORRHAGE

Hemorrhage into the genitourinary tract is a problem often seen with certain malignancies. It requires vigilant anticipation and specialized care. Specific antineoplastic agents, such as cyclophosphamide and ifosfamide, are associated with this complication. Management differs according to the site of the process, tumor involvement, and status of the patient.

MANAGEMENT OR INTERVENTION

1. Hemorrhagic cystitis
   Catheter drainage and continuous irrigation
   Intravesical cautery
   Intravesical therapy with formalin
2. Refractory bleeding
   Cystotomy with instillation of phenol and ligation of the bladder vessels
   In severe cases, urinary diversion and removal of the organ to stop life-threatening bleeding are necessary

CAUSATIVE AGENTS

Cyclophosphamide, ifosfamide, L-asparaginase, actinomycin D, mitomycin C, mithramycin, 6-mercaptopurine, anticoagulants

PATHOLOGIC PROCESS

Toxic metabolites of certain chemotherapeutic agents have direct effect on urethral surface; high concentrations of these metabolites can cause erosion of the bladder mucosal system, leading to microscopic and gross bladder hemorrhage

DIFFERENTIAL DIAGNOSES

Chemotherapeutic agents, tumor involvement, prostate disorders

PATIENT ASSESSMENT

Clinical examination, urinalysis, cystoscopy, urinary irrigation and drainage.

TOXICITY GRADING

	0	1	2	3	4
Hematuria	No change	Microscopic	Gross	Gross + clots	Obstructive uropathy

CHAPTER 28: PULMONARY AND CARDIOVASCULAR COMPLICATIONS OF CANCER THERAPY

Matthew Volm, Howard Hochster

PULMONARY COMPLICATIONS OF CANCER THERAPY

Pulmonary complications arising from the administration of antineoplastic drugs range from asymptomatic, mild abnormalities (detected by chest radiograph or pulmonary function tests) to fatal pulmonary fibrosis. The incidence and severity of pulmonary toxicity depends on the characteristics of the responsible drug as well as host factors. It is useful to consider three major syndromes that may result from the pharmacologic treatment of cancer: 1) acute drug reactions (usually hypersensitivity), 2) noncardiogenic pulmonary edema, and 3) interstitial pneumonitis/pulmonary fibrosis. Table 28-1 provides a list of the drugs associated with pulmonary complications [1].

HYPERSENSITIVITY PNEUMONITIS/ACUTE DRUG REACTIONS: METHOTREXATE, PROCARBAZINE, AND VINCA ALKALOIDS

Acute hypersensitivity pneumonitis with dyspnea, cough, and a variety of symptoms (eg, fever, chills, malaise, arthralgias, rash, pleuritic chest pain, and headache) may be seen with the administration of methotrexate, procarbazine, and bleomycin. Peripheral blood eosinophilia and diffuse pulmonary infiltrates are characteristic. The incidence is highest in patients receiving methotrexate, occurring in approximately 8% of patients [2]. Withdrawal of the drug and the administration of steroids may produce rapid resolution of symptoms, and the overall prognosis is good, although approximately 10% of patients may develop pulmonary fibrosis.

Acute respiratory distress with the administration of vinca alkaloids is unusual, occurring in fewer than 1% of patients, but it may be fatal. Many of the reported reactions have occurred when the vinca alkaloid was administered concurrently with mitomycin. The rapid administration of steroids is likely beneficial.

NONCARDIOGENIC PULMONARY EDEMA: CYTARABINE

High-dose cytarabine, given as consolidation treatment for a variety hematologic malignancies (usually 3.0 gm/m² every 12 h for 8–12 doses), may result in noncardiogenic pulmonary edema. Patients present with dyspnea and physical and radiographic signs of pulmonary edema, but they lack other signs of heart failure. This complication appears related to the cumulative dose of cytarabine, occurring in 10% to 12% of patients receiving 12 to 18 g/m² compared with 21% to 32% of patients receiving 24 to 26 g/m² [3].

Much more rarely, the syndrome occurs in association with teniposide, methotrexate (including intrathecal administration), and cyclophosphamide. The mechanism underlying the syndrome is unknown but has been postulated to be via central nervous system effects on pulmonary capillary permeability. Treatment is supportive; close attention to volume status and the judicious use of diuretics and supplemental oxygen are mainstays. There is a suggestion that high-dose intravenous methylprednisolone may be beneficial. In spite of the high reported incidence, the outcome is usually favorable, and most patients do not require ventilatory support.

INTERSTITIAL PNEUMONITIS/PULMONARY FIBROSIS: BLEOMYCIN, MITOMYCIN, NITROSOUREAS, ALKYLATING AGENTS, AND METHOTREXATE

Bleomycin

The pulmonary toxicity of bleomycin has been studied extensively. The fundamental insult appears to be oxidant damage to pulmonary endothelial cells and type I pneumocytes, resulting in an inflammatory exudate within alveoli and a subsequent fibrotic reaction that may permanently impair diffusion and reduce lung volumes. The activation of various cytokines, particularly tumor necrosis factor α and transforming growth factor β, may also be important. In reported series, the incidence of clinically significant lung injury ranges from 2% to 40%, depending on several factors that are listed in Table 28-2 [4,5].

Patients typically present with dyspnea and, occasionally, a nonproductive cough. Dry rales and a pleural friction rub may be present on examination, and low-grade fever may be present. Chest radiograph typically reveals diffuse interstitial infiltrates but may be normal and, rarely, may show pulmonary nodules that can cavitate and be mistaken for metastases.

On pulmonary function tests, the earliest change is a decrease in diffusing capacity (D_LCO) followed by a loss of lung volumes consistent with a restrictive pattern. Mild subclinical toxicity may not predict for the development of clinically significant fibrosis, and loss of lung function may occur suddenly long after treatment has been discontinued. Therefore, the usefulness of serial D_LCOs is limited. Although the routine use of D_LCO to detect subclinical toxicity is

---

Table 28-1. Commonly Used Anti-Cancer Drugs Associated with Pulmonary Toxicity

Antibiotics
Bleomycin, mitomycin
Nitrosoureas
Carmustine (BCNU), lomustine (CCNU), semustine (methyl-CCNU)
Alkylating agents
Busulfan, cyclophosphamide, chlorambucil, melphalan
Antimetabolites
Methotrexate, cytarabine
Miscellaneous
Procarbazine, etoposide, vinblastine, vindesine

Table 28-2. Risk Factors for Pulmonary Toxicity from Bleomycin

Increased cumulative dose (> 400 U there is a 10% incidence of fibrosis)
Increased age (especially > 70 y)
Supplemental oxygen
Prior or concurrent radiotherapy to the chest
Renal dysfunction (concurrent cisplatin administration)
Concurrent administration of other drugs with pulmonary toxicity
Administration of hematopoietic growth factors or other cytokines (controversial, under investigation)
Bolus administration (some evidence that continuous infusion schedules result in less pulmonary toxicity, but data are limited and inconsistent)

---

controversial, it is important to recognize early clinical signs and symptoms of bleomycin toxicity (eg, dyspnea, dry cough, fine rales, and the development of subtle reticulonodular infiltrates on chest radiograph) [6,7]. Bleomycin should be discontinued when any of these signs or symptoms is present until drug toxicity can be reasonably excluded as a cause of the finding.

Because the treatment of bleomycin-induced pulmonary toxicity is unsatisfactory and its morbidity and mortality are substantial, it is imperative to recognize the risk factors for its development and to weigh the risks and benefits of treatment for all patients. Toxicity is most common after cumulative doses of 400 to 450 U of bleomycin have been administered, but fatal toxicity has been reported with cumulative doses as low as 50 U. Subclinical renal impairment, as associated with the administration of cisplatin, may significantly heighten the risk of bleomycin-induced pulmonary toxicity.

The potential of granulocyte colony-stimulating factor (G-CSF) and granulocyte–macrophage colony stimulating factor (GM-CSF) to increase the inflammatory or fibrotic response to bleomycin in the lung remains a significant question. Several small case series suggest that G-CSF or GM-CSF enhances bleomycin toxicity, particularly when given as part of the ABVD regimen (doxorubicin, bleomycin, vinblastine, and dacarbazine) for Hodgkin's disease [8]. A retrospective analysis of patients who received bleomycin for germ cells tumors, however, showed an equal incidence of pulmonary toxicity regardless of whether patients received G-CSF [9]. Nonetheless, caution should be exercised in the administration of cytokines to patients who have received bleomycin. Whether continuous infusion schedules reduce the pulmonary toxicity of bleomycin when compared with IV bolus schedules remains an unanswered question.

Withdrawal of bleomycin is the mainstay of management of bleomycin-induced pulmonary toxicity. Although steroids are commonly given and clearly can produce clinical responses, their overall efficacy in preventing progressive fibrosis has not been documented. Tapering of steroids may result in a recurrence of symptoms and should be done slowly. Mortality is reported to be as high as 30% among patients who develop bleomycin-induced pulmonary toxicity. Patients who survive may require long-term supplemental oxygen and may benefit from a formal program of pulmonary rehabilitation.

Mitomycin

In contrast to bleomycin, mitomycin-induced pulmonary toxicity is not dose dependent. The incidence of mitomycin-induced pulmonary toxicity is 3% to 12%, with mortality as high as 50% [10]. The clinical presentation is similar to that caused by bleomycin. Treatment includes the withdrawal of mitomycin and the administration of steroids.

Nitrosoureas

Carmustine (BCNU) is associated with dose-dependent pulmonary fibrosis that occurs in 20% to 30% of patients and may become clinically evident many years after treatment. Toxicity is rare in patients who receive less than 960 mg/m^2 but is seen in 30% to 50% of patients when the cumulative dose is greater than 1500 mg/m^2 [11]. Symptoms include dyspnea, dry cough, and bibasilar rales. Histologically, fibrosis predominates, and the inflammatory picture seen early in bleomycin toxicity is usually absent. Mortality is reported to be 24% to 90%. Steroids may be beneficial. Pulmonary toxicity resulting from other nitrosoureas, lomustine (CCNU) and semustine (methyl-CCNU) has rarely been reported.

Alkylating Agents

Pulmonary toxicity occurs with several alkylating agents but is most often associated with busulfan, occurring in approximately 4% of patients [12]. The onset of the typical symptoms of dyspnea, cough, and a low-grade fever may occur up to 10 years after the administration of busulfan. Although a clear dose-response curve has not been demonstrated, a threshold for toxicity may exist at a cumulative dose of approximately 500 mg. Steroids administered concurrently with busulfan do not appear to decrease the risk of fibrosis and are minimally effective in halting its progression. Mortality is approximately 50%.

Cyclophosphamide is reported to cause pulmonary toxicity similar to that of busulfan, but the incidence is less than 1%. The syndrome may be precipitated by the withdrawal of steroids that are commonly included in combination drug regimens for hematologic malignancies. Case reports of pulmonary toxicity resulting from melphalan or chlorambucil are rare.

HIGH-DOSE REGIMENS REQUIRING BONE MARROW OR PERIPHERAL-BLOOD STEM CELL SUPPORT

The use of high-dose chemotherapy regimens requiring bone marrow or peripheral-blood stem cell support has increased dramatically in the past decade. Although multiple organs are susceptible to nonhematologic toxicity from high-dose therapy, the lungs are often at greatest risk. The likelihood of developing pulmonary toxicity depends on several factors: 1) the conventional-dose chemotherapy the patient has received, 2) the particular drugs used in the high-dose regimen, 3) whether the hematopoietic graft is allogeneic or autologous, and 4) the patient's exposure to radiation. The differential diagnosis of pulmonary abnormalities in the setting of high-dose therapy is complex and includes both infectious and noninfectious complications. The most serious complications are associated with allogeneic transplant in which high doses of alkylating agents and/or total-body irradiation are employed and prolonged immune suppression is required [13]. The STAMP V regimen (cyclophosphamide, thiotepa, and carboplatinum), commonly used before autologous stem cell transplants in breast cancer, produces a decrease in DLCO of more than 20% in 32% of patients; 11% of patients have symptomatic pneumonitis that appears to respond to prednisone [14].

For a summary of syndromes occurring with chemotherapy, see Table 28-3.

PULMONARY COMPLICATIONS OF RADIOTHERAPY

Due to the focal nature of radiation therapy, pulmonary complications tend to be less severe than those resulting from chemotherapy [15]. Nonetheless, approximately 5% to 15% of patients who receive radiation to the chest develop pulmonary complications, and significant morbidity and rarely mortality are seen.

The changes that result from radiation have been studied extensively and are well characterized histopathologically, although the precise mechanisms of damage are not yet defined. Six to 12 weeks following exposure to ionizing radiation, an exudate is seen in pulmonary alveoli, followed quickly by an infiltration of inflammatory cells and sloughing of epithelial cells from alveolar walls. These changes may be asymptomatic and resolve completely or may be associated with the clinical picture of acute radiation pneumonitis. Subsequently, the exudate is organized, and to varying degrees, progressive fibrosis of alveolar septa occurs. The syndrome of acute pneumonitis is usually followed by some degree of pulmonary fibro-

Table 28-3. Summary of Pulmonary Syndromes Resulting from Chemotherapy

Syndrome (Drugs)	Clinical Presentation	Treatment Guidelines
Hypersensitivity pneumonitis/acute drug reactions (methotrexate, procarbazine and vinca alkaloids)	Dyspnea, cough, and a variety of symptoms (including fever, chills, malaise, arthralgias, rash, pleuritic chest pain, and headache) in a patient who is receiving chemotherapy; peripheral blood eosinophilia may occur	Discontinue offending drug; the administration of steroid (usually prednisone 1–2 mg/kg/d) is beneficial; acute drug reactions involving vinca alkaloids may require intravenous steroids and aggressive bronchodilator therapy; prognosis is usually good, although occasional patients with hypersensitivity pneumonitis go on to develop pulmonary fibrosis
Noncardiogenic pulmonary edema (cytarabine; rarely methotrexate, cyclophosphamide, and teniposide)	Dyspnea and respiratory failure in a patient who is receiving high-dose cytarabine; rales may be present on examination	Discontinue offending drug; pay close attention to volume status and the judicious of diuretics to maintain a "dry" weight are important; prognosis is good
Interstitial pneumonitis/pulmonary fibrosis (bleomycin, mitomycin, nitrosoureas, alkylating agents, and methotrexate)	Dyspnea and, occasionally, a nonproductive cough and low-grade fever; presentation may be weeks, months, or years after chemotherapy; dry rales and a pleural friction rub may be present on examination	Prednisone 1–2 mg/kg/d may relieve symptoms of pneumonitis but does not appear to prevent the development of fibrosis; tapering should be done slowly because symptoms may be exacerbated by steroid withdrawal; outcome is often poor, chronic low-flow oxygen, bronchodilators and formal pulmonary rehabilitation may be required; cor pulmonale is a common late complication

sis, whereas pulmonary fibrosis may occur months following radiation without any antecedent clinical pneumonitis. Injury to pulmonary capillary endothelial cells and type II surfactant-producing pneumocytes, as well as the activation of various cytokines, appears to be important in inducing and sustaining the fibrotic reaction. Risk factors for the development of radiation toxicity are summarized in Table 28-4.

Because of the large number of variables, the occurrence of pulmonary toxicity can be difficult to predict. Although chronic obstructive pulmonary disease is not a risk per se, baseline pulmonary function obviously has important implications regarding the degree of radiation fibrosis that may be tolerated.

Acute Radiation Pneumonitis

Dyspnea that occurs 2 to 3 months following the completion of chest radiation is usually the chief complaint of patients with acute radiation pneumonitis. Rarely, symptoms occur as early as 1 month following radiation, and sometimes the development of symptoms may occur as late as 6 months after radiation. A cough with scant, occasionally pink-tinged sputum may be present, although frank hemoptysis is unusual. Fever may be present. Physical examination is usually unremarkable, although occasionally moist rales or a pleural friction rub is detectable over the irradiated area. The earliest radiographic change associated with acute pneumonitis is a hazy "ground glass" appearance to the irradiated area. As the pneumonitis progresses, patchy infiltrates with varying degrees of consolidation are seen.

Corticosteroids are the mainstay of treatment for acute radiation pneumonitis. No controlled clinical trials have been conducted to document their efficacy, but animal data and nonrandomized series suggest a benefit. Although steroids clearly may produce symptomatic improvement, it is unclear whether their use during acute radiation pneumonitis reduces the severity of subsequent fibrosis. It is common practice to begin prednisone, 1 mg/kg/d, once the diagnosis of radiation pneumonitis is reasonably certain. Prednisone is administered at this dose for 2 to 3 weeks and then tapered very slowly over several additional weeks. Tapering too rapidly may cause relapse of symptoms.

Chronic Pulmonary Fibrosis

Radiologic evidence of fibrosis is seen in most patients who received chest radiation regardless of whether they experienced acute radiation pneumonitis. Radiation changes (linear streaking in mild cases; frank consolidation in more severe cases) are usually confined to the area irradiated but may be more extensive. It is sometimes difficult to determine whether the radiographic abnormality represents fibrotic changes or recurrent malignancy, and biopsy may be necessary to answer the question.

Corticosteroids appear to be of no benefit once fibrosis has developed, and treatment is supportive. In severe cases, the development of cor pulmonale and heart failure are consequences that may result in significant morbidity and mortality.

CARDIOVASCULAR COMPLICATIONS OF CANCER THERAPY

The use of chemotherapy in the cancer patient produces a wide range of direct and indirect cardiovascular effects. Significant concerns regarding the use of such agents in an older population—many of whom bear the overlapping risk factors for cancer and cardiovascular disease—should be under constant consideration at the time of therapy and, even more critically, at the time of toxic events. The role of

Table 28-4. Factors Influencing the Development of Radiation Pneumonitis and Fibrosis

Factor	Influence
Total dose	In whole lung irradiation, there is a threshold and a steep dose-response curve once the threshold is met
Volume irradiated	The higher the volume irradiated, the greater the risk
Fractionation and rate	Increased rate of irradiation and decreased fractionation; increased risk
Chemotherapy	Concurrent or prior chemotherapy, especially with drugs with established pulmonary toxicity; increased risk
Supplemental oxygen	Increases pulmonary toxicity

Table 28-5. Predisposing Cardiovascular Conditions in the Cancer Patient

Cardiac conditions
    Atherosclerotic heart disease
    Valvular heart disease
    Congestive heart failure
    Diastolic dysfunction
Vascular events
    Dehydration (diarrhea or diuretics)
    Anemia
Metabolic complications (predisposing to arrhythmia)
    Hyponatremia
    Hypernatremia
    Hypocalcemia
    Hypercalcemia
    Hypomagnesemia

Table 28-6. Cardiac Complications of Anticancer Drugs

Agent	Cardiac Effect
Chemotherapeutic	
Amsacrine	Arrhythmias
Anthracyclines	Arrhythmias; congestive cardiomyopathy; pericardial effusion
Anthrapyrazoles	Congestive cardiomyopathy
Bleomycin	Raynaud's phenomenon
Cyclophosphamide	Acute congestive heart failure; hemorrhagic myocarditis; pericardial effusions
5-Fluorouracil	Myocardial ischemia; arrhythmias
Mitoxantrone	Congestive cardiomyopathy
Taxol	Arrhythmias (bradycardia); electrocardiogram changes; ischemia
Vinca alkaloids	Angina; Raynaud's phenomenon
Biologic response modifier	
Interferon α	Hypotension; tachycardia
Interferon β	Hypotension
Interferon γ	Hypotension
Interleukin-1 α	Hypotension
Interleukin-2	Congestive heart failure; hypotension; arrhythmias; ischemia
Interleukin-4	Congestive heart failure
Tumor necrosis factor	Hypotension; ischemia
GM-CSF	Hypotension; pericardial effusion
Radiation therapy	Congestive heart failure; coronary artery disease; pericarditis/effusion

GM-CSF—granulocyte–macrophage colony-stimulating factor.
Adapted from Speyer and Freedberg [20].

underlying cardiovascular disease predisposing to more significant and even life-threatening toxicity should similarly be under constant consideration. Cardiovascular complications of chemotherapy fall into the following major categories: general cardiovascular concerns, anthracycline cardiomyopathy, other cardiomyopathies, anginal syndromes, arrhythmias, and pericardial disease.

GENERAL CARDIOVASCULAR CONCERNS

Some of the general cardiovascular factors to be considered when caring for the oncology patient include underlying ischemic heart disease, valvular heart disease, idiopathic hypertrophic subaortic stenosis (IHSS) or asymmetrical septal hypertrophy, diastolic dysfunction, existing arrhythmia, and use of diuretics. However, the use of chemotherapeutic agents that produce significant diarrhea and electrolyte loss (*eg*, fluoropyrimidines and irinotecan), probably cause the most frequent acute cardiovascular problems in everyday practice (*ie*, dehydration and hypotension). Electrolyte loss may produce additional complications, such as exacerbation of mental status change, ileus, and cardiac arrhythmias. Hypomagnesemia, resulting from cisplatin-induced tubular dysfunction, may predispose to ventricular arrhythmias. Furthermore, repletion of whole-body potassium stores may be difficult until normal total-body magnesium levels are restored, due to continuing renal potassium wasting.

Table 28-5 lists some underlying cardiovascular diseases that predispose to vascular instability and complications. Treatment of these problems should be directed to rapid resuscitation with physiologic electrolyte solutions and/or blood products. Stat analysis of blood chemistries should direct the physician to repletion of electrolytes and the use of appropriate intravenous solutions. Volume depletion may also occur as a general complication in elderly or cachectic patients with decreased intake of fluids, particularly in the setting of diuretics. The practice of prescribing diuretics in an attempt to alleviate patient discomfort from mild peripheral edema should be discouraged, particularly in the elderly cancer patient. The use of diuretic agents may result in dehydration due to inadequate fluid intake (especially during periods of warmer ambient temperature), in the setting of fevers, or in conjunction with altered mental status. Dehydration from any of these causes may precipitate unstable angina and myocardial infarction. In the setting of IHSS or diastolic dysfunction, volume depletion and reduction of preload may precipitate overt congestive heart failure. Here, the physician must correctly administer fluids and blood products rather than diuretics.

Chemotherapy-induced anemia is also an important factor in exacerbating anginal syndromes or producing high-output cardiac failure. Acute anemia should be treated with transfusion of packed red blood cells, whereas chronic anemia may be treated with blood products or the use of recombinant human erythropoietin (Procrit [Ohio Biotechnology, New Brunswick, NJ] and Epogen [Amgen, Thousand Oaks, CA]) 5000 to 10,000 U SQ three times per week or 20,000 U weekly. Many patients will have improved exercise tolerance and a greater sense of well-being with the use of growth factors preventing chronic anemia. These common problems must be considered in the differential diagnosis prior to diagnosing more direct cardiac complications of cancer therapy.

Biologic therapies may also have considerable cardiovascular consequences in cancer patients, particularly when given at higher doses (Table 28-6). Interleukin-2 is the cytokine most widely known for its cardiovascular effects when given on the common high-dose schedules (12 MU IV every 8 h). When given in this dose and schedule, a full 70% of patients will require ICU-level care with the use of pressor agents for development of hypotension, shock, and pulmonary edema, presumably due to capillary leak syndrome. Additional effects, including angina and myocardial infarction, have been reported [16]. Other biologics that may produce hypotension and cardiovascular collapse include the interferons and GM-CSF. Interleukin-4 has been associated with direct cardiac toxicity and pathologic myocardial changes in both humans and animals [17].

ANTHRACYCLINE CARDIOMYOPATHY

The most well-known and feared cardiac complication of chemotherapy is anthracycline-induced cumulative cardiomyopathy [18,19]. This complication has been the subject of considerable research and is reviewed in detail elsewhere [20,21]. Although anthracyclines such as doxorubicin generally act as DNA-damaging agents (as intercalating agents and through inhibition of topoisomerase II), they have a unique damaging effect on myocardium through a mechanism based on accelerated production of free radicals [22]. The four-ring chromophore moiety of the anthracycline is easily reduced to a semiquinone through a "red-ox" cycle that simultaneously induces the formation of oxygen and peroxide free radicals. Under normal conditions, free radical damage is limited by cellular defenses, including superoxide dismutase, catalase, and glutathione peroxidase. However, myocardium possesses less of these enzymes than other tissues. These myocardial enzymatic defenses become overwhelmed in the presence of ferric (Fe^{+3}) cations that form a stable, noncovalent complex with doxorubicin, thereby increasing the rate of free radical formation several hundred–fold. These free radicals then cause widespread membrane damage by lipid peroxidation. Subcellular targets include the nuclear and cellular membranes and, in the myocardium, the sarcoplasmic reticulum. This damage to the myocyte sarcolemma results in decreased bound calcium and decreased contractility via the actin–myosin complex.

Clinically, the result of this free radical damage to the myocardium is a global cardiomyopathy, resulting in biventricular congestive heart failure (CHF). This cumulative process has been reported to result in a 5% to 10% incidence of clinical CHF at a cumulative doxorubicin dose of 450 to 500 mg/m² in retrospective studies [18,23]. This figure, however, has been underestimated due to inconsistent cardiac monitoring and the retrospective nature of these studies. In the more recent prospective studies that have required consistent gated pool monitoring of cardiac function every one to two cycles, the true incidence of clinical CHF at a cumulative doxorubicin dose of 450 to 500 mg/m² is 20% to 25% [20,24–26]. Also, using the common definition of cardiac toxicity based on gated heart-pool scanning to quantitate the left ventricular ejection fraction (LVEF) (*ie*, 10% drop from baseline LVEF or fall in LVEF to < 50%), the incidence of cardiac toxicity is approximately 35% at a cumulative doxorubicin dose of 450 mg/m² in these same studies. The cumulative dose for development of cardiomyopathy varies according to anthracycline. These clinical changes are associated with pathognomonic electron micrographic findings described by Billingham and coworkers [27] and are quantitated on a scale form 0 to 3 (Table 28-7).

In practice, patients should have baseline LVEF determination at a cumulative doxorubicin dose of 300 and 450 mg/m² and every cycle thereafter until LVEF criteria for cardiac toxicity dictate discontinuing doxorubicin. Alternatively, many oncologists have not exceeded a lifetime cumulative doxorubicin dose limitation of 450 mg/m². It should be borne in mind that cardiac toxicity may progress for up to 2 months after the last dose of doxorubicin and some patients with falling LVEF may go on to develop clinical CHF. Some risk factors associated with development of CHF include prior myocardial infarction and age greater than 65 years.

Although these considerations have dictated the clinical boundaries of doxorubicin use in the past, anthracycline cardiomyopathy may now largely be prevented through the use of dexrazoxane (ICRF-187, Zinecard [Pharmacia and Upjohn, Kalamazoo, MI],

Table 28-7. Histopathologic Scale of Doxorubicin Cardiomyopathy

Grade	Description
0	Within normal limits
1	Less than 5% of cells with early changes (myofibrillar loss and distended sarcoplasmic reticulum)
1.5	Small groups of cells (5%–15%) involved with definitive changes (marked myofibrillar loss and/or vacuolization)
2	Groups of cells (16%–25%) involved with definitive changes (marked myofibrillar loss and/or vacuolization)
2.5	Groups of cells (26%–35%) involved with definitive changes (marked myofibrillar loss and/or vacuolization)
3	Diffuse cell damage (> 35%) with marked change, including degeneration of organelles, mitochondria, and nucleus and loss of contractile elements

Cardioxane [Eurocenter, Amsterdam, Holland]). Prospective randomized studies conducted at New York University [28], the National Cancer Institute (NCI) [26] (in children), and in industry-sponsored multicenter studies [25,2931] have demonstrated the efficacy of this bisdioxopiperazine compound. Dexrazoxane is converted intracellularly to a bidentate chelator analogue of EDTA. This form of the drug is able to strip the Fe^{+3} cations from the Fe^{+3}:doxorubicin complex, thereby preventing cardiomyopathy. In these prospective randomized placebo and nonplacebo controlled clinical trials dexrazoxane has been shown to prevent anthracycline-induced cardiac toxicity based on clinical CHF, LVEF, and biopsy criteria. As approved in the United States, the drug is administered at a dose of 500 mg/m² (ratio of 10:1 to doxorubicin) over 15 minutes beginning 30 minutes prior to doxorubicin administration. Using this dose and schedule, no clinically significant myelosuppression was found for dexrazoxane together with the FAC regimen (fluorouracil, doxorubicin, and cyclophosphamide).

Nearly all trials have shown that dexrazoxane does not change the response rate seen with doxorubicin. However, because of concern raised in one multicenter breast cancer trial [25,29], the drug has been approved for use in the United States beginning after a cumulative doxorubicin dose of 300 mg/m² has been reached in those patients continuing with the drug. In practice, it would be reasonable to begin use of dexrazoxane as soon as there is evidence of antitumor activity for doxorubicin, assuming it is the oncologist's goal to continue doxorubicin until evidence of tumor progression. For example, in the New York University study, which used dexrazoxane at the dose of 1000 mg/m² and started treatment from the first cycle, 15% of all women treated with dexrazoxane were able to tolerate cumulative doxorubicin doses in excess of 1000 mg/m² and several doses at more than 2000 mg/m², with the major cause of treatment termination being progression (rather than cardiac toxicity) [24].

Other strategies for abrogation of anthracycline cardiomyopathy have been also investigated. Less cardiotoxic analogs, such as 4'-epidoxorubicin (epirubicin), have been developed. This agent is widely used in Europe as the anthracycline of choice due to its somewhat improved toxicity profile. Epirubicin is also cardiotoxic via the same mechanisms as doxorubicin, although at a reduced level. Dexrazoxane also provides cardiac protection against epirubicin-induced cardiomyopathy when administered in a ratio of 10:1 [32]. Another approach has been the use of prolonged (durations of up to 96 h) infusion of doxorubicin. This method avoids the higher peak concentrations of doxorubicin produced by bolus administration, allowing tolerance of a somewhat greater cumulative dose [33]. Others have suggested that weekly administration may also lower the risk of cardiomyopathy [34]. Most recently, doxorubicin packaged in pegylated-liposomes (Doxil; Sequus Pharmaceuticals, Menlo Park, CA) has been approved for the treatment of Kaposi's sarcoma. This compound has significantly different pharmacokinetics compared with free drug, with effective circulation time of weeks. It also produces a very different toxicity spectrum compared with doxorubicin. To date, animal studies have not shown an association with cardiotoxicity. Human studies are limited, but patients with Kaposi's sarcoma often have exceeded normally cardiotoxic doses of free doxorubicin (500–1000 mg/m^2) without evidence of cardiac toxicity by LVEF. A study comparing endomyocardial biopsies in these patients with age-matched controls receiving equal doses of doxorubicin showed a median score of 0.50 for Doxil compared with 2.25 for the doxorubicin treated group [35]. Additionally, in 29 women with breast cancer receiving a median of 550 mg/m^2, the median biopsy score was 0 (range 0.0–1.5) [36].

OTHER CARDIOMYOPATHIES

Mitoxantrone, an anthracenedione compound, is structurally similar to the anthracyclines but lacks their characteristic daunosamine sugar moiety. The cardiac toxicity of mitoxantrone is not related to the free radical mechanism described for the anthracyclines. Clinically, however, this cardiomyopathy presents in a similar fashion to doxorubicin, although at a reduced incidence based on equitoxic cumulative dosing. At a cumulative dose of 160 mg/m^2, approximately 5% of patients may develop CHF; therefore, cumulative dosing should be limited, especially in patients with prior anthracycline exposure.

Other agents associated with cardiomyopathy include drugs causing direct myocardial injury. This has been documented most commonly with high-dose alkylating agents, particularly cyclophosphamide, in the setting of bone marrow transplantation or stem cell rescue. Effects associated with high-dose alkylating agents include acute hemorrhagic myocarditis, CHF, and death [37]. The majority of patients receiving doses of 120 to 240 mg/kg over 1 to 4 days have electrocardiogram changes consisting of a decrease in the QRS voltage associated with an asymptomatic decrease in systolic function [38]. This is usually reversible unless hemorrhagic myocarditis occurs. Postmortem and animal-model studies suggest that direct endothelial injury results in capillary microthrombosis and interstitial fibrin deposition.

Radiation therapy may also cause cardiomyopathy due to dose-related interstitial myocardial fibrosis. This long-term complication results from capillary and microcirculatory damage, exudation of fibrin, and eventual fibrosis [39]. Doses greater than 6000 cGy and treatment with a single anterior-posterior portal have been associated with increased risk of this complication, which may occur 5 to 20 years after radiation. This form of biventricular myocardial failure should be differentiated from radiation-induced chronic pericarditis by echocardiography.

ANGINAL SYNDROMES

5-Fluorouracil (5-FU) is the chemotherapy drug associated with the highest reported incidence of myocardial ischemia. The proposed mechanism is by direct induction of coronary artery spasm. Clinically, 5-FU produces angina with typical symptoms, electrocar-

diogram changes, and response to nitroglycerin, although some patients studied have had normal coronary angiograms, even with ergonovine [40]. Moreover, there have been reports of patients who, after experiencing an anginal syndrome during 5-FU, have successfully been reexposed at lower doses without significant subsequent toxicity [41].

In a review of 1000 patients receiving 5-FU, a 4.5% incidence of cardiac ischemia or arrhythmia was noted in patients with a history of coronary artery disease versus a 1.1% incidence of cardiac toxicity in those patients with no previous cardiac history [42]. This association is more striking in those patients who receive a continuous infusion of 5-FU and in those patients who receive concomitant cisplatin [43,44]. Akhtar and coworkers [45], noted an 8% incidence of cardiac side effects in patients without cardiac history who were treated with 96-hour 5-FU infusion in combination with mitomycin-C or cisplatin. These side effects included angina (5 patients), palpitations (3 patients), diaphoresis (2 patients), and syncope (1 patient). There was no relationship between cardiotoxicity and age, sex, tumor, or drug combination.

ARRHYTHMIAS

Bone Marrow Transplantation

Cardiovascular toxicity has been reported to be related to the infusion of cryopreserved grafts for use in bone marrow transplantation. Keung and coworkers [46] noted an 82% incidence of transient cardiac arrhythmias, including sinus bradycardia and complete heart block, although all the patients remained asymptomatic. Another study, however, did not find a relationship between cryopreserved cell administration and cardiac arrhythmias in 44 consecutive patients [47].

The etiology of cardiac toxicity associated with graft infusion is probably multifactorial and may include underlying defects in cardiac conduction, electrolyte abnormalities, cell lysis products of the infusate, mechanical effects of a large volume load, and cardiotoxic effects of the cryopreservative dimethyl sulfoxide.

5-Fluorouracil

5-FU has been associated with arrhythmia as well as anginal syndromes. The incidence of cardiac side effects has been estimated at 5% to 8%, with arrhythmias accounting for approximately half of these episodes (see Anginal Syndromes section). Although most of the documented cases have included ventricular arrhythmias, a prospective evaluation of the specific nature and incidence of these arrhythmias with the use of Holter monitors remains to be performed.

Paclitaxel

Intravenous infusion of paclitaxel (Taxol) was initially associated with a high incidence of bradyarrhythmias [48]. As a result initial NCI-sponsored studies eliminated all patients with cardiac risk factors and required cardiac monitoring. With these precautions, a reassessment of the 3400 patients in the NCI database demonstrated only a 0.29% incidence of grade 4 or 5 cardiac toxicity, including heart block (4 patients), atrial arrhythmias (3 patients), ventricular tachycardia (9 patients), and myocardial infarction within 14 days of Taxol infusion (7 patients) [49]. Ten of these patients had prior cardiac risk factors. At present, routine cardiac monitoring for Taxol administration is not recommended, although it may be considered for patients with known cardiac conditions.

Cisplatin

Cisplatin induces renal tubular dysfunction, resulting in urinary magnesium and potassium loss. These electrolyte abnormalities may result in prolongation of the QT interval and subsequent ventricular arrhythmia. Oral supplementation with both magnesium (eg Slow-Mag 64 mg twice daily) and potassium salts may be necessary chronically.

PERICARDIAL DISEASE

Pericardial disease with a malignant pericardial effusion causing tamponade and CHF should always be considered in the cancer patient. Routine chest radiograph may demonstrate a clearly enlarged and symmetric cardiac shadow. The presence of pericardial disease should be confirmed with echocardiography. This complication has been associated with malignant mediastinal adenopathy, resulting in lymphatic obstruction and pericardial tumor involvement, most commonly in patients with non–small cell lung cancer and breast cancer. Pericardial effusion has also been associated with the use of anthracyclines [50] and high-dose cyclophosphamide [38] generally in the setting of other manifestations of cardiac toxicity. Radiation-induced acute and chronic pericarditis has also been described. Acute pericarditis is dose related, with an estimated 10% to 15% incidence reported in patients with Hodgkin's disease who received greater than 40 Gy to the mediastinum [51]. A smaller proportion of these patients will go on to develop long-term, chronic constrictive pericarditis due to radiation-induced fibrosis. More modern radiation techniques should result in an incidence of less than 2.5% for these complications [52].

REFERENCES

1. Twohig K, Matthay R: Pulmonary effects of cytotoxic agents otherthan bleomycin. *Clin Chest Med* 1990, 11:31–54.

2. Lehne G, Lote K: Pulmonary toxicity of cytotoxic and immunosuppressive agents: a review. *Acta Oncol* 1990, 29:113–124.

3. Anderson B, Cogan B, Keating M, *et al.*: Subacute pulmonary failure complicating therapy with high-doseara-C in acute leukemia. *Cancer* 1985, 56:2181–2184.

4. Crooke S, Bradner W: Bleomycin: a review. *J Med* 1976, 7:333–428.

5. Jules-ElyseeK, White D: Bleomycin-induced pulmonary toxicity. *Clin Chest Med* 1990, 11:1–20.

6. Comis R: Bleomycin pulmonary toxicity: current statusand future directions. *Semin Oncol* 1992, 19(suppl 5):64–70.

7. Comis R: Detecting bleomycin pulmonary toxicity: a continuedconundrum. *J Clin Oncol* 1990, 8:765–767.

8. Lei K, Leung W, Johnson P: Serious pulmonary complications in patients receiving recombinantgranulocyte colony-stimulating factor during BACOP chemotherapy foraggressive non-Hodgkin's lymphoma. *Br J Cancer* 1994, 70:1009–1013.

9. Saxman S, Nichols C, Einhorn L: Pulmonarytoxicity in patients with advanced-stage germ cell tumors receivingbleomycin with and without granulocyte colony stimulating factor. *Chest* 1997, 111:657–660.

10. Buzdar A, Legha S, Luna M, *et al.*: Pulmonary toxicity of mitomycin. *Cancer* 1980, 45:236–244.

11. Weinstein A, Deiner-West M, Nelson D, *et al.*: Pulmonary toxicity of carmustine inpatients treated for malignant glioma. *Cancer Treat Rep* 1986, 70:943–946.

12. Gibson S, Comis R: The pulmonary toxicity ofantineoplastic agents. *Semin Oncol* 1982, 9:34–51.

13. Chan C, Hyland R, Hutcheon M: Pulmonary complications following bone marrowtransplantation. *Clin Chest Med* 1990, 2:323–332.

14. Abdel-Razeq H,Overmoyer B, Pohlman B, *et al.*: Pulmonary toxicity of STAMP V preparative regimen in high-dose chemotherapy (HDC) and autologousbone marrow transplantation (ABMT) for breast cancer [abstract]. *Proc Annu Meet Am Soc Clin Oncol* 1997, 16:100.

15. Rosiello R, Merrill W: Radiation-induced lung injury. *Clin Chest Med* 1990, 11:65–71.

16. Nora R, Abrams J, Tait N, *et al.*: Myocardial toxic effects during IL-2 therapy. *J Natl Cancer Inst* 1989, 81:59–63.

17. Trehu EG, Karp DD, Atkins MB: Possible myocardial toxicity associated with Interleukin-4 therapy. *J Immunother* 1993, 14:348–351.

18. Von Hoff D, Layard M, Basa P, *et al.*: Risk factors for doxorubicin-induced congestive heart failure. *Ann Intern Med* 1979, 91:710–717.

19. Von Hoff D, Rozencweig M, Layard M, *et al.*: Daunomycin-induced cardiotoxicity in children and adults: a review of 110 cases. *Am J Med* 1977, 62:200–208.

20. Speyer J, Freedberg R: *Clinical Oncology.* New York: Churchill Livingstone, Inc.; 1995.

21. Hochster H, Wasserheit C, Speyer J: Cardiotoxicity and cardioprotection during chemotherapy. *Curr Opinion Oncol* 1995, 7:304–309.

22. Gianni L, Myers C: The role of free radical formation in the cardiotoxicity of anthracycline. In *Cancer Treatment and the Heart.* Edited by Muggia F, Green M, Speyer J. Baltimore: The Johns Hopkins University Press; 1992:9–46.

23. Bristow M, Mason J, Billingham M, *et al.*: Dose-effect and structure-function relationships in doxorubicin cardiomyopathy. *Am Heart J* 1981, 102:709–718.

24. Speyer J, Green M, Zeleniuch-Jacquotte A, *et al.*: ICRF-187 permits longer treatment with doxorubicin in women with breast cancer. *J Clin Oncol* 1992, 10:117–127.

25. Swain S, Whaley F, Gerber M, *et al.*: Cardioprotection with dexrazoxane for doxorubicin-containing therapy in advanced breast cancer. *J Clin Oncol* 1997, 15:1318–1332.

26. Wexler L, Andrich M, Venzon D, *et al.*: Randomized trial of the cardioprotective agent ICRF-187 in pediatric sarcoma patients treated with doxorubicin. *J Clin Oncol* 1996, 14:362–372.

27. Billingham M, Mason J, Bristow M, *et al.*: Anthracycline cardiomyopathy monitored by morphologic changes. *Cancer Treat Rep* 1978, 62:865–872.

28. Speyer J, Green M, Kramer E, *et al.*: Protective effect of the bispiperazine ICRF-187 against doxorubicin induced cardiac toxicity in women with advanced breast cancer. *N Engl J Med* 1988, 319:745–752.

29. Swain S, Whaley F, Gerber M, *et al.*: Delayed administration of dexrazoxane provides cardioprotection for patients with advanced breast cancer treated with doxorubicin-containing therapy. *J Clin Oncol* 1997, 15:1333–1340.

30. Gams R: Prospective data management in the conduct of large multicenter clinical trials [abstract]. *Proc Am Assoc Cancer Res* 1994, 35:A1151.

31. Lopez M, Vici P, Lauro LD, *et al.*: Randomized prospective clinical trial of high-dose epirubicin and dexrazoxane in patients with advanced breast cancer and soft tissue sarcomas. *J Clin Oncol* 1998, 16:1–7.

32. Sorensen B, Bastholt L, Mirza M, *et al.*: The cardioprotector ADR-529 and high-dose epirubicin given in combination with cyclophosphamide, 5-fluorouracil, and tamoxifen: a phase I study in metastatic breast cancer. *Cancer Chemother Pharmacol* 1994, 34:439–443.

33. Legha S, Benjamin R, Mackay B, *et al.*: Reduction of doxorubicin cardiotoxicity by prolonged continuous intravenous infusion. *Ann Intern Med* 1982, 96:133–139.

34. Torti F, Bristow M, Howes A, *et al.*: Reduced cardiotoxicity of doxorubicin delivered on a weekly schedule: assessment by endomyocardial biopsy. *Ann Intern Med* 1983, 99:745–749.

35. Berry G, Billingham M, Alderman E, *et al.*: Reduced cardiotoxicity of Doxil in AIDS Kaposi's sarcoma patients compared to a matched control group of cancer patients given doxorubicin [abstract]. *Proc Annu Meet Am Soc Clin Oncol* 1996, 15:A843.

36. Fonseca G, Valero V, Buzdar A, *et al.*: Decreased cardiac toxicity by TLC D-99 in the treatment of metastatic breast carcinoma [abstract]. *Proc of ASCO* 1995, 14:A99.

37. Gottdeiner J, Appelbaum F, Ferrans V, *et al.*: Cardiotoxicity associated with high-dose cyclophosphamide therapy. *Arch Intern Med* 1981, 141:758–763.

38. Cazin B, Gorin N, Laporte J, *et al.*: Cardiac complications after bone marrow transplantation: a report on a series of 63 consecutive transplantations. *Cancer* 1986, 57:2061–2069.

39. Stewart JR FL: Radiation-induced heart disease: an update. *Cardiovasc Dis* 1984, 27:27–35.

40. Freeman N, Costanza M: 5-fluorouracil associated carciotoxicity. *Cancer* 1988, 61:36–45.

41. Weidmann B, Teipel A, Niederle N: The syndrome of 5-Fluorouracil cardiotoxicity: an elusive cardiopathy. *Cancer* 1994, 73:2001–2002.

42. Labianca R, Beretta G, Clerici M, *et al.*: Cardiac toxicity of 5-FU: a study of 1083. *Tumor* 1982, 68:505–510.

43. Forni MD, Malet-Martino M, Jaillais P, *et al.*: Cardiotoxicity of high-dose continuous infusion fluorouracil: a prospective clinical study. *J Clin Oncol* 1992, 10:1795–801.

44. Ensley J, Kish J, Tapazoglou E, *et al.*: 5-fluorouracil infusions associated with an ischemic cardiotoxicity syndrome. *Proc ASCO* 1986, 5:142.

45. Akhtar S, Salim K, Bano Z: Symptomatic cardiotoxicity with high-dose 5-Fluorouracil infusion: a prospective study. *Oncology* 1993, 50:441–444.

46. Keung YK, Lau S, Elkayam U, *et al.*: Cardiac arrythmia after infusion of cryopreserved stem cells. *Bone Marrow Transplantation* 1994, 14:363–367.

47. Lopez-Jimenez J, Munoz A, Hdez-Madrid A, *et al.*: Cardiovascular toxicities related to the infusion of cryopreserved grafts: results of a controlled study. *Bone Marrow Transplantation* 1994, 13:789–793.

48. Rowinsky E, McGuire W, Guarnieri T, *et al.*: Cardiac disturbances during the administration of Taxol. *J Clin Oncol* 1991, 9:1704–1712.

49. Arbuck S, Strauss H, Rowinksy E, *et al.*: A reassessment of cardiac toxicity associated with Taxol. *Monogr Natl Cancer Inst* 1993, 15:117–130.

50. Bristow M, Thompson P, Martin R, *et al.*: Early anthracycline cardiotoxicity. *Am J Med* 1978, 65:823–832.

51. Lawmore-Luria H, Kohn K, Pasternack R: Radiation heart disease. *J Cardiovasc Med* 1993, 8:113–125.

52. Tarbell N, Thompson L, Mauch P: Thoracic irradiation in Hodgkin's disease: disease control and long-term complications. *Int J Radiat Oncol Biol Phys* 1990, 18:275–282.

CHAPTER 29: NEUROTOXICITIES
David Schiff

The concept of neurologic toxicity is of major importance in the ability to treat malignancy with radiation and chemotherapy. In many cases, neurotoxicity represents the dose-limiting toxicity of antineoplastic treatments. There is no specific therapy available to reverse or prevent most of the neurotoxicities discussed in this chapter, although some are self-limited or spontaneously improve. Furthermore, most neurotoxicities are dose related. Recognition that a neurologic problem may be related to treatment rather than to the underlying malignancy will sometimes obviates the need for unnecessary diagnostic studies and alleviates the anxiety of patients and families. It may also permit the offending agent to be discontinued while neurotoxicity is still reversible or relatively mild. Thus, it is imperative that the clinician who is caring for patients receiving these treatment modalities has an understanding of the neurologic complications, timing, and relationship to total dose and route of administration. Although constraints do not permit a discussion of all cancer treatment modalities, we will address the more common causes of neurotoxicity and the most common therapeutic agents currently in usage. More encyclopedic data are available in excellent recent reviews [1,2].

NEUROTOXICITIES OF VARIOUS CHEMOTHERAPEUTIC AGENTS

ALKYLATING AGENTS
Chlorambucil
Overdose has been associated with transient encephalopathy and status epilepticus. Conventional doses have rarely been associated with seizures.

Cyclophosphamide
This agent uncommonly produces hyponatremia, which can produce encephalopathy and seizures. Otherwise, it has no neurotoxicity in conventional doses.

Ifosfamide
Up to 25% of patients receiving ifosfamide experience central neurotoxicity. Risk factors for encephalopathy and seizures may include 1) high-dose, renal, or hepatic dysfunction; 2) low serum albumin; and 3) prior exposure to cisplatin [3]. Typically, delirium, stupor, mutism, or catatonia not associated with focal neurologic deficits occur within a few days of receiving ifosfamide. Brain scans are normal, but electroencephalography (EEG) generally demonstrates a diffusely slow background. Although overt seizures are rare, nonconvulsive status epilepticus has been reported [4], and intravenous diazepam has been reported to improve the encephalopathy [5]. The mechanism of ifosfamide neurotoxicity is unknown, although ifosfamide's metabolite chloracetaldehyde may be neurotoxic. A few patients have been treated with methylene blue, which blocks mitochondrial production of chloracetaldehyde from ifosfamide; results have been mixed, and this treatment is not presently routine. Patients typically recover completely from the syndrome but may redevelop the syndrome if retreated at the same dose. High-dose ifosfamide (14 gm/m^2) has produced a syndrome of acute, painful distal paresthesias, numbness lasting several days, or both [6].

Melphalan
Melphalan is not associated with neurotoxicity.

Mechlorethamine
Mechlorethamine commonly produces confusion, headache, lethargy, and seizures when given in high doses in preparation for bone marrow transplantation (BMT). Long-term follow-up of some of these patients revealed dementia with ventriculomegaly on computed tomography (CT) and background slowing on EEG [7].

Thiotepa
Thiotepa has occasionally been associated with myelopathy when administered intrathecally for leptomeningeal carcinomatosis [8].

Busulfan
High doses of this lipophilic agent in preparation for BMT produce seizures in approximately 10% of patients, leading some physicians to administer prophylactic anticonvulsants [9].

Table 29-1. Chemotherapy producing seizures*	
Busulfan	Methotrexate
Ifosfamide	Paclitaxel
Cisplatin	L-asparaginase
Cyclosporine	Cytarabine
Tacrolimus	Etoposide
Vincristine	Chlorambucil
Cyclophosphamide	Mechlorethamine

*Must be distinguished from seizures related to parenchymal or leptomeningeal metastases, electrolyte disturbances, hypoxia, and other causes.

Table 29-2. Chemotherapy producing acute encephalopathy*	
Cisplatin	Clardribine
Ifosfamide	Pentostatin
Cyclophosphamide	Cyclosporine
Procarbazine	Tacrolimus
Hexamethylmelamine	Vincristine
Methotrexate	Etoposide
Cytarabine	Paclitaxel
5-Fluorouracil	Interferons
Fotofur	5-Azacytidine
Fludarabine	Interleukin-2

*Must be distinguished from other causes of acute encephalopathy, including parenchymal and leptomeningeal metastases, paraneoplastic syndromes, electrolyte disturbances, sepsis, psychoactive medications, hypoxia, and other causes.

Table 29-3. Chemotherapy producing dementia*
Methotrexate
Interferon-α
BCNU
Fludarabine
Pentostatin
Cladribine
Carmofur

*Radiation-induced dementia, paraneoplastic encephalomyelitis, brain metastases and other causes of dementia must be excluded.

Nitrosoureas

Carmustine (BCNU) is the prototype and most frequently used drug in this family of lipid-soluble alkylating agents that cross the blood–brain barrier. BCNU in its usual intravenous doses of 200 mg/m² causes no neurotoxicity, although high-dose intravenous BCNU (600–2000 mg/m²) as preparation for BMT has been linked to subacute irreversible necrotizing encephalopathy [10]. Intracarotid BCNU, which has been largely abandoned, reliably produced eye pain and headache and, at higher doses, ipsilateral leukoencephalopathy and retinal toxicity [2].

Cisplatin

The ability to limit nephrotoxicity of this agent with aggressive hydration has rendered neurologic symptoms the dose-limiting toxicity. Cumulative doses of approximately ≥ 400 mg/m² generally produce a large-fiber sensory neuropathy characterized by decreased sensation of light touch, vibration, and proprioception as well as diminished deep tendon reflexes; the resulting sensory ataxia may be disabling [11,12]. Although neuropathy may worsen for a few weeks following the last cycle of cisplatin, it eventually improves in most cases. The adrenocorticotropic analogue Org 2766 and the sulfhydryl compound amifostine appear to offer some protection against the development of this complication but have not been approved for this indication [13,14]. High-frequency hearing loss and tinnitus are also common with cisplatin. Occasionally, transient Lhermitte's phenomenon (an electric shock-like sensation down the spine and sometimes into the extremities precipitated by neck flexion) is seen several weeks to months after receiving cisplatin. This phenomenon is presumably due to dorsal-column demyelination but is generally not associated with more serious symptoms or signs of myelopathy. Rare patients have developed cortical blindness or other stroke-like phenomena shortly after receiving cisplatin; fortunately, this generally resolves spontaneously.

Carboplatin

Although carboplatin shares very similar antineoplastic activity with cisplatin, it carries virtually no neurotoxicity. Like cisplatin, it has rarely caused a microangiopathic hemolytic anemia with cerebral infarction.

Mitomycin

Like platinum compounds, it may cause thrombotic microangiopathy with resulting strokes.

Procarbazine

Intravenous administration of this agent, which readily crosses the blood–brain barrier, is associated with prolonged somnolence; consequently, procarbazine is given orally. Patients receiving standard doses (up to 150 mg/m²/d) occasionally complain of lethargy, nightmares, depression, anxiety, or hallucinations. Procarbazine also produces a reversible sensory neuropathy in 10%–20% of patients characterized by distal lower extremity paresthesias and diminished deep tendon reflexes. Transient myalgias have also been observed [15]. Because procarbazine is an MAO inhibitor, patients are advised to avoid tyramine-rich foods, antidepressants, and sympathomimetic drugs so as not to develop hypertensive crisis; fortunately, this interaction is clinically uncommon [1]. Procarbazine can produce a disulfiram-like reaction with ethanol and may produce synergistic central nervous system (CNS) depression when given with CNS depressants such as phenothiazines, antihistamines, narcotics, and centrally acting antihypertensive medicines [16].

Dacarbazine

High doses of dacarbazine can cause transient headaches. Otherwise, no neurotoxicity has been reported.

Temozolomide

No neurotoxicity has been associated with this promising agent for melanoma and gliomas.

Hexamethylmelamine

Prolonged oral administration of this agent, whose mechanism of action is uncertain, has produced sensorimotor peripheral neuropathy [17].

DNA STRAND BREAKAGE AGENTS

Bleomycin

Bleomycin is not associated with neurotoxicity.

TOPOISOMERASE I INHIBITORS

Topotecan

Topotecan and irinotecan have not been reported to produce significant neurotoxicity. However, their use is occasionally associated with headache or lethargy.

Table 29-4. Chemotherapy producing cerebellar dysfunction*
Cytarabine
5-Fluorouracil
Cyclosporine
Procarbazine
Hexamethylmelamine
Vincristine

*Must be distinguished from cerebellar metastases, hydrocephalus, paraneoplastic cerebellar degeneration, ataxia from spinal cord compression, and non-malignant causes of ataxia.

Tables 29-5. Chemotherapy producing myelopathy*
Intrathecal methotrexate
Intrathecal cytarabine
Intrathecal Thiotepa

*The clinical setting is usually obvious.

Table 29-6. Chemotherapy producing neuropathy	
Vincristine	Teniposide
Cisplatin	Etoposide
Paclitaxel	Cytarabine
Docetaxel	5-Azacytidine
Suramin	Cladribine
Hexamethylmelamine	Fludarabine
Misonidazole	Interferon
Procarbazine	

TOPOISOMERASE II INHIBITORS

The DNA intercalating agents daunorubicin, doxorubicin, idarubicin, and mitoxantrone have no neurotoxic effects when administered intravenously.

Etoposide

Etoposide may cause a sensory neuropathy in high doses for BMT, especially in patients previously exposed to vincristine [18] and may synergistically produce neuropathy with vincristine [19]. Myeloablative doses frequently result in transient worsening of focal neurologic symptoms approximately 10 days after treatment in patients with primary brain tumors [20].

Teniposide

Teniposide has no neurotoxicity of its own. It has been suggested, however, to predispose to severe vincristine neuropathy [21].

ANTIMETABOLITES

Methotrexate

This antifolate agent, which interferes with thymidylate synthetase, produces several forms of neurotoxicity depending on the dose and route of administration. Intrathecal or intra-Ommaya methotrexate produces aseptic meningitis lasting a few days in up to 10% of patients, generally with onset within several hours of administration. Cerebrospinal fluid (CSF) pleocytosis is present, which raises the concern of infection, but the timing is too rapid for iatrogenic bacterial meningitis, and cultures are negative [22]. Rarely, patients receiving intrathecal methotrexate have developed paraplegia with spinal cord necrosis for which there is no specific treatment [23]. Intrathecal methotrexate overdoses have sometimes been successfully treated with ventriculolumbar perfusion or leucovorin rescue [24]. High-dose intravenous methotrexate (several g/m^2) occasionally causes encephalopathy or stroke-like transient focal deficits of uncertain pathogenesis. The most feared methotrexate complication is a delayed cerebral leukoencephalopathy that may be associated with dementia, spasticity, hemiparesis, ataxia, and coma. This syndrome may occur several months to years after either intrathecal or high-dose intravenous methotrexate, particularly in patients who also received cranial irradiation (radiation prior to methotrexate appears more toxic than the reverse sequence) [25–28]. Cerebral white matter appears hypodense on CT and T2-hyperintense on magnetic resonance imaging (MRI); cortical calcifications and cerebral atrophy may also be present [29,30]. No treatment for this complication is available. The potential for this complication often limits the combined use of methotrexate and radiotherapy.

Among the purine antagonists, mercaptopurine and 6-thioguanine are not associated with neurotoxicity. However, fludarabine, cladribine and pentostatin are associated with neurotoxicity.

Fludarabine

High doses of fludarabine (≥ 125 mg/m^2/d for 5 d) have resulted in severe CNS toxicity. At these dose levels, approximately 50% of patients developed mental status changes several weeks after treatment. These changes then progressed to produce coma, spasticity, cortical blindness, and optic neuritis. Brain MRI and autopsy showed widespread demyelination [31]. At lower doses, similar cases have been rarely reported, but neurotoxicity is much less; somnolence, peripheral neuropathy, and visual changes have been reported [32]. Occasional patients have had reversible clinical syndromes with neuroimaging abnormalities [33].

Cladribine

A high incidence of paraparesis has been noted several weeks following treatment with 7- to 14-day continuous infusions of 0.3–0.5 mg/m^2/d after a several-week delay [34]. At doses of approximately 20 mg/m^2/d administered by continuous infusion for 5 days, severe axonal sensorimotor peripheral neuropathy, with prominent proximal lower extremity weakness noted [35]; similar doses given as a bolus do not have this effect [36].

Pentostatin

Standard doses in the range of 4–5 mg/m^2/wk occasionally produce lethargy. Sedative and hypnotic agents should be used with caution. At higher doses, encephalopathy, seizures, and coma may occur [32].

Cytarabine

Cytarabine (ara-C) is a pyrimidine antagonist that crosses the blood–brain barrier and blood–CSF barrier fairly poorly, and it has no neurotoxicity at its usual intravenous doses of 100–200 mg/m^2. In doses of 3 g/m^2, ara-C achieves significant CNS levels and is capable of producing distinctive neurotoxicity. Up to 20% of patients receiving 3 g/m^2 twice daily over 4 to 6 days will develop cerebellar dysfunction and sometimes encephalopathy and lethargy. Hepatic or renal dysfunction, age > 50 years, and increasing cumulative doses of ara-C may increase the risk of developing this syndrome, which usually resolves within a few weeks of drug discontinuation [37]. MRI and CSF examination are unremarkable. High-dose ara-C also rarely causes a poorly characterized sensorimotor peripheral neuropathy. Ara-C is sometimes given intrathecally for leptomeningeal leukemia or lymphoma. Like methotrexate, it occasionally causes aseptic meningitis, encephalopathy, seizures, and rarely, necrotizing myelopathy.

Gemcitabine

Although related to cytarabine, gemcitabine produces little or no neurotoxicity. It occasionally produces lethargy and has rarely been reported to cause confusion.

5-Fluorouracil

5-Fluorouracil (5-FU) is the prototypic fluorinated pyrimidine. Other members of this class of agents include floxuridine, carmofur, and fotofur, which are all are capable of producing CNS dysfunction. 5-FU produces cerebellar dysfunction consisting of ataxia, nystagmus, dysmetria, and scanning speech. This toxicity is uncommon at conventional doses and usually resolves within a few days of discontinuing the agent. Rechallenged patients may have a recrudescence of symptoms. Concomitant use of allopurinol increases the likelihood of this syndrome. Levamisole and 5-FU produce unique neurotoxicity as described under Levamisole on page 356. Other agents in this class sometimes produce cerebellar syndromes or encephalopathy [1,2].

TUBULIN-INTERACTIVE AGENTS

Vincristine

Vincristine's antineoplastic effect is based on its inhibition of microtubule formation, which interferes with the mitotic apparatus. It also interferes with neuronal axonal transport, accounting for its neurotoxicity. Vincristine reliably produces a dose-dependent peripheral neuropathy that is usually its dose-limiting toxicity. The physician may notice absent ankle reflexes and generalized hyporeflexia before the patient voices complaints. Patients typically notice paresthesias in the fingers and toes, which may be painful. As neuropathy worsens, these symptoms progress proximally, and sensory deficits (especially to pinprick and cold) become evident. With severe vincristine neuropathy, distal weakness with wrist and foot drop ensues. Autonomic neuropathy, manifesting as constipation and abdominal pain, is common. Preexisting neuropathy may accentuate the neurotoxicity of vincristine, and patients with hereditary motor and sensory neuropathy (Charcot–Marie–Tooth disease) seem particularly prone to this [38]. Electromyography demonstrates an axonal neuropathy but are generally not necessary given the typical presentation [39]. Rare complications include syndrome of inappropriate antidiuretic hormone, cranial mononeuropathies, and seizures. Other vinca alkaloids (including vinblastine, vindesine, and vinorelbine) are much more myelosuppressive than vincristine; although they occasionally produce neuropathy, hematotoxicity usually precedes this complication.

Paclitaxel

The most common neurologic side effect of this agent is sensory polyneuropathy, which usually involves all sensory modalities and produces prominent dysesthesias and paresthesias. Risk of developing neuropathy correlates with the increasing of both individual and cumulative doses. Neuropathy may be dose limiting, especially when colony-stimulating factors mitigate hematotoxicity. Neuropathy does not always worsen with additional cycles and usually resolves following cessation of therapy [40]. Patients previously receiving cisplatin may develop symptoms more readily [41]. Proximal weakness occasionally occurs as well. Not surprisingly, patients receiving concurrent paclitaxel and cisplatin develop more severe neuropathy; prior paclitaxel exposure appears to predispose to developing neuropathy from vinorelbine. Nerve growth factors are undergoing clinical trials to determine whether they protect against paclitaxel neuropathy. Docetaxel produces a similar neuropathy [42,43]. Other uncommon toxicities of paclitaxel include seizures and a transient confusional state several days after receiving the agent [44]. Finally, high-dose paclitaxel sometimes produces transient stupor or coma, attributed to the soporific effects of the Cremophor [44] or alcohol in the vehicle.

HORMONAL AGENTS

Corticosteroids

Cancer patients (particularly those with hematologic malignancies, brain tumors, or spinal cord compression) often receive dexamethasone, prednisone, or other corticosteroids. Neurologic complications figure prominently among these agents' many side effects. Corticosteroid myopathy occurs in many patients treated for more than a couple of weeks and ranges from mild to severe. Its severity increases with dose, and it is more common in patients receiving 9-α-fluorinated corticosteroids (eg, dexamethasone). Patients often note difficulty rising from the toilet or couch as an early symptom. Neck flexor weakness is an early physical finding suggesting the diagnosis of myopathy as opposed to neuropathy or myelopathy; painless symmetric proximal extremity weakness with preserved reflexes and sensation are the norm. The serum creatine phosphokinase is normal in steroid myopathy, which is in contrast to inflammatory myopathies like polymyositis and dermatomyositis, and EMG is usually normal as well.

Typical cases require no diagnostic studies, and generally improve if steroids can be tapered; when this is impossible, switching to a nonfluorinated compound may help. Steroid-associated psychiatric symptoms are common and may include euphoria, depression, and frank psychosis. Tapering the medication, implementing symptom-targeted psychoactive medications, or both are helpful. Insomnia is common, and it is preferable to avoid giving steroids in the evening. The half-life of dexamethasone allows for twice-daily dosing in most patients. Steroids frequently cause tremor as well as blurry vision from refractive changes in the lens, and their long-term administration may lead to avascular necrosis of the hip (which sometimes simulates lumbar radiculopathy) and epidural lipomatosis (which rarely has produced symptomatic spinal cord compression). [1,2]

Tamoxifen

In usual doses (20 mg/d), tamoxifen has minimal neurotoxicity. Occasionally, it is associated with headaches and rarely with a reversible optic neuropathy characterized by visual loss and disk edema [16]. The use of high-dose tamoxifen is being explored because of its potential ability to reverse the multidrug resistance phenotype and to inhibit protein kinase C. Tamoxifen crosses the blood–brain barrier, and doses > 150 mg/m^2 twice daily have caused reversible cerebellar ataxia, tremor, hyperreflexia, and dizziness [45].

Aminoglutethimide

This antiadrenal agent is related to the hypnotic glutethimide Doriden, and produces ataxia, nystagmus, and lethargy in doses – 1500 mg/d [46].

Leuprolide

This gonadotropin-releasing hormone analogue occasionally produces dizziness and headache. It may also lead to a temporary flare of bone pain and spinal cord compression, which can be blocked by concomitantly giving flutamide [47]. Pseudotumor cerebri may rarely occur with this agent.

Flutamide

Flutamide, an androgen receptor antagonist, is not associated with any neurologic complications.

Progestins

Progestins such as megestrol acetate produce no major neurotoxicity but may cause headaches, anxiety, insomnia, and dizziness. The estrogen diethylstilbestrol and the androgen danazol can cause the same symptoms.

BIOLOGIC AGENTS

Interferon-α

This agent is commonly associated with neuropsychiatric symptoms, including depression, lack of motivation, personality change, cognitive slowing, and memory impairment. Patients sometimes appear parkinsonian, with bradykinesia and micrographia. These problems may be dose limiting but usually resolve following drug discontinuation [52,53]. The pathophysiology is unknown. Apart from lowering the dose or providing a drug holiday, no specific treatment is available. Occasionally, antidepressants have been of benefit, and the use of naltrexone in preventing these symptoms is being studied. Patients with brain metastases may develop increased intracranial pressure while receiving interferon-α, and consequently, it is advised that patients be screened with brain CT or MRI prior to treatment.

Interleukin-2

Interleukin-2 can acutely cause dose-dependent behavioral changes characterized by confusion, drowsiness, and inattention. These changes typically resolve following cessation of treatment. As with interferon-α, patients with brain metastases may develop increased cerebral edema [53]. Rare patients have developed contrast-enhancing multifocal cerebral lesions associated with mental status changes and focal neurologic deficits. The neuroimaging abnormalities (which may resemble metastases, abscesses, or the posterior hemispheric abnormalities seen in cyclosporin toxicity or eclampsia) typically resolve spontaneously; most patients have recovered fully [54]. Interleukin-2 has also been associated with carpal tunnel syndrome, probably from vascular leak producing interstitial edema in the carpal tunnel. Such patients do not generally require nerve conduction studies [55].

All-*trans*-retinoic acid

The main neurotoxicity of all-*trans*-retinoic acid (ATRA), a differentiation agent, is a headache that typically occurs several hours after oral administration. When mild, the headache can be managed with standard analgesics. ATRA can produce pseudotumor cerebri (increased intracranial pressure associated with papilledema and a normal brain scan); such patients require dose reduction or cessation of ATRA in addition to brain CT or MRI, a lumbar puncture (to document increased pressure and exclude other causes such as leptomeningeal metastases), and close ophthalmologic follow-up. Myalgias also occur. *Cis*-retinoic acid has a similar side effect profile.

Levamisole

This immunostimulatory drug is used in conjunction with 5-FU to decrease the risk of recurrence in patients with Dukes' C colon carcinoma . Occasional patients have developed confusion and ataxia associated with multifocal contrast-enhancing white-matter lesions suggestive of brain metastases that have spontaneously resolved. Brain biopsy has shown active demyelination. Typically, symptoms have ensued approximately 4 months after starting chemotherapy and begin to improve several weeks after discontinuing treatment. Allopurinol may increase the risk of developing the syndrome. Some patients have been treated with corticosteroids, although others have recovered fully without their use [56].

Bone marrow transplantation

Bone marrow transplantation is now commonly used for hematologic malignancies and aplastic anemia; its use in solid tumors is undergoing study. Neurologic complications occur in more than 50% of patients [57]. Toxic-metabolic encephalopathy and mild peripheral neuropathy are common. Immunologic alterations predispose patients to a variety of neurotropic infections as well as neuromuscular disease (*eg*, polymyositis and myasthenia gravis). Of most relevance are the neurologic complications associated with immunosuppressive therapy. Although azathioprine has no neurotoxicity, both cyclosporine and tacrolimus (FK 506) produce significant, sometimes dose-limiting neurotoxicity. Each may cause tremulousness, confusion, seizures, cortical blindness, and headaches. MRIs frequently show transitory parietooccipital white-matter signal changes. Cyclosporine levels are frequently but not invariably toxic when symptoms begin. Hypomagnesemia and hypocholesterolemia have been suggested as risk factors for developing the syndrome. Treatment consists of stopping or decreasing the offending agent in addition to anticonvulsants if needed; complete recovery is the rule [58,59].

SUPPORTIVE CARE AGENTS

Ondansetron and granisetron

Ondansetron and granisetron are 5-HT3–receptor antagonists that are highly effective in chemotherapy-induced nausea and vomiting. Headache occurs in up to 20% of patients, although it is rarely severe.

Filgrastim

Headaches (mild to moderate) occur in 39% of normal controls given filgrastim (G-CSF). Bone pain occurs in the majority of patients, and fatigue is also sometimes noted [60]; sargramostim (GM-CSF) has similar side effects. A single case of recurrent encephalopathy and status epilepticus has been linked to filgrastim [61].

Erythropoietin

This agent sometimes induces severe hypertension. Several cases of hypertensive encephalopathy with posterior white-matter changes on MRI have been associated with erythropoietin use [62].

MISCELLANEOUS AGENTS

Hydroxyurea

Hydroxyurea does not cause neurotoxicity.

L-asparaginase

The enzyme L-asparaginase capitalizes on the inability of acute lymphoblastic leukemia cells to synthesize asparagine by cleaving asparagine in the bloodstream, thereby depleting the tumor of this essential amino acid. CNS dysfunction was a frequent side effect in the past when higher doses were given; between 25% and 50% of patients developed encephalopathy ranging from drowsiness to delirium to frank coma within several days of treatment. More recently, as doses have been reduced, the main complication has been cortical vein or dural sinus thrombosis, presumably through a decrease in antithrombotic proteins and an increase in thrombin activity. Symptoms may include headache, seizures, encephalopathy, and hemiparesis [1]. MRI may demonstrate the venous thrombosis as well as venous infarction. Corticosteroids are sometimes beneficial symptomatically, and anticonvulsants should be used as needed. Some patients have been treated with fresh frozen plasma or heparin, but the benefit of these agents is unproven.

Mitotane

Most patients treated with this antiadrenal drug develop some degree of neurotoxicity [48]. Mood disorders and a mild axonal peripheral neuropathy are the rule, whereas confusion, ataxia, dysarthria, and parkinsonism are fairly common.

Suramin

This agent, capable of blocking interactions between various growth factors and their receptors, occasionally produces a Guillain–Barré–like, acute, severe, sensorimotor peripheral neuropathy that sometimes results in quadriplegia [49]. Electrophysiologic studies reveal conduction block suggestive of demyelination; also reminiscent of Guillain-Barré syndrome is the elevated CSF protein. A milder stocking-and-glove sensorimotor polyneuropathy on EMG/NCV that is suggestive of axonal damage has also been reported [50]. Risk neuropathy appears to be a function of both the increasing plasma suramin complications and the duration of the suramin infusion [50,51], although most patients have gradually recovered. Plasmapheresis has not been of benefit.

NEUROLOGIC TOXICITY OF RADIATION THERAPY
Intracranial complications

Radiation complications are classically subdivided depending on their timing of onset relative to radiotherapy into acute, early-delayed (subacute), and late-delayed reactions. Acute radiation reactions are rarely seen now. They typically ensue when patients receive large radiation fractions, particularly in the setting of large brain masses with cerebral edema. Such patients sometimes develop headache, nausea, fever, encephalopathy, and worsening of focal neurologic deficits within hours of starting radiotherapy; herniation and death sometimes occurs. Presumably, radiation opens the blood–brain barrier and worsens cerebral edema. Consequently, patients with large tumors or multiple brain metastases are usually pretreated with dexamethasone 8 to 16 mg daily, 1 to 3 days before radiotherapy, and are often given relatively small radiation fractions (≤ 200 cGy) for the first few days of treatment. When such symptoms do occur, they generally respond to increased dexamethasone [1].

Early-delayed radiation reactions take multiple forms. Uncommonly, patients having undergone whole-brain radiotherapy 1 to 4 months previously (especially children with acute lymphoblastic leukemia) develop somnolence with or without headache and nausea. Such patients may sleep 18 to 20 hours daily for a few weeks. Corticosteroids usually ameliorate these symptoms and may be preventive if given during radiotherapy [63]. Another syndrome affects brain tumor patients who may develop symptoms of clinical tumor progression (headaches, fatigue, and worsening of focal symptoms) several weeks following conclusion of radiotherapy. Imaging studies may also suggest progression, but a subset of these patients will experience spontaneous clinical and radiographic improvement over the next few months, demonstrating that radiation reactions may simulate tumor progression [64]. Although nuclear imaging studies (eg, SPECT and PET scans) are sometimes used to differentiate tumor progression from radiation reaction (radiation reactions are usually hypometabolic and tumor progression hypermetabolic), they are not completely reliable. The clinical setting, time, and sometimes biopsy help distinguish these possibilities. Finally, focal cerebral symptoms may occur a few months after the brain has been unavoidably included in radiation ports for extracranial tumors (eg, carcinoma of the head and neck) [1].

Delayed cerebral radiation damage may be focal or diffuse. Focal delayed radiation damage is called radionecrosis and may present with symptoms of a mass lesion associated with a contrast-enhancing mass with surrounding edema that is radiographically indistinguishable from tumor on CT or MRI [65]. It may occur as quickly as a few months or as late as two decades following radiotherapy, although most commonly ensues after 9 to 12 months; it tends to occur in white matter. The pathology reveals a combination of vascular damage with hyalinized vessels and fibrinoid necrosis as well as demyelination.

The risk of radionecrosis is related to the total dose of radiation, fraction size, and treatment volume, with larger total dose, fractions, and treatment volumes increasing the risk [66]. As a rough guideline, 5000 cGy in 25 fractions to a focal port carries minimal risk of producing radionecrosis, 6000 cGy in 30 fractions produces a 5% to 15% risk, and 7000 cGy in 35 fractions produces a 50% risk. Techniques for giving large radiation boosts to small intracranial targets (eg, interstitial brachytherapy and stereotactic radiosurgery) frequently produce radionecrosis; 50% of patients undergoing brachytherapy for malignant gliomas develop symptomatic radionecrosis requiring reoperation. No noninvasive test reliably distinguishes radionecrosis from intracranial tumor, although positron emmission tomography (PET), single-

photon-emmission computed tomography (SPECT), and MRI spectroscopy have their adherents. Radiation necrosis may respond favorably to corticosteroids, although in some cases it requires debulking or proves fatal. Anecdotal reports have suggested that anticoagulation [67] or hyperbaric oxygen therapy [68] are beneficial, but these have not been confirmed.

Diffuse cerebral radiation damage often manifests as the presence of cerebral atrophy, ventriculomegaly, and low-attenuation periventricular white-matter changes on CT scan or T2-hyperintense changes on MRI. Occasionally, small focal areas of contrast enhancement may be seen [69]. Such changes will be seen in more than 50% of patients receiving 3000 cGy in 10 fractions or 5000 cGy in 25 fractions within a few years of undergoing whole-brain radiotherapy. Many of these patients will display short-term memory problems, and some develop more severe dementia or additional problems with gait and urinary incontinence reminiscent of normal-pressure hydrocephalus [70]. These changes are most problematic in young children (who on average "lose" 20–25 IQ points following whole brain radiotherapy) and patients aged > 50 or 60 years and are a major reason why patients with primary brain tumors are generally treated with focal rather than whole brain radiation ports. Patients requiring whole-brain radiotherapy with a relatively good prognosis are often treated with 4000 cGy in 20 to 22 fractions rather than 3000 cGy in 10 fractions to decrease the risk of this complication. Administration of methotrexate either intravenously or intrathecally increases the risk of diffuse radiation damage.

Radiation's effect on extracerebral tissue within the cranium and neck also occasionally results in neurologic toxicity. Of the cranial nerves, the optic nerve is most radiosensitive, and radiation doses encompassing the optic nerve that are capable of producing cerebral radionecrosis may produce decreased visual acuity with a similar time course. Radiation accelerates the development of atherosclerosis, and it is not rare to see carotid artery stenosis producing strokes and transient ischemic attacks in relatively young patients who have received radiation to their great vessels. Patients with this complication are candidates for endarterectomy or antiplatelet therapy. Irradiation of the hypothalamus and pituitary sometimes results in delayed neuroendocrine dysfunction. Growth hormone secretion is particularly vulnerable, and children receiving cranial radiation should be followed for this possibility. In adults, sexual dysfunction is relatively common as is hypothalamic hypothyroidism; hypercortisolism, however, is rare [37].

Finally, the carcinogenic effects of radiation may result in secondary intracranial neoplasms [2]. Patients receiving low-dose scalp irradiation for dermatologic conditions have a several-fold increased incidence of meningiomas (which are more likely to be multiple or biologically malignant than in the general population) as well as an increased incidence of gliomas. Survivors of acute lymphoblastic leukemia who underwent prophylactic cranial irradiation have a 22.6-fold increased incidence of brain tumors, primarily astrocytomas. Higher doses of cranial radiation also predispose to the development of intracranial or calvarial sarcomas.

SPINAL CORD AND PERIPHERAL NERVE COMPLICATIONS

As in the brain, multiple types of radiation injury to the spinal cord may be seen. By far, the type of most concern is chronic progressive radiation myelopathy. Any patient whose spinal cord has been included in radiation ports (a common occurrence with lung or head and neck cancer as well as spinal tumors) is at potential risk for this complication. The pathologic changes are similar to cerebral radionecrosis, as are the risk factors of increasing total dose, fraction size, and length of spinal cord irradiated. Symptoms typically begin 9 to 15 months following radiotherapy and include ascending sensory symptoms, pain (usually less prominent than in epidural metastasis), and spasticity. Examination reveals a progressive myelopathy that may have a hemicord localization. The myelopathy may progress over months to paraplegia or quadriplegia or may stabilize at any point, although objective improvement is exceptional. The differential diagnosis includes epidural spinal cord compression (which rarely produces a hemicord syndrome), intramedullary spinal cord metastasis, and other causes of myelopathy. MRI is useful in excluding these other possibilities; the picture in chronic progressive radiation myelopathy is variable and may include parenchymal T2 hyperintensity, cord atrophy or swelling, and focal contrast enhancement. Corticosteroids may be of symptomatic benefit, but no treatment has been demonstrated to alter the course of this condition [72].

Transient radiation myelopathy is a relatively common phenomenon among patients undergoing radiation to the neck for head and neck cancer, lung cancer, or Hodgkin's disease. Affected patients report Lhermitte's phenomenon several weeks to months after conclusion of radiotherapy. The physical examination and MRI are normal, and symptoms generally resolve within a few months. The pathophysiology is presumed to be dorsal column demyelination.

Two other radiation complications in the spinal cord are fortunately quite rare. An acute transverse myelopathy developing over hours to days presumably has a vascular pathogenesis. A lower motor neuron syndrome rarely develops in patients having received lumbosacral spine or pelvic radiation several months earlier. This is characterized by subacute progressive leg weakness, atrophy, and fasciculations, with normal sensation and bowel/bladder function. Neuroimaging and CSF studies are unremarkable, and the clinical course is variable [1].

Peripheral nerves are relatively radioresistant but are occasionally damaged, most commonly in the brachial or lumbosacral plexus. This typically occurs several months to a few years following radiation. The clinical presentation includes peripheral nerve weakness and numbness progressing slowly and is usually not associated with severe pain (differentiating it from neoplastic plexopathy, which is typically quite painful) [73]. Electrophysiologic studies may reveal abnormal repetitive "myokymic" discharges that are relatively specific for radiation damage. Neuroimaging is normal in radiation plexopathy but is mandatory to exclude tumor recurrence or the development of a secondary radiation-induced sarcoma.

REFERENCES

1. Posner JB: *Neurologic Complications of Cancer*. Philadelphia: FA Davis Co.; 1995.

2. Rottenberg DA: *Neurological Complications of Cancer Treatment*. Stoneham, MA: Butterworth-Heineman; 1991.

3. Miller LJ, Eaton VE. Ifosfamide-induced neurotoxicity: a case report and review of the literature [review]. *Ann Pharmacother* 1992, 26:183–187.

4. Wengs WJ, Talwar D, Bernard J: Ifosfamide-induced nonconvulsive status epilepticus. *Arch Neurol* 1993, 50:1104–1105.

5. Simonian NA, Gilliam FG, Chiappa KH: Ifosfamide causes a diazepam-sensitive encephalopathy . *Neurology* 1993, 43:2700–2702.

6. Patel SR, Forman AD, Benjamin RS: High-dose ifosfamide-induced exacerbation of peripheral neuropathy. *J Natl Cancer Inst* 1994, 86:305–306.

7. Sullivan KM, Storb R, Shulman HM, *et al.*: Immediate and delayed neurotoxicity after mechlorethamine preparation for bone marrow transplantation. *Ann Int Med* 1982, 97:182–189.

8. Gutin PH, Levi JA, Wiernik PH, Walker MD: Treatment of malignant meningeal disease with intrathecal thiotepa: a phase II study. *Cancer Treatment Rep* 1977, 61:885–887.

9. Vassal G, Deroussent A, Hartmann O, *et al.*: Dose-dependent neurotoxicity of high-dose busulfan in children: a clinical and pharmacological study. *Cancer Res* 1990, 50:6203–6207.

10. Burger PC, Kamenar E, Schold SC, *et al.*: Encephalomyelopathy following high-dose BCNU therapy. *Cancer* 1981, 48:1318–1327.

11. Roelofs RI, Hrushesky W, Rogin J, Rosenberg L: Peripheral sensory neuropathy and cisplatin chemotherapy. *Neurology* 1984, 34:934–938.

12. Siegal T, Haim N: Cisplatin-induced peripheral neuropathy: frequent off-therapy deterioration, demyelinating syndromes, and muscle cramps. *Cancer* 1990, 66:1117–1123.

13. van der Hoop RG, Vecht CJ, van der Burg ME, *et al.*: Prevention of cisplatin neurotoxicity with an ACTH(4-9) analogue in patients with ovarian cancer . *New Engl J Med* 1990, 322:89–94.

14. Mollman JE, Glover DJ, Hogan WM, Furman RE: Cisplatin neuropathy: risk factors, prognosis, and protection by WR-2721. *Cancer* 1988, 61:2192–2195.

15. Weiss HD, Walker MD, Wiernik PH. Neurotoxicity of commonly used antineoplastic agents (second of two parts) [review]. *New Engl J Med* 1974, 291:127–133.

16. Dorr RT, Von Hoff DD: *Cancer Chemotherapy Handbook*, ed 2. Norwalk, CT: Appleton & Lange; 1994.

17. Foster BJ, Harding BJ, Leyland-Jones B, Hoth D: Hexamethylmelamine: a critical review of an active drug [review]. *Cancer Treatment Rev* 1986, 13:197–217.

18. Imrie KR, Couture F, Turner CC, *et al.*: Peripheral neuropathy following high-dose etoposide and autologous bone marrow transplantation. *Bone Marrow Transplantation* 1994, 13:77–79.

19. Thant M, Hawley RJ, Smith MT, *et al.*: Possible enhancement of vincristine neuropathy by VP-16. *Cancer* 1982, 49:859–864.

20. Leff RS, Thompson JM, Daly MB, *et al.*: Acute neurologic dysfunction after high-dose etoposide therapy for malignant glioma. *Cancer* 1988, 62:32–35.

21. Griffiths JD, Stark RJ, Ding JC, Cooper IA: Vincristine neurotoxicity enhanced in combination chemotherapy including both teniposide and vincristine. *Cancer Treatment Rep* 1986, 70:519–521.

22. Geiser CF, Bishop Y, Jaffe N, *et al.*: Adverse effects of intrathecal methotrexate in children with acute leukemia in remission. *Blood* 1975, 45:189–195.

23. Gagliano RG, Costanzi JJ: Paraplegia following intrathecal methotrexate: report of a case and review of the literature. *Cancer* 1976, 37:1663–1668.

24. Spiegel RJ, Cooper PR, Blum RH, *et al.*: Treatment of massive intrathecal methotrexate overdose by ventriculolumbar perfusion. *New Engl J Med* 1984, 311:386–388.

25. Bleyer WA: Neurologic sequelae of methotrexate and ionizing radiation: a new classification. *Cancer Treatment Rep* 1981, 65(suppl 1):89–98.

26. Rubinstein LJ, Herman MM, Long TF, Wilbur JR: Disseminated necrotizing leukoencephalopathy: a complication of treated central nervous system leukemia and lymphoma. *Cancer* 1975, 35:291–305.

27. Allen JC, Rosen G, Mehta BM, Horten B: Leukoencephalopathy following high-dose iv methotrexate chemotherapy with leucovorin rescue. *Cancer Treatment Rep* 1980, 64:1261–1273.

28. Shapiro WR, Allen JC, Horten BC: Chronic methotrexate toxicity to the central nervous system. *Clin Bull* 1980, 10:49–52.

29. Matsumoto K, Takahashi S, Sato A, *et al.*: Leukoencephalopathy in childhood hematopoietic neoplasm caused by moderate-dose methotrexate and prophylactic cranial radiotherapy: an MR analysis. *Int J Radiat Oncol Biol Phys* 1995, 32:913–918.

30. Peylan-Ramu N, Poplack DG, Pizzo PA, *et al.*: Abnormal CT scans of the brain in asymptomatic children with acute lymphocytic leukemia after prophylactic treatment of the central nervous system with radiation and intrathecal chemotherapy. *New Engl J Med* 1978, 298:815–818.

31. Warrell RPJ, Berman E: Phase I and II study of fludarabine phosphate in leukemia: therapeutic efficacy with delayed central nervous system toxicity. *J Clin Oncol* 1986, 4:74–79.

32. Cheson BD, Vena DA, Foss FM, Sorensen JM: Neurotoxicity of purine analogs: a review. *J Clin Oncol* 1994, 12:2216–2228.

33. Cohen RB, Abdallah JM, Gray JR, Foss F: Reversible neurologic toxicity in patients treated with standard-dose fludarabine phosphate for mycosis fungoides and chronic lymphocytic leukemia. *Ann Int Med* 1993, 118:114–116.

34. Beutler E: Cladribine (2-chlorodeoxyadenosine) . *Lancet* 1992, 340:952–956.

35. Vahdat L, Wong ET, Wile MJ, *et al.*: Therapeutic and neurotoxic effects of 2-chlorodeoxyadenosine in adults with acute myeloid leukemia. *Blood* 1994, 84:3429–3434.

36. Larson RA, Mick R, Spielberger RT, *et al.*: O'Brien SM, Ratain MJ. Dose-escalation trial of cladribine using five daily intravenous infusions in patients with advanced hematologic malignancies. *J Clin Oncol* 1996, 14:188–195.

37. Baker WJ, Royer GLJ, Weiss RB: Cytarabine and neurologic toxicity [review]. *J Clin Oncol* 1991, 9:679–693.

38. Graf WD, Chance PF, Lensch MW, *et al.*: Severe vincristine neuropathy in Charcot-Marie-Tooth disease type 1A. *Cancer* 1996, 77:1356–1362.

39. Casey EB, Jellife AM, Le QP, Millett YL: Vincristine neuropathy: clinical and electrophysiological observations. *Brain* 1973, 96:69–86.

40. Forsyth PA, Balmaceda C, Peterson K, *et al.*: Prospective study of paclitaxel-induced peripheral neuropathy with quantitative sensory testing. *J Neurooncol* 1997, 35:47–53.

41. Cavaletti G, Bogliun G, Marzorati L, *et al.*: Peripheral neurotoxicity of taxol in patients previously treated with cisplatin . *Cancer* 1995, 75:1141–1150.

42. Hilkens PH, Verweij J, Stoter G, *et al.*: Peripheral neurotoxicity induced by docetaxel . *Neurology* 1996, 46:104–108.

43. New PZ, Jackson CE, Rinaldi D, *et al.*: Peripheral neuropathy secondary to docetaxel (Taxotere) . *Neurology* 1996, 46:108–111.

44. Perry JR, Warner E: Transient encephalopathy after paclitaxel (Taxol) infusion. *Neurology* 1996, 46:1596–1599.

45. Trump DL, Smith DC, Ellis PG, *et al.*: High-dose oral tamoxifen, a potential multidrug-resistance-reversal agent: phase I trial in combination with vinblastine. *J Natl Cancer Inst* 1992, 84:1811–1816.

46. Lipton A, Santen RJ. Proceedings: medical adrenalectomy using aminoglutethimide and dexamethasone in advanced breast cancer. *Cancer* 1974, 33:503–512.

47. Huben RP. Hormone therapy of prostatic bone metastases. *Adv Exp Med Biol* 1992, 324:305–316.

48. du RH, Krempf M, Mussini JM, *et al.*: Neurotoxicity of mitotane therapy of adrenocortical carcinoma (5 cases) and Cushing's syndrome (7 cases) [French]. *Presse Medicale* 1987, 16:951–954.

49. La Rocca RV, Meer J, Gilliatt RW, *et al.*: Suramin-induced polyneuropathy. *Neurology* 1990, 40:954–960.

50. Chaudhry V, Eisenberger MA, Sinibaldi VJ, *et al.*: A prospective study of suramin-induced peripheral neuropathy. *Brain* 1996, 119:2039–2052.

51. Bowden CJ, Figg WD, Dawson NA, *et al.*: A phase I/II study of continuous infusion suramin in patients with hormone-refractory prostate cancer: toxicity and response. *Cancer Chemother Pharmacol* 1996, 39:1–8.

52. Meyers CA, Scheibel RS, Forman AD: Persistent neurotoxicity of systemically administered interferon-α. *Neurology* 1991, 41:672–676.

53. Forman AD: Neurologic complications of cytokine therapy [review]. *Oncology* 1994, 8:105–110.

54. Karp BI, Yang JC, Khorsand M, *et al.*: Multiple cerebral lesions complicating therapy with interleukin-2. *Neurology* 1996, 47:417–424.

55. Puduvalli VK, Sella A, Austin SG, Forman AD: Carpal tunnel syndrome associated with interleukin-2 therapy. *Cancer* 1996, 77:1189–1192.

56. Hook CC, Kimmel DW, Kvols LK, *et al.*: Multifocal inflammatory leukoencephalopathy with 5-fluorouracil and levamisole. *Ann Neurol* 1992, 31:262–267.

57. Swoboda K, Wen PY: Neurologic complications of bone marrow transplantation. In *Office Practice of Neurology*. Edited by Samuels MA, Feske S. New York: Churchill Livingstone; 1996:944–949.

58. Small SL, Fukui MB, Bramblett GT, Eidelman BH: Immunosuppression-induced leukoencephalopathy from tacrolimus (FK506). *Ann Neurol* 1996, 40:575–580.

59. Wijdicks EF, Wiesner RH, Krom RA: Neurotoxicity in liver transplant recipients with cyclosporine immunosuppression. *Neurology* 1995, 45:1962–1964.

60. Stroncek DF, Clay ME, Petzoldt ML, *et al.*: Treatment of normal individuals with granulocyte-colony-stimulating factor: donor experiences and the effects on peripheral blood CD34+ cell counts and on the collection of peripheral blood stem cells . *Transfusion* 1996, 36:601–610.

61. Kastrup O, Diener HC: Granulocyte-stimulating factor filgrastim and molgramostim induced recurring encephalopathy and focal status epilepticus [letter]. *J Neurol* 1997, 244:274–275.

62. Delanty N, Vaughan C, Frucht S, Stubgen P: Eythropoietin-associated hypertensive posterior leukoencephalpathy. *Neurology* 1997, 49:686–689.

63. Mandell LR, Walker RW, Steinherz P, Fuks Z: Reduced incidence of the somnolence syndrome in leukemic children with steroid coverage during prophylactic cranial radiation therapy: results of a pilot study [review]. *Cancer* 1989, 63:1975–1978.

64. Watne K, Hager B, Heier M, Hirschberg H: Reversible oedema and necrosis after irradiation of the brain: diagnostic procedures and clinical manifestations. *Acta Oncologica* 1990, 29:891–895.

65. Morris JG, Grattan-Smith P, Panegyres PK, *et al.*: Delayed cerebral radiation necrosis. *Q J Med* 1994, 87:119–129.

66. Sheline GE, Wara WM, Smith V: Therapeutic irradiation and brain injury [review]. *Int J Radiat Oncol Biol Phys* 1980, 6:1215–1228.

67. Glantz MJ, Burger PC, Friedman AH, *et al.*: Treatment of radiation-induced nervous system injury with heparin and warfarin . *Neurology* 1994, 44:2020–2027.

68. Chuba PJ, Aronin P, Bhambhani K, *et al.*: Hyperbaric oxygen therapy for radiation-induced brain injury in children. *Cancer* 1997, 80:2005–2012.

69. Peterson K, Clark HB, Hall WA, Truwit CL: Multifocal enhancing magnetic resonance imaging lesions following cranial irradiation. *Ann Neurol* 1995, 38:237–244.

70. DeAngelis LM, Delattre JY, Posner JB: Radiation-induced dementia in patients cured of brain metastases. *Neurology* 1989, 39:789–796.

71. Arlt W, Hove U, Muller B, Reincke M, *et al.*: Frequent and frequently overlooked: treatment-induced endocrine dysfunction in adult long-term survivors of primary brain tumors. *Neurology* 1997, 49:498–506.

72. Schultheiss TE, Stephens LC: Invited review: permanent radiation myelopathy [review]. *Brit J Radiol* 1992, 65:737–753.

73. Jaeckle KA. Nerve plexus metastases [review]. *Neurol Clin* 1991, 9:857–866.

CHAPTER 30: EVALUATION OF QUALITY OF LIFE IN CANCER CLINICAL TRIALS

Bernard F. Cole, Richard D. Gelber, Shari Gelber

Quality of life is an important consideration when making treatment decisions [1–3]. The choice of one treatment option over another for an individual patient may hinge on how the treatments affect quality of life. Therefore, it is important that the practicing oncologist have a thorough understanding of the potential impacts that treatments can have on quality of life in general as well as an understanding of the individual patient's needs and preferences. To help address these issues, the evaluation of quality of life is taking on an increasingly larger role in cancer clinical research. In particular, patient-oriented quality-of-life assessments are frequently being included in clinical trials as study endpoints for treatment comparisons. The purpose of this chapter is to provide an overview of the most common methods used in cancer clinical trials for the evaluation of quality of life.

HISTORICAL BACKGROUND

Early measures of quality of life in cancer focused on quantifying a patient's physical functioning. The Karnofsky Performance Status (KPS) measure, introduced in 1948 [4,5], is generally considered to be the first measure of physical functioning and has been widely used in cancer clinical research. KPS is measured on an 11-point scale from 0% to 100% (in 10% increments) in which 0% denotes death, 100% denotes normal function, and other values denote the approximate percentage of normal physical performance. The KPS assessment is made by the clinician. In 1960, the Eastern Cooperative Oncology Group (ECOG) converted the KPS into a six-point scale, often called the Zubrod scale [6].

Subsequent efforts in quality-of-life evaluation incorporated patients' perspectives of their illnesses and therapeutic regimens. For example, in 1971, Izsak and Medalie [7] developed a multidimensional scale that measured physical, social, and psychological variables in cancer patients. The scale was tailored to specific cancers and designed to assist clinicians in determining rehabilitation needs and evaluating patient progress. In 1975, a trial for patients with acute myelogenous leukemia used a six-level assessment of quality of life, ranging from "hospital stay throughout illness" to "no symptoms, normal life" [8]. The assessments were based on patient reports of their symptoms and functioning.

The modern era of quality of life assessment in cancer clinical trials research is generally cited to have begun in 1976 when Priestman and Baum [9] studied breast cancer treatment. They used 10 questions to assess patients' general feeling of well being, mood, level of activity, pain, nausea, appetite, ability to perform housework, social activities, general level of anxiety, and overall treatment assessment. Their results indicated that this instrument could be used to assess the subjective benefit of treatment in individual women, to detect changes over time, and to compare different treatments within a clinical trial.

MEASURING QUALITY OF LIFE

Many instruments are available for descriptively measuring quality of life in clinical trials. In general, these can be divided into two main categories: general quality-of-life instruments and disease-specific quality-of-life instruments. Examples of general instruments include the SF-36 [10], the Sickness Impact Profile [11], the SCL-90-R [12], and the World Health Organization Quality-of-Life Assessment Instrument [13], which is currently being developed. Each of these instruments includes general questions relating to a patient's health and functioning, and they can be applied in a wide range of disease settings. Table 30-1 presents a list of instruments that are cancer-specific. These instruments include specific items that are relevant for cancer patients.

Regardless of the instrument used, the goal is to provide measures of quality of life in various domains and, usually, an overall measure of global quality of life. The three most frequently measured domains are physical, social, and mental health. Other domains include disease symptoms, pain, general health perceptions, vitality, and role functioning. The last column of Table 30-1 shows the domains assessed by the cancer-specific quality-of-life instruments. Each quality-of-life instrument usually includes several individual questions or items that pertain to a particular domain, and the domain score (also called scale score) is obtained by summarizing the responses from the associated items (ie, average of the item responses). Each instrument has its own rules regarding the computation of the domain scores, and these rules are established after careful testing. The second column of Table 30-1 shows the total number of items used in each cancer-specific instrument. Each item is generally measured on a Likert scale or a linear

Table 30-1. Cancer-Specific Quality-of-Life Measurement Instruments

Instrument	Items, *n*	Domains Assessed
Breast Cancer Chemotherapy Questionnaire (BCQ) [14]	30	Attractiveness, fatigue, physical symptoms, inconvenience, emotional, hope social support
Cancer Rehabilitation Evaluation System (CARES) [15]	93–132	Physical, psychosocial, medical interaction, marital, sexual, symptom- and treatment-specific items
European Organization for Research and Treatment of Cancer scale (EORTC: QLQ-C30) [16]	42	Five functional scales (physical, role, cognitive, emotional, social), three symptom scales (fatigue, pain, nausea), disease-specific items, global quality of life
Functional Assessment of Cancer Therapy (FACT) [17]	36–40	Physical, social/family, relationship with doctor, emotional, functional, well-being, disease-specific items
Functional Living Index — Cancer (FLIC) [18]	22	Psychological, social, disease symptoms, global well-being, treatment and disease issues, physical functioning
International Breast Cancer Study Group Quality of Life Questionnaire (IBCSG-QL) [19]	10	Physical well-being, mood, fatigue, appetite, coping, social support, symptoms, overall health
Linear Analogue Self Assessment (LASA) (Priestman and Baum [9])	25	Physical, psychological, social
Quality of Life Index (QLI) [20]	5	Physical activity, daily living, health perceptions, psychological, social support, outlook on life

analogue self-assessment (LASA) scale. The Likert scale is a categorical scale consisting of a limited choice of clearly defined responses. The most frequently employed scales use either four or five categories. In contrast, the LASA scale is an unmarked line, usually 10 cm long, with text at either end describing the extremes of the scale. Patients are asked to place a mark on the line in a position that best reflects his or her response.

MEASURING PATIENTS' PREFERENCES AND UTILITIES

In addition to measuring descriptive quality of life, there are methods for measuring a patient's preference, or utility, for particular health states. These methods attempt to measure how a patient might value one health state compared with another based on the quality-of-life attributes of the health states. For example, two patients might report similar symptoms with similar frequency and duration, but they may differ on how important these symptoms are in their daily lives. Descriptive quality-of-life instruments will correctly provide similar scores for the two patients, whereas a measurement of preference or utility will differentiate them.

Utility is measured on an interval scale from zero to one, where zero denotes a health state that is as bad as death, and one denotes a health state as good as best possible health. Values between zero and one denote degrees between these extremes. A simple interpretation of a utility for a specific health state (eg, state A) is that the utility represents the amount of time in a state of perfect health for which a patient values equally as one unit of time in state A. For example, suppose that state A has a utility of 0.7; the patient then values one month in state A as being equivalent to 0.7 months of perfect health. This interpretation leads to the idea of quality-of-life–adjusted time, which can be obtained by multiplying a health state duration by its utility coefficient. For example, if a patient experiences six months of toxicity and has a utility weight of 0.8 for time with toxicity, then the quality-adjusted time spent with toxicity is 4.2 months. This adjustment allows treatments that have different impacts on quality of life to be compared in a meaningful way.

Classically, utility assessment is carried out using interview techniques. The "standard gamble" technique gives patients a choice between a chronic health state with certainty or an uncertain health state that is either perfect health (with probability p), or death (with probability 1-p). The probability p is varied until the patient is indifferent between the certain and the uncertain choice, and the final p is taken as the utility value. The "time trade-off" technique gives patients a choice between living for a certain amount of time in a state of less than perfect health or a shorter amount of time in a state of perfect health. The duration of the perfect health state is varied until the patient expresses indifference in the choice. The utility is then taken as the ratio of the final health state durations. For a detailed overview of utility assessment, see Bennett and Torrance [21].

These interview techniques are cumbersome to use in practice. Fortunately, there are procedures for obtaining utility data from quality-of-life instruments. Generally, these procedures were developed by administering both the instrument and the interview to a study sample and building a statistical model for predicting the utility value from the instrument responses. Instruments that can be used for this purpose include the EuroQol [22], Health Utilities Index (HUI) [23], and Spitzer's Quality of Life Index (QLI) [20,24].

STUDY DESIGN IN CLINICAL TRIALS

As a "gold standard" study design, the authors propose a cancer clinical trial including the following outcomes: 1) usual clinical endpoints such as progression-free survival and overall survival, (2) usual assessment of toxicity/adverse event frequency and grade, 3) measurements of the timing and duration of all toxicities and adverse events, 4) longitudinal assessment of quality of life using a general instrument and a specific instrument, 5) a procedure for estimating patient utility or preference, and 6) a procedure for estimating health care cost. By including all of these components in a clinical trial, it becomes possible to address the clinical benefits of a new therapy as well as its impact on quality of life and whether it is cost effective.

Of course, due to constrained resources, few studies will include all of these components. In addition, clinical trials that began in the 1980s or early 1990s will generally not include components for measuring quality of life or utility because methods for assessment were not as well established as they are today. To fill this potential gap, researchers use other methods to address pressing clinical issues. The best approach is to launch a smaller study that collects quality-of-life and utility data from a group of patients. Such a study can be longitudinal or cross-sectional. The advantage of the cross-sectional design is that the study can be completed more quickly. The disadvantage is that longitudinal effects on quality of life cannot be estimated. Inferior ancillary study designs include those that use proxy data for subjective quality-of-life domains.

Another approach that is described in more detail later is to retrospectively evaluate the duration of major health states that are thought to impact quality of life (eg, toxicity, disease progression). By combining clinical-outcome data with patient-level, cycle-by-cycle toxicity data (both of which are typically collected in cancer clinical trials), it is often possible to obtain estimates of durations of the health states. Utility weights can then be assigned to the health states, and this health-state utility model can be used to compare treatments in terms of quality-adjusted time. The utility weights can be estimated from a secondary cross-sectional study or they may be left unspecified. In the latter case, the results of the analysis should be displayed for a wide variety of choices for the utility weight values, not for just one or two arbitrary selections.

For new clinical trials currently being designed, it is critical that quality-of-life components be prospectively incorporated. At a minimum, a general quality-of-life instrument should be administered longitudinally; however, a disease-specific instrument will likely have better sensitivity to changes in quality of life. The timing of assessments should be designed to measure quality of life for the various clinical health states that a patient might experience both during and after therapy (eg, treatment-related toxicity, disease progression). For randomized studies, a baseline assessment should take place prior to treatment randomization. In addition, patients should be able to self-report troublesome adverse events and symptoms and their durations using a diary. These data could be used to validate the physician-reported adverse-event data typically collected. The diary idea is particularly appealing from a quality-of-life perspective because it is likely that a patient will self-report a particular adverse event that is causing him or her some distress and, therefore, represents a decrement in quality of life. As a result, diary data are useful for estimating the duration of time spent with adverse events—an outcome necessary for a health-state utility model.

ANALYSIS OF QUALITY OF LIFE DATA

Once data have been collected in a clinical trial or perhaps in a secondary cross-sectional study, the next step is to analyze the data to make inferences about the quality-of-life treatment effect. A number of standard statistical procedures are available. The most common approach is a *t* test or an analysis of variance (with repeated measures if the data are longitudinal). These procedures compare the mean quality-of-life scores across the treatment groups. In the longitudinal setting, the analysis can evaluate trends over time and test for a treatment by time interaction. The interaction test evaluates whether quality-of-life score changes differ over time according to treatment group. Analysis of variance can adjust the treatment comparison for other factors that may differ across the treatment groups. This is particularly important if the factors influence (confound) the quality-of-life assessments. For example, prognosis, demographic outcomes, and health care institution are potential confounders. A helpful visual display of this information can be obtained by plotting the (adjusted) mean quality-of-life scores over time according to treatment group.

The main difficulty in analyzing quality-of-life scores is missing data. Assessments may be missing more often when a patient's quality of life is deteriorating. For example, a patient was not feeling well and, therefore, was unable to concentrate on the form. Missing data that are related to the actual (unobserved) quality-of-life score are called nonignorable missing data. This term reflects the notion that the missing data cannot be ignored in the analysis. Therefore, an appropriate analysis of quality-of-life data will give a thorough description of the pattern of missing data. In particular, the rates of missing data across treatment groups are important statistics. If the rates of missing data are similar across treatment groups, then it is likely that the estimation bias within each treatment group will be balanced by the estimation bias in the other treatment groups. In other words, the biases will likely cancel, and the difference in quality-of-life scores between two treatments will be an accurate estimate of the treatment effect. If the pattern of missing assessment differs across the treatment groups, then the situation becomes more complex. If the higher rate of missing data is observed in the treatment group that has the lower quality-of-life scores, then the difference in quality of life scores is likely to be an underestimate of the true treatment effect. If this estimate is large in magnitude and statistically significantly different from zero, then the analysis gives a meaningful result. New statistical procedures are currently being developed to better analyze quality-of-life data that is nonignorably missing [25], but these approaches are not yet widely applied. These methods require additional assumptions concerning the mechanism of missing data.

COMBINING QUALITY AND QUANTITY OF LIFE

An endpoint that is increasingly being used in cancer clinical research is quality-of-life–adjusted survival time. Generally, this endpoint represents a patient's survival time weighted by the quality of life experienced, in which the weightings are based on utility values. Because utility is measured on a scale from zero to one, the quality-adjusted survival time is measured in the same time units as overall survival. The main advantage of a quality-adjusted endpoint is that it allows treatments that differ in their quality-of-life effects and their effects on survival to be compared in a metric that accounts for both of these differences. This is a common issue in cancer clinical research in which a new therapy may improve overall or progression-free survival but is also associated with more toxicity.

One approach to evaluating quality-adjusted survival time is the Quality-adjusted Time Without Symptoms or Toxicity method (Q-

TWiST) [26]. Q-TWiST evaluates treatments by computing the time spent in a series of clinical health states that may differ in terms of quality of life. Each health state is then weighted by a utility value to adjust the health-state duration according to its value in terms of quality of life.

The three steps involved in a Q-TWiST analysis are briefly described below. To make the procedure more concrete, we also provide a specific example that compares high-dose interferon α-2b administered for 1 year versus clinical observation for the adjuvant therapy of malignant melanoma. These data are obtained from 280 patients who participated in the ECOG clinical trial EST1684 [27,28]. The original report of this study indicated that high-dose interferon improved overall survival and relapse-free survival, but the regimen was also associated with significant toxicity that may cause a decrement in quality of life [27]. A Q-TWiST analysis was used to evaluate the clinical benefits after adjusting for the toxicity associated with high-dose interferon [28].

Step 1: Define Clinical Health States
The first step in the analysis is to define quality-of-life–oriented health states that are relevant for the disease setting and the treatments being studied. Typically, the health states reflect changes in clinical status that may be associated with changes in quality of

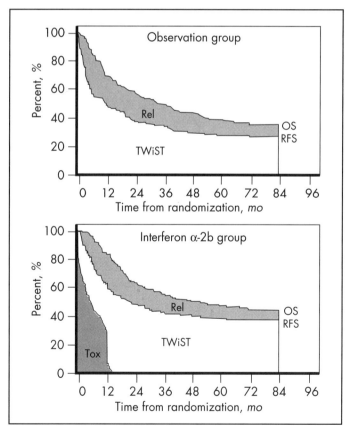

FIGURE 30-1.

Partitioned survival plots for the Eastern Cooperative Oncology Group trial. Rel—time following disease relapse; Tox—time with severe or life-threatening side effects of treatment toxicity; TWiST—time without severe or life-threatening treatment toxicity and without disease relapse.

Table 30-2. Mean Time for the Components of Q-TWiST Restricted to 84 Months of Median Follow-up in the ECOG Trial EST1684

Treatment Group	Treatment Group		Difference, *m*	95% CI, *m*	*P* (2-sided)
	Observation, *m*	Interferon α-2b, *m*			
Tox	0.0	5.8	5.8	5.0–6.7	< 0.001
TWiST	30.0	33.1	3.1	-4.8–11.0	0.400
Rel	12.4	10.4	-2.0	-6.2–2.3	0.400
OS	42.4	49.3	7.0	-0.6–14.5	0.070
RFS	30.0	38.9	8.9	0.8–17.0	0.030

CI—confidence interval; OS—overall survival; Rel—time following disease relapse; RFS—relapse-free survival; Tox—time with severe or life-threatening side effects of treatment toxicity; TWiST—time without severe or life-threatening treatment toxicity and without disease relapse.

life. For example, one health state may be associated with toxicity due to therapy, whereas another health state may be associated with disease progression. Usually, the health-state model includes a state of best possible health (given that the patient was diagnosed with cancer) represented by toxicity related to all time spent without treatment and without disease progression. Different health states may be defined for different treatment regimens when appropriate. For example, if two chemotherapy regimens are being compared and one of the regimens has a different toxicity profile than the other, then separate health states can be used to account for this in the model.

For example, in the ECOG trial comparing high-dose interferon versus observation for malignant melanoma, the following health states were defined: Tox represents all time with severe or life-threatening side effects of high-dose interferon, TWiST represents all time without severe or life-threatening treatment toxicity and without symptoms of disease relapse, and Rel represents all time following disease relapse. These health states reflect the major clinical changes in quality of life that are important for evaluating the impact of high-dose interferon.

Step 2: Partitioning Overall Survival

The second step in the analysis is to estimate the times at which patients make transitions from one health state to the next. This is accomplished by partitioning the overall survival time into the time spent in each of the health states. Kaplan–Meier survival curves are plotted for each health-state transition time and time to death on the same graph. A separate graph is used for each treatment group.

For example, using the health states Tox, TWiST, and Rel, one would plot the overall survival curve, a curve corresponding to the end of treatment toxicity (and the beginning of TWiST), and a curve corresponding to the disease relapse (indicating the end of TWiST and the beginning of Rel). This technique allows one to visualize the

health state durations as a portion of the overall survival time and compare them across the treatment groups. Most importantly, this procedure provides estimates of the mean duration of each health state. These estimates are derived from the areas between the curves. In the example, the mean duration of toxicity is given by the area under the toxicity curve, the mean duration of TWiST is the area between the relapse-free survival (RFS) curve and the toxicity curve, and the mean duration of Rel is the area between the overall survival (OS) curve and the relapse-free survival curve.

Figure 30-1 shows the partitioning of overall survival into the health states according to treatment group in the ECOG study. For each graph, the area beneath the overall survival curve is partitioned into the health states Tox, TWiST, and Rel as indicated. This partitioning was restricted to the median follow-up interval of 84 months. Table 30-2 shows the mean health state durations, the mean survival time, and the mean relapse-free survival time within the first 84 months from randomization in the study. The results indicate that patients in the interferon group experienced more time in TWiST and less time in Rel as compared with the observation group; however, the interferon group also experienced more time with severe or life-threatening toxicity.

Step 3: Comparing the Treatments

The third step is to compare the treatments using a weighted sum of the health-state durations. For example, in the Tox, TWiST, and Rel health-state model, the quality-adjusted survival endpoint (Q-TWiST) is defined by the equation Q-TWiST = (u_{Tox} × Tox) + TWiST + (u_{Rel} × Rel) in which Tox, TWiST, and Rel denote the mean time spent in each of the respective health states and u_{Tox} and u_{Rel} represent the utility weightings assigned to the states Tox and Rel, respectively.

Q-TWiST is calculated separately for each treatment group, and the treatment effects are obtained by subtracting the Q-

Table 30-3. Mean Q-TWiST Within 84 Months of Median Follow-up in the ECOG Trial for Arbitrary Sets of Utility Weight Values

Utility Values		Treatment Group		Difference, *m*	95% CI, *m*	*P* (2-sided)
u_{Tox}	u_{Rel}	Observation, *m*	Interferon α-2b, *m*			
0.5	0.5	36.2	41.2	5.0	-2.4–12.5	0.20
0.9	0.4	34.9	42.5	7.6	0.0?–15.1	0.05

CI—confidence interval; u_{Rel}—utility weighting assigned to the time following disease relapse; u_{Tox}—utility weighting assigned to the time with severe or life-threatening side effects of treatment toxicity.

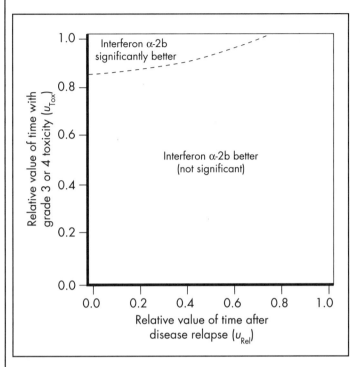

FIGURE 30-2.

Threshold utility analysis for the Eastern Cooperative Oncology Group trial. u_{Rel}—utility weighting assigned to the time following disease relapse; u_{Tox}—utility weighting assigned to the time with severe or life-threatening side effects of treatment toxicity.

TWiST estimate for one treatment group from the Q-TWiST estimate for another treatment group. If data are available for the utility weightings, then these data can be incorporated into the analysis, and the estimated treatment effects can be tested for statistical significance. In the case in which utility data are not available, the treatment comparison can still be evaluated by computing the treatment effect for varying values of the utility weights. In the case in which two utility weights are unknown and two treatments are being compared (A versus B), the treatment comparison can be plotted across all possible values of the utility weights in a two-dimensional graph called a threshold plot. A solid line can be used to illustrate the set of utility weight pairs for which the two treatments have equal amounts of Q-TWiST on average. This "threshold line" will separate the utility space into two regions that correspond to "greater Q-TWiST on average for treatment A" and "greater Q-TWiST on average for treatment B." Dashed lines can be used to plot a confidence region for the threshold line. The confidence region will indicate pairs of utility-weight values for which treatment A gives significantly more Q-TWiST than treatment B and vice versa. This allows an examination of how the treatment effect is influenced by the values of the utility weightings.

Table 30-3 shows the computation of Q-TWiST for two possible selections of the utility weights u_{Tox} and u_{Rel}. Figure 30-2 illustrates the threshold plot for the treatment comparison. Note that in this case, the interferon group experienced more quality-adjusted time than the control group, regardless of the utility values used. Therefore, the threshold line does not appear on the graph. However, the upper 95% confidence band for the threshold line does appear in the graph, so that the utility space is divided into two regions corresponding to "interferon is significantly better ($P < 0.05$)" and "interferon is better but the comparison is not statistically significant ($P \geq 0.05$)."

The Q-TWiST analysis of the ECOG trial indicates that high-dose interferon can be beneficial for patients even after accounting for its side effects. However, the magnitude of the benefit for an individual patient depends on his or her utility weight values for the health states Tox and Rel. This is illustrated in Table 30-3 and the threshold plot in Figure 30-2. For example, the results indicate that for patients with a low utility weight for toxicity, there may be a quality-adjusted (Q-TWiST) benefit for high-dose interferon, but the comparison is not statistically significant. The optimal treatment for an individual patient is also influenced by the disease stage and nodal status (*see* Kirkwood *et al.* [27] for a full description).

DISCUSSION

In this chapter, we provided an overview of the basic components of quality-of-life research in cancer clinical trials, and there are a number of excellent references for further reading. In particular, the large volume edited by Spilker [29] is a thorough reference covering quality-of-life measurement, analysis, cross-cultural and cross-national issues, health policy issues, and pharmacoeconomics. This book is particularly well suited to the quality-of-life researcher who is involved with study design and analysis. Another, more compact reference is the chapter by Gelber and Gelber [30]. This chapter reviews methods used in clinical research and provides more detail regarding statistical analysis methods.

We also provided an example illustrating the use of quality-of-life-adjusted survival time (Q-TWiST) in cancer clinical research. The Q-TWiST analysis of the ECOG trial EST1684 improved the clinical usefulness of the information obtained from the clinical trial. Moreover, the evaluation illustrates the need to consider quality-adjusted survival comparisons in clinical research and develop better ways to evaluate patient preferences for incorporation in the decision-making process.

The use of assessment tools and procedures similar to those described in this chapter is becoming increasingly important in cancer clinical research. At a minimum, future clinical trials should carefully collect data regarding toxicity grade and duration in addition to the usual clinical outcomes. The longitudinal use of a quality-of-life instrument is also strongly recommended, as is the tracking of individual health care costs over the course of a study. With these components in place, we can expect to have a meaningful evaluation of the treatments being compared in terms of clinical outcome, quality of life, and cost.

ACKNOWLEDGMENTS

Partial support for this work was provided by Grant #PBR-53 from the American Cancer Society.

REFERENCES

1. Schumacher M, Olschewski M, Schulgen G: Assessment of quality of life in clinical trials. *Stat Med* 1991, 10:1915–1930.

2. Cox DR, Fitzpatrick R, Fletcher AE, *et al.*: Quality of life assessment: can we keep it simple? *J R Stat Soc A* 1992; 155:353–393.

3. Gelber RD, Goldhirsch A, Hürny C, *et al.*: Quality of life in clinical trials of adjuvant therapies. *J Natl Cancer Inst Monogr* 1992, 11:127–135.

4. Karnofsky DA, Abelmann WH, Craver LF, Burchenal JH: The use of nitrogen mustards in the palliative treatment of carcinoma. *Cancer* 1948, 1:634.

5. Yates JW, Chalmer B, McKegney FP: Evaluation of patients with advanced cancer using the Karnofsky Performance Status. *Cancer* 1980, 45:2220–2224.

6. Zubrod CG, Schneiderman M, Frei E, *et al.*: Appraisal of methods for the study of chemotherapy in man. *J Chron Dis* 1960, 11:7.

7. Izak FC, Medalie JH: Comprehensive follow-up of carcinoma patients. *J Chron Dis* 1971, 24:179–191.

8. Burge PS, Prankerd TA, Richards JD, *et al.*: Quality and quantity of survival in acute myeloid leukemia. *Lancet* 1975, 2:621–624.

9. Priestman TJ, Baum M: Evaluation of quality of life in patients receiving treatment for advanced breast cancer. *Lancet* 1976, 1:899–900.

10. Ware JE Jr: The SF-36 health survey. In *Quality of Life and Pharmacoeconomics in Clinical Trials*, ed 2. Edited by Spilker B. Philadelphia: Lippincott-Raven Publishers; 1996:337–345.

11. Damiano AM: The sickness impact profile. In *Quality of Life and Pharmacoeconomics in Clinical Trials*, ed 2. Edited by Spilker B. Philadelphia: Lippincott-Raven Publishers; 1996:347–354.

12. Derogatis LR, Derogatis MF: SCL-90-R and the BSI. In *Quality of Life and Pharmacoeconomics in Clinical Trials*, ed 2. Edited by Spilker B. Philadelphia: Lippincott-Raven Publishers; 1996:323–335.

13. Szabo S: The World Health Organization quality of life (WHOQOL) assessment instrument. In *Quality of Life and Pharmacoeconomics in Clinical Trials*, ed 2. Edited by Spilker B. Philadelphia: Lippincott-Raven Publishers; 1996:355–362.

14. Levine MN, Guyatt GH, Gent M: Quality of life in stage II breast cancer: an instrument for clinical trials. *J Clin Oncol* 1988, 6:1789–1810.

15. Ganz PA, Schag CAC, Lee JJ, *et al.*: The CARES: a generic measure of health-related quality of life for patients with cancer. *Qual Life Res* 1992, 1:19–29.

16. Aaronson NK, Bullinger M, Ahmedzai S: A modular approach to quality-of-life assessment in cancer clinical trials. *Recent Results Cancer Res* 1988, 111:231–249.

17. Cella DF, Bonomi AE: The functional assessment of cancer therapy (FACT) and functional assessment of HIV infection (FAHI) quality of life measurement system. In *Quality of Life and Pharmacoeconomics in Clinical Trials*, ed 2. Edited by Spilker B. Philadelphia: Lippincott-Raven Publishers; 1996:203–214.

18. Clinch JJ: The functional living index—cancer: ten years later. In *Quality of Life and Pharmacoeconomics in Clinical Trials*, ed 2. Edited by Spilker B. Philadelphia: Lippincott-Raven Publishers; 1996:215–225.

19. Hürny C, Bernhard J, Gelber RD, *et al.*: Quality of life measures for patients receiving adjuvant therapy for breast cancer. *Eur J Cancer* 1992, 28:118–124.

20. Spitzer WO, Dobson AJ, Hall J, *et al.*: Measuring the quality of life of cancer patients. *J Chron Dis* 1981, 34:585–597.

21. Bennett KJ, Torrance GW: Measuring health state preferences and utilities: rating scale, time trade-off and standard gamble techniques. In *Quality of Life and Pharmacoeconomics in Clinical Trials*, ed 2. Edited by Spilker B. Philadelphia: Lippincott-Raven Publishers; 1996:253–265.

22. Kind P: The EuroQoL instrument: an index of health-related quality of life. In *Quality of Life and Pharmacoeconomics in Clinical Trials*, ed 2. Edited by Spilker B. Philadelphia: Lippincott-Raven Publishers; 1996:191–201.

23. Feeny DH, Torrance GW, Furlong WJ: Health utilities index. In *Quality of Life and Pharmacoeconomics in Clinical Trials*, ed 2. Edited by Spilker B. Philadelphia: Lippincott-Raven Publishers; 1996:239–252.

24. Weeks J, O'Leary J, Fairclough D, *et al.* The 'Q-tility index': a new tool for assessing health-related quality of life and utilities in clinical trials and clinical practice. *Proc Am Soc Clin Oncol* 1994, 13:436.

25. Proceedings of the Workshop on Missing Data in Quality of Life Research in Cancer Clinical Trials: practical and methodological issues: July 1-3, 1996, Bad Horn, Switzerland. *Stat Med* 1998, 17:511–796.

26. Gelber RD, Cole BF, Gelber S, Goldhirsch A: The Q-TWiST method. In *Quality of Life and Pharmacoeconomics in Clinical Trials*, ed 2. Edited by Spilker B. Philadelphia: Lippincott-Raven Publishers; 1996:437–444.

27. Kirkwood JM, Hunt Strawderman M, Ernstoff MS, *et al.*: Interferon alpha-2b adjuvant therapy of high-risk resected cutaneous melanoma: the Eastern Cooperative Oncology Group Trial EST1684. *J Clin Oncol* 1996, 14:7–17.

28. Cole BF, Gelber RD, Kirkwood JM, *et al.* Quality-of-life-adjusted survival analysis of interferon alfa-2b adjuvant treatment of high-risk resected cutaneous melanoma: an Eastern Cooperative Oncology Group Study. *J Clin Oncol* 1996, 14:2666–2673.

29. Spilker B (ed): *Quality of Life and Pharmacoeconomics in Clinical Trials*, ed 2. Philadelphia: Lippincott-Raven Publishers; 1996.

30. Gelber R, Gelber S: Quality-of-life assessment in clinical trials. In *Recent Advances in Clincial Trial Design and Analysis*. Edited by Thall PF. Norwell, MA: Kluwer Academic Publishers; 1995.

CHAPTER 31: SYSTEMIC MANIFESTATIONS
David F. McDermott, Susan A. Sajer, Michael B. Atkins

Surgery, radiation therapy, and chemotherapy are the traditional modalities used for the treatment of cancer. These treatments, used either alone or in combination, can cure approximately 50% of all patients with cancer. The other 50% (those that eventually succumb to their disease) represent greater than 500,000 patients annually in the United States. These sobering statistics have prompted the continued search for new treatment approaches.

Over the past decade, advances in the fields of biotechnology and immunology have led to the development of numerous novel cancer therapies. These biologic response modifiers have included vaccines, monoclonal or polyclonal antibodies, adoptively transferred cells, specifically immunostimulatory cytokines, growth factors, selective growth-factor inhibitors, and angiogenesis inhibitors. At the same time, advances in pharmacology have resulted in more efficacious chemotherapeutic agents.

This chapter focuses on several systemic side effects associated with these new therapies, including fatigue, flu-like syndrome, and capillary leak syndrome as well as infectious, hemodynamic, and allergic/immune-mediated complications. The side effects observed with FDA-approved agents are discussed in the context of their approved indications (Table 31-1). Some of the material discussed may be applicable to other biologic and chemotherapeutic agents currently under investigation.

CONSTITUTIONAL EFFECTS: FLU-LIKE SYNDROME

Constitutional effects, often described as an influenza-like syndrome, including fever, chills, malaise, myalgias, arthralgias, headache, and occasionally nausea, vomiting, diarrhea, nasal congestion, dizziness, and light-headedness, were described in reports from early human interferon α trials that used crude preparations of interferon. These effects were initially thought to be related to contaminants in the interferon preparations. When these symptoms persisted with highly purified interferon preparations and later with recombinant interferon, they were believed to be directly related to interferon. Subsequent studies have demonstrated that interferon α is intrinsically pyrogenic, that is, capable of inducing prostaglandin E_2 (PGE_2) synthesis (in the rat hypothalamus)—and a direct role for interferon in producing constitutional symptoms has been postulated (Fig. 31-1) [1]. With the use of other recombinant proteins, such as aldesleukin and sargramostim, the flu-like syndrome was observed again, suggesting that a common mechanism was involved. Aldesleukin and sargramostim stimulate lymphocytes or monocytes to release or generate the secondary cytokines interleukin-1 (IL-1), tumor necrosis factor (TNF), interleukin-6 (IL-6), and interferon γ, which are believed to mediate the fever and many of the constitutional effects associated with aldesleukin or sargramostim administration. The PGE_2 released in response to various pyrogenic primary or secondary cytokines is believed to be the ultimate mediator of many of the flu-like symptoms.

All patients receiving standard high-dose aldesleukin therapy, most patients receiving interferon α-2 therapy, and some patients receiving sargramostim or oprelvekin (IL-11) therapy develop the flu-like syndrome. These side effects are dose related, occur 1 to 6 hours after a dose, are more common with bolus administration, and resolve spontaneously within 24 hours of a single dose administra-

Table 31-1. FDA-Approved Agents, Indications, and Systemic Side Effects

Agent	Indications	Systemic Side Effects
Aldesleukin (IL-2 or Proleukin)	Metastatic renal cell carcinoma and melanoma	Flu-like and capillary-leak syndromes; fatigue; and infectious, hemodynamic and allergic/immune-mediated complications
Bacillus Calmette-Guerin (BCG, TICE, or TheraCys)	Carcinoma in situ of the bladder	Flu-like syndrome, infectious and allergic/immune-mediated complications
Dacarbazine (DTIC)	Metastatic melanoma, Hodgkin's disease	Flu-like syndrome
Docetaxel (Taxotere)	Second-line therapy in locally advanced or metastatic breast cancer	Allergic/immune-mediated complications and capillary-leak syndrome
Epoetin α (erythropoietin, Epogen, or Procrit)	Anemia secondary to chemotherapy in patients with nonmyeloid malignancies	Hemodynamic complications
Filgrastim (G-CSF or Neupogen)	Patients with nonmyeloid malignancies receiving myelosuppressive chemotherapy associated with a significant incidence of severe neutropenia and fever	Allergic/immune-mediated complications
Interferon α-2 (IFN α-2a or Roferon A; interferon α-2b or Intron A)	Hairy cell leukemia; AIDS-related Kaposi's sarcoma; High-risk melanoma	Flu-like syndrome; fatigue; and infectious, hemodynamic and allergic/immune-mediated complications
Levamisole hydrochloride (Ergamisol)	Adjuvant treatment in combination with 5-FU after surgical resection of Dukes' stage C colon cancer	Flu-like syndrome and allergic/immune-mediated complications
Oprelvekin (IL-11 or Neumega)	Prevention of severe thrombocytopenia following myelosuppressive chemotherapy in patients with nonmyeloid malignancies	Flu-like syndrome and fluid retention
Paclitaxel (Taxol)	Second-line treatment in metastatic carcinoma of the breast and ovary	Allergic/immune-mediated complications
Rituximab (IDEC-C2B8 antibody, CD 20 antibody, or Rituxan)	B-cell NHL that is relapsed or refractory, low-grade or follicular, and CD 20–positive	Flu-like syndrome and hemodynamic complications
Sargramostim (GM-CSF or Prokine)	Myeloid reconstitution after autologous BMT for NHL, ALL, and Hodgkin's disease; BMT engraftment failure or delay	Flu-like and capillary-leak syndromes; fatigue; infectious, hemodynamic, and allergic/immune-mediated complications

ALL—acute lymphoblastic leukemia; BMT—bone marrow transplantation; 5-FU—5-fluorouracil; G-CSF—granulocyte colony-stimulating factor; GM-CSF—granulocyte–macrophage colony-stimulating factor; IL—interleukin; NHL—non-Hodgkin's lymphoma.

tion. When administered repeatedly, tachyphylaxis often develops, with symptoms subsiding over time. Pretreatment with nonsteroidal antiinflammatory agents appears to lessen the febrile response, and with symptomatic therapy, this or other constitutional effects are rarely dose limiting. High fevers occurring after several days of treatment or recurring after resolution of the early fevers are unusual and should prompt a search for an infectious source and, if indicated, institution of appropriate antibiotic therapy. Interestingly, despite the relatively frequent occurrence of flu-like symptoms (eg, arthralgia, myalgia, fatigue, nausea, and headache), clinically significant fevers have not been reported with IL-11 administration [2]. The recently approved monoclonal antibody CD 20 (rituximab) has also been reported to produce a flu-like syndrome. Frequent side effects include fever, chills, nausea, asthenia, and headache. As with the cytokines, these side effects were more frequent and severe following the initial antibody infusion. These symptoms were usually controlled with diphenhydramine and acetaminophen and, if necessary, by temporarily halting the antibody infusions [3].

Constitutional effects occur in up to 33% of patients receiving levamisole. Symptoms generally occur on the day of treatment, range from mild and transient to severe and progressive, and necessitate discontinuation of therapy in up to 2% of patients [4,5]. Intravenous administration of epoetin α can cause transient flushing or a flu-like syndrome: however, these symptoms have not been observed with subcutaneous administration [6,7]. Intravesical administration of BCG causes a flu-like syndrome in up to 60% of patients. Symptoms usually begin 6 to 12 hours after a dose, may persist for 1 to 2 days, and typically parallel the severity of the associated cystitis. Unlike the aforementioned cytokines and rituximab, symptoms are far more common after several doses of BCG than after the initial dose. Symptoms persisting beyond 2 days often indicate systemic BCG infection and warrant prompt institution of antituberculous therapy [8,9]. The etiologic mechanisms for the constitutional effects produced by levamisole, epoetin α and BCG

administration are unclear but may also be related to secondary cytokine release.

A flu-like syndrome may also occur with the administration of systemic chemotherapy, especially high-dose dacarbazine (DTIC) therapy, docetaxel, or combination chemotherapy with cytosine arabinoside (ara-C) and cisplatin (CDDP). More than one third of patients treated with docetaxel and up to 50% of patients treated with dacarbazine develop flu-like symptoms [10,11,12]. With dacarbazine, the symptoms typically last for several days and often recur with successive treatments [11]. Although the mechanism of this toxicity is unknown, it is tempting to hypothesize cytokine release as an important mediator.

FATIGUE

Chronic fatigue is the most important dose-limiting toxicity of interferon-α therapy and can be dose limiting in patients receiving aldesleukin and sargramostim therapy. Fatigue usually begins with the initial constitutional effects; however, tachyphylaxis to fatigue does not occur. Instead, with repeated doses, the fatigue may persist or increase in severity, ultimately resulting in a decrease in the patient's performance status. Although there is wide individual variation in tolerance, most patients can tolerate interferon at 3 to 10 mU/d for prolonged periods. With intermittent schedules two to three times per week, tolerance is better and fatigue may be mild or even unnoticed. At doses higher than 20 mU, most patients require a 50% or greater dose reduction during the first 2 to 4 weeks of daily therapy or the first 8 to 12 weeks of intermittent therapy. Doses of more than 100 mU are rarely tolerated for more than 1 to 2 weeks, if given daily, or 4 to 8 weeks, if given intermittently. Fatigue is most severe at doses of greater than 20 mU/d, in elderly patients, and in patients with a poor performance status. In some patients, evening administration of interferon improves tolerance [1].

Fatigue, weakness, and malaise occur in up to 50% of patients receiving high-dose aldesleukin therapy. Unlike many of the other toxic manifestations of aldesleukin therapy that resolve quickly after discontinuation of aldesleukin therapy, the fatigue may persist for several weeks after administration of the last dose.

Fatigue occurring with sargramostim has been reported infrequently (< 5%), perhaps because it is difficult to distinguish from the fatigue associated with high-dose chemotherapy, bone marrow transplantation, or other intercurrent illnesses common to most clinical settings in which sargramostim is used. Rosenfeld and colleagues [13] reported fatigue in patients with myelodysplasia receiving sargramostim at doses of 60 to 250 µg/m²/d subcutaneously or by 2-hour intravenous infusion for 14 days. One of 18 patients treated by the intravenous route and 4 of 19 patients treated by the subcutaneous route had a decrease in ECOG performance status of two grades. One patient receiving 125 µg/m²/d subcutaneously required a dose reduction because of fatigue. Physicians should thus be aware that some patients receiving sargramostim (especially at doses > 250 µg/m²/d may develop significant fatigue requiring dose modification. Fatigue has also been reported in less than 5% of patients treated with levamisole, 7% to 33% of patients treated with BCG (in association with the flu-like syndrome), many patients treated with IL-11, and rarely, if ever, with filgrastim and epoetin-α treatment. With none of these agents was fatigue dose limiting.

The pathogenesis of the fatigue associated with biologic therapy is unclear but may be part of the broad constellation of central nervous system (CNS) toxicity observed with these agents. Dinarello [14]

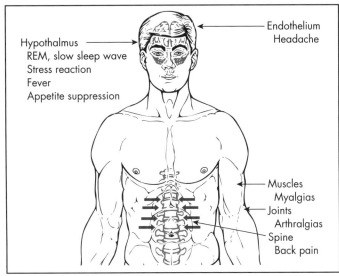

FIGURE 31-1.

Many symptoms of flu-like syndrome are mediated by the effects of prostaglandin E₂ (PGE₂ *arrows*) on muscle, causing myalgias; joints, causing arthralgias; the spine causing back pain; vascular endothelium, causing headache; and the hypothalamus, eventually resulting in slow-wave sleep, pituitary stress hormone release, fever, and appetite suppression.

suggests that fatigue may be related to the direct effects of either IL-1 or secondarily released PGE_2 from paraventricular endothelial cells on neurons and glial cells exposed to systemic circulation in the organ vasculosum laminar terminalis (OVLT) of the hypothalamus (Fig 31-2). In experimental systems, IL-1 administration rapidly induces fever, sleep, and the release of a variety of neuropeptides. Although IL-1 does not cross the blood–brain barrier, glial and possibly neural cells synthesize IL-1 and other neurotransmitters, which then may interact with receptors distributed throughout the brain, including the sleep center where a rapid change from REM to slow-wave activity occurs. IL-1 also may act as a cofactor in synaptic transmission with low concentrations of IL-1 actually augmenting γ-aminobutyric acid-a (GABAa) receptor function. To what extent these effects of IL-1 or unknown effects of other secondary cytokines contribute to the fatigue associated with biologic response modifier therapy remains to be elucidated.

INFECTIOUS COMPLICATIONS

Bacteremia and sepsis have occurred with unusual frequency in patients receiving aldesleukin therapy. In clinical trials with high-dose bolus aldesleukin, bacteremia occurred in 10% to 20% of treatment courses and was often related to central intravenous catheters. *Staphylococcus aureus* was the most common pathogen isolated, accounting for 65% of cases, followed by *Staphylococcus epidermidis,*

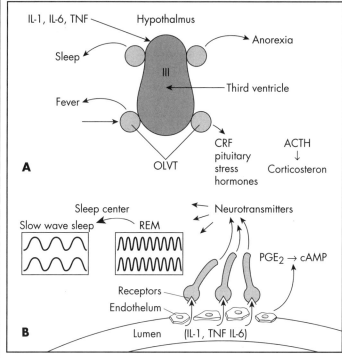

FIGURE 31-2.

In fatigue, cytokines such as IL-1, IL-6, and TNF act on the organ vasculosum lamina terminalis (OVLT) located around the third ventricle in the hypothalamus, triggering a variety of phenomena (A). B, In the OVLT cytokines react with receptors on either vascular endothelial cells producing PGE_2 or directly together with PGE_2 on receptors on neurons and glial cells that lie at the other side of loose junctions. Neurons and glial cells trigger cyclic AMP and other neurotransmitters that affect the sleep center, producing slow-wave sleep pattern detectable on electroencephalograms. Similar mechanisms may be responsible for anorexia, fever, and pituitary stress hormone release.

Escherichia coli, and polymicrobial infection. Patients at highest risk for infection included those with grade 2 or greater skin toxicity with skin desquamation, skin colonization at the catheter site with *S. aureus*, and an indwelling central venous catheter. The bacteremias were often severe, with a large number of positive blood cultures, persistent bacteremia for an average of 2.5 days after institution of appropriate antibiotic therapy, and significant clinical sequelae. Of 20 patients with bacteremia described by Klempner and Snydman [15] two died of sepsis, three developed thrombophlebitis, one developed probable septic arthritis, one had a septic arterial aneurysm at an arterial line site, and one had peritonitis and probable meningitis. Other types of nosocomial infections, such as pneumonia, decubital ulcer, or urinary tract infections, were rarely seen in these aldesleukin recipients.

The management of bacteremia and sepsis associated with aldesleukin therapy requires prompt recognition and initiation of appropriate antibiotic therapy. Optimal intravenous catheter care should be practiced to decrease the risk for infection, with catheters being removed after each 5-day course of therapy. Surveillance cultures of the catheter site should be performed twice per week. Prophylactic antibiotic therapy with oxacillin, cephalosporins, or quinolones has decreased the incidence of bacteremia significantly and should be used in all patients with central venous catheters. When sepsis is suspected, blood samples should be obtained from both catheter and peripheral sites and empiric intravenous antibiotic therapy instituted while culture results are awaited. Vancomycin is the antibiotic of choice because gram-positive bacteremia is very common; however, about 10% of infection may be due to gram-negative organisms and thus broader coverage may be indicated in some patients. If the infection is catheter related, the catheter should be removed as soon as possible. Klempner and Snydman [15] suggested that the unusually high incidence of bacterial infections associated with aldesleukin administration is related to a severe aldesleukin–induced impairment in neutrophil chemotaxis.

Brosman and Lamm [6] reviewed complications of intravesical BCG therapy in 1254 patients treated over 15 years. The majority of patients had been treated with the TICE strain, although patients were also treated with the Connaught, Pasteur (Armand Frappier), and Glaxo strains. The strains appeared similar in toxicity. Overall, granulomatous involvement of various organs occurred in less than 5% of patients. Granulomatous prostatitis was reported in 1.3% of patients, although if routine prostate biopsy specimens were obtained in asymptomatic patients, the incidence might have been as high as 25% [7]. In most cases, cultures for active BCG infections were negative. Epididymitis–orchitis occurred in 0.2%, renal granulomas in 0.1%, BCG pneumonitis or hepatitis in 0.9%, BCG bone marrow involvement with subsequent cytopenia in 0.1%, and sepsis in 0.4%. Death from disseminated BCG infections, "BCGosis," occurred in 7 patients (0.6%). Most patients who developed sepsis or BCGosis showed signs of increasingly severe reactions, with each dose of BCG manifested by higher and more prolonged fevers. In all fatal cases and in most septic cases, intravascular dissemination of BCG was believed to have occurred as a result of traumatic catherization or absorption through an inflamed, friable, bleeding urothelium. The use of isoniazid alone appears ineffective in preventing death from BCG sepsis. Two patients treated with multiple antituberculous agents, including cycloserine, have survived.

In general, there is a much higher incidence of systemic BCG infections in patients treated with intralesional BCG or immunosuppressed patients treated with intradermal BCG. One patient who had a history of intradermal BCG therapy developed activation of dormant BCG infection after immunosuppression with systemic chemotherapy. Because similar activation has not been reported in patients who have received intravesical BCG, routine antituberculous prophylaxis is not recommended for patients treated with intravesical BCG who later require systemic chemotherapy. Finally, not all granulomatous lesions are infectious. Orihuela and coworkers [9] reported several cases of culture-negative pelvic lymphadenitis, hepatic granulomas, and pulmonary lesions, which were believed to be immune in origin.

Interferon α-2 therapy has been associated with reactivation of herpes simplex infections in up to 10% of patients within the first several days of treatment. These infections generally clear within 10 days, even while patients continue receiving interferon. Disseminated herpes has not been reported [16]. Because interferon has antiviral properties and has been used to treat herpetic infections, this reactivation of herpes simplex is difficult to explain.

Levamisole has only been associated with infections in patients who develop levamisole-induced neutropenia or agranulocytosis, which occurs in less than 2% of patients.

HEMODYNAMIC COMPLICATIONS

Although hypotension is the most frequent dose-limiting side effect of aldesleukin therapy, it is rarely observed with sargramostim, rituximab, and interferon α-2 therapy, and rarely, if ever, with IL-11, filgrastim, BCG, and levamisole therapy. Nearly all patients receiving high-dose aldesleukin therapy by intermittent bolus injection for 5 days develop hypotension (Fig. 31-3). Approximately 75% of these patients require pressure support to continue aldesleukin therapy safely. Within 2 to 4 hours after the

initial dose of aldesleukin, vasodilation occurs, with a decrease in systemic vascular resistance and mean arterial pressure, and a compensatory increase in heart rate and cardiac index. The increase in cardiac index is not fully compensated, as evidenced by renal hypoperfusion, resulting in a prerenal state. These changes are identical to the changes observed during the early phases of septic shock. With aldesleukin therapy, the lowered systemic vascular resistance does not return to baseline until up to 5 days after the completion of therapy. In addition to the effects on vascular resistance, aldesleukin induces a capillary leak syndrome, resulting in third-space accumulation of fluid and worsening of the hypotension. The exact pathway by which aldesleukin exerts an effect on vascular smooth muscle remains to be defined, although nitric oxide is believed to be the final and pivotal mediator in this process. In most patients, the hypotension can be safely managed without disruption of aldesleukin therapy by the judicious use of intravenous fluids and the institution of pressor support with dopamine or phenylephrine [17].

Hemodynamic complications of sargramostim are much less frequent and less carefully studied. A first-dose reaction characterized by transient hypotension, hypoxemia, flushing tachycardia, musculoskeletal pain, rigors, leg spasms, dyspnea, nausea, and vomiting has been observed with molgramostim (nonglycosylated, E. coli-derived sargramostim) but rarely with sargramostim (glycosylated, yeast–derived sargramostim). This reaction appears to be more common with doses of 5 μg/kg/d or more, high-peak serum sargramostim levels and intravenous administration. Continuous infusion of molgramostim may decrease the frequency and severity of this reaction. This reaction is limited to the first dose of each treat-

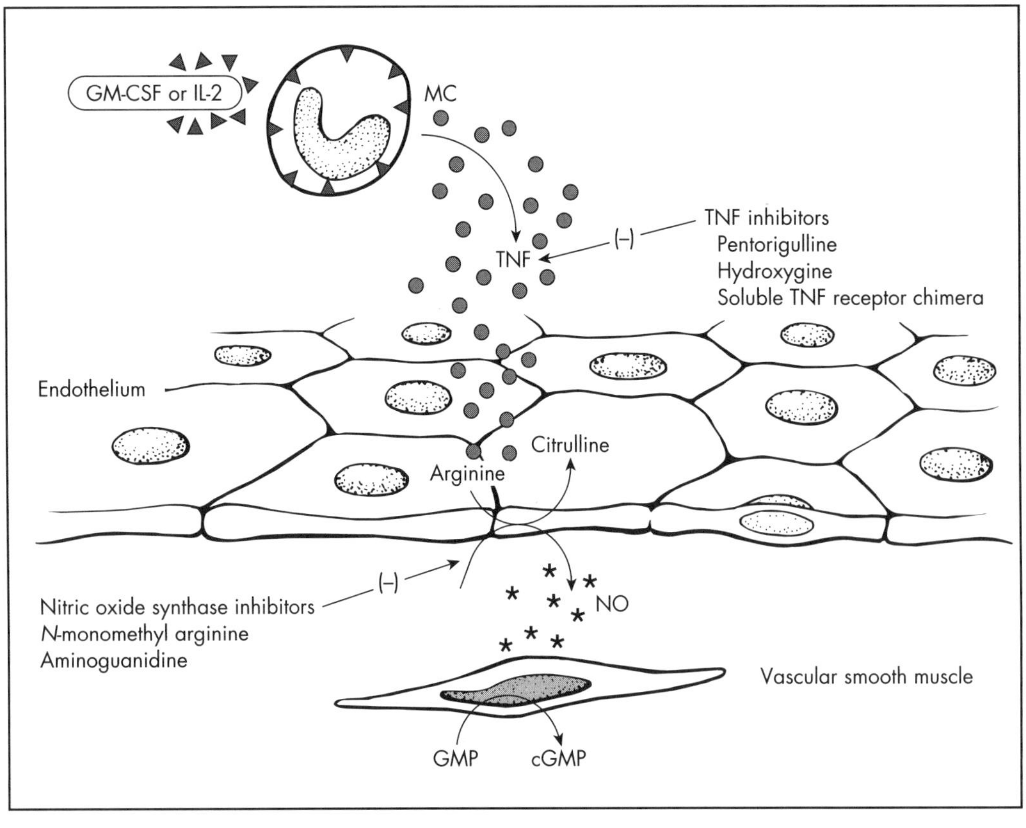

FIGURE 31-3.

In hypotension, IL-2 and GM-CSF interact with receptors on mononuclear cells, causing release of secondary cytokines, such as TNF, which exert direct effects on vascular endothelium primarily through the stimulation of nitric oxide synthetase resulting in the conversion of arginine to citrulline releasing nitric oxide (NO). Nitric oxide then exerts direct effects on vascular smooth muscles, which are mediated through cyclic GMP, resulting in smooth muscle relaxation, decreased peripheral vascular resistance, and hypotension.

ment cycle and thus is not dose limiting. The mechanism of the first dose reaction is unclear but appears unrelated to TNF [18,19]. Hypotension also may occur late during a course of therapy and be related to vasodilation and the capillary leak syndrome, similar to what has been reported with aldesleukin [19,20].

Rituximab infusion is associated with mild to moderate hypotension in 10% to 15% of patients. This usually occurs during administration of the antibody in conjunction with other acute systemic manifestations and usually can be effectively managed by slowing or interrupting the infusion and supportive measures, including administration of intravenous saline [3].

Hypotension has occurred in up to 6% of patients with cancer treated with interferon α. It is generally mild and easily managed with intravenous fluids. Rarely, dose modifications are required [21].

Hypertension has been noted rarely in cancer patients treated with epoetin α. The hypertension has been associated with a significant increase in hematocrit, often in a patients with preexisting hypertension. Epoetin α should not be administered to patients with uncontrolled hypertension [4].

CAPILLARY LEAK SYNDROME (FLUID RETENTION)

The capillary leak (or vascular leak) syndrome was initially described in trials that used high-dose aldesleukin and lymphokine-activated killer (LAK) cells but has subsequently been observed in most patients

receiving high-dose aldesleukin, many patients receiving IL-11, and in approximately 10% of patients receiving sargramostim at a dosage of 250 μg/m^2/d by 2-hour infusion (Fig. 31-4). This syndrome is a common dose-limiting side effect of therapy with these cytokines and consists of a generalized increase in vascular permeability with fluid extravasation into the tissues. Clinical manifestations usually begin within 24 hours of the initiation of aldesleukin therapy and progress from mild facial and ankle edema to anasarca with weight gain in excess of 5% to 10% of baseline body weight due to fluid retention. Ascites occurs in some patients, especially those with extensive hepatic metastases, whereas pleural or pericardial effusions occur in approximately 50% of aldesleukin recipients. IL-11 has been reported to produce demonstrable fluid retention, including peripheral edema (63%), dyspnea (48%), and pleural effusions (18%) in a large percentage of patients. In patients with preexisting pleural or pericardial effusions, aldesleukin, IL-11, or sargramostim may aggravate localized fluid retention. Because of the high risk for cerebral edema when there is disruption of the blood–brain barrier, patients with brain metastases should not receive aldesleukin or sargramostim therapy [22,23].

The capillary leak syndrome also has been observed in patients receiving docetaxel, particularly in cumulative doses of more than 400 mg/m^2. Corticosteroids decrease the severity and delay the onset of this syndrome and are now used routinely in ongoing trials with docetaxel [10].

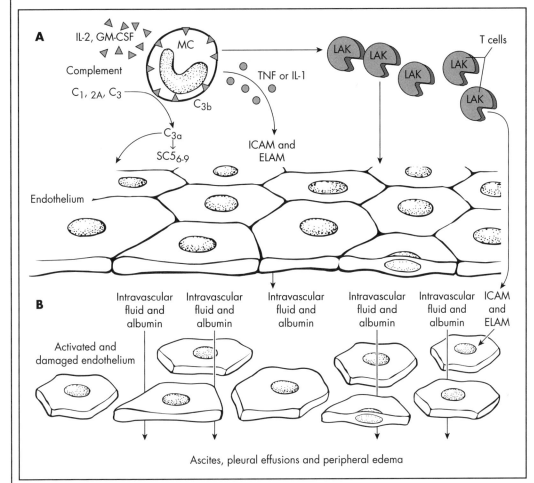

FIGURE 31-4.

In capillary leak syndrome, *A*, multiple mechanisms for producing vascular leak syndrome are displayed: IL-2 ± GM-CSF interact with mononuclear cells resulting in activation of nonspecific LAK cells, release of TNF and IL-1, and complement activation. LAK cells and activated complement can damage endothelium directly. TNF and IL-1 lead to increased adhesion molecule expression enhancing binding of activated cells. *B*, These processes lead to loss of integrity of endothelial surface and extravasation of intravascular fluid and albumin into third spaces, resulting in ascites, pleural effusion, and peripheral edema.

Diffuse or focal pulmonary infiltrates, observed in 40% of patients treated with aldesleukin, may result in significant dyspnea, hypoxia, and, in less than 5% of cases, the need for short-term ventilatory support. The development of pulmonary edema is more common in patients with marginal pulmonary reserve (*ie*, patients with pretreatment FEV_1 of ≤ 2.0 L) and in those whose treatment is complicated by bacteremia. The extent of peripheral edema or the amount of weight gain does not correlate with or predict the development of pulmonary infiltrates. Because the extravasation of fluid into the alveoli occurs in the setting of a normal pulmonary capillary wedge pressure, the pulmonary infiltrates are most likely caused by an increased capillary permeability rather than fluid overload or left ventricular dysfunction [24]. A similar syndrome has been reported in the setting of bone marrow transplantation with the use of high-dose cytosine arabinoside or a combination of high-dose busulfan, etoposide, and carmustine [25,26].

The management of the capillary leak syndrome is often complicated by other treatment side effects, especially hypotension. Symptomatic fluid retention limits the amount of fluid that can be administered to support the blood pressure, and hypotension precludes the use of diuretics to reverse fluid retention. Severe cardiovascular or pulmonary toxicity is an indication to withhold doses of aldesleukin or sargramostim, or to decrease the dose of sargramostim. Diuretics can be safely administered and are indicated, once therapy has been completed and blood pressure has normalized, to assist in the clearance of excess retained fluid. Side effects resolve rapidly after the discontinuation of therapy, with most patients reverting to their baseline weight in 4 to 5 days after completing a course of treatment.

Although the pathogenesis of the capillary leak syndrome is uncertain, most likely a combination of factors are involved. Direct endothelial injury is mediated by aldesleukin–activated leukocytes (natural killer [NK] or LAK cells in particular) or their oxidative products. Both aldesleukin and sargramostim activate peripheral blood mononuclear cells to release secondary cytokines, including TNF and IL-1. These secondary cytokines may worsen the process by inducing various adhesion molecules necessary for the attachment of activated leukocytes to the endothelium. On the other hand, these cytokines, especially IL-1, may at the same time render the endothelium less susceptible to cell-mediated injury. Finally, aldesleukin treatment is associated with systemic complement activation and high plasma concentrations of anaphylatoxins such as C_{3a}, which have potent effects on vascular permeability [22].

ALLERGIC AND IMMUNE-MEDIATED COMPLICATIONS

Biologic therapy alters the immune system in a variety of ways, including alteration of tumor antigen expression, stimulation of immune effector cells, enhancement of humoral immunity, and the release of secondary cytokines. This immunomodulation is most likely responsible for both the beneficial effects and toxic effects of biologic therapy. Not surprisingly, a number of allergic and immune-mediated side effects have been observed in patients treated with aldesleukin, interferon, and, less commonly, sargramostim, filgrastim, BCG, and levamisole (Fig. 31-5).

Allergic reactions are common and frequently occur at the local site of administration. When aldesleukin, interferon α-2, sargramostim, oprelvekin, or filgrastim are administered subcutaneously, self-limited erythematous cutaneous reactions occur at the injection site. Similarly, when BCG is administered intravesically, a self-limited cystitis occurs in 60% to 90% of patients [9,27]. Acute serious hypersensitivity reactions, such as urticaria, angioedema, bronchoconstriction, and anaphylaxis, have rarely been observed with aldesleukin, interferon α-2, sargramostim, filgrastim, epoetin α, rituximab, levamisole, and BCG.

A "recall reaction" to iodinated radiographic contrast medium occurs in approximately 10% of patients undergoing routine intravenous contrast studies for follow-up of previous aldesleukin therapy. Reactions usually occur at least 1 month after initial exposure to aldesleukin and contrast medium. Typical reactions begin 1 to 4 hours after reexposure to radiographic contrast medium and consist of fever, chills, rash, diarrhea, nausea, vomiting, urticaria, dyspnea, weakness, and hypotension. Reactions appear to be more common in patients receiving intraarterial rather than systemic aldesleukin therapy or concomitant administration of aldesleukin and radiographic contrast material. A similar hypersensitivity reaction (including pruritus, erythema, edema, and hypotension) has been reported to cytotoxic chemotherapy agents in patients with metastatic melanoma who have previously received regimens that combine aldesleukin with cisplatin-based cytotoxic chemotherapy [28]. This recall reaction may be related to enhancement by aldesleukin of an immune response to radiographic contrast material or chemotherapy agent, followed by an anamnestic response on reexposure to the contrast

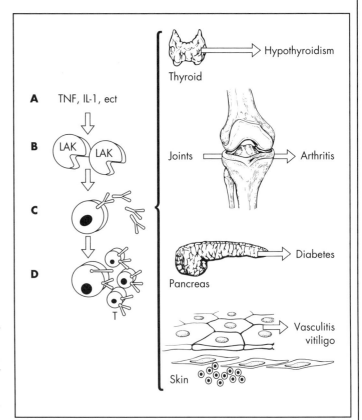

FIGURE 31-5.

Potential mechanisms for cytokine-induced autoimmune reactions include *A*, release of secondary cytokines, such as TNF and IL-1; *B*, generation of LAK cells; *C*, synthesis of specific autoantibodies; and *D*, activation and proliferation of specific autoreactive cytotoxic T cells. These substances either nonspecifically (*A, B*) or specifically (*C, D*) interact with end organs, such as thyroid gland, joints, pancreas, or skin, causing dysfunction. Mechanism *D* is the most likely process involved.

material [24]. Early trials with paclitaxel and docetaxel have reported a high incidence of infusion-related hypersensitivity reactions characterized by dyspnea, bronchospasm, and hypotension. Premedication with dexamethasone (a now routine practice) has significantly decreased the incidence and severity of such reactions [29–31].

Many of these agents, but especially aldesleukin and interferon, have been associated with the development or exacerbation of preexisting autoimmune or chronic inflammatory diseases. Both aldesleukin and interferon have been associated with the development or exacerbation of preexisting autoimmune thyroiditis, hemolytic anemia, immune thrombocytopenia purpura (ITP), rheumatoid arthritis, psoriasis, vasculitis, inflammatory bowel disease, and nephritis [1,24]. sargramostim has been associated with reactivation of ITP, autoimmune thyroiditis, rheumatoid arthritis, and hemolysis, whereas filgrastim has been associated with exacerbations of preexisting eczema, psoriasis, and vasculitis [18,32]. Although BCG vaccination and intralesional BCG administration have been associated with erythema nodosum, cutaneous vasculitis, and generalized Shwartzman reaction, these side effects have not been reported with intravesical BCG treatment [9]. Symoens and colleagues [33] reported a higher frequency of levamisole-induced leukopenia and agranulocytosis in patients with rheumatic diseases (4.9%) when compared with patients with cancer (2%). However, these results are difficult to interpret because leukopenia and agranulocytosis occur frequently in patients with rheumatic diseases in the absence of levamisole therapy. The agranulocytosis appears to be related to antigranulocyte antibodies and circulating immune complexes [4]. A cutaneous necrotizing vasculitis has also been reported with levamisole therapy [33]. The mechanisms involved in the development of autoimmune and inflammatory diseases with biologic therapy are complex and as yet poorly defined. In some cases the administered cytokine may play a direct role in the pathogenesis of disease.

Enhanced production of autoantibodies to insulin, thyrotropin, platelets, and other antigens has been reported after biologic therapy, and it is likely that, as our experience with biologic agents grows, numerous other autoantibodies will be detected. Many of these autoantibodies may be associated with the development of autoimmune disease. For example, after high-dose aldesleukin therapy, 10% to 20% of patients develop a thyroiditis that is often associated with increased serum titers of antithyroid antibodies. Patients typically present with hypothyroidism approximately 8 to 10 weeks after the initiation of treatment. Frequently a transient period of hyperthyroidism or even thyrotoxicosis precedes the hypothyroidism. Thyroid dysfunction is more frequent in women, patients with antithyroid antibodies or subclinical evidence of thyroiditis pretreatment, and patients receiving prolonged and repeated courses of aldesleukin, particularly in

association with interferon α. The thyroid abnormalities resolve spontaneously 4 to 10 months after treatment is completed. Similarly, patients treated with interferon α-2 may develop antithyroid antibodies and associated thyroid abnormalities. Treatment should be discontinued in patients whose thyroid function cannot be normalized with drug therapy [1,34]. Aldesleukin and interferon α–related thyroid dysfunction may be related to a direct toxic effect of activated NK or LAK cells on thyrocytes, an inhibition of thyroglobulin production by secondary cytokines, such as IL-1 and TNF, a direct or indirect stimulation of humoral immunity to thyroid autoantigens, or reactivation of preexisting T-cell clones directed against thyroid autoantigens, resulting in autoimmune thyroiditis [32].

Vitiligo has been reported to develop frequently following aldesleukin therapy [32]. Interestingly, its appearance is virtually restricted to patients with metastatic melanoma, implying some requirement for tumor antigen presentation. In addition, vitiligo appears to occur more commonly in patients responding to therapy, implying some cross-reactivity between antigens expressed on tumor cells and melanocytes. Furthermore, it suggests that aldesleukin therapy is able to induce immune responses against antigens to which the host has been previously tolerated.

Both neutralizing and nonneutralizing antibodies against aldesleukin, sargramostim, and interferon α-2 but not filgrastim and epoetin α have been observed. The clinical significance of these antibodies remains unclear, but in several cases the development of neutralizing antibodies to interferon was associated with disease relapse [1]. Many factors influence the frequency, magnitude, and importance of antibody induction, including underlying disease, treatment schedule, cumulative dose, treatment duration, route of administration, blood sampling time, source of protein, and assay methods. For interferon α-2, the underlying disease plays an important role in frequency of antibody formation, with the highest incidence occurring in patients treated for Kaposi's sarcoma (5%) and renal cell carcinoma (32%–38%) [35]. In addition, interferon-neutralizing antibodies occur more frequently with interferon α-2a than interferon α-2b perhaps because of different purification techniques. Despite numerous systemic aldesleukin trials, neutralizing antibodies to aldesleukin develop uncommonly. The low incidence of aldesleukin antibodies may be related to the short duration of standard high-dose aldesleukin therapy. As new studies with long-term administration of low-dose aldesleukin therapy are now underway, the incidence and clinical significance of aldesleukin antibody formation may become significant. In addition, a case report and in vitro studies suggest that interferon may act synergistically with aldesleukin in inducing a humoral response, with the resultant production of high titers of antialdesleukin antibodies [36].

REFERENCES

1. Quesada JR, Talpaz M, Rios A, *et al.*: Clinical toxicity of interferons in cancer patients: a review. *J Clin Oncol* 1988, 4:234–243.

2. Isaacs C, Robert NJ, Bailey A: Randomized placebo-controlled study of recombinant human interleukin-11 to prevent chemotherapy-induced thrombocytopenia in patients with breast cancer receiving dose-intensive cyclophosphamide and doxorubicin. *J Clin Oncol* 1997, 15:3368–3377.

3. Maloney DG, Grillo-Lopez AJ, White CA, *et al.*: IDEC-C2B8 (Rituximab) anti-CD20 monoclonal antibody therapy in patients with relapsed low-grade non-Hodgkin's lymphoma. *Blood* 1997, 90:2188–2195.

4. Parkinson DR, Jerry LM, Shibata HR, *et al.*: Complications of cancer immunotherapy with levamisole. *Lancet* 1977, 1:1129–1132.

5. Quirt IC, Shelly WE, Pater JL, *et al.*: Improved survival in patients with poor-prognosis malignant melanoma treated with adjuvant levamisole: a phase III study by the National Cancer Institute of Canada Clinical Trials Group. *J Clin Oncol* 1991, 9:729–735.

6. Spivak JL: Recombinant human erythropoietin and the anemia of cancer. *Blood* 1994, 84:997–1004.

7. Miller CB, Platanias LC, Mills SR, *et al.*: Phase I-II trial of erythropoietin in the treatment of cisplatin-associated anemia. *JNCI* 1992, 84:98–103.

8. Brosman SA, Lamm DL: The preparation, handling and use of intravesical bacillus Calmette-Guérin for the management of stage Ta, T1, carcinoma in situ and transitional cell cancer. *J Urol* 1990, 144:313–315.

9. Orihuela E, Herr HW, Pinsky CM, Whitmore WF: Toxicity of intravesical BCG and its management in patients with superficial bladder tumors. *Cancer* 1987, 60:326–333.

10. Cortes JE, R Pazdur: Docetaxel. *J Clin Oncol* 1995, 13:2643–2655.

11. Beusa JM, Mouridsen HT, van-Oosterom AT, *et al.*: High-dose DTIC in advanced soft-tissue sarcomas in the adult: a phase II study of the EORTC Soft Tissue and Bone Sarcoma Group. *Ann Oncol* 1991, 2:307–309.

12. Margolin K, Doroshow J, Leong L, *et al.*: Combination chemotherapy with cytosine arabinoside (ara-C) and cis-diamminedichloroplatinum (CDDP) for squamous cancers of the upper aerodigestive tract. *Am J Clin Oncol* 1989, 12:494–497.

13. Rosenfeld CS, Sulecki M, Evans C, Shadduck RK: Comparison of intravenous versus subcutaneous recombinant human granulocyte-macrophage colony-stimulating factor in patients with myelodysplasia. *Exp Hematol* 1991, 19:273–277.

14. Dinarello CA: Interleukin-1 and interleukin-1 antagonism. *Blood* 1992, 77:1627–1652.

15. Klempner MS, Snydman DR: Infectious complication associated with interleukin-2. In Atkins MB, Mier JW (eds): *Therapeutic Applications of Interleukin-2*. New York: Marcel Dekker, 1993: 409–424.

16. Sherwin SA, Knost JA, Fein S, *et al.*: A multiple-dose phase I trial of recombinant leukocyte A interferon in cancer patients. *JAMA* 1982, 248:2461–2466.

17. Gaynor ER, Fisher RI: Hemodynamic and cardiovascular effects of aldesleukin. In Atkins MB, Mier JW, (eds) *Therapeutic Applications of Interleukin-2*. New York: Marcel Dekker, 1993: 381–387.

18. ASCO Ad Hoc Colony-Stimulating Factor Guideline Expert Panel: American Society of Clinical Oncology recommendations for the use of hematopoietic colony-stimulating factors: evidence-based, clinical practice guidelines. *J Clin Oncol* 1994, 12:2471–2508.

19. Cebon J, Lieschke GJ, Bury RW, Morstyn G: The dissociation of sargramostim efficacy from toxicity according to route of administration: a pharmacodynamic study. *Br J Haematol* 1992, 80:144–150.

20. Lieschke GJ, Cebon J, Morstyn G: Characterization of the clinical effects after the first dose of bacterially synthesized recombinant human granulocyte-macrophage colony-stimulating factor. *Blood* 1989, 74:2634–2643.

21. Jones GJ, Itri LM: Safety and tolerance of recombinant interferon alpha-2a (Roferon-A) in cancer patients. *Cancer* 1986, 57:1709–1715.

22. Mier JW: Pathogenesis of the aldesleukin-induced vascular leak syndrome. In Atkins MB, Mier JW (eds): *Therapeutic Applications of Interleukin-2*. New York: Marcel Dekker, 1993: 363–380.

23. Lieschke GJ, Burgess AW: Granulocyte colony-stimulating factor and granulocyte-macrophage colony-stimulating factor. *N Engl J Med* 1992, 327:28–35.

24. Margolin KA: The clinical toxicities of high-dose aldesleukin. In Atkins MB, Mier JW (eds): *Therapeutic Applications of Interleukin-2*. New York: Marcel Dekker, 1993: 331–362.

25. Woods WG, Ramsay NK, Weisdorf DJ, *et al.*: Bone marrow transplantation for acute lymphoblastic leukemia utilizing total body irradiation followed by high doses of cytosine arabinoside: lack of superiority over cyclophosphamide-containing conditioning regimens. *Bone Marrow Transplant* 1990, 6:9–16.

26. Takahashi H, Sekiguchi H, Kai S, *et al.*: Recurrent pulmonary edema in a patient with acute lymphoblastic leukemia after syngeneic bone marrow transplantation. *Rinsho Ketsueki* 1992, 33:354–359.

27. Lamm DL, Stogdill VD, Stogdill BJ, Crispen RG: Complications of bacillus Calmette-Guérin immunotherapy in 1278 patients with bladder cancer. *J Urol* 1986, 135:272–274.

28. Heywood GR, Rosenberg SA, Weber JS: Hypersensitivity reactions to chemotherapy agents in patients receiving chemoimmunotherapy with high-dose interleukin-2. *J Natl Cancer Inst* 1995, 87:915–922.

29. Weiss R, Donehower RC, Wiernik PH, *et al.*: Hypersensitivity reactions from Taxol. *J Clin Oncol* 1990, 8:1263–1269.

30. Wanders J, Schrijvers D, Bruntush U, *et al.*: The EORTC-ECTG experience with acute hypersensitivity reactions (HSR) in Taxotere studies [abstract]. *Pro Am Soc Clin Oncol* 1993:73.

31. Gennari A, Salvadori B, Tognoni A, Conte PF: Rapid intravenous infusion premedication with dexamethasone prevents hypersensitivity reactions to paclitaxel [letter]. *Ann Oncol* 1996, 7:978–979.

32. Atkins MB: Autoimmune disorders induced by interleukin-2 therapy. In Atkins MB, Mier JW (eds): *Therapeutic Applications of Interleukin-2*. New York: Marcel Dekker, 1993:389–408.

33. Symoens J, Veys E, Mielants M, Pinals R: Adverse reactions to levamisole. *Cancer Treat Rep* 1978, 62:1721–1730.

34. Schultz M, Muller R, von zur Muhlen A, Brabant G: Induction of hyperthyrodism by interferon-alpha-2B. *Lancet* 1989, 1:1452.

35. Figlin RA: Biotherapy in clinical practice. *Semin Hematol* 1989, 26(suppl):15–24.

36. Kirchner H, Korfer A, Evers P, *et al.*: The development of neutralizing antibodies in a patient receiving subcutaneous recombinant and natural interleukin-2. *Cancer* 1990, 67:1862–1864.

FLU-LIKE SYNDROME

Patients undergoing biologic therapy with aldesleukin, interferon α-2, sargramostim, oprelvekin, rituximab, and less frequently, BCG and levamisole develop a flu-like syndrome consisting of fever, chills, malaise, myalgias, arthralgias, headache, and occasionally nausea, vomiting, diarrhea, nasal congestion, dizziness, and light-headedness. For aldesleukin, interferon α-2, and sargramostim these side effects are dose related, occur 1–6 h after a dose, are more common with bolus administration, and resolve spontaneously within 24 h of administration of a single dose. With repeated daily doses (8 h for aldesleukin, daily for interferon α, oprelvekin, rituximab, sargramostim) there is a tendency to tachyphylaxis, with symptoms subsiding over time; however, with intermittent treatment, tachyphylaxis usually does not occur. With BCG, these side effects occur 6–12 h after intravesical administration, and resolve within 1–2 d. The severity tends to parallel the intensity of the local reaction. With levamisole, side effects typically occur on the days of treatment. With epoetin α, the flu-like syndrome has occurred with IV but not SC administration. With any of these agents, fevers that occur after several days of therapy or that recur after resolution of early fevers are unusual and an infectious cause should be sought. Rarely are these constitutional symptoms dose limiting [1–3,5–8,23,24].

CAUSATIVE AGENTS
Interferon α, aldesleukin, sargramostim, oprelvekin, rituximab, BCG, levamisole, occasionally cytotoxic chemotherapy

PATHOLOGIC PROCESS
Release or generation of secondary cytokines (*eg* IL-1, TNF, IL-6) by lymphocytes or monocytes in response to aldesleukin and sargramostim; PGE_2 probably directly responsible for interferon-related constitutional symptoms; mechanism of levamisole and BCG toxicity is unclear, but may also be related to secondary cytokine release

DIFFERENTIAL DIAGNOSES
Coexisting viral, bacterial, or fungal infection, paraneoplastic syndromes

PATIENT ASSESSMENT
Rule out infections or neoplastic causes, especially if symptoms progress and are not closely related to administration of above agents.

TOXICITY GRADING

	0	1	2	3	4
Fever in absence of infection	None	37.1°–38.0°C 98.7°–100.4°F	38.1°–40.0°C 100.5°–104.0°F	> 40.0°C > 104.0°F for < 24 h	> 40.0°C > 104.0°F for 24 h or accompanied by hypotension
Nausea	None	Able to eat reasonable intake	Intake significantly decreased but can eat	No significant intake	—
Vomiting	None	1 episode in 24 h	2–5 episodes in 24 h	6–10 episodes in 24 h	> 10 episodes in 24 h or requiring parenteral support
Diarrhea	None	Increase of 2–3 stools/d over pretreatment	Increase of 4–6 stools/d, nocturnal stools, moderate cramping	Increase of 7–9 stools/d, incontinence, or severe cramping	Increase of ≥ 10 stools/d, grossly bloody diarrhea, or need for parenteral support
Headache	None	Mild, no treatment required	Moderate non-narcotic treatment	Severe narcotics required	—
Sinus congestion	None	Mild, no treatment required	Moderate	—	—
Chills, rigors	None	Mild, < 30 min, resolves spontaneously	Moderate, < 30 min, requires intervention	—	—
Myalgia, arthralgia	None	Mild	Moderate	Severe	Intractable

MANAGEMENT

Agent	Dose	Maximum Dose	Action	Guidelines
Acetaminophen (Tylenol)	650 mg q 4 h PO or PR	4000 mg/d	Inhibits prostaglandin synthesis	Begin prior to the first dose of IL-2 or IFN and continue until completing treatment
Indomethacin (Indocin)	25 mg q 6 h PO or PR	200 mg/d	Inhibits prostaglandin synthesis	Begin prior to first dose of IL-2 and continue until completion of treatment; PRN fever with acetaminophen
Diphenhydramine (Benadryl)	25–50 mg PO or IV q 8 h prn	400 mg/d	H_1 receptor antagonist	For fever, malaise, chills secondary to hypersensitivity reaction (especially with BCG)
Prochlorperazine (Compazine)	10 mg PO or IV, 25 mg PR q 6 h prn	40 mg/d	Dopamine receptor antagonist; affects the chemoreceptor trigger zone and vomiting center	For nausea and vomiting
Meperidine (Demerol)	25–50 mg IM or IV q 4 h prn	—	Central nervous system opioid agonist	For severe chills and rigors
Loperamide Hydrochloride (Imodium)	4 mg followed by 2 mg after each unformed stool prn diarrhea	16 mg/d	Slows intestinal motility	For diarrhea
Diphenoxylate Hydrochloride with atropine sulfate (Lomotil)	2 tablets q 6 h or 10 mL q 6 h prn (2.5–5.0 mg diphenoxylate Hcl and 0.025–0.05 mg atropine sulfate)	20 mg diphenoxylate HCl/d	Slows intestinal motility	For severe diarrhea

CHRONIC FATIGUE

The fatigue syndrome accompanying interferon α-2, aldesleukin, sargramostim, and oprelvekin therapy varies considerably from mild to severe and, in some cases, defines the maximum tolerated dose. Fatigue is dose-related and is often less when intermittent schedules and lower doses are used. Although individual variation in tolerance is wide, fatigue is often more profound in older patients or those with poor performance status.

MANAGEMENT OR INTERVENTION

1. Evening administration of interferon may reduce fatigue or improve tolerance
2. Moderate or severe fatigue with decreased performance status often improves with a 50% dose reduction of interferon α-2 or sargramostim; if no improvement, reduce drug doses an additional 10% of starting dose or discontinue therapy until fatigue resolves

TOXICITY GRADING SCALE

0	1	2	3	4
Asymptomatic	Symptomatic	Symptomatic, in bed < 50% of day	Symptomatic, in bed > 50% of day but not bedridden	Bedridden

CAUSATIVE AGENTS

Interleukin-2, interferon α-2, sargramostim, oprelvekin

PATHOLOGIC PROCESS

Unclear, but may be part of the broad constellation of CNS toxicity observed with these agents; may be related to IL-1 or other cytokine release [14]

DIFFERENTIAL DIAGNOSES

Anemia; comorbid illness, especially chronic infections, thyroid dysfunction, hepatitis, renal dysfunction; tumor progression; other medications, particularly antiemetics, analgesics, sedatives, cytotoxic chemotherapy

PATIENT ASSESSMENT

Obtain hemoglobin, hematocrit, liver function tests, serum electrolytes (calcium), thyroid function tests, TSH, BUN, and creatinine; review other medications; assess for tumor progression.

INFECTIOUS COMPLICATIONS

In patients receiving aldesleukin therapy bacteremia occurs in 10%–20%. The majority of these infections are related to the use of an indwelling intravenous catheter and occur toward the end of a course of aldesleukin treatment. If unrecognized or if institution of appropriate antibiotic therapy is delayed, these infections can be fatal. Antibiotic prophylaxis with several agents has greatly reduced both the incidence and severity of infections. Although uncommon, systemic BCG infections do occur and in rare cases have been fatal. Most septic and fatal cases are related to intravasation of intravesically instilled BCG, often from traumatic catheterization or instrumentation [8,27].

Interferon therapy has been associated with reactivation of herpes simplex infections in up to 10% of patients within the first several days of treatment. These infections generally clear within 10 d even while interferon therapy continues. Disseminated herpes has not been reported [16]. Levamisole has only been associated with infections in patients who develop levamisole-induced agranulocytosis or neutropenia.

CAUSATIVE AGENTS
Aldesleukin, interferon α-2, BCG

PATHOLOGIC PROCESS
Aldesleukin infections: probably related to severely impaired neutrophil chemotaxis, resulting either directly or indirectly from aldesleukin administration; **Systemic BCG infections**: most likely related to intravascular disseminiation of BCG through an inflamed, friable, or bleeding urothelium; **Interferon α-2 therapy**: mechanism involved with reactivation of herpes simplex infections is unclear

DIFFERENTIAL DIAGNOSES
Flu-like syndrome associated with biologic agents, unrelated infectious process, drug reaction, paraneoplastic syndrome

PATIENT ASSESSMENT
Aldesleukin: obtain blood cultures from central venous catheter site and peripherally, examine central venous catheter site and skin for generalized reactions, check for lapse in antipyretic administration, assess fever pattern with prior doses; **Interferon α-2**: evaluate lesions, obtain herpes virus culture; **BCG**: rule out other infections causes, culture bacterial strains and biopsy of affected sites.

MANAGEMENT OR INTERVENTION

Aldesleukin
1. Optimal intravenous catheter management; remove after ≤ 7 d
2. Surveillance cultures of intravenous catheter twice weekly
3. Prophylactic antibiotics (ciprofloxacin, 250 mg PO bid; cefazolin sodium, 250–500 mg IV q 8 h; or oxacillin, 500 mg IV q 6 h) for patients requiring central venous catheters
4. Prompt recognition of infections and initiation of appropriate antibiotics after obtaining cultures. Because of high risk for *S. aureus*, vancomycin hydrochloride, 1 g 12 h (dose adjusted for impaired renal failure) is empiric drug of choice; broader coverage may be indicated in some patients—particularly those with a history of urinary tract infections, biliary colic, abdominal discomfort, or neutropenia
5. Removal of intravenous catheter once infection is suspected or confirmed

Interferon α-2
Acyclovir, 200 mg PO 5 ×/d to manage pain associated with herpes labialis infection

BCG
1. Avoid use of BCG in immunosuppressed patients because of risk of systemic infection
2. Postpone BCG treatment until concurrent febrile illness, urinary tract infection, or gross hematuria resolves
3. Delay BCG dose for 7–14 d after traumatic catherization, biopsy, or transurethral resection
4. For fevers greater than 100°F or bladder-irritative symptoms lasting longer than 24 h and gross hematuria, administer isoniazid, 300 mg PO × 3 d; repeat isoniazid with subsequent administrations
5. Discontinue BCG if patient continues to have fevers while receiving isoniazid, recurrent elevations in liver function tests (related to isoniazid), or signs of prostatitis, orchitis, etc.
6. For systemic BCG infection, therapy should include: isoniazid 300 mg PO daily, rifampin 600 mg PO daily, and ethambutol 1200 mg PO daily for at least 6 mo. For patients with life-threatening BCG sepsis or "BCGosis," administer cycloserine 250–500 mg PO bid for first 3 d of treatment

TOXICITY GRADING

0	1	2	3	4
None	Minor, localized, antibiotics not required	Minor, antibiotics required	Severe, major organ infection	Disseminated, life-threatening

HEMODYNAMIC COMPLICATIONS

Hypotension is the most frequent dose-limiting side effect of high-dose aldesleukin therapy, particularly when administered by intermittent intravenous bolus. The sequence of hemodynamic effects is characterized by an initial vasodilatory phase occurring 2–4 h after a dose of aldesleukin, during which the systemic vascular resistance falls but vascular integrity is maintained. Subsequently, the capillary leak syndrome with third-space accumulation of fluid often develops. The decreased systemic vascular resistance persists until the completion of therapy [17].

Hemodynamic complications of GM-CSF are much less frequent and less carefully studied. A first-dose reaction, characterized by transient hypotension, hypoxemia, flushing, tachycardia, musculoskeletal pain, rigors, leg spasms, dyspnea, nausea, and vomiting has been observed with molgramostim (nonglycosylated, *E. coli*–derived GM-CSF) but rarely with sargramostim (glycosylated, yeast- derived GM-CSF). This reaction is limited to the first dose of each treatment cycle and is not dose limiting. The mechanism of the first reaction dose is unclear but appears unrelated to TNF [18,19]. Hypotension also may occur late during a course of therapy and be related to vasodilation and the capillary leak syndrome, similar to what has been reported with aldesleukin [19,20].

Hypotension has occurred in up to 6% of patients with cancer treated with interferon α-2. It is generally mild and easily managed with intravenous fluids. Rarely are dose modifications required [21]. Rituximab infusion is associated with mild to moderate hypotension in 10%–15% of patients. This usually occurs during administration of the antibody in conjunction with other acute systemic manifestations and usually can be effectively managed by slowing or interrupting the infusion and supportive measures, including administration of intravenous saline [3]. The mechanism is most likely a hypersensitivity reaction, although secondary cytokine release cannot be excluded. Hypertension has been noted rarely in cancer patients treated with epoetin α. The hypertension has been associated with a significant increase in hematocrit often in a patient with preexisting hypertension. Epoetin α should not be administered to patients with uncontrolled hypertension [6].

CAUSATIVE AGENTS
Aldesleukin, sargramostim, interferon α-2, epoetim α, rituximab

PATHOLOGIC PROCESS
Decreased systemic vascular resistance and consequent hypotension are most likely related to a release of the secondary cytokine TNF; TNF is also responsible for the similar hemodynamic changes observed in early septic shock—may exert its effect on vascular smooth muscle through the synthesis of nitric oxide; mechanism of the first dose sargramostim reaction is unclear, but appears to be unrelated to TNF [15]

DIFFERENTIAL DIAGNOSES
Bacterial sepsis; hypovolemia secondary to over-aggressive diuresis; vomiting, diarrhea, or bleeding; cardiac dysfunction; concomitant medications

PATIENT ASSESSMENT
Hemoglobin, hematocrit, ECG, BUN/creatinine; evaluate for infection, review daily weight.

MANAGEMENT OR INTERVENTION

Aldesleukin
1. Administer normal saline for a weight gain of between 5%–10% of baseline weight over the 5-d course of aldesleukin therapy
2. In patients with preexisting essential hypertension, therapy with antihypertensive agents should be stopped
3. For hypotension, administer up to 3 normal saline fluid boluses (250 mL each); once weight reaches > 5% of baseline, initiate pressors rather than continue fluid boluses
4. If hypotension persists despite adequate fluid replacement, begin dopamine hydrochloride, 2–8 µg/kg/min; titrate dose to maintain a systolic BP 80–100 mm Hg; monitor for occurrence of atrial tachyarrhythmias—if they occur, and hypotension persists, change to phenylephrine hydrochloride
5. Phenylephrine hydrochloride, 0.1–2.0 µg/kg/min, may be used alone or with dopamine for persistent hypotension
6. Hold dose of aldesleukin if patient remains hypotensive despite pressors or if high doses of pressors are required to maintain blood pressure

Sargramostim
1. Symptomatic management of first-dose effect includes oxygen therapy, intravenous fluids for hypotension, NSAIDs for musculoskeletal pains, and morphine sulfate reserved for severe pain;
2. Prehydration may decrease incidence and severity of hypotension

TOXICITY GRADING

0	1	2	3	4
None or no change	Changes requiring no therapy (including transient orthostatic hypotension)	Requires fluid replacement only	Requires pressors, resolves within 48 h of stopping the agent	Requires pressors for > 48 h after stopping the agent

CAPILLARY LEAK SYNDROME

The capillary leak (vascular leak) syndrome is a common dose-limiting side effect of aldesleukin and occasionally sargramostim therapy. The administration of high-dose aldesleukin and, less frequently, sargramostim and oprelvekin, results in a generalized increase in vascular permeability and fluid extravasation into the tissues. The capillary leak syndrome is often first manifested as mild facial and ankle edema within 24 h of the initiation of treatment. It may subsequently progress to anasarca during the course of treatment. Weight gain equivalent to 5%–10% of baseline body weight due to fluid retention, ascites (especially in patients with extensive hepatic metastases), pulmonary edema, and pleural and pericardial effusions are commonly observed. The development of pulmonary edema is more frequent in patients with marginal pulmonary reserve (*ie*, in patients with a pretreatment FEV_1 of ≤ 2.0 L) and in those whose treatment is complicated by bacteremia. Edema of the CNS occurs as well and can be fatal in patients with brain metastases. The capillary leak syndrome occurs to some degree in all patients receiving standard high-dose aldesleukin therapy, but only rarely in patients receiving sargramostim in doses ≤ 250 $\mu g/m^2/d$ or 6 $\mu g/kg/d$, and although more frequent, it is usually mild in patients receiving oprelvekin. The development of these potentially life-threatening side effects often contributes to decisions to withhold aldesleukin doses or otherwise limit the intensity or duration of a course of immunotherapy. Side effects resolve rapidly after the discontinuation of therapy, with most patients reverting to their baseline weight in 4 to 5 days after completion of a course of therapy [22,23].

CAUSATIVE AGENTS

Aldesleukin, sargramostim, oprelvekin

PATHOLOGIC PROCESS

Uncertain, but most likely a combination of several factors; direct endothelial injury mediated by aldesleukin activated leukocytes (NK and LAK cells, in particular), or their oxidative products; secondary cytokine release, TNF, and IL-1, which may induce various adhesion molecules necessary for attachment of activated leukocytes to endothelium) or systemic complement activation with resultant high plasma concentrations of anaphylatoxins such as C3a, which have potent effects on vascular permeability

DIFFERENTIAL DIAGNOSES

Bacterial sepsis; tumor progression with malignant effusions; IVC compression or thrombosis; hepatic dysfunction; congestive heart failure

PATIENT ASSESSMENT

Rule out infection; check radiograph, ECG, LFTs, albumin; evaluate for tumor progression with IVC compression; rule out IVC or other deep vein thrombosis.

MANAGEMENT OR INTERVENTION

Aldesleukin

1. Select patients carefully. Patients should have no evidence of cardiac disease or brain metastases, adequate pulmonary reserve ($FEV_1 \geq 2.0$ L or $\geq 75\%$ of predicted for height and age), no significant pleural or pericardial effusions, and ECOG performance status of 0–1
2. Administer normal saline intravenously to limit weight gain to 5%–10% of baseline weight over 5-d course of aldesleukin
3. Give oxygen therapy for symptomatic pleural effusions or pulmonary edema
4. For severe cardiovascular or pulmonary compromise, hold aldesleukin until symptoms have resolved; for life-threatening complications, dexamethasone, 10 mg IV q 6 h may be given
5. Once treatment has been completed and blood pressure is normal off pressors, begin diuresis with furosemide, 20–40 mg PO or IV daily until edema has resolved and patient has returned to baseline weight

Sargramostim and oprelvekin

1. Select patients carefully. Patients should have no evidence of cardiac disease or brain metastases, adequate pulmonary function and no significant pleural or pericardial effusions
2. Give oxygen therapy for symptomatic pleural effusions or pulmonary edema
3. Reduce dose for moderate cardiovascular or pulmonary compromise
4. For severe cardiovascular or pulmonary compromise, hold sargramostim and oprelvekin therapy until symptoms have resolved; for life-threatening complications, dexamethasone, 10 mg IV q 6 h may be given

TOXICITY GRADING

	0	1	2	3	4
Weight gain	< 5%	5%–9.9%	10.0%–19.9%	20%–29.9%	$\geq 30\%$
Pulmonary	None or no change	Asymptomatic, with abnormality in PFTs	Dyspnea on exertion	Dyspnea at rest	Severe symptoms not responsive to treatment, requiring intubation
Pericardial	None	Asymptomatic effusion, no intervention required	Pericarditis (rub, chest pain, ECG changes)	Symptomatic effusion; drainage required	Tamponade; drainage urgently required

ALLERGIC AND IMMUNE-MEDIATED COMPLICATIONS

Patients treated with aldesleukin, interferon α, rituximab, and less commonly, sargramostim, oprelvekin, filgrastim, levamisole, and BCG, may develop a variety of allergic and immune-mediated side effects. Although relatively common, local injection site reactions (cystitis with BCG, erythematous skin lesions at SC injection sites with the other agents) are generally self-limited. Acute serious hypersensitivity reactions, such as urticaria, angioedema, bronchoconstriction, and anaphylaxis have rarely been observed with these agents. Many of these agents have been associated with the development or exacerbation of preexisting autoimmune or chronic inflammatory diseases (eg, immune thrombocytopenia purpura, autoimmune hemolytic anemia, vitiligo, psoriasis, rheumatoid arthritis, vasculitis, thyroiditis, inflammatory bowel disease). In most cases, therapy must be discontinued.

Both neutralizing and nonneutralizing antibodies against aldesleukin, sargramostim, and interferon α-2 have been observed. The clinical significance of these antibodies remains unclear, but in several cases the development of neutralizing antibodies to interferon was associated with disease relapse [1,35]. The development of autoantibodies to insulin, thyroid peroxidase, platelets, and other antigens has been described, and many of these autoantibodies may be associated with the development of autoimmune disease. For example, thyroiditis, which is seen in 10%–20% of patients undergoing high-dose aldesleukin therapy, is frequently associated with the development of antithyroid antibodies.

Unusual recall reactions to iodinated contrast medium and cytotoxic chemotherapy have occurred in patients receiving aldesleukin therapy. As many as 10% of patients undergoing routine IV contrast studies during follow-up for previous aldesleukin therapy and 50% of patients receiving combination cisplatin-based chemotherapy with aldesleukin therapy develop such reactions. These reactions usually occur at least 1 mo after initial exposure to aldesleukin and contrast medium or on second or subsequent chemotherapy cycles. Typical reactions begin 1–4 h after reexposure to the agent and consist of fever, chills, rash, diarrhea, nausea, vomiting, urticaria, dyspnea, weakness, and hypotension; resolution is within 24 hours. Reactions appear to be more common in patients who receive aldesleukin and radiographic contrast medium simultaneously [28,32].

CAUSATIVE AGENTS
Aldesleukin, interferon α-2, BCG, levamisole, sargramostim, filgrastim

PATHOLOGIC PROCESS
Poorly defined: release of secondary cytokines may induce expression of HLA-DR antigens on cells, eg, thyrocytes. These cells are then rendered competent to present cell-specific antigens, eg, thyroglobulin, to autoreactive T lymphocytes already present in the host. In some cases, administered cytokine may play a direct role in pathogenesis. Recall reaction may be related to enhancement by aldesleukin of an immune response to radiographic contrast material, followed by an anamnestic response on reexposure to the contrast material.

DIFFERENTIAL DIAGNOSES
Allergic reactions or side effects of other medications, comorbid illnesses

PATIENT ASSESSMENT
Varies according to problem.

MANAGEMENT OR INTERVENTION
1. Avoid biologic therapy or administer with great caution in patients with history of autoimmune or chronic inflammatory disease
2. Manage acute serious allergic reactions in a standard way with antihistamines, epinephrine, and, in some cases, corticosteroids
3. Discontinue therapy if severe reactions develop
4. Avoid or significantly decrease "recall reaction" to iodinated contrast medium by pretreatment with antipyretics and antihistamines
5. Because of the relatively high frequency of thyroiditis, monitor thyroid function for patients on aldesleukin or interferon α-2 therapy
6. BCG cystitis may be treated symptomatically with phenazopyridine hydrochloride, 200 mg PO tid, propantheline bromide, 15 mg PO before meals and 30 mg PO qhs, oxbutynin hydrochloride, 5 mg PO tid

TOXICITY GRADING

0	1	2	3	4
None	Transient rash, drug fever < 38°C, 100.4°F	Urticaria, drug fever > 38°C, 100.4°F, mild bronchospasm	Serum sickness, bronchospasm, requires parenteral meds	Anaphylaxis

Immune-mediated complications may be graded using standard toxicity grading criteria for the affected organ or organs.

Tissue wasting is a common and often devastating sequela of the cancer-bearing state. This loss in body mass can result in multiorgan derangements, including impaired immune function, impaired locomotive capacity, and ultimately impaired respiratory function. As little as 5% reduction in lean body mass has been associated with increased mortality in cancer patients. Numerous factors contribute to produce wasting and malnutrition in these patients (Table 34-1). Advances in understanding of these factors as well as improvements in nutrient delivery methods and availability of immunostimulatory nutrients and growth factors offer exciting potential modalities for specific treatment of cancer-related wasting.

CAUSES

The factors that produce malnutrition in the cancer patient are well-known. Gastrointestinal obstruction from tumor, perioperative gastrointestinal tract dysfunction, and the oral and esophageal mucositis that often complicates chemotherapy or radiation represent physical impediments to nutrient intake. In addition, anorexia or a decreased desire for food is a common finding in cancer-bearing states. The causes of the anorexia may be direct actions of tumor-related mediators on the hypothalamic satiety centers or result indirectly from depression, nausea, or vomiting. Gastrointestinal fistula formation as well as diarrhea and malabsorption can result not only from direct influences of certain tumors but can complicate surgical, chemotherapeutic, or radiation treatment plans. The effects of such malabsorption on nutritional status are obvious (Fig. 32-1).

Even without clear physical reasons, and often at low tumor burdens, the cancer-bearing state may be associated with a syndrome of anorexia, weight loss, anemia, and severe lean tissue wasting. Although the mechanisms underlying this syndrome of cancer

cachexia remain elusive, the alterations in substrate handling that characterize this syndrome are well described [1] (Table 32-2) and are summarized briefly.

Glucose

Carbohydrate-related changes of the tumor-bearing state can be characterized by increases in glycolysis, anaerobic glycolysis by the tumor and certain host tissues, and insulin resistance. The increased glycolysis results in host glycogen depletion and is accompanied by an increase in liver gluconeogenesis. The resultant drain on body energy store is thought to be responsible, in part, for wasting of peripheral tissues.

Protein

The protein-specific changes associated with cancer cachexia are characterized by an increased peripheral skeletal muscle breakdown, decreased skeletal muscle protein synthesis, and an increased hepatic acute phase protein synthesis. The net result is an increased peripheral wasting. These protein metabolic changes often occur despite

Table 32-1. Causes of Malnutrition in Cancer Patients

Poor intake	Stress of surgery, chemotherapy, or radiation therapy
Anorexia	Perioperative intestinal dysfunction
Gastrointestinal dysfunction	Diarrhea
Blockage	Vomiting
Diarrhea	Anorexia
Malabsorption	Malabsorption
Altered substrate cycles	

Table 32-2. Changes in Substrate Handling in the Cancer Patient

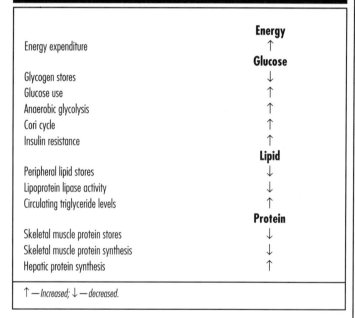

	Energy
Energy expenditure	↑
	Glucose
Glycogen stores	↓
Glucose use	↑
Anaerobic glycolysis	↑
Cori cycle	↑
Insulin resistance	↑
	Lipid
Peripheral lipid stores	↓
Lipoprotein lipase activity	↓
Circulating triglyceride levels	↑
	Protein
Skeletal muscle protein stores	↓
Skeletal muscle protein synthesis	↓
Hepatic protein synthesis	↑

↑ —Increased; ↓ —decreased.

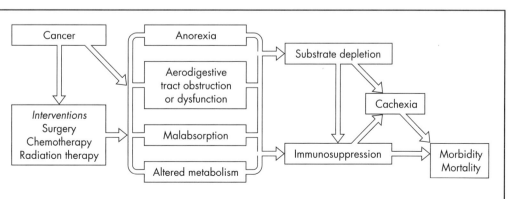

FIGURE 32-1.

Causes of malnutrition and cachexia in oncology patients.

decreased food intake, indicating an aberration in the normal mechanisms of protein preservation during starvation in these patients.

Fat

Central to the lipid-related changes in cancer is a decreased activity of lipoprotein lipase, which is a membrane-bound enzyme pivotal in triglyceride uptake by the peripheral adipocytes. The result is poor disposal of circulating triglycerides, peripheral lipid depletion, and hypertriglyceridemia. There also may be increased lipolysis, with the effect of loss of peripheral lipid stores, which is characteristic of the tumor-bearing state.

Vitamins

Patients with neoplastic disease are at a high risk for deficiency of vitamins. This deficiency results from a combination of poor intake, poor absorption, and increased requirements. Because of the limited stores of water-soluble vitamins within the body, deficiencies of these are more common and may occur even after relatively short-term dietary deprivation. Deficiency of fat-soluble vitamins usually results only after prolonged dietary deficiency or is related to compromised fat or bile absorption.

Vitamins may have a role in the prevention of cancers. Deficiencies of certain vitamins have been linked to an increased risk for malignancies. For example, deficiency of folate has been linked to increased risk of cancers of the esophagus, colon, bronchus, and cervix [2]. Therefore, experimental and clinical studies have sought to determine if vitamin supplementation may prevent development of cancer in high-risk groups. Administration of retinoids and β-carotene, which are synthetic analogues and precursors of vitamin A, have shown promise in the prevention of epithelial tumors [3,4]. In ulcerative colitis, an inflammatory condition that predisposes to colon cancer, folate supplementation has been shown to decrease the incidence of colonic neoplasia [5]. Although the definitive mechanisms by which each of these vitamins protects against tumor are incompletely defined, all of these vitamins have been shown to enhance anticancer immune function. Vitamins C and E and β-carotenes also have been shown to have antioxidant properties, whereas retinoids and folate have major roles in regulation of the cell cycles of normal and neoplastic cells. Further discussion of vitamins as a cancer prevention modality are beyond the scope of this chapter; interested readers are referred to reviews for a discussion of these issues [6,7]. This chapter concentrates on vitamin supplementation as it may relate to treatment of malnutrition.

ASSESSMENT

The simplest and most frequently used measures of nutritional status are the anthropometric measurements of weight, weight loss, arm circumference, and triceps skinfold thickness. Of these, weight loss has been found to be the most useful, with weight loss of more than 5% correlating with poor outcome. Arm circumference and triceps skinfold thickness are not good independent predictors of morbidity or mortality and therefore have limited use.

Circulating levels of serum proteins decrease with malnutrition and have been proposed as clinical markers of malnutrition. The most useful serum protein has been albumin, levels of which have been found to correlate inversely to complications. Because this protein has a circulating half-life on the order of 30 days, decreased circulating levels of this protein are a good index of persistent malnutrition but may not reflect acute changes. Measurements of prealbumin (half-life, 2 to 3 d) have been advocated as a better reflection of acute changes in nutritional status. Costs of measuring proteins other than albumin, however, are still too high to consider using them as routine in assessment of the cancer patient.

Urinary creatinine excretion has been advocated as a parameter of nutritional status because creatinine excretion in normal subjects is related to lean tissue mass. Patients with a creatinine-to-height ratio of less than 60% ideal as determined by standard tables usually are considered severely malnourished. In cancer-bearing states, however, nitrogen excretion often does not correlate with lean tissue mass. Nitrogen excretion has been found to persist at high levels even as wasting progresses, indicating persistent catabolic influences and rendering the creatinine-to-height ratio of little use in assessing nutrition reserve in this population. Nitrogen excretion is indicative of the level of catabolism and may guide efforts in repletion.

Immune parameters also have been touted as a criterion for malnutrition. These include delayed hypersensitivity skin testing and determination of total lymphocytic counts. Three problems exist for using such parameters in cancer patients, however. Immunosuppression can be a primary consequence of malignancy. Second, host immune function may be altered by other disease-related conditions, such as infection, hemorrhage, or cirrhosis. Third, iatrogenic factors, such as chemotherapeutic agents or surgical procedures, also may alter host immune function.

More sophisticated assessments of nutritional status, such as isotopic measurements of body composition or protein metabolism, are much too costly and complicated to be used routinely in the assessment of the cancer patient and are relegated to the research arena. Of the above-mentioned parameters, the major correlates to outcome are weight loss [8] and albumin levels. In fact, there are studies showing that a clinical history and clinical assessment are as good as any laboratory or physical parameter in predicting outcome [9]. Nevertheless, certain clinical findings should alert the clinician to significant nutrition and need for repletion, particularly if major surgical or chemotherapeutic intervention is planned (Table 32-3). These include weight loss of greater than 10%, weight loss of greater than 0.5 kg/week, evidence of muscular weakness, and serum albumin less than 3.2 g/dL [10]. A simple grading scale for the degree of malnutrition using these simple clinical and laboratory parameters is presented in Table 32-4.

Table 32-3. Assessment of Malnutrition in Cancer Patients

Absolute Indicators of Malnutrition	Relative Indicators of Malnutrition
Weight loss > 10%	Immune parameters
Weight loss of 0.5 kg/wk	Anergy in delayed hypersensitivity testing
Clinically evident muscular weakness	T cell numbers < 1500/mL
Serum albumin < 3.2 g/dL	Decreased complement levels
	Hypoproteinemia
	Thyroxine-binding prealbumin
	Transferrin
	Retinol binding protein
	Creatinine:height ratio < 60% ideal
	Negative nitrogen balance
	Clinical
	Stomatitis
	Gastrointestinal dysfunction

Table 32-4. Toxicity Scale for Malnutrition

Grade	Degree of Malnutrition	Clinical Findings	Laboratory Findings
0	None	No weight loss	Normal albumin Normal transferrin level Reactive delayed hypersensitivity skin test
1	Mild	Weight loss < 5%	Albumin < 3.5 Decreased transferrin level
2	Moderate	5%–10% weight loss	< 5 mm reactivity on skin test Albumin < 3.2
3	Severe	Weight loss > 10% Muscular weakness	Nonreactive skin test Albumin < 2.7

In the clinical consideration of cancer patients, all patients should be assessed for vitamin deficiency. The most common symptoms for deficiencies of the various vitamins are summarized in Table 32-5. The patient history should be evaluated for risk factors predisposing to vitamin insufficiency. Dietary history should look specifically for poor oral intake. Assessment should be made for signs and symptoms of intestinal or biliary obstruction, symptoms of pancreatic insufficiency or fat malabsorption, or past history of intestinal resection. Any of these conditions may result in deficiencies of fat-soluble vitamins [11] because bile and fats are important for absorption of these vitamins. Vitamin B_{12} deficiency also may result from disease or resection of the terminal small bowel because this vitamin is absorbed in this region. Patients on long-term antibiotic therapy or mechanical bowel cleansing also may develop deficiencies of vitamins normally produced by the intestinal flora, such as biotin and vitamin K. Although laboratory tests for deficiencies of individual vitamins are available (*see* Table 32-5), their routine use in the screening of asymptomatic patients is discouraged.

TREATMENT

Strategies with the aim to treat malnutrition associated with cancer-bearing states must be directed at repleting lean tissue losses that have already occurred and preventing further loss of vital tissues. Such strategies have to overcome two basic obstacles. First are the physical factors that prevent intake or absorption of nutrients and second are the alterations in host metabolic substrate handling that predispose to tissue wasting. Clinical and experimental strategies that

Table 32-5. Symptoms of Vitamin Deficiencies and Assays for Confirmation of Deficiencies

	Fat-Soluble Vitamins		
Vitamin	**Symptoms of Deficiency**	**Toxicity**	**Test for Deficiency**
A	Night blindness, conjunctival xerotosis, hyperkeratosis, immune dysfunction, increased cerebrospinal fluid pressure, anemia, hepatosplenomegaly, anorexia	Dry mucous membranes, hepatic fibrosis, anemia, pseudotumor cerebri, headache, vomiting, diplopia	Optic dark adaptation, plasma retinol level, retinol-binding protein
D	Osteomalacia, bone fractures	Nephrocalcinosis, renal insufficiency, metastatic calcifications	Plasma calcidiol levels, plasma calcitriol levels
E	Hemolytic anemia, neuromuscular damage, brain stem demyelination	Nausea, headache, fatigue	Blood total tocopherols
K	Bleeding disorder	Hemolytic anemia, vomiting, anaphylaxis	Prothrombin time
	Water-Soluble Vitamins		
C	Anorexia, irritability, weight loss, hemorrhage, anemia	Nausea, vomiting, diarrhea, hemolysis	Plama vitamin C level
Thiamine	Peripheral neuropathy, congestive heart failure, cardiomegaly, edema, confusion, ataxia, nystagmus	Anaphylaxis	Urinary thiamine level
Riboflavin (B_2)	Stomatitis, glossitis, dermatitis	None	Erythrocyte riboflavin content
Niacin	Dermatitis, diarrhea, dementia, anorexia	Flushing	Urinary niacin
B_6	Anemia, stomatitis, irritability	Liver injury, ataxia, peripheral neuropathy	Tryptophan loading test
Folate	Macrocytic anemia, leukopenia	Renal damage	Serum or RBC folate levels
B_{12}	Megaloblastic anemia, peripheral neuropathy, confusion, memory loss, dementia	None	Serum holotranscobalamin II level, serum B_{12} level

Table 32-6. Potential Treatments of Malnutrition in Cancer Patients

Eradication of tumor	Growth factors
Increasing nutrient intake	Anabolic steroids
Enteral supplementation	Insulin
IV supplementation	Growth hormone
Specific nutrient administration	Insulin-like growth factors
Nucleotides	Pharmacologic agents
Specific amino acids	Megestrol
Polyunsaturated free fatty acids	Metoclopramide
	Dronabinol

have been devised and practiced can be divided into four main categories: elimination of tumor, increasing nutrient intake, use of growth factors, and use of pharmacologic agents (Table 32-6). Elimination of tumor, whether by surgery, chemotherapy, or radiation is paramount and may reverse many of the derangements associated with cancer cachexia.

Increasing Nutrient Intake

Total Parenteral Nutrition in the Surgical Patient

Since the landmark report of Dudrick and coworkers in 1965 showing that high caloric IV feeding alone can provide long-term sustenance for patients, total parenteral nutrition (TPN) has become a widely used part of the clinical armamentarium. In cancer patients at least 19 studies examining this modality have been published and reviewed [12]. Although the majority are negative studies that do not show improvements in outcome parameters even with aggressive feeding, most studies are flawed by poor control groups, small sample sizes, and heterogeneity of patient population. These shortcomings are discussed at length in the metanalysis of this literature by Detsky and coworkers [12]. A number of these studies are sufficiently well executed to deserve further discussion (Table 32-7).

Muller and colleagues examined patients with TPN undergoing gastric or esophageal surgery and found that parenteral feedings for 10 days (*n* = 66) significantly reduced the rate of mortality and major

postoperative complications when compared with control patients undergoing customary oral feedings (*n* = 59) [13]. A subsequent study by the Veterans Affairs Study Group [14] examined patients (*n* = 395) undergoing abdominal or thoracic surgery. Although no overall differences existed between the groups in terms of morbidity or mortality in this study of 7 to 10 days of preoperative TPN, in subset analysis, for patients with severe malnutrition as defined by clinical parameters (weight loss > 20%, serum albumin < 2.9), there was an advantage in preoperative TPN. Fan and coworkers [15] published a trial in which patients undergoing hepatectomy for hepatocellular carcinoma were randomized to receive or not receive preoperative TPN; they found patients receiving TPN to have a significantly lower complication rate. This may yet be another trial demonstrating the use of nutritional support in a severely malnourished patient population because patients suffering from hepatocellular carcinoma generally have cirrhosis and poor baseline nutritional status.

Lacking further evidence, a reasonable recommendation is that in preoperative patients with greater than 10% weight loss, preoperative aggressive nutritional supplementation is reasonable, whether by the enteral or parenteral route. If the decision is to use the parenteral route, at least a 7- to 10-day course of TPN is warranted. There is no evidence that any shorter course has clinical efficacy, and TPN is certainly not without complications (Table 32-8). A more recent randomized, controlled trial evaluated the effect of early postoperative TPN on outcome of patients undergoing surgery for upper gastrointestinal cancers and found no benefit to TPN. The patients randomizing to postoperative TPN actually had a higher infection rate compared with controls [16]. Routine postoperative parenteral nutritional feeding therefore is not justified. Only in patients with prolonged intestinal dysfunction or with severe malnutrition should TPN be used. Typical orders for initiating TPN are outlined in Table 32-9.

Total Parenteral Nutrition in the Chemotherapy Patient

Common adverse effects of chemotherapy include anorexia, emesis, diarrhea, and intestinal mucosal sloughing that leads to malabsorption. These effects and the fact that chemotherapy patients tend to have more advanced disease and larger tumor burdens make this group attractive to treat with parenteral nutrition. Despite our clinical prejudice that supplemental nutrient administration should

Table 32-7. Major Studies of Nutritional Support in Cancer Patients

First Author	Year	Reference	Feeding	Patient Population	Findings
Parenteral nutrition					
Mullin	1980	*Ann Surg* 192:604	TPN—10 d preoperatively	Gastrointestinal surgery patients (*n*=145)	Improved survival, reduced complications
Muller	1982	*Lancet* 1:68[13]	TPN—10 d preoperatively	Esophageal and gastric resections (*n*=125)	Improved survival, reduced complications
VA Cooperative Group	1991	*N Engl J Med* 325:525[14]	TPN—7–10 d preoperatively	Gastrointestinal and thoracic surgery (*n*=117)	Reduced complications in severely malnourished subset
Brennan	1994	*Ann Surg* 220:436[16]	TPN—postoperatively	Upper gastrointestinal malignancies (*n*=117)	No benefit
Fan	1994	*N Engl J Med* 331:1547[15]	TPN—preoperatively	Liver surgery patients	Improved survival
Enteral Nutrition					
Evans	1987	*J Clin Oncol* 5:113	Oral diet counseling and supplementation	Chemotherapy patients for lung or colon cancer (*n*=192)	Improved caloric intake, no change in clinical parameters

TPN—Total parenteral nutrition.

Table 32-8. Common Complications of Total Parenteral Nutrition

Complication	Frequency, %
Central line–related	
Pneumothorax	1–3
Thrombophlebitis*	1–2
Brachial plexus injury	0.5–1
Carotid or subclavian artery injuries	0.25–0.5
Overall	4–15
Infectious	
Line sepsis	2–10
Metabolic	
Electrolyte abnormalities	
Hyperglycemia (including hyperglycemic hyperosmotic coma)	
Hyperkalemia	
Hypomagnesemia	
Hypophosphatemia	
Acid-base disturbances	
Most commonly hyperchloremic metabolic acidosis	
Congestive heart failure	
Altered liver function	
Overall†	5–10

*Clinically apparent thrombophlebitis, angiographically evident thrombophlebitis may be 25% to 30% in select populations.
†Severe metabolic complications.

Table 32-9. Typical Orders for Total Parenteral Nutrition

Makeup of Typical Total Parenteral Nutrition Solution (per 1000 mL)

Nutrients	
Mixed amino acid	50 g
Dextrose	250 g
Electrolytes	
Calcium gluconate	4.6 mEq
Magnesium sulfate	8 mEq
Potassium chloride	22.4 mEq
Potassium phosphate	12 mM
Sodium acetate	18 mEq
Sodium chloride	33.5 mEq
Trace elements (per day)	
Zinc	5 mg
Copper	2 mg
Manganese	0.5 mg
Chromium	10 µg
Multivitamins (per day)	
Vitamin A	1mg
Ergocalciferol (vitamin D)	5 µg
Vitamin E	10 mg
Thiamine	3 mg
Riboflavin	3.6 mg
Niacinamide	40 mg
Dexpanthenol	15 mg
Pyridoxine HCl	4 mg
Biotin	60 µg
Cyanocobalamin	5 µg
Folic acid	400 mg
Ascorbic acid	100 mg
Fat emulsions	500 mL of 10% solution twice a week (4% of total nonprotein calories)

Medical Orders Relating to Start of Total Parenteral Nutrition

Start infusion at 40 mL/h
Maximum incremental increase should be 40 mL/h
Routine catheter care
Infuse total parenteral nutrition via pump
Vital signs q 6 h
Urine by dipstick q 6 h
Stat glucose for > 2+ and call house officer
Strict input and output
Weight 3 times/week
Routine blood tests
3 times/week: Electrolytes, liver function tests, glucose
Once weekly: Prothrombin time, CBC, platelet count, cholesterol, triglyceride, transferrin

improve clinical status of these patients and animal experimental data suggesting that TPN improves outcome from chemotherapy, no clinical data exist to support this. A multitude of studies have been performed and are summarized by McGeer and coworkers [17]. The conclusions of this position paper by the American College of Physicians were that TPN in the mildly malnourished medical oncology patient may be more harmful than helpful, likely owing to catheter sepsis in this immunosuppressed population. Further, in the severely malnourished person, more data needs to be gathered before a conclusion of the risk-to-benefit ratio of TPN can be determined.

Total Parenteral Nutrition in Radiation Therapy Patients

There have been relatively few studies examining the efficacy of nutritional supplementation and the results of radiation therapy for cancer. They can be described as small, poorly controlled studies that are inconclusive and have been reviewed [18]. Based on current clinical data, no conclusion with regard to intravenous nutritional supplement in this population can be made.

Enteral Feedings

The majority of studies concerning aggressive nutritional supplementation and the cancer patient are performed using parenteral nutrition. Certainly, in patients with nonfunctional gastrointestinal tracts, the intravenous route represents the only option. When the enteral route is an option, however, there is clear evidence that this route is preferable from an immunologic and metabolic standpoint. Animal and human data indicate that feeding by the intravenous route particularly suppresses host immunologic function. Only one prospective study of adequate sample size has examined the use of enteral feedings in the treatment of cancer patients. In a study of 192 patients with unresectable colorectal or lung cancer, patients were randomized to three groups: nutritional intake without restriction, dietary counseling, and dietary counseling and enteral defined formula supplementation if goals of 1.7 to 1.95 times resting energy expenditure were not reached [19]. No difference in clinical outcome could be discerned among the groups in this study. It must be noted, however, that aggressive tube feedings were not pursued in this study. Studies examining aggressive enteral feeding protocols for preoperative, chemotherapy, or radiation therapy patients are still largely lacking, and this is an active area of research. There is certainly a large selection of enteral supplements available for the nutritional treatment of the cancer patient (*see* Table 32-9).

Specific Nutrients

In addition to strategies that improve total caloric and nitrogen intake there are also strategies aimed at delivering specific nutrients at high concentrations to the patients. These clinical strategies are based on experimental studies that demonstrate some nutrients to have particularly potent trophic or stimulatory effects on components of the host defense mechanism. Most of these strategies must be considered experimental.

Nucleotides

Nucleotides are essential components of cellular RNA and DNA. Dietary deficiency of nucleic acids alters host cellular immunity, as measured by natural killer cell activity, T cell response to mitogens, and macrophage cytokine release. Exogenous administration of polynucleotides enhances natural killer cell activity and release of cytokines. One randomized trial on the use of nucleic acids on cancer patients has been performed. In a placebo-controlled trial of patients undergoing resection of breast cancer, there was enhanced survival in polyadenylic acid–treated postmenopausal patients [20]. Further studies need to be performed to verify these results and examine whether similar effects on patients with other tumor types exist. Even before such studies are performed, however, tube feedings supplemented with nucleotides are already commercially available (Table 32-10).

Amino Acids

GLUTAMINE

The amino acid glutamine is a primary nitrogenous substrate used by the gastrointestinal tract. It appears to be a particularly potent trophic factor for intestinal mucosa. Specific use of this amino acid

has two goals in mind: improvement of gut barrier function and improvement of intestinal absorptive capacity. For this reason trials are underway to examine the efficacy of adding this amino acid to parenteral and enteral feedings. Preliminary studies from bone marrow transplant patients have not shown a major beneficial role for this amino acid in protecting against complications [21]. Trials in other cancer populations are underway.

ARGININE

Arginine is another amino acid with established immunostimulatory effects. Administration of high doses of this amino acid to cancer patients enhances in vitro parameters of lymphocyte function, including natural killer cell activity, lymphocyte response to stimulation, and increased T helper cell numbers [22]. Whether this translates to improved outcome during cancer therapy is uncertain. Active trials examining the use of this amino acid in the treatment of cancer patients are in progress.

Polyunsaturated Free Fatty Acids

Composition of the dietary fat also seems to have a major effect on host immune function. In particular, the contents of unsaturated free fatty acids appear to be a major determinant of lymphocyte function and macrophage cytokine production. Experimental studies have documented that diets containing fish oils that are high in n-3 fatty acids can enhance not only measured host immune function but can protect against infection and sepsis. The effects of fish oils or the manipulations of the dietary fats on tumor-bearing states remain unexplored. The findings from studies on sepsis and infection as well as the prevalence of infection in the cancer-bearing populations encourage these lines of investigation.

Vitamins

The causes of vitamin deficiency in cancer patients can be classified into three broad categories: altered intake, altered absorption and metabolism, and increased requirements. These causes contribute to the frequency of vitamin deficiency in this population.

There are many causes of poor vitamin intake. Mechanical obstruction of the oral-digestive tract by certain malignancies is an

Table 32-10. Common Oral Nutritional Supplements

Product	Calories/mL	Nonprotein calories:gN	Osmolality	Tube/Oral	Taste	Cost	Advantage
Isocal	1.06	167:1	300	Both	Fair	+	Isotonic, tolerated well orally, inexpensive
Isocal HCN	2.00	145:1	690	Both	Fair	++	Useful in fluid restriction
Ensure	1.06	153:1	470	Both	Good	+	Taste suitable for oral supplement, inexpensive, low residue/can be used for bowel preparation
Ensure Plus	1.50	146:1	690	Both	Fair	++	Useful in fluid restriction, low residue
Sustacal HC	1.50	134:1	650	Both	Good	++	Low sodium content
Isosource HN	1.20	116:1	330	Both	Fair	++	Low residue
Specialty Formulas							
Pulmocare	1.50	125:1	520	Tube	Poor	+++++	Low nonprotein caloric content may be beneficial for patients with pulmonary compromise
Impact	1.00	71:1	375	Tube	Poor	+++++	Contains arginine, fish oils, nucleotides: suggested to improve immune function
Elemental Formulas							
Vivonex TEN	1.00	149:1	630	Tube	Poor	+++++	Elemental/predigested, low fat, low residue
Criticare HN	1.06	148:1	650	Tube	Poor	++++	Elemental/predigested, low fat, low residue

obvious cause. During treatment, patients may be kept without oral intake either for diagnostic testing or therapeutic interventional procedures. Anorexia, nausea, and vomiting related to either tumor or treatment are other causes. Vitamins, by definition, must be obtained from dietary or parenteral routes. Fat-soluble vitamins (see Table 32-5) usually are stored in high amounts within the body; unless patients have other causes for deficiencies or poor intake is prolonged (> 3 months) it is unusual for patients to manifest a clinically significant deficiency of these vitamins. Water-soluble vitamins are more prone to deficiencies from short-term deprivation because, with the exception of vitamin B_{12}, water-soluble vitamins are stored in limited amounts within the body. Assessment of deficiency or empiric supplementation should be considered for any patient with mechanical obstruction of the oral-digestive tract.

Altered dietary fat content can have profound effects on the absorption of fat-soluble vitamins. Other alterations in fat absorption, such as exocrine pancreatic insufficiency, also could result in deficiency of fat-soluble vitamins. Additionally, these fat-soluble vitamins depend on bile acids for absorption. Any interruption of the enterohepatic circulation of bile affects body stores of these vitamins. Therefore, any patient who has biliary obstruction, external biliary drainage or fistula, or resection of the terminal ileum should be assessed clinically for deficiencies of vitamins A, E, D, and K. Many vitamins are manufactured partly by the bacterial flora in the gastrointestinal tract, but this source of vitamins is particularly importantly for vitamin K. In any patient submitted to removal of a significant portion of the large intestine or who undergoes mechanical or antibiotic clearance of intestinal bacterial flora, exogenous supplementation with vitamin K may be necessary.

Patients with cancer may have an increased requirement for certain vitamins. In studies measuring levels of vitamins, patients with cancer may have a deficiency despite intakes judged adequate by recommended daily allowances (RDA) for normal people. In one study of vitamin C nearly half of the patients with cancer had a deficiency of intracellular vitamin C when their leukocytes were assayed [23]. Stressed patients have particularly high niacin requirements [24]. Folate deficiency is also more common in patients with malignancy. More systematic studies are necessary before determining if an RDA for cancer patients should be adopted. Therapeutic interventions for cancer also can increase vitamin requirements. It is well accepted that surgical stress increased requirements for certain vitamins important for protein synthesis and wound healing, including vitamin C. Certain chemotherapeutic agents have been definitively documented to increase the requirements for vitamins. The use of the 5-fluorouracil, for example, has been shown to increase the need for niacin [25].

Patients with clinically evident deficiencies of specific vitamins should be repleted according to the guidelines in Table 32-11. The assays listed in Table 32-5 allow confirmation of deficiencies of individual vitamins. Empiric supplementation with the RDAs of each vitamin through the use of multisupplement tablets for patients with no symptoms of vitamin deficiency is recommended for cancer patients undergoing therapy because this is more cost-effective than using the various assays to document subclinical deficiency. All patients on TPN should receive vitamin supplementation. The doses to be added to the TPN are elaborated in Table 32-9. Fat-soluble vitamins bind to the plastics on intravenous administration equipment, and bioavailability of the administered vitamins may be significantly lower than that intended. Additionally, certain vitamins, such as vitamin A, are light sensitive and should be added to the TPN solution immediately before administration or kept in shielded bags. Even with these precautions, only 25% to 30% of the administered parenteral dose reaches the patient.

Growth Factors

Advances over the last century have uncovered the important roles that peptide growth factors and steroids play in growth and development. It was not until recently, however, with widespread application of molecular biologic techniques, that large-scale production of many growth factors was possible. Peptide hormones, such as insulin, growth hormone, and insulin-like growth factor, are available in large quantities and, along with anabolic steroids, represent potential therapeutic modalities for cancer cachexia. Although many studies have been performed examining the potential roles of growth factors in the cancer patient, their role in the clinical treatment of this population is poorly defined.

Insulin

This pancreatic hormone has major anabolic and catabolic effects. It promotes amino acid and carbohydrate uptake by many tissues, increases use of glucose for glycogen synthesis and lipogenesis and protein synthesis, and decreases gluconeogenesis and lipolysis. In these ways, insulin is a major determinant of normal metabolism and growth. Clinicians have long attempted to harness the tissue-sparing effects of this polypeptide in the treatment of catabolic disease. The three major clinical studies in the injured population involved either burn or trauma patients. In these populations, infusions of high doses of insulin along with high glucose intravenous feedings produced laboratory measures of protein sparing, such as decreased urinary nitrogen excretion or decreased 3-methyl histidine excretion. These studies were difficult to interpret because the treatment populations had significantly higher caloric intakes than the control populations.

Table 32-11. Recommended Daily Allowances of Various Vitamins and Treatment Recommendations for Deficiences

Vitamin	Male RDA*	Female RDA	Treatment for Deficiency
Fat-Soluble Vitamins			
A	3300 U	2600 U	100,000 U/day x 3 d, then 50,000 U/day x 2 weeks
D	200 U	200 U	1000–10,000 U/d orally or 10,000 U IM
E	10 mg	8 mg	40–50 mg/d orally or IM
K	80 µg	65 µg	10–15 mg SQ or IV q day x 3 d
Water-Soluble Vitamins			
C	60 mg	60 mg	100–250 mg tid orally, IM, or IV
Thiamine	1.5 mg	1.1 mg	5–10 mg tid or 5–100 mg IM/IV
Riboflavin	1.7 mg	1.3 mg	5–30 mg/d orally or 50 mg IM
Niacin	19 mg	15 mg	10–50 mg tid orally or IM
B_6	2.0 mg	1.6 mg	10–20 mg q day x 3 weeks, then 3–5 mg q day orally, or 30–600 mg IV or IM
Folate	200 µg	180 µg	1–5 mg/d orally, IV
B_{12}	2.0 µg	2.0 µg	1 mg IM q day x 7 days, then weekly

RDA — Recommended daily allowance for age 25 to 50.

In addition, two possible complications associated with high-dose insulin infusions have deterred clinical use. First, when high doses of insulin are employed, life-threatening hypoglycemia is a possible complication. In some studies, monitoring of serum glucose has been as frequent as every hour [26]. Second, high-dose insulin and glucose infusions may produce marked increases in lipogenesis. Such an increase in lipogenesis may manifest sufficient increases of carbon dioxide production to overcome pulmonary reserve and product respiratory compromise and failure. An increased lipogenesis also may lead to fatty liver formation and hepatic dysfunction. High-dose insulin alone is unlikely to be a clinically useful adjunct to nutritional supplementation.

Growth Hormone

Growth hormone is a 191–amino acid polypeptide secreted by the anterior pituitary gland and is a prime stimulus for growth during puberty. In adults, this hormone also is released in an intermittent pulsatile pattern that may be important in normal homeostasis. The actions of this hormone are complex but can be summarized briefly as protein anabolic lipolytic and gluconeogenic. It appears that this hormone redirects the body to use lipids as fuel in preference to proteins and is thus an attractive agent in the treatment of the catabolic patient. Despite these clear theoretic advantages, proving clinical use of growth hormone in the injured patient has been difficult.

The majority of clinical nutritional studies performed before the availability of synthetic human growth hormone in the mid-1980s were performed in orthopedic or burn patients. Since then numerous preclinical studies and three clinical studies in cancer patients have been performed (Table 32-12). A most impressive clinical testimony to the potent influences of growth hormone on nitrogen accrual is the study of Jiang and coworkers [27] demonstrating that even in the setting of hypocaloric feedings, growth hormone can produce positive nitrogen balance in patients after surgery for intraabdominal tumor. Although these studies in cancer patients as well as a majority of studies in other clinical populations provided evidence for improved nitrogen retention with growth hormone administration, none has provided evidence that this is accompanied by improved clinical outcome. This situation likely is due to the small sample sizes in all studies performed to date and the short follow-up in these studies. A large randomized trial of this hormone in the cancer patient is imperative because the cost of this hormone is not inconsequential.

More recently, combination therapy consisting of growth hormone and insulin has been studied as adjuncts to nutritional supplementation. Preliminary studies in cancer patients [28] have shown that daily injections of growth hormone for 3 days followed by a constant infusion of insulin acutely promotes skeletal muscle and whole body nitrogen retention at doses of insulin that are of a long magnitude less than the previously discussed clinical studies of insulin alone. The mechanisms of the hormone interaction and whether this or other combinations of growth factors will be clinically useful await future studies.

Insulin-Like Growth Factor 1

Insulin-like growth factor 1 (IGF-1), originally isolated and called somatomedin-C, is an intermediary hormone that mediates many of the actions of growth hormone. IGF-1 exerts many of the effects of insulin, including hypoglycemia and inhibition of lipolysis. In vitro, IGF-1 stimulates protein synthesis, and in vivo this hormone inhibits proteolysis. With synthesis of this molecule by recombinant techniques, potentially limitless quantities are now available, facilitating in vivo studies and making large-scale clinical trials possible. Studies of this hormone as nutritional adjunct in animals have been encouraging. Results of initial clinical studies should be available in the near future.

Anabolic Steroids

Androgenic steroids have long been known to have potent anabolic activities. Pharmacologic modifications of the natural androgens have been performed with the aim to reduce their androgenic actions, increase the ease of administration, and enhance their anabolic actions. Such efforts have resulted in production of a class of synthetic compounds referred to as anabolic steroids.

These compounds have been tested in the clinical setting for a long time. As early as 1944, Abels and coworkers found testosterone propionate to enhance nitrogen balance in three patients with gastric

Table 32-12. Major Studies of Growth Factors in Cancer Patients

First Author	Year	Reference	Agent	Patient Population	Findings
Growth Hormone					
Ward	1986	*Ann Surg* 206:56	hGH	GI surgery patients (n=16)	Increased fat oxidation, decreased protein oxidation
Jiang	1989	*Ann Surg* 210:513[27]	hGH	GI surgery patients (n=18)	Increased protein synthesis
Douglas	1990	*Br J Surg* 77:785	hGH	Total parenteral nutrition patients (n=25)	Reduced protein loss
Growth Hormone and Insulin					
Wolf	1992	*Ann Surg* 216:280[28]	hGH and insulin	GI surgery patients (n=28)	Reduced protein loss
Anabolic Steroids					
Abels	1944	*J Clin Endocrinol Metab* 4:198[29]	Testosterone	Gastric cancer (n=5)	Improved nitrogen balance
Johnston	1963	*Br J Surg* 50:924	Methandienone	GI surgery (n=25)	Improved nitrogen balance
Young	1982	*J Paren Ent Nutr* 7:221	Nandrolone decanoate	Perioperative patients (n=24)	Decreased plasma amino acids
Hansell	1989	*J Paren Ent Nutr* 13:349[30]	Stanozolol	Colorectal surgery (n=60)	Improved nitrogen balance

hGH—Human growth hormone; GI—gastrointestinal.

cancer [29]. Since then, the clinical use of anabolic steroids has been examined in diverse clinical populations, including at least three other studies in cancer patients. The study of Hansell and coworkers [30] deserves particular mention because it is the only study of even moderate size [30]. In this study, 60 colorectal surgery patients were randomized to receive or not receive stanozolol along with either hypocaloric or eucaloric supplementation. Improved nitrogen balance was noted only in the group with hypocaloric nutrition. The studies on cancer patients are summarized in Table 34-10. Although a number of studies have shown an improvement in serum or urine parameters of nitrogen retention, no study to date has shown an improvement in any clinical outcome parameter. This may again be the result of inadequate sample sizes in the studies. Additionally the varied nutritional regimens and the steroid preparations used make this literature particularly difficult to decipher. One must conclude that the question of whether anabolic steroids have any role as an adjunct to clinical nutrition remains unanswered. Certainly, a large trial, possibly in a multicenter fashion, is necessary to evaluate use of these compounds by clinical outcome.

Another major obstacle to using anabolic steroids in the clinical setting is the significant side effects of these compounds. Virilization is a potential side effect, often manifest by hirsutism, acne, clitoral hypertrophy, voice coarsening, and male pattern baldness. Alternatively, peripheral conversion of testosterone and androstenedione to estradiol and estrone may result in "feminizing" effects, such as gynecomastia. Other potential detrimental effects include hypogonadism; lipoprotein abnormalities, including increased low-density lipoprotein; sleep apnea; and hepatic complications, including development of hepatocellular carcinoma.

Nutritional Support and Growth Factors

A major goal of aggressive nutritional support is growth of normal tissues. A commonly voiced concern in nutritional support of the cancer patient, however, is disproportional growth of the neoplastic tissues. Such concerns are fueled by animal studies documenting disproportionately enhanced tumor growth by nutritional support. No clinical study in patients corroborates these animal models. Using stable isotope methods, Mullen and colleagues could not demonstrate an increased synthetic rate in tumor tissues compared to normal tissues [31].

A major theoretic obstacle to routine use of growth factors in the clinical setting is fear that growth factors may stimulate cancer growth. Animal and in vivo studies have linked growth hormone to development of certain lymphoid malignancies [32]. IGF-1 has been shown to be a stimulus for in vitro growth of breast tumors [33] and lung tumors [34]. Data also exist that show that growth hormone administration in rats actually decreased the number of tumor metastases in a transplantable adenocarcinoma model in rodents [35]. The relative influences of the mitogenic effects of growth factors compared with their beneficial influence on host cancer surveillance through improvements in immunocompetence remain to be determined. Further, if certain growth factors are capable of shifting tumors into the proliferative phase, such action may render tumors more sensitive to radiotherapy or chemotherapy. Therapeutic investigations using this treatment strategy are currently underway in myeloid leukemia, in which colony-stimulating factors are being administered as priming agents to stimulate acute myeloid leukemic blast cells to become more sensitive to cell cycle–specific chemotherapy. No human study has examined the effects of growth factors on cancer appearance or growth. These studies will not only be interesting but also will be necessary before accepting growth factor therapy as a routine clinical modality. Trials of growth factors as adjuncts to chemotherapy or radiotherapy will undoubtedly be an area of fruitful future investigation.

Pharmacologic Agents

In addition to the various growth factors and anabolic steroids many pharmacologic agents have been proposed as potential agents for enhancing weight gain during treatment for malignancy. Following are three that have undergone the most extensive trials.

Megestrol Acetate (Megace)

Megestrol acetate is a synthetic progestational agent used in the therapy of advanced breast cancer. In this population, the clinical observation was made that this agent improved appetite and weight gain. Although the relative importance of the central nervous system appetite-stimulating effects of this compound versus the metabolic effects of megestrol on peripheral tissue metabolism are still being debated, clinical trials of this compound as a nutritional adjunct in cancer patients have begun. In one study, 89 patients with various tumor types were studied in a randomized, placebo-controlled study [36]. The patients receiving megestrol had a significantly improved appetite and food intake. Although clinical use of this medication as a modality in the treatment of disease-related malnutrition is far from proven, megestrol holds promise in such a capacity and is under investigation for a variety of disease states [37].

Cyproheptadine (Periactin)

Cyproheptadine (Periactin) is an antihistamine that has been tested in the cancer population because the compound enhances appetite in humans without cancer. Early trials had suggested that cyproheptadine may increase appetite in tumor-bearing humans, but more recent studies have failed to verify this. In a randomized, blinded, placebo trial involving 295 patients with advanced malignancy, there was no improvement in anorexia or weight gain [38]. There is no role for this medication in the clinical treatment of cancer cachexia.

Metoclopramide (Reglan)

Primary effects of tumor-bearing states as well as effects of treatment may produce alterations in intestinal motility. The most prominent treatment-related factors are postsurgical ileus and intestinal dysmotility associated with narcotic administration. Metoclopramide has been proposed as an agent to alleviate intestinal dysmotility in these and other cancer-related situations. Although metoclopramide improves gastric emptying following gastrointestinal surgery and in select cancer-bearing states, whether administration of this medication can have an impact on any clinically measurable nutritional parameter remains undetermined. Future prospective trials with defined nutritional end points are necessary to ascertain the use of this agent in clinical practice.

Dronabinol (Marinol)

Whether from disease or treatment, nausea and vomiting are a significant part of the clinical course of cancer patients. Nausea and vomiting can be a prime reason for reduced food intake. Strategies for improving nutritional status have been directed at mitigating nausea and vomiting. Dronabinol, the major active ingredient of the marijuana plant, is an effective agent in treating of otherwise refractory nausea and vomiting. This reduction in nausea is likely the mechanism of improved appetite that was noted in early studies using this medication. A small (n = 42) single-arm trial evaluating this medication with appetite and weight loss as clinical parameters has been performed. Administration of dronabinol improved appetite and reduced the rate of weight loss [39]. Further controlled trials are needed to ascertain the efficacy of this medication in the nutritional treatment of cancer patients.

Other Agents

As the mechanisms of the anorexia and altered substrate cycles associated with cancer-bearing states are better understood, many other agents emerged as potential therapeutic modalities for cancer cachexia. For example, as the causative roles of cytokines such as tumor necrosis factor and interleukin-1 in mediating the anorexia and metabolic changes in cancer are elucidated, agents such as specific antibodies against these cytokines or pharmacologic agents such as pentoxyifylline that block the effects of these cytokines may emerge as useful modalities in clinical treatment of cachexia [40]. However, these must be regarded as experimental agents.

CONCLUSION

It is agreed that progressive nutritional depletion is often a major clinical feature of the cancer patient, at times dominating the clinical manifestations of the disease. Many strategies have been investigated in efforts to improve the nutritional status of the cancer patient. TPN can improve caloric intake and nitrogen balance of the patient, particularly those with dysfunctional gastrointestinal tracts. Pharmacologic agents may improve gastrointestinal dysmotility and attenuate nausea. Growth factors also may improve nitrogen and protein balance. Except in severely malnourished people none of these modalities alone have thus far been shown to improve clinical outcome.

A combination of the aforementioned strategies will likely prove most fruitful in the treatment of cancer patients; therefore, studies combining the various modalities are necessary. Areas of the greatest promise for future research include studies of the multitude of recombinant growth factors that are becoming available and studies of the gastrointestinal tract as the primary route of aggressive nutritional supplementation. In the meantime, a practical strategy can be recommended from available data (Table 32-13). Elimination of tumor is still of paramount importance, and effective responses to anticancer therapy are associated with more dramatic response to nutritional support. Patients with greater than 10% weight loss are likely to benefit from 7 to 10 days of aggressive intravenous nutritional support before major therapy (Fig. 32-2). Narcotic use should be minimized. Medications that attenuate nausea and gastrointestinal dysmotility should be considered as supplemental agents in the nutritional therapy of the cancer patient.

Table 32-13. Current Recommendations for Nutritional Support in Cancer Patients

Elminate tumor
Maintain adequate oral intake as possible
Consider TPN or tube feedings for patients with > 10% weight loss
In patients with > 10% weight loss, consider 7–10 d of TPN before surgical therapy
Minimize narcotic use
Consider medications that attenuate nausea and gastrointestinal dysmotility as supplemental agents in nutritional therapy

TPN — Total parenteral nutrition.

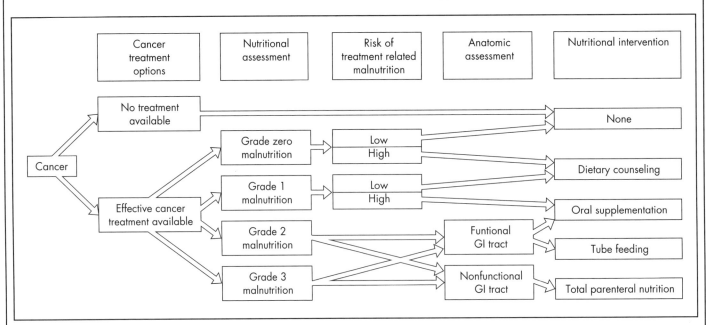

FIGURE 32-2.
The treatment of malnutrition in cancer patients.

REFERENCES

1. van Eys J: Nutrition and cancer: physiologic interrelationships. *Ann Rev Nutr* 1985, 5:435–461.

2. Butterworth CE: Folate deficiency and cancer. In *Micronutrients in Health and Disease Prevention.* Edited by Bandich A, Butterworth CE. New York: Marcel Dekker, 1991:165–183.

3. Creagan ET, Moertel CG, O'Fallon JR, *et al.*: Failure of high dose vitamin C (ascorbic acid) therapy to benefit patients with advanced cancer. *N Engl J Med* 1979, 301:687–690.

4. Moertel CG, Fleming TR, Creagan ET, *et al.*: High dose vitamin C versus placebo in the treatment of patients with advanced cancer who have had no prior chemotherapy. *N Engl J Med* 1985, 312:137–141.

5. Lashner BA, Heidenreich PA, Su GL, *et al.*: Effect of folate supplementation on the incidence of dysplasia and cancer in chronic ulcerative colitis: a case control study. *Gastroenterology* 1989, 97:255–259.

6. Michels KB, Willet WC: Vitamins and cancer: a practical means of prevention. In *Important Advances in Oncology 1994.* Edited by DeVita VT, Hellman S, Rosenberg SA. Philadelphia: JB Lippincott, 1994:85–114.

7. Willet WC: Micronutrients and cancer risk. *Am J Clin Nutr* 1995, 59:1162S–1165S.

8. Dewys WD, Begg C, Lavin PT, *et al.*: Prognostic effect of weight loss prior to chemotherapy in cancer patients: Eastern Cooperative Study Group. *Am J Med* 1980, 69:491–497.

9. Baker JP, Detsky AS, Wesson DE, *et al.*: Nutritional assessment: a comparison of clinical judgment and objective measurements. *N Engl J Med* 1982, 306:969–972.

10. Hill GL: Malnutritional and surgical risk: guidelines for nutritional therapy. *Ann R Coll Surg Engl* 1987, 69:263–265.

11. Baker SJ, Kumar S, Swaminathan SP: Excretion of folic acid in bile. *Lancet* 1965, 1:685.

12. Detsky AS, Baker JP, O'Rourke K, Goel V: Perioperative parenteral nutrition: a meta-analysis. *Ann Intern Med* 1987, 107:195–203.

13. Muller JM, Brenner U, Dienst C, Pichlmaier H: Preoperative parenteral feeding in patients with gastrointestinal carcinoma. *Lancet* 1982, 1:68–71.

14. Perioperative total nutrition in surgical patients: the Veterans Affairs Total parenteral Nutrition Cooperative Study Group. *N Engl J Med* 1991, 325:525–532.

15. Fan ST, Lo CM, *et al.*: Perioperative nutritional support in patients undergoing hepatectomy for hepatocellular carcinoma. *N Engl J Med* 1994, 331:1547–1552.

16. Brennan MF, Pisters PWT, Posner M, *et al.*: A prospective randomized trial of total parenteral nutrition after major pancreatic resection for malignancy. *Ann Surg* 1994, 220:436–444.

17. Parenteral nutrition in patients receiving cancer chemotherapy: American College of Physicians. *Ann Intern Med* 1989, 110:734–736.

18. Heys SD, Park KG, Garlick PJ, Eremin O: Nutrition and malignant disease: implications for surgical practice. *Br J Surg* 1992, 79:614–623.

19. Chlebowski RT: Nutritional support of the medical oncology patient. *Hematol Oncol Clin North Am* 1991, 5:147–160.

20. Lacour J: Clinical trials using polyadenylic-polyuridylic acid as an adjuvant to surgery in treating different human tumors. *J Biol Resp Modif* 1985, 4:538–543.

21. Ziegler TR, Young LS, Benfell K, *et al.*: Clinical and metabolic efficacy of glutamine-supplemented parenteral nutrition after bone marrow transplantation: a randomized, double-blind, controlled study. *Ann Intern Med* 1992, 116:821–828.

22. Daly JM, Reynolds J, Thom A, *et al.*: Immune and metabolic effects of arginine in the surgical patient. *Ann Surg* 1988, 208:512–523.

23. Soukop M, Calman KC: Nutritional support in patients with malignant disease. *J Human Nutr* 1979, 33:179–188.

24. Inculet RI, Norton JA, Nichoald GE, *et al.*: Water-soluble vitamins in cancer patients on parenteral nutrition: a prospective study. *J Paren Ent Nutr* 1987, 11:243–249.

25. Aksoy M: Thiamin status of patients treated with drug combinations containing 5-fluorouracil. *Eur J Cancer* 1980, 16:1041–1055.

26. Hinton P, Allison SP, Littlejohn S, Lloyd J: Insulin and glucose to reduce catabolic response to injury in burned patients. *Lancet* 1971, 1:767–769.

27. Jiang ZM, He GZ, Zhang SY, *et al.*: Low-dose growth hormone and hypocaloric nutrition attenuate the protein-catabolic response after major operation. *Ann Surg* 1989, 210:513–524.

28. Wolf RF, Pearlstone DB, Newman E, *et al.*: Growth hormone and insulin reverse net whole body and skeletal protein catabolism in cancer patients. *Ann Surg* 1992, 216:280–290.

29. Abels JC, Young NF, Taylor HC: Effects of testosterone and of testosterone propionate on protein formation in man. *J Clin Endocrinol Metab* 1944, 4:198–201.

30. Hansell DT, Davies JW, Shenkin A, *et al.*: The effects of an anabolic steroid and peripherally administered intravenous nutrition in the early postoperative period. *J Paren Ent Nutr* 1989, 13:349-358.

31. Mullen JL, Buzby GP, Gertner MH, *et al.*: Protein synthesis dynamics in human gastrointestinal malignancies. *Surgery* 1980, 87:331–338.

32. Rogers PC, Kemp D, Rogol A, *et al.*: Possible effects of growth hormone on development of acute lymphoblastic leukemia. *Lancet* 1977, 1:434–435.

33. Lippman ME, Dickson RB, Bates S, *et al.*: Autocrine and paracrine growth regulation of human breast cancer. *Breast Cancer Res Treat* 1986, 7:59–70.

34. Nakanishi Y, Mulshine JL, Kasprzyk PG, *et al.*: Insulin-like growth factor can mediate autocrine proliferation of human small cell lung cancer line in vitro. *J Clin Invest* 1988, 82:354–359.

35. Donoway RB, Torosian MH: Growth hormone inhibits tumor metastases. *Surg Forum* 1989, 40:413-415.

36. Tchekmedyian NS, Hickman M, Siau J, *et al.*: Megestrol acetate in cancer anorexia and weight loss. *Cancer* 1992, 69:1268–1274.

37. Tchekmedyian NS, Hickman M, Heber D: Treatment of anorexia and weight loss with megestrol acetate in patients with cancer or acquired immunodeficiency syndrome. *Semin Oncol* 1991, 18:35–42.

38. Kardinal CG, Loprinzi CL, Schaid DJ, *et al.*: A controlled trial of cyproheptadine in cancer patients with anorexia and/or cachexia. *Cancer* 1990, 65:2657–2662.

39. Plasse TF, Gorter RW, Krasnow SH, *et al.*: Recent clinical experience with dronabinol. *Pharmacol Biochem Behav* 1991, 40:695–700.

40. Espat NJ, Moldawer LL, Copeland EM: Cytokine-mediated alterations in host metabolism prevent nutritional repletion in cachectic cancer patients. *J Surg Oncol* 1995, 58:77–82.

MALNUTRITION

Tissue wasting is a common and often devastating sequela of the cancer-bearing state. This loss in body mass can result in multi-organ derangements including impaired immune function, impaired locomotive capacity, and, ultimately, impaired respiratory function. As little as a 5% reduction in lean body mass has been associated with increased mortality in patients with cancer. Numerous factors contribute to produce wasting and malnutrition in patients with cancer. Recent advances in our understanding of these factors, as well as improvements in nutrient delivery methods and availability of immunostimulatory nutrients and growth factors offer exciting potential modalities for specific treatment of cancer-related wasting.

CAUSATIVE FACTORS

Poor intake: anorexia, gastrointestinal dysfunction (blockage, diarrhea, malabsorption); altered substrate cycles; stress of surgery, chemotherapy, or radiation therapy: peri-operative intestinal dysfunction, diarrhea, vomiting, anorexia, malabsorption

PATHOLOGIC PROCESS

Gastrointestinal obstruction from tumor, perioperative gastrointestinal tract dysfunction, oral or esophageal mucositis complicating chemotherapy or radiation therapy, anorexia, depression, nausea, vomiting, gastrointestinal fistula formation, diarrhea, malabsorption

PATIENT ASSESSMENT

Absolute indicators of malnutrition: weight loss >10%, weight loss of 0.5 kg/wk, clinically evident muscular weakness, serum albumin < 3.2 g/dl; **Relative indicators of malnutrition:** immune parameters—anergy in delayed hypersensitivity testing, T-cell numbers < 1500 /ml, decreased complement levels; hypoproteinemia—thyroxine-binding prealbumin, transferrin, retinol-binding protein; creatinine-height ratio < 60% ideal; negative nitrogen balance; clinical—stomatitis, GI dysfunction.

MANAGEMENT

1. Eradication of tumor
2. Increasing nutrient intake
   a. Enteral supplementation
   b. Intravenous supplementation
   c. Specific nutrient administration
      i. Nucleotides
      ii. Specific amino acids
      iii. Polyunsaturated free fatty acids
3. Growth factors
   a. Anabolic steroids
   b. Insulin
   c. Growth hormone
   d. Insulin-like growth factors
4. Pharmacologic agents
   a. Megestrol
   b. Cyproheptadine
   b. Metoclopramide
   c. Dronabinol

TOXICITY GRADING

	0	1	2	3
Degree of malnutrition	None	Mild	Moderate	Severe
Clinical findings	No weight loss	Weight loss < 5%	5–10% weight loss	> 10% weight loss, muscular weakness
Laboratory findings	Normal albumin, normal transferrin level, reactive delayed hypersensitivity skin test	Albumin < 3.5, decreased transferrin level, < 5 mm reactivity on skin test	Albumin < 3.2, nonreactive skin test	Albumin < 2.7

Data collection for clinical trials may be addressed using a variety of methods that depend on the type of clinical trial. Pharmaceutically supported and cooperative-group trials generally have very specific data-collection requirements with preprinted or online computerized forms. Individuals responsible for data collection have an opportunity to attend workshops that are offered periodically throughout the year or as new clinical trials are opened for accrual. These trials are also closely monitored by clinical site monitors, the sponsors, or the cooperative group so data queries, corrections, and suggestions are made on a frequent basis. It is, however, the specific institution's or facility's responsibility to maintain data prospectively. Because these two groups have well documented data management systems and educational programs for individuals new to clinical trials, this chapter will address the management of clinical trial data from a systems perspective, with particular attention paid to institutionally developed clinical trials.

PRESTUDY

Data management and collection actually begins when the idea for a new clinical trial is discussed. At the inception of the idea and the formation of the research questions, it is important that the issue of data collection be addressed. Generally, this process is best addressed collaboratively by members of the research team—the principle investigator, clinical research coordinator, data manager, outpatient/inpatient representative, and biostatistician. It is important that the various disciplines involved in study implementation be included; however, the process should be well developed so that it is streamlined and efficient. The most important question to keep in mind is what data are necessary to answer the proposed research questions. In today's cost-containment environment, it is essential that data collection be kept to a minimum because increased resources may not be a possibility. Also, it should be kept in mind that all data collected should be an important component of the study analysis; if they will not be, then these data are probably unnecessary.

As the clinical trial continues to make its way through the various regulatory and approval systems, the research team should be refining the data-collection process. These efforts will facilitate the implementation of the clinical trial because prior to accrual of the first participant, the research team will be well aware of all data to be collected. This information is essential because the clinical research coordinator needs to educate all members of the health care team who will be responsible for the care of the research participant. Data collection must be a team effort in order to be successful. It is also important that all members of the health care team are aware of their role and responsibility in the data-collection process.

In order to avoid hours of nonproductivity and frustration when making decisions about data collection for a specific clinical trial, the development of a systematic approach is essential. A methodology that is often successful is the development of a generic package of data-collection forms that meet the needs of most studies. These forms should be developed by representatives involved in the research process (eg, investigators in medical, surgical, and radiation oncology; coordinators; data managers; biostatisticians, information systems specialists; laboratory representatives; programmers; and so on). Once the forms have been developed by this group, they should be reviewed by all key investigators, and the necessary changes should be made for each prior to clinical trial implementation . These generic forms will not meet every potential data issue but should cover the

most frequently collected data. If one's system is computerized, then the computer screens should be identical to the data-collection forms, thus facilitating the process of data entry and quality control. Suggested forms include the following:

- Registration
- Prior history
- Laboratory
- Status change
- Radiation history
- Surgical history
- Physician notes
- Physician examination
- Medical history
- History of hospitalization
- Extent of disease
- History of drug administration
- Clinical response
- Postoperative complications
- Concomitant measures
- Adverse events
- CTB

The selection of forms needed will depend on the types of clinical trials implemented at one's institution. Some of these forms are self-explanatory and are used primarily for study specific data collection.

Registration and status-change forms provide information that is beneficial because they contain information such as name, date of birth, on-study date, date of diagnosis, and so on. The clinical-response form can be used as a part of the case-report form binder or study record but can also be printed, signed, and dated by the investigator as the clinical response is finalized. There are a multitude of uses for the data-collection forms; one merely needs to think creatively as well as from a cost-containment and efficiency perspective.

STUDY IMPLEMENTATION

At the time of study implementation, the selected data forms should be reviewed one final time at the clinical trail's implementation meeting. This review will familiarize all members of the research team with the data collection forms and allow for any last-minute concerns or questions regarding the data to be collected. It is, however, the primary responsibility of the clinical research coordinator (or data manager) to collect the actual data. Data collection is only done in an accountable manner if one individual is primarily responsible. This person can delegate certain components to others, but one person must be responsible for ensuring accountability. In order to prevent unnecessary delays, the data manager is provided with an individual study calendar at the time a participant is enrolled on study. This calendar serves as the template for data collection. It specifies such things as physician visits, treatment dates, blood studies, radiology studies, and other necessary monitoring studies. The data manager should be notified of all changes in the calendar so that it can be used as a guide to collect data as it becomes available. Depending on the institution, information (eg, tests results, history, physical examination, pathology, and so on) may be accessed from computer data, whereas other data items may need to be obtained from the medical record. It is also possible, with the availability of information systems, to download specific data points, such as lab results, directly onto the computerized laboratory forms within the clinical research database. All downloaded data must be verified to ensure accuracy. This verification should be done on a daily basis with documented procedures in place.

All data should be collected on a prospective basis whenever possible; however, there may be delays while awaiting dictation, pathology reports, and so on. The data manager should maintain either a paper or computerized log of what items are missing on specific dates for each patient. This log should be reviewed at least weekly, and missing items should be retrieved as soon as they become available. This prevents incomplete or inaccurate data sets at the conclusion of the study.

Review of all participant data should be done on a routinely scheduled basis by the investigator, clinical research coordinator, and other members of the research team. This facilitates quality research as well as quality care of the participants. Data review will provide the study team with possible positive or negative study trends (eg, potential problems with white blood cell counts, adverse events, tolerance of drugs, unexpected side effects) and will keep everyone aware of the status of the data or trend. Data review also provides an opportunity for modifications to the study if the ongoing data is indicative of a problem or trend.

QUALITY ASSURANCE

In order to ensure quality research, it is essential that an internal auditing and/or quality assurance system be developed. Institutionally developed studies are rarely audited except on rare occasions by the Food and Drug Administration (FDA), National Institution of Health (NIH), or National Cancer Institute (NCI). Occasionally, there are other regulatory agencies that may become involved. Processes must be in place to ensure that quality research is being conducted. A plan needs to be developed so that a specific number of clinical trials are audited on a routine basis. The number will depend on the size of the institution, number of clinical trials, and participant accrual. If possible, the clinical trial and the study participants should be selected randomly. A suggestion is to develop a process so that the clinical trials and participants are randomly selected by the computer. The study or studies should be audited by individuals who are not directly involved. The audit team should consist of an investigator, a clinical research coordinator, and a regulatory representative or another member of the research team. It is essential that study and regulatory compliance be reviewed. The audit findings should be documented and then reviewed with the investigator and the specific research team involved in the audited clinical trial. An institution may have additional mechanisms for reporting the findings. All documentation of findings must be filed within the department along with any corrective action plans, depending on the audit findings. Additionally, procedures for the audit process and outcome need to be developed.

DATA MONITORING

Monitoring of data can become an insurmountable task as the number of participants and clinical trials increase. It is important that a system be developed either on paper or computerized to track data are required to be collected on each participant, particularly when participants are in the follow-up phase of the clinical trial. Follow-up participants are monitored less frequently and can often be forgotten without an adequate system for tracking. This information can be viewed on a monthly basis to determine what data requirements are necessary throughout the next month to maintain a prospective system. It also provides information regarding ongoing missing data points. Over several months, missing data points may require a plan of action to prevent a participant from being lost to follow-up or significant data from being forgotten. This system is vital if the institution has an active outreach program for participation in their clinical trials.

The monthly report can provide whatever information is important to the specific institution. One suggestion is to develop the report so that individualized reports can be distributed to each clinical research coordinator/data manager, outreach site, or both. This provides the individual with information that is specific for their studies. The report should provide information such as the study number, patient ID, and the specific type of data to be collected that month. Once the data has been collected, the report will be updated manually or entered into the computerized database by the main institution. This provides an excellent mechanism for keeping track of the data status for all clinical trials on a daily basis. It also facilitates data retrieval from outreach sites because it will provide information for each investigator and participant at each specific facility. This information will provide a mechanism for determining the outreach sites where data need to be collected. When the institution sends a data manager to the outreach institution, data can be collected for all active studies by the same individual. This provides for an efficient system because data collection in outreach institutions is a costly and labor-intensive endeavor.

EDUCATION

Clinical research is very specialized, and there are no readily formal mechanisms available to learn the process. This is especially true for investigator-developed clinical trials. As mentioned previously, pharmaceutically sponsored and cooperative-group trials have formalized this process. Institutionally developed clinical trials have their own unique needs, and there needs to be a mechanism in place to provide ongoing education for seasoned clinical research coordinators and data managers as well as new coordinators and data managers. One suggestion is to develop self-directed educational resources. This may be done on the Internet, with a manual, video, or combination of methods. Individuals also need to be mentored and monitored closely for a designated period of time. Orientation and education needs to be consistent for everyone, and documentation of such should be in each staff members' file upon satisfactory completion of specific data-management educational resources. Individuals involved in clinical trial data collection need to be updated periodically as regulations change that have an impact on data collection. This may be the only opportunity these individuals have for ongoing education; therefore, there should be an ongoing educational process for individuals involved in clinical trial research.

Organizations are beginning to certify individuals as clinical research coordinators and data managers. These organizations (eg, Society of Clinical Research Associates [SoCRA] and Association of Clinical Research Professionals [ACRP]) also have formal training programs that are available prior to the certification exam, but they may not meet an institution's individual needs. Certification and membership in these organizations provides individuals involved with clinical trials a network for education and problem resolution.

This is an excellent opportunity for clinical research coordinators and data managers to obtain support and mentorship outside of their institution.

CONCLUSION

The management of clinical trial data collection is essential for quality research. This can be best accomplished with the education of staff, a mechanism for determining specific data requirements per study, and an organized mechanism for monitoring data.

Centralization of clinical trial coordination and data management, when possible, can facilitate these processes and ensure institutional consistency. If these mechanisms are in place, data collection can be done efficiently within the institutions as well as in the outreach locations. It also helps to demystify clinical trial research because it provides individuals with a concrete knowledge base to use in performing their role. The positive outcome of an effective data-management process can increase entry onto clinical trials because the management of participants on a clinical trial is no longer a time-consuming, frustrating experience.

Note: Page numbers followed by f indicate figures; page numbers followed by t indicate tables.